PULMONARY HYPERTENSION

Collected Reprints (1961-2015)

By

William C. Roberts, MD

and

Colleagues

ISBN: 979-8-88862-144-8
Printed in the United States of America on acid-free paper.

Preface

Systemic hypertension is the most common cardiovascular disease. In contrast, pulmonary hypertension is far less common. There are 80 drugs for treatment of systemic hypertension and <5 for pulmonary hypertension. The causes of primary pulmonary hypertension are precapillary or capillary and consist of pulmonary arterial obstruction (thrombus, embolus, neoplasm), primary pulmonary hypertension (etiology unclear), and alterations in the bellows breathing mechanism (scleroderma, crucification, etc.). The causes of secondary pulmonary hypertension are left-sided cardiac disease (coronary artery disease, mitral stenosis, etc.). Collected here are a variety of conditions causing primary and secondary hypertension.

—William C. Roberts, MD

Table of Contents

*Articles are numbered based on WCR's CV.

Increased Bronchial Collateral Circulation in a Patient with Transposition of the Great Vessels and Pulmonary Hypertension*

ROLAND FOLSE, M.D., WILLIAM C. ROBERTS, M.D. *and* WILLIAM P. CORNELL, M.D.

Bethesda, Maryland

It is well established that patients with cyanotic congenital heart disease characterized by diminished pulmonary blood flow have increased collateral circulation to the lungs through enlarged bronchial arteries. The incidence, stimuli for development and structural arrangement of these collateral vessels are not well understood.

Large bronchial vessels are commonly found in patients with stenotic lesions in the right side of the heart or the pulmonary artery producing an intracardiac right to left shunt such as is seen in tetralogy of Fallot, pulmonic stenosis with atrial septal defect or tricuspid atresia. In these patients the pulmonary artery pressure and blood flow are diminished. Intravascular thromboses in the pulmonary vascular bed, presumably secondary to capillary stasis and polycythemia, may further diminish the pulmonary blood flow and thus further the need for bronchial collaterals.[1] Likewise, in patients with complete absence or atresia of the pulmonary arteries, communications arising directly from the aorta persist from fetal life and are essential not only for the nourishment of the pulmonary structures but also for supplying the lungs with desaturated blood in order to provide for exchange of gases.[2]

Bronchial collaterals may also develop in acyanotic patients. For example, the congenital absence of one main pulmonary artery is associated with enlarged bronchial arteries to that lung.[3] In other diseases, additional mechanisms may lead to increased collateral circulation to the lungs. Patients without heart disease, such as those with pulmonary infarction, bronchiectasis, tuberculosis, emphysema or lung tumors, may have increased bronchial blood flow to the diseased portions of the lungs.

It has not been generally appreciated that patients with cyanotic congenital heart disease and pulmonary hypertension may also have extensive collateral circulation to the lungs. This communication describes an infant with complete transposition of the great vessels, a ventricular septal defect and pulmonary hypertension, who also had markedly increased pulmonary collateral blood flow.

Clinical Summary

T. N., a fourteen month old male infant, had been cyanotic since birth. His early growth and development were somewhat retarded and he had frequent respiratory infections but no episodes of severe cyanosis or squatting. He was described as being an active child with some limitation due to fatigability. There was no history of heart failure.

On examination the patient was moderately cyanotic at rest and had evidence of clubbing of the digits. He was somewhat small for his age, his weight being in the tenth percentile on the anthropometric chart. The heart was enlarged to both the right and left sides of the sternum. There was a lift over the lower left sternal area, but no thrill was palpable. The second sound at the base was slightly accentuated and was thought to be single. There was a soft, grade 1–6 early systolic murmur heard along the lower left sternal border. The hematocrit was 75 per cent and the hemoglobin 21.5 gm. per 100 ml. The electrocardiogram demonstrated right atrial enlargement, right axis deviation and right ventricular hypertrophy (Fig. 1). Cardiac fluoroscopy revealed enlargement of both ventricles with narrowing of the base of the heart. The horizontal course of tortuous vessels in the hilar regions suggested the presence of prominent bronchial arteries.

At catheterization the pulmonary artery was not

* From the Clinic of Surgery, National Heart Institute and Department of Pathologic Anatomy, the Clinical Center, National Institutes of Health, Bethesda, Maryland.

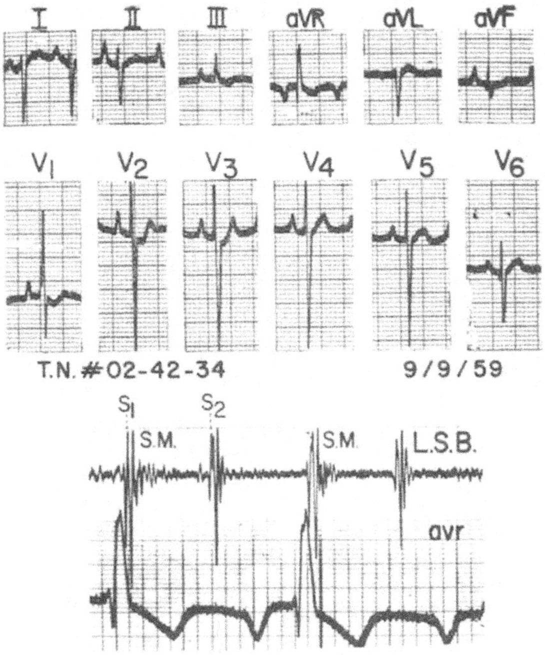

FIG. 1. Electrocardiogram and phonocardiogram. S.M. = systolic murmur; L.S.B. = left sternal border.

entered. The systemic arterial oxygen saturation was 43 per cent under general anesthesia. *A selective right ventricular angiocardiogram* (Fig. 2) was performed which demonstrated that the aorta arose from the anatomic right ventricle. The left ventricle and pulmonary artery were not opacified in the early films. Large bronchial arteries were seen to arise from the descending aorta and appeared to be equally distributed to all parts of both lungs. The right main pulmonary artery visualized well in the later films, suggesting that it was filled by communications with the bronchial arteries. Because of the lack of prominent pulmonary vascularity on the roentgenogram of the chest and the presence of extremely prominent collateral vessels, it was believed that the patient had complete transposition of the great vessels with associated pulmonic stenosis and would, therefore, benefit from a subclavian-pulmonary artery anastomosis.

At operation the pulmonary artery, which was approximately the same size as the aorta, was observed to arise from the left ventricle and in a position directly posterior to the aorta. Pressures measured simultaneously in the pulmonary artery and aorta were equal. A large number of dilated bronchial arteries and veins were present in the hili of the lungs, in the interlobar fissures and along the subpleural surface of the lungs. Because of the high pressure in the pulmonary artery, an anastomosis was not performed. Postoperatively, the patient became

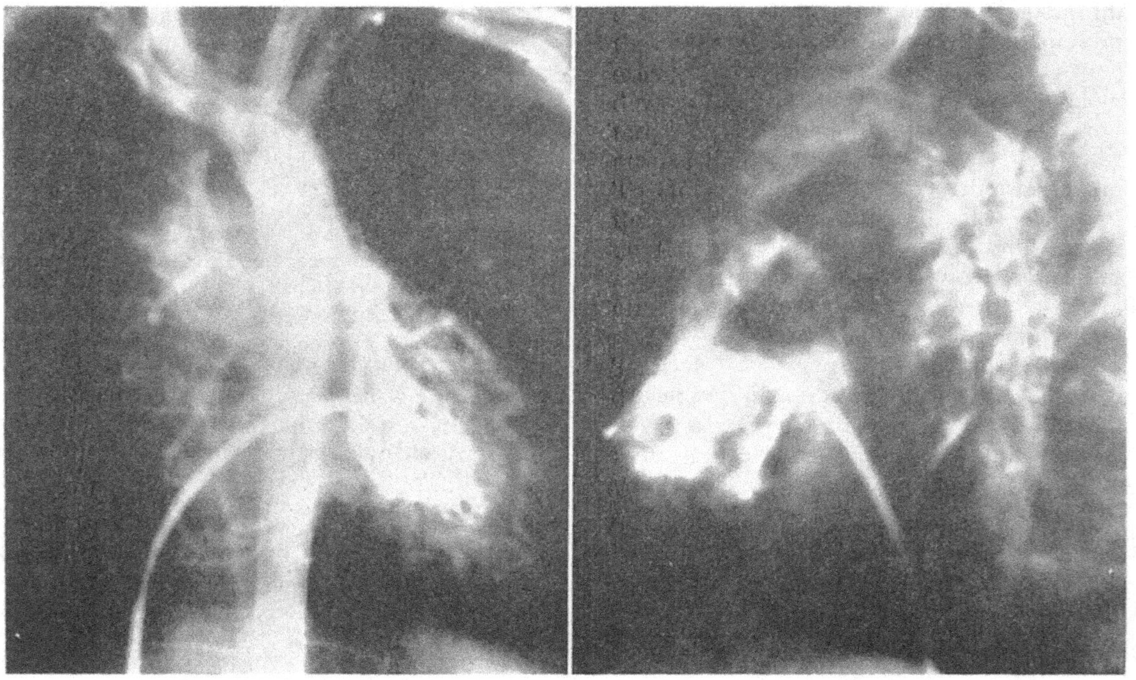

A B

FIG. 2. Selective right ventricular angiocardiogram demonstrating complete transposition of the great vessels and large bronchial arteries arising from the descending thoracic aorta. A, posteroanterior view; B, lateral view.

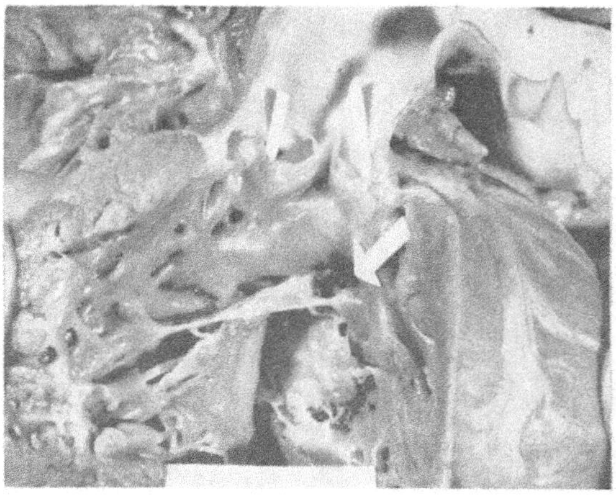

FIG. 3. The right ventricle, aortic valve and aorta are opened. The aorta lies anteriorly and arises exclusively from the right ventricle. The coronary arteries arise from the aorta (narrow white pointers). A ventricular septal defect (thick white arrow) is located immediately inferior to the supraventricular muscle. Note the large size of the coronary arteries.

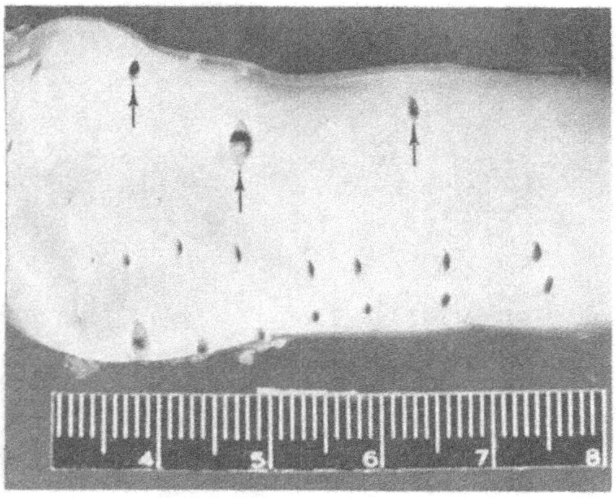

FIG. 4. Descending thoracic aorta demonstrating the markedly dilated ostia (arrows) of the bronchial arteries.

progressively more cyanotic, and his condition gradually deteriorated until he died eighteen hours after operation.

PATHOLOGIC FINDINGS

Necropsy confirmed the operative finding of complete transposition of the great vessels. The aorta arose exclusively from the right ventricle (Fig. 3) and the pulmonary trunk from the left ventricle. The ascending aorta lay directly anterior to the pulmonary trunk. Both ventricles were hypertrophied; the left measured 0.1 cm. and the right, 0.9 cm. in greatest thickness. A ventricular septal defect was present immediately inferior to the supraventricularis muscle (Fig. 3). Both atria were dilated, the right more than the left. The atrial appendages were normally situated. A valvular-competent foramen ovale was present. The venae cavae entered the right atrium, and the pulmonary veins entered the left atrium in a normal manner. The atrioventricular valves were normally developed. The pulmonic valve lay posteriorly and joined the anterior mitral leaflet in a manner similar to the connections between the mitral and aortic valves in a normal heart. The cusps of the pulmonic and aortic valves were delicate and pliable and there was no evidence of stenosis. Three large bronchial arteries arose directly from the descending thoracic aorta (Fig. 4) and coursed along the posterior aspect of the lower trachea and main bronchi before entering the hili of the lungs (Fig. 5). No atherosclerotic changes were present in the pulmonary artery or aorta. The ostia of the coronary arteries arose from the two posterior sinuses of Valsalva (Fig. 3).

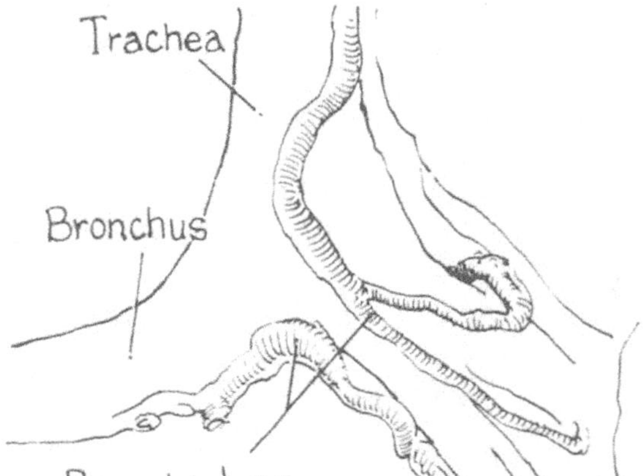

FIG. 5. Diagram (traced from the original photograph of this area) illustrating the large bronchial arteries coursing along the posterior aspect of the lower trachea and main bronchi before entering the hili of the lungs.

Microscopically, in the sections from the hili of the lungs many dilated, thick-walled bronchial arteries surrounding the bronchi were seen (Fig. 6A). Also, there was proliferation of the intima of some bronchial arteries (Fig. 6B), a finding which has not received attention in the past. Many dilated bronchial veins were seen in the subpleural areas of the lungs, particularly the hilar regions. Sections from the main pulmonary arteries showed the elastic fibers arranged in an orderly fashion similar to those found in a fetal pulmonary artery (Fig. 7). This picture is noted in the lungs of patients in whom pulmonary hypertension has been present from birth and in whom the normal transition to the adult type of pulmonary artery has not taken place.[4] The elastic and muscular pulmonary arteries were dilated, and the latter showed medial hypertrophy and occasional intimal thickening. The lumina of the pulmonary arterioles were narrowed by intimal proliferation (Fig. 8).

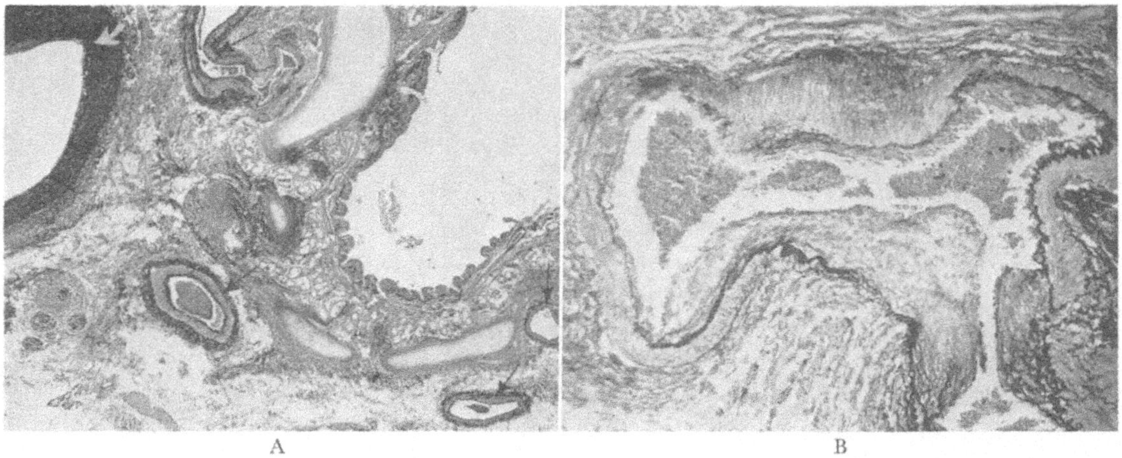

Fig. 6. A, photomicrograph of lung in hilar region demonstrating thick-walled, dilated bronchial arteries (black arrows) surrounding a bronchus. There is intimal thickening in addition to medial hypertrophy of the bronchial artery in the uppermost portion of the figure. A large elastic pulmonary artery (white arrow) of the fetal type is present in the left upper corner of the figure. (Elastic van Giesson stain, original magnification × 17.) B, close-up view of the large bronchial artery appearing in A. Note the marked intimal proliferation and medial hypertrophy. (Elastic van Giesson stain, original magnification × 120.)

Comments

It was demonstrated early in experiments on dogs by Mathes and associates[5] that bronchial collateral circulation to the lungs will develop following obstruction of the pulmonary artery. Liebow et al.[6] have traced the pathway of development of collateral vessels from the bronchial artery to the pulmonary artery to the pulmonary capillaries, with drainage directly into the pulmonary veins or into the azygos system by way of the bronchial veins.

There are few documented reports in the literature of augmentation of the bronchial circulation in association with transposition of the great vessels. The combination of complete transposition of the great vessels with pulmonary hypertension and enlarged bronchial arteries in particular, has not been well described previously. The case of transposition of the great vessels which Cockle[7] described in 1863 had enlarged bronchial vessels and probably a normal or increased pulmonary artery pressure, since there was no stenosis of the pulmonic valve and the pulmonary artery was larger than the aorta. Also, no obstruction of the pulmonary valve was noted in pathologic findings of the patient with complete transposition in whom Cudkowicz et al.[8] demonstrated extensive bron-

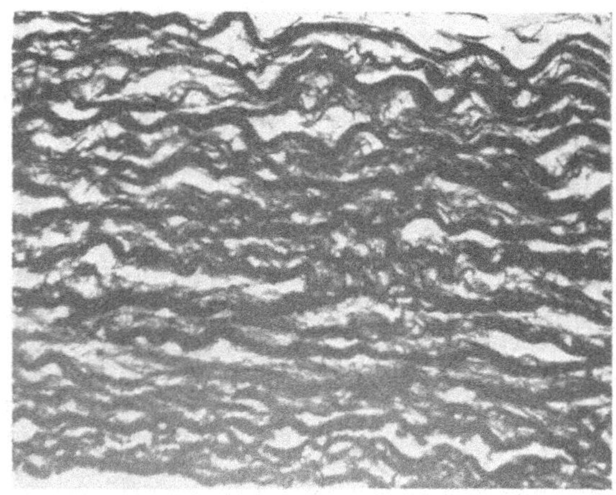

Fig. 7. Photomicrograph of main pulmonary artery demonstrating the aorta-like fetal configuration of the elastic lamellae. (Elastic van Giesson stain, original magnification × 450.)

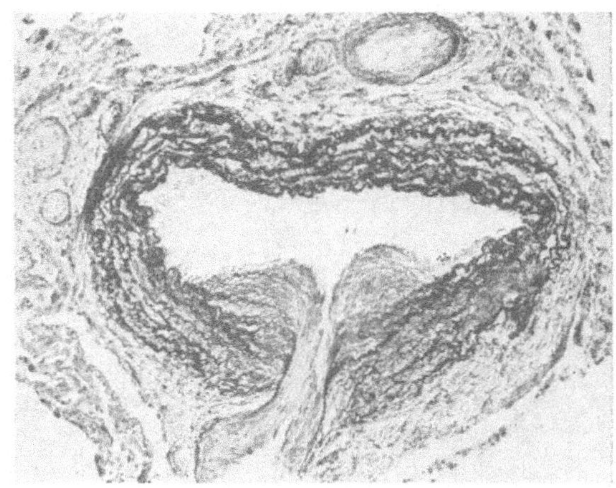

Fig. 8. Photomicrograph of pulmonary artery demonstrating marked intimal proliferation and narrowing at the junction of an arteriolar branch. (Elastic van Giesson stain, original magnification × 155.)

chial collateral circulation by injection technics. The pulmonary arteries were dilated and communicated freely with the vasa vasorum supplied by the bronchial arteries.

Bronchopulmonary arterial communications may be found in patients with single ventricle and pulmonary hypertension as in the case reported by Heath,[9] in which bronchial collaterals were prominent in the adventitia of large arteries, surrounding the bronchi and along the visceral pleura. In a similar case illustrated by Liebow,[10] proliferated bronchial arteries were demonstrated to communicate with tortuous pulmonary vessels. In the lungs of patients with Eisenmenger's complex, collateral channels in the form of angiomatoid lesions may connect the pulmonary and bronchial circulations.[11] Similar lesions have been reported in patients with patent ductus arteriosus with pulmonary hypertension[12,13] and in those with atrial septal defect and pulmonary hypertension;[14] these vessels may divert blood to the alveolar capillaries.

It appears, therefore, that there is a wide spectrum of malformations in which collateral channels to the lungs may develop. The presence of reduced pulmonary blood flow or the absence of elevated pulmonary vascular resistance should not be suspected in a patient with cyanotic congenital heart disease merely because of the existence of enlarged bronchial vessels. Catheterization of the pulmonary artery is difficult or impossible in patients with transposition of the great vessels, single ventricle, truncus arteriosus and other complicated forms of cyanotic heart disease; therefore, the use of right- and left-sided angiocardiography would be valuable in assessing the size of the pulmonary artery, the relative amount of pulmonary blood flow and in estimating the pulmonary artery pressure.

In the patient reported herein a right ventricular angiocardiogram was performed, but because of the presence of complete transposition of the great vessels only the aorta was opacified; the pulmonary artery could not be visualized. As this case illustrates, the clinical picture associated with cyanotic heart disease and pulmonary hypertension may be confused with that associated with obstruction to pulmonary flow secondary to obstruction in the right ventricular outflow tract or at the pulmonary valve. The reduced pulmonary vascularity on the roentgenogram in this patient was suggestive of a reduced pulmonary artery pressure. The closely split second heart sound heard at the base resulted from the presence of equal pressures in the great vessels rather than from an obstruction to right ventricular outflow. The very soft systolic murmur probably indicated that only a small amount of blood passed across the ventricular septal defect, due to the equal ventricular pressures. Accordingly, it is essential that a thorough angiographic and hemodynamic evaluation of the pulmonary vascular bed precede any operative procedure designed to increase pulmonary blood flow in patients with transposition of the great vessels.

Summary

The clinical, diagnostic and pathologic findings in a fourteen month old infant with complete transposition of the great vessels, ventricular septal defect and pulmonary hypertension with increased bronchial collateral circulation are presented. It is emphasized that the presence of increased bronchial collateral blood flow is not necessarily associated with decreased pulmonary blood flow due to obstruction to right ventricular outflow, but may also be associated with pulmonary hypertension and elevation of pulmonary vascular resistance. Thus, the presence of enlarged bronchial vessels should not indicate that the patient will benefit from an operation designed to increase the pulmonary blood flow. The importance of right and left ventricular angiocardiograms in the preoperative assessment of the pulmonary vascular bed is discussed.

References

1. Rich, A. R. A hitherto unrecognized tendency to the development of widespread vascular obstruction in patients with congenital pulmonary stenosis (tetralogy of Fallot). *Bull. Johns Hopkins Hosp.*, 82: 389, 1958.
2. Tobin, C. E. The bronchial arteries and their connections with other vessels in the human lung. *Surg. Gynec. & Obst.*, 95: 741, 1957.
3. Tabakin, B. S., Hanson, J. S., Adhikari, P. K. and Miller, D. B. Physiologic studies in congenital absence of the left main pulmonary artery. *Circulation*, 22: 1107, 1960.
4. Heath, D., DuShane, J. W., Wood, E. H. and Edwards, J. E. The structure of the pulmonary trunk at different ages and in cases of pulmonary hypertension and pulmonary stenosis. *J. Path. Bact.*, 77: 443, 1959.
5. Mathes, M. E., Holman, E. and Reichert, F. L. A study of the bronchial, pulmonary, and lymphatic circulations of the lung under various pathologic conditions experimentally produced. *J. Thoracic Surg.*, 1: 339, 1932.
6. Liebow, A. A., Hales, M. R., Harrison, W.,

Bloomer, W. E. and Lindskog, G. E. The genesis and functional implications of collateral circulation to the lungs. *Yale J. Biol. & Med.*, 22: 637, 1950.

7. Cockle, J. Case of transposition of the great vessels of the heart. *Tr. Med.-Chir. Soc. London*, 46: 193, 1863.
8. Cudkowicz, L. and Armstrong, J. B. Injection of the bronchial circulation in a case of transposition. *Brit. Heart J.*, 14: 374, 1952.
9. Heath, D. Cor triloculare biatriatum. *Circulation*, 15: 701, 1957.
10. Liebow, A. A. Pathology of the Heart, Chap. 15. Edited by Gould, S. E. Springfield, Ill., 1960. Charles C Thomas.
11. Brewer, D. B. and Heath, D. Pulmonary vascular changes in Eisenmenger's complex. *J. Path. Bact.*, 77: 141, 1959.
12. Brewer, D. B. Fibrous occlusion and anastomosis of the pulmonary vessels in a case of pulmonary hypertension associated with patent ductus arteriosus. *J. Path. Bact.*, 70: 299, 1955.
13. Dammann, J. F., Jr., Berthrong, M. and Bing, R. J. Reverse ductus: a presentation of the syndrome of patency of the ductus arteriosus with pulmonary hypertension and a shunting of blood flow from pulmonary artery to aorta. *Bull. Johns Hopkins Hosp.*, 92: 128, 1953.
14. Rossall, R. E. and Thompson, H. Formation of new vascular channels in the lungs of a patient with secondary pulmonary hypertension. *J. Path. Bact.*, 76: 593, 1958.

The histologic structure of the pulmonary trunk in patients with "primary" pulmonary hypertension

*William C. Roberts, M.D.**
Bethesda, Md.

The etiological factors involved in idiopathic or "primary" pulmonary hypertension (PPH) remain unknown. Recent studies[1,2] have suggested that in a small proportion of patients with this condition the pulmonary hypertension may have been present from birth, although in most the hypertension of the lesser circulation is acquired later in life. The present report describes the microscopic structure of the elastic tissue in the media of the pulmonary trunk in five patients with proved PPH, in an attempt to determine the congenital or acquired basis for this disease.

Material and methods

Five patients who had PPH were studied. Each had severe pulmonary arterial hypertension as determined by cardiac catheterization (Table I), and at autopsy none had congenital cardiac anomalies. All five patients fulfilled the criteria generally accepted for the diagnosis of PPH, i.e., hypertension of the lesser circulation, absence of primary cardiac anomalies, and absence of significant parenchymal disease of the lungs. In sections of the lungs from Patient 5 (Table I), multiple cholesterol granulomata of undetermined etiology were found. These granulomata, however, had no apparent association with the pulmonary arteries, and, thus, were not believed to have played a role in the production of the pulmonary hypertension. At autopsy, all five patients had dilatation of the right ventricle, right atrium, pulmonic valve "ring," and pulmonary trunk, hypertrophy of the right ventricle, and atherosclerosis of the pulmonary arteries. The hypertensive pulmonary vascular changes in each of the patients were of Grade 5/6 severity (classification of Heath and Edwards[3]). Four of the five patients were females. The age range was 8 to 29 years.

Transverse blocks of the pulmonary trunk and ascending aorta were removed

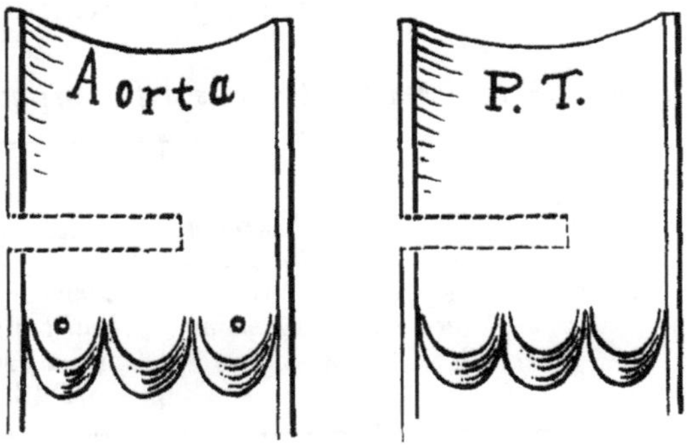

Fig. *1.* Diagram of the pulmonary trunk (*P.T.*) and ascending aorta, illustrating the site from which sections for histologic study were obtained.

From the Pathologic Anatomy Department, Clinical Center, National Institutes of Health, Bethesda, Md.
Received for publication May 30, 1962.
*Present address: Department of Medicine, The Johns Hopkins Hospital, Baltimore 5, Md.

from sites 1 cm. above the respective semilunar valves (Fig. 1), fixed in 10 per cent formalin, and embedded in paraffin in the usual way. The histologic characteristics of the elastic tissue were studied in both vessels in sections cut 6 micra thick and stained by Van Gieson's method for elastic fibrils. In each instance the tissue of the pulmonary trunk was designated as "aortic" or "adult-pulmonary" in type (Table I). This classification is based on the studies of Heath and associates.

Results

The aortic or fetal configuration of the elastic fibers of the pulmonary trunk was present in one, and the normal adult-pulmonary configuration was present in three of the five patients in this study (Table I). In Patient 4 the configuration was neither adult-pulmonary nor aortic in type, but intermediate (transitional) between these two. The aorta was normal in all five patients. Photomicrographs of transverse sections of the media of the pulmonary trunk and ascending aorta in each of the five patients are shown in Figs. 2-6.

Discussion

In the normal newborn infant the pressure in the pulmonary trunk is similar to that in the aorta.[5] Shortly thereafter, however, the pressure in the former falls considerably, whereas the pressure in the latter changes slightly. Coincident with the changes in the pressure in the lesser circulation after birth, a change in the configuration of the elastic tissue in the media of the pulmonary trunk occurs. According to Heath and associates,[4] at birth the configuration of the elastic tissue in the pulmonary trunk is similar to that in the ascending aorta (Fig. 7). During the first few months of extrauterine life, the elastic fibrils in the pulmonary trunk decrease in number, become irregular, fragmented, shortened, and frequently clumped or club shaped. By 6 months of age the configuration of the elastic tissue in the pulmonary trunk is distinctly different from that in the aorta, and by the end of the second year the adult-pulmonary type of elastic configuration of the media is established (Fig. 8). The configuration of the elastic tissue in the aorta does not change from birth to adulthood. Its media consists of long, uniform, tightly packed, parallel elastic fibrils. When pulmonary hypertension is acquired later in life, as in some patients with atrial septal defect (Fig. 9) or rheumatic mitral stenosis (Fig. 10), the configuration of the elastic tissue in the pulmonary trunk is unchanged from the normal adult-pulmonary type. On the other hand, when pulmonary hyper-

Table I. *Data from five patients with "primary" pulmonary hypertension*

Patient	*Age (yr.), race, sex*	*Length of illness from onset of symptoms (yr.)*	*Cardiac catheterization*			*Type configuration of elastica in media of pulmonary trunk*
			*Pulmonary arterial pressure (mm. Hg) S/D (M)**	*Brachial arterial pressure (mm. Hg)*	*Index, pulmonary blood flow (L./min./M.²)*	
1. A54–32	29, W, F	5	120/40		1.52	Adult-pulmonary
2. A56–160	22, W, M	3	88/54 (61)	100/60 (75)	1.50	Adult-pulmonary
3. A57–215	25, W, F	2½	90/34	96/74		Adult-pulmonary
4. A58–21	8, W, F	2	190/100 (130)	90/55 (60)		Transitional
5. A60–219	16, W, F	2†	192/5‡	138/90 (123)	2.14	Aortic (fetal)

*S/D (M) Systolic/diastolic (mean).
†Died during cardiac catheterization procedure.
‡Right ventricular pressure. Pulmonary artery not entered, but pulmonary valve normal at autopsy.

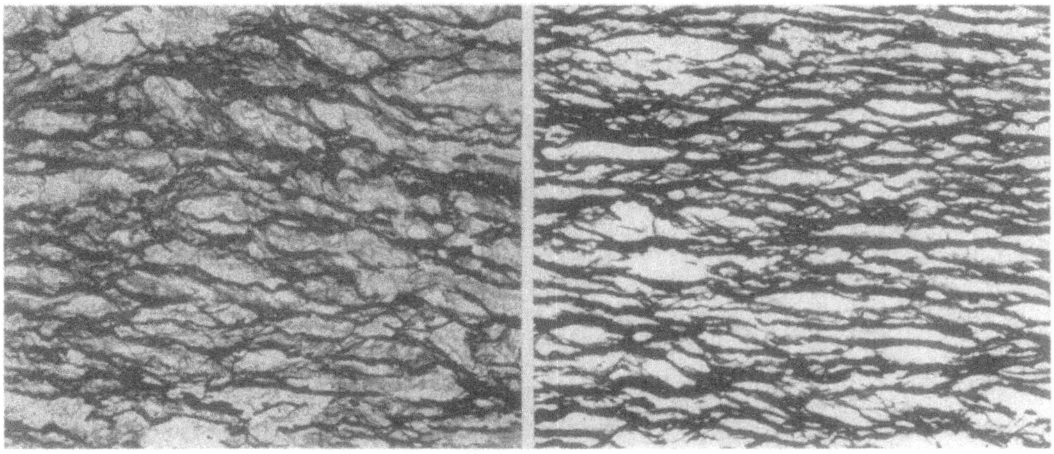

Fig. 2. Case 1. Pulmonary trunk (*left*); ascending aorta (*right*). The configuration of the elastic fibers of the pulmonary trunk resembles that of the adult-pulmonary type. Elastic tissue stains; ×155.

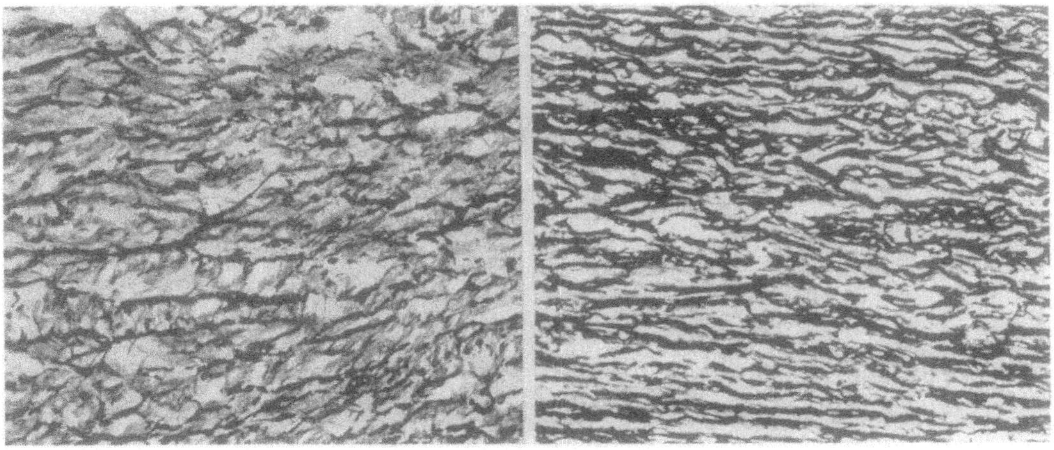

Fig. 3. Case 2. Pulmonary trunk (*left*); ascending aorta (*right*). The elastic fibers of the pulmonary trunk are of the adult-pulmonary type. Elastic tissue stains; ×155.

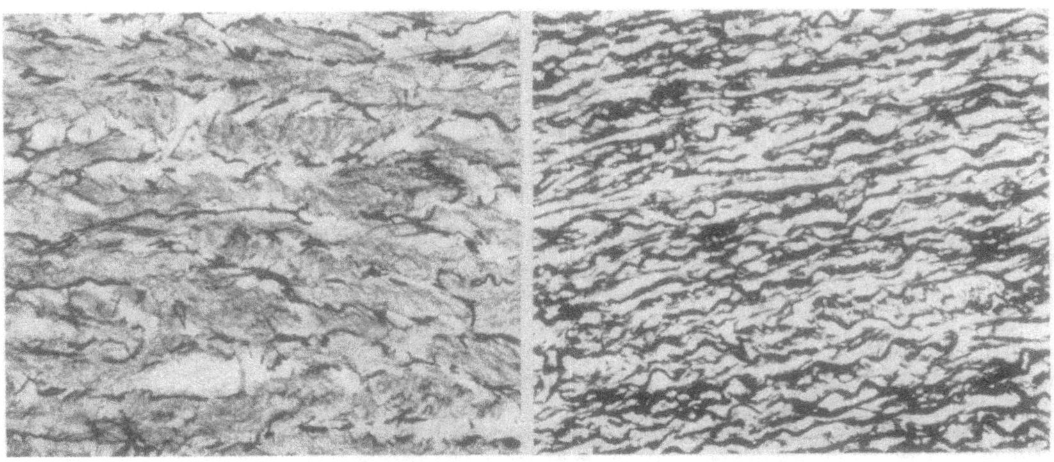

Fig. 4. Case 3. Pulmonary trunk (*left*); ascending aorta (*right*). The elastic fibers of the pulmonary trunk have an adult configuration. Elastic tissue stains; ×155.

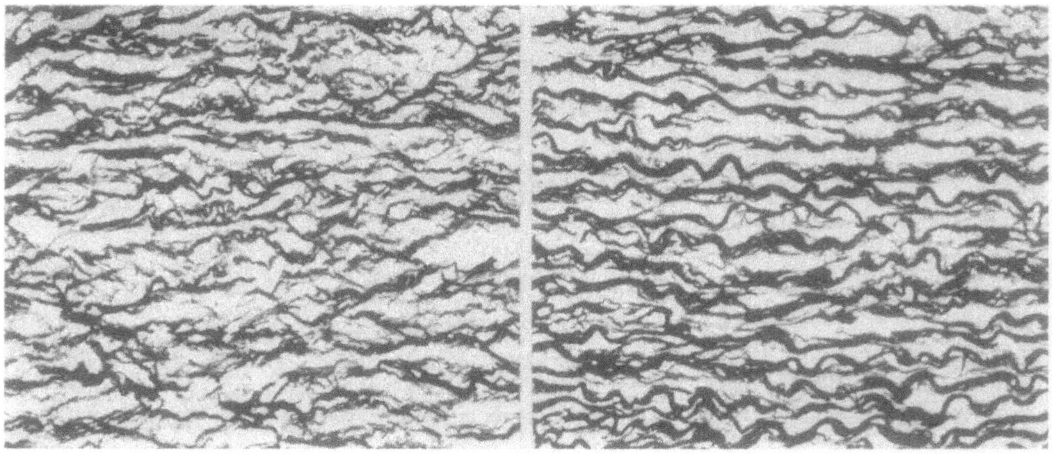

Fig. *5*. Case 4. Pulmonary trunk (*left*); ascending aorta (*right*). The configuration of the elastica of the pulmonary trunk is transitional, being neither fetal nor adult-pulmonary in type. Elastic tissue stains; ×155.

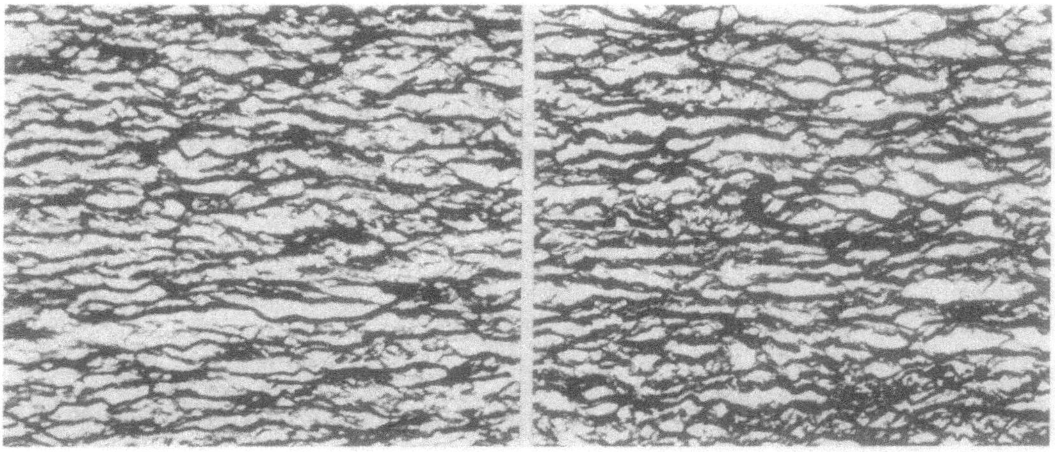

Fig. *6*. Case 5. Pulmonary trunk (*left*); ascending aorta (*right*). The configuration of the elastic fibers of the pulmonary trunk is of the fetal type, being indistinguishable from that of the ascending aorta. Elastic tissue stains; ×155.

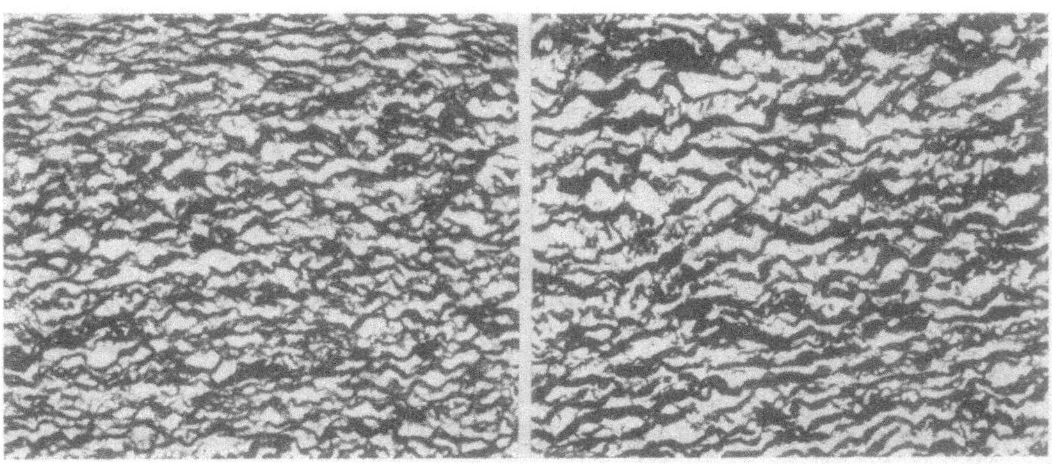

Fig. *7*. Control pulmonary trunk (*left*) and ascending aorta (*right*) in a 19-hour-old newborn infant. The configuration of the elastic tissue of each is similar. Elastic tissue stains; ×155.

Fig. *8*. Control pulmonary trunk (*left*) and ascending aorta (*right*) in a 20-year-old woman. The media of the pulmonary trunk has considerably fewer elastic fibrils than does the media of the ascending aorta. The configuration of the elastica of the pulmonary trunk is of the normal adult-pulmonary type. Elastic tissue stains; ×155.

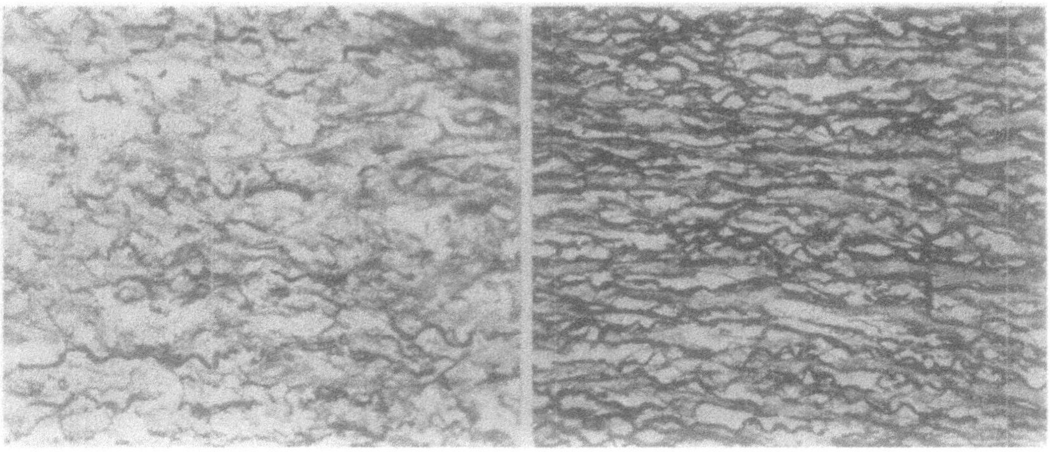

Fig. *9*. Pulmonary trunk (*left*) and ascending aorta (*right*) in a 31-year-old woman with an atrial septal defect and secondary pulmonary hypertension. The configuration of the elastica of the pulmonary trunk is of the normal adult type, indicating that the hypertension of the lesser circulation was acquired later in life. Elastic tissue stains; ×155.

tension is present from birth, as in patients with large ventricular septal defect (Fig. 11) or widely patent ductus arteriosus, the fetal, aortic-like configuration of the elastic tissue in the pulmonary trunk persists.[4]

The presence of the adult-pulmonary configuration in three of the five patients with PPH in this study may be interpreted as indicating that pulmonary hypertension was acquired in these cases. The finding of a definite aortic-like, fetal, configuration of elastic tissue in one patient in this study suggests that pulmonary hypertension was present from birth in this instance, and the transitional configuration in the other patient may be indicative of pulmonary hypertension of milder degree from birth. The results of this study are similar to those reported by Heath and Edwards[1] and by Farrar and associates.[2] The former investigators found an adult-pulmonary configuration of the elastica in the pulmonary trunk in five, and a transitional configuration in one of six patients with PPH.

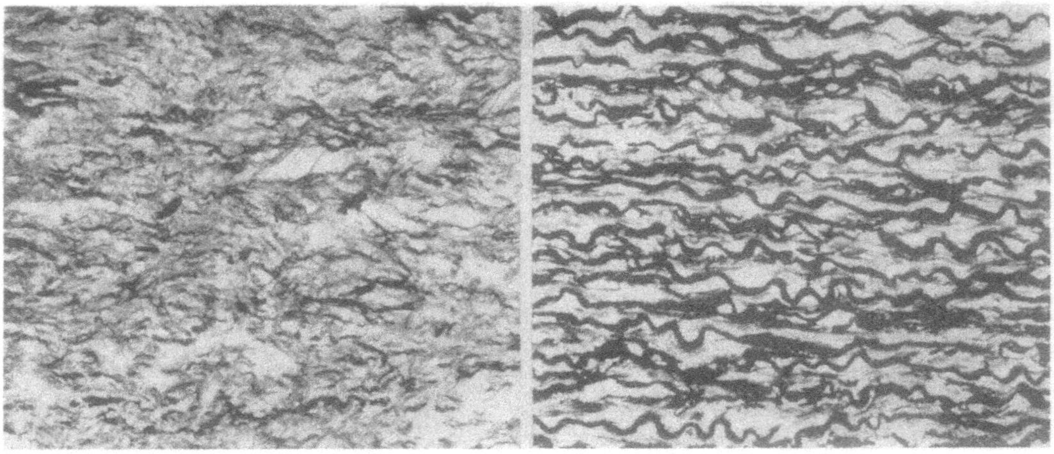

Fig. *10*. Pulmonary trunk (*left*) and ascending aorta (*right*) in a 32-year-old woman with rheumatic mitral stenosis and secondary pulmonary hypertension. The configuration of media of the pulmonary trunk is of the adult-pulmonary type, indicating that the pressure in the pulmonary arterial circuit was at one time normal, and that the hypertension was acquired. Elastic tissue stains; ×155.

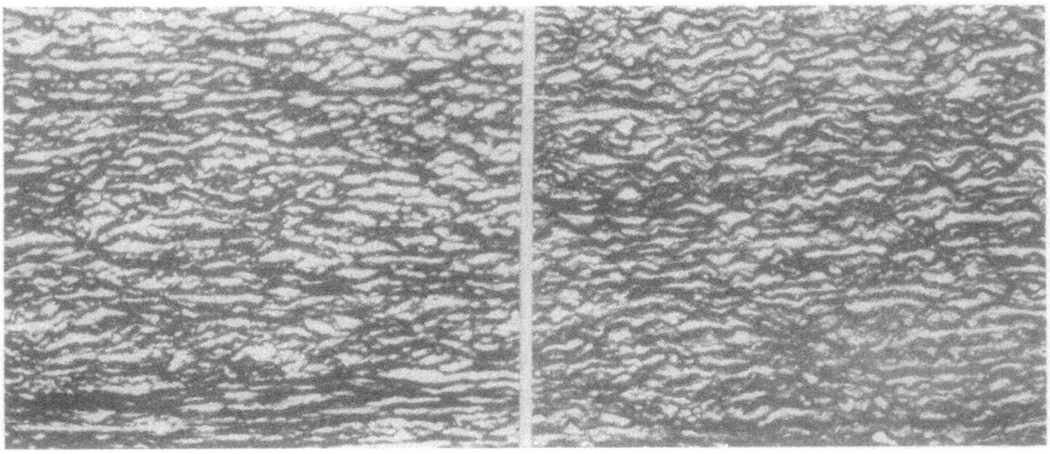

Fig. *11*. Pulmonary trunk (*left*) and ascending aorta (*right*) in an 8-year-old boy with a large ventricular septal defect and pulmonary hypertension. The aortic-like or fetal configuration of the elastica of the pulmonary trunk would indicate that the pulmonary hypertension was present from birth. Elastic tissue stains; ×155.

Farrar and associates found an adult-pulmonary configuration of the pulmonary trunk in two, and a transitional configuration in one of three patients with PPH studied at autopsy.

From the data in Table I, it would be impossible to make a definite correlation between the type of configuration of elastic tissue in the pulmonary trunk and the age, length of illness, pulmonary arterial pressure, or pulmonary blood flow in these patients. The pulmonary arterial pressure, however, appears to be slightly higher in those patients with the aortic or transitional type of pulmonary trunk. The conclusions of Heath and Edwards[3] would indicate that one (Patient 5, Table I), and possibly two (Patient 4, Table I), of the five patients in this study had pulmonary hypertension for periods of 16 and 8 years, respectively.

I wish to thank Dr. Eugene Braunwald, Chief, Cardiology Branch, National Heart Institute, for his helpful suggestions during the preparation of this manuscript and for his allowing me free use of the cardiac catheterization data. In addition, I wish to express my appreciation to Dr. Jesse Edwards, Professor of Pathology, Mayo Foundation, and Graduate School, University of Minnesota, for reviewing the histologic sections.

REFERENCES

1. Heath, D., and Edwards, J. E.: Configuration of elastic tissue of pulmonary trunk in idiopathic pulmonary hypertension, Circulation **21**:59, 1960.
2. Farrar, J. F., Reye, R. D. K., and Stuckey, D.: Primary pulmonary hypertension in childhood, Brit. Heart J. **23**:605, 1961.
3. Heath, D., and Edwards, J. E.: The pathology of hypertensive pulmonary vascular disease. A description of six grades of structural changes in the pulmonary arteries, with special reference to congenital cardiac septal defect, Circulation **28**:533, 1958.
4. Heath, D., DuShane, J. W., Wood, E. H., and Edwards, J. E.: The structure of the pulmonary trunk at different ages and in cases of pulmonary hypertension and pulmonary stenosis, J. Path. & Bact. **77**:443, 1959.
5. Barcroft, J.: Researches on pre-natal life, Springfield, Ill., 1946, Charles C Thomas, Publisher, p. 292.

Acute Severe Mitral Regurgitation Secondary to Ruptured Chordae Tendineae

Clinical, Hemodynamic, and Pathologic Considerations

By William C. Roberts, M.D., Eugene Braunwald, M.D., and Andrew G. Morrow, M.D.

THE MAJORITY of patients with severe mitral regurgitation have enlarged left atria, atrial fibrillation, a history of acute rheumatic fever, and a gradual onset of symptoms of cardiac decompensation that may persist for many years. This report describes 10 patients with severe mitral regurgitation caused by rupture of one or more chordae tendineae, and contrasts the clinical, radiographic, hemodynamic, and pathologic findings in these patients with those commonly noted in patients with the more usual form of mitral regurgitation. Thus, the majority of the patients with ruptured chordae tendineae had little left atrial enlargement, were in sinus rhythm, and had not had a history of acute rheumatic fever. The symptoms of cardiac decompensation generally appeared abruptly, and were usually present for only several months before they led to the patient's death or necessitated operative treatment. An appreciation of this relatively pure, acute form of mitral regurgitation is important in the understanding of the wide range of physiologic, pathologic, and clinical findings that may accompany this valvular lesion.

Description of Patients

A summary of the clinical, electrocardiographic, hemodynamic and pathologic findings in the individual patients is presented in table 1.

History. The 10 patients ranged in age from 17 to 54 years. Six were women. Only one patient (L. L.) had a history suggestive of acute rheumatic fever, and none had a history of chorea or chest trauma. Six patients had a definite history of bacterial endocarditis, and each had been asymptomatic and fully active prior to the onset of the infection. Pregnancy appeared to have played a role in the appearance of the bacterial endocarditis in three patients; A. L. and A. A. developed the infection shortly after parturition, while patient R. H. developed pyogenic endometritis after an abortion which in turn was followed by bacterial endocarditis. In two patients each *alpha streptococcus* and *staphylococcus aureus* were the organisms responsible for the endocarditis, and in one patient each the causative organisms were *streptococcus faecalis* and *staphylococcus albus.* The onset of cardiac decompensation was abrupt in nine patients and was progressive thereafter, while in patient V. C., who did not have a history of bacterial endocarditis, symptoms developed more slowly. In seven patients the period of time from the onset of symptoms of cardiac failure to autopsy or operation was less than 16 months, while in the other three patients the interval ranged from 5 to 8 years. Seven patients had no knowledge of heart murmurs before the onset of bacterial endocarditis or cardiac failure. Three patients, two of whom had a history of bacterial endocarditis, were known to have had precordial murmurs for periods ranging from 12 to 43 years before operation or death. In one of these patients, the murmur may have resulted from the presence of associated partial anomalous pulmonary venous connection and a small atrial septal defect.

Each of the patients complained of easy fatigability, exertional and nocturnal dyspnea, and all but one had pedal edema. All were treated with digitalis and salt restriction, but despite these measures they were severely disabled and considered to be in functional classes III or IV.

Physical Examination. Each of the 10 patients had prominent right ventricular and less prominent left ventricular lifts as well as easily papable apical systolic thrills. The sound of pulmonic valve closure was accentuated in all patients, and a third heart sound was almost always audible. In every patient, a blowing pansystolic murmur of at least grade IV/VI intensity was heard over the entire precordium, loudest over the cardiac apex, with radiation to the left axilla. In two patients the murmur at the cardiac apex was of whistling or

From the Clinic of Surgery and the Cardiology Branch, National Heart Institute, National Institutes of Health, Bethesda, Maryland.

cooing quality, and in two others the systolic murmur was also audible over the entire vertebral column.[1] In five patients the systolic murmur along the lower left sternal border became louder during inspiration. Seven patients had short, low-pitched, mid-diastolic flow murmurs at the apex, and two patients had high-pitched, blowing, diastolic murmurs along the left sternal border. The liver was palpable and tender in the majority of the patients, and pulsated during systole in three of them.

Electrocardiograms (Fig. 1). Eight patients had sinus rhythm, and two had atrial fibrillation; in one of the latter this arrhythmia appeared shortly before death. Right axis deviation was present in five patients, and left axis deviation in one. Four patients had first-degree atrioventricular block. Right ventricular hypertrophy was present in seven patients and left ventricular hypertrophy as well in three. Seven patients exhibited the peaked P waves characteristic of right atrial enlargement, and one had left atrial enlargement.

Roentgenograms (Fig. 2). Some degree of cardiac enlargement was evident on the chest roentgenograms of all 10 patients. The left atrium was mildly or moderately enlarged in eight patients, and markedly enlarged in only the two patients who had been symptomatic for the longest times, 5 and 8 years. Both ventricles were considered to be enlarged in all 10 patients. Calcification in the region of the mitral valve was detected in only one patient (L. L.). Angiographic studies with left ventricular injection in each of two patients (A. F. and L. S.) showed near-normal sized left atria which expanded strikingly during ventricular systole, but there was no evidence of prolapse of a mitral valve leaflet into the left atrium.

Hemodynamic Findings (Fig. 3). All nine patients who underwent right heart catheterization had markedly elevated pulmonary arterial and right ventricular systolic pressures, ranging from 61 to 110 mm. Hg. The mean left atrial pressures were elevated to between 15 and 32 mm. Hg in eight patients, and within normal limits (11 mm. Hg) in the ninth. The v-wave peaks were abnormally elevated in all nine patients and ranged from 23 to 66 mm. Hg (average, 45 mm. Hg). The left ventricular end-diastolic pressure was normal ($\leqq$ 12 mm. Hg) in six of the eight patients in whom it was measured, and was markedly elevated (20 and 27 mm. Hg) in two. The

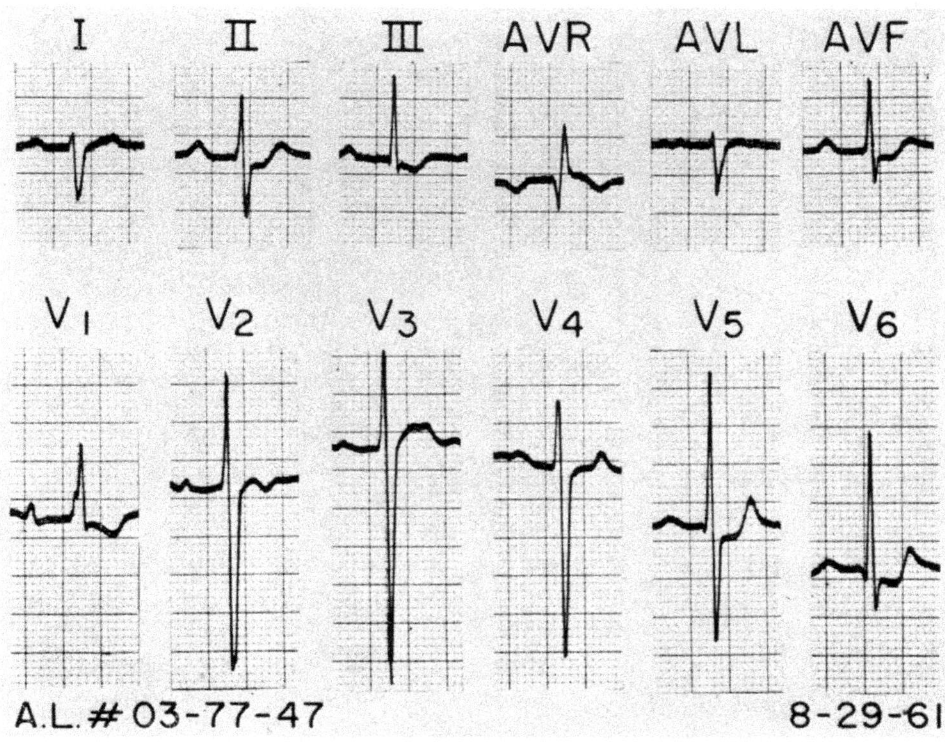

Figure 1

Electrocardiogram of patient A.L. Right axis deviation, right atrial enlargement, right ventricular hypertrophy, and possible left ventricular hypertrophy are present, although mitral regurgitation had been present for only 16 months.

Table 1

Clinical, Electrocardiographic, Hemodynamic, and Pathologic Data from the 10 Patients with Ruptured Mitral Chordae Tendineae

Patient no. (sex)	Age at death or at operation / Length of symptoms	History of bacterial endocarditis (organism)	Electro-cardiogram	Hemodynamic data: PA s/d (mean) (mm. Hg)	LA mean—v wave (mm. Hg)	LV s/d (mm. Hg)	Cardiac index (L./min./M.²)	Pulmonary vascular resistance (dynes sec. cm.⁻⁵)	LA size at operation (O) at autopsy (A)
1. V.C. 01-21-66 (M)	41 yr. / 5 yr.	—	AF, RAD, RAE, RVH, LVH	110/40 (67)	32—39*		1.4	1217	Dilated (A)
2. A.A. 01-71-62 (F)	37 yr. / 7 mo.	—	NSR, RAE, RVH		24—52	92/27			"Normal" (A)
3. A.L. 03-77-47 (F)	19 yr. / 16 mo.	+ Streptococcus Group D	NSR, RAD, RAE, RVH, First-degree HB	70/30 (45)	15—36	100/10	1.7	950	"Normal" (A)
4. R.H. 03-99-19 (F)	24 yr. / 5 mo.	+ Enterococcus	NSR, RAE, First-degree HB	72/32 (54)	27—66	108/11	1.5	1000	"Normal" (A)
5. P.H. 04-94-07 (F)	29 yr. / 5 yr.	+ Staphylococcus albus	NSR, RAD, RAE, RVH, LVH	105/40 (70)	15—35		1.6	2000	"Normal" (A)
6. B.F. 04-85-25 (F)	21 yr. / 13 mo.	+ Staphylococcus aureus	NSR, RAD, RAE, RVH, LVH	65/28† ↓ 32/11 (16)‡	11—23† ↓ 6—11‡	100/9†	1.4† ↓ 3.0‡	1100† ↓ 179‡	"Normal" (O)
7. J.W. 04-87-16 (M)	54 yr. / 8 yr.	+ Alpha strepto-coccus	NSR, RVH, LAE, First-degree HB	70/27 ↓(37)† 44/20 (28)‡	15—32† ↓ 7—10‡	90/11† ↓ 95/5‡	2.8‡	382‡	Dilated (O)
8. L.L. 05-45-40 (M)	53 yr. / 9 mo.	—	AF, LAD	61/25† ↓(39) 29/10 (17)‡	22—56† ↓ 10—21‡	81/9† ↓ 119/9‡	0.9† ↓ 3.2‡	1070† ↓ 94‡	"Normal" (O)
9. A.F. 05-78-22 (M)	48 yr. / 7 mo.	—	NSR, Nonspecific T-wave changes	84/30	25—65	100/20	1.8	609	"Normal" (O)
10. L.S. 05-99-23 (F)	17 yr. / 5 mo.	+ Staphylococcus aureus	NSR, RVH, RAE, RAD, First-degree HB	71/41 (51)	24*	86/12			"Normal" (A)

*Pulmonary arterial wedge pressures.

†Before operation.

‡Several months after operation.

Abbreviations: PA, pulmonary arterial pressure; LA, left atrial pressure; LV, left ventricular pressure; s/d (mean), systolic/diastolic (mean) pressures; AF, atrial fibrillation; RBBB, right bundle-branch block; NSR, normal sinus rhythm; RVH, right ventricular hypertrophy; RAE, right atrial enlargement; LVH, left ventricular hypertrophy; LAE, left atrial enlargement; LAD, left axis deviation; HB, heart block. "Normal," near normal size or only moderately dilated.

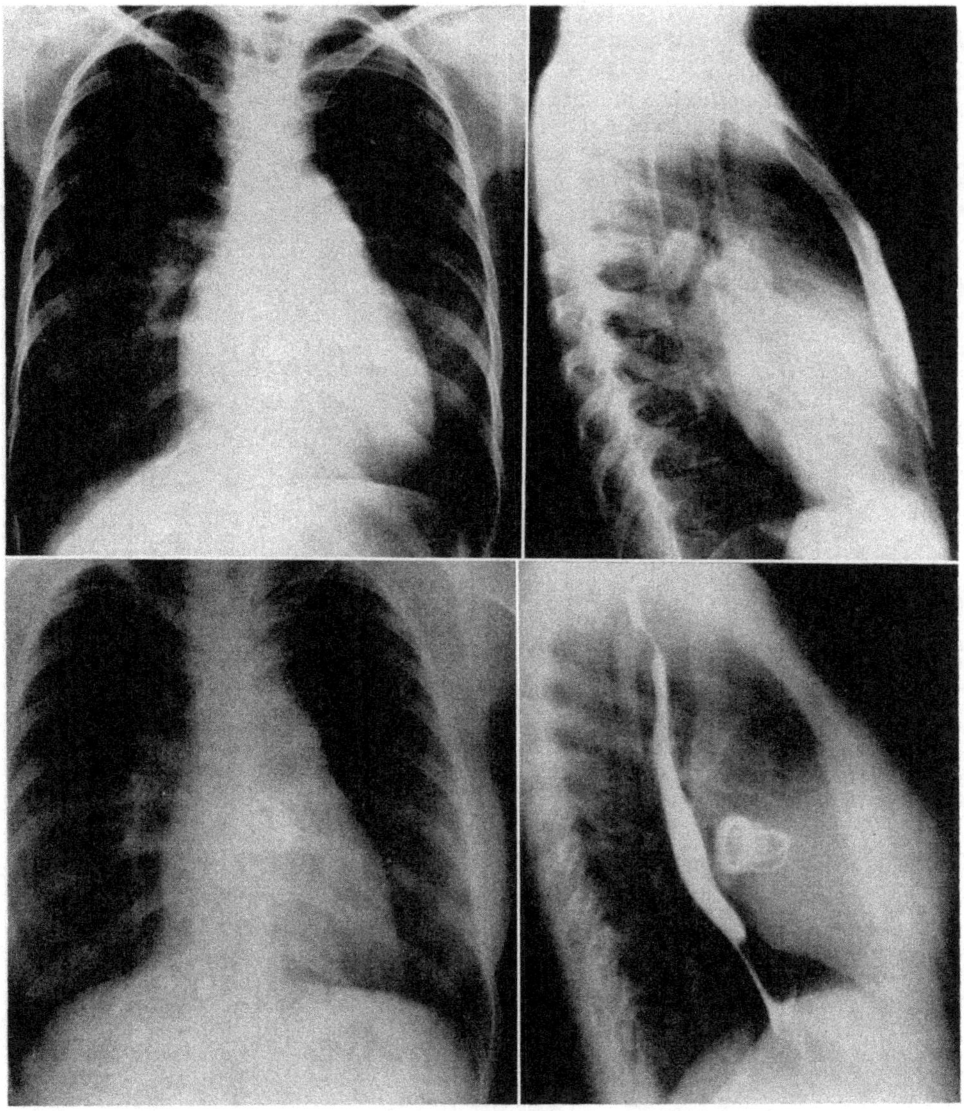

Figure 2

Roentgenograms obtained preoperatively (upper) *and 7 months postoperatively* (lower) *in patient B.F. This patient had had severe mitral regurgitation for 13 months before operation, but there was only minimal left atrial enlargement.*

cardiac output was markedly reduced in each of the seven patients in whom it was measured, and ranged from 0.9 to 1.8 L./min./M.^{2}, with an average of 1.5 L./min./M.^{2}. Pulmonary vascular resistance was calculated in seven patients and ranged from 609 to 2,000 with an average of 1135 dynes sec. cm.$^{-5}$. Indicator-dilution curves recorded from a systemic artery following injection into the left ventricle or left atrium in seven patients showed the prolonged descending limb characteristic of severe mitral regurgitation.

Pathologic Findings (Figs. 4-11). The mitral valves and chordae tendineae were examined in six patients at necropsy. In the other four patients the mitral valve was examined after it had been surgically excised with the chordae tendineae and papillary muscles intact. One patient died of heart failure, one from a complication of cardiac catheterization, three following mitral annuloplasty, and one following Starr-Edwards mitral valve replacement.

Ruptured chordae tendineae were responsible for mitral regurgitation in every patient, and in six of them the rupture was clearly the result of bacterial endocarditis. Active endocarditis was present in two patients (R. H. and L. S.); it involved the posterior half of the aortic leaflet of the mitral valve in one (fig. 6); and both anterior and posterior leaflets in the other patient. All chordae that had inserted into these portions of the valve had been destroyed. Organisms, however, were not found in sections of the valves of either of these patients. In six patients most or all of the chordae to one half of the anterior leaflet of the mitral valve were ruptured, in one patient all of the chordae that had been attached to the posterior leaflet were involved, and in three patients several chordae from both leaflets were destroyed. With the exception of the two patients with active endocarditis, there were no essential differences between the pathologic findings in the patients with and those without a history of bacterial endocarditis. Although some fibrous thickening of the mitral leaflet adjacent to the ruptured chordae was usually evident, the remaining mitral valve leaflets, commissures, and remaining chordae showed no apparent abnormalities. The aortic valve was normal in the six autopsied patients. In the other four patients, no abnormalities of the aortic valve were detected at the time of operation. The tricuspid and pulmonic valves also were normal in the hearts examined at necropsy.

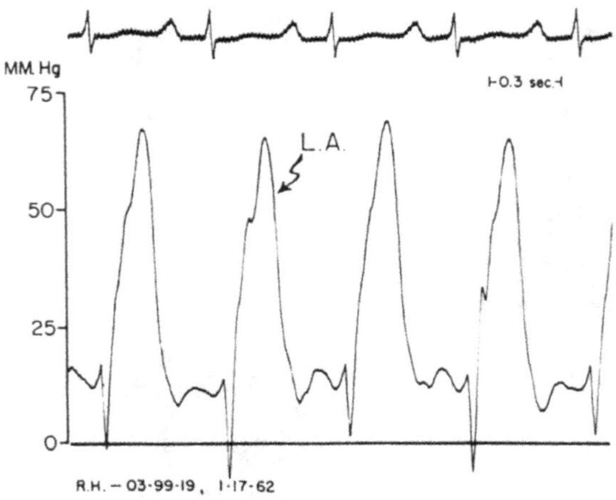

Figure 3

Left atrial pressure tracing in patient R.H., who had had mitral regurgitation for only 5 months.

The left atrial chamber was near normal size, or only moderately enlarged, in the six autopsied patients, and in each of them the left atrial wall was considerably thickened. In two of the patients, who had had symptoms for 5 and 8 years, the left atrium was severely dilated. Jet lesions were present on the endocardial surface of the left atrium in all 10 patients, their location depending upon the position of the ruptured chordae. The right

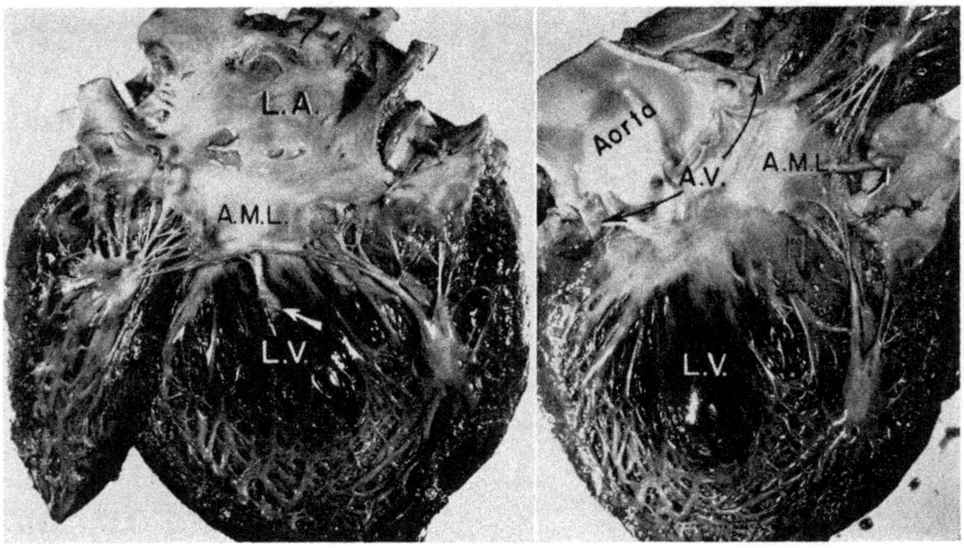

Figure 4

Photographs of heart of patient 2 (A.A.). Left. *The left atrium (L.A.), mitral valve, and left ventricle (L.V.) are seen. The ruptured chorda* (arrow), *which is club-shaped, arises from the midportion of the anterior mitral leaflet (A.M.L.). The nonruptured chordae are normal. The left atrium is not dilated, but the left ventricle is considerably dilated.* Right. *The anterior mitral leaflet (A.M.L.) is now seen from the ventricular aspect. The aortic valve (A.V.) is normal.*

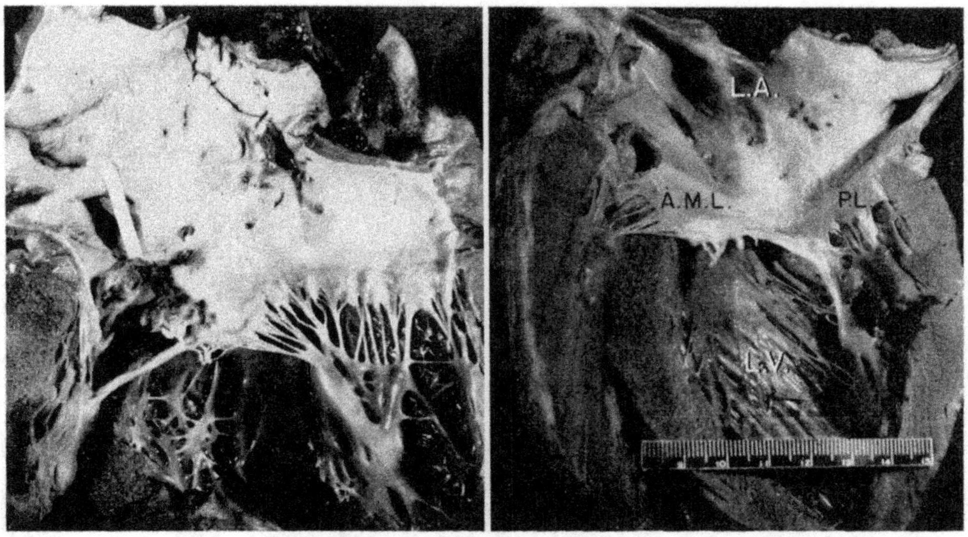

Figure 5

Photographs of opened left atrium (L.A.), mitral valve, and left ventricle (L.V.) of patient 3 (A.L.) left, *and patient 5 (P.H.)* right. *Chordae tendineae that had attached to the anterior (A.M.L.) and posterior (P.L.) mitral leaflets adjacent to the anterolateral commissure are absent in the heart of patient 3* (left). *The arrow points to the site of jet lesion in the left atrium in this patient. All chordae tendineae from the posterior portion of the anterior mitral leaflet (A.M.L.) are severed in patient 5* (right). *The nonruptured chordae in each patient are normal, and in neither is the left atrium dilated.*

ventricle was dilated and hypertrophied in the six patients studied at necropsy.

On microscopic examination, there were no Aschoff bodies in sections of the heart from any of the six autopsied patients, and sections of the left atrial walls disclosed severe hypertrophy of the myocardial fibers and marked thickening of the endocardium (fig. 8). Histologic examination of sections from the lungs of the six autopsied patients disclosed grade 3/6 hypertensive pulmonary vascular changes in each (classification of Heath and Edwards[2]). Three patients had ossific nodules scattered in the lungs. Examples of microscopic changes in the lungs of two patients are shown in figures 9 and 10. The pulmonary vascular changes in patients R. H. and A. A. were particularly noteworthy, since these patients had had clinical evidence of mitral regurgitation for only 5 and 7 months, respectively, before death. There was severe centrolobular hepatic congestion in each of the six autopsied patients, an example of which is shown in figure 11.

Discussion

In the past, the conditions considered to be responsible for ruptured chordae tendineae of the mitral valve included rheumatic fever,[3-5] trauma,[6] so-called spontaneous rupture,[7] and bacterial endocarditis involving either diseased or normal valves.[5, 8-10] Most authors have considered that chordal rupture occurs predominantly in previously diseased valves. In the National Institutes of Health collection of almost 150 hearts with acquired mitral valvular disease, there are only two with ruptured mitral chordae, and in both patients this was clearly of secondary importance in the resultant regurgitation. On the other hand, we have encountered the 10 patients, described in this report, who had ruptured mitral chordae involving a valve that otherwise appeared not to be grossly diseased. Critical review of earlier reports, including published photographs of ruptured mitral chordae, indicated numerous instances of ruptured mitral chordae in valves that also did not appear grossly abnormal,[4, 5, 7, 10-17] although some of the authors had considered that rheumatic heart disease was the underlying process. Although bacterial endocarditis tends to affect obviously malformed or previously diseased valves most often, and chronic rheumatic involvement might thus predispose to chordal rupture, it seems entirely possible that the marked thickening and shortening of the chordae tendineae of a rheumatic valve may actually serve to protect these structures from rupture. On the basis of the experience with the patients described in this report, as well as the many published illustrations of ruptured chordae in valves that do not appear grossly abnormal, it is suggested that bacterial endocarditis occurring in hearts without detectable anatomic valvular abnormalities is an important cause of chordal rupture.

Immediately following rupture of a single chorda in the dog, the left atrial pressure, particularly the v-wave peak, rises abruptly, a systolic thrill and murmur become detectable in this chamber, and the left atrial appendage begins to balloon during each ventricular systole.[18, 19] The animals rapidly develop congestive cardiac failure, and their course is usually one of rapid progression. From the hemodynamic point of view, the

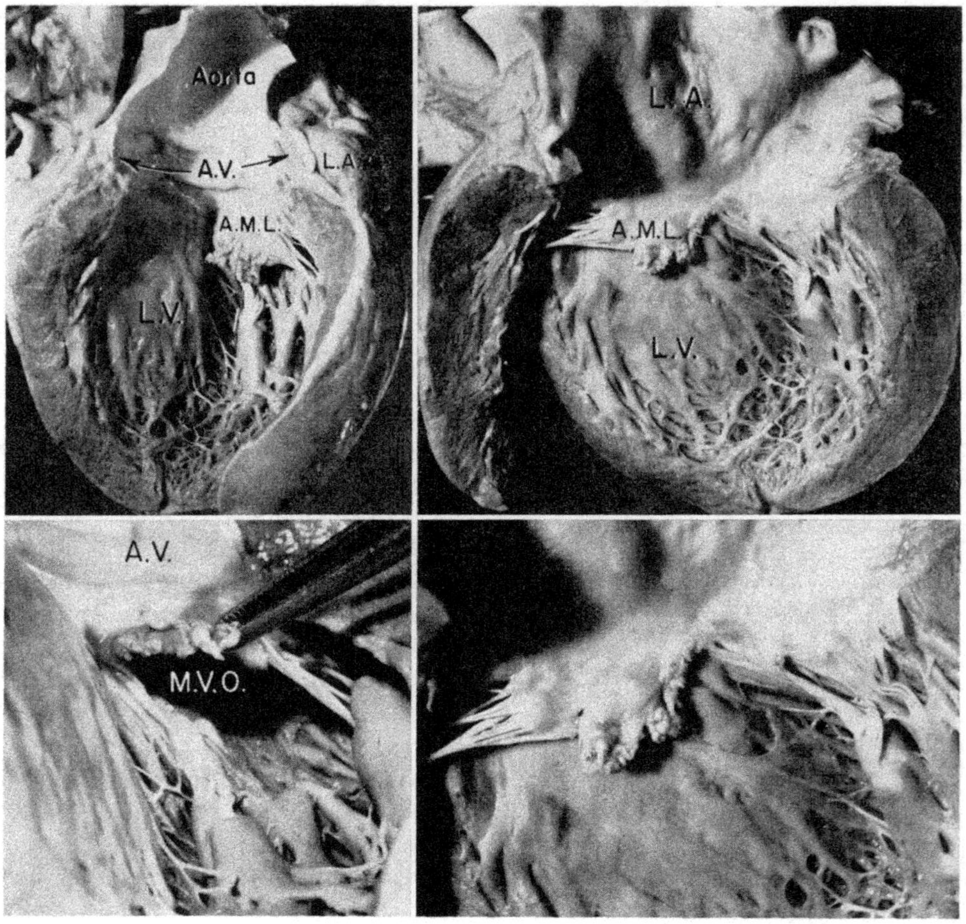

Figure 6

Photographs of heart of patient 4 (R.H.). Upper left. *The mitral valve is exposed by opening the left ventricle (L.V.), aortic valve (A.V.), and aorta. All chordae tendineae that had attached to the posterior portion of the anterior mitral leaflet (A.M.L.) are severed. The endocarditis that ruptured the chordae is active. The aortic valve is normal. L.A.A., left atrial appendage.* Lower left. *The size of the incompetent mitral valve orifice (M.V.O.) is apparent from this view. A.V., aortic valve cusps.* Upper right. *The left atrium (L.A.), mitral valve, and left ventricle (L.V.) are opened. The nonruptured mitral chordae are normal. A.M.L., anterior mitral leaflet.* Lower right. *Close-up of the ruptured mitral chordae of the anterior leaflet.*

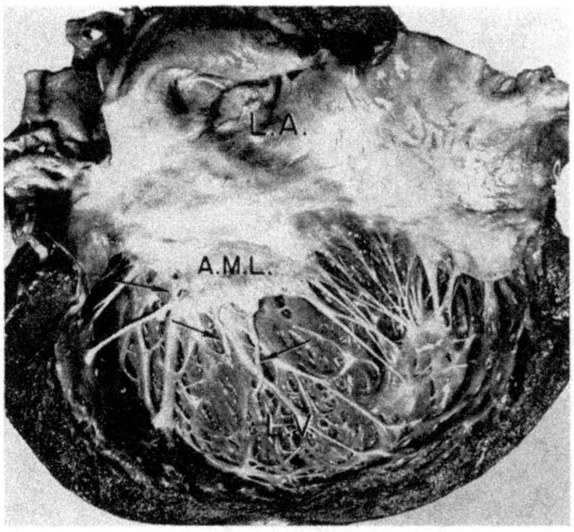

Figure 7

Photograph of heart of patient 1 (V.C.). The left atrium (L.A.), mitral valve, and left ventricle (L.V.) are opened. Both chambers are considerably dilated as is the mitral valve annulus. This patient had known mitral regurgitation for at least 5 years. At least three chordae tendineae (arrows) *from the anterior mitral leaflet (A.M.L.) are severed and each of these is thickened as is a portion of this leaflet. The non-ruptured chordae are elongated, but otherwise normal. The posterior leaflet is normal.*

regurgitation produced suddenly in experimental animals more closely resembles the mitral regurgitation that developed acutely in the patients described herein than the regurgitation observed in patients with chronic rheumatic mitral regurgitation. In the latter condition, the regurgitation usually develops gradually, and sufficient time is available for the usual adjustments to this lesion to take place. In addition, the myocardium of the left atrium and of the left ventricle may also be affected by the rheumatic process. In the present group of patients with ruptured mitral chordae tendineae, however, the myocardium and pulmonary vascular bed were presumably normal at the time the chordae ruptured, and the resultant clinical, hemodynamic, and anatomic abnormalities may be attributed entirely or almost entirely to the mechanical defect.

The unusual hemodynamic and clinical features of the majority of patients described herein may be emphasized by comparing them with other groups of patients having severe mitral regurgitation. Patients with se-

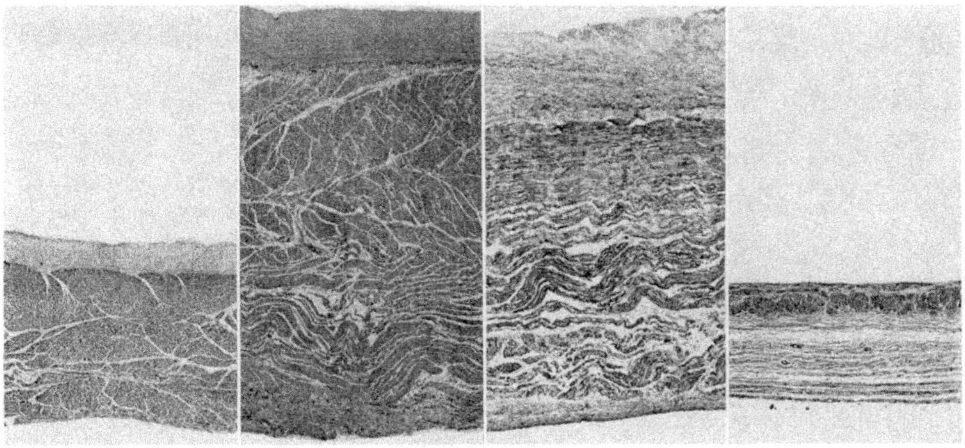

Figure 8

Photomicrographs of sections of posterior wall of left atrium in four patients each taken from a site approximately 3 cm. above the mitral annulus. Left. *Left atrial wall in 30-year-old woman dying of acute leukemia (for control). The endocardium is above, the epicardium, below.* Mid-left. *Left atrial wall in patient 4 (R.H.) showing marked thickening. This patient died 5 months after the onset of cardiac decompensation.* Mid-right. *Left atrial wall in patient 5 (P.H.) who lived for 5 years after the onset of cardiac decompensation. The endocardium is thicker, but the myocardium is thinner than in patient R.H.* Right. *Left atrial wall of a patient with mitral regurgitation, a giant left atrium, and normal left atrial pressures. The myocardial fibers are extremely elongated and thinned. The smooth muscle immediately beneath the endocardium is hypertrophied. Hematoxylin and eosin stains, original magnification in each* × *20.*

vere mitral regurgitation were previously separated into three major groups on the basis of obvious differences in atrial compliance.[20] I. A group with the sudden development of mitral regurgitation in whom there was mild to moderate enlargement of the left atrium, striking elevation of the mean left atrial pressure, of the left atrial v wave, the pul-

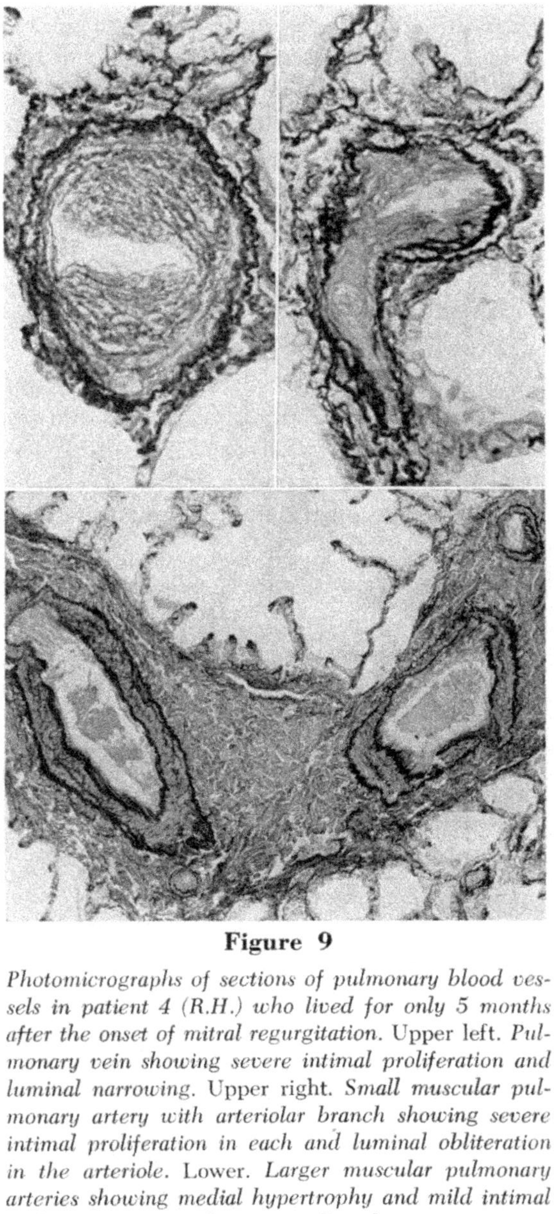

Figure 9

Photomicrographs of sections of pulmonary blood vessels in patient 4 (R.H.) who lived for only 5 months after the onset of mitral regurgitation. Upper left. *Pulmonary vein showing severe intimal proliferation and luminal narrowing.* Upper right. *Small muscular pulmonary artery with arteriolar branch showing severe intimal proliferation in each and luminal obliteration in the arteriole.* Lower. *Larger muscular pulmonary arteries showing medial hypertrophy and mild intimal proliferation. An adjacent small pulmonary artery is markedly narrowed by intimal fibrosis. Elastic tissue stains; original magnification × 340 (two upper), × 125 (lower).*

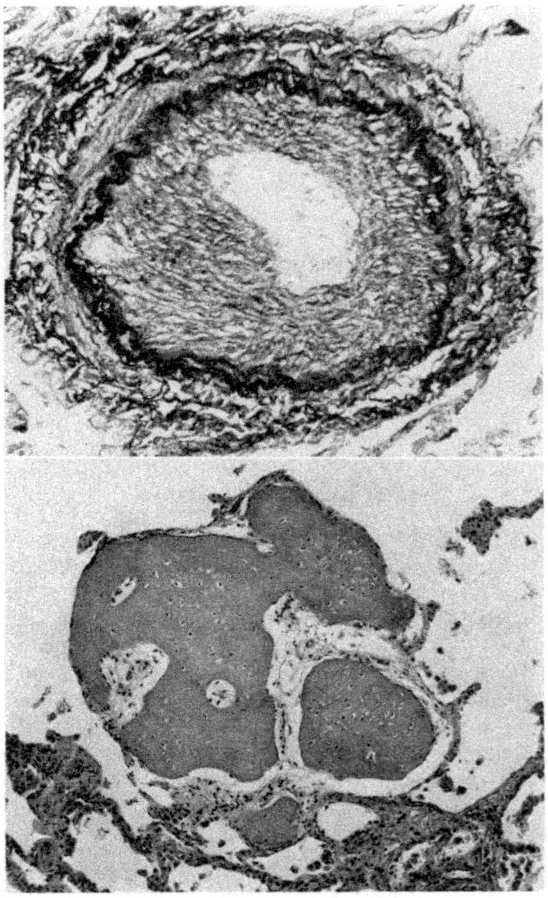

Figure 10

Photomicrographs of sections of lung in patient 2 (A.A.), who survived 7 months after the onset of mitral regurgitation. Upper. *Pulmonary vein showing severe intimal fibrosis.* Lower. *Ossific nodule. These "lung bones" were seen in sections of lungs in three of the six autopsied patients. Elastic tissue stain (upper), hematoxylin and eosin stain (lower); original magnification × 210 (upper), × 135 (lower).*

monary vascular resistance, and in whom severe right heart failure was often present. II. A group who had normal left atrial and pulmonary arterial pressures, normal pulmonary vascular resistance, a low cardiac output, huge left atria, atrial fibrillation, a history of acute rheumatic fever, and a long-standing history of heart failure (the syndrome of severe mitral regurgitation with normal left atrial pressure).[20] III. The largest number of patients with severe mitral regurgitation lies between these two extremes, and they exhibit both gross left atrial enlargement and an

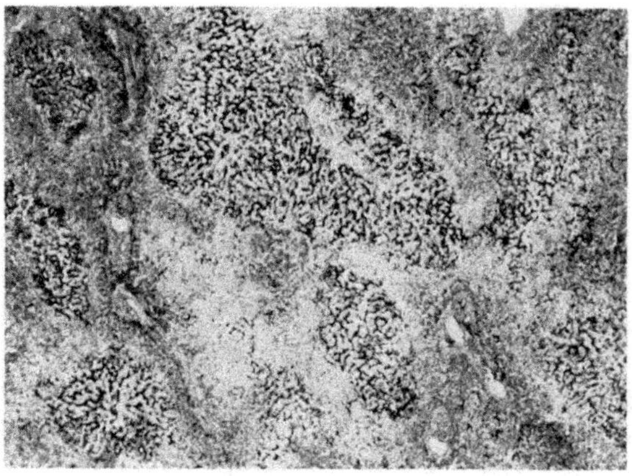

Figure 11

Photomicrograph of section of liver in patient 4 (R.H.), showing massive centrolobular necrosis (dark areas). The few remaining hepatic cells are located adjacent to the portal areas. Similar degrees of hepatic congestion and necrosis were seen in each of the six autopsied patients in this series. Phosphotungstic-acid hematoxylin stain, original magnification × 32.

elevated left atrial pressure. Thus, the patients with the syndrome of severe mitral regurgitation with normal left atrial pressure represent one end of the spectrum of mitral regurgitation, and the seven patients described in this report whose cardiac failure progressed rapidly represent the opposite end.

The severe pulmonary vascular changes observed in these patients with ruptured chordae tendineae are interpreted as anatomic expressions of the markedly elevated left atrial and pulmonary arterial pressures. The advanced pulmonary vascular changes, in association with little or no left atrial enlargement, contrasts sharply with the absence of these changes in patients with huge left atria secondary to long-standing mitral regurgitation.[20] As a consequence of the abnormalities in the pulmonary vascular bed, right ventricular hypertrophy was always present in the patients with acute mitral regurgitation and relatively small left atria, whereas right ventricular hypertrophy is rare in the patients with extremely dilated left atria.[21]

It is likely that the rapidity with which regurgitation develops is the primary determinant of hemodynamic, pathologic, and clinical changes observed in patients with severe mitral insufficiency. It is apparent that the walls of the left atria, and of the pulmonary vessels, were far less compliant in the nine patients with ruptured chordae tendineae who developed heart failure rapidly than in the group of patients with severely dilated left atria and normal left atrial pressures described previously.[20] Long-standing, gradually developing mitral regurgitation would appear, in some instances, to alter the elastic properties of the left atrial wall and, thereby, displace the atrial pressure-volume curve to make this chamber more compliant, so that a normal pressure may exist in a greatly enlarged atrium. Mitral regurgitation was present for only 5 to 16 months in seven of the eight patients in this series with normal or only moderately enlarged left atria. In contrast, symptoms of cardiac decompensation had been present for 5 to 8 years in the two patients with ruptured chordae tendineae who had very large left atria. Additional support for the view that the atrial compliance may increase as a late development in the course of mitral regurgitation was gained from observations in a 9-year-old patient with congenital mitral regurgitation in whom serial catheterization studies were carried out.[22] He was in sinus rhythm and exhibited slight disability at the time his left atrial pressure was grossly elevated (mean, 25; v peak, 45 mm. Hg). Subsequently, the patient developed cardiac failure, atrial fibrillation, and roentgenographic evidence of further increase in size of the left atrium. These changes were accompanied by a decline of left atrial pressure (mean, 15; v peak, 24 mm. Hg). Thus, in this patient a decrease in the mean left atrial pressure and the atrial v-wave peak pressure occurred in the face of an increase in the left atrial size, further substantiating the notion that the elastic properties of the left atrial wall had been altered.

In other reports of patients with ruptured mitral chordae tendineae, the left atrial chamber is usually described as being quite dilated. This finding was present in the six patients with ruptured mitral chordae reported by Menges et al.,[12] and the five described in detail by Osmundson et al.[5] These patients had been symptomatic for a number of years and, in general, the size of the left atrium correlated with the duration of the illness. In contrast, the heart of the first reported patient with ruptured mitral chordae, described by Corvisart in 1812,[23] was not grossly enlarged, but this patient survived for only 10 days after the onset of cardiac symptoms. Similarly, in the patient with ruptured mitral chordae reported by Frothingham and Hass,[7] who had been symptomatic for only 8 months, the left atrium was apparently not enlarged. In the patients described in these reports and others,[4, 10, 11, 13–16] a good correlation existed between left atrial size and the presence or absence of atrial fibrillation. The patients with atrial fibrillation were generally those with symptoms of cardiac disease for several years and very large left atria. The presence of atrial fibrillation in all of the patients with markedly dilated left atrial chambers, but normal atrial pressures,[20] and the absence of this arrhythmia in the patients with ruptured chordae tendineae, as well as in the child with congenital mitral regurgitation discussed above, suggest the possibility that the process that increases atrial compliance may be related to the development of atrial fibrillation.

Operative treatment was undertaken in seven of the 10 patients described herein. Mitral annuloplasty, with or without insertion of artificial chordae, which was originally utilized in this clinic for repair of ruptured chordae, was attempted in two patients, but each of them died in the immediate postoperative period. Mitral valve replacement with a Starr-Edwards prosthesis was carried out in the other five patients, and four have shown considerable improvement. The fifth died 2 weeks after operation of severe pulmonary infection including pulmonary abscess and empyema. Total valve replacement appears to be the most effective operative method for correcting ruptured chordae, although others[12, 15, 16, 17, 24] have reported good results with mitral plication and insertion of artificial chordae tendineae.

Since, with any given magnitude of regurgitant flow, the atrial pressure varies inversely with the compliance of the atrium, the extent to which the atrial pressure can be expected to decline following a corrective operation will also vary inversely with atrial compliance. Accordingly, the clinical and hemodynamic benefits of operation may be expected to be greatest in patients with relatively small left atria and high left atrial pressures. This may be illustrated by two patients in this series who have had postoperative catheterization following mitral valve replacement. B. F., a 21-year-old woman, was completely bedridden immediately before operation, although she had been well until 13 months earlier, when bacterial endocarditis was soon followed by the development of mitral regurgitation. At the time of the operation she weighed only 33 Kg. Preoperatively, the left atrial (mean, 11; v peak, 23 mm. Hg) and pulmonary arterial (65/28, mean 38 mm. Hg) pressures were elevated, roentgenographically the left atrium was only mildly enlarged, and on a standard oral sodium tolerance test she was unable to excrete any sodium.[25] Following replacement of the mitral valve with a Starr-Edwards prosthesis, she has been entirely asymptomatic. Seven months after operation she weighed 50 Kg. and the pulmonary arterial wedge (mean, 6; v peak, 11 mm. Hg) and pulmonary arterial (32/11, mean 16 mm. Hg) pressures were normal, the heart was smaller roentgenographically (fig. 2), and her sodium tolerance had become normal. J. W., a 54-year-old man, also was incapacitated before operation. He was emaciated, in severe cardiac failure, and the mean left atrial pressure was 15 with v waves of 32 mm. Hg, and the pulmonary arterial pressure was 70/27 mm. Hg. Twelve months after replacement of his mitral valve, the left atrial mean pressure had fallen to 7, the v waves to 10 mm. Hg, and the pulmonary arterial pressure to 44/20 mm. Hg. This patient has improved symptomatically, but he continues to accumulate fluid despite diuretic therapy, presumably consequent to persistent "relative" tricuspid regurgitation, and his heart had remained enlarged. Although this man also developed severe mitral regurgitation following rupture of chordae tendineae as a consequence of bacterial endocarditis, 8 years had elapsed from the onset of the valvular regurgitation until the valve was replaced, and the left atrium dilated during this interval. It is suspected that the left atrial pressures were greatly elevated immediately following the mitral chordal rupture, but as the left atrial chamber dilated the left atrial pressures decreased to levels approaching normal.

Summary and Conclusions

This report describes the clinical, radiographic, hemodynamic, and pathologic findings in 10 patients, in each of whom ruptured mitral chordae tendineae were responsible for severe mitral regurgitation. In six patients, the chordal rupture was the result of proved bacterial endocarditis, and in the other four, although the cause was not determined, it is considered that bacterial endocarditis may have been the etiologic factor in them as well. Only one of the patients had a history suggestive of acute rheumatic fever. From examination of the mitral valves at autopsy, or after operative excision, no gross abnormalities of the valves were apparent, other than the ruptured chordae and mild thickening of the adjacent leaflet. The signs and symptoms of mitral regurgitation appeared abruptly in all but one patient and were unrelenting thereafter. Eight patients had sinus rhythm and two had atrial fibrillation. Each of the latter had had symptoms of cardiac decompensation for several years, and their left atria were markedly enlarged. The left atrial chamber in the other eight patients was of near normal size or only moderately enlarged. The interval from the onset of symptoms of mitral regurgitation to operation in the two patients with dilated left atria averaged $6\frac{1}{2}$ years, whereas the interval in the eight patients with near normal or only moderately dilated left atria averaged 15 months. In all patients the pulmonary arterial and the left atrial pressures, particularly the v-wave peak, were elevated. The cardiac index was low, and the calculated pulmonary vascular resistance was elevated in the seven patients in whom it was measured. Mitral annuloplasty was performed in two patients, with insertion of artificial chordae, but both died in the early postoperative period. Replacement of the mitral valve with a Starr-Edwards prosthesis was performed in five patients, with considerable improvement in four. The fifth died of a pulmonary complication 2 weeks after operation.

The distinctive clinical and hemodynamic findings in the majority of these patients, i.e., the rapid progression of heart failure, sinus rhythm, normal-sized or only moderately enlarged left atria, and the greatly elevated pressures in the pulmonary artery and left atrium are attributed to the sudden onset of the mitral regurgitation. These findings are contrasted to those in patients with chronic rheumatic mitral regurgitation, whose disability progresses slowly and who exhibit atrial fibrillation, marked left atrial enlargement, and sometimes normal pulmonary arterial and left atrial pressures. It is proposed that the majority of patients with ruptured chordae cannot sustain the acutely imposed hemodynamic burden for periods of time sufficient to allow the increase in left atrial compliance so frequently observed in patients with chronic rheumatic mitral regurgitation.

References

1. Perloff, J. K., and Harvey, W. P.: Auscultatory and phonocardiographic manifestations of pure mitral regurgitation. Progr. Cardiovas. Dis. **5**: 172, 1962.
2. Heath, D., and Edwards, J. E.: The pathology of hypertensive pulmonary vascular disease. A description of six grades of structural changes in the pulmonary arteries with special reference to congenital cardiac septal defects. Circulation **18**: 533, 1958.
3. Frew, H. W. O.: Rupture of the chordae tendineae following scarlet fever. Glasgow M. J. **115**: 195, 1931.
4. Bailey, O. T., and Hickman, J. B.: Rupture of mitral chordae tendineae. Clinical and pathologic observations on seven cases in which there was no bacterial endocarditis. Am. Heart J. **28**: 578, 1944.
5. Osmundson, P. J., Callahan, J. A., and Edwards, J. E.: Ruptured mitral chordae tendinae. Circulation **23**: 42, 1961.
6. Barber, H.: The effects of trauma, direct and

indirect, on the heart. Quart. J. Med., n.s., **13:** 137, 1944.

7. Frothingham, C., and Hass, G. M.: Rupture of normal chordae tendineae of the mitral valve. Am. Heart J. **9:** 492, 1934.
8. Libman, E., and Friedberg, C. K.: Subacute Bacterial Endocarditis. London, Oxford University Press, 1941, 108 pp.
9. Saphir, O.: Endocarditis. *In* Gould, S. E., Editor: Pathology of the Heart. Springfield, Illinois, Charles C Thomas Publisher, 1953, p. 707.
10. Hepper, N. G. G., Burchell, H. B., and Edwards, J. E.: Cardiac Clinic CXLVI. Mitral insufficiency in healed, unrecognized bacterial endocarditis. Proc. Staff Meet., Mayo Clinic **31:** 659, 1956.
11. Perrin, A., Froment, R., and Pasquier, J.: Insuffisances mitrales par luxation de la petite valve et rupture de cordages. (A propos de 5 observations anatomo-cliniques simulant le retrecissement aortique). Arch. mal. coeur **54:** 82, 1961.
12. Menges, H., Jr., Ankeney, J. L., and Hellerstein, H. K.: The clinical diagnosis and surgical management of ruptured mitral chordae tendineae. Circulation **30:** 8, 1964.
13. Miller, R., Jr., and Pearson, R. J., Jr.: Mitral insufficiency simulating aortic stenosis. Report of an unusual manifestation of Marfan's syndrome. New England. J. Med. **260:** 1210, 1959.
14. Shapiro, H. A., and Weiss, D. R.: Mitral insufficiency due to ruptured chordae tendineae simulating aortic stenosis. New England J. Med. **261:** 272, 1959.
15. January, L. E., Fisher, J. M., and Ehrenhaft, J. L.: Mitral insufficiency resulting from rupture of normal chordae tendineae. Report of a surgically corrected case. Circulation **26:** 1329, 1962.
16. Wolnisty, C., and Freidman, S. L.: Mitral insufficiency secondary to ruptured chordae tendineae. Report of surgically corrected case. J.A.M.A. **188:** 687, 1964.
17. Morris, J. D., Penner, D. A., and Brandt, R. L.: Surgical correction of ruptured chordae tendineae. J. Thor. & Cardiov. Surg. **48:** 772, 1964.
18. Haller, J. A., Jr., and Morrow, A. G.: Experimental mitral insufficiency. An operative method of chronic survival. Ann. Surg. **142:** 37, 1955.
19. Haller, J. A., Jr., and Morrow, A. G.: Experimental mitral insufficiency. Surgery **38:** 518, 1955.
20. Braunwald, E., and Awe, W. C.: The syndrome of severe mitral regurgitation with normal left atrial pressure. Circulation **27:** 29, 1963.
21. Best, P. V., and Heath, D.: The right ventricle and small pulmonary arteries in aneurysmal dilatation of the left atrium. Brit. Heart J. **26:** 312, 1964.
22. Carney, E. K., Braunwald, E., Roberts, W. C., Aygen, M., and Morrow, A. G.: Congenital mitral regurgitation. Clinical, hemodynamic, and angiocardiographic findings in nine patients. Am. J. Med. **33:** 223, 1962.
23. Corvisart, J. N.: An Essay on the Organic Diseases of the Heart and Great Vessels. (Translated by Jacob Gates) Boston, Bradford and Read, 1812, 344 pp.
24. McGoon, D. C.: Repair of mitral insufficiency due to ruptured chordae tendineae. J. Thor. & Cardiov. Surg. **39:** 357, 1960.
25. Braunwald, E., Plauth, W. H., Jr., and Morrow, A. G.: A method for the detection and quantification of impaired sodium excretion: Results of an oral sodium tolerance test in normal subjects and in patients with heart disease. Circulation **32:** 223, 1965.

Familial Occurrence of Primary Pulmonary Hypertension

HENRY S. KINGDON, MD, PhD; LAWRENCE S. COHEN, MD; WILLIAM C. ROBERTS, MD; AND EUGENE BRAUNWALD, MD, BETHESDA, MD

A NUMBER of studies of primary pulmonary hypertension have suggested that this disease may occur in a familial form.[1-8] In a previous communication from this laboratory, a family in which five members in three generations had primary pulmonary hypertension was described.[9] It is the purpose of this report to describe a kindred in which primary pulmonary hypertension was present in two siblings and their father. Complete postmortem examinations were performed on the father and on one of the siblings.

Clinical Descriptions

CASE 1.—Patient 1 (No. 01-32-09) was referred to the National Heart Institute in 1956 at the age of 22 years with the chief complaint of progressive exertional dyspnea of two years' duration. He had immigrated to the United States at the age of 16 years, and at that time results of his physical examination was reported as being normal. One year prior to admission a chest roentgenogram showed an enlarged heart, and six months later a single episode of hemoptysis occurred. He was treated with digitalis and was put on a low salt diet. At the time of admission he was able to climb only one flight of stairs.

Physical examination revealed mild distension of the jugular veins, a lift of the right ventricle, a widely split second heart sound with a markedly accentuated pulmonic component, and a grade 3/6 harsh, high-pitched, holosystolic murmur maximal in the fourth intercostal space at the left sternal border. Results of examination of the lungs were normal. The liver was palpable just below the right costal margin. There was no clubbing, cyanosis, or edema.

Results of the urinalysis and white blood count (WBC) were normal. The hemoglobin level was 17.9 gm/100 cc and the hematocrit reading was 56%. The routine blood chemical determinations were all within normal limits. The chest roentgenogram exhibited gross cardiac enlargement, prominence of the main pulmonary artery, enlargement of the right ventricle, but no left atrial enlargement. The electrocardiogram showed normal sinus rhythm, right ventricular hypertrophy, a right ventricular conduction defect, and right atrial enlargement. Cardiac catheterization demonstrated a pulmonary artery pressure of 88/54 mm Hg, a mean right atrial pressure of 13 mm Hg, a mean pulmonary artery wedge pressure of 6 mm Hg, and no evidence of an intracardiac shunt.

Several weeks after discharge the patient became stranded in his automobile and died after considerable exertion related to his efforts to free the automobile. The heart and lungs were examined at the National Heart Institute. The heart weighed 420 gm; the right ventricle was markedly dilated and hypertrophied, and the right atrium was slightly dilated as well. The foramen ovale was closed, and there were no interatrial or interventricular communications. The valves were normal. The main, medium, and small pulmonary arteries had a marked degree of atherosclerosis, both on gross and microscopic examinations. The larger vessels were dilated. Severe occlusive vascular disease, graded as 5/6 by the system of Heath and Edwards[10] was present in the smallest muscular branches of the pulmonary arteries (Fig 1). The pathologic diagnoses were primary pulmonary hypertension with hypertrophy and dilatation of the right side of the heart.

CASE 2.—Patient 2 (No. 06-45-63), the sister and only sibling of patient 1, was referred to the National Heart Institute in 1965 at the age of 27 years with the chief complaint of exertional dyspnea. Her first pregnancy at the age of 24 years

Received for publication April 28, 1966; accepted Aug 23.

From the Cardiology Branch and the Clinic of Surgery, National Heart Institute, Bethesda.

Reprint requests to the Cardiology Branch, National Heart Institute, Bethesda, Md 20014 (Dr. Braunwald).

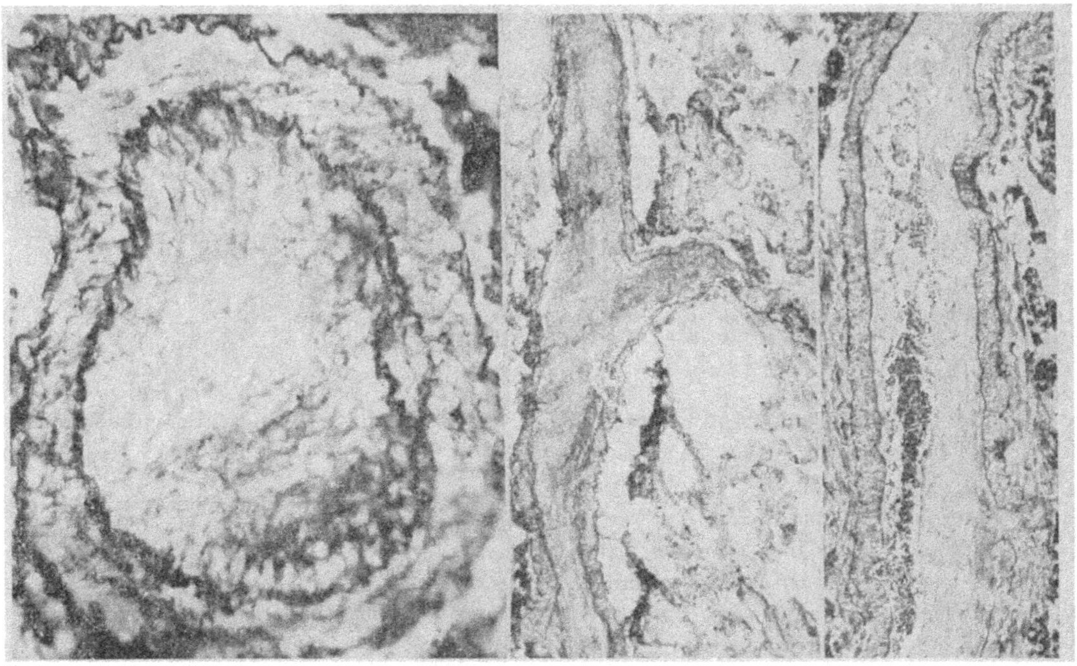

Fig 1.—Photomicrographs of pulmonary arteries in patient 1. *Left,* Cross section of small muscular pulmonary artery with hypertrophied media and lumen completely obliterated by fibrous intimal proliferation. *Center,* Longitudinal section of small muscular pulmonary artery with fibrous obliteration of its lumen. *Right,* Longitudinal section of another muscular pulmonary artery with partially obstructed lumen. This patient also had plexiform lesions in his lungs (elastic tissue stains, slightly reduced from ×400 [left], ×90 [center], and ×99 [right]).

was complicated by the development of ankle edema. Her second pregnancy, one year later, was marked by severe dyspnea as well as edema. Between the second pregnancy and her admission she suffered from progressive exertional dyspnea, fatigue, and ankle edema, which necessitated hospitalization 11 months prior to admission. However, her condition improved when she was treated with digitalis, diuretics, and dietary salt restriction.

Physical examination revealed prominent atrial (*a*) waves in the jugular venous pulse, a lift of the right ventricle, a palpable pulmonary artery, the shock of pulmonary valve closure, a fixed, widely split second heart sound with a markedly accentuated pulmonic component, a third heart sound along the left sternal margin, and a grade 2/6 systolic ejection murmur at the base of the heart. Examination of the lungs was normal. A tender liver edge was felt 8 cm below the right costal margin, and a spleen tip was palpable below the left costal margin. There was mild pretibial edema, but no cyanosis or clubbing.

Results of urinalysis and WBC were normal. The hemoglobin level was 16.5 gm/100 cc and the hematocrit reading was 53%. The routine blood chemical determinations were within normal limits. The chest roentgenogram demonstrated enlargement of the right ventricle, prominence of the main pulmonary artery, and hilar and peripheral pulmonary arteries which appeared to be normal. The ECG showed normal sinus rhythm with first degree atrioventricular block, right axis deviation, right ventricular hypertrophy, and right atrial enlargement.

Cardiac catheterization demonstrated a pulmonary artery pressure of 90/30 mm Hg, a right ventricular pressure of 90/8 mm Hg, a right atrial mean pressure of 4 mm Hg, a pulmonary artery wedge pressure of 4 mm Hg, and no evidence of an intracardiac shunt. There was no change in the pulmonary artery pressure after a ten-minute period breathing 100% O_2. She was discharged on anticoagulants, and there has been little change in her clinical condition.

Case 3.—Patient 3 (Autopsy No. A-66-8), the father of patients 1 and 2, died in 1957 at the age of 56 years. He was apparently well until two years prior to his death when he suffered an injury to his legs in a power mower accident. One year prior to his death he was hospitalized for six weeks because of pleurisy and pneumonia. He then developed progressively increasing shortness of breath, and this was his major symptom at the time of his death.

Physical examination by W. R. Tench, MD, of Clearwater, Florida, five months prior to death revealed cyanosis, diaphoresis, increased respiratory rate, distended neck veins with prominent *a* waves, a widely split second heart sound with an accentuated pulmonic component, and a third heart sound. Examination of the lungs was normal. A tender liver edge was felt 8 cm below the right costal margin. The left leg was larger than the right and was edematous. There was no clubbing.

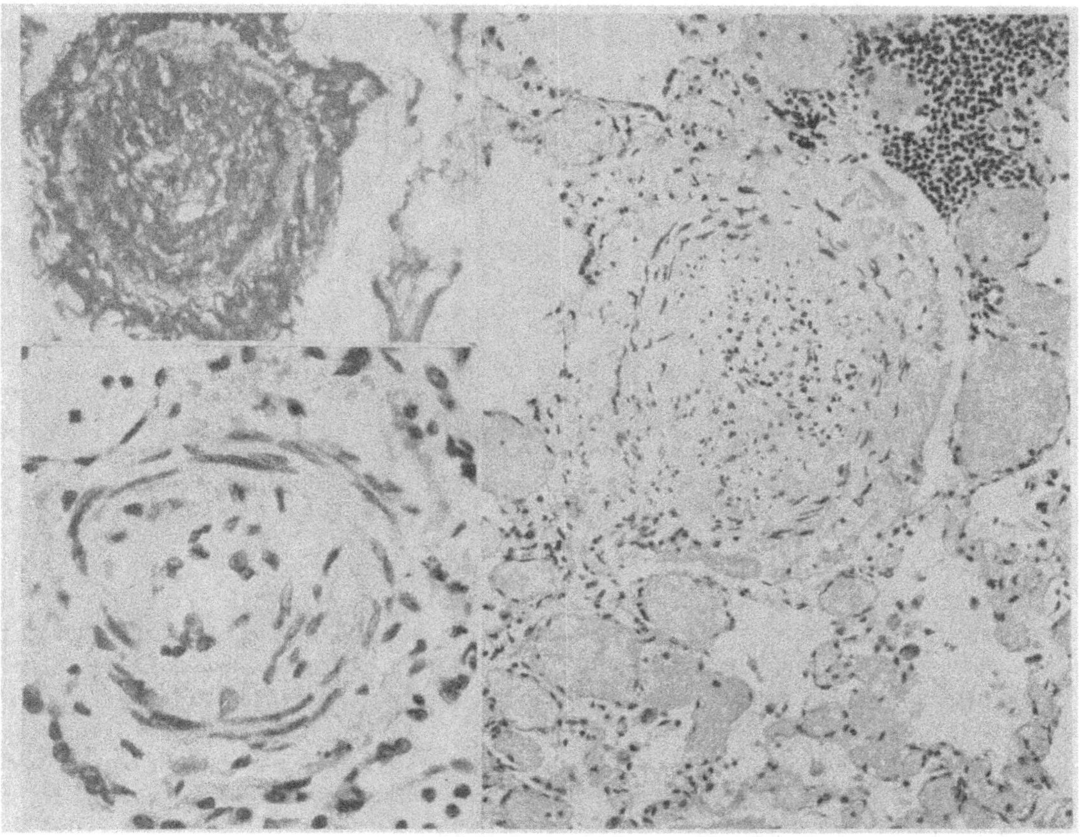

Fig 2.—Photomicrographs of small pulmonary arteries in patient 3. *Bottom left,* Pulmonary arteriole with lumen narrowed by cellular intimal proliferation (hematoxylin and eosin stain, ×400). *Upper left,* A small muscular pulmonary artery with complete obliteration of its lumen (elastic tissue stain, ×235). *Right,* A larger muscular pulmonary artery with obliterated lumen and surrounded by markedly dilated vascular channels. This patient also had plexiform-type vascular lesions within his lung (hematoxylin and eosin stain, ×160).

The ECG showed right axis deviation, right ventricular hypertrophy, and right atrial enlargement. During the following months cyanosis and hepatomegaly increased progressively up to the time of his death.

Postmortem examination was carried out at the Morton F. Plant Hospital and the microscopic sections of the lung were reviewed at the National Heart Institute. The right atrium and right atrial appendage were markedly dilated. The right ventricular wall measured 8 mm in thickness and the trabeculi were prominent. The tricuspid valve ring was dilated and measured 16 cm in circumference. In contrast, the mitral valve was only 9.5 cm in circumference. All valves were normal. Both the left and right coronary arteries were patent throughout. The myocardium was grossly normal, and there were no intracardiac shunts.

The cut surface of the lungs revealed the parenchyma to be firm. Section of the pulmonary vascular tree revealed arteries that were widely dilated to a point approximately 2 cm from the pleural surface. On microscopic section, these arteries showed some intimal thickening with plaque formation. In contrast, the smaller vessels showed grade 5/6 pulmonary hypertensive changes[10] (Fig 2). The pathologic diagnoses were primary pulmonary hypertension with hypertrophy and dilatation of the right ventricle and atrium, and congestive heart failure of the right side.

The two children and the mother of patient 2 have been examined recently and are apparently well. There is no history of heart disease in any of the other members of the family, except that the mother of patient 3 died at the age of 59 years of an illness thought to be cardiac in origin.

Comment

Although it has been suspected that genetic transmission may occur in primary pulmonary hypertension,[1-8] firm documentation of the disease occurring in several generations has been lacking. The previous report from this laboratory of a kindred in which five members in three generations were affected lent support to the idea that primary pulmonary hypertension might be inheritable.[9]

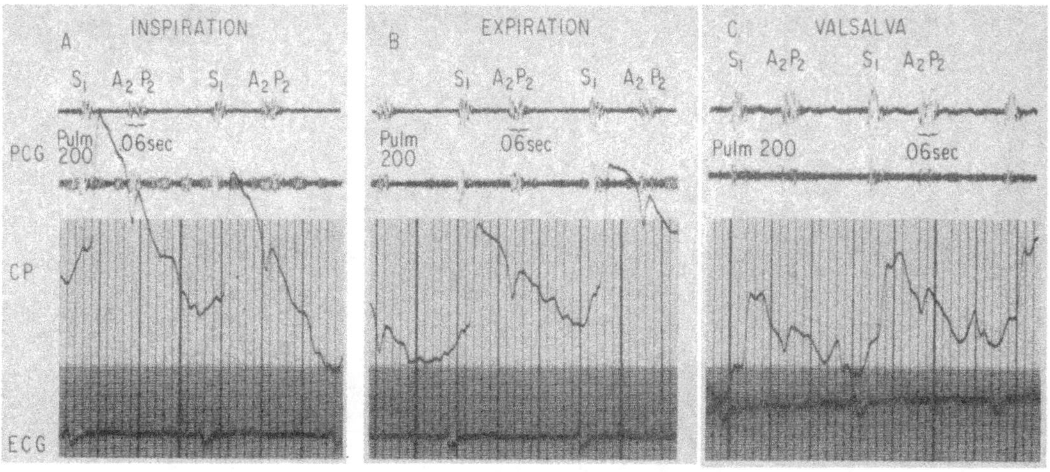

Fig 3.—Phonocardiogram of patient 2. Fixed splitting of the second heart sound is demonstrated in both phases of respiration and with the Valsalva maneuver.

Since then, two further families with primary pulmonary hypertension have been reported.[11,12] The present report of primary pulmonary hypertension in a man and his only two offspring provides further evidence that this disease may be familial. Our previous report included gross autopsy examinations in three generations of a kindred, and the present report included gross and microscopic examinations in members of two generations.

As with the first family which we studied,[9] genetic anticipation may be suspected, since the disease became manifest at an earlier age in the offspring. Genetic anticipation can also be invoked in the family of Parry and Verel [12]; the mother died at age 49 years, and the daughters at ages 26 and 27 years. It may be that families with this disease previously have been overlooked because of the genetic anticipation, with the parent assumed to have a form of heart disease more common in the middle-aged adult population. This in fact was the case in the present family; prior to autopsy the father's illness had been attributed to pulmonary embolization.

The etiology of primary pulmonary hypertension remains obscure, and debate has continued over whether there is an intrinsic defect in the pulmonary arterioles or whether all instances regarded as primary are, in fact, due to multiple minute emboli, as suggested by Rosenberg.[13] Several other etiologies seem possible. There may be a heretofore unrecognized genetically determined hypercoagulable state leading to multiple small emboli or an inherited deficiency in a component of the plasma fibrinolytic system which would ordinarily lyse any in vivo pulmonary thromboses. Finally, it has been suggested that a hypersensitive immune mechanism may be involved.[14]

All three patients described in this report demonstrated a widely split second heart sound. In patients 1 and 2 this was documented by phonocardiography, and in addition, the splitting was found not to vary with respiration (Fig 3). This finding is at variance with the generally accepted statement that the second heart sound is closely split in primary pulmonary hypertension.[15-17] A possible explanation for this finding is that all three patients were in heart failure of the right side at the time of examination, a state which could have prolonged the ejection period of the right ventricle, and delayed the pulmonic component of the second heart sound. Under these circumstances, the decline of intrapleural pressure occurring during inspiration would not necessarily be accompanied by augmentation of right ventricular stroke volume. The demonstration of a widely split second heart sound in these three patients suggests that this finding cannot be used to exclude the diagnosis of primary pulmonary hypertension.

Summary

A family is reported in which a man and his only two offspring had primary pulmonary hypertension. The diagnosis was based on clinical examination, hemodynamic studies, and gross and microscopic pathologic examinations. The possibility that genetic anticipation occurred is considered.

George H. Christ, MD, Clearwater, Fla, referred patient 2 to us for the study and supplied the clinical and pathological information presented in case 3.

REFERENCES

1. Clarke, R.C., et al: On Certain Abnormalities, Congenital and Acquired, of Pulmonary Artery, *Quart J Med* **21**:51-69, 1927.

2. Lange, F.: Die essentielle Hypertonie der Lungenstrombahn und ihr familiäres Vorkommen, *Deutsche Med Wschr* **72**:322-326, 1948.

3. Dresdale, D.T.; Michtom, R.J.; and Schultz, M.: Recent Studies in Primary Pulmonary Hypertension Including Pharmacodynamic Observations on Pulmonary Vascular Resistance, *Bull NY Acad Med* **30**: 195-207, 1954.

4. Van Epps, E.F.: Primary Pulmonary Hypertension in Brothers, *Amer J Roentgen* **78**:471-482, 1957.

5. Coleman, P.N.; Edmunds, A.W.B.; and Tregillus, J.: Primary Pulmonary Hypertension in Three Sibs, *Brit Heart J* **21**:81-88, 1959.

6. Fleming, H.: Primary Pulmonary Hypertension in Eight Patients Including Mother and Her Daughter, *Aust Ann Med* **9**:18-28, 1960.

7. Cahen, P., et al: Hypertension pulmonaire primitive chez la mère et al fille, *Arch Mal Coeur* **54**: 95-101, 1961.

8. Van Bogaert, A., et al: Familial Primary Pulmonary Hypertension, *Arch Mal Coeur* **54**:1185-1203, 1961.

9. Melmon, K.L., and Braunwald, E.: Familial Pulmonary Hypertension, *New Eng J Med* **269**:770-775, 1963.

10. Heath, D., and Edwards, J.E.: The Pathology of Hypertensive Pulmonary Vascular Disease: A Description of Six Grades of Structural Changes in the Pulmonary Arteries With Special Reference to Congenital Cardiac Septal Defects, *Circulation* **18**: 533-547, 1958.

11. Boiteau, G.M., and Libanoff, A.J.: Primary Pulmonary Hypertension: Familial Incidence, *Angiology* **14**:260-264, 1963.

12. Parry, W.R., and Verel, D.: Familial Primary Pulmonary Hypertension, *Brit Heart J* **28**:193-198, 1966.

13. Rosenberg, S.A.: A Study of the Etiological Basis of Primary Pulmonary Hypertension, *Amer Heart J* **68**:484-489, 1964.

14. Farrar, J.F.: Idiopathic Pulmonary Hypertension, *Amer Heart J* **66**:128-135, 1963.

15. Wood, P.: *Diseases of the Heart and Circulation*, ed 2, Philadelphia: J. B. Lippincott Company, 1956, p 843.

16. Levine, S.A., and Harvey, W.P.: *Clinical Auscultation of the Heart*, ed 2, Philadelphia: W. B. Saunders Company, 1959, p 516.

17. McCusick, V.A.: *Cardiovascular Sound in Health and Disease*, Baltimore: The Williams & Wilkins Company, 1958, p 430.

Gaucher's Disease of the Lung Causing Severe Pulmonary Hypertension with Associated Acute Recurrent Pericarditis

By William C. Roberts, M.D., and Donald S. Fredrickson, M.D.

SUMMARY

The clinical and pathological features of a 30-year-old man with Gaucher's disease are described. He had severe pulmonary hypertension resulting from obstruction of pulmonary capillaries by Gaucher cells. Acute recurrent pericarditis of unknown etiology terminally led to hemopericardium and cardiac tamponade.

Additional Indexing Words:

Cerebral involvement   Cor pulmonale   Anemia
Elastic fibers   Bronchial constriction   Ruptured pericardial vessels

GAUCHER'S DISEASE is a familial disorder characterized by accumulation in reticuloendothelial cells of glucocerebrosides, compounds containing sphingosine, fatty acid, and glucose in equimolar amounts. The storage cells, called Gaucher cells, have a characteristic appearance, and their increasing numbers in the liver, spleen, lymph nodes, and bone marrow are responsible for most of the clinical manifestations of the disorder.[1] Although nearly all patients have hepatosplenomegaly, Gaucher cells in marrow aspirates, and an abnormally high concentration of non-tartrate-inhibitable serum acid phosphatase, at least two forms of Gaucher's disease exist clinically. They probably represent expression of different mutations. In the *infantile* or *acute* form, the children have a characteristic stereotyped appearance (strabismus, opisthotonus, retracted lips and often spastic and flexed extremities), and death generally occurs before 2 years of age. The *adult* or *chronic* form comprises the majority of cases of Gaucher's disease. It may be detected at any age, usually because of hepatosplenomegaly. Neurological signs rarely if ever occur, osseous lesions are often pronounced, and hematological abnormalities associated with hypersplenism, skin pigmentation, and pingueculae usually develop. It is relatively common amoung Ashkenazi Jews, in contrast to the infantile form, which is very rarely seen in a Jewish child. Death in the infantile form is usually related to the cerebral involvement and cachexia, and, in the adult form, to anemia or superimposed infection. The present report describes an adult patient with Gaucher's disease followed for 25 years, who developed severe pulmonary hypertension, recurrent acute pericarditis, and finally hemorrhagic cardiac tamponade. Pulmonary hypertension, which has not been documented previously in a patient with Gaucher's disease, resulted from the plugging of alveolar capillaries by Gaucher cells.

Report of Patient

A.K. (02-62-62), a 30-year-old lawyer, died at the National Heart Institute on January 3, 1962. He had been followed from age 5 to age 16 years (1936-1947) by Dr. Siegfried J. Thannhauser, who described this patient's course during this interval in detail in his monograph on the lipidoses (patient 48).[2] This patient was the younger of two male children of parents who were both Ashkenazi Jews. A single bone marrow aspiration in the mother, who came from Palestine, showed no abnormality. The father, who came from Lithuania, died at age 32 of an

From the Laboratory of Pathology, Clinic of Surgery and Laboratory of Molecular Diseases, National Heart Institute, National Institutes of Health, Bethesda, Maryland.

acute myocardial infarct. The patient's oldest sibling is normal. Between the ages of 9 and 12 months, the patient was taken to physicians with a question of retarded growth and abdominal enlargement. At age 4 years hepatosplenomegaly was established and Gaucher cells were discovered in the sternal marrow. By age 7 years the spleen had become so large (7 pounds; patient weighed 35 pounds) that abdominal discomfort and dyspnea resulted, and it was therefore removed. For the next 20 years he led an outwardly normal life. He was an excellent student, and was admitted to the bar. Throughout his school life, however, he had repeated episodes of bone pain and fractures, some spontaneous and others associated with minor

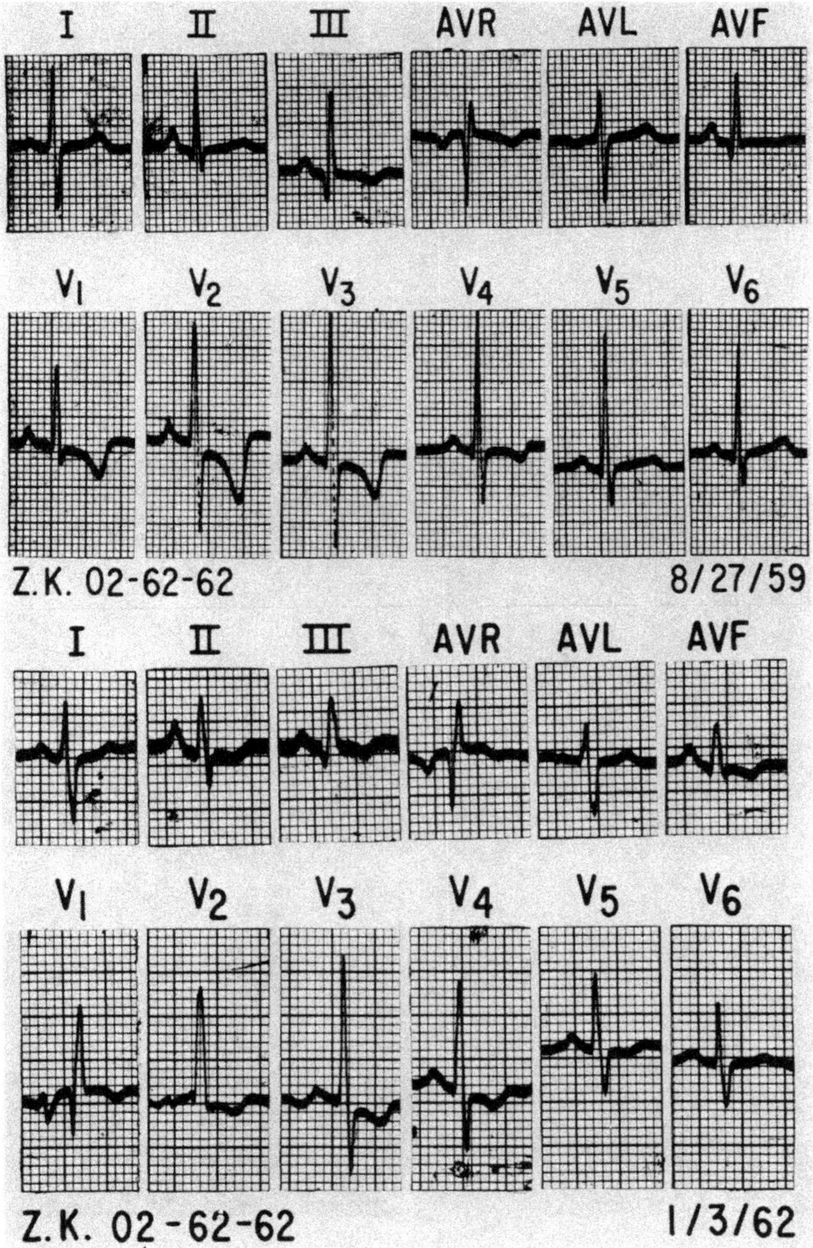

Figure 1

Electrocardiograms. Upper. *Recorded 29 months before death.* Lower. *Recorded 1 hour before death at the time of massive hemopericardium.*

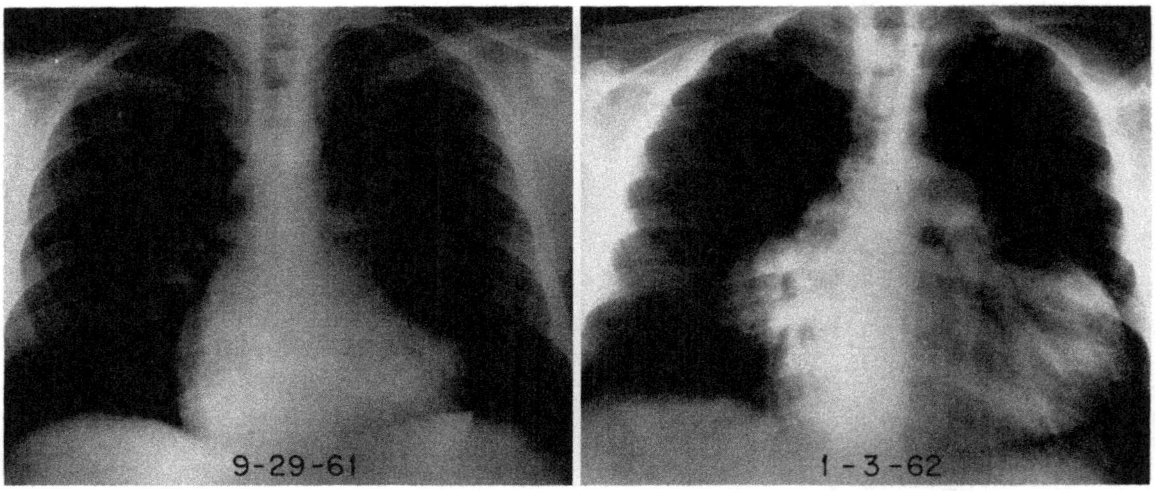

Figure 2

Chest roentgenograms. Left. *Two months before death.* Right. *Day of death, demonstrating massive pericardial effusion.*

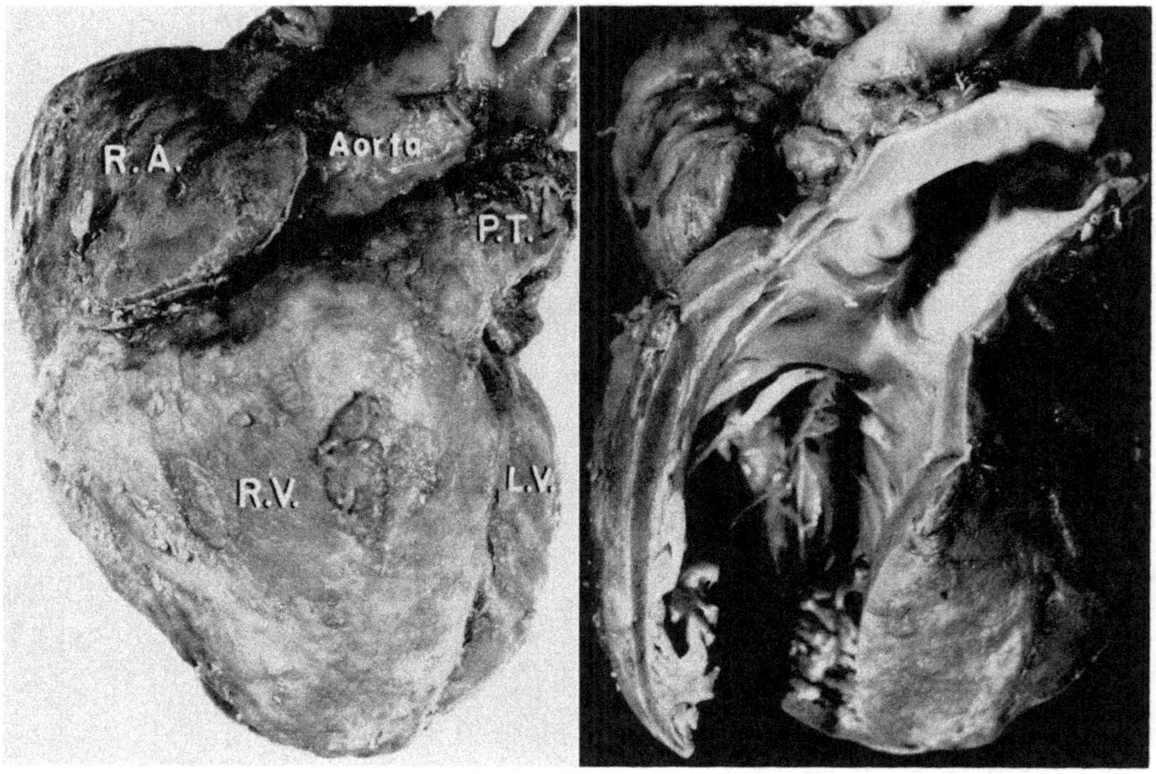

Figure 3

Exterior of heart (left) *and opened right ventricle and pulmonary trunk* (right). *The right ventricle (R.V.) is markedly hypertrophied; the left ventricle (L.V.) is small. Atheromata are present in the pulmonary trunk (P.T.). R.A. = right atrium.*

trauma, eventually leading to permanent deformities of the left hip and leg.

The patient was first seen by one of us (D.S.F.) in August 1959. His only complaints during the previous 5 years were easy fatigability and rare bone pain. Five days earlier he had fainted while lifting a heavy table. On examination, the liver was enormous, extending to the iliac crest. The skin had a sallow yellow color with duskiness over the tibias, and each eye had small pingueculae. The pulmonic second sound was markedly accentuated, but there was no precordial murmur or rub. The blood pressure was 120/80 mm Hg. The axillary, cervical, supraclavicular and inguinal lymph nodes were not enlarged. No abnormalities were detected on neurological examination.

The electrocardiogram (fig. 1) showed right axis deviation, right atrial and right ventricular hypertrophy, and the chest roentgenogram (fig. 2) showed a large right ventricle and pulmonary trunk. The blood hematocrit was 46%, white blood cell count, 18,000 mm^3 with 48 neutrophils, 49 lymphocytes and 3% monocytes; serum acid phosphatase, 3.08 Bessey-Lowry units (upper limit of normal = 0.6), 0.15 being tartrate-inhibitable, Bromsulphalein retention in 45 minutes, 11%; total serum bilirubin, 0.7 mg per 100 ml; total cholesterol, 135 mg per 100 ml with free cholesterol 46; phospholipids 176; and triglycerides, 192 mg per 100 ml (upper limit of normal for triglyceides = 150 mg per 100 ml).

Fifteen months later (November 1960) he had the first episode of acute lower substernal and precordial pain, which worsened with inspiration and movement and lasted 18 hours. Several days later the pain reappeared and a loud precordial friction rub was heard as well as a ventricular gallop. Six similar episodes of anterior chest pain occurred during the next 13 months. A pericardial friction rub was audible on each occasion, sometimes accompanied by a pleural friction rub. Atrial flutter occurred during four of these episodes. He was afebrile and had normal erythrocyte sedimentation rates during each episode. On one occasion the antistreptolysin-O titer was 500 units. His last acute illness began 7 days before death with the onset of a severe, nonproductive, hacking cough. He was brought to the hospital 2 hours before death, and at this time was severely dyspneic, cyanotic, and had tachycardia, distended neck veins, pulsus paradoxus (20 mm Hg), and a white blood cell count of 31,000 mm.^{3} Chest roentgenogram showed an enormous cardiac silhouette, a massive increase in size as compared to his previous x-rays (fig. 2). Pericardiocentesis yielded 150 ml of blood. Shortly thereafter asystole occurred.

At autopsy (A62-4), 600 ml of blood was found in the pericardial sac; the pericardial surfaces were "shaggy" and contained numerous acute and chronic inflammatory cells and vascular channels, but no Gaucher cells. The left pleural space contained 600 ml of serosanguineous fluid, but the pleural surfaces were normal. The heart weighed 500 g; the right ventricle and atrium were markedly hypertrophied (fig. 3) and contained focal fibrous scars. The cardiac valves were normal and coronary arteries were within the range of normal for this age. The lungs together weighed 850 g, and showed evidence of pulmonary edema. The walls of both small and large pulmonary arteries were thickened and contained atheromata. The histological sections of lung disclosed the presence of numerous Gaucher cells plugging the lumina of alveolar capillaries throughout the lung (fig. 4). In addition, Gaucher cells were seen occasionally in the alveolar spaces. The pulmonary arterioles, muscular arteries, and elastic arteries showed changes characteristic of severe (grade V/VI) hypertensive pulmonary vascular disease (classification of Heath and Edwards[3]) (fig. 5). Plexiform lesions were present throughout all lobes of both lungs (fig. 5). The liver, bone marrow, and lymph nodes contained massive numbers of Gaucher cells. The liver weighed 8.1 kg, and its architecture was disrupted by infiltrates of Gaucher cells, hemopoietic elements, and fibrous tissue. Analysis of the liver revealed 77 mg of chloroform-soluble glycolipids per gm of dry weight (normal < 10 mg per g). The

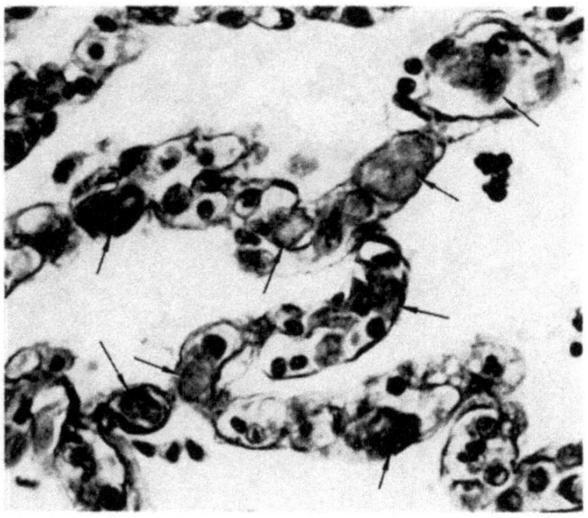

Figure 4

Pulmonary alveolar capillaries occluded by Gaucher cells (arrows). *Periodic acid-Schiff stain;* × *780.*

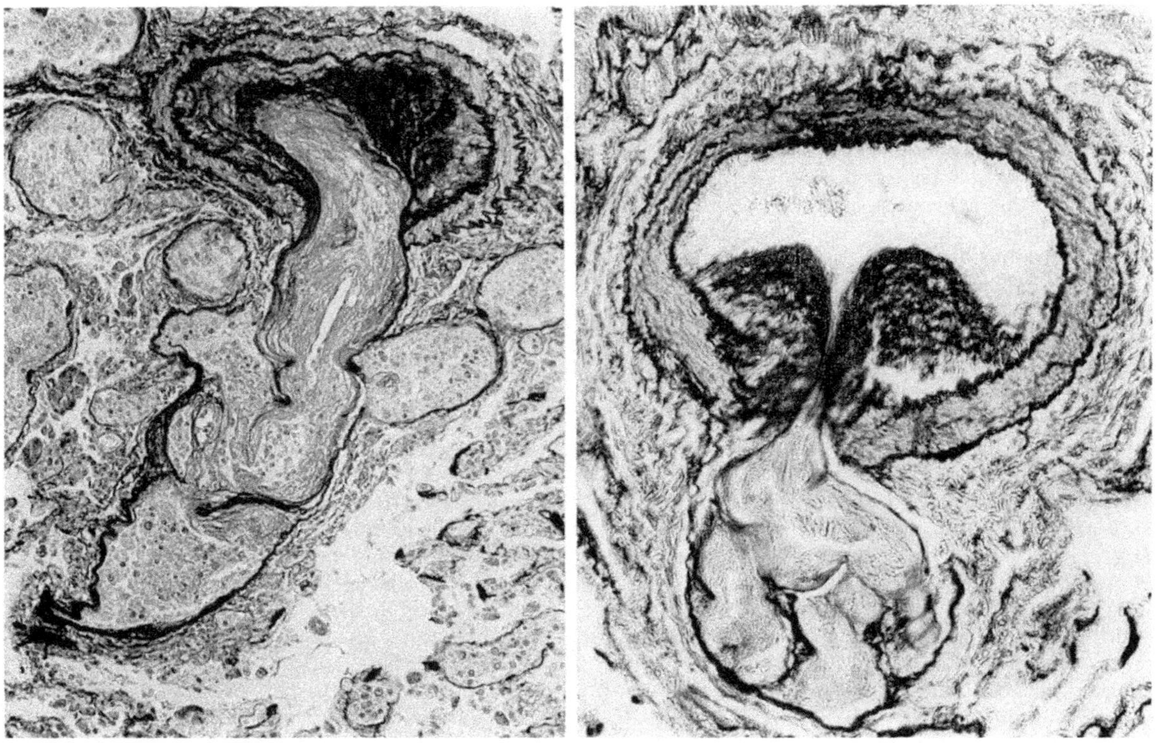

Figure 5

Muscular pulmonary arteries, each demonstrating changes indicative of severe pulmonary hypertension. Left. *The muscular artery and its branching arteriole shows extensive intimal proliferation. Numerous large thin-walled dilated vessels surround the obstructed arteriole.* Right. *Classical plexiform lesion arising from a muscular artery, which has hypertrophied media and intimal fibrous proliferation at the site of origin of the plexiform lesion. Elastic-van Gieson stains;* × *150 (left),* × *195 (right).*

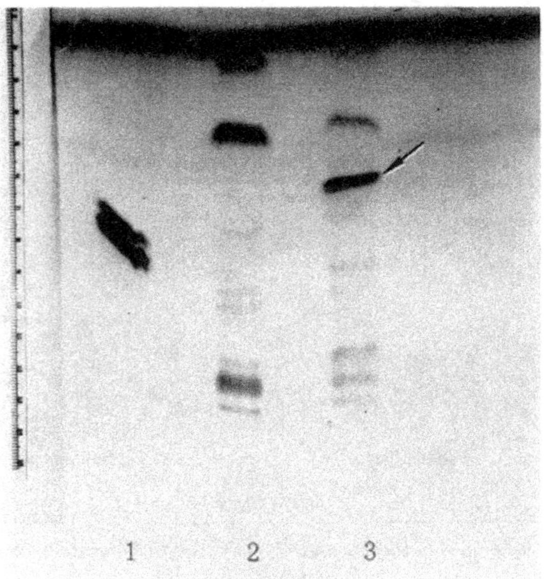

abdominal lymph nodes were enlarged (up to 3 cm in diameter) and were virtually replaced by Gaucher cells. The thoracic lymph nodes were not enlarged.

Figure 6

Thin-layer chromatography of the chloroform-soluble glycolipids prepared from lung according to the technique of Mårtensson et al.[4] *Extracts representing equal amounts of wet lung tissue are chromatographed in lanes 2 (control) and 3 (patient A.K.). Chromatographed in lane 1 is a mixture of galactocerebrosides obtained from beef spinal cord. The arrow designates a dense band of material in the lung of A.K. having an Rf comparable to glucocerebrosides. Note the absence of significant amounts of this material in the control extract. Chromatographs were developed in one dimension in chloroform/methanol/*H_2O *(65/25/4) and the spots identified by spraying with an acid solution of anisaldehyde and heating 20 minutes for 120.°*

The glycolipids from a sample of frozen lung from patient A. K. and from a control were extracted and partially purified according to the technique of Mårtensson and associates.[4] The control patient (I. D., A56-217) was a 12-year-old boy who had idiopathic left ventricular hypertrophy. His pulmonary arterial pressure was 16/9 mm Hg, and his left ventricular pressure was 130/10 mm Hg. The cerebroside contents of the lungs were compared qualitatively by thin-layer chromatography (fig. 6). The lung from A. K. contained massive amounts of material having the chromatographic behavior of glucocerebrosides relative to the control.

Comments

In 1933 Merklen and associates reported the finding of Gaucher cells in the sputum of a 51-year-old man with this disease.[5] In 1937 Myers described Gaucher cells in the alveolar walls and sacs and in the hilar and mediastinal lymph nodes of an 8-year-old girl who died of Gaucher's disease.[6] In addition to pleurisy this child had signs of bronchial constriction, which were attributed to compression on these structures by the enlarged hilar lymph nodes. In 1948 Groen and Garrer described an "especially accentuated" pulmonic second sound, diffuse crepitant pulmonary rales, bilateral pleural effusions, cardiomegaly, and dilatation of the pulmonary trunk in a 48-year-old woman who died of Gaucher's disease after repeated attacks of severe dyspnea with extreme cyanosis.[7] An autopsy was not performed but these authors speculated that the clinical picture of cor pulmonale and pulmonary hypertension resulted from "obstruction in the smaller circulation . . . due to an accumulation of Gaucher cells in the lungs." In 1950 Kaiser described a miliary pattern on chest roentgenogram in a patient with Gaucher's disease.[8] Subsequently, this miliary-type appearance had been described in other patients with this disease.[1, 9–12] The 3-year-old child (case VII) reported by Levin died from "massive hemoptysis" and necropsy disclosed "numerous Gaucher cells in the lungs."[9] The patient reported by Jackson and Simon was also a 3-year-old girl who died of severe respiratory distress.[12] The lungs of this child on chest roentgenogram also demonstrated a miliary pattern, and at autopsy "enormous numbers of Gaucher cells" were present in the alveolar septa and spaces.

Although Gaucher cells have been described in alveolar septa, their location within the alveolar capillaries has not been previously described. In the present patient, obstruction to these capillaries by Gaucher cells appears to have been the cause of his severe pulmonary hypertension. The configuration of the elastic fibers in the pulmonary trunk were of the adult type, indicating that the pulmonary hypertension was acquired and not present at birth.[13] There is no mention of the cardiovascular or pulmonary systems in the description of this patient during childhood by Thannhauser.[2] When first seen at this clinic 29 months before his death, he demonstrated signs of severe pulmonary hypertension.

The cause of the acute recurrent pericarditis was never determined. Although a wide variety of inflammatory cells were present, no Gaucher cells were identified in the pericardium. Since this patient's pericardium was exceedingly vascular and since he experienced uncontrollable coughing during his last several days, the terminal hemopericardium and cardiac tamponade may have resulted from rupture of one or several of the pericardial vessels during the coughing episodes. Hemopericardium with cardiac tamponade has been described previously in a patient with Gaucher's disease.[14] This 59-year-old woman, however, also had an adenocarcinoma, probably primary in the lung, and malignant cells were found in the aspirated pericardial and pleural fluids. Zlotnick and Groen in 1961 described massive pericardial calcification in a 46-year-old woman who died of Gaucher's disease.[15] The cause of the pericardial calcification was not determined although "hemorrhagic diathesis . . . secondary to unrecognized hemorrhage into the pericardial cavity, with organization and deposition of calcium" was suggested. No Gaucher cells were described in her pericardium at necropsy, but interestingly these cells were found in her lungs.

This patient had had an accentuated pulmonic second sound, but electrocardiogram did not indicate ventricular hypertrophy.

Acknowledgment

The authors wish to acknowledge the invaluable participation of Dr. Eugene Braunwald and other members of the Cardiology Branch of the National Heart Institute in the clinical management of patient A. K.

References

1. Fredrickson, D. S.: Cerebroside Lipidosis: Gaucher's Disease in the Metabolic Basis of Inherited Disease, ed. 2. New York, The Blakiston Division-McGraw-Hill Book Co., 1966, p. 565.
2. Thannhauser, S. J.: Lipidoses: Diseases of the Intracellular Lipid Metabolism, ed. 3. New York, Grune & Stratton, 1958, 600 pp.
3. Heath, D., and Edwards, J. E.: The pathology of hypertensive pulmonary vascular disease: A description of six grades of structural changes in the pulmonary arteries with special reference to congenital cardiac septal defects. Circulation **18:** 533, 1958.
4. Mårtensson, E., Percy, A., and Svennerholm, L.: Kidney glycolipids in late infantile metachromatic leucodystrophy. Acta Pediat Scand **55:** 1, 1966.
5. Merklen, P., Waitz, R., and Warter, J.: Un cas de maladie de Gaucher ã dèterminations osseuses, avec cellules de Gaucher dans les crachats. Bull Soc Med Hop Paris **49:** 36, 1933.
6. Myers, B.: Gaucher's disease of the lungs. Brit Med J **2:** 8, 1937.
7. Groen, J., and Garrer, A. H.: Adult Gaucher's disease, with special reference to the variations in its clinical course and the value of sternal puncture as an aid to its diagnosis. Blood **3:** 1221, 1948.
8. Kaiser, A.: Morbus Gaucher-specifische lungeninfiltration unter dem bilde einer miliar-Tb. Mschr Kinderheilk **98:** 252, 1950.
9. Levin, B.: Gaucher's disease: Clinical and roentgenologic manifestations. Amer J Roentgen **85:** 685, 1961.
10. Maccioni, L., and Cappelli, B.: Le alterazioni polmonari nel morbo di Gaucher ad evoluzione cronica. Policlinico **69:** 157, 1962.
11. Pratesi, V.: Un casodi malattia di Gaucher a prevalente localizzazione polmonare. Riv Clin Pediat **72:** 396, 1963.
12. Jackson, D. C., and Simon, G.: Unusual bone and lung changes in a case of Gaucher's disease. Brit J Radiol **38:** 698, 1965.
13. Roberts, W. C.: The histologic structure of the pulmonary trunk in patients with "primary" pulmonary hypertension. Amer Heart J **65:** 230, 1963.
14. Rosenfeld, S., and Epstein, S.: Gaucher's disease complicated by metastatic carcinoma presenting symptoms of recurrent pericardial tamponade with secondary acute renal failure. New York J Med **61:** 4080, 1961.
15. Zlotnick, A., and Groen, J. J.: Observations on a patient with Gaucher's disease. Amer J Med **30:** 637, 1961.

Pulmonary Parenchymal Cholesterol-Ester Granulomas in Patients with Pulmonary Hypertension*

D. LUKE GLANCY, M.D., PAUL D. FRAZIER, D.D.S.† and WILLIAM C. ROBERTS, M.D.

Bethesda, Maryland

Granulomas containing acicular crystals, usually identified histologically as cholesterol, were found at necropsy in the lungs of twelve patients. A review of the clinical records and the pathologic study of the hearts and pulmonary vessels of these patients at necropsy showed that each of them had had pulmonary hypertension. Two had severe parenchymal pulmonary disease; cholesterol pneumonia was found in one and sarcoidosis in the other. Of the remaining ten patients, none of whom had significant parenchymal pulmonary disease, five had congenital cardiac malformations with shunts, two had valvular lesions, predominantly mitral stenosis, and three had primary pulmonary hypertension. The crystals, obtained by microdissection from the pulmonary granulomas of one patient, were identified by x-ray diffraction analysis as cholesteryl palmitate and/or stearate, and not free cholesterol. Possible causes of the cholesterol-ester granulomas were discussed. Pulmonary hypertension appears to be most important in the pathogenesis since it was the only factor recognized in all twelve patients, and since these granulomas have not been observed at necropsy in the lungs of any patient at the National Heart Institute who did not have pulmonary hypertension.

SINCE the work of Parker and Weiss [1] and later of Edwards and associates [2–5], it has been appreciated that anatomic changes occur in the lungs of most patients with severe pulmonary hypertension. When pulmonary hypertension is the result of a shunt, changes are observed in the arterioles, and in the muscular and elastic arteries of the lungs [2–5]. When pulmonary hypertension is due to an acquired cardiac lesion (for example, mitral stenosis), changes are observed not only in the pulmonary arteries and arterioles but also in the pulmonary capillaries, veins and lymphatics, and in the pulmonary parenchyma itself. The pulmonary veins and alveolar capillaries become dilated [1], the veins develop fibrous intimal thickening and there is dilatation of the perivascular, peribronchial and interlobular septal lymphatics [5–7]. Parenchymal changes include edema [1,6] and fibrous thickening of the interlobular septums, hyperplasia of the alveolar lining cells [1,7,8], accumulation of numerous hemosiderin-laden macrophages in the alveoli with focal fibrous thickening of alveolar walls [9], focal calcification of bronchial cartilage, formation of ossific nodules in the lungs [6–9] and an increase in smooth muscle in the walls of distal air passages [8–10].

During the past twelve years we have observed on histologic examination granulomas containing acicular crystals in the lungs of twelve patients with pulmonary hypertension. We failed to find any description of similar granulomas in publications describing the pulmonary histology of patients with pulmonary hypertension [1–10]. This report summarizes the clinical and necropsy features of the twelve patients we observed with pulmonary hypertension and describes the granulomas we saw in the pulmonary parenchyma. Also described

* From the Section of Pathology, Clinic of Surgery, National Heart Institute and the Laboratory of Histology and Pathology, National Institute of Dental Research, National Institutes of Health, Bethesda, Maryland. Requests for reprints should be addressed to D. Luke Glancy, M.D., at the Section of Pathology. Manuscript received August 28, 1967.

† Present address: Department of Biological Structure, University of Washington, Seattle, Washington 98105.

are the methods used for isolating the crystals and the x-ray diffraction technics employed in identifying them.

CLINICAL AND NECROPSY OBSERVATIONS

Pertinent clinical and pathologic data concerning the twelve patients appear in Table I. Four patients (Cases 3, 6, 7 and 11) had congenital cardiac disease with central shunts and increased pulmonary blood flow. Another patient (Case 1) had a shunt, but at the time of cardiac catheterization, four months before death, pulmonary blood flow was less than systemic blood flow. Three patients (Cases 2, 8 and 12) had primary or idiopathic pulmonary hypertension, and two (Cases 4 and 5) had rheumatic cardiac disease with predominant mitral stenosis. Two patients had chronic cor pulmonale: one (Case 9) had a systemic illness and extensive interstitial pulmonary fibrosis, and the other (Case 10) had pulmonary sarcoidosis. In eight of ten patients in whom cardiac catheterization was performed, pulmonary arterial pressures equaled or nearly equaled systemic arterial pressures. Two patients (Cases 5 and 12) had only moderate pulmonary hypertension, but in one (Case 12) pulmonary vascular resistance was markedly elevated (72 per cent of systemic).

Only one (Case 6) of the twelve patients had had hemoptysis. No patient was known to have ingested mineral oil, to have used nose drops containing oil or to have undergone bronchography. The serum total cholesterol was measured in two patients: in one (Case 1) it was 83 and in the other (Case 9) 243 and 164 mg. per 100 ml.

Only two patients (Cases 9 and 10) had

TABLE I
DATA IN TWELVE PATIENTS WITH PULMONARY CHOLESTEROL-ESTER GRANULOMAS

Case No.	Patient No.	Age (yr.) and Sex	Diagnosis	PA Pressure (mm. Hg)	BA Pressure (mm. Hg)	P/S Flow	Anatomic Grade of HPVD (0–6)*
1	A55-21	33, M	PDA, VSD	106/64	132/52 (FA)	0.9	5
2	A60-219	16, F	PPH	192/5 (RV)	138/90	1.0	5
3	A61-209	24, F	Double outlet RV, VSD, stenotic RPA	72/18	90/58	2.7	0 (R)† 2 (L)
4	A63-99	46, F	MS, MI, AS, AI	96/50	116/60	1.0	3
5	A65-140	52, F	MS, MI, AS, AI, TS, TI	54/21	150/55	1.0	3
6	A65-212	38, M	CT, VSD, Ligated LPA	83/20	102/65	2.1	0 (R)‡
7	A66-25	8½, F	ASD, VSD	85/42	95/60	1.5	1
8	A66-190	27, F	PPH	90/40	111/75	1.0	5
9	A61-168	58, F	Cor pulmonale, CHD	...	...	...	2
10	A67-19	40, F	Sarcoidosis, cor pulmonale	...	...	...	3
11	A67-116	8, M	Taussig-Bing, VSD, PDA	70/2 (RV)§	...	§	4
12	A65-75	39, F	PPH	50/30	96/73	0.54¶	3

NOTE: PA = pulmonary artery; BA = brachial artery; P/S = pulmonary/systemic; HPVD = hypertensive pulmonary vascular disease; PDA = patent ductus arteriosus; VSD = ventricular septal defect; FA = femoral artery; PPH = primary pulmonary hypertension; RV = right ventricle; RPA = right pulmonary artery; MS = mitral stenosis; MI = mitral insufficiency; AS = aortic stenosis; AI = aortic insufficiency; TS = tricuspid stenosis; TI = tricuspid insufficiency; CT = corrected transposition; LPA = left pulmonary artery; ASD = atrial septal defect; CHD = coronary heart disease.

* Classification of Heath and Edwards [*4*].

† The right main pulmonary artery was stenotic. There were no changes of hypertensive pulmonary vascular disease in the right lung (R), but there were grade 2/6 changes in the left lung (L).

‡ The left main pulmonary artery, having been mistaken for a patent ductus arteriosus, was ligated fourteen years before death. The lumens of the left pulmonary arteries were small and partially obliterated by organized thrombus. The pulmonary arteries of the right lung (R), which received all of the right ventricular output, were dilated, but showed no changes of hypertensive pulmonary vascular disease.

§ Performed elsewhere at age seven months. There was no valvular or subvalvular pulmonic stenosis, and the pulmonary trunk arose from both ventricles above a large ventricular septal defect, suggesting that right ventricular, left ventricular and pulmonary arterial systolic pressures were equal. The narrow subaortic infundibulum, small aorta, large pulmonary trunk and arteries, and the chest roentgenograms and angiocardiograms suggest that pulmonary blood flow was much greater than systemic.

¶ Large right to left shunt through a patent foramen ovale.

clinical or roentgenographic evidence of chronic pulmonary parenchymal disease, and the incidence of preceding respiratory illness in the other ten patients was no greater than would be expected for patients with severe cardiac disease: one patient (Case 4) had had pneumonia three years before death, and another (Case 5) thirty-four years before death; two patients (Cases 6 and 7) with left to right shunts had had frequent respiratory tract infections; and one patient (Case 12) had a history of asthmatic attacks in childhood but the timed vital capacity one week before death was normal. At necropsy, each of three patients (Cases 1, 2 and 12) had hypertrophied bronchial smooth muscle and a few inflammatory cells, including eosinophils in one (Case 12), in the bronchi. Otherwise, except for the crystal granulomas and the usual changes of hypertensive pulmonary vascular disease, the lungs of these ten patients were unremarkable. The causes of death varied: one patient (Case 1) died during a cardiac operation and four patients (Cases 3, 5, 6 and 7) following cardiac operations; two patients (Cases 2 and 11) died suddenly, presumably of cardiac arrhythmias;) one patient (Case 4) died of a complication of cardiac catheterization; one patient (Case 8) died of progressive cardiac failure; two patients (Cases 9 and 10) died of chronic pulmonary insufficiency and cor pulmonale; and one patient (Case 12) of coronary arterial occlusion.

In none of the twelve patients were the pulmonary granulomas detectable on roentgenographic or gross examinations of the lungs. On microscopic examination the granulomas appeared as acicular spaces surrounded by macrophages, epithelioid cells and foreign body giant cells (Fig. 1 through 4). Frequently, a dense collection of mononuclear cells, predominantly lymphocytes, surrounded the granulomas (Fig. 2, 3 and 4), and many of them were clearly in small, distal air spaces, some of which were lined by cuboidal epithelium (Fig. 1 and 3A). Focal, microscopic-sized, interstitial scars surrounded many of the granulomas, which were never found in pulmonary vessels. A few foamy macrophages were observed in occasional alveoli in all patients, and collections of these cells were frequently found adjacent to the granulomas (Fig. 1 and 2C). Various stages from collections of foamy macrophages to well organized granulomas surrounding acicular spaces could be found (Fig. 1 and 4B). Hemosiderin granules were visible in many foamy macrophages and in granulomas. In one patient (Case 10) the granulomas with acicular spaces could be distinguished from the tubercles of sarcoidosis, and a few of each type of granuloma contained calcium.

Acicular clefts were easily found on histologic examination of the lungs of the two patients (Cases 9 and 10) with chronic pulmonary parenchymal disease, and in the lungs of the three patients (Cases 1, 2 and 8) with the most severe anatomic changes of hypertensive pulmonary vascular disease. In the other patients, only 1 to 8 granulomas per patient were found on reviewing six to eighteen histologic sections of lung. The granulomas were found in one patient (Case 11) only after additional blocks of the lungs were cut and examined because foamy macrophages were noted in the original sections. In another patient (Case 8) most of the granulomas were near the hilus of each lung, but in the remaining patients they were scattered throughout the lungs. The elastic pulmonary arteries of each patient contained atheromas, and the right ventricle of each was hypertrophied.

Following fixation of the pulmonary tissue in 10 per cent formalin and routine processing procedures the acicular spaces within the granulomas were empty because the crystals, soluble in xylene and alcohol, had dissolved. Doubly refractile crystals, however, could be detected in the spaces in frozen sections of formalin-fixed or fresh tissue examined by polarized light (Fig. 2E and 4D). The crystals did not stain for fat by oil red O or cholesterol by the Schultz modification of the Liebermann-Burchardt reaction, but other portions of the granulomas and the surrounding foamy macrophages frequently showed positive fat and cholesterol staining (Fig. 4).

IDENTIFICATION OF THE CRYSTALS

In frozen sections of the lungs of one patient (Case 2), the doubly refractile crystals were identified under a polarizing light microscope, and the granulomas containing them were circled with a fine dissecting needle. The remainder of the tissue was removed from the slide leaving the crystal granulomas, which were then placed in special lead-free glass capillaries (0.3 mm. diameter, 0.1 mm. wall thickness) for x-ray diffraction. Samples of cholesterol (Δ^5-cholesten-3β-ol), cholesteryl palmitate (Δ^5-

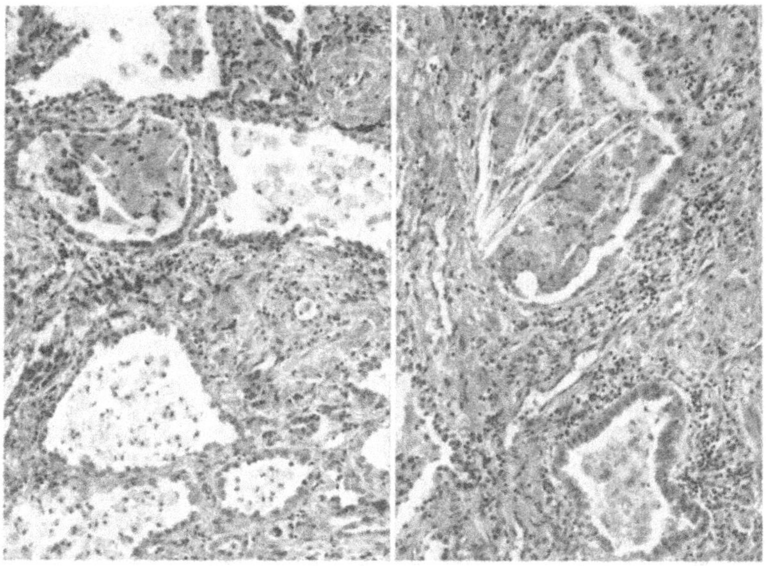

FIG. 1. Case 1. Specimen of lung. Foamy macrophages are in alveoli lined by cuboidal epithelium. The alveolar septums are thickened, fibrotic and contain mononuclear cells. In two alveoli, acicular spaces are surrounded by giant cells and debris. Hematoxylin and eosin stains; original magnification of each × 160.

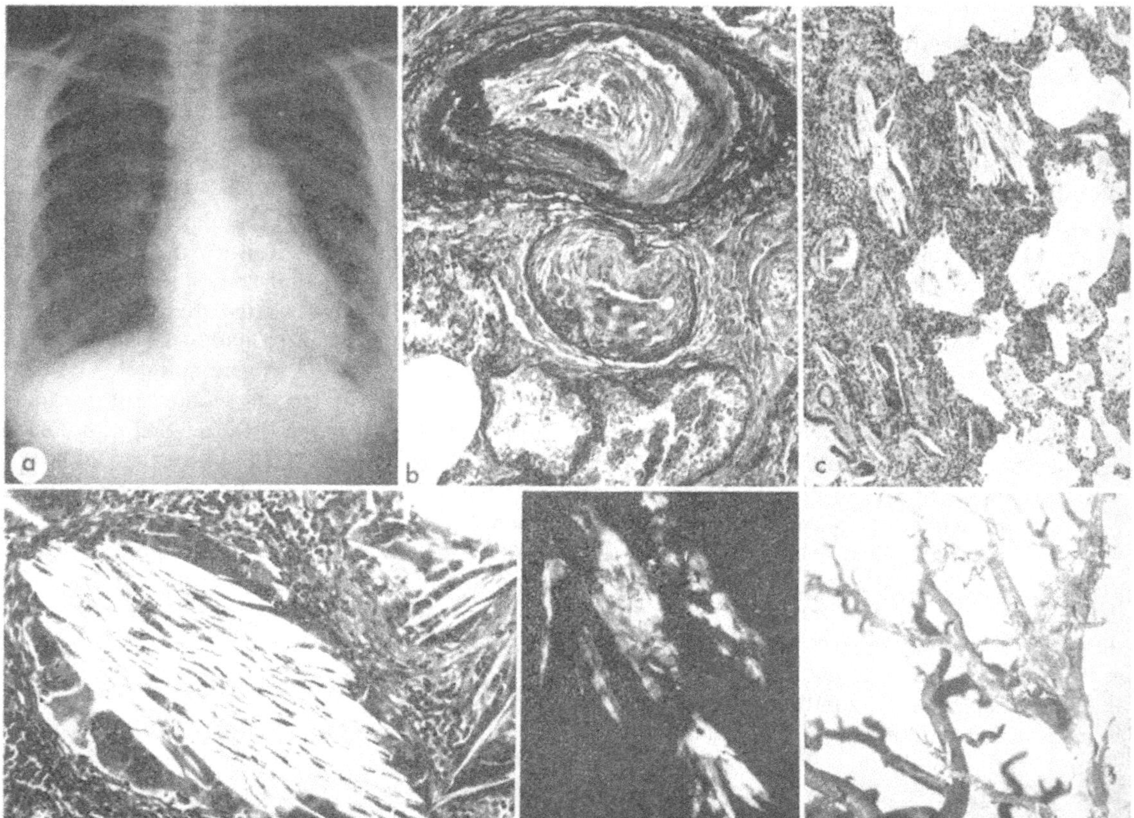

FIG. 2. Case 2. *a*, chest roentgenogram showing clear lungs, but enlargement of the heart, pulmonary trunk and proximal pulmonary arteries. *b*, obliterative intimal proliferation in a muscular pulmonary artery and in an arteriole. The thin-walled vascular spaces below the arteriole are part of an angiomatoid lesion. Elastic tissue stain, original magnification × 167. *c*, foamy macrophages within alveoli, and granulomas containing acicular spaces. The interstitial tissue is thickened, fibrotic and infiltrated by mononuclear cells. Hematoxylin and eosin stain; original magnification × 99. *d*, pulmonary acicular spaces surrounded by multinucleated giant cells. Hematoxylin and eosin stain; original magnification × 210. *e*, frozen section of pulmonary parenchymal granuloma photographed with polarized light showing birefringent crystals. Oil red O stain; original magnification × 330. *f*, corrosion cast of pulmonary arteries showing abrupt narrowing of the smaller vessels.

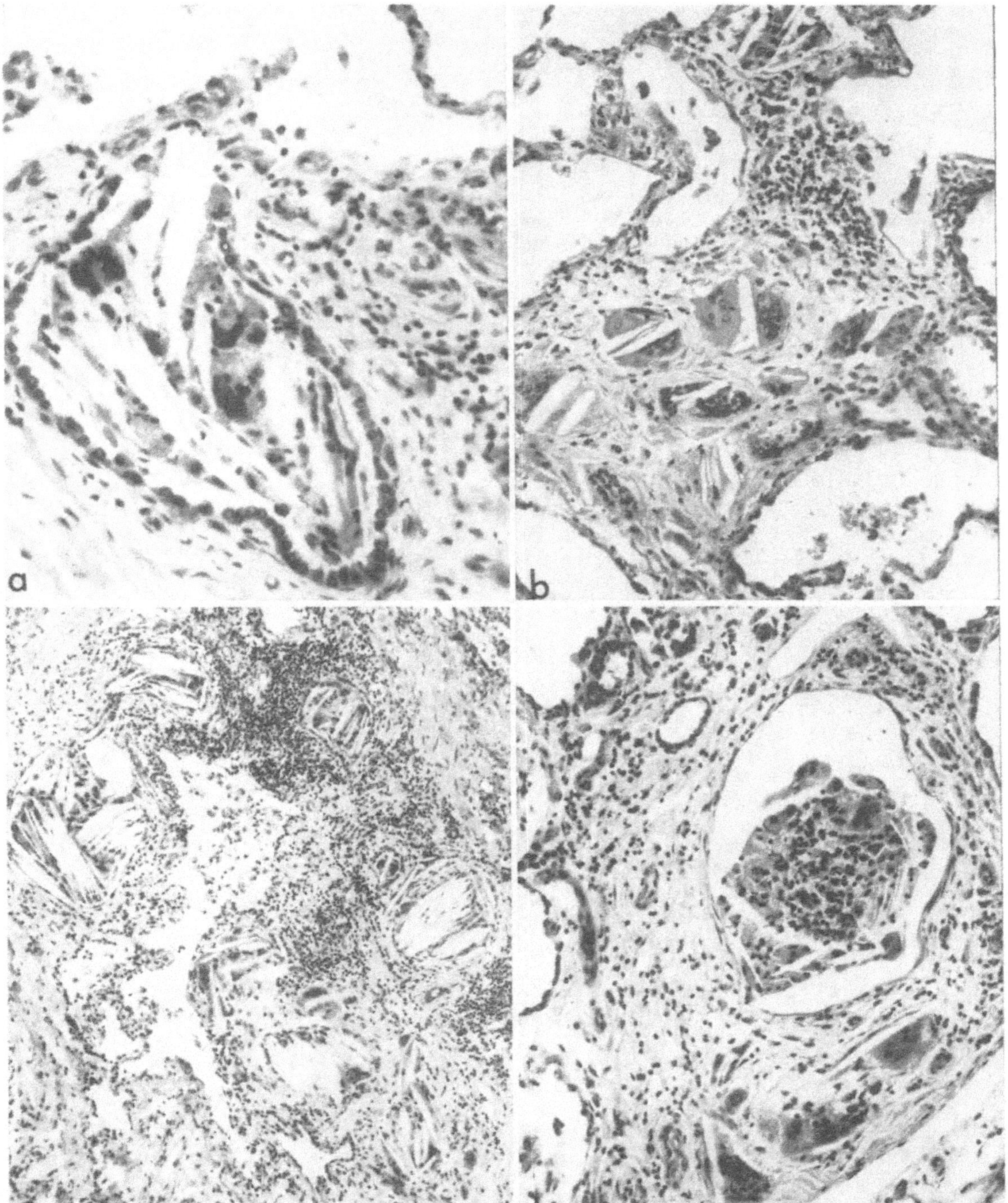

FIG. 3. Pulmonary parenchymal granulomas. The cholesterol-ester crystals have dissolved, leaving acicular spaces. *a*, Case 4. Original magnification × 251. *b*, Case 5. Original magnification × 160. *c*, Case 6. Original magnification × 82. *d*, Case 7. Original magnification × 160. All sections stained with hematoxylin and eosin.

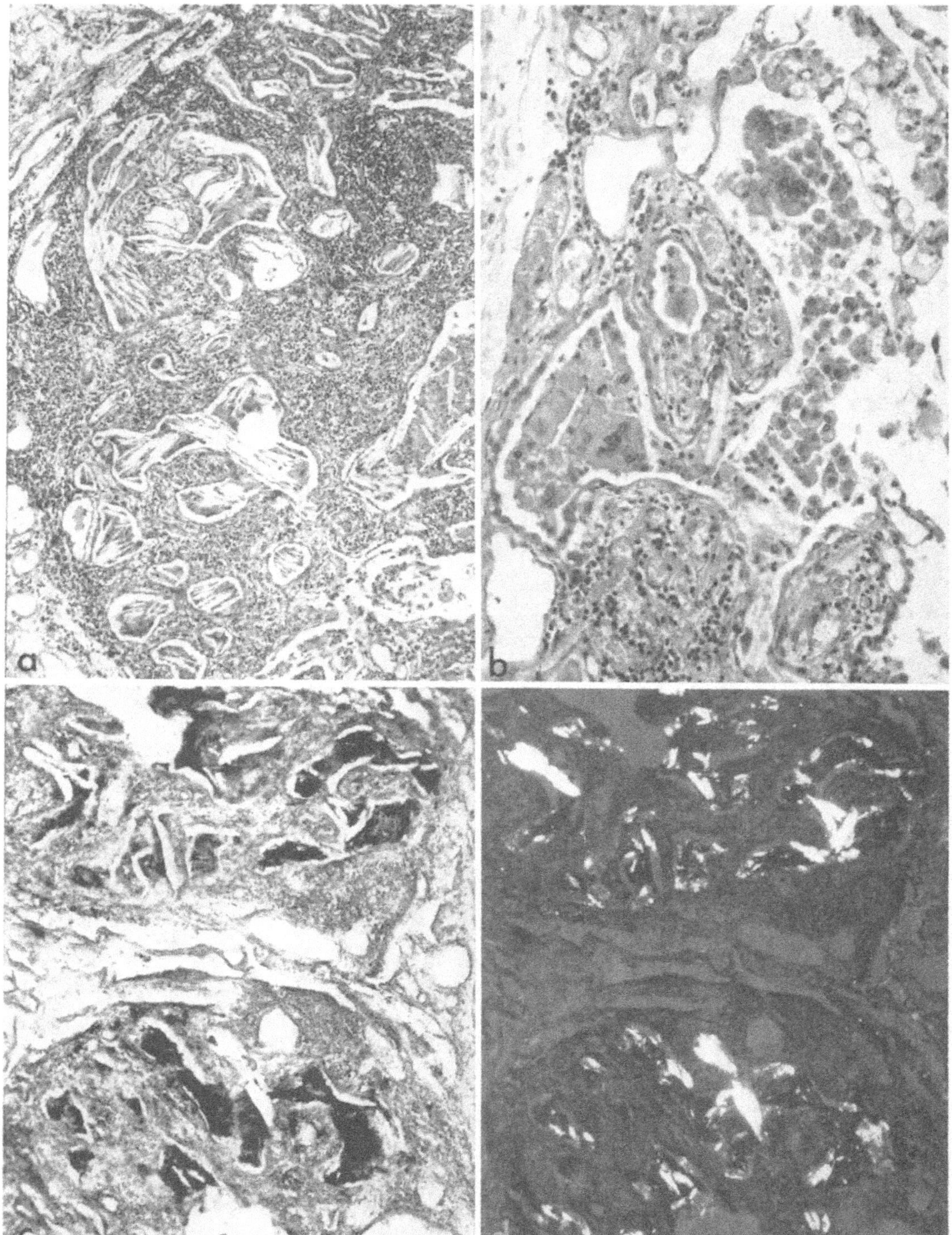

FIG. 4. Case 8. *a*, an unusually large number of acicular spaces surrounded by interstitial fibrous tissue containing lymphocytes. Hematoxylin and eosin stain; original magnification × 63. *b*, intra-alveolar macrophages. The alveolus on the left shows cuboidalization of the alveolar lining cells; the macrophages within it have fused, and small acicular spaces are seen. Hematoxylin and eosin stain; original magnification × 160. *c*, oil red O stain of a frozen section of pulmonary granulomas. The dark staining material is lipid within macrophages and giant cells. *d*, the same field photographed with polarized light. The cholesterol-ester crystals are birefringent and do not take the oil red O stain. Original magnification × 63.

Table II
X-RAY DIFFRACTION d-SPACING DATA

Cholesterol*		Cholesteryl Stearate*		Cholesteryl Stearate†		Cholesteryl Palmitate*		Cholesteryl Palmitate†		Lung Tissue	
d (Å)	I	d (Å)	I	d (Å)	I_1	d (Å)	I	d (Å)	I_1	d (Å)	I_2
33.6	100	...	...	25.63	35	21.24	13	26.40	40	25.23	S
16.8	12	...	...	18.18	45	...	...	17.50	25	17.50	S
13.87	5	...	...	13.85	5	13.37	7	13.14	5	...	...
...	...	...	...	10.95	15	10.27	10	10.27	5	...	...
(6)	...	9.45	20	9.39	15	9.30	13	9.39	5	9.39	MS
8.36	5	...	...	8.48	5	...	...	8.35	5	8.63	W
...	...	7.60	20	7.64	10	7.59	20	7.65	10	7.52	S
(6)	...	7.13	10	7.23	10	7.13	3	7.12	5	7.03	W
6.24	12	6.08	100	6.13	100	6.08	100	6.13	100	6.07	VS
5.74	21	...	...	5.80	30	5.81	13	5.86	20	5.80	W
(2)	...	5.57	40	5.57	20	5.57	20	5.55	20	...	...
5.25	6	5.33	10	5.33	30	5.32	7	5.33	5	(2)	VW
5.23	17	4.97	50 (b)	4.95	40 (b)	5.08	10	5.05	5	...	...
5.09	20	...	...	...	...	4.88	10	4.88	5	4.90	W
4.90	21	4.65	60	4.65	50	4.64	40	4.65	25	4.65	S
...	...	4.48	10	4.45	30	4.45	3	4.42	5	...	...
(16)	...	...	...	...	...	4.20	40	...	...	...	...
...	...	4.15	100 (b)	4.15	70 (b)	4.16	73	4.15	50 (b)	4.12	VS
...	...	3.80	80	3.80	70	3.80	87	3.80	35	3.79	VS
		3.54	10	...	...	3.55	7	...	...	...	...
...	...	3.24	5 (b)	...	...	...	...	...	...	(1)	VW
...	...	3.11	5	...	...	...	...	...	...	...	...
...	...	3.02	5	...	...	(7)	...	...	...	...	...
...	...	2.49	5	...	...	...	...	...	...	2.82	MS
...	...	2.40	5	...	...	...	...	...	...	...	...
...	...	2.33	5	...	...	...	...	...	...	...	...
...	...	2.25	20	...	...	2.26	13	...	...	...	...
...	...	1.88	5	...	...	(4)	...	...	...	...	...

Note: I = intensity. I_1 = intensity determined by microdensitometer tracing. I_2 = intensity determined by visual comparison. VS = very strong, S = strong, MS = medium strong, W = weak, VW = very weak. ( ) = indicate the number of lines present with relative intensities less than 5. (b) = broad line.

* Data for cholesterol, cholesteryl stearate and cholesteryl palmitate taken from ASTM Cards No. 7-742, 10-543, and 15-1004, respectively.

† Standards obtained from Sigma Chemical Co., St. Louis, Mo. 63118.

cholesten-3β-ol-3-hexadecanoate) and cholesteryl stearate (Δ^5-cholesten-3β-ol-3-octadecanoate) of high purity served as standards for comparison.* Diffraction patterns were recorded in a Debye-Scherrer type powder camera (114.50 mm. diameter) using V-filtered Cr radiation. Exposure time at 40 kv. and 10 ma. was eighteen hours for the standards, but the tissue preparations required ninety-six hours to give satisfactory line intensities, because of the small quantities of crystalline material.

The diffraction lines on the photographs were measured and the Bragg angles calculated and converted to interplanar d-spacing values by use of appropriate tables [*11*]. The relative intensities of the reflections from the standards were determined to the nearest multiple of 5 from a microdensitometer tracing. Because the diffraction patterns from the lung samples were generally weaker, it was necessary to estimate their line intensities visually. The interplanar d-spacing values, expressed in ångstroms, of the pulmonary crystals and their relative intensities of reflection are compared in Table II with those of the standards and with the listings [*12*] of the American Society for Testing and Materials (ASTM).

Comparison of the diffraction lines from the tissue preparations with those from the standards indicates that the crystalline material is not free cholesterol, and suggests that it is either cholesteryl palmitate, cholesteryl stearate or a mixture of the two (Fig. 5). Published d-spacing values

* Sigma Chemical Co., 3500 De Kalb Street, St. Louis, Missouri 63118.

and relative intensities for other cholesterol esters differ significantly from those obtained for the pulmonary crystals of this patient.

The characteristic lines and many of the minor reflections of the pulmonary crystals agree with those of the ASTM listing for cholesteryl palmitate (Table II), and ordinarily this would be more than enough evidence to make positive identification [*13,14*]. The difficulty, however, is that the stearate and palmitate esters of cholesterol have nearly identical diffraction patterns. The differences between cholesterol and the esters are easily seen (Fig. 5), but it is impossible to distinguish between the stearate and palmitate patterns visually, and even careful measurements of the diffraction lines (Table II) fail to show sharp differences in d-values. Under these conditions the relative intensities are important. When a mixture is present or isomorphic substitution has occurred, however, the intensity relationships are no longer useful because of the effects of substituted atoms and/or peak superimposition on relative intensity. Isomorphic substitution also will cause diffraction line shifts (change in d-values). Although the possibility that some or all the crystalline material obtained from our patient might be cholesteryl stearate could not be excluded, the x-ray diffraction pattern most closely corresponds with that of cholesteryl palmitate, and the concentration of the palmitic acid ester of cholesterol in serum and in erythrocytes is approximately ten times that of the stearic acid ester [*16*].

Except for cholesterol, differences were observed between the d-values and relative intensities of the standards and the ASTM data. This difference is not surprising because different patterns have been observed for the same compound, depending upon the local conditions during crystallization [*15*].

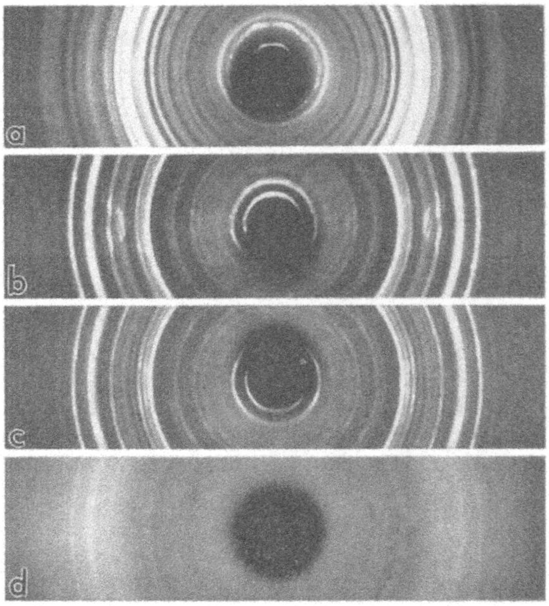

FIG. 5. X-ray diffraction patterns. *a*, cholesterol standard. *b*, cholesteryl stearate standard. *c*, cholesteryl palmitate standard. *d*, the pattern obtained from the pulmonary granulomas of patient (Case 2). Here the lines are less intense than those of the standards because of the small quantity of crystalline material. The spacings of the characteristic diffraction lines of the pulmonary crystals (*d*) have a one to one correspondence with those of the palmitate standard (*c*), but also correspond with those of the stearate standard (*b*). Thus, the pulmonary crystals are composed of one or both of these cholesterol esters. The diffraction pattern of the cholesterol standard (*a*) is clearly different from the other three.

COMMENTS

The strongest evidence of a relationship between cholesterol-ester granulomas and pulmonary hypertension is our failure to observe them in patients without pulmonary hypertension. Since granulomas with cholesterol-like crystals rarely occur in the lungs and have not been described except in pulmonary parenchymal disease, an association with pulmonary hypertension, either direct or indirect, is clearly indicated in these patients.

The cholesterol-ester granulomas probably arose from focal collections of lipid-laden macrophages, since these cells were found in the lungs of all twelve patients, they were most conspicuous in areas adjacent to the granulomas and were seen in aggregates suggesting early granuloma-formation (Fig. 1, 3D and 4B). The source of lipid within these macrophages, however, is uncertain. Erythrocytes [*16*], plasma and pulmonary tissue [*17,18*] contain lipids, including cholesterol and its esters, which might be phagocytized by macrophages and subsequently crystallize. Said and associates [*19*] suggest that alveolar septal cells and alveolar macrophages synthesize fatty acids and phospholipids.

Extravasation of erythrocytes into alveoli is common in patients with mitral stenosis [*7–9,20*] and pulmonary hemosiderosis occurs in patients with severe pulmonary arterial disease associated with intracardiac shunts or primary pulmonary hypertension [*4,5*]. Several observations, however, make erythrophagocytosis an unsatisfactory explanation for the genesis of the lipid-laden macrophages and cholesterol-ester granulomas. First, although many of the macrophages and granulomas contained hemosiderin, not all of them did. Second, the pulmonary hemosiderosis was only mild to moderate in eleven of our patients and absent in one patient, whereas many patients with severe pulmonary hemosiderosis have neither foamy macrophages nor cholesterol-ester granulomas. Third, although mitral stenosis is the most frequent cause of severe pulmonary hemosiderosis, intra-alveolar hemorrhage in these subjects appears to result more from pulmonary venous than from pulmonary arterial hypertension [*7,20*]. If erythrophagocytosis led to the formation of pulmonary cholesterol-ester granulomas, they should have been found in many more patients with mitral stenosis and in some with only mildly elevated pulmonary arterial pressures. Finally, hemosiderin-laden macrophages appear following the introduction of blood into the lungs of rabbits, but lipid-laden macrophages and granulomas do not [*21*].

Necrosis of pulmonary parenchyma is another potential source of cholesterol and its esters. Infarcts, however, were not observed in the lungs of any of our patients, and cholesterol-laden macrophages are not found around pulmonary infarcts [*22,23*].

Embolic cholesterol crystals surrounded by granulomatous reaction have been observed in the systemic arteries of patients with atherosclerotic aortas [*24*], and similar granulomas have been found in the pulmonary arteries [*24*] and parenchyma [*25*] of rabbits following intravenous injections of suspensions of cholesterol and its esters. The granulomas in our patients may have resulted from embolization of cholesterol and cholesterol esters originating from deposits in the intima of the elastic pulmonary arteries. Embolic foreign material may traverse the wall of the embolized pulmonary artery and the resulting granulomatous reaction may eventually lie within the parenchyma [*26*]. All the cholesterol-ester granulomas that we examined were extravascular, and this is evidence against their being embolic in origin. Also, pulmonary arterial atherosclerosis was minimal in some patients.

An infectious etiology for the granulomas is unlikely, and stains for bacteria (Brown and Brenn), fungi (methenamine silver) and acid-fast bacteria (Ziehl-Neelsen) revealed no organisms. The histologic findings in our patients are unlike granulomas caused by the aspiration of mineral oils, vegetable oils or exogenous animal fats [*27–30*], and none of our patients had a clinical history or roentgenographic features to suggest aspiration pneumonitis. No evidence was found for an abnormality of lipid metabolism to account for the accumulation of cholesterol esters. None of the twelve patients had any of the physical stigmata of hypercholesterolemia, and the serum total cholesterol was not elevated in the two patients in whom it was measured. Cholesterol-like crystals occur in pulmonary granulomas in patients with histiocytosis X [*31*] and in alveoli of patients with pulmonary alveolar proteinosis [*32*], but none of these crystals have been identified by x-ray diffraction, and none of our patients had clinical, roentgenographic or pathologic evidence of these diseases.

Two patients (Cases 9 and 10) had severe pulmonary parenchymal disease both clinically and pathologically. The history of two years of pulmonary disease and the histologic findings of extensive interstitial pulmonary fibrosis, severe inflammation and obstruction of the smaller branches of the bronchial tree, numerous intra-alveolar foamy macrophages, and acicular clefts predominantly in degenerating inflammatory debris and fibrous tissue (Fig. 6), rather than in true granulomas, suggest that one patient (Case 9) had a condition which has been called "cholesterol pneumonia" [*29*], "chronic pneumonitis of the cholesterol type" [*33,34*], "foam cell pneumonia" [*35*], "endogenous lipoid pneumonia" [*30,37*] and "golden pneumonia." Cholesterol pneumonia occurs most frequently as "obstructive pneumonitis" [*22,29,36*] distal to a carcinoma, but it also has been observed in suppurative processes, such as infected bronchiectasis and pulmonary abscess [*22,23,29,33*], focally in pulmonary tuberculosis [*23,33*], in pneumoconiosis due to bauxite fumes [*37*], in a necrotizing granulomatosis and angiitis of the lungs resembling Wegener's granulomatosis [*34*], and, as in one of our patients (Case 9), in subjects with no other recognizable pulmonary disease [*23,31,33,34,38–40*]. One report [*41*] describes cholesterol pneumonia in the lower lobe of the left lung which had always been perfused at systemic pressures by an aberrant pulmonary artery arising from the thoracic aorta. Cholesterol pneumonia, which is said to be the most common lipoid pneumonia [*29*], is usually a localized process,

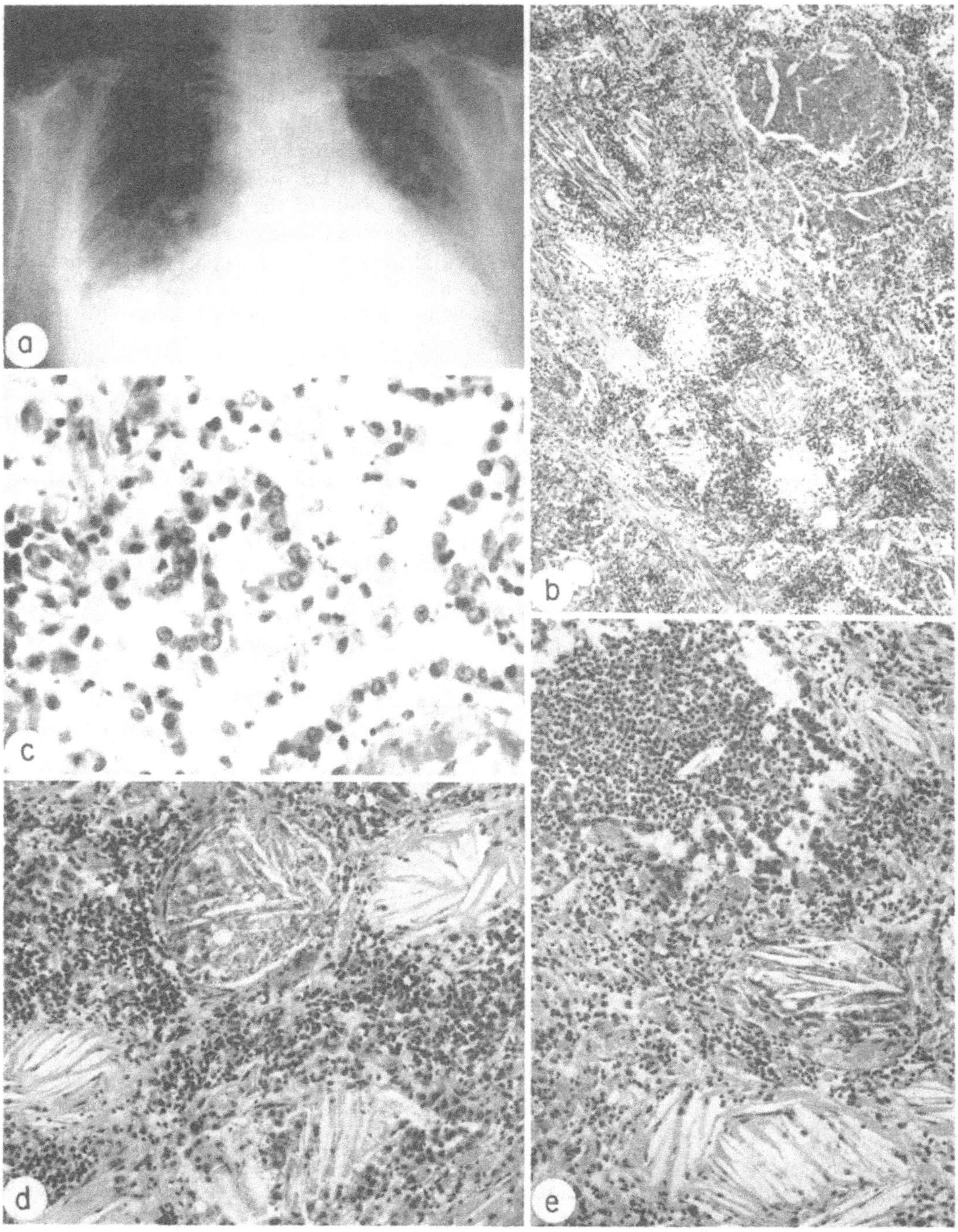

FIG. 6. Case 9. *a*, chest roentgenogram showing cardiomegaly, bilateral pleural effusions and diffuse pulmonary infiltrates, which are most prominent in the lower lobes. *b*, section of lung showing complete destruction of the parenchyma by cholesterol crystals, inflammatory cells and fibrous tissue. *c*, another area of lung showing cuboidalization of alveolar lining cells and intra-alveolar foamy macrophages. *d*, interstitial lymphocytes, plasmacytes, macrophages and polymorphonuclear neutrophiles surround acicular spaces, which are enclosed by fibrous tissue or degenerating inflammatory debris. *e*, another area of lung showing a distal air space (upper part of photo) lined by cuboidal epithelium and filled with polymorphonuclear leukocytes. One collection of acicular spaces is surrounded by necrotic debris, but others (lower portion of photo) are surrounded by fibrous tissue. Hematoxylin and eosin stains; original magnification × 63 (*b*), × 400 (*c*), × 160 (*d* and *e*).

Fig. 7. Lipoid pneumonia in a twenty-four month-old female BALB/c mouse (courtesy of Dr. Thelma B. Dunn). *a*, in the center of the field is a bronchus filled with inflammatory cells, mostly lymphocytes. Toward the pleura (upper portion of photo) all alveoli are filled with foamy macrophages. Hematoxylin and eosin stain; original magnification × 63. *b*, acicular clefts in and between intra-alveolar foamy macrophages. Hematoxylin and eosin stain; original magnification × 476.

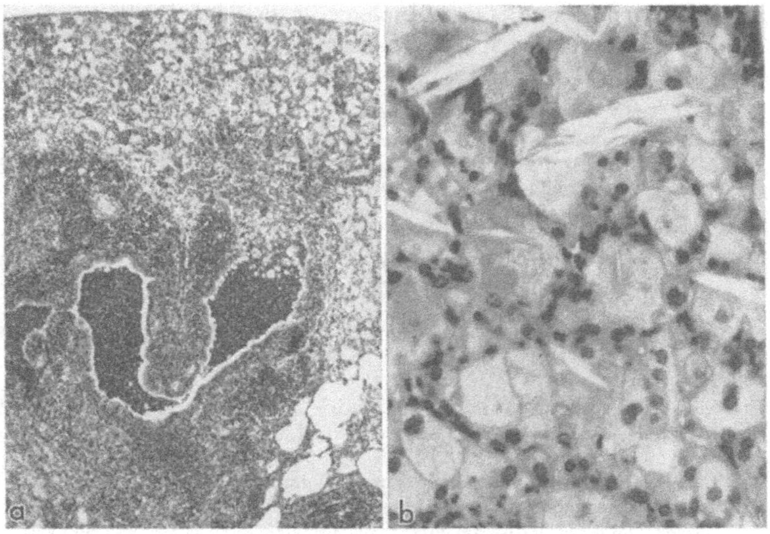

and it frequently progresses to severe interstitial fibrosis of the involved segment or lobe. We have studied microscopic sections of the lungs from three patients with the idiopathic type of cholesterol pneumonia at the Armed Forces Institute of Pathology [*42*]. The histologic changes were similar to those in one of our patients (Case 9), one of the few patients with the idiopathic form who has been examined at necropsy. The pulmonary involvement was unusual because every lobe was severely involved, in contrast to the localized involvement in other recorded cases.

The extensive fibrosis of sarcoidosis in one of our patients (Case 10) may have led to obstruction of the smaller branches of the bronchial tree, with the accumulation of foamy macrophages and subsequent formation of cholesterol-like granulomas. Similar changes have not been reported in sarcoidosis, but have been observed in other granulomatous diseases [*23,33,34*], and bronchial obstruction was thought to be important in the pathogenesis of idiopathic cholesterol pneumonia [*34*].

In the other ten patients in this study, pulmonary parenchymal changes were limited to microscopic areas of fibrosis around some of the widely scattered cholesterol-ester granulomas. Inflammation of small bronchi was minimal in three patients and absent in the other seven, and no patient had an obstructed major bronchus. None of the ten patients had had chronic pulmonary disease clinically or pulmonary infiltrates roentgenographically. These facts suggest that the cause of the cholesterol-ester granulomas in these patients was different from the cause in patients with cholesterol pneumonia, all of whom have had severe, pulmonary parenchymal disease clinically, roentgenographically and pathologically demonstrable. Even if a common etiology and pathogenesis were assumed, the apparent predilection of the cholesterol-ester granulomas for the lungs of patients with pulmonary hypertension would not be explained.

Lesions closely resembling cholesterol pneumonia have been produced experimentally in rabbits [43], rats [*37,44*] and hamsters [*45*], and occur spontaneously in old BALB/c mice (Fig. 7) [*46*]. We have no reports, however, of granulomas containing cholesterol-like crystals in the lungs of man or animals in the absence of severe, pulmonary parenchymal disease.

In recent years x-ray diffraction analysis has been used to identify crystalline substances found in autopsy and surgical specimens [*47–53*]. We have found no previous reports of its use to identify organic pulmonary crystals. This technic is more precise than histochemical procedures, and we were able to determine that the pulmonary crystals were cholesterol palmitate and/or stearate and not free cholesterol, which has been the identification usually made by histologic technics of any substance producing acicular clefts in tissues. We cannot explain why the palmitate and/or stearate rather than some other ester of cholesterol or free cholesterol itself should occur in the lungs of patients with pulmonary hypertension.

Acknowledgment: We wish to thank Commander Elias G. Theros, USNMC, USN, who allowed us to examine the histologic sections of lung of three patients with cholesterol pneumonia whose records were in the files of the Armed Forces Institute of Pathology, Washington, D.C. Dr. Thelma B. Dunn, Laboratory of Pathology, National Cancer Institute, allowed us to photograph the sections of lung shown in Figure 7, and offered helpful suggestions during the preparation of this manuscript. Mr. Larry D. Ent provided technical assistance.

REFERENCES

1. PARKER, F., JR. and WEISS, S. The nature and significance of the structural changes in the lungs in mitral stenosis. *Am. J. Path.*, 12: 573, 1936.
2. EDWARDS, J. E. Structural changes of the pulmonary vascular bed and their functional significance in congenital cardiac disease. *Proc. Inst. Med. Chicago*, 18: 134, 1950.
3. EDWARDS, J. E. Functional pathology of the pulmonary vascular tree in congenital cardiac disease. *Circulation*, 15: 164, 1957.
4. HEATH, D. and EDWARDS, J. E. The pathology of hypertensive pulmonary vascular disease. A description of six grades of structural changes in the pulmonary arteries with special reference to congenital cardiac septal defects. *Circulation*, 18: 533, 1958.
5. WAGENVOORT, C. A., HEATH, D. and EDWARDS, J. E. Pathology of the Pulmonary Vasculature, p. 146. Springfield, Ill., 1964. Charles C Thomas.
6. GOUGH, J. Correlation of radiological and pathological changes in some diseases of the lung. *Lancet*, 1: 161, 1955.
7. HARRIS, P. and HEATH, D. The Human Pulmonary Circulation. Its Form and Function in Health and Disease, p. 215. Baltimore, 1962. Williams & Wilkins Co.
8. SPENCER, H. Pathology of the Lung, p. 487. New York, 1962. The Macmillan Co.
9. LENDRUM, A. C., SCOTT, L. D. W. and PARK, S. D. S. Pulmonary change due to cardiac disease with special reference to haemosiderosis. *Quart. J. Med.*, 19: 249, 1950.
10. LIEBOW, A. A. Cardiopulmonary disease. In: Pathology of the Heart, 2nd ed., p. 940. Edited by Gould, S. E. Springfield, Ill., 1960. Charles C Thomas.
11. Tables for Conversion of X-ray Diffraction Angles to Interplanar Spacing. U.S. Department of Commerce, National Bureau of Standards. Washington, D.C., 1950. U.S. Government Printing Office.
12. ASTM Publication No. PDIS-160: Index (Organic) to the Powder Diffraction File. Philadelphia, 1966. American Society for Testing and Materials.
13. AZAROFF, L. V. and BUERGER, M. J. The Powder Method in X-Ray Crystallography. New York, 1958. McGraw-Hill Book Co., Inc.
14. BUNN, C. W. Chemical Crystallography. Oxford, 1961. Clarendon Press.
15. PARSONS, J., BEHER, W. T. and BAKER, G. D. X-Ray diffraction powder data and index for the steroids. *Henry Ford Hosp. M. Bull.*, 6: 365, 1958.
16. HANAHAN, D. J., WATTS, R. M. and PAPPAJOHN, D. Some chemical characteristics of the lipids of human and bovine erythrocytes and plasma. *J. Lipid Res.*, 1: 421, 1960.
17. DEUEL, H. J., JR. The Lipids, vol. 2, p. 787. New York, 1955. Interscience Publishers, Inc.
18. TOMBROPOULOS, E. G. Fatty acid synthesis by subcellular fractions of the lung. *Science*, 146: 1180, 1964.
19. SAID, S. I., KLEIN, R. M., NORRELL, L. W. and MADDOX, Y. T. Metabolism of alveolar cells. Histochemical evidence and relation to pulmonary surfactant. *Science*, 152: 657, 1966.
20. WOOD, P. Diseases of the Heart and Circulation, 2nd ed., p. 523. Philadelphia, 1956. J. B. Lippincott Co.
21. STRASSMAN, G. Formation of hemosiderin in the lungs. An experimental study. *Arch. Path.*, 38: 76, 1944.
22. SPENCER, H. Pathology of the Lung, p. 398. New York, 1962. The Macmillan Co.
23. WADDELL, W. R., SNIFFEN, R. C. and SWEET, R. H. Chronic pneumonitis. Its clinical and pathologic importance. Report of ten cases showing interstitial pneumonitis and unusual cholesterol deposits. *J. Thoracic Surg.*, 18: 707, 1949.
24. FLORY, C. M. Arterial occlusions produced by emboli from eroded aortic atheromatous plaques. *Am. J. Path.*, 21: 549, 1945.
25. HIRSCH, E. F., NAILOR, R. and BAUER, F. C., JR. Atherosclerosis v. The serum and plaque lipids in experimental hypercholesterolemia, with a comparison of plaque structure and lung granulomas caused by cholesterol esters. *Arch. Path.*, 64: 117, 1957.
26. VON GLAHN, W. C. and HALL, J. W. The reaction produced in the pulmonary arteries by emboli of cotton fibers. *Am. J. Path.*, 25: 575, 1949.
27. PINKERTON, H. Oils and fats. Their entrance into and fate in the lungs of infants and children. A clinical and pathological report. *Am. J. Dis. Child.*, 33: 259, 1927.
28. PINKERTON, H. The reaction to oils and fats in the lung. *Arch. Path.*, 5: 380, 1928.
29. MCDONALD, J. R. and HODGSON, C. H. The problem of lipoid pneumonia or granuloma of the lung. *M. Clin. North America*, 38: 989, 1954.
30. SUNDBERG, R. H., KIRSCHNER, K. E. and BROWN, M. J. Evaluation of lipoid pneumonia. *Dis. Chest*, 36: 594, 1959.
31. FORSEE, J. H. and BLAKE, H. A. Pulmonary cystic changes in xanthomatosis. *Ann. Surg.*, 139: 76, 1954.
32. ROSEN, S. H., CASTLEMAN, B. and LIEBOW, A. A. Pulmonary alveolar proteinosis. *New England J. Med.*, 258: 1123, 1958.
33. ROBBINS, L. L. and SNIFFEN, R. C. Correlation between the roentgenologic and pathologic findings in chronic pneumonitis of the cholesterol type. *Radiology*, 53: 187, 1949.
34. FIENBERG, R. Necrotizing granulomatosis and angiitis of the lungs and its relationship to chronic pneumonitis of the cholesterol type. *Am. J. Path.*, 29: 913, 1953.
35. CHIARI, H. Über chronische abszedierende Schaumzellenpneumonie. *Langenbecks Arch. klin. Chir.*, 268: 125, 1951.

36. McDonald, J. R., Harrington, S. W. and Clagett, O. T. Obstructive pneumonitis of neoplastic origin. An interpretation of one form of so-called atelectasis and its correlation according to presence or absence of sputum. *J. Thoracic Surg.*, 18: 97, 1949.
37. Gross, P., Brown, J. H. U. and Hatch, T. F. Experimental endogenous lipoid pneumonia. *Am. J. Path.*, 28: 211, 1952.
38. Engle, R. L. Giant cell foreign body reaction to non-cholesterol lipid plate crystals. A case report with chemical studies. *Am. J. Path.*, 27: 317, 1951.
39. Roggatz, J. Fremdkörperriesenzellen in der Lunge. *Frankfurt Ztschr. Path.*, 74: 331, 1965.
40. Adams, W. E. Chronic nonspecific suppurative pneumonitis. *Surgery*, 22: 723, 1947.
41. Claggett, O. T. and McDonald, J. R. Bronchiectasis and lipoid pneumonitis associated with a large aberrant pulmonary artery. *Proc. Staff Meet. Mayo Clin.*, 20: 1, 1945.
42. Theros, E. G. Personal communication.
43. Waddell, W. R., Sniffen, R. C. and Whytehead, L. L. The etiology of chronic interstitial pneumonitis associated with lipid deposition. An experimental study. *J. Thoracic Surg.*, 28: 134, 1954.
44. Bernick, S. and Alfin-Slater, R. B. Pulmonary infiltration of lipid in essential fatty-acid deficiency: progressive changes. *Arch. Path.*, 75: 13, 1963.
45. Herrold, K. M. Fibrosing alveolitis and atypical proliferative lesions of the lung. An experimental study in Syrian hamsters. *Am. J. Path.*, 50: 639, 1967.
46. Dunn, T. B. Personal communication.
47. Prien, E. L. and Frondel, C. Studies in urolithiasis. I. The composition of urinary calculi. *J. Urol.*, 57: 949, 1947.
48. Kennard, O. The use of x-ray diffraction methods in some clinical problems. In: Proceedings of the Second International Symposium on X-ray Microscopy and X-ray Microanalysis, p. 525. Amsterdam, 1960. Elsevier Publishing Co.
49. Parsons, J. and Eurs, F. J. X-ray diffraction analysis of crystals in pathology. *Am. J. Clin. Path.*, 32: 405, 1959.
50. Parsons, J. The application of x-ray diffraction to medical problems. In: Advances in X-ray Analysis, vol. 3, p. 349. Edited by Muller, W. M. New York, 1960. Plenum Press.
51. Howell, R. R., Eanes, D. E. and Seegmiller, J. E. X-ray diffraction studies of the tophaceous deposits in gout. *Arthritis & Rheumat.*, 6: 97, 1963.
52. Frazier, P. D., Lietman, P. S. and Seegmiller, J. E. Identification of l-cystine crystals in bone marrow by X-ray diffraction. *J. Lab. & Clin. Med.*, 65: 108, 1965.
53. Lietman, P. S., Frazier, P. D., Wong, V. G., Shalton, D. and Seegmiller, J. E. Adult cystinosis. A benign disorder. *Am. J. Med.*, 40: 511, 1966.

SCIMITAR SYNDROME ASSOCIATED WITH PATENT DUCTUS ARTERIOSUS, AORTIC COARCTATION AND IRREVERSIBLE PULMONARY HYPERTENSION

D. LUKE GLANCY, NINA S. BRAUNWALD, KEVIN P. O'BRIEN, AND WILLIAM C. ROBERTS

The Section of Pathology and the Surgery and Cardiology Branches, National Heart Institute, National Institutes of Health, Bethesda, Maryland

Received for publication July 29, 1968

The scimitar syndrome receives its name from the scimitar-like, roentgenographic appearance of an anomalous vein connecting most or all of the right pulmonary veins with the inferior vena cava (1). The venous abnormality is usually associated with other anomalies of the right lung. Since it was first recognized (2) in 1836, this congenital malformation has been observed in over 70 patients (3, 4), but hemodynamic data together with detailed morphologic study at necropsy have been presented in only one of them (1). This report describes the clinical, hemodynamic, and necropsy findings in a boy with patent ductus arteriosus and preductile aortic coarctation, a complex of malformations not previously found in association with the scimitar syndrome.

Report of Patient

A seven-year-old boy (C.C. #07-39-01) entered the National Heart Institute for evaluation of cardiomegaly, first noted at age two months, and a precordial murmur, discovered at age three years. During infancy he had gained weight slowly, had frequent respiratory infections, and had developed dyspnea and cyanosis with exertion. At age three years he had been given digoxin, and thereafter his respiratory infections and symptoms had steadily decreased. Examination (age seven) revealed a bulging precordium, a prominent left parasternal lift, and a loud pulmonic closure sound. A grade 3/6 continuous murmur beneath the left clavicle, a grade 2/6 basal systolic ejection murmur, and a grade 2/6 mid-diastolic rumble at the lower left sternal border were heard. Femoral arterial pulsations were full, but delayed. The electrocardiogram and chest roentgenograms are shown in Figures 1 and 2, respectively.

At cardiac catheterization (Table I) oxygen step-ups were found high in the inferior vena cava and in the pulmonary artery. Pulmonary blood flow was calculated to be twice systemic flow, and the pulmonary resistance to be approximately one third of systemic resistance. A 13 mm Hg pressure gradient was measured across the junction of an anomalous right pulmonary vein with the inferior vena cava at the level of the diaphragm. Pressures in the pulmonary artery and descending aorta,

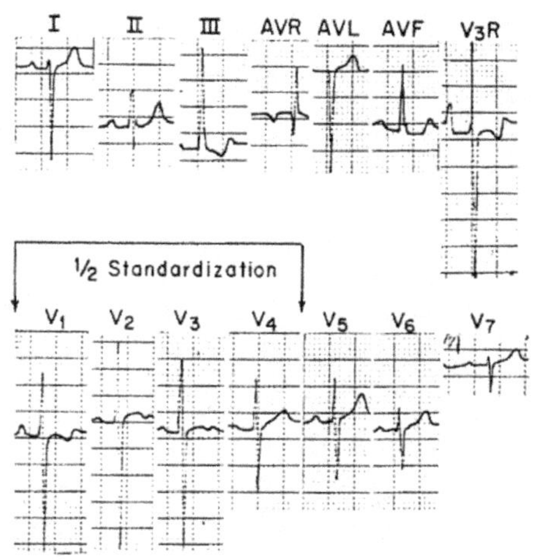

FIG 1. Electrocardiogram showing right axis deviation, right ventricular hypertrophy and right atrial enlargement.

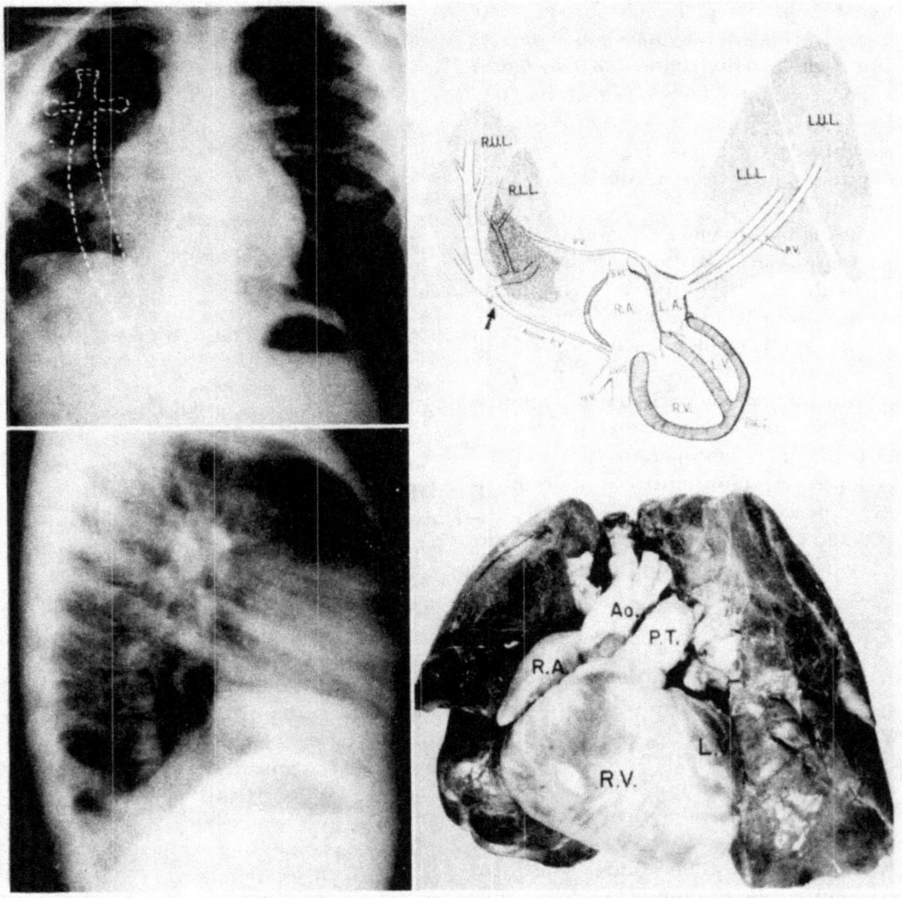

FIG. 2. *Upper left:* Posteroanterior chest roentgenogram. The right lung is small; the right diaphragm is elevated; and the heart is shifted to the right. Within the blade of the scimitar (dashed lines) is a long, anomalous, pulmonary vein which descends in the interlobar fissure to connect with the inferior vena cava. The pulmonary trunk is prominent. *Lower left:* Lateral roentgenogram showing the elevated right hemidiaphragm and the retrosternal space filled by the large right ventricle. *Upper right:* Diagram of the heart, lungs, and pulmonary veins (P.V.). The right lung has no middle lobe, but the right lower lobe (R.L.L.) has an extra segment (dark stippling) on its medial surface. All veins from the left upper (L.U.L.) and left lower (L.L.L.) lobes and a small vein from the R.L.L. connect with the left atrium (L.A.) normally. All right upper lobe (R.U.L.) and most R.L.L. veins connect with an anomalous vein (Anom. P.V.) which empties into the inferior vena cava (I.V.C.) just below the right atrium (R.A.) and above the hepatic veins (H.V.). The anomalous vein appears to be compressed (arrow) as it emerges through a notch on the inferomedial surface of the lung, and its extrapulmonary segment is narrower than its intrapulmonary segment. L.V. = left ventricle; R.V. = right ventricle; S.V.C. = superior vena cava. *Lower right:* Anterior view of the heart and lungs at necropsy. The left lung is larger than the right. The right ventricle (R.V.) is massively hypertrophied and forms the apex of the heart. A white fibrous plaque, so-called soldier's patch, is on its epicardial surface. The right atrial appendage (R.A.) and pulmonary trunk (P.T.) are dilated. Ao. = aorta; L.V. = left ventricle.

ntered from the pulmonary artery, were identical. Cinearteriograms following an ortic root injection showed narrowing of the aortic isthmus and filling of the pulmonary artery from the aorta distal to the oarctation. A 30 mm Hg peak systolic pressure gradient was measured across the oarctation.

On August 23, 1967, the aortic coarctaion was resected; its lumen measured 1.5 nm in diameter (Fig 5). A patent ductus rteriosus, which was distal to the coarctaion and 0.75 cm in diameter, was closed with sutures and divided. At the end of the operation the pulmonary arterial pressure was 70/40 and systemic arterial pressure, 5/70 mm Hg. Postoperatively, the child developed respiratory distress, intermittent ever, anemia, leukocytosis, and changing pulmonary infiltrates. Despite antibiotics nd adrenal corticosteroids, the dyspnea radually worsened, and he died eight veeks after operation.

The pulmonary and cardiac findings at ecropsy (A67-251) are illustrated in Figres 2–5. The left lung was of normal size, ad two lobes, and its bronchi, arteries nd veins had normal distributions and onnections. In contrast, the right lung vas small and had abnormalities of lobaion, bronchial distribution, arterial suply, and venous connections. The right lung had no middle lobe. The lower lobe ad an extra segment on its medial surace, which was partially separated from the rest of the lower lobe by pleura. A bronchus, arising from the main bronchus to the right lower lobe just distal to its origin, supplied both the extra segment nd a portion of the upper lobe. The right pulmonary artery was of normal size nd divided into three branches: large ones to the upper and lower lobes and a smaller one to the extra segment. A systemic artery arising from the aorta at the level of the diaphragm entered the posterior basal segment of the right lower lobe. Histologically, it was an elastic artery. The

TABLE I

Cardiac Catheterization Data

Site	Pressure (mm Hg)	Oxygen Saturation (%)
Superior vena cava		67
Inferior vena cava, low		73
Inferior vena cava, high		79
Anomalous pulmonary vein	17	93
Right atrium	4	77
Right ventricle	96/4	78
Pulmonary artery	96/60	83
Descending aorta	96/60	92
Left radial artery	126/69	94

pulmonary venous connections are described in Figures 2 and 3.

All segments of both lungs were consolidated and hemorrhagic. Virtually every alveolus was filled with erythrocytes and/or edema fluid. Large mononuclear cells were present in most alveoli. Many contained hemosiderin, many had foamy cytoplasm, a few had phagocytosed erythrocytes, and an occasional multinucleated cell was seen. Pleural veins and lymphatics were dilated, and the interlobular septae were edematous.

In every segment of both lungs there were grade 4/6 [Heath and Edwards classification (5)] changes of hypertensive pulmonary arterial disease: medial hypertrophy; intimal proliferation, which was most severe in the medium-sized muscular arteries; numerous plexiform lesions; and occasional dilatation lesions. Small infarcts were present in both lungs. The configuration of the elastic fibers in the media of the pulmonary trunk and ascending aorta were identical, suggesting that pulmonary hypertension had been present from birth (6).

Most of the cardiac mass was right ventricle. Although hypertrophied, the left ventricle was much smaller than the right ventricle. The right atrium and pulmonary trunk were dilated; their walls were thicker than normal; and the intima of the pulmonary trunk contained small deposits

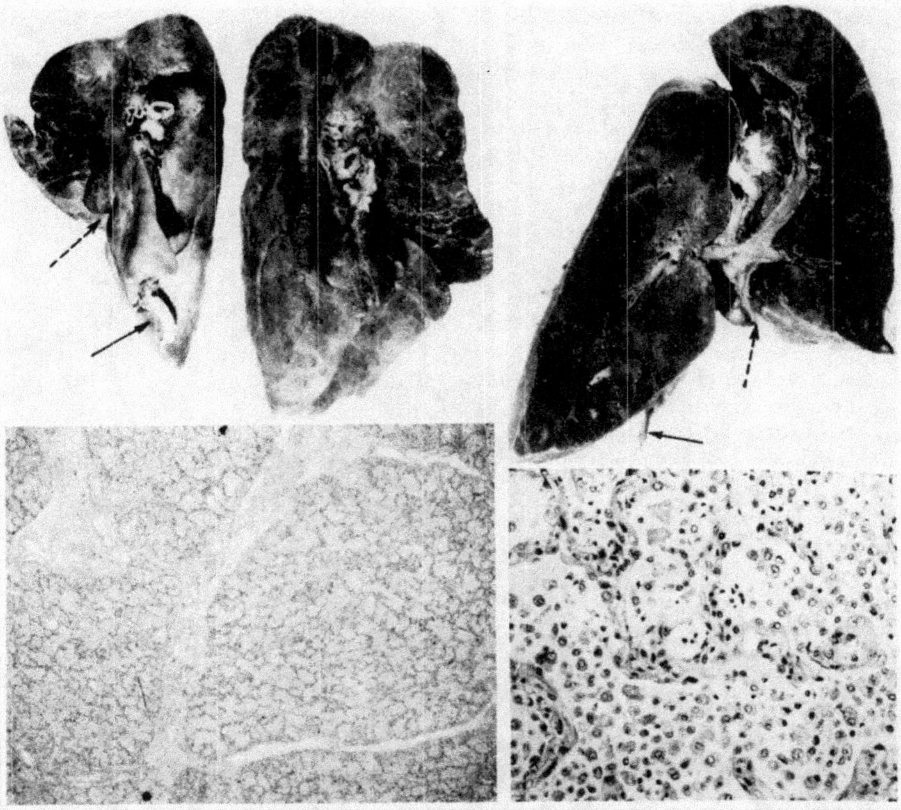

FIG 3. The lungs. *Upper left:* Medial surface of the lungs. The right lung is much smaller than the left. The solid arrow indicates the systemic artery which enters the posterior basal segment of the right lower lobe; and the dashed arrow, the notch through which the anomalous vein left the lung to connect with the inferior vena cava. The extra right lower lobe segment is between the two arrows. *Upper right:* The lateral portion of the right lung has been cut away. The parenchyma of both lobes is consolidated and hemorrhagic. The anomalous pulmonary vein and several of its larger branches lie in the interlobar fissure. The solid arrow indicates the systemic artery; and the dashed arrow, the anomalous vein where it is compressed as it leaves the lung. *Lower left:* Histologic section of lung in which every alveolus is filled with blood and/or edema fluid. Many alveoli also contain large mononuclear cells. Two dilated lymphatics are on the right, and an edematous interlobular septum is in the middle of the field (H and E; × 19). *Lower right:* A higher power photomicrograph (periodic acid-Schiff; × 147) showing alveoli containing numerous large mononuclear cells, occasional multinucleated forms, and a few polymorphonuclear neutrophils.

of lipid. The aortic valve was congenitally bicuspid, but otherwise normal. The aortic lumen at the site of anastomosis measured 6.5 mm in diameter.

COMMENTS

The essential component of the scimitar syndrome is an anomalous vein which connects most or all of the right pulmonary veins with the inferior vena cava. Other components which are frequently present are listed in Table II. Almost one fourth of the patients have had other congenital cardiovascular anomalies. Atrial septal defect has been the most common, and coarctation of the aorta has been reported

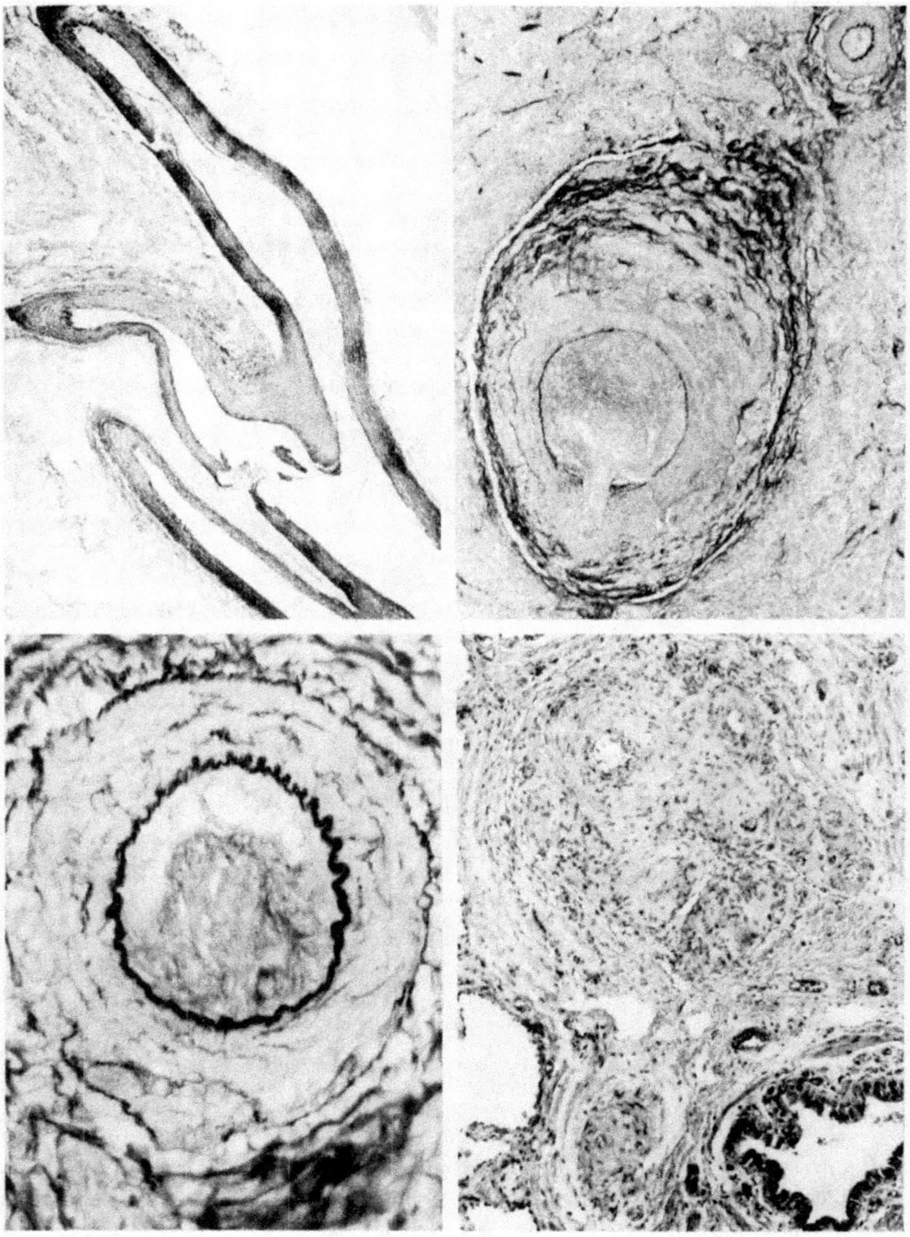

FIG. 4. Photomicrographs of arteries in the lungs. *Upper left:* Elastic tissue stain (× 22) of the systemic artery as it branches on entering the right lower lobe. The arterial media is composed primarily of elastic tissue. *Upper right:* A medium-sized, muscular, pulmonary artery. The adventitia is thickened by fibroelastic tissue; the media is hypertrophied; and the lumen, including the orifice of a small branch, is completely obliterated by fibrous intimal proliferation. A small muscular artery with medial hypertrophy and intimal proliferation is seen in the upper right corner of the field (elastic tissue stain; × 83). *Lower left:* A small, muscular, pulmonary artery with marked medial hypertrophy and a lumen almost completely obliterated by fibro-cellular intimal proliferation (elastic tissue stain; × 356). *Lower right:* A plexiform lesion with marked medial hypertrophy and cellular intimal proliferation of both the parent muscular artery (upper left) and its branches (H and E; × 88).

only once previously (7). Congenital anomalies outside the cardiopulmonary system, such as hemivertebrae, double ureter, uterine duplication, and omphalocele, have occasionally been observed (1, 3). Two thirds of the patients have been females.

TABLE II

SCIMITAR SYNDROME

1. Connection of most or all of the right pulmonary veins to the inferior vena cava via an anomalous vein.
2. Small right lung associated with:
   a. Deficient or abnormal lobation.
   b. Anomalous distribution of bronchi.
   c. Bronchial diverticula or cysts.
   d. Diaphragmatic elevation or anomaly.
   e. Rightward cardiac displacement.
3. Hypoplasia of the right pulmonary artery.
4. Branches of the upper abdominal or lower thoracic aorta supply part of the right lung.
5. Congenital cardiac disease (20 – 25%):
   a. Atrial septal defect.
   b. Patent ductus arteriosus.
   c. Tetralogy of Fallot.
   d. Ventricular septal defect.
   e. Coarctation of the aorta.

In the absence of other cardiovascular anomalies, patients with the scimitar syndrome usually have normal or only mildly elevated pulmonary arterial pressures, and 56/26 mm Hg is the highest recorded (8). This finding is not surprising since the left-to-right shunt occurs proximal to the tricuspid valve as in atrial septal defect, is usually small, and in some patients cannot be detected by oxygen series (3). Only one reported patient has had a shunt greater than 50% of pulmonary blood flow (4), and in him coexisting mitral stenosis, by elevating the pressure in the normally draining pulmonary veins, probably encouraged flow through the anomalous vein. Four patients, including ours, have had

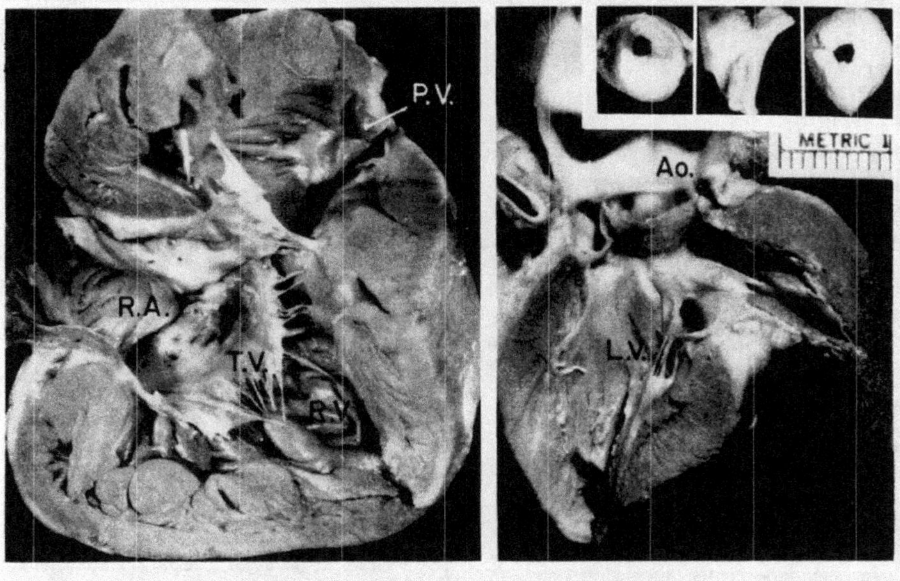

FIG 5. The heart. *Left:* The opened right atrium (R.A.), tricuspid (T.V.) and pulmonic (P.V.) valves, and massively hypertrophied right ventricle (R.V.). *Right:* The opened left ventricle (L.V.), aortic valve, and aorta (Ao.). Although its wall is thicker (1.5 cm) than normal, the left ventricle is dwarfed by the right. (Both pictures were taken from the same distance.) The aortic valve is congenitally bicuspid. The posterior cusp is intact; the anterior cusp has been cut. *Inset:* The resected aortic coarctation: proximal (left), lateral and distal (right) aspects. The lumen measures 1.5 mm in diameter. The ruler measures only the coarctation specimen.

moderate or severe pulmonary hypertension (1, 9, 10), and each of them had patent ductus arteriosus. In our patient and two others (1, 9) with patent ductus and pulmonary hypertension, a pressure gradient was measured between the anomalous vein and the inferior vena cava. Venous obstruction of one lung can cause pulmonary arterial hypertension (11) and may have contributed to the pulmonary hypertension in these patients. At least one reported patient with the scimitar syndrome and obstruction of the anomalous vein, however, did not have pulmonary arterial hypertension (12). Pulmonary parenchymal disease, hypoplasia or absence (13) of the right pulmonary artery, or multiple pulmonary arterial branch stenoses (9) could potentiate pulmonary hypertension in patients with the scimitar syndrome.

In our patient the large patent ductus arteriosus probably was the most important factor in the development of severe pulmonary hypertension and obliterative arterial disease. When he was catheterized at age seven, a moderate-sized left-to-right shunt was demonstrated, but most of this was probably obligatory shunting via the anomalous vein. Bidirectional shunting may have been present through the ductus, and indicator dilution curves from the right side of the heart with sampling from the femoral artery might have been the best method for uncovering the right-to-left component, which at the time of catheterization must have been small since the oxygen saturation was only 2% higher in radial arterial blood than in simultaneously obtained descending aortic blood. Despite overall pulmonary/systemic flow and resistance ratios which seemed favorable for operation, the patient had irreversible obliterative pulmonary arterial disease. Like most patients with Eisenmenger's syndrome, he did not tolerate closure of the communication between systemic and pulmonary circulations, and extensive intra-alveolar hemorrhage resulted in death.

SUMMARY

The clinical, hemodynamic and necropsy findings are presented in a seven-year-old boy with the scimitar syndrome, patent ductus arteriosus, preductile aortic coarctation and severe pulmonary hypertension, and hemodynamic findings in patients with the scimitar syndrome are discussed.

REFERENCES

1. Neill, C. A., Ferencz, C., Sabiston, D. C. and Sheldon, H.: The familial occurrence of hypoplastic right lung with systemic arterial supply and venous drainage "scimitar syndrome." Bull. Hopkins Hosp., 107: 1, 1960.
2. Cooper, G.: Case of malformation of the thoracic viscera: Consisting of imperfect development of right lung, and transposition of the heart. London Med. Gaz., 18: 600, 1836.
3. Kiely, B., Filler, J., Stone, S. and Doyle, E. F.: Syndrome of anomalous venous drainage of the right lung to the inferior vena cava. A review of 67 reported cases and three new cases in children. Amer. J. Cardiol., 20: 102, 1967.
4. Kalke, B. R., Carlson, R. G., Ferlic, R. M., Sellers, R. D. and Lillehei, C. W.: Partial anomalous pulmonary venous connections. Amer. J. Cardiol., 20: 91, 1967.
5. Heath, D. and Edwards, J. E.: The pathology of hypertensive pulmonary vascular disease. A description of six grades of structural changes in the pulmonary arteries with special reference to congenital cardiac septal defects. Circulation, 18: 533, 1958.
6. Heath, D., Wood, E. H., Du Shane, J. W. and Edwards, J. E.: The structure of the pulmonary trunk at different ages and in cases of pulmonary hypertension and pulmonary stenosis. J. Path. Bact., 77: 443, 1959.
7. Steinberg, I.: Roentgen diagnosis of anomalous pulmonary venous drainage of right lung into inferior vena cava. Report of three new cases. Am. J. Roentgen., 81: 280, 1959.
8. Frye, R. L., Marshall, H. W., Kincaid, O. W. and Burchell, H. B.: Anomalous pulmonary venous drainage of the right lung into the inferior vena cava. Brit. Heart J., 24: 696, 1962.
9. Yonehiro, E. G., Hallman, G. L. and Cooley,

D. A.: Anomalous pulmonary venous return from a hypoplastic right lung to the inferior vena cava (scimitar syndrome): Report of successful correction and review of surgical treatment. Cardiov. Res. Cent. Bull. (Houston), **4:** 106, 1965–66.

10. Jue, K. L., Amplatz, K., Adams, P., Jr. and Anderson, R. C.: Anomalies of the great vessels associated with lung hypoplasia. The scimitar syndrome. Amer. J. Dis. Child., **111:** 35, 1966.

11. Ferencz, C. and Dammann, J. F., Jr.: Significance of the pulmonary vascular bed in congenital heart disease. Part V. Lesions of the left side of the heart causing obstruction of the pulmonary venous return. Circulation, **16:** 1046, 1957.

12. Kaplan, S. quoted by Neill, C. A., et al in reference 1.

13. Hollis, W. J.: The scimitar anomaly with absent right pulmonary artery. Amer. J. Cardiol., **14:** 262, 1964.

Giant right atrium in rheumatic mitral stenosis

Atrial enlargement restricted by mural calcification

*William C. Roberts, M.D.**
J. O'Neal Humphries, M.D.
Andrew G. Morrow, M.D.
Bethesda and Baltimore, Md.

In most patients with rheumatic mitral stenosis or regurgitation some degree of left atrial enlargement is evident, and when the left atrium becomes greatly dilated, the right atrial chamber is usually also quite large, even though the tricuspid valve leaflets and chordae tendineae may be anatomically normal. Enormous dilatation of the right atrium with only slight and quite disproportionate enlargement of the left atrium has not been reported in patients with acquired mitral valve disease. These were the unusual findings, however, in 3 patients recently studied by us. A description of the clinical and pathologic observations in these three patients is presented in the report which follows.

Patients studied

Pertinent clinical and necropsy features in the 3 patients are summarized in Table I. All had histories of acute rheumatic fever and long-standing symptoms of cardiac dysfunction. In each mitral commissurotomy had been performed 6 to 9 years previously. Left atrial thrombi had been encountered at mitral commissurotomy in Patients Nos. 1 and 2, but none had had a systemic embolus. Before commissurotomy, Patients 1 and 2 had pure mitral stenosis; Patient No. 3, in addition to severe mitral stenosis, had a blowing systolic murmur compatible with tricuspid regurgitation, although there was no jugular venous distention, hepatomegaly, ascites, or subcutaneous edema. This patient had had this murmur at least since he was 19 years old, at which time he was suspected of having a pulmonary embolus. Angiography at that time, in addition to showing poor filling of the pulmonary arteries to the lower lobes, also showed a hugely dilated right atrium and a normal-sized left atrium. Mitral commissurotomy was performed at age 33, and a systolic thrill was palpated over the right atrium at that time.

Each of the 3 patients was improved by mitral commissurotomy, but symptoms of cardiac dysfunction recurred two (Patients 1 and 3) to nine years (Patient 2) later. Severe right-sided congestive cardiac failure with dependent subcutaneous edema, ascites, pleural effusion, a large and pulsatile liver, and progressive deterioration occurred in each patient, almost certainly the result of restenosis of the mitral valve and concomitant development or worsening of tricuspid regurgitation. Precordial murmurs typical of tricuspid regurgitation were

From the Section of Pathology and the Clinic of Surgery, National Heart Institute, Bethesda, Md., and the Division of Cardiology, Department of Medicine, The Johns Hopkins University and Hospital, Baltimore, Md.
Received for publication March 19, 1969.
*Reprint requests to: Dr. Roberts, Building 10A, Room 3E30, National Institutes of Health, Bethesda, Md. 20014.

Table I. *Giant right atrium and nearly normal-sized left atrium in mitral stenosis*

Patient	*Age, sex*	*Length of symptoms (yr.)*	*Cardiac valvular lesions*	*ECG*	*Age at cardiac cath. (yr.)*	*PA*	*Pressures (mm. Hg)*				*SA*	*LA-LV mean gradient*	*CO/CI*	*Heart weight (Gm.)*
							RV†	*RA*	*LA*	*LV*†				
1, M. V.	57, F	24	MS	AF										680
A65-36			TR*	RVH	57		52/15	m15	m19	118/12	118/61	8	4.6/3.1	
								v22	v29					
2, E. L.	32, F	11	MS	AF	22	53/32	55/7	m4	m17		120/65		3.3/1.9	
A65-149			TR*	RVH				v5	v23					560
					29	36/20	36/4		m15	96/6	116/72	5	3.5/2.0	
									v22					
					32	59/41	59/17	m23	m26				2.3/1.3	
								v36						
3, J. S.	39, M	26	MS	AF	19	73/45	73/0				125/62			
JHH 36136			TR	RVH	33	64/22	72/0	m9		135/6	135/65	15	3.4/2.0	850
				RBBB				v18	v28					
					38	82/32	83/12	m25		118/8	123/79		6.0/3.5	
								v35						

Abbreviations: Cath., Catheterization; PA, pulmonary artery; RV, right ventricle; RA, right atrium; LA, left atrium; LV, left ventricle; SA, systemic artery; CO, cardiac output; CI, cardiac index; MS, mitral stenosis; TR, tricuspid regurgitation; AF, atrial fibrillation; RVH, right ventricular hypertrophy; RBBB, right bundle branch block; m, mean; v, v wave.

*TR was not present before mitral commissurotomy.

†Systolic and end-diastolic pressures.

audible in each patient after the recurrence of symptoms of cardiac dysfunction. Reoperation was carried out in 2 patients; in Patient 1 the tricuspid valve was replaced, another mitral commissurotomy was performed, and a portion of the redundant right atrial wall was resected; in Patient 3 the mitral valve was replaced and a tricuspid annuloplasty performed. In both patients severe tricuspid regurgitation was evident at operation. Patient No. 2 died before reoperation was performed. Patient No. 1 died 10 days postoperatively of inadequate cardiac output, probably the result of operatively induced mitral regurgitation, and Patient No. 3 died 4 months postoperatively from consequences of prosthetic mitral stenosis resulting from interference to ball movement by the left ventricular wall.

Necropsy in each patient disclosed a large heart, an enormous right atrium, a mildly dilated left atrium, diffuse calcific deposits of the left atrial and atrial septal walls, and mitral valve leaflets, but no calcification of the right atrial walls. The tricuspid valve leaflets and chordae tendineae were thickened and fibrous in each patient. All 3 patients had extensive pulmonary vascular and parenchymal changes, and congestion of all viscera, including severe centrolobular hepatic necrosis, hemorrhage, and fibrosis. Various clinical and necropsy findings of particular interest are illustrated in Figs. 1 through 7.

Discussion

Extreme, enormous, or giant-sized dilatation of the left atrium (probably greater than 1,000 ml. capacity; normal less than 150 ml.[1,2]) has been discussed for years.[1,3-8] These reports indicate that enormous left atrial dilatation nearly always occurs in patients with mitral valvular disease. The mitral lesion may be pure regurgitation, pure stenosis, or a combination of the two, and there is some controversy as to which of these functional alterations is most frequently associated with a giant-sized left atrium. Also, the reason that one patient with mitral dysfunction has a huge left atrium and another with a similar functional abnormality has only minimal left atrial dilatation has not been resolved.

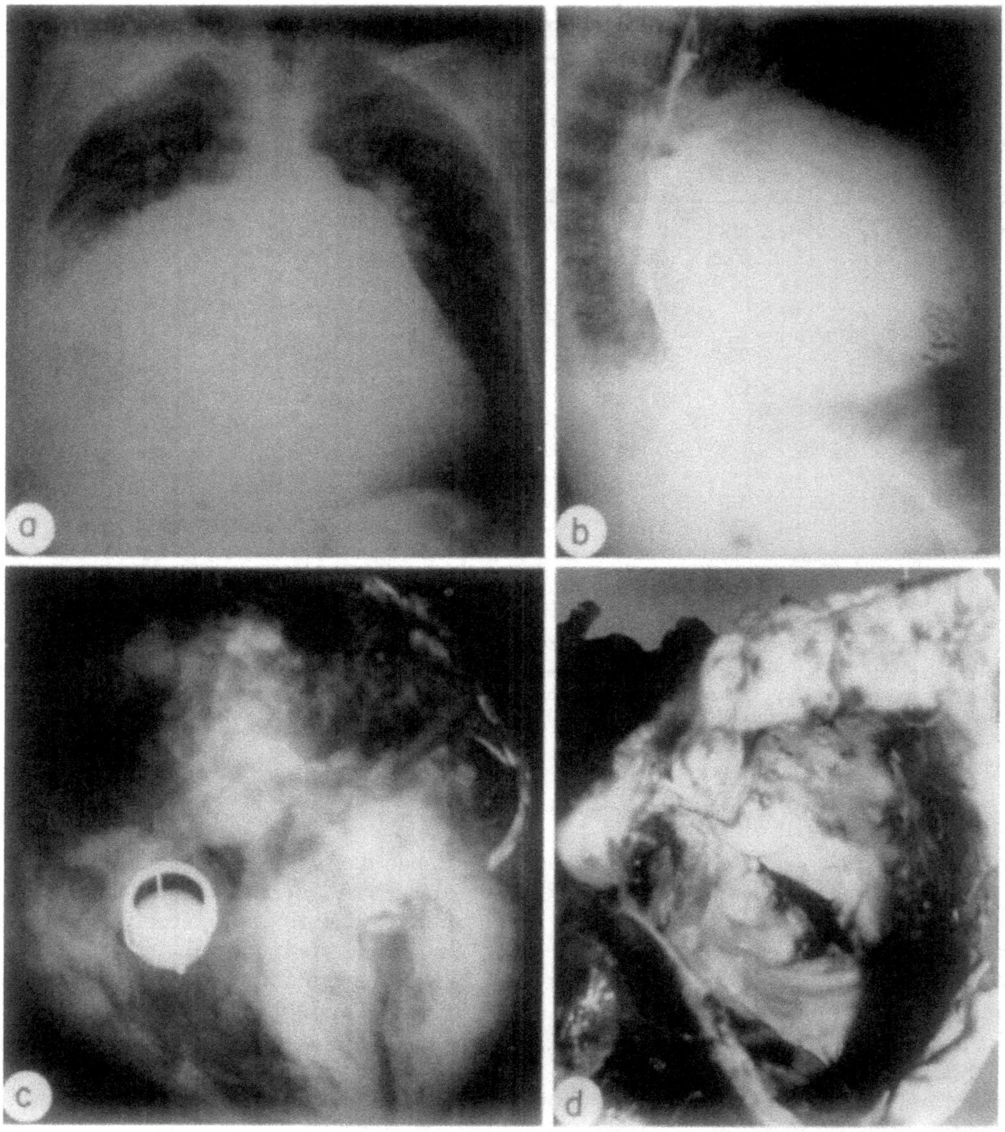

Fig. *1*. Patient 1 (Table I). *a* and *b*, Chest roentgenograms taken 3 weeks before death. The huge right atrium forms the right border of the heart on the posteroanterior view. *c*, Radiograph of the heart specimen. The left atrial wall is calcified. Much of the right atrial wall was excised at operation. The tricuspid valve was replaced with a Starr-Edwards prosthesis, and a mitral commissurotomy was also done. *d*, Opened left atrium showign its calcified wall which also is focally covered by thrombi.

Nearly all patients with enormous left atria have histories of acute rheumatic fever or chorea, and it has been suggested that they have more severe attacks of, or more relapses of, acute rheumatic fever than do patients with similar valvular lesions and less left atrial dilatation. Since rheumatic fever always involves the left atrial wall,[9] it is reasonable to speculate that if the inflammatory process was severe or occurred repeatedly the atrial wall would be more damaged, consequently more compliant or elastic, and, therefore, more easily dilated by increased intra-atrial pressure. Although nearly all patients with chronic rheumatic mitral disease have abnormal left atrial walls, the degree of myocardial destruction and fibrosis appears to be far worse in the subjects with dilated left atria than in those with smaller sized chambers.

Patients with giant-sized left atria and

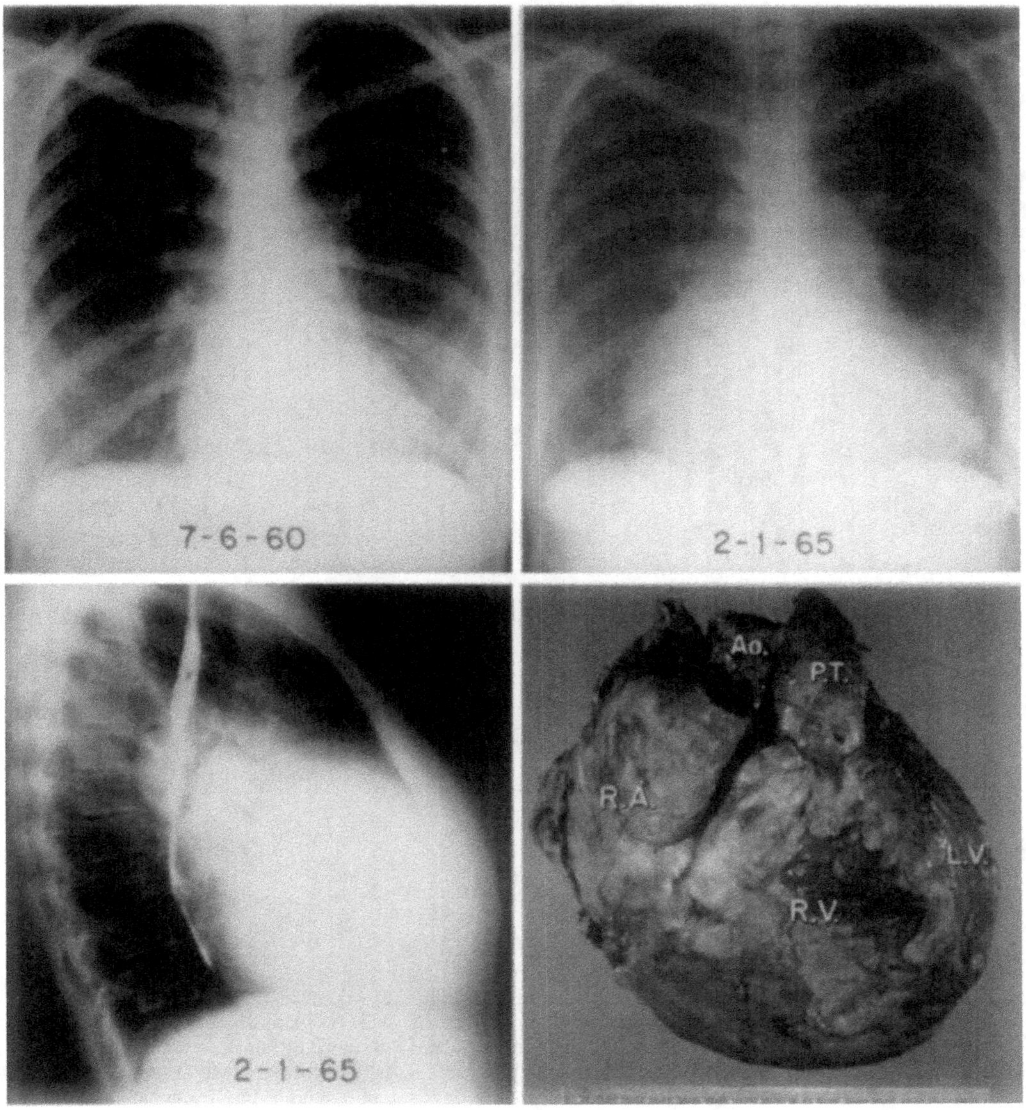

Fig. 2. Patient No. 2. *Upper* and *lower left:* Chest roentgenograms taken on the dates shown. The patient died Aug. 13, 1965. *Lower right:* Anterior surface of heart. The left atrium is not visible anteriorly but the right atrium (*R.A.*) is very large. *R.V.*, Right ventricle; *L.V.*, left ventricle; *P.T.*, pulmonary trunk; *Ao*, aorta.

severe mitral valvular disease usually have only slightly elevated or even normal left atrial, pulmonary venous, pulmonary arterial and right ventricular pressures.[10] In contrast, these pressures are usually quite high in subjects with only mildly dilated or normal-sized left atria and severe mitral valvular disease.[11] The small left atrium is less compliant, and reflects its elevated pressure to the lung and to the right ventricle, whereas the hugely dilated left atrium is readily compliant and "absorbs" the pressure energy. In most patients with giant left atrium the right atrium is also dilated, but is never as large as the left.[1,6] Right atrial dilatation occurs as the result of tricuspid regurgitation, which may be either organic or functional in type and with or without accompanying tricuspid stenosis. Stretching of the atrial septum by the dilatation of the left atrium probably contributes to the dilatation of the right atrium also.

Many reports have described the occurrence of giant left atrium in patients with mitral valvular disease, but the oc-

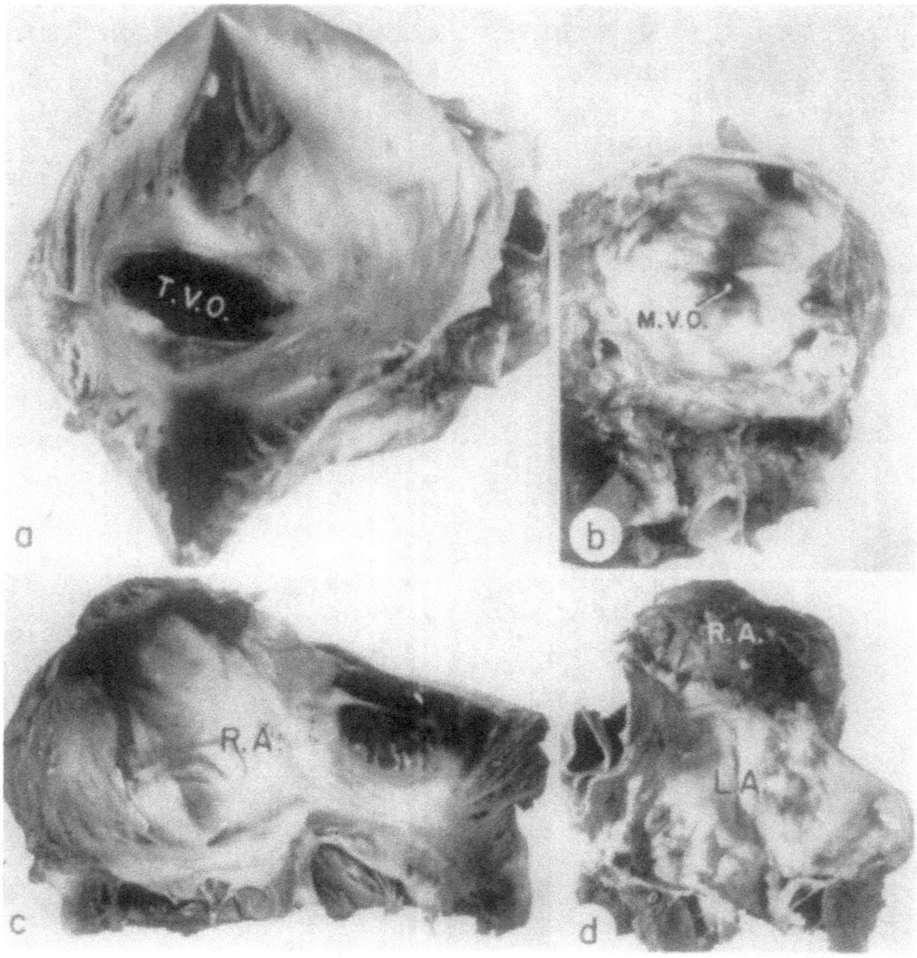

Fig. *3*. Heart in Patient No. 2. *a* and *b* were photographed at the same magnification; in *a* the huge right atrium has been partially opened showing the dilated tricuspid valve orifice (*T.V.O.*), and in *b* the only slightly dilated left atrium has been partially opened showing the stenotic mitral valve orifice (*M.V.O.*). *c* and *d* likewise were taken at the same magnification and show a huge right atrium (*R.A.*) in *c* compared to an only slightly dilated left atrium (*L.A.*) in *d*. The left atrial wall contains many deposits of calcium. The tricuspid leaflets are only slightly thickened, not enough in themselves to account for the tricuspid regurgitation.

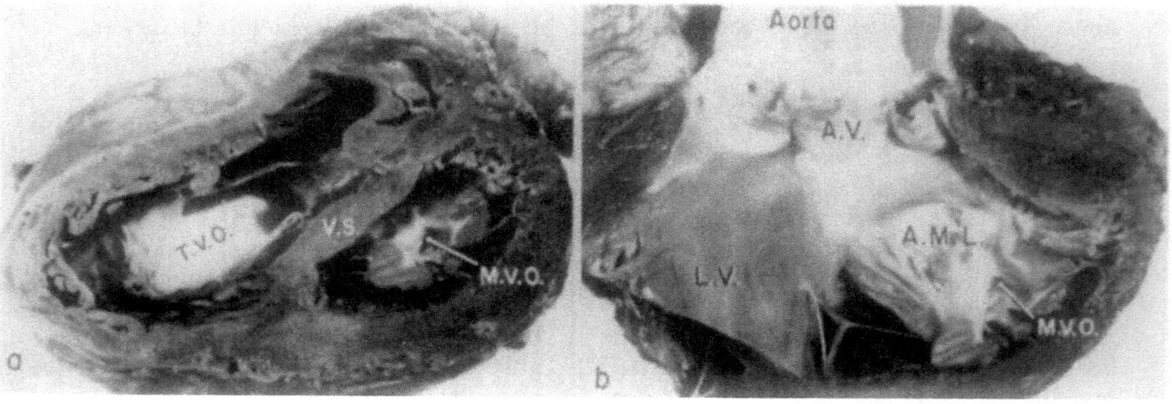

Fig. *4*. Heart in Patient No. 2. *a*, The caudal portions of the ventricles have been removed. The right ventricular cavity is much larger than the left, and the mitral valve orifice (*M.V.O.*) is severely stenotic. The tricuspid valve orifice (*T.V.O.*), in contrast, is greatly dilated. *b*, Opened aorta, normal aortic valve (*A.V.*) and left ventricular outflow tract (*L.V.*). The mitral leaflets insert directly into the papillary muscles. The cause of the left ventricular dilatation is uncertain. *A.M.L.*, Anterior mitral leaflet.

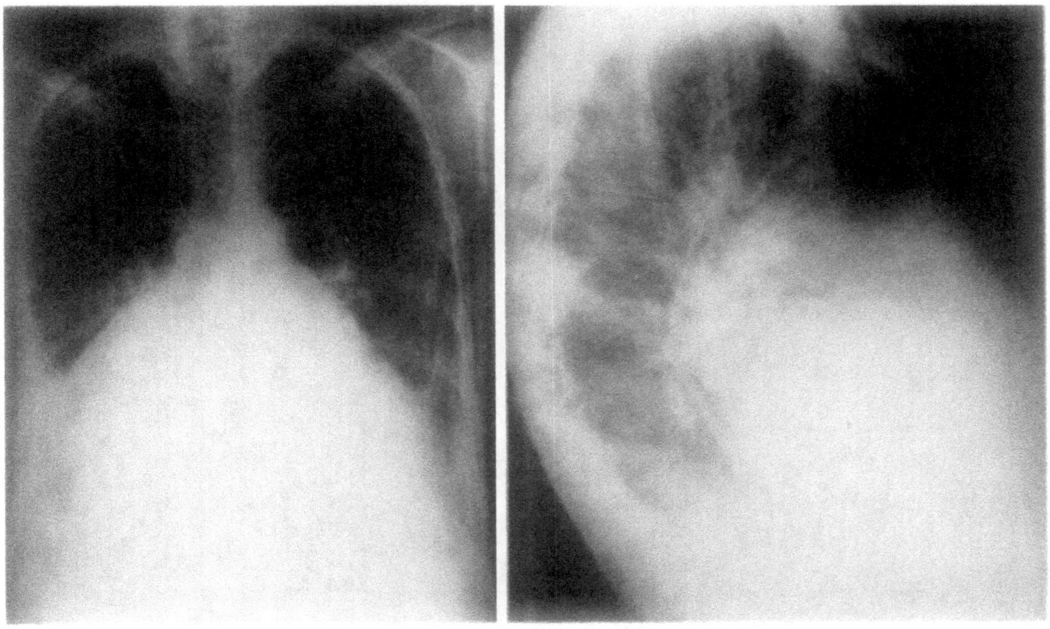

Fig. 5. Chest roentgenograms in Patient No. 3 taken 5 months before death.

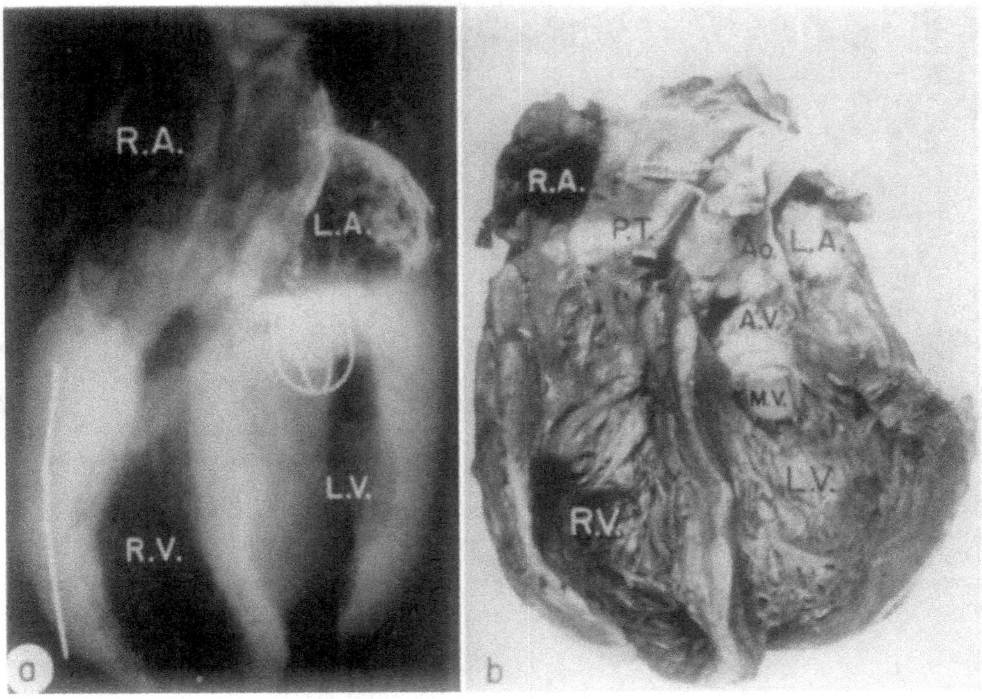

Fig. 6. Heart of Patient No. 3. *a*, Radiograph of excised heart, showing large calcific deposits in the left atrial (*L.A.*) wall. The mitral valve has been replaced with a Starr-Edwards prosthesis. *R.A.*, Right atrium; *R.V.*, right ventricle; *L.V.*, left ventricle. *b*, Opened right ventricle, pulmonary trunk (*P.T.*), left ventricle (*L.V.*), aortic valve (*A.V.*), and aorta (*Ao.*). Both ventricles are greatly enlarged. *M.V.*, Mitral valve prosthesis.

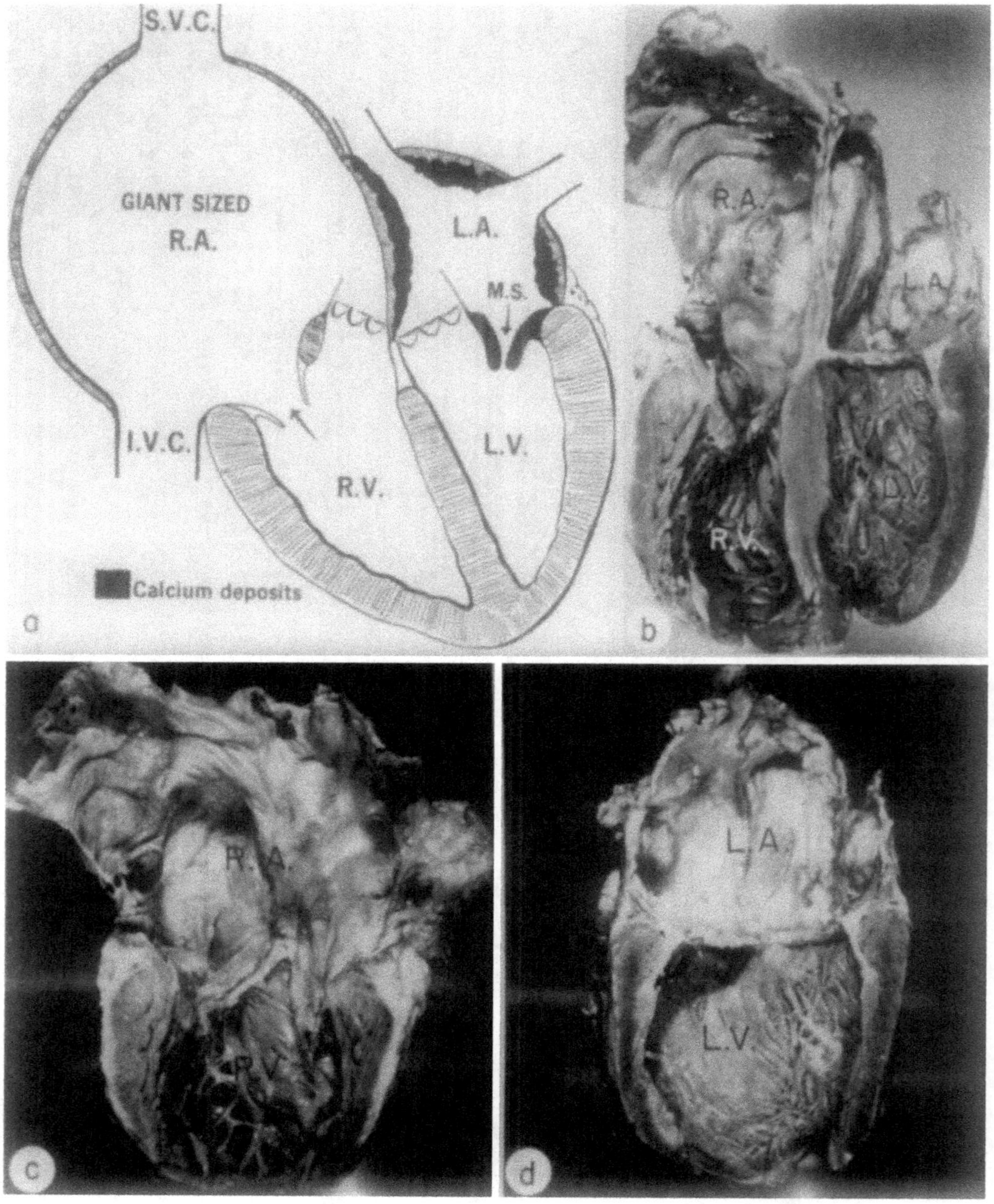

Fig. 7. Heart of Patient No. 3. *a*, Diagram. *S.V.C.*, Superior vena cava; *I.V.C.*, inferior vena cava; *R.A.*, right atrium; *R.V.*, right ventricle; *L.A.*, left atrium; *M.S.*, mitral stenosis; and *L.V.*, left ventricle. *b*, Longitudinal section of heart again showing the calcified left atrial wall and the huge right atrium. *c* and *d* are taken at the same magnification. *c*, Opened right atrium and right ventricle and *d* opened left atrium and left ventricle. The mitral prosthesis has been removed.

currence of a giant-sized right atrium with only a slightly dilated left atrium has not been specifically described. Taussig[12] noted enormous (capacity 2,150 ml.) dilatation of the right atrium and a normal-sized (capacity 100 ml.) left atrium in a 43-year-old woman with mitral and tricuspid stenosis and regurgitation, probably of rheumatic etiology, although the patient may have had the Marfan syndrome. The left atrial wall was free of calcific deposits and the heart weighed 505 grams. The cause of this unusual type of atrial dilatation is unknown.

In each of the 3 present patients the left atrial wall was calcified, the left atrium was only mildly dilated, but the right atrial cavity was huge. The hemodynamic and anatomic findings suggest that the calcium deposits in the left atrial wall prevented this chamber from dilating, decreased its compliance, and caused the elevated left atrial pressure to be immediately reflected to the pulmonary vessels and right ventricle, leading to tricuspid regurgitation of progressive severity. It seems likely that the calcification of the left atrium was the result of organization of thrombi, and in two of the patients thrombi were found at the initial operation. Each of the three patients had severe, nearly pure, mitral stenosis. Had significant or pure mitral regurgitation been present it appears unlikely that left atrial thrombi would have formed, since significantly sized left atrial thrombi have not been found, in our experience, in patients with severe mitral regurgitation.

Summary

Attention is called to the occurrence of a giant-sized right atrium and a nearly normal-sized left atrium in 3 adult patients with rheumatic mitral stenosis. In each patient the left atrial wall was calcified, probably the result of organization of intra-atrial thrombus, and the calcific deposits prevented the left atrium from dilating. All patients also had tricuspid regurgitation, which certainly contributed to the development of enormous right atrial dilatation, although other undetermined factors were probably operative also.

REFERENCES

1. Rogers, W. R., and Wittels, B.: Extreme bilateral atriomegaly. Review of the literature and report of a case, Circulation **15**:434, 1957.
2. Liu, C. K., Piccirillo, R. T., and Ellestad, M.: Distensibility of the postmortem human left atrium in nonrheumatic and rheumatic heart disease, Am. J. Cardiol. **13**:232, 1964.
3. Daley, R., and Franks, R.: Massive dilatation of the left atrium, Quart. J. Med. **18**:81, 1949.
4. Kent, E. M., Fisher, D. L., Ford, W. B., and Neville, J. F., Jr.: Mitral valve surgery and left heart catheterization in giant left atrium, Arch. Surg. **73**:503, 1956.
5. Parmley, L. F.: Congenital atriomegaly, Circulation **25**:553, 1962.
6. DeSanctis, R. W., Dean, D. C., and Bland, E. F.: Extreme left atrial enlargement. Some characteristic features, Circulation **29**:14, 1964.
7. Best, P. V., and Heath, D.: The right ventricle and small pulmonary arteries in aneurysmal dilatation of the left atrium, Brit. Heart J. **26**:312, 1964.
8. Bishop, L. F., and Howard, E. J.: Massive left atriomegaly, Dis. Chest. **49**:179, 1966.
9. Gross, L.: Lesions of the left auricle in rheumatic fever, Am. J. Path. **11**:711, 1935.
10. Braunwald, E. B., and Awe, W. C.: The syndrome of severe mitral regurgitation with normal left atrial pressure, Circulation **27**:29, 1963.
11. Roberts, W. C., Braunwald, E., and Morrow, A. G.: Acute severe mitral regurgitation secondary to ruptured chordae tendineae. Clinical, hemodynamic, and pathologic considerations, Circulation **33**:58, 1966.
12. Taussig, B. L.: A case of tricuspid stenosis with enormous dilatation of the right auricle, Am. Heart J. **14**:744, 1937.

Pulmonary Parenchymal Ossific Nodules in Idiopathic Hypertrophic Subaortic Stenosis

L. MAXIMILIAN BUJA, MD
and WILLIAM C. ROBERTS, MD, FACC
Bethesda, Maryland

Attention is called to the occurrence of pulmonary parenchymal ossific nodules in 2 siblings, both young adults, with idiopathic hypertrophic subaortic stenosis. This association has not been described previously.

Ossific nodules in the pulmonary parenchyma frequently are observed radiographically and morphologically in patients with rheumatic mitral valvular disease, especially stenosis.[1–3] Similar nodules have been observed rarely in patients with interstitial pulmonary fibrosis (Hamman-Rich syndrome)[4] and in at least 1 patient with each of the following conditions: left atrial myxoma, constrictive pericarditis, systemic hypertension, coronary arterial disease and aortic regurgitation.[5,6] This report describes pulmonary ossific nodules in 2 siblings with idiopathic hypertrophic subaortic stenosis. The association of such nodules with this entity has not been recorded previously, and we did not observe them at autopsy examination of the lungs of 7 other patients with idiopathic hypertrophic subaortic stenosis.

Case Reports

Case 1. At age 26, this man was asymptomatic when examined at the National Heart Institute, Bethesda, Md. A grade 2–3/6 systolic murmur was heard over the left sternal border and apex. Electrocardiogram showed sinus rhythm, biatrial enlargement and T wave abnormalities. Chest roentgenograms (Fig. 1) showed cardiomegaly and multiple densities throughout both lung fields. (These lesions were reported to have been observed on a chest roentgenogram taken 5 years earlier.) Repeated radiograms during the subsequent 7 years showed no increase in the number or size of the pulmonary parenchymal nodules. Results of the histoplasmin skin test were positive; those of skin tests for blastomycosis, coccidiomycosis and tuberculosis were negative. On cardiac catheterization the intravascular pressures (mm Hg) were right atrial mean 3; right ventricular 35/3; pulmonary arterial 35/24; left atrial mean 16, with *a* waves 26 and *v* waves 20; simultaneous left ventricular and brachial arterial 150/26 and 120/70, respectively, yielding a 30 mm Hg peak systolic gradient at rest which increased to 85 mm Hg with provocation (ouabain). The cardiac index was 2.1 liters/min per m^2.

At age 33 (6 months before death) exertional and nocturnal dyspnea and atrial fibrillation developed. Three weeks before death the patient was again hospitalized. The precordial systolic murmur was now only intermittently audible. Electrocardiogram showed atrial fibrillation and intraventricular conduction defect. The rhythm reverted to normal after transthoracic electrical countershock.

From the Section of Pathology, National Heart and Lung Institute, National Institutes of Health, Bethesda, Md. 20014. Manuscript received December 30, 1968, accepted February 25, 1969.

Address for reprints: Dr. William C. Roberts, Section of Pathology, National Heart and Lung Institute, National Institutes of Health, Bethesda, Md. 20014.

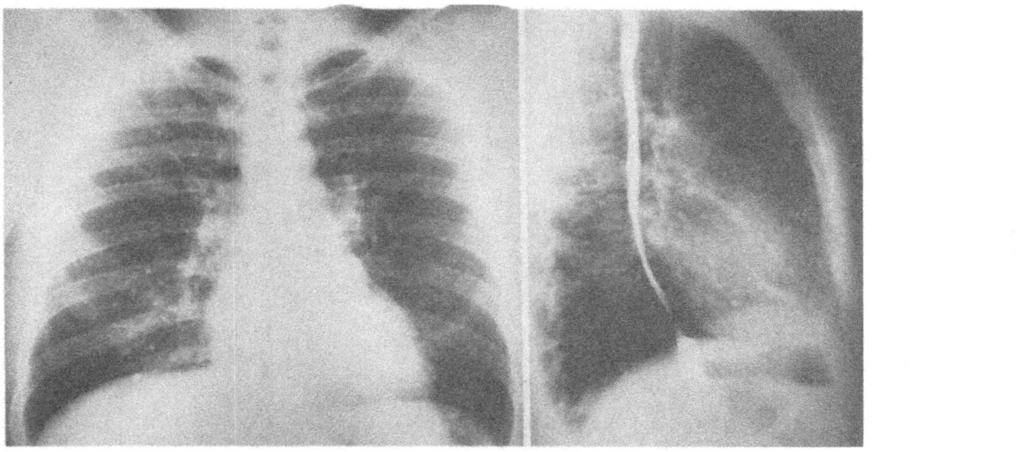

Figure 1. Case 1. Chest roentgenograms taken at age 26. Anteroposterior **(left)** and lateral **(right)** views.

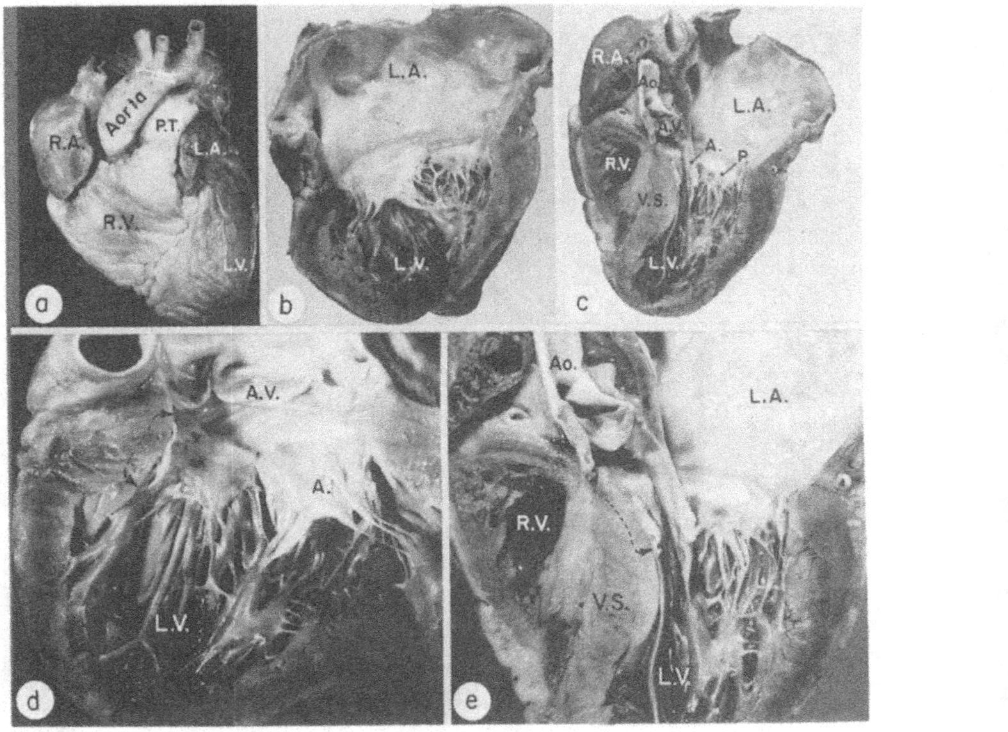

Figure 2. Case 1. Heart at autopsy. **a,** exterior view. All chambers are enlarged L.A. = left atrium; L.V. = left ventricle; P.T. = pulmonary trunk; R.A. = right atrium; R.V. = right ventricle. **b,** open left side showing dilated left atrium, focally thickened mitral leaflets and chordae and hypertrophied left ventricle. A thrombus is present at the apex of the left ventricle. **c,** coronal section. The ventricular septum (V.S.) is thicker than the free wall of the left ventricle. A close-up view of the outflow tract is shown in **e.** A. and P. = anterior and posterior mitral leaflets, respectively; Ao. = aorta. **d,** opened aorta, aortic valve (A.V.) and left ventricle. The endocardium in the outflow tract is thickened, and this thickening corresponds to similar thickening on the ventricular aspect of the anterior mitral leaflet (A.). The aortic valve is normal.

Repeat catheterization showed the pulmonary arterial pressure to be 52/25; mean pulmonary arterial wedge 22, with *a* waves 24 and *v* waves 26; and simultaneous left ventricular and brachial arterial pressures 120/26 and 120/80 mm Hg, respectively. A 33 mm Hg gradient was provoked by isoproterenol. The cardiac index was 2.0 liters/min per m^2. Six days after catheterization atrial fibrillation recurred, and 4 days later sudden unilateral hemiparesis appeared. The next day the left femoral arterial pulse was absent, and the patient died.

At necropsy the left external iliac, right internal iliac and left internal carotid arteries were completely occluded by thromboembolic material, as were several small mesenteric arteries. A thrombus (1.5 by 1.5 by 1.5 cm) was present in the apex of the left ventricle. Several renal and splenic infarcts were present.

The heart (Fig. 2) weighed 450 g. The ventricular septum was 2.7 cm thick, and the left ventricular free wall was 1.3 cm thick. An endocardial plaque was present in the left ventricular outflow tract. The mitral valve leaflets and several chordae tendineae were thickened. The left atrium was dilated, and the endocardium of its posterosuperior wall was thickened. There was narrowing of the lumens of the anterior descending (25 to 50 percent), left circumflex (50 to 75 percent) and left marginal (90 percent) coronary arteries.

The lungs together weighed 1,050 g. On postmortem radiograms and plastic (vinyl) cast preparations (Fig. 3) circumscribed nodules measuring between 0.1 to 0.6 cm were observed in all lobes. The ossific nodules (Fig. 3) consisted of mature lamellar bone with osteocytes and bone marrow but no iron or sim-

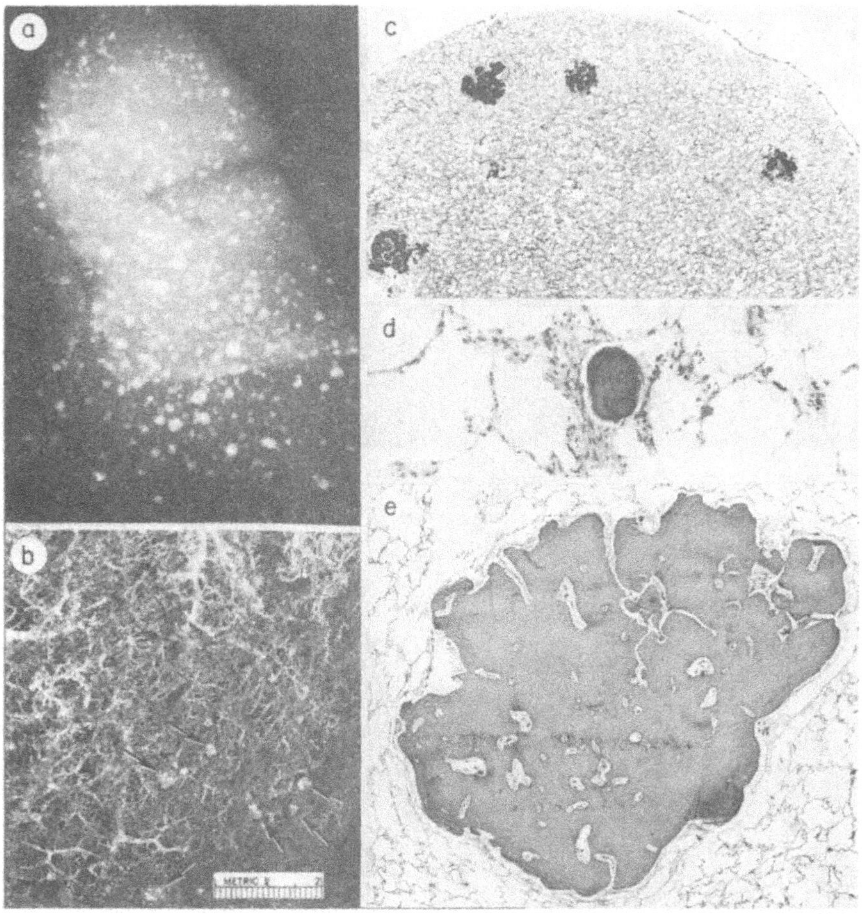

Figure 3. Case 1. Lung at autopsy. **a,** postmortem radiograph of left lung showing numerous pulmonary parenchymal ossific nodules. **b,** a plastic (vinyl) cast preparation of right lung demonstrating normal pulmonary arteries. Pulmonary ossific nodules are indicated by arrows. **c,** photomicrograph of lung showing four ossific nodules. Elastic van Gieson, × 6, reduced by 39 percent. **d,** minute ossific nodule located entirely within an alveolus. Hematoxylin and eosin stain, × 160, reduced by 39 percent. **e,** more usual-sized ossific nodule consisting of mature, lamellar bone with osteocytes in lacunae and spaces containing bone marrow. Hematoxylin and eosin, × 20, reduced by 39 percent.

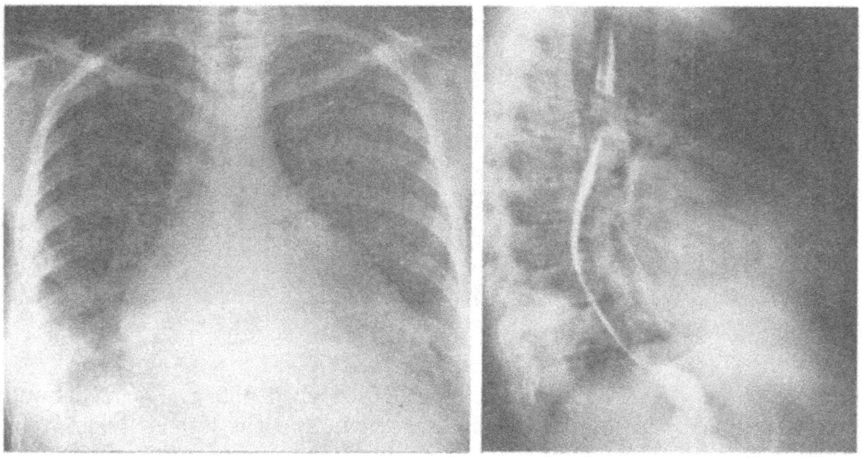

Figure 4. Case 2. Chest roentgenograms taken at age 25. Anteroposterior (left) and lateral (right) views.

ple calcium salts (Prussian blue and Von Kossa stains).* Hemosiderin-laden macrophages were present in a few alveoli. No microorganisms were seen. The capillaries were congested, and the interlobular septa were edematous. The pulmonary blood vessels were normal histologically.

* The Von Kossa method stains the phosphate and carbonate ions of calcium phosphate and carbonate molecules that remain in tissue after the calcium has been removed to facilitate histologic sectioning. The method is positive only for simple molecules and is negative once the calcium phosphate and carbonate are formed into the complex crystals of mature bone. Thus, the stain is positive only in areas of recent calcific deposition or areas of bone destruction.

Case 2. This 26 year old woman was the sister of the patient in Case 1. She had had exertional and nocturnal dyspnea and persistent dependent subcutaneous edema for 3 years before she was examined at the National Heart Institute at age 25. A grade 3/6 blowing systolic murmur was heard over the apex, left axilla and left sternal border. The feet were edematous. Electrocardiogram showed atrial fibrillation, left ventricular hypertrophy with strain, left ventricular conduction delay and an occasional premature contraction. Chest roentgenograms (Fig. 4) showed left atrial enlargement and right pleural effusion. On cardiac catheterization the intravascular pressures (mm Hg) were right atrial mean 10; right ventricular

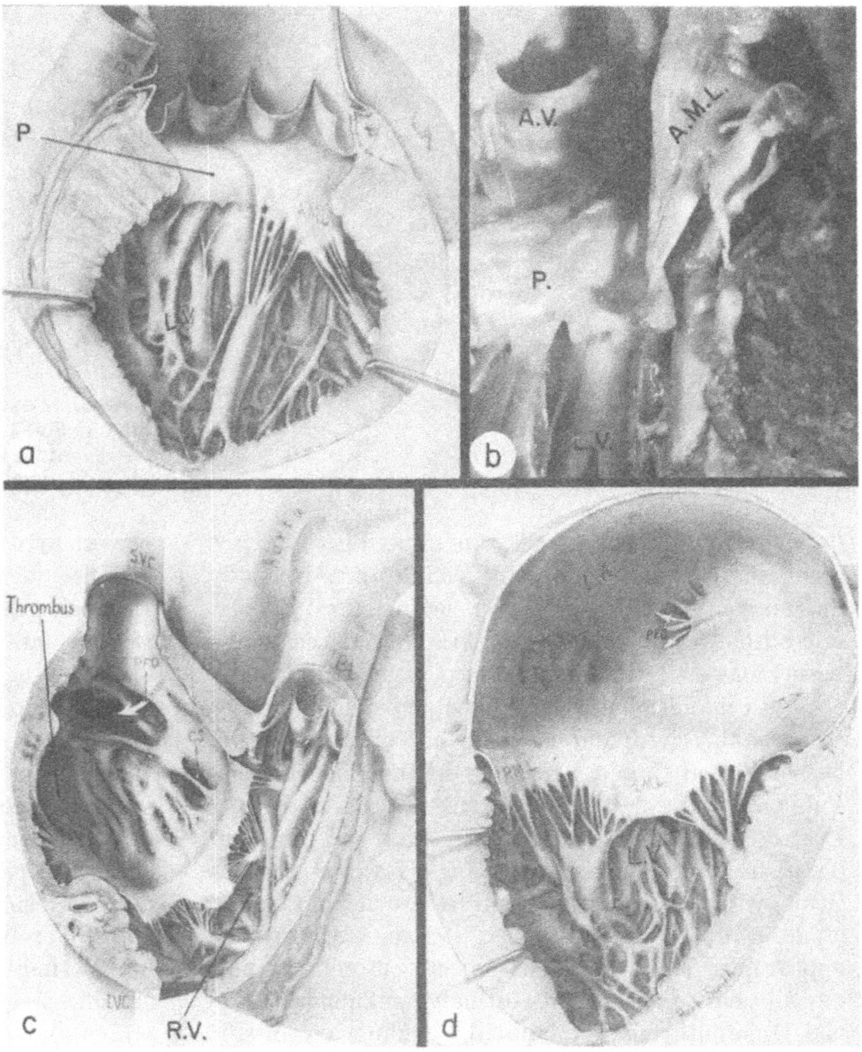

Figure 5. Case 2. Heart at autopsy. **a,** drawing of opened aorta and hypertrophied left ventricle (L.V.). A thick endocardial plaque (P) covers the left ventricular aspect of the cephalad portion of the ventricular septum which is severely hypertrophied. The anterior leaflet of the mitral valve (A.M.L.) and some of the chordae tendineae are thickened. P.A. = pulmonary trunk; L.A. = left atrium. **b,** a close-up of an actual photograph of the left ventricular outflow tract. A.V. = aortic valve. **c,** drawing of the opened right side of the heart. The right atrium is dilated and contains a thrombus. The fossa ovale region is probe-patent but valvular-competent (P.F.O.). The tricuspid valve is normal, and the right ventricular (R.V.) cavity is very small. S.V.C. = superior vena cava; C.S. = ostium of coronary sinus; I.V.C. = inferior vena cava. **d,** drawing of opened left atrium (L.A.), thickened mitral valve and left ventricle. The left atrium is dilated. P.M.L. = posterior mitral leaflet.

50/8; pulmonary arterial 40/25; left atrial mean 19—with v waves 23; left ventricular 103/2; and aortic 95/55. The cardiac index was 1.8 liters/min per m^2. Symptoms of cardiac dysfunction progressed, and she died with severe congestive heart failure 1 year later at another hospital.

At autopsy the heart weighed 350 g and was very similar to the heart of the patient's brother (Case 1). The cephalad portion of the ventricular septum was disproportionally thickened, and an endocardial plaque present in the left ventricular outflow tract corresponded to fibrous thickening of the ventricular aspect of the anterior mitral leaflet (Fig. 5). The left atrium was dilated, and the aortic valvular cusps were normal. An antemortem thrombus was present in the right atrium. The coronary arteries appeared normal.

The lungs showed changes of severe chronic pulmonary congestion and pulmonary hypertension. The alveolar septa were focally but extensively thickened; many alveoli contained hemosiderin-laden macrophages; parenchymal cholesterol granulomas were frequent;[7] acute pneumonia was present in the right lower lobe; large areas of atelectasis were present bilaterally; the visceral pleura over the lower lobes was thick; and many ossific nodules, similar to those seen in the lungs in Case 1, were found throughout the pulmonary parenchyma (Fig. 6).

The muscular pulmonary arteries and arterioles showed medial hypertrophy and intimal proliferation. A few smaller pulmonary arteries contained organized thromboemboli. The lumens of the pulmonary veins also were severely narrowed by fibrous intimal tissue.

Discussion

Differential diagnosis: The pulmonary parenchymal nodules observed in these 2 cases were similar radiographically and morphologically to those seen in patients with rheumatic mitral valvular disease.[1–3] Such nodules consist of mature lamellar bone. They measure 0.1 to 1.0 cm in diameter and are located within the pulmonary parenchyma, often purely intra-alveolar. They may be present in any lobe, most frequently the lower lobes, and they may contain

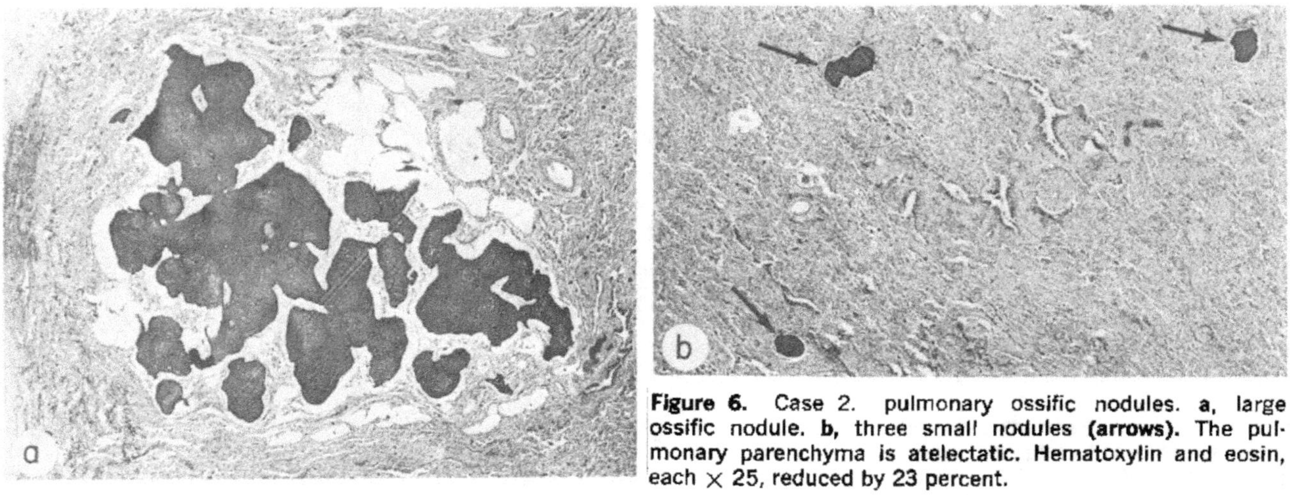

Figure 6. Case 2. pulmonary ossific nodules. **a,** large ossific nodule. **b,** three small nodules **(arrows).** The pulmonary parenchyma is atelectatic. Hematoxylin and eosin, each × 25, reduced by 23 percent.

bone marrow or iron or calcium salts. They are free of microorganisms. The ossific nodules are distinctly different morphologically from pulmonary alveolar microliths,[8] pulmonary corpora amylacea[9] and branching interstitial pulmonary bone occasionally observed in older patients.[1] Pulmonary ossific nodules, corpora amylacea and alveolar microliths have not been reported to occur together in the same patient. Pulmonary alveolar microlithiasis presents a distinctive roentgenographic appearance similar to that produced by acute pulmonary edema. However, the patients with pulmonary microliths are asymptomatic at least initially despite the striking radiographic appearance. Later in these subjects chronic cor pulmonale may develop. Interestingly, pulmonary alveolar microlithiasis is familial.[8] Pulmonary ossific nodules as occurred in each of our 2 cases have not been reported previously in more than 1 member of a single family. Pulmonary corpora amylacea are not visible radiographically, and there is no evidence that they produce pulmonary dysfunction.

The nodules observed on chest roentgenograms of patients with healed histoplasmosis, miliary tuberculosis, chickenpox or some pneumoconioses may simulate the radiographic appearance of pulmonary parenchymal ossific nodules. The nodules in the lungs of Patient 1 were diagnosed radiographically during life as healed histoplasmosis.

Mechanism of formation of pulmonary parenchymal ossific nodules: The mechanism of formation is speculative. The only finding that appears to be common to patients with these nodules is pulmonary venous hypertension, but the exact relation of the increased pressure to the ossific nodules is unknown.[2,3,5] Pulmonary nodules have been observed in patients with[3,5] and without[2] overt congestive cardiac failure. Organization of pulmonary edema fluid to form osteoid and finally bone has been suggested as a possible mechanism of formation of the pulmonary parenchymal ossific nodules.[2,3,5] Development of the ossific nodules by transformation of intraalveolar hemosiderin deposits also has been suggested[10] but seems unlikely. Ossific nodules may be observed in portions of lung entirely free from hemosiderin deposits, and ossific nodules have not been described in subjects with idiopathic pulmonary hemosiderosis, a condition that produces the largest deposition of iron in the alveolar spaces.[11] The ossific nodules were not observed at various stages of formation in either of our 2 patients. Indeed, whether the nodules were large or small, their morphologic features were similar. This fact suggests that all of the ossific nodules in an individual patient formed at the same time. Ossific nodules have been observed experimentally in rabbits given irradiation to the lungs 1 to 2 months before sacrifice.[12]

Relation of ossific nodules to degree of cardiac dysfunction: Although pulmonary venous hypertension occurred in our 2 cases, neither the number nor the size of the pulmonary ossific nodules was proportional to the degree of rise in pulmonary venous pressure. Patient 2 had severe cardiac failure for several years with extensive pulmonary parenchymal and vascular changes of chronic congestion. In contrast, Patient 1 was asymptomatic until 6 months before death, and his lungs were virtually normal except for the presence of numerous ossific nodules. Although Patient 2 had far more evidence of chronic pulmonary congestion than did Patient 1, she had far fewer ossific nodules. However, at autopsy the hearts of both patients were strikingly similar although the degree of cardiac dysfunction was quite different.

Acknowledgment

We thank Doctors Eugene Braunwald and Stephen E. Epstein for use of the clinical information in the 2 cases described.

References

1. **Wells HG, Dunlap CE:** Disseminated ossification of the lungs. Arch Path (Chicago) 35:420–426, 1943
2. **Fleming HA, Robinson CLN:** Pulmonary ossification with cardiac calcification in mitral valve disease. Brit Heart J 19:532–538, 1957
3. **Galloway RW, Epstein EJ, Coulshed N:** Pulmonary ossific nodules in mitral valve disease. Brit Heart J 23:297–307, 1961
4. **Ventura JC:** Disseminated nodular pulmonary ossification with Hamman-Rich syndrome. J Lancet 86:60–63, 1966
5. **Epstein EJ, Chapman R, Coulshed N, et al:** Pulmonary ossific nodule formation in the absence of mitral valve disease. A report of four cases. Amer Heart J 65:816–825, 1963
6. **Hudson REB:** Cardiovascular Pathology, Vol. I. Baltimore, Williams & Wilkins, 1961, p 1015
7. **Glancy DL, Frazier PD, Roberts WC:** Pulmonary parenchymal cholesterol-ester granulomas in patients with pulmonary hypertension. Amer J Med 45:198–210, 1968
8. **Sosman MC, Dodd GD, Jones WD, et al:** The familial occurrence of pulmonary alveolar microlithiasis. Amer J Roentgen 77:947–1012, 1957
9. **Michaels L, Levine C:** Pulmonary corpora amylacea. J Path Bact 74:49–56, 1957
10. **Ellman P, Gee A:** Pulmonary hemosiderosis. Brit Med J 2:384–390, 1951
11. **Soergel KH, Sommers SC:** Idiopathic pulmonary hemosiderosis and related syndromes Amer J Med 32:499–511, 1962
12. **Engelstad RB:** Über die Wirkungen der Röntgenstrahlen auf die Lungen. Acta Radiol (Stockholm) 15: Suppl 19:1–93, 1934

Stenosis of the right pulmonary artery: A complication of acute dissecting aneurysm of the ascending aorta

L. Maximilian Buja, M.D.
Nayab Ali, M.D.
Ross D. Fletcher, M.D.
William C. Roberts, M.D.
Washington, D. C.

Common complications of acute dissecting aortic aneurysm include external rupture with fatal hemorrhage, dissection and occlusion of major branches of the aorta, and aortic regurgitation.[1-5] Although lesions of the pulmonary vessels may complicate nondissecting (syphilitic, arteriosclerotic, Marfan's) thoracic aneurysms,[6-10] pulmonary vascular lesions caused by acute dissecting aortic aneurysm have not been described. This has recently been observed by us and is the subject of this report.

Case report

A. W., a 57-year-old man, who had a history of systemic hypertension, developed severe persistent precordial chest pain 17 hours before death. When hospitalized 9 hours before death, the patient's blood pressure was 180/120 mm. Hg, and an atrial diastolic gallop was audible. No precordial murmur was heard. An anteroposterior chest roentgenogram showed minimal cardiomegaly and a widened mediastinum. The electrocardiogram (ECG) disclosed sinus tachycardia (120 beats per minute), left ventricular hypertrophy, left atrial enlargement, S-T segment elevation in Leads V_{1-3}, and S-T segment depression with T wave inversion in Leads I, aV_L, and V_{5-6}. Two hours before death, the chest pain worsened and hypotension (100/70 mm. Hg) and ventricular tachycardia appeared. Sinus rhythm and hypertension (170/130 mm. Hg) returned after an intravenous injection of lidocaine. The ECG was unchanged except for the presence of small Q waves in Leads II, III, and aV_F. One hour before death, complete heart block appeared and the patient lost consciousness. Resuscitative efforts including attempted transvenous pacing were unsuccessful.

At autopsy an acute medial dissection of the ascending thoracic aorta (Type II of De Bakey and associates[5]) was found (Figs. 1 and 2), and it had ruptured into the pericardial cavity. The aneurysm contained a large hematoma which narrowed the aortic lumen. Extravasated blood also was present in the adventitia of the ascending and transverse portions of the aorta, pulmonary trunk, right and left main pulmonary arteries, and left atrium (superior wall). Extravasated blood also surrounded the proximal right and left coronary arteries, and the lumen of the right coronary artery was slightly compressed by the adventitial blood. The lumen of the right main pulmonary artery was narrowed > 75 per cent by the adventitial hematoma (Fig. 3). This obstructed artery was located between the left atrium (inferior) and aortic arch (superior). The heart weighed 550 grams. The left ventricle was hypertrophied but not dilated.

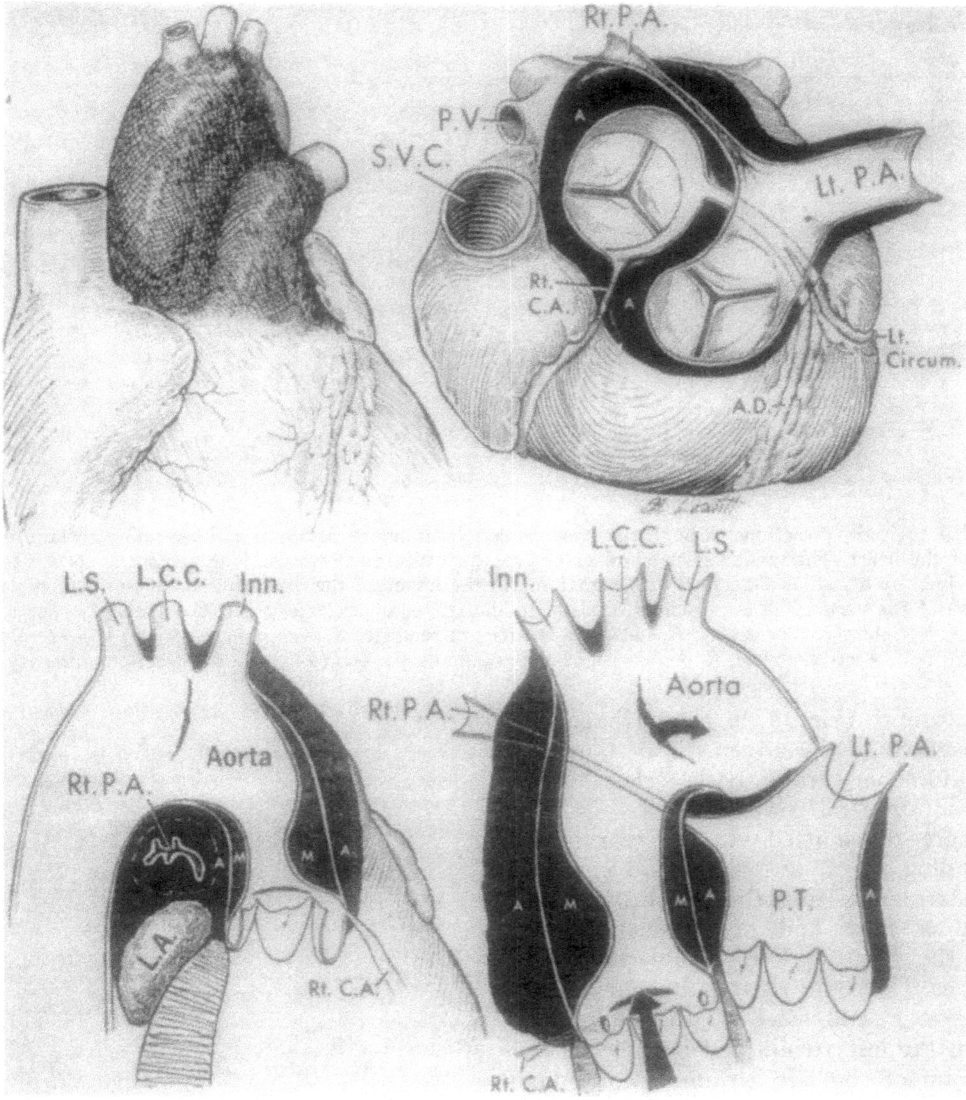

Fig. *1*. Drawing of heart and great vessels. External view of anterior surface (top left), superior view with cross section of great vessels (top right), and lateral (bottom left) and frontal (bottom right) views of longitudinal sections. Extensive hematoma is present in the adventitia (*A*) of the ascending and transverse aortas, pulmonary trunk (*P.T.*), and right and left main pulmonary arteries (*Rt. P.A.* and *Lt. P.A.*). The lumen of the right main pulmonary artery is severely compressed by the adventitial hematoma (*A*) as the artery passes between aorta and left atrium (*L.A.*). The lumen of the proximal right coronary artery (*Rt. C.A.*) also is narrowed by the adventitial hematoma. The ascending aorta is involved by an acute medial dissection with proximal and distal tears (bottom left and right). Medial hematoma (*M*) in the lumen of the dissecting aneurysm narrows the lumen of the ascending aorta. *A.D.* = left anterior descending coronary artery; *Lt. Circum.* = left circumflex coronary artery; *Inn.* = innominate artery; *L.C.C.* = left common carotid artery; *L.S.* = left subclavian artery; *S.V.C.* = superior vena cava; and *P.V.* = pulmonary vein.

The lumens of the coronary arteries were narrowed < 50 per cent by arteriosclerotic plaques. No foci of myocardial fibrosis or necrosis were present.

Comments

Severe obstruction of the right main pulmonary artery in this patient probably occurred in the following manner. The aortic aneurysm, which originally had dissected through only a part of the media, ruptured through the entire aortic media at a site just above the aortic valve. At this level the ascending aorta and pulmonary trunk share a common investment, visceral

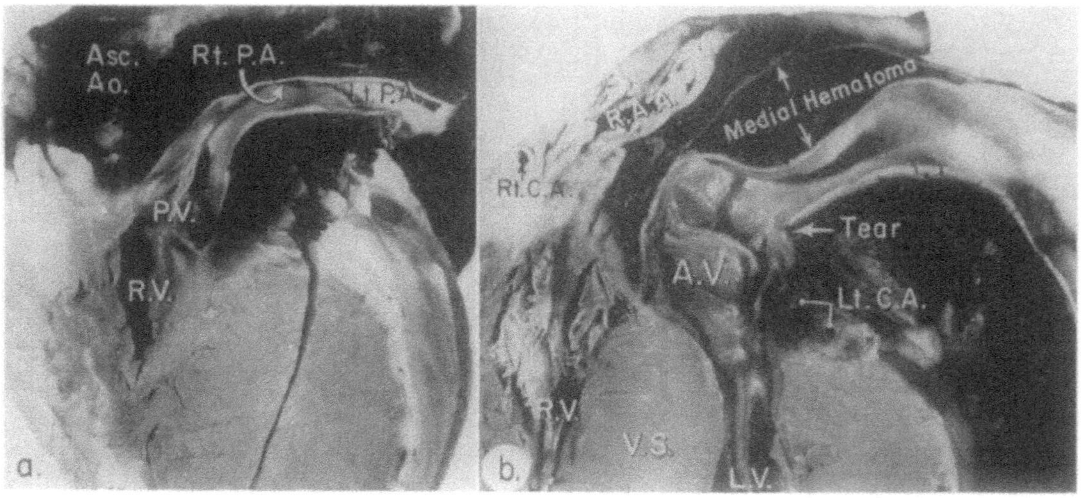

Fig. 2. Longitudinal sections through the great vessels (pulmonary trunk, *a*, and ascending aorta, *b*) and the base of the heart. The great vessels show extensive adventitial hemorrhage. The ascending aorta (*Asc. Ao.*) is involved by a medial dissection with hematoma in the lumen of the dissecting aneurysm. A complete tear (arrow) of the aortic wall is present just distal to the left coronary artery (*Lt. C.A.*). *A.V.* = aortic valve; *Rt. C.A.* = right coronary artery; *R.A.A.* = right atrial appendage; *R.V.* = right ventricle; *V.S.* = ventricular septum; *L.V.* = left ventricle; *Rt. P.A.* = right main pulmonary artery; *Lt. P.A.* = left main pulmonary artery.

pericardium (Fig. 4).[11] Hemorrhage was propagated in the adventitia of the aorta and pulmonary trunk, both enclosed in the common visceral pericardium, by systemic pressure transmitted via the tear in the ascending aorta, and the blood extended in this manner into the adventitia of the distal ascending and transverse aortas, and into the right and left main pulmonary arteries. Only the right pulmonary artery was compressed since it was located between the left atrium and aorta. The epicardium of the left atrium is continuous with the adventitia of the right pulmonary artery (Fig. 4), and this connection accounts for extravasated blood in the left atrial wall superiorly. The hematoma in the false channel of the aortic dissecting aneurysm probably formed when blood flow slowed severely. This hematoma narrowed the true lumen of the aorta nearly 50 per cent.

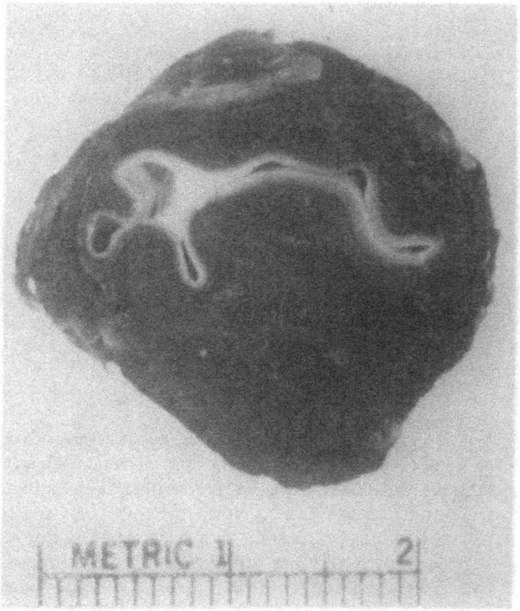

Fig. 3. Cross-section of the right main pulmonary artery showing severe luminal compression by adventitial hematoma. Histologic examination showed that the media of this vessel was normal and that the hematoma was entirely in the adventitia.

Summary

Attention is called to the occurrence of severe obstruction of the right main pulmonary artery as a consequence of acute dissection of the ascending aorta. The pulmonary arterial obstruction appears to have resulted from compression of this artery by an adventitial hematoma which extended from the ascending aorta after medial rupture of the aortic dissecting aneurysm. This complication of acute dissecting aortic aneurysm has not been described previously.

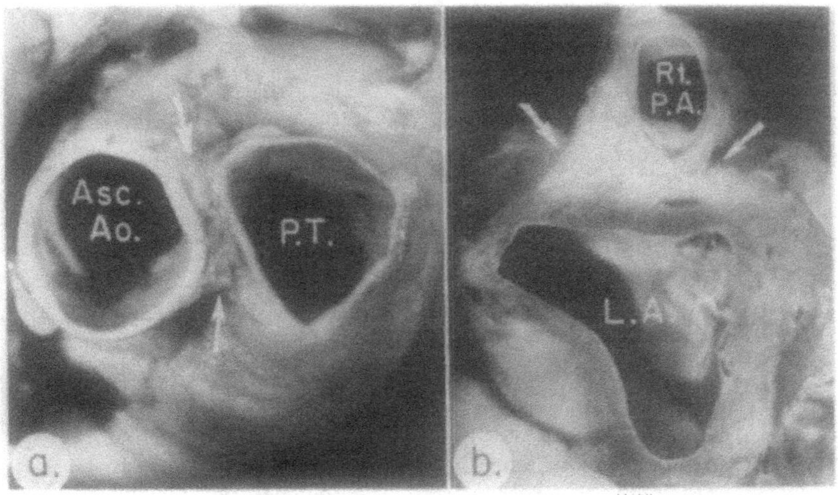

Fig. *4*. Normal heart. Superior view, *a*, of cross section of pulmonary trunk (*P.T.*) and ascending aorta (*Asc. Ao.*), and lateral view, *b*, of longitudinal section through the right main pulmonary artery (*Rt. P.A.*) and left atrium (*L.A.*). In *a*, the common investment by visceral pericardium (arrows) of the ascending aorta and pulmonary trunk is shown. In *b*, the relationship of the right main pulmonary artery to the left atrium and and continuity of the adventitia of the artery with the visceral pericardium of the atrium are shown.

REFERENCES

1. Shennan, T.: Dissecting aneurysms. Medical Research Council, Special Report Series No. 193, London, 1934, H. M. Stationary Office.
2. Hirst, A. E., Jr., Johns, V. J., Jr., and Kime, S. W., Jr.: Dissecting aneurysm of the aorta: A review of 505 cases, Medicine (Balt.) **37**:217, 1958.
3. Gore, I., and Seiwert, V. J.: Dissecting aneurysm of the aorta, pathological aspects: An analysis of 85 cases, Arch. Path. (Chicago) **53**:121, 1952.
4. Lindsay, J., Jr., and Hurst, J. W.: Clinical features and prognosis in dissecting aneurysm of the aorta: A reappraisal, Circulation **35**:880, 1967.
5. De Bakey, M. E., Henly, W. S., Cooley, D. A., Morris, G. C., Jr., Crawford, E. S., and Beall, A. C., Jr.: Surgical management of dissecting aneurysms of the aorta, J. Thorac. Cardiovasc. Surg. **49**:130, 1965.
6. Nicholson, R. E.: Syndrome of aortic aneurysm rupture into the pulmonary artery: Review of literature with report of two cases, Ann. Intern. Med. **19**:286, 1943.
7. Mark, H., Aaron, R. S., Elias, K., Hurwitt, E. S.: Rupture of aortic aneurysm into left pulmonary artery: Attempt at surgical correction, Amer. J. Cardiol. **1**:757, 1958.
8. Pearson, J. R., and Nichol, E. S.: The syndrome of compression of the pulmonary artery by a syphilitic aortic aneurysm resulting in chronic cor pulmonale, with report of a case, Ann. Intern. Med. **34**:483, 1951.
9. Bevin, A. G., Rojas, R. H., and Stansel, H. C., Jr.: Aneurysm of the ascending aorta causing obstruction of the left pulmonary artery, J. Thorac. Cardiovasc. Surg. **52**:245, 1966.
10. Yacoub, M. H., Braimbridge, M. V., and Gold, R. G.: Aneurysm of the ascending aorta presenting with pulmonary stenosis, Thorax **21**:236, 1966.
11. Goss, C. M., editor: Gray's anatomy, ed. 28, Philadelphia, 1966, Lea & Febiger, Publishers, pp. 545, 574.

Diffuse Fibrotic Lung Disease: A Correlative Study

Jack D. Fulmer, M.D.; William C. Roberts, M.D.;** and Ronald G. Crystal, M.D.**

Diffuse fibrotic lung disease is a complex, clinically protean disorder which we view through a number of separate monitors: morphologic, physiologic, and biochemical. Our laboratory has undertaken a large scale, multidisciplinary study of the etiology, pathogenesis, pathophysiology, and therapy of this disorder (Fig 1). This paper will present correlative clinical, physiologic, and pathologic data in a selected group of patients with diffuse fibrotic lung disease. Biochemical approaches to this disorder are described elsewhere in this volume.[1]

Material and Methods

Twenty patients (ten men, ten women, mean age 50 years) have been evaluated. Thirteen patients had open lung biopsy either prior to or during their evaluation at NIH. All patients presented initially with dyspnea, and all had a radiographic pattern of diffuse infiltrative process. Seventeen patients had idiopathic fibrotic lung disease; the remainder had fibrotic lung disease associated with collagen-vascular disease. Vital capacity (VC) and total lung capacity (TLC) are widely distributed with a range between 28 and 84 percent predicted for VC and 44 to 86 percent predicted for TLC (Fig 2). Most patients have reduced VC and TLC, but an occasional patient with histologic evidence of fibrotic disease will have a normal VC and/or TLC. The diffusing capacity ($D_{L_{CO}}$) was consistently reduced in all patients (range 14 to 70 percent predicted). The ratio of forced expiratory volume in one second (FEV_1) to forced vital capacity was normal in all but one patient in whom there was a borderline reduction. Residual volume to total lung capacity ratio ranged from 20 percent to 52 percent (Fig 2). Analysis of the static volume-pressure relationships demonstrates that compliance is reduced in the majority of the patients (Fig 3).

Maximum expiratory flow volume curves, dynamic compliance, maximum flow-static recoil curves, upstream resistance and single breath oxygen test (ΔN_2 750-1250) were performed in all patients as monitors of airway time constants and mechanics. Independently, and in a single blind fashion, one of us (WCR) reviewed the histopathology and graded the small airways as to whether they were normal or exhibited varying degrees of obstruction from either bronchioli-

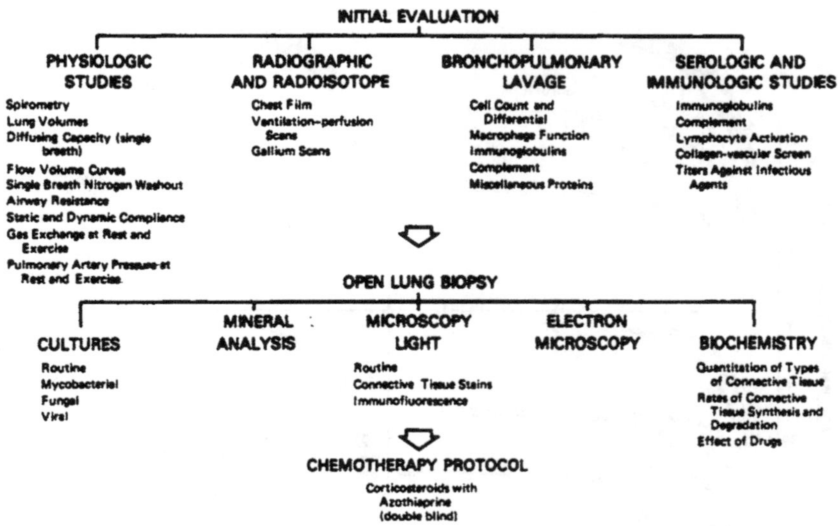

FIGURE 1. Protocol for the National Heart and Lung Institute, Intramural Division, Section on Pulmonary Biochemistry, Pulmonary Branch fibrotic disease study.

tis of peribronchial fibrosis and narrowing. A significant percentage of these physiologic and morphologic parameters were abnormal in these patients (Table 1). These data suggest agreement between the physiologic and morphologic data, and thus indicate that obstructive disease of airways is a feature of this disorder.

The volume-pressure data in these patients were analyzed using the peak transpulmonary pressure, slope of the volume-pressure curve and its position along the pressure axis. These parameters were compared to the severity of fibrosis (graded by WCR) on the open lung biopsy specimen. There was correlation between peak transpulmonary pressure and severity of fibrosis, but there was no correlation between slope or position of the pressure-volume curve with severity of fibrosis nor was there correlation between maximum transpulmonary pressure, slope or position of the pressure-volume curve with degree of interstitial cellularity, alveolar cellularity or obstruction of airways. These data suggest that the relationship between factors associated with lung distensibility and factors which govern pressure-volume characteristics in patients are complex and likely interdependently related to chest wall strength, airways disease, location and amount of fibrosis, and amount of lung destruction.

Complete gas exchange studies were performed in 17 patients. All exhibited progressive arterial hypoxemia (PaO_2, range 38-60 mm Hg) and widening of the alveolar-arterial oxygen gradient (range 40-100 mm Hg) with graded exercise. There was no apparent correlation with severity of disease on biopsy with response to exercise. Five patients have been followed for up to nine months with serial lung volumes, diffusing capacity, and gas exchange studies. All five patients have subjectively worsened with no change in lung volumes, diffusing capacity or resting PaO_2. Preliminary longitudinal data suggest that quantitation of the rate of change of PaO_2 with oxygen consumption is a sensitive correlate with severity of breathlessness even in situations where TLC, D_{LCO} and resting PaO_2 remain stable.

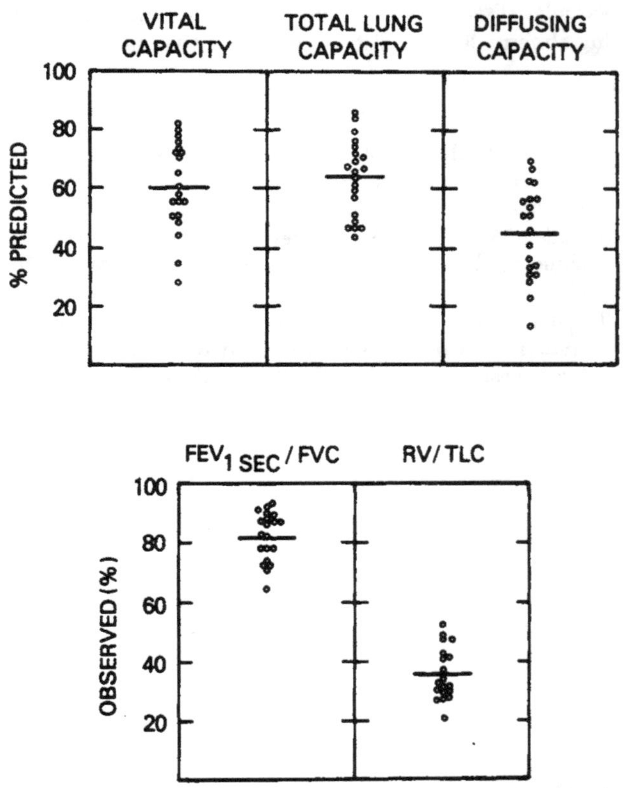

FIGURE 2. Lung volumes, simple mechanics and diffusing capacity in patients with pulmonary fibrosis of unknown etiology. Vital capacity, total lung capacity and diffusing capacity are expressed as percent predicted. Forced expiratory volume (1 sec)/forced vital capacity (FEV_1/FVC) and residual volume/total lung capacity (RV/TLC) are expressed as percentage of observed. Patients are represented by open circles.

RESULTS

The diagnostic usefulness of the change in dead-space to tidal volume ratio (V_D/V_T) with exercise has been debated.[2,3] Eighty percent of patients studied exhibited an abnormal response in V_D/V_T with exercise. Correla-

Table 1—*Comparison between Physiologic Monitors of Airway Mechanics and Histopathologic Evidence of Airway Obstruction*

Physiologic Parameter	% Abnormal	Comparison with Pathology
Maximum expiratory flow volume curve	45	good
Dynamic compliance	59	good
Upstream resistance	32	poor
Single breath oxygen test	80	good

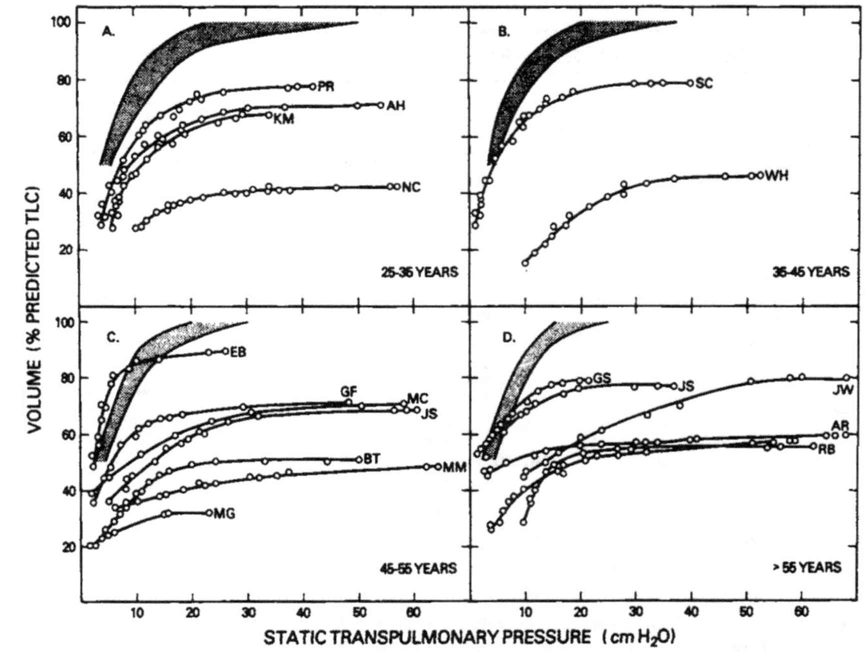

FIGURE 3. Static volume-pressure curves in patients with pulmonary fibrosis of unknown etiology. (A) Patients 25-35 years old; (B) 35-45 years old; (C) 45-55 years old; and (D) >55 years old. Lung volumes are presented as percent predicted total lung capacity (TLC). The shaded areas are normals matched for age.

tion of these data with evidence of pulmonary vascular disease on open lung biopsy was poor while correlation with evidence of obstruction of airways was good. These data suggest that distribution of ventilation is an important determinant in the V_D/V_T and emphasize the possible error in this test in diagnosis of pulmonary vascular disease.

In summary, correlative physiologic, pathogenic and clinical data are presented which suggest the following: 1) obstructive disease of airways with increased resistance to air flow is present in a significant percentage of patients with diffuse fibrotic lung disease; 2) although the peak transpulmonary pressure correlated with the degree of fibrosis, the lack of correlation of other parameters of the volume-pressure curve with the histopathology casts doubt on the usefulness of the volume-pressure relationships as a long-term monitor of diffuse fibrotic disease; 3) exercise physiologic testing with quantitation of the rate of change in PaO_2 with oxygen consumption appears to be the most sensitive correlate to clinical severity of disease; 4) the dead space-to-tidal volume ratio during exercise correlates poorly with evidence of pulmonary vascular disease, but appears to correlate well with evidence of obstruction of airways. The value of this test in the diagnosis of pulmonary vascular disease must be interpreted in light of co-existing abnormalities of distribution of ventilation.

REFERENCES

1 Hance AJ, Horwitz AL, Cowan MJ, et al: Biochemical approaches to the investigation of fibrotic lung disease. Chest 69:257-261, 1976

2 Nadel JA, Gold WM, Burgess JH: Early diagnosis of chronic pulmonary vascular obstruction. Am J Med 44:16-25, 1968

3 Williams HM, Adler JJ, Colp C: Pulmonary function studies as an aid in the differential diagnosis of pulmonary hypertension. Am J Med 47:378-383, 1969

Intravenous Injection of Talc-Containing Drugs Intended for Oral Use

A Cause of Pulmonary Granulomatosis and Pulmonary Hypertension

ERNEST N. ARNETT, M.D.
Bethesda, Maryland

WILLIAM E. BATTLE, M.D.
JOHN V. RUSSO, M.D.†
Washington, D.C.

WILLIAM C. ROBERTS, M.D.
Bethesda, Maryland

Clinical and morphologic features are described in two patients known to have repeatedly injected intravenously talc-containing drugs intended for oral use. In one patient severe pulmonary hypertension developed; the talc granulomas in him were located predominantly within the pulmonary arteries. The second patient had normal pulmonary arterial pressures, and the talc granulomas in him were located predominantly in the pulmonary interstitium. Of 19 previously described patients with pulmonary talc granulomas, 12 had morphologic evidence of pulmonary hypertension (in three of severe degree); in each, talc granulomas were located predominantly within the pulmonary arteries. In those without signs of pulmonary hypertension, granulomas were located predominantly in the pulmonary interstitium. Why there are differences in the distribution of the talc granulomas is unclear. It is clear, however, as demonstrated by one of our patients, that severe pulmonary hypertension may be a consequence of intravenous injection of drugs intended for oral use.

The usual causes of pulmonary hypertension include left-sided cardiac disease, left-to-right vascular shunts, pulmonary parenchymal disease, various hypoventilation syndromes and primary pulmonary vascular disorders [1]. Among the latter causes of chronic pulmonary hypertension, repeated pulmonary emboli and primary pulmonary hypertension are the most common [2]. Recently, we encountered two young men each of whom over a several-year period had repeatedly injected into his veins one or more drugs intended for oral administration. Both had extensive pulmonary talc granulomas, one had severe pulmonary hypertension. Although talc granulomas in the lungs are a well recognized consequence of intravenous injection of drugs intended for oral use, the occurrence of severe pulmonary hypertension from this mechanism is not well known. The present report, therefore, calls attention to a new cause of pulmonary hypertension and summarizes previous reports on patients with pulmonary talc granulomas after intravenous injections of various drugs.

CASE REPORTS

Case 1. A 22 year old black man, a drug addict since age 15, was well until age 17 (five years before death) when he began to note dyspnea while participating in sports. At age 18 he was classified 4F by the Selective Service. By age 19 he was no longer able to participate in vigorous

From the Section of Pathology, National Heart & Lung Institute, National Institutes of Health, Bethesda, Maryland, the Georgetown Medical Service, District of Columbia General Hospital, and the Washington Hospital Center, Washington, D.C. Requests for reprints should be addressed to Dr. William C. Roberts, Bldg. 10A, Rm. 3E30, NIH, Bethesda, Maryland 20014.
Manuscript accepted October 1, 1975.
* Present address: Section of Cardiology, Department of Medicine, Rush-Presbyterian-St. Lukes Medical Center, Chicago, Illinois 60612.

† Present address: 2001 I Street, N.W., Washington, D.C. 20006.

physical activities because of severe exertional dyspnea. He never had nocturnal dyspnea, orthopnea, chest pain, palpitations, syncope, peripheral edema, a known precordial murmur or acute rheumatic fever. During his last seven years he took intravenously both heroin and phenmetrazine hydrochloride tablets (Preludin ®) ("BAM").

He was in his usual state of health until seven days before his death when exertional dyspnea and fatiguability increased considerably. He continued to take drugs intravenously until three days before death. He was admitted to D.C. General Hospital (the first hospitalization in his life) 8 hours before death. On examination, he appeared chronically ill, confused and restless; his breathing was rapid (34 breaths a minute). The blood pressure was 90/70 mm Hg, heart rate 140/min and the pulse was weak. The nail beds were mildly cyanotic. The jugular venous pulse was elevated; a and v waves were equally prominent. There was a prominent parasternal lift and systolic thrill, most intense at the fourth left intercostal space. The second heart sound split persistently and moved physiologically. The pulmonic valve closure-sound was loud and palpable, and both third and fourth heart sounds were present. A grade 4/6 blowing pansystolic murmur was heard over the entire precordium, loudest along the lower left sternal border. The lungs were clear. The liver was enlarged and tender. There was no subcutaneous edema.

The electrocardiogram (Figure 1) showed sinus tachycardia, right atrial enlargement, right axis deviation and right ventricular hypertrophy. Chest roentgenograms (Figure 2) showed right ventricular enlargement and prominent central pulmonary arteries. There was no evidence of pulmonary venous hypertension. The blood hemoglobin was 13 g/100 ml, the hematocrit value 42 per cent and the white blood cell count 8,000/mm^3. The arterial blood pH was 7.45, oxygen tension (pO_2) 67 mm Hg and carbon dioxide tension (pCO_2) 28 mm Hg. Digitalis, diuretics and oxygen were administered; cardiac arrest occurred, however, and resuscitative attempts were unsuccessful.

At necropsy, the heart weighed 550 g; both right-sided cardiac chambers and valve rings were dilated. The right ventricular wall was markedly hypertrophied (up to 1.0 cm thick) (Figure 3). In contrast, both left atrial and left ventricular cavities were of normal size, and their walls were of normal thickness. The mitral and aortic valves, and the coronary arteries were normal. No foci of myocardial necrosis or fibrosis were observed.

Except for emphysematous blebs in the apical portions of the lower lobes, the pulmonary parenchyma grossly appeared normal. The large pulmonary arteries were thickened, and their intimal surfaces contained many elevated yellow plaques. Histologic examination of sections of lung revealed many granulomas with giant cells containing refractile amorphous material. A few granulomas were located in the pulmonary interstitium, but most were within lumens of pulmonary arteries (Figure 4). The media of most of the muscular pulmonary arteries was severely hy-

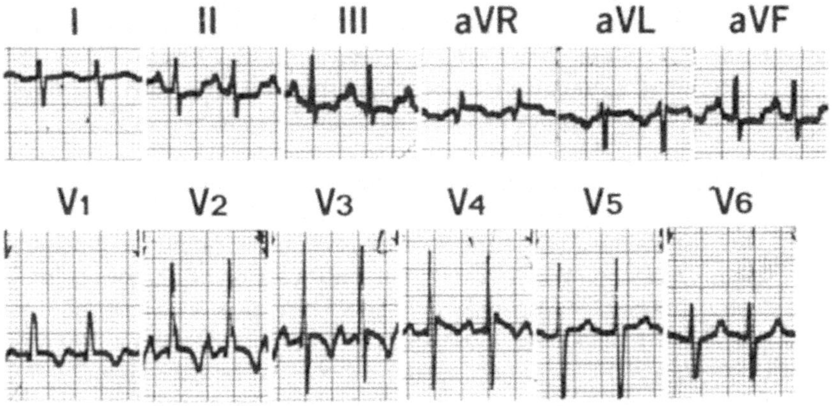

Figure 1. Case 1. Electrocardiogram shortly before death.

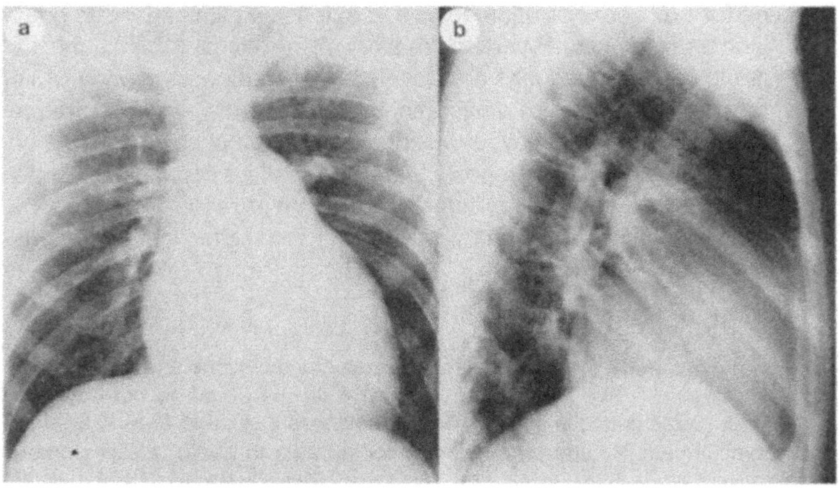

*Figure 2. Case 1. Posteroanterior **(a)** and lateral **(b)** chest roentgenograms shortly before death. The heart is large and the pulmonary arteries centrally are dilated. Marked right ventricular enlargement is apparent on the lateral film.*

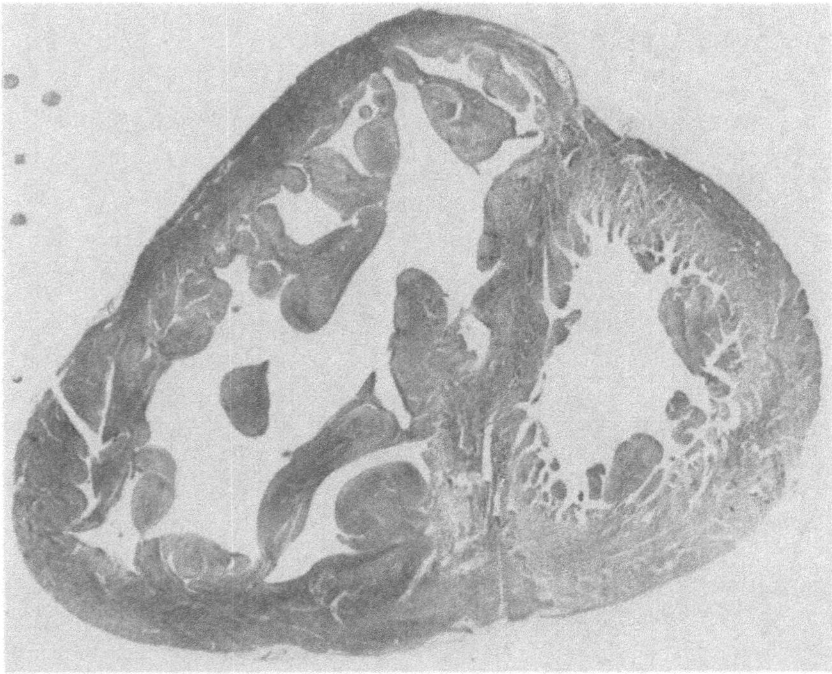

Figure 3. *Case 1. Transverse section of the cardiac ventricles. The right ventricular cavity is dilated and its wall is markedly thickened. In contrast the left ventricular cavity size and wall thickness are normal.*

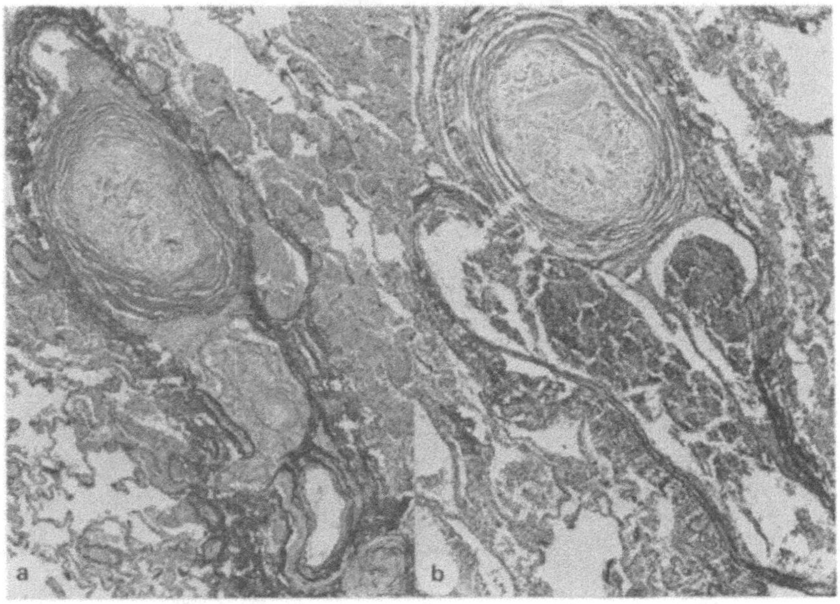

Figure 4. *Case 1. Histologic sections of lung. This patient had severe pulmonary hypertension and predominantly intravascular granulomas. Two muscular pulmonary arteries totally occluded by granulomas are shown. One **(a)** is adjacent to a plexiform lesion, and the other **(b)** is adjacent to a dilated thin-walled artery. Large giant cells and refractile material are present within the lumens of the vessel. Elastic van Gieson stains; original magnification on each × 55, reduced by 30 per cent.*

pertrophied, but some arteries showed medial atrophy; the former had very narrow lumens; the latter, dilated lumens. The obstruction in some vessels resulted entirely from collections of giant cells containing refractile material (Figure 4); in other arteries, the obstruction appeared to result primarily from fibrous tissue (Figures 5, 6 and 7). Although a single section from each of six paraffin blocks of lung tissue only suggested their presence, serial sections (every 5 μ) of one paraffin block disclosed numerous plexiform (angiomatoid) lesions (Figures 6 and 7).

Case 2. A 23 year old white man was apparently well until April 9, 1972, when he had the first of several episodes of hemoptysis. On June 20, 1972, he noted fever, chills, malaise and anorexia, and on July 3 he was hospitalized. On admission, he related that he had been an intravenous drug addict for at least five years. In addition to injecting heroin and methadone intravenously, he also had frequently injected intravenously dissolved methylphenidate (Ritalin®) tablets. On examination, he was dehydrated and febrile (103.8°F orally). A left-sided pleural friction rub and bibasilar coarse rhonchi were audible. The heart was not enlarged. A grade 2/6 systolic murmur was audible along the left lower sternal border, and it increased in intensity with inspiration. The spleen and lymph glands in the cervical, axillary and inguinal regions were palpable.

Blood and sputum cultures grew Staphylococcus aureus and chest roentgenograms showed bilateral pulmonary infiltrates which cleared with oxacillin therapy. The

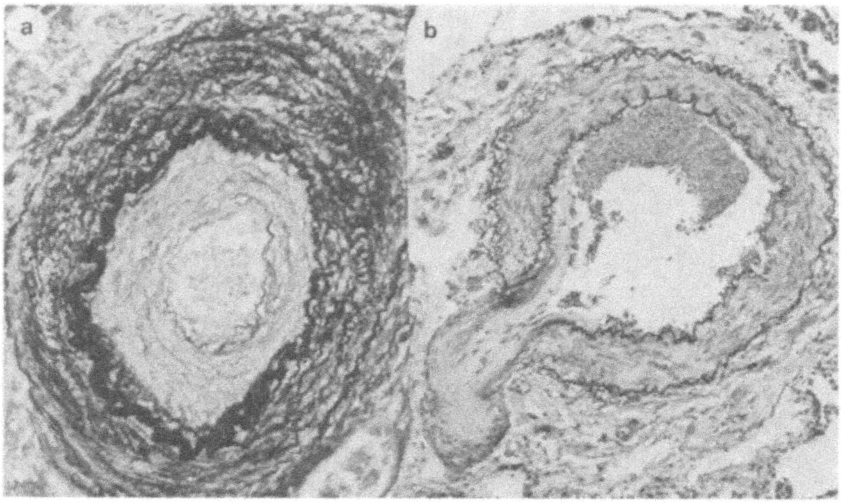

Figure 5. *Case 1. Pulmonary arteries with marked medial hypertrophy* ***(a** and **b)*** *and fibrous intimal proliferation* ***(a).*** *In* ***b,*** *a narrowed arteriole arises from the muscular artery. Elastic tissue stains; original magnification × 220* ***(a)*** *and × 140* ***(b),*** *reduced by 30 per cent.*

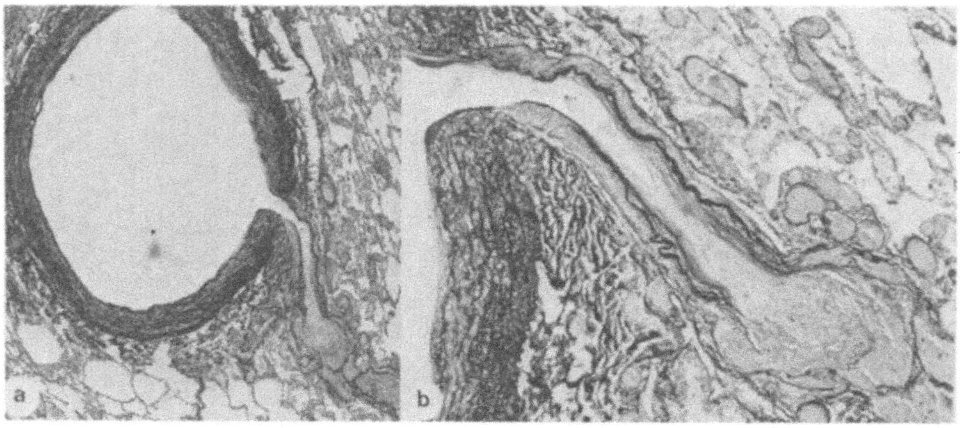

Figure 6. *Case 1. Plexiform lesion arising from a muscular pulmonary artery shortly after it branches from a large artery. Elastic van Gieson stains; original magnification × 26* ***(a)*** *and × 90* ***(b),*** *reduced by 23 per cent.*

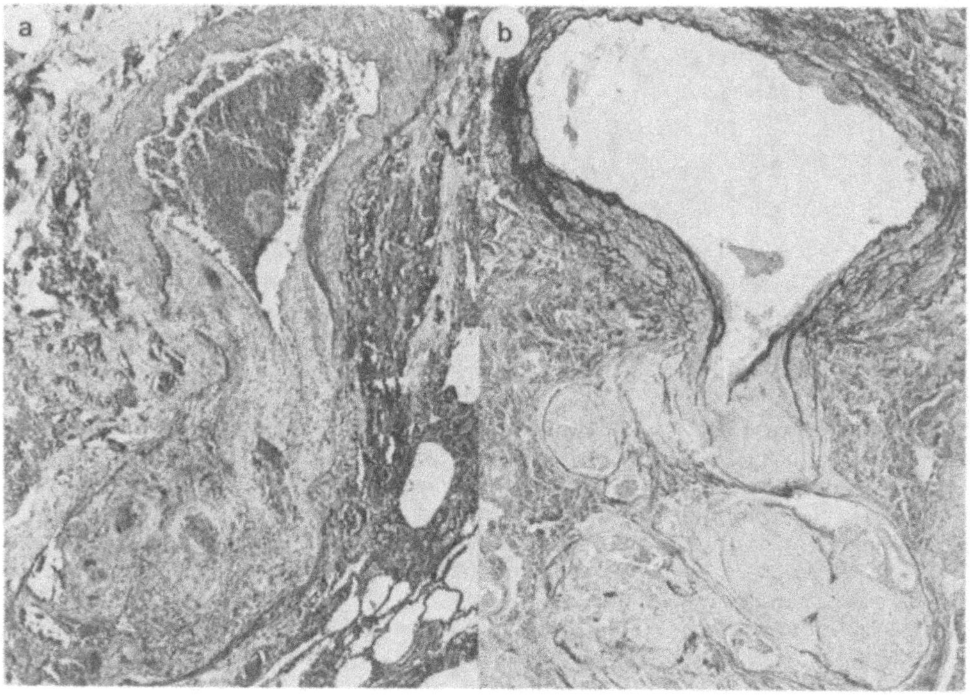

Figure 7. *Case 1. Obliterated pulmonary arteries.* ***a,*** *Small muscular pulmonary artery with lumen totally occluded by granulomas associated with refractile material.* ***b,*** *Plexiform lesion, an anatomic indicator of severe pulmonary hypertension, arising from a pulmonary artery. Elastic tissue stains; original magnification × 54* ***(a)*** *and × 70* ***(b),*** *reduced by 20 per cent.*

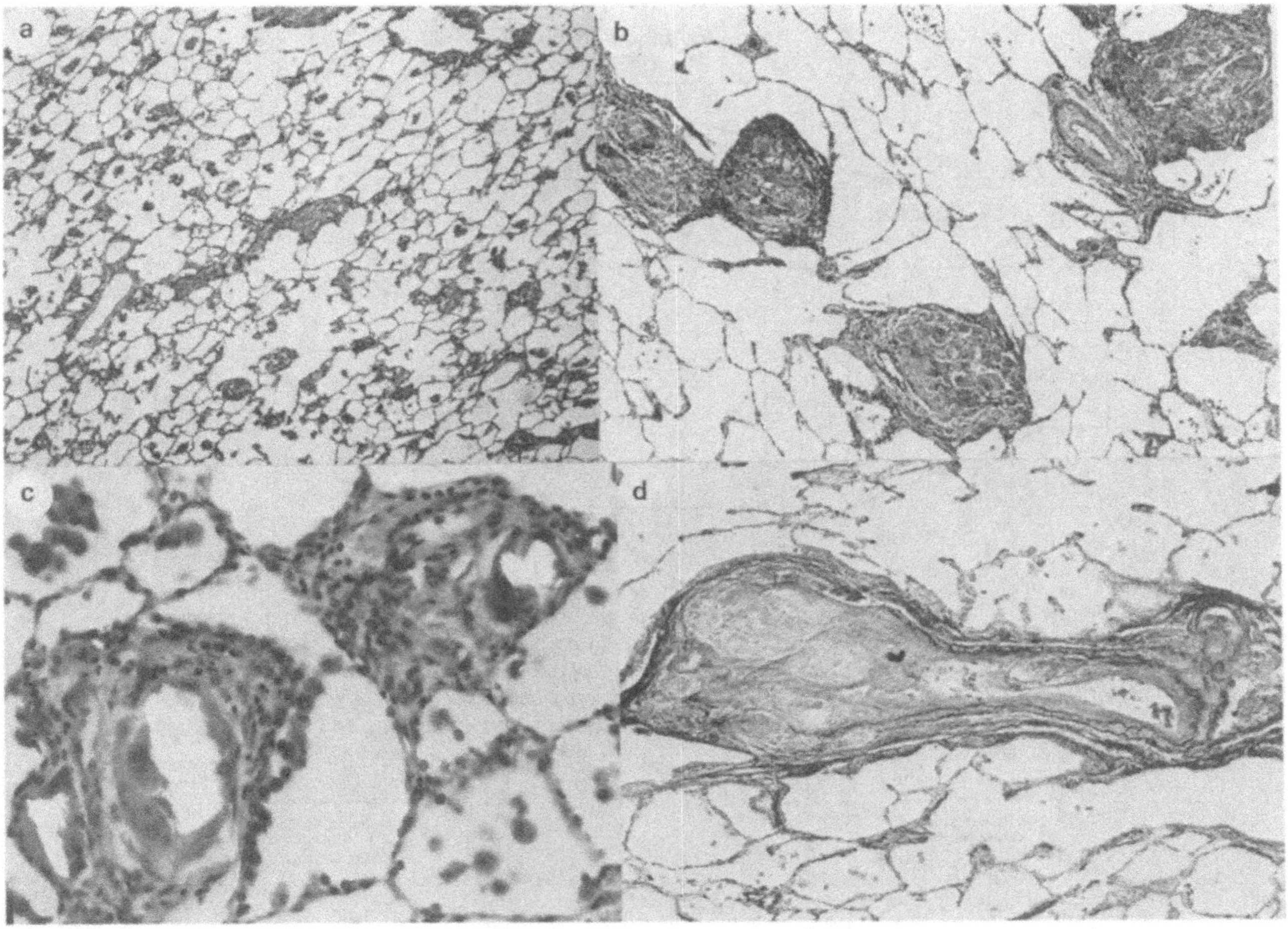

Figure 8. *Case 2. Histologic sections from the excised left lower lobe of lung. Interstitial talc granulomas are shown in **a, b** and **c** at progressively higher magnifications. The refractile talc is best seen in **c.** Intra-arterial granuloma, an unusual occurrence in this patient **(d)**. Hematoxylin and eosin stains **(a, b** and **c)**; elastic van Gieson stain **(d)**; original magnification × 16 **(a)**, × 54 **(b)**, × 160 **(c)** and × 80 **(d)**, reduced by 20 per cent.*

working diagnosis was staphylococcal tricuspid valve endocarditis with septic embolic pneumonia.

Recovery was uneventful until August 2, when hemoptysis (100 ml) occurred. Bronchoscopy on August 8 revealed persistent bleeding from the bronchus of the lower lobe of the left lung. On August 10, right heart catheterization disclosed normal ventricular and pulmonary arterial pressures, and pulmonary arteriography revealed two ovoid densities in the left lower lobe behind the heart, each approximately 2.5 cm in diameter. These densities filled during the venous phase of the injection. On August 23 the lower lobe of the left lung was excised. Blood cultures thereafter remained sterile without antibiotic therapy; the patient had no further pulmonary complaints and no further findings appeared. The patient was discharged on September 18. Thereafter, he was seen on several occasions in the Emergency Room requesting a methylphenidate prescription. The last such visit was in April 1973.

Examination of the excised lung revealed an inflamed aneurysm of a pulmonary artery which had eroded into the lumen of an adjacent bronchus. Histologically, numerous talc granulomas were observed (Figure 8). Most of the granulomas were located in the pulmonary interstitium. A few were located in the lumens of pulmonary arteries causing severe narrowing of the lumen of an occasional vessel. The walls of the pulmonary arteries were normal and no plexiform or dilatation lesions were observed despite examination of numerous histologic sections of lung.

COMMENTS

Among drug (excluding alcohol) addicts, the exact per cent who inject intravenously tablets intended for oral use is uncertain [3,4]. As shown in Figure 9, however, it is probably about 1 per cent of nonalcoholic drug addicts. Among intravenous drug addicts (Figure 10), all appear to inject opiates and probably none inject only tablets. It is probable that only a small percentage of the opiate addicts frequently also inject tablets intravenously [5]. Pulmonary talc granulomas do not result from intravenous injection of opiates alone (Figure 10) because these drugs are diluted by maltose, lactose and quinine, called "fillers," all of which are readily soluble. Foreign-body reactions consequently are not a consequence of

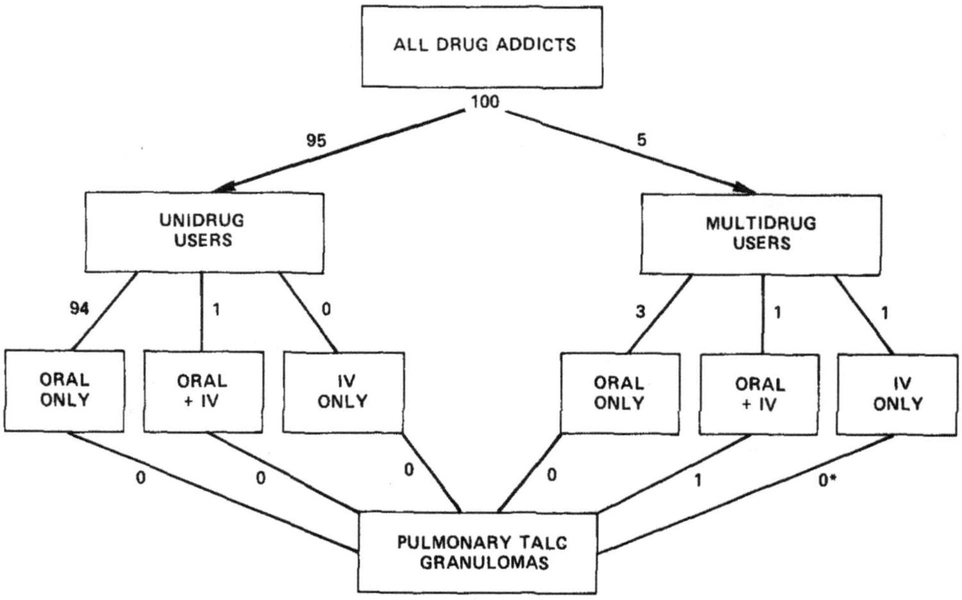

Figure 9. *Among all persons who abuse drugs, those who use only one drug constitute the great majority, and those who abuse many drugs, the minority. Virtually all intravenous drug abusers appear to fall into the "multidrug" group, but again they constitute the minority of this group. Talc granulomas form only in multidrug users because the intravenous injectors of tablets intended for oral use also usually use intravenous opiates and/or ingest drugs orally as well.*

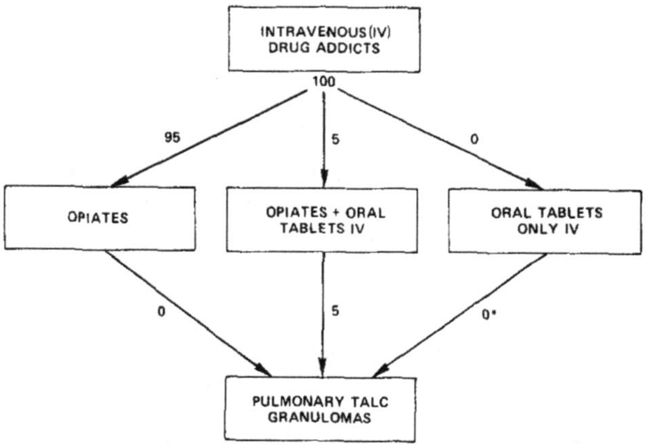

Figure 10. *The intravenous use of drugs intended for oral use is relatively uncommon and appears limited to addicts who also inject opiates. Thus, of all intravenous drug users, pulmonary talc granulomas develop in only about 5 per cent, i.e., those who also inject oral tablets.*

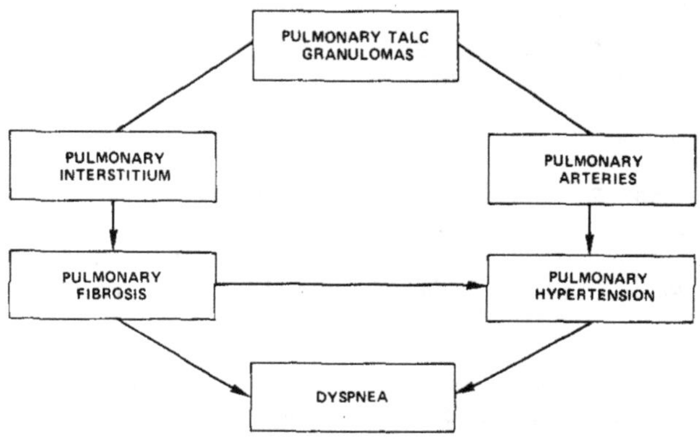

Figure 11. *Pulmonary talc granulomas may be located in pulmonary interstitium or in lumens of pulmonary arteries. In the patients with predominantly intravascular talc granulomas pulmonary hypertension may develop whereas in those with predominantly interstitial granulomas interstitial fibrosis may develop. The most frequent symptom among patients with pulmonary talc granulomas, regardless of the location of the granulomas in their lungs, is dyspnea.*

Table I) intravenous injection of opiates alone [5]. The intravenous injection of oral tablets, however, has added another complication to intravenous addiction (Table I), namely, arterial obstruction by foreign material—talc (Figures 10 and 11). Most tablets (including phenmetrazine and methylphenidate) contain talc which is used to hold the components of the medication together in tablet form [6]. When these talc-containing drugs are injected into blood vessels rather than swallowed, foreign-body granulomatous reactions occur. The injection of these talc-containing drugs into a peripheral artery may cause ischemic necrosis of portions of the distal extremities [7]. The more common practice of injecting these drugs into peripheral veins results in foreign-body granulomas in the lungs.

Of 19 patients reported on with morphologically-confirmed (lung biopsy or necropsy) pulmonary talc granulomas, 17 were known to have repeatedly injected intravenously medications intended for oral use [8–21]. Six different medications were reported to be associated with pulmonary granulomas (Table

TABLE I Pulmonary Complications of Intravenous Drug Addiction

	Opiates IV	Opiates IV and Oral Tablets IV
Acute pulmonary edema	+	+
Acute pneumonia	+	+
Spontaneous		
Aspiration		
Septic pulmonary emboli		
Pulmonary infarction		
Pulmonary abscess	+	+
Atelectasis	+	+
Talc granulomas	0	+

TABLE II Pulmonary Talc Granulomas in Drug Addicts: Tablets Frequently Injected Intravenously

Methylphenidate (Ritalin®)
Methadone
Tripelennamine (Pyribenzamine®)
Propoxyphene (Darvon®)
Phenmetrazine (Preludin®)
Amphetamines

II), and all contained talc. In each of the 19 patients, the foreign material present in the granulomas was morphologically consistent with talc; in several, x-ray diffraction studies positively identified the material as talc [9–11]. In addition, when various components of drugs associated with these granulomas are injected into experimental animals, only talc produces granulomas [22]. Thus, talc, long known to cause foreign-body granulomatous reactions when applied to serosal surfaces and similar granulomatous reactions in the lungs when inhaled over prolonged periods [23,24], also produces foreign-body granulomas when injected intravenously as part of a dissolved oral medication.

The reaction to talc, however, is variable. In some patients, as demonstrated by our second patient (Case 2), widespread granulomas develop in the interstitium of the lung but relatively few in the pulmonary arteries. In other patients this interstitial reaction may eventually lead to interstitial pulmonary fibrosis. Three of the 19 patients reported on with pulmonary talc granulomas had clinical evidence of restrictive lung disease; in each, interstitial pulmonary fibrosis was found [14,21]. Other patients, after intravenous injection of oral medications, have talc granulomas as demonstrated by our first patient (Case 1), predominantly within the lumens of small pulmonary arteries rather than in the interstitium. The result in these patients rather than interstitial pulmonary disease is pulmonary arterial hypertension. In addition to our patient (Case 1), nine of 11 necropsy patients reported on with pulmonary talc granulomas had morphologic evidence of pulmonary arterial hypertension (Table III): right ventricular hypertrophy (eight patients); medial hypertrophy of muscular pulmonary arteries (four patients); and fibrous intimal proliferation in these vessels and plexiform (angiomatoid) lesions (three patients). In addition, three of eight living patients with known pulmonary talc granulomas after intravenous injection of oral drugs had medial hypertrophy of muscular pulmonary arteries in biopsy specimens of lung [12,19]. Thus, of 21 patients with pulmonary talc granulomas, 13 had morphologic evidence of pulmonary hypertension, and four of the 13 had morphologic changes indicative of *severe* pulmonary hypertension.

Why the pulmonary talc granulomas in some patients are located predominantly in the interstitium

TABLE III Pulmonary Talc Granulomas in Drug Addicts: Reported Necropsy Observations

	Reference	Year	Age (yr) and Sex	Heart Weight (g)	RVH*	Muscular Pulmonary Arteries: Medial Hypertropy	Fibrous Intimal Thickening	Plexiform Lesions
1	Spain	1950	–,M	–	+	0	0	0
2	Wendt	1964	32,F	720	+	+	+	+
3	Burton	1965	25,M	400	+	0	0	0
4	Butz	1969	29,M	375	+	+	+	+
5	Hahn	1969	30,M	–	–	0	0	0
6	Hahn	1969	28,F	–	–	+	0	0
7	Bainborough	1970	35,F	–	+	0	0	0
8	Douglas	1971	52,M	–	+	0	0	0
9	Lewman	1972	30,M	440	+	+	+	+
10	Genereau	1974	52,M	–	+	0	0	0
11	Genereau	1974	32,M	–	0	0	0	0

*RVH = right ventricular hypertrophy (>0.5 cm thick).

and in others, predominantly in the lumens of the pulmonary arteries is unclear. The total amount of injected talc must be important, but quantity may not be the only factor. Both of our patients repeatedly injected oral drugs over a several year period. It is unlikely that the type of tablet injected played an important role since each of the four patients with morphologic evidence of severe pulmonary hypertension (and predominantly intravascular granulomas) injected a different talc-containing drug (propoxyphene, methylphenidate, tripelennamine and phenmetrazine). Conceivably, there are differences in the talc itself, or possibly, people react differently to injections of identical talc.

REFERENCES

1. Wagenvoort CA, Heath D, Edwards JE: The Pathology of the Pulmonary Vasculature. Springfield, Ill., Charles C Thomas, 1964, p. 491.
2. Wagenvoort CA, Wagenvoort N: Primary pulmonary hypertension. A pathologic study of the lung vessels in 156 clinically diagnosed cases. Circulation 42: 1163, 1970.
3. Fraser HF: Patterns of abuse of narcotics: an historical view. Drug Abuse, Proceedings of the International Conference (Zarafonetis CJD, ed), Philadelphia, Lea & Febiger, 1972, p 141.
4. Chambers CD, Taylor WJR: Patterns of "cheating" among methadone maintenance patients. Drug Abuse, Current Concepts and Research (Keup W, ed), Springfield, Ill., Charles C Thomas, 1972, p 328.
5. Siegel H, Bloustein P: Continuing studies in the diagnosis and pathology of death from intravenous narcotism. J. Forensic Sci 15: 179, 1970.
6. Vinocur M, Director Pathology and Toxicology, Boehringer Ingelheim Laboratories, Elmsford, New York: Personal communication, 1975.
7. Lindell TD, Porter JM, Langston C: Intra-arterial injections of oral medications. A complication of drug addiction. N Engl J Med 287: 1132, 1972.
8. Spain DM: Patterns of pulmonary fibrosis as related to pulmonary function. Ann Intern Med 33: 1150, 1950.
9. Wendt VE, Puro HE, Shapiro J, Mathews W, Wolf PL: Angiothrombotic pulmonary hypertension in addicts. "Blue velvet" addiction. JAMA 188: 755, 1964.
10. Burton JF, Zawadzki ES, Wetherell HR, Moy TW: Mainliners and blue velvet. J Forensic Sci 10: 466, 1965.
11. Butz WC: Pulmonary arteriole foreign body granulomata associated with angiomatoids resulting from the intravenous injection of oral medications, e.g., propoxyphene hydrochloride (Darvon®). J Forensic Sci 14: 317, 1969.
12. Hahn HH, Schweid AI, Beaty HN: Complications of injecting dissolved methylphenidate tablets. Arch Intern Med 123: 656, 1969.
13. Hopkins GB, Taylor DG: Pulmonary talc granulomatosis. A complication of drug abuse. Am Rev Respir Dis 101: 101, 1970.
14. Szwed JJ: Pulmonary angiothrombosis caused by "blue velvet" addiction. Ann Intern Med 73: 771, 1970.
15. Bainborough AR, Jericho KWF: Cor pulmonale secondary to talc granulomata in the lungs of a drug addict. Can Med Assoc J 103: 1297, 1970.
16. Douglas FG, Kafilmont KJ, Patt NL: Foreign particle embolism in drug addicts. Ann Intern Med 75: 865, 1971.
17. Lewman LV: Fatal pulmonary hypertension from intravenous injection of methylphenidate (Ritalin) tablets. Human Pathol 3: 67, 1972.
18. Vevaina JR, Civantos F, Viamonte M, Avery WG: Emphysema associated with talcum granulomatosis in a drug addict. South Med J 67: 113, 1974.
19. Gottlieb LS, Boylen TC: Pulmonary complications of drug abuse. West J Med 120: 8, 1974.
20. Schofferman J, Billesdon J, Hall R: Microangiopathic hemolytic anemia. Another complication of drug abuse. JAMA 230: 721, 1974.
21. Genereux GP, Emson HE: Talc granulomatosis and angiothrombotic pulmonary hypertension in drug addicts. J Can Assoc Radiol 25: 87, 1974.
22. Puro HE, Wolf PL, Skirgaudas J, Vazquez J: Experimental production of human "blue velvet" and "red devil" lesions. JAMA 197: 1100, 1966.
23. Eiseman B, Seelig MG, Womack NA: Talcum powder granuloma: a frequent and serious postoperative complication. Ann Surg 126: 820, 1947.
24. Miller A, Teirstein AS, Bader ME, Selikoff IJ: Talc pneumoconiosis. Significance of sublight microscopic mineral particles. Am J Med 50: 395, 1971.

Idiopathic Pulmonary Fibrosis

Clinical, Histologic, Radiographic, Physiologic, Scintigraphic, Cytologic, and Biochemical Aspects

Moderator: RONALD G. CRYSTAL, M.D. *Discussants:* JACK D. FULMER, M.D.; WILLIAM C. ROBERTS, M.D.; MORTON L. MOSS, M.D.; BRUCE R. LINE, M.D.; and HERBERT Y. REYNOLDS, M.D., F.A.C.P.; Bethesda, Maryland

Idiopathic pulmonary fibrosis is a fatal disorder that starts as an alveolitis and progresses to interstitial fibrosis. Correlative morphologic, physiologic, and biochemical studies in 29 patients have shown that the inflammatory process is best followed by serial bronchoalveolar lavage and ^{67}Ga citrate scanning, and the fibrotic process is best followed by quantitation of the exercise-induced drop in arterial oxygen tension per unit of oxygen consumed. Although biopsies in idiopathic pulmonary fibrosis seem to show increased amounts of fibrotic tissue, biochemical studies suggest that the disease is probably one of collagen rearrangement rather than collagen increase. Perhaps because of this, peripheral lymphocytes of these patients recognize collagen as "non-self" and, when exposed to it in vitro, produce lymphokines and cell lysis. The fibrotic process is probably irreversible, but the inflammatory and immune processes that cause it may be amenable to therapy if diagnosed early.

DR. RONALD G. CRYSTAL*: Forty one years ago, Hamman and Rich (1) described the clinical and morphologic features of four patients with progressive, rapidly fatal, diffuse pulmonary fibrosis. Clinicians soon began to diagnose this illness antemortem, and by 1957 more than 50 cases had appeared in the literature under the heading "Hamman-Rich syndrome" (2, 3). However, as more cases were described, it became apparent that the fulminating course of the original patients of Hamman and Rich manifested only part of the spectrum of the disorder now known as idiopathic pulmonary fibrosis (4-35).

More commonly, patients with idiopathic pulmonary fibrosis present with the insidious onset of breathlessness, sometimes after a flulike illness. It affects slightly more men than women; most patients are between the ages of 40 and 70 years, although the disease is sometimes found in children and young adults (36, 37). Almost all patients develop late inspiratory rales in the lower lung fields, clubbing of the fingers and occasionally the toes, and evidence of pulmonary hypertension. Although the inevitably fatal course of the disease can progress as rapidly as that described by Hamman and Rich, some patients can have the disorder for 15 to 20 years. However, this slower course is unusual; the average life span of a patient with idiopathic pulmonary fibrosis is only 47 months from the onset of symptoms (26).

In the early 1950s, as investigators developed the sophisticated tools to evaluate pulmonary disorders, Austrian and associates (38) described the "classic" physiologic concept of idiopathic pulmonary fibrosis. In general, patients have reduced lung volumes, reduced diffusing capacity, a normal forced expiratory volume in 1 sec/forced vital capacity ($FEV_1\%$), and arterial hypoxemia that worsens with exercise. These investigators coined the term "alveolar-capillary block," suggesting that the hypoxemia of idiopathic pulmonary fibrosis was secondary to an anatomic barrier to oxygen due to a thickened alveolar interstitium (38). This term was popular in the literature until 1962, when Finley, Swenson, and Comroe (39) presented data suggesting that the major cause of hypoxemia in these patients was not a diffusion barrier to oxygen, but rather was secondary to ventilation-perfusion mismatching. Clinicians had only recently adjusted to this new concept when it was challenged. Using sophisticated methods, Wagner and associates (40) showed that most of the hypoxemia in idiopathic pulmonary fibrosis is indeed secondary to ventilation-perfusion imbalance. With exercise, however, approximately 20% is due to a diffusion barrier to oxygen. Thus, our understanding of this phenomenon has come full circle. We will see later that, although ventilation-perfusion mismatching is

* Chief, Pulmonary Branch, National Heart, Lung, and Blood Institute.

► An edited transcription of a Combined Clinical Staff Conference at the Clinical Center, Bethesda, Maryland, 13 November 1975, by the National Heart, Lung, and Blood Institute, National Institutes of Health, U.S. Department of Health, Education, and Welfare.

Table 1. Classification of the Fibrotic Lung Disorders

Known Cause	Unknown Cause
Occupational and environmental* inhalants	Idiopathic pulmonary fibrosis
Drug reactions	Associated with a collagen-vascular disease†
Physical agents	Not associated with any known disorder
Infectious disorders	Associated with pulmonary arteritis‡
Cardiac disease	Sarcoidosis
Pulmonary vascular disease	Ankylosing spondylitis
Neoplastic disease	Congenital; familial
	Eosinophilic granuloma
	Idiopathic pulmonary hemosiderosis
	Alveolar microlithiasis
	Goodpasture's syndrome
	Alveolar proteinosis

* Including the group of disorders termed extrinsic allergic alveolitis; the fibrotic form is called chronic hypersensitivity pneumonitis.

† Including rheumatoid arthritis, progressive systemic sclerosis, systemic lupus erythematosus, dermatomyositis-polymyositis, Sjögren's syndrome, and the mixed connective tissue syndrome, but excluding patients with necrobiotic nodules or vasculitis.

‡ Including periarteritis nodosa; Wegener's granulomatosis; rheumatoid arthritis with necrobiotic nodules; and rheumatoid arthritis, progressive systemic sclerosis, and polymyositis-dermatomyositis with arteritis.

critically important in idiopathic pulmonary fibrosis, we are just beginning to understand what causes it.

For years, the morphologic features of idiopathic pulmonary fibrosis described by Hamman and Rich were accepted as definitive: a diffuse interstitial fibrosis with mononuclear cell infiltration (1, 2). It took the pioneering efforts of Scadding and Hinson (6, 18) and Liebow and co-workers (15, 21, 22) to point out that the spectrum of idiopathic pulmonary fibrosis was much broader and included marked intraalveolar cellularity as part of the histologic spectrum of the disease. Although most investigators have abandoned the designations "desquamative interstitial pneumonitis" (many intraalveolar cells with little interstitial disease) and "usual interstitial pneumonitis" (interstitial cellularity and fibrosis with little intraalveolar cellularity), these concepts remain important as probably representing the stages in the development of idiopathic pulmonary fibrosis (18, 29, 30, 33, 35).

As more clinicians recognized the importance of idiopathic pulmonary fibrosis, it became clear that many of these patients have serologic abnormalities that are associated with the collagen-vascular disorders. The physiologic and histologic features of idiopathic pulmonary fibrosis were noted in patients with rheumatoid arthritis (4, 25, 28, 33, 41-56), progressive systemic sclerosis (38, 52-66), polymyositis-dermatomyositis (65-80), and systemic lupus erythematosus (52-56, 81-85). As the association of these disorders became more evident, patients with idiopathic pulmonary fibrosis were screened with this in mind, and three groups emerged: those with a defined collagen-vascular disorder (41-85); those with serologic abnormalities that are seen in collagen-vascular disorders but that did not meet the criteria for a defined collagen-vascular disorder (33, 86-99); and those with no serologic abnormalities associated with the collagen-vascular disorders. Thus, for convenience, idiopathic pulmonary fibrosis is now categorized as "associated with a collagen-vascular disorder" (group 1) or "not associated with any known disorder" (groups 2 and 3) (Table 1). It is important to note, however, that with few exceptions, the two categories are identical. The major exceptions are that a small percentage of patients with rheumatoid arthritis have pulmonary necrobiotic nodules (46-48), and some patients with systemic lupus erythematosus, rheumatoid arthritis, progressive systemic sclerosis, or dermatomyositis-polymyositis have pulmonary arteritis (46, 48, 72, 84, 100). Even if these patients have pulmonary fibrosis, their disease is not considered to be idiopathic pulmonary fibrosis, and they will be excluded from our discussion. Likewise, patients with the lymphoproliferative form of Sjögrens syndrome (101), polyarteritis nodosa (102), Wegener's granulomatosis (103), and ankylosing spondylitis (104) clearly have a disorder different from idiopathic pulmonary fibrosis, and they will not be discussed.

Because idiopathic pulmonary fibrosis falls into the group of fibrotic lung disorders of unknown cause (Table 1), clinicians have tended to consider it a diagnosis of exclusion. However, as we will point out, this disorder has clearly defined clinical, histologic, radiographic, physiologic, scintigraphic, cytologic, and biochemical features that, taken as a whole, describe a characteristic and specific clinical entity. To give an overview of the current concepts of idiopathic pulmonary fibrosis, we will first present the general clinical, pathologic, and radiographic findings in 29 patients with this disorder. This will serve to place in context the newer physiologic, diagnostic, investigative, and therapeutic concepts that will follow.

Clinical Aspects of Idiopathic Pulmonary Fibrosis

Dr. Jack D. Fulmer*: A brief description of the clinical findings in this group of 29 patients will help to define idiopathic pulmonary fibrosis and its manifestations. Although these findings are not limited to this disorder, when considered in the setting of the whole clinical entity, they help to establish idiopathic pulmonary fibrosis as a specific and characteristic disease.

Eighty percent of the patients under discussion had idiopathic pulmonary fibrosis without any other associated disorder; the rest had a defined collagen-vascular disorder. Nationwide statistics are not available, but we think these relative percentages probably reflect only the pattern of our referrals. At least some manifestations of idiopathic pulmonary fibrosis are relatively common in rheumatoid arthritis (25, 33, 45-51) and progressive systemic sclerosis (33, 58, 61-63), so there are probably more patients with idiopathic pulmonary fibrosis associated with a collagen-vascular disorder than our patient population reflects.

The average age of all patients was 51.8 years. However, the group with associated collagen-vascular disorders were generally younger. There was a slightly higher percentage of men than women (1.1:1) in our idiopathic pulmonary fibrosis population, but in the group with collagen-vascular disorders women predominated. These age and sex distributions reflect the typical findings for idiopathic pulmonary fibrosis found in the literature (12, 13, 17). With the

* Chief, Clinical Service, Pulmonary Branch, National Heart, Lung, and Blood Institute.

Table 2. Clinical, Laboratory, and Physiologic Findings in Patients with Idiopathic Pulmonary Fibrosis

Presenting Symptoms	Percent of Patients	Laboratory	Percent of Patients	Physiologic Studies	Mean Values*
Breathlessness	100	↑ Sedimentation rate	94†	Vital capacity	61.7 ± 2.9‡
Cough	86	+ Antinuclear antibodies	7†		
Systemic§	48†	+ Rheumatoid factor	14†	Total lung capacity	62.9 ± 2.9‡
		+ Cryoimmunoglobulins	41†		
		+ Lupus erythematosus preparations	3†	Residual volume/	
				total lung capacity	34.4 ± 1.6‖
Physical		Abnormal serum protein			
Tachypnea	46	electrophoresis		FEV$_1$%**	97.6 ± 2.3‡
Clubbing	72	↑ $\alpha 2$ macroglobulins	22		
Chest findings		↑ γ globulins	17	Diffusing capacity††	46.8 ± 3.5‡
Normal	14	Serum immunoglobulins			
Rales	65	↑ IgG	4		
Ronchi or bronchovesicular		↑ IgA	39		
sounds	21	↑ IgM	9		
Cardiac findings		Serum complement (C50) ↓	6†		
Normal	30	Polycythemia	3		
Augmented P$_2$	70				

* Mean ± SEM.
† These data refer only to patients with idiopathic pulmonary fibrosis with no associated collagen-vascular disorder; of the 29 patients with idiopathic pulmonary fibrosis, three had rheumatoid arthritis, one had systemic lupus erythematosus, one had a mixed collagen-vascular disease, and one had progressive systemic sclerosis.
‡ Percent predicted.
§ Systemic symptoms included flulike illness, fatigue, joint symptoms, fever, or weight loss.
‖ Percent observed.
** Forced expiratory volume in 1 sec/forced vital capacity.
†† Single breath, carbon monoxide.

exception of age and sex and the specific systemic abnormalities of each collagen-vascular syndrome in the group with associated collagen-vascular disorders, the manifestations of idiopathic pulmonary fibrosis in both groups were identical (49, 85) (Table 2).

The duration of symptoms from onset to evaluation at the NIH ranged from 0.5 to 10 years, but averaged 2.9 years. In the most extensive study of the natural history of idiopathic pulmonary fibrosis (26), the mean survival of patients was 4 years, with a range of 0.4 to 20 years. Although most of our patients are still alive, the relative number that have died would suggest that they are following a similar natural history.

The onset of idiopathic pulmonary fibrosis is usually associated with breathlessness, characteristically first noted during exercise (6, 17, 30). Most patients also noted a nonproductive cough early in the course of the disease, and about half noted constitutional symptoms such as a flulike illness, fatigability, weight loss, or arthralgias (Table 2).

In contrast to other pulmonary disorders associated with clubbing (105, 106), patients with idiopathic pulmonary fibrosis with clubbing rarely have hypertrophic osteoarthropathy. Excluding clubbing and varied constitutional symptoms, all of the clinical manifestations of idiopathic pulmonary fibrosis were limited to the chest. Early in the course of the disease, the chest examination may be normal. Later, in midcourse, the typical patient with idiopathic pulmonary fibrosis will have tachypnea (46%), harsh, dry rales at both bases (65%), and findings consistent with pulmonary hypertension (70%). Occasionally, patients will have only diffuse bronchovesicular breath sounds or rhonchi, or both. Although cardiac examination findings can be normal for years, the usual progression includes the development of a right ventricular heave and eventual right-sided failure (13). About 20% of the patients with idiopathic pulmonary fibrosis eventually die from a cardiovascular disorder, but most succumb to primary respiratory failure, often precipitated by infection (26).

Most patients with idiopathic pulmonary fibrosis have resting arterial hypoxemia that worsens with exercise. Polycythemia, however, is almost never seen (13), in marked contrast to other hypoxic states such as chronic obstructive lung disease or congenital heart disease (107). Almost all patients with idiopathic pulmonary fibrosis have an elevated sedimentation rate (94%). As pointed out by Dr. Crystal, idiopathic pulmonary fibrosis is definitely associated with abnormalities of the immune system (33, 86-98). However, of the routine studies available, none are specific for this disorder. Excluding patients with definable collagen-vascular disorders, abnormalities in antinuclear antibodies, rheumatoid factor, and γ-globulins are not as prominent in our group of patients as one would expect from reviewing the literature (compare Table 2 with References 88, 89). In addition, although an association had made between chronic hepatitis and idiopathic pulmonary fibrosis (108), none of our patients had liver function abnormalities. It is not generally recognized that many have circulating cryoimmunoglobulins (Table 2, Reference 33). The specific immunoglobulins involved have not been characterized as yet. There are other, probably much more important abnormalities of the immune system that are almost universal in idiopathic pulmonary fibrosis, and these will be discussed later.

The average patient with idiopathic pulmonary fibrosis had a total lung capacity of 62.9% predicted and a diffusing capacity of 46.8% predicted. However, two patients had normal lung volumes and one patient a normal diffusing capacity, even though they had morphologic evidence of mild to moderate fibrosis. Thus, although a

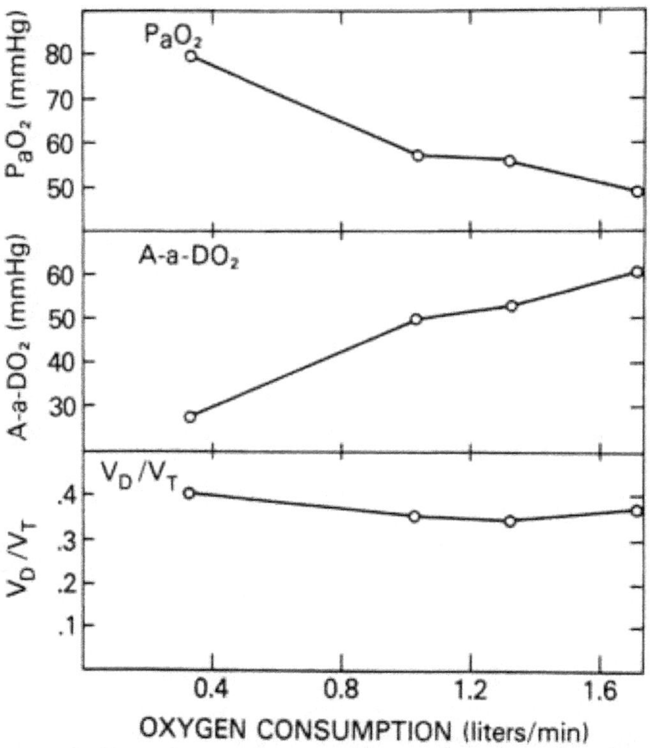

Figure 1. Gas exchange data from a 42-year-old man with idiopathic pulmonary fibrosis taken at rest and during treadmill exercise (see also Figures 2, 5c and d). **Top.** Progressive decrease in arterial oxygen tension (Pao_2) with exercise. **Middle.** Progressive increase in alveolar-arterial oxygen difference ($D[A\text{-}a]o_2$) with exercise. **Bottom.** Dead space to tidal volume ratio (VD/VT) is abnormally high and does not decrease with progressive exercise. Oxygen consumption is proportional to power output.

reduced total lung capacity and diffusing capacity are the physiologic hallmarks of the disease, it is not mandatory that both be abnormal. Likewise, the average patient with idiopathic pulmonary fibrosis has resting arterial hypoxemia (69.3 mm Hg), but four of our patients have normal resting arterial oxygen tension (Pao_2). It is important to point out that a decreased diffusing capacity does not implicate a defect in oxygen diffusion but rather signifies a reduction of available alveolar-capillary bed (109).

Interestingly, 21% of our patients had decreased Pao_2 values when they rose from the supine to the upright position, in direct opposition to what occurs in normal individuals. In idiopathic pulmonary fibrosis, the reversal of position-dependent changes in Pao_2 is probably associated with alterations in pulmonary hemodynamics, causing greater ventilation-perfusion imbalance in the upright position (110).

It is generally thought that the hypoxemia of idiopathic pulmonary fibrosis is related to ventilation-perfusion mismatching, although limitation to oxygen diffusion may be present, especially during exercise (40). As we will discuss later, much of the ventilation-perfusion mismatching may be related to abnormalities in ventilation. However, the latter is not due to abnormalities in the large airways because almost all patients with idiopathic pulmonary fibrosis have normal values for $FEV_1\%$ (Table 2) and airway resistance by body plethysmography (111).

Even though the resting Pao_2 can be normal in idiopathic pulmonary fibrosis, the resting alveolar-arterial oxygen gradient ($D[A\text{-}a]o_2$) is almost invariably abnormal (97% of the patients). Even more sensitive physiologic monitors of idiopathic pulmonary fibrosis are the fall in Pao_2 and the widening of $D(A\text{-}a)o_2$ with exercise, findings that are universal in these patients (Figure 1, *Top and Middle*) (12, 30, 38).

Physiologic shunt at rest (as measured by 100% O_2) can be significant in idiopathic pulmonary fibrosis but usually develops late in the course of the disease (38, 39). Of our population, the four patients with the mildest disease had a physiologic shunt of less than 6%, whereas the four patients with the most advanced disease had a shunt of 15% to 30%. Thus, although physiologic shunt is generally not a significant cause of hypoxemia early in the disease, it becomes a major problem in the care of patients very late in their course, because even with very high inspired oxygen concentrations, they do not achieve adequate oxygenation.

Another characteristic of idiopathic pulmonary fibrosis is the increased physiologic dead space found in 60% of the patients even at rest (7, 12, 112). Whereas normal persons waste (that is, ventilate nonfunctional regions of lung) less than one third of their total ventilation, patients with idiopathic pulmonary fibrosis will often have dead space to tidal volume ratios (V_D/V_T) of greater than 0.4. In normal individuals the efficiency of ventilation improves with exercise (that is, the V_D/V_T falls) (113, 114); in more than 90% of patients with idiopathic pulmonary fibrosis it stays constant or may increase (Figure 1, *bottom*).

Also characteristic of idiopathic pulmonary fibrosis is the volume-pressure curve (Figure 2) that expresses the mechanical properties of lung and is usually discussed in terms of its position, shape, and slope (115). Typically,

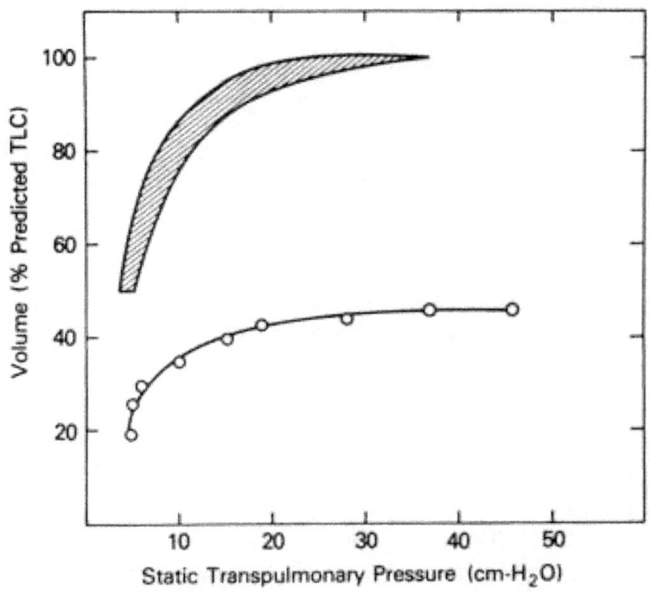

Figure 2. Volume-pressure relations of a 42-year-old man with idiopathic pulmonary fibrosis (see also Figures 1, 5c and d) showing a curve (○—○) that is shifted down and to the right of normal (*shaded area*). The volume data is presented as percentage of predicted total lung capacity (*TLC*).

patients with idiopathic pulmonary fibrosis have a volume-pressure curve shifted downward and to the right, whereas patients with emphysema have a curve shifted upward and to the left (112, 116). The reasons for these findings are controversial, but the curve graphically illustrates that after a certain point patients with idiopathic pulmonary fibrosis take in little volume of air, and to do so requires a large negative transpulmonary pressure. Although such a volume-pressure curve is not specific for idiopathic pulmonary fibrosis (it is seen in any infiltrative disease of lung) (115), taken in context, it helps to characterize the disorder.

Histologic Observations in Idiopathic Pulmonary Fibrosis

Dr. William C. Roberts*: This section will summarize our histologic observations from open lung biopsies in 29 patients with idiopathic pulmonary fibrosis and discuss the significance of some of these changes. There were no histologic differences between the groups with idiopathic pulmonary fibrosis and idiopathic pulmonary fibrosis associated with collagen-vascular disorders (12, 48).

The anatomic distribution of idiopathic pulmonary fibrosis is heterogeneous, a finding easily visualized with low power views of the biopsies (Figures 3*A*, 4*A*). Yet this same local heterogeneity is usually seen in multiple samples throughout the lung at postmortem evaluation of idiopathic pulmonary fibrosis, suggesting open lung biopsy specimens are, in general, representative of the disease process.

The major histologic abnormalities of idiopathic pulmonary fibrosis are listed in Table 3 and illustrated in Figures 3 and 4. A characteristic histologic feature of all biopsies was the apparent increased amounts of fibrous tissue in the alveolar septae. The distribution of this fibrous tissue, however, varied: in 23% of the patients it was focal, and most of the alveolar septae appeared normal; in another 23% there were more areas of the lung biopsy with apparently increased fibrous tissue than areas of normal-appearing lung; and in the remaining 54% most or all alveolar septae appeared thickened by fibrous tissue, the pulmonary architecture was considerably distorted, and the amount of area occupied by air appeared less than that occupied by tissue. Many patients had considerable peribronchiolar fibrosis and fibrous thickening of the interlobular septae and visceral pleura.

Inflammatory cells, mainly lymphocytes, macrophages, and plasma cells, were always seen in areas of increased fibrous tissue. A feature of idiopathic pulmonary fibrosis that is not often recognized is that eosinophils and neutrophils are present as well (2, 18, 29, 35). The number of mononuclear cells in the interstitium was quite variable: 13% of patients had considerable numbers, 54% had moderate numbers, and 33% were judged to have scattered cells. The normal lung has almost no inflammatory cells in the interstitium or alveolus, so the observation of even scattered interstitial inflammatory cells is important.

In many areas where the alveolar septae were thickened, the air side was lined by large cuboidal-shaped cells, often associated with collections of cells free in the alveolar sacs. The former has been referred to as "cuboidalization of alveolar lining cells" (19, 24, 117) and the latter as "desquamation" (15). Some degree of cuboidalization and desquamation was observed in all biopsies.

Normally, the epithelial surfaces of alveoli are covered by two types of cells: the alveolar type I cell (also called the type I pneumocyte, type A epithelial cell, small alveolar cell, or membranous pneumocyte) and the alveolar type II cell (also called the type II pneumocyte, large alveolar cell, granular pneumocyte, or vacuolated alveolar cell) (118). The type II cell is particularly important for its production of the material that lowers alveolar surface tension (119). The type I cell covers more than 90% of the alveolar surface area and is not visible by light microscopy; the type II cell covers the remaining surface area and is visible by light microscopy. Even though the vast majority of the epithelial surface is composed of type I cells, there are ordinarily 1.5 to 2 type II cells for every type I cell (118). In idiopathic pulmonary fibrosis, however, this ratio increases since the cuboidalization of the alveolar epithelial surface is most likely due to loss of type I cells and proliferation of type II cells. This change in alveolar epithelial cells is not specific for idiopathic pulmonary fibrosis because it occurs in most conditions associated with alveolar injury, including causes of pulmonary venous hypertension such as mitral stenosis (19, 117, 120, 121).

The term "desquamated" cells was originally used to describe free-floating cells within alveolar spaces, as these cells were thought to be alveolar type II cells that had been sloughed from the epithelial surface (15). As more patients with idiopathic pulmonary fibrosis were studied using electron microscopy, it became apparent that the term "desquamated" is probably improper because many of these cells are macrophages (29, 120, 122, 123). All of our patients with idiopathic pulmonary fibrosis have desquamated cells in alveoli. The relative numbers of these cells, however, varied (large in 7%, moderate in 43%, and only a few in 50%). The amount of "desquamation" varies not only from patient to patient, but also within the limited area of the same open lung biopsy specimen (Figure 3). This finding strengthens the concept that "desquamative interstitial pneumonitis" and "usual interstitial pneumonitis" are simply parts of the same disease rather than specific disease entities. Desquamative interstitial pneumonitis most likely represents early idiopathic pulmonary fibrosis, whereas usual interstitial pneumonitis represents the later stages of the disease (6, 18, 24, 29, 30, 33, 35). Since the morphology of both can appear in the same patient at the same time (Figure 3), it is probable that part of the heterogeneity of idiopathic pulmonary fibrosis within the same biopsy represents the same disease process at different stages.

Although idiopathic pulmonary fibrosis is classically considered a disorder of alveoli, 80% of the biopsies showed peribronchiolar fibrous tissue or peribronchial mononuclear inflammatory cells, or both. Many of the airway lumina contained cellular debris or mucus, or both (Figures 3*E*, 4*C*). In open lung biopsy specimens of normal lung, the

* Chief, Pathology Branch, National Heart, Lung, and Blood Institute.

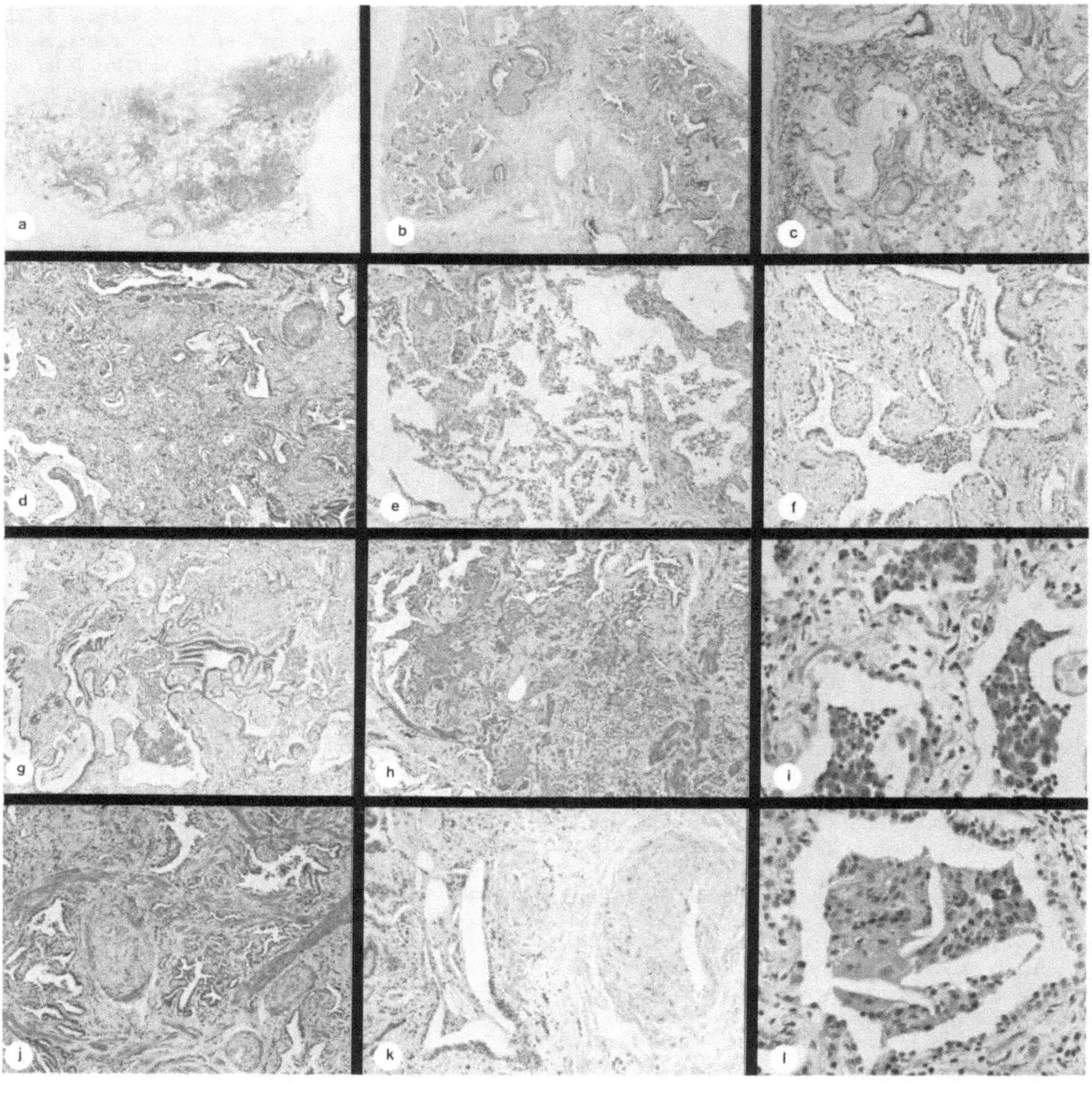

Figure 3. Twelve photomicrographs from a lung biopsy showing typical histologic features of idiopathic pulmonary fibrosis in a 66-year-old man who was symptomatic for 12 months before the biopsy was done. **a.** Longitudinal section of the entire biopsy. Some areas are quite scarred, others relatively normal. (Hematoxylin and eosin; original magnification, × 9.) **b.** Portion of thickened area showing marked distortion of pulmonary parenchyma, loss of alveolar space, marked increase in fibrous tissue, and "desquamation" in some air spaces. (Movat; original magnification, × 40.) **c.** Area encompassing a portion of that shown in *b*. There is both medial hypertrophy and intimal fibrous proliferation of the arteries. The latter produced luminal narrowing. The interlobular septae show increased fibrous tissue in some sites and edema fluid in others. The black represents elastic fibers. (Elastic van Gieson; original magnification, × 40.) **d.** Masson trichome stain showing huge amounts of fibrous tissue (*stained blue*). The arteries have narrowed lumina. Debris is present in some air spaces (original magnification, × 54). **e.** Area of lung with only mild increase in fibrous tissue but "desquamation" in alveolar sacs. (Hematoxylin and eosin; original magnification, × 80.) **f.** Close-up showing marked thickening of alveolar septae by fibrous tissue. Three cholesterol clefts are present in one alveolar space. (Movat; original magnification, × 130.) **g.** The alveolar spaces and airways here are filled with desquamated cells and mucinous material. There is smooth muscle proliferation in the alveolar septae, and the lumina of the arteries are narrowed. (Hematoxylin and eosin; original magnification, × 155.) **h.** Area showing alveoli packed with desquamated cells. The smooth muscle is prominent. (Movat; original magnification, × 80.) **i.** Periodic acid-Schiff (PAS) stain showing that the cytoplasm of the desquamated cells in the alveolar spaces is PAS-positive. The alveolar septae in this area appear edematous and also contain increased fibrous tissue. There is proliferation of the alveolar lining cells ("cuboidalization") (original magnification, × 360). **j.** Close-up showing proliferation of smooth muscle in the alveolar septae. The arteries have thick walls and narrowed lumina. (Movat; original magnification, × 80.) **k.** Close-up showing multiple cholesterol clefts in an alveolar space and an adjacent pulmonary artery with a narrowed lumen. (Movat; original magnification, × 140.) **l.** Close-up of cholesterol granuloma in an alveolus. The cholesterol clefts are indicative of pulmonary hypertension (124). (Hematoxylin and eosin; original magnification, × 380.)

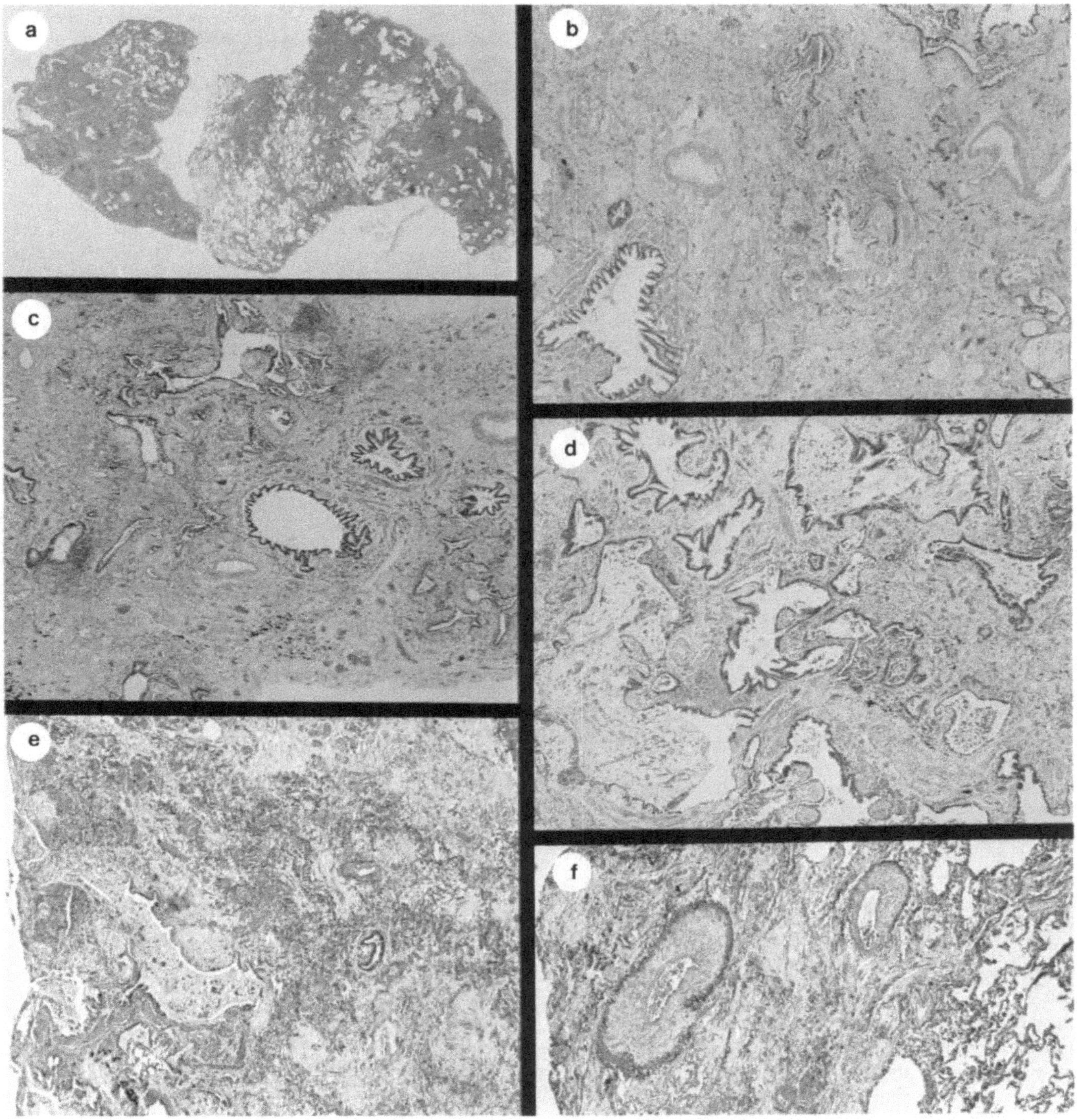

Figure 4. Lung biopsy in a 67-year-old man who had symptoms of respiratory insufficiency for only 6 months before this biopsy was obtained. **a.** Low-power view of the entire biopsy, which was in two pieces. Most of the pulmonary parenchyma is markedly thickened by fibrous tissue. Only a small area of near-normal lung remains. (Hematoxylin and eosin; original magnification, × 4.) **b.** Section showing loss of air space and replacement by fibrous tissue. A cholesterol granuloma is present in the air space near the center of the field. (Hematoxylin and eosin; original magnification, × 35.) **c.** Another area showing several airways, some of which are narrowed and others dilated. (Hematoxylin and eosin; original magnification, × 35.) **d.** Close-up of many dilated airways, some of which are filled with mucinous material. (Hematoxylin and eosin; original magnification, × 54.) **e.** Marked "condensation" of elastic fibers (*stained black*) in a subpleural location. (Movat; original magnification, × 54.) **f.** Another subpleural scar showing two pulmonary veins with narrowed lumina due to severe fibromuscular intimal proliferation. The lung parenchyma at the right is relatively intact. (Movat; original magnification, × 54.)

diameter of the small airways is always larger than the adjacent pulmonary artery. Using this as a criterion, 70% of the patients had narrowed airways and 30%, normal or dilated airways. All of those with dilated airways had narrowed airways in other areas of the biopsy.

Cholesterol-ester clefts were found in air spaces in 43% of our patients (Figure 3*G*). In a previous study (124), we suggested that these lesions indicate pulmonary hypertension. As a correlate of this finding, 70% of our biopsies showed thickening of the walls of the muscular pulmonary arteries by both medial hypertrophy and fibrous intimal proliferation. All patients with cholesterol clefts had these

Table 3. Histologic Observations from Open Lung Biopsies in 29 Patients with Idiopathic Pulmonary Fibrosis

Finding	Percent of Patients	Mild	Moderate	Severe
		←	%	→
Alveolar septal fibrosis	100	23	23	54
Interstitial inflammation	97	33	54	13
Alveolar "desquamation"	100	50	43	7
Cuboidalization of alveolar lining cells	100	33	27	40
Narrowed airways	70			
Normal or dilated airways	30			
Cholesterol-ester clefts	43			
Thickened pulmonary arteries	70			
Smooth-muscle proliferation	83			
Cystic changes	53			
Lymphoid nodules	50			
Granulomas	0			
Arteritis	0			

pulmonary arterial changes consistent with pulmonary hypertension. It also was noted that all of the patients with the more severe degree of interstitial fibrosis had concomitant pulmonary arterial changes.

Increased amounts of smooth muscle were seen in the interstitium in 83% of the patients. Smooth muscle proliferation is a recognized phenomenon in patients with idiopathic pulmonary fibrosis (125), but it is not clear whether this represents smooth muscle cells or rather increased numbers of interstitial mesenchymal cells with actin filaments, such as those described by Kapanci and associates (126).

Collections of lymphocytes in the lung parenchyma, some with centrally located histiocytes, were observed in half of the biopsies. This apparent increase in the number of parenchymal cells with the potential for immune competence may have significance in relation to the immune system abnormalities in idiopathic pulmonary fibrosis that will be discussed later.

Patients with idiopathic pulmonary fibrosis do not have arteritis, granulomas, or evidence of minerals in the lung (24, 102, 127-129). This important distinguishing feature of idiopathic pulmonary fibrosis is one of the major justifications for lung biopsy in these patients, because the presence of any of these abnormalities rules out idiopathic pulmonary fibrosis and indicates other possible disorders such as polyarteritis, extrinsic allergic alveolitis, or silicosis, all of which call for different therapeutic approaches.

The Chest X ray in Idiopathic Pulmonary Fibrosis

Dr. Morton L. Moss*: A detailed review of the chest X rays of this group of patients with idiopathic pulmonary fibrosis showed six radiographic patterns. The dominant patterns were reticular, reticulonodular, and ground glass (Figure 5). Seen less often were localized linear densities, nodular densities, and so-called "ill-defined" densities. In general, the radiographic findings of idiopathic pulmonary fibrosis involved both lungs equally but were predominant in the lower lung zones. Occasionally, these abnormalities were lobar or confined to the upper lung zones.

Reticular pattern refers to the netlike appearance of linear or curvilinear densities, or both, that are probably derived from the interstitial septal fibrosis and inflammation (130). The random orientation of the reticular net differentiates it from pulmonary vascular markings that are radially distributed from the hila. The reticular pattern can vary because of the thickness of the linear or curvilinear densities themselves, or because of the size of the translucent air spaces. These variables yield overall reticular patterns that can be defined as having fine, medium, or coarse textures. In general, the texture was fine early in the disease, with densities of less than 1 mm in width. As the disease progressed the texture coarsened, and the densities often were several millimeters in diameter. "Honeycombing," seen late in the disease, refers to a coarse reticular pattern with the translucencies measuring 0.5 cm to 1.0 cm in diameter (131, 132) (Figure 5*a*).

A reticulonodular pattern results from the superimposition of nodular densities (representing alveolitis, superimposition of thickened interstitium, or interstitium on end) on a reticular pattern (Figure 5*b*) (131). A ground glass pattern typically has a homogeneous, hazy appearance, probably resulting from an alveolitis (Figure 5*c*) (130). When this pattern surrounds airways, air bronchograms can be found, even though the lung is functional and not consolidated (Figure 5*d*) (130).

Less often, patients with idiopathic pulmonary fibrosis had localized areas of linear, nodular, or "ill-defined" densities either alone, in combination with each other, or in combination with the three more widespread patterns of reticular, reticulonodular, or ground glass densities. The isolated linear densities were often in the form of Kerley-B lines. Localized linear densities are probably an early form of the reticular pattern, while nodular and ill-defined densities are localized areas of alveolitis. The nodular densities are usually discrete 0.2- cm to 1.0-cm shadows, while ill-defined densities are poorly marginated and range from 1 cm to large amorphous densities of 4 cm to 5 cm.

Evaluation of the X rays of patients who have been followed from the onset of symptoms suggested that the radiographic evolution of idiopathic pulmonary fibrosis in our series was in general agreement with the data of Livingstone and co-workers (13). X rays of patients in the early course of disease showed localized linear, nodular, or "ill-defined" densities or a ground glass pattern, probably representing the alveolitis of idiopathic pulmonary fibrosis. With progression of the disease, reticular and reticulonodular patterns began to appear. In later stages the diaphragms were elevated, the pulmonary arteries were dilated, and a coarse reticular pattern developed. Terminal stages usually showed coarse reticulation often associated with cystic lesions and bullae. The cystic lesions were usually seen in the upper zones (132), although the bullae were randomly distributed. No matter how extensive their disease, patients with idiopathic pulmonary fibrosis seldom had fissure displacement or mediastinal shift. Occasionally, there was pleural thickening but never pleural effusion.

To evaluate the chest X ray as a tool in the diagnosis and

* Staff Radiologist, Diagnostic Radiology, Clinical Center.

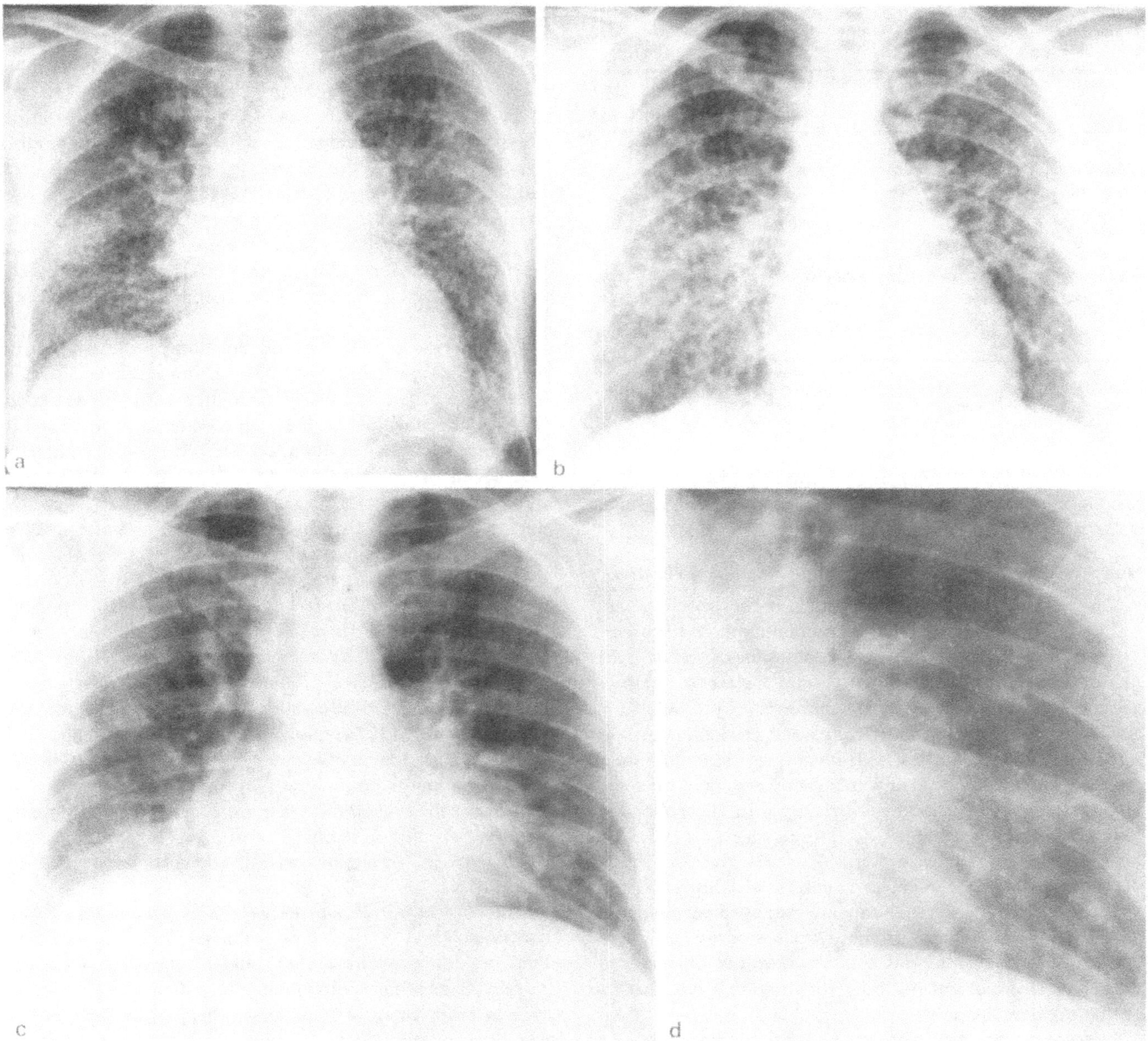

Figure 5. Three dominant radiographic patterns seen in patients with idiopathic pulmonary fibrosis. **a.** Coarse reticular pattern in a 56-year-old woman with symptoms for 4 years. Typical "honeycombing" is seen in the left lower lung field. **b.** Reticulonodular pattern in a 31-year-old woman with a 6-month history of progressive breathlessness after a flulike illness. **c.** Ground glass pattern in a 42-year-old man with symptoms for 2 years. **d.** A close-up of the left lower lung field of the X ray in panel C showing the homogeneous hazy appearance with air bronchograms.

staging of idiopathic pulmonary fibrosis, we graded the films of these patients as to the type and extensiveness of roentgenographic pattern and compared these data with the morphologic and physiologic findings. These comparisons showed a positive correlation between roentgenographic patterns indicating alveolitis and morphologic findings of marked cellularity. Furthermore, the honeycombing seen on chest X ray correlated well with the morphologic finding of cystic lesions accompanying severe fibrosis. Interestingly, there was a poor correlation between the degree of fibrosis seen on lung biopsy and the severity of disease estimated by chest film. However, this was not too surprising because the radiographic correlate of the fibrotic process can be masked by concomitant alveolitis. Furthermore, the chest X ray can, on rare occasion, be normal with morphologic evidence of fibrotic disease. In general, there was good agreement between the radiographic estimate of lung volume and the physiologic determination of lung volume by inert gas or body plethysmography. There was, however, no correlation between the degree of reduction in other physiologic variables and the radiologic estimate of severity of disease.

These comparisons would suggest that the chest X ray is useful in early idiopathic pulmonary fibrosis for a rough estimation of disease activity (for example, alveolitis). In midcourse idiopathic pulmonary fibrosis, X rays are not as reliable as physiologic and morphologic evaluations to gauge severity of disease and degree of fibrosis. They are

Table 4. Comparison of the Laboratory Evaluation of Idiopathic Pulmonary Fibrosis and the Degree of Fibrosis Found on Open Lung Biopsy Specimens

Physiologic Study	Correlation with Histopathology*
Chest X ray	Poor
Vital capacity	Poor
Total lung capacity	Poor
Diffusing capacity	Poor
Coefficient of retraction	Good
Resting arterial oxygen tension (Po_2)	Poor
Resting alveolar-arterial oxygen gradient ($D[A\text{-}a]o_2$)	Poor
Change in arterial Pao_2 and $D(A\text{-}a)o_2$ with exercise	Good

* The degree of fibrosis on the open lung biopsy specimens of 18 patients with idiopathic pulmonary fibrosis were graded as noted in Table 3. These rankings were compared with the physiologic values using a Spearmen rank correlation: poor = $P > 0.05$; good = $P < 0.05$.

of value again in later stages of disease for detecting cystic lesions and severe fibrosis (for example, coarse reticular pattern).

New Physiologic Concepts of Idiopathic Pulmonary Fibrosis

Dr. Fulmer: From the discussions of the histologic and radiographic features of idiopathic pulmonary fibrosis, a general pattern of the disease process emerges. It most likely begins as an alveolitis (ground glass or nodular appearance radiographically; inflammatory cells and "desquamation" seen histologically) and gradually develops into alveolar septal fibrosis (reticular or reticulonodular appearance radiographically; increasing numbers of alveolar septae appear fibrotic histologically). In all probability, idiopathic pulmonary fibrosis is a reversible process in the alveolitis stage, but once fibrosis occurs the anatomical derangements of the alveolar-capillary bed are such that affected portions of parenchyma are damaged permanently.

Therefore, assessment of the overall progression of disease must include methods that monitor the fibrotic process. This is important not only for prognosis but also for evaluating new therapies.

In common practice, patients with idiopathic pulmonary fibrosis are followed by four variables: the chest X ray, lung volumes (vital capacity or total lung capacity, or both), diffusion capacity, and resting arterial oxygen tension (12, 17, 133, 134). However, in our group of patients, none of these variables correlate with the degree of fibrosis determined histologically (Table 4). This, however, is not as surprising as it appears. As described earlier, the chest X ray, lung volumes, diffusing capacity, or resting Po_2 can be normal in patients with moderate degrees of fibrosis. In addition, there is often no overall correlation between the clinical severity of the disease (for example, what the patient feels) and any of these variables. Even the resting alveolar-arterial oxygen gradient, which was abnormal in 97% of our patients, does not correlate with the degree of fibrosis on the biopsy specimens (Table 4).

If the chest X ray, lung volumes, diffusing capacity, and resting arterial oxygen tension do not correlate with the degree of fibrosis in idiopathic pulmonary fibrosis, what physiologic tools can be used to stage and follow the fibrotic process? The two most useful variables are the volume-pressure curve for staging fibrosis (mild, moderate, or severe; *see* Table 3), and the exercise study to both stage and follow the fibrotic process.

To establish the usefulness of the static deflation volume-pressure curve in idiopathic pulmonary fibrosis (Figure 2), we correlated the degree of fibrosis on open lung biopsy with the slope ($\Delta V/\Delta P$) (115) and position (defined as the static transpulmonary pressure at 70% total lung capacity) of the curve; the maximum static transpulmonary pressure (Pst max) (116); and Pst max/observed total lung capacity (the coefficient of retraction) (135).

Comparison of $\Delta V/\Delta P$ and position of the curve with the morphologic grading of fibrosis showed that although a decreased slope is usually associated with the degree of fibrosis, the position of the volume-pressure curve (shift to right or left) does not correlate with the morphologic assessment of the degree of fibrosis. In contrast, Pst max did correlate with the degree of fibrosis; that is, as the degree of fibrosis increased, more transpulmonary pressure was required to achieve full inspiration. However, Pst max is not the perfect variable for staging the fibrosis of idiopathic pulmonary fibrosis because normal young persons can often develop large negative transpulmonary pressures (135, 136). The coefficient of retraction also correlates with the degree of fibrosis but more clearly separates patients with idiopathic pulmonary fibrosis from normal persons (135). Our current data suggest, however, that although the coefficient of retraction is useful for staging idiopathic pulmonary fibrosis, it may not be as useful in following the disease process because if patients improve without a major increase in lung volumes, the coefficient of retraction usually does not change significantly.

The lack of correlation between static monitors of lung function (chest X ray, lung volumes, diffusing capacity, Pao_2, volume-pressure curves) and progression of the disease explains what is obvious to the patient: as the disease evolves from early to midcourse, the patient feels fine at rest but invariably gives a history of breathlessness and fatigue with exercise. The physiologic correlate of this may be the decrease in Pao_2 with exercise that is always found (Figure 2). It is difficult, however, to quantitate exercise studies in these patients because the maximum amount of work they can do depends not only on their pulmonary status but also on their cardiovascular system, muscle

Table 5. Physiologic Evaluation of Airways in Patients with Idiopathic Pulmonary Fibrosis

Study	Patients with Abnormal Results
	%
$FEV_1\%$*	0
Airway resistance by body plethysmography	0
Dynamic compliance	70
Maximum expiratory flow-volume curves	45
Maximum flow-static recoil curve	31

* Forced expiratory volume in 1 sec/forced vital capacity.

strength, efficiency of muscle use, and willingness to achieve maximum effort (114). To obviate these problems, we have "normalized" the change in Pa_{O_2} and $D(A\text{-}a)\,O_2$ during exercise (Figure 2) to the relative amount of work done. The latter is directly proportional to oxygen consumption ($\dot{V}O_2$), so we have used $\Delta PO_2/\Delta\dot{V}O_2$ and $\Delta(D[A\text{-}a]O_2)/\Delta\dot{V}O_2$ to correlate with the degree of fibrosis in open lung biopsy specimens. There is a significant correlation between both exercise variables and degree of fibrosis (Table 4), and thus these measurements are extremely useful in staging the degree of fibrosis in idiopathic pulmonary fibrosis. We have also used the $\Delta PO_2/\Delta\dot{V}O_2$ and $\Delta(D[A\text{-}a]O_2)/\Delta\dot{V}O_2$ obtained in serial exercise studies to follow several patients for more than 1.5 years; so far the data show that this quantitative approach to exercise physiology is a sensitive and objective method of following the temporal changes in the fibrotic process (Figure 6).

As we discussed earlier, the major cause of hypoxemia in idiopathic pulmonary fibrosis has been attributed to ventilation-perfusion imbalance (40). Because air flow mechanics ($FEV_1\%$, airway resistance by body plethysmography) are usually normal in these patients (38, 39, 111), the abnormalities in distribution of ventilation have been ascribed to regional alterations in compliance (39). However, in other diseases such as asthma, recent data suggest that small airways disease, undetectable by $FEV_1\%$ and plethysmography methods, can result in significant ventilation-perfusion mismatching that causes hypoxemia (137-139). Nevertheless, when tests of small airways function such as dynamic compliance (140), maximum expiratory flow-volume curves (141), and maximum flow-static recoil curves (115, 142) are used to evaluate patients with idiopathic pulmonary fibrosis, a significant number show abnormal results (143, 144) (Table 5). This physiologic evidence of small airway disease correlates well with the morphologic observations that the small airways in idiopathic pulmonary fibrosis have peribronchiolar fibrosis and inflammation and that 70% of the patients with this disease show narrowed airways (Table 3). The clear association of abnormal physiologic function of small airways with the morphologic evidence of disease of these airways suggests that at least part of the ventilation abnormalities, and hence hypoxemia, of idiopathic pulmonary fibrosis may be due to small airways disease.

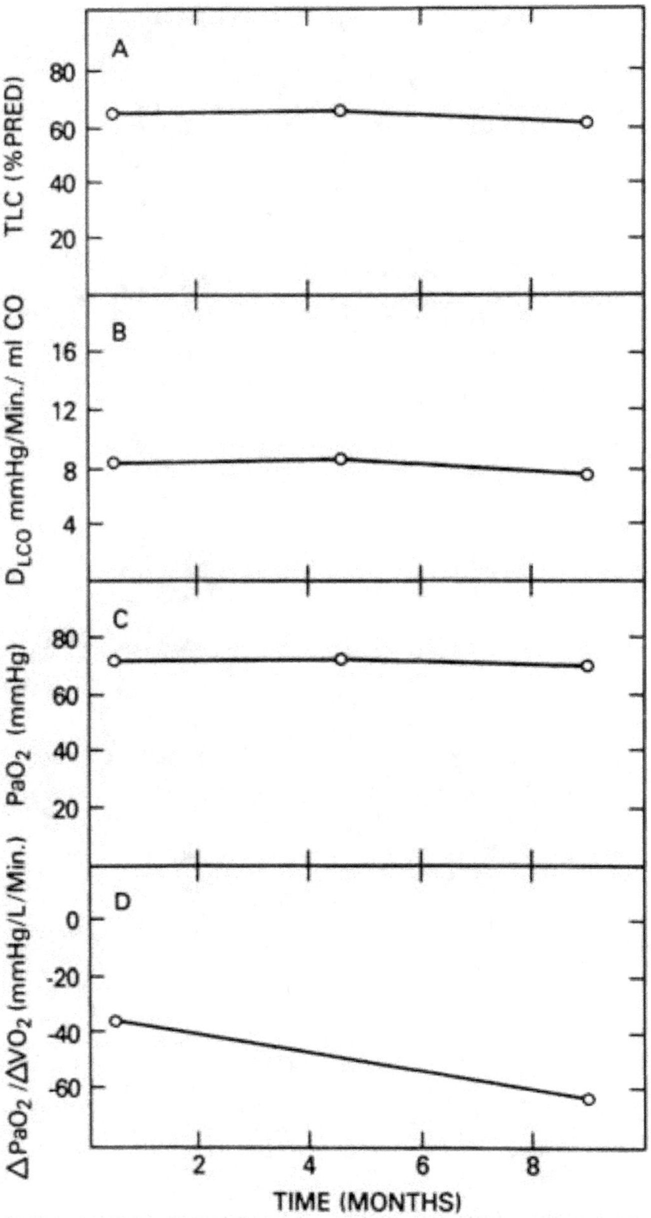

Figure 6. Temporal changes. A. In total lung capacity (*TLC*). B. In diffusing capacity (DLco). C. In resting oxygen tension (Po_2). D. Change in Pa_{O_2} with exercise ($\Delta Pa_{O_2}/\Delta\dot{V}O_2$) in a 65-year-old woman with idiopathic pulmonary fibrosis. Over a 9-month period the patient developed progressive exertional breathlessness. The only objective finding was a further decrease in the $\Delta Pa_{O_2}/\Delta\dot{V}O_2$ on serial exercise testing.

Nuclear Scanning in Idiopathic Pulmonary Fibrosis

Dr. Bruce R. Line*: Nuclear scanning methods are useful in evaluating a chronic lung disorder such as idiopathic pulmonary fibrosis. Isotopic methods provide information about regional pulmonary function in terms of temporal and spatial tracer distribution images, in contrast to the static structural data provided by the standard chest X ray.

Three nuclear scanning methods are being used to study idiopathic pulmonary fibrosis: macroaggregated albumin labeled with technetium-99m (Tc-99m MAA) to evaluate lung perfusion; xenon-133 (^{133}Xe) or xenon-127 (^{127}Xe)† gas to evaluate ventilatory function; and gallium-67 citrate (^{67}Ga) to quantitate lung inflammation and hence the "alveolitis" of the disease.

The pulmonary capillary bed effectively filters particulate matter greater than 10 μm in diameter. After intravenous injection, particles of Tc-99m MAA (10 to 50 μm) mix with the right ventricular blood pool and are trapped in the pulmonary microcirculation. This microembolization produces little hemodynamic stress because fewer than one in 2000 capillaries are occluded (145, 146). The albumin particles are broken down and later consumed by the pulmonary reticuloendothelial system. The scintigraphic image obtained just after injection reflects the distribution of the

* Research Analyst, Division of Computer Research and Technology, and Clinical Associate, Department of Nuclear Medicine, Clinical Center.

† The recent availability of ^{127}Xe has resulted in a significant improvement in the quality of ventilation scans.

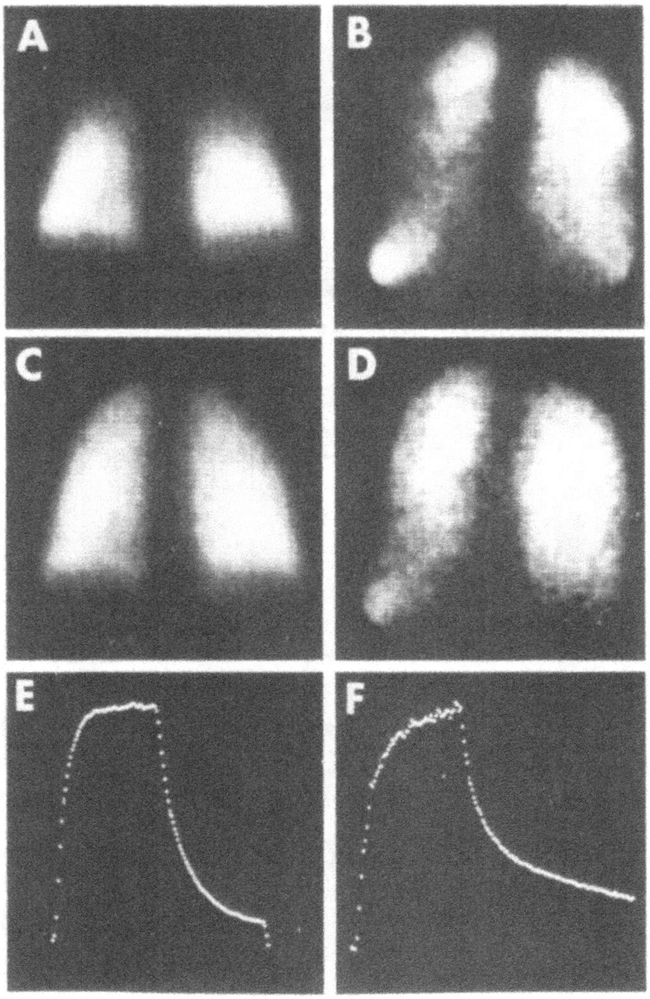

Figure 7. Perfusion and ventilation scans in a normal 57-year-old man (*A, C, E*) and a 48-year-old man with idiopathic pulmonary fibrosis (*B, D, F*). **A.** Normal perfusion scan with basal tracer prominence. **B.** Idiopathic pulmonary fibrosis perfusion scan; inhomogeneous pattern with marked upward shift. **C.** Normal equilibrium phase ventilation scan. **D.** Idiopathic pulmonary fibrosis equilibrium phase ventilation scan showing decreased tracer in the lower lung zones. **E.** Full thorax count profile of ventilation study showing normal wash-in, equilibrium, and wash-out phases. **F.** Rounded profile in idiopathic pulmonary fibrosis suggesting prolonged airspace time constants. The scans in A-D are all posterior views; the count profiles in E-F are also derived from posterior views.

right ventricular output. Because pulmonary blood flow is influenced by gravitational forces (147), a patient studied in the upright position normally shows little tracer in the upper lung zones with an increasing gradient of tracer intensity toward the lung base (Figure 7*A*). Excluding cardiac and diaphragmatic impressions, normal lung images show convex margins and have bilateral symmetry (148). Defects in tracer homogeneity may be related to a loss of capillary perfusion such as may accompany vasoconstriction in response to alveolar hypoxia (149) (pneumonia, asthma), parenchymal destruction (150) (idiopathic pulmonary fibrosis, emphysema), or pulmonary vascular occlusion (148) (embolic or thrombotic disease). Regional decreases in tracer localization may also be secondary to displacement of normal parenchyma by pleural fluid masses and bullae. In idiopathic pulmonary fibrosis, two basic findings appear in the perfusion scan: nonsegmental inhomogeneities and increased perfusion to the upper lung zones (Figure 7*B*).

These nonsegmental inhomogeneities are probably due to the localized loss of capillary bed and are usually seen in the lower lobes. Comparison of the chest X ray and the Tc-99m MAA scan shows correlation between areas of compromised perfusion and areas of reticular, reticulonodular, or ground glass densities, or a combination of these. Patients with idiopathic pulmonary fibrosis can also have nonsegmental inhomogeneities of the perfusion scan in radiographically normal areas, suggesting that a local deficit in capillary perfusion may be present before abnormalities are seen on the chest film.

Pulmonary hypertension has been associated with an upward shift in the gradient of capillary perfusion and a corresponding increase in apical tracer in upright perfusion images (110, 151). This has proven valuable in substantiating the diagnosis of pulmonary hypertension in patients with idiopathic pulmonary fibrosis.

The patency of airways and the functional integrity of alveoli can be assessed using the ventilation scan (152, 153). In comparison to the perfusion scan, which reflects the static distribution of macromolecules trapped in the pulmonary capillary bed, the ventilation scan is more complex, as it measures the dynamic bronchoalveolar distribution of a tracer gas. In the ventilation study, the patient rebreathes a mixture of tracer and air ("wash-in" phase) until the radioactivity measured over the chest stays constant ("equilibrium" phase). The patient then breathes room air until all of the radioactive gas leaves the lungs ("wash-out" phase).

The equilibrium picture of ^{127}Xe distribution reflects the relative proportion of lung that is being ventilated. For example, little radioactivity would be detected over areas of pneumonia or noncommunicating bullae. Patients with idiopathic pulmonary fibrosis have patchy, nonsegmental areas of decreased ventilation, reflecting regions of airway obstruction or alveolar destruction (Figures 7*C, D*). The equilibrium scintigraphs have been useful for detecting marginally functional parenchyma and indicating the presence of noncommunicating cysts or bullae in patients with idiopathic pulmonary fibrosis.

If the count rates over the lung fields are summed and plotted versus time, a curve is generated describing the rate of tracer accumulation or release from the lung. Patients with normal airways and alveoli will have a curve that is nearly "square," indicating rapid wash-in, flat equilibrium, and rapid wash-out phases (Figure 7*E*). With dysfunction of airways or alveoli, or both, the wash-in and wash-out phases are prolonged, so that the curve is rounded. About 70% of our patients showed a spectrum of abnormal curves, reflecting a slowness to come to equilibrium (Figure 7*F*). Regions of decreased compliance (for example, interstitial fibrosis) produce fast wash-in and wash-out phases. Therefore studies yielding prolonged phases indicate areas of increased compliance (such as the cystic areas of idiopathic pulmonary fibrosis) or airway dysfunction (such as the small airway disease of idiopathic pulmonary fibrosis).

The equilibrium phase (representing the total ventilated volume in each lung region) and the wash-out phase (representing the change in count rate per unit time in each region) may be combined to indicate the relative volume exchanged in each lung area per unit time (154, 155). This is computed in approximately one thousand small areas of the lung to generate a picture of dynamic regional ventilation. Whereas normal patients have homogeneous patterns of dynamic volume exchange, patients with idiopathic pulmonary fibrosis show disparity between lung zones, reflecting cystic areas or small airway disease (Figures 8*A* and *B*).

The data from the ventilation and perfusion scans can be combined to produce an image of the relative ventilation-perfusion ratio of each small region of the lung fields. In idiopathic pulmonary fibrosis, there is a general patchiness to the ventilation-perfusion matching throughout the lung. In addition, there is often a shift in perfusion to the upper lobes (reflecting pulmonary hypertension) so that areas of relatively low ventilation-perfusion ratios are seen in the upper zones (Figures 8*C* and *D*). This image has been used to estimate the proportion of regions with low ventilation-perfusion ratios such as functional shunt, as well as the proportion of areas of high ventilation-perfusion ratios such as areas of wasted ventilation. These findings support the concept that a significant portion of hypoxemia in patients with idiopathic pulmonary fibrosis is due to ventilation-perfusion mismatching (39, 40) and also confirm that the high dead space to tidal volume ratio found at rest in many of these patients (7, 12, 112) is well founded on anatomic grounds.

As discussed in the sections on the histology and radiology of idiopathic pulmonary fibrosis, alveolar inflammation is probably an early manifestation of the disease process. Whereas physiologic methods can detect the fibrotic process (coefficient of retraction, exercise $\Delta Po_2/\Delta \dot{V}o_2$), it has been extremely difficult to evaluate alveolar inflammation in this disease without resorting to repeated lung biopsies. Gallium-67 scanning has been investigated as a means to follow the alveolitis of idiopathic pulmonary fibrosis because studies have shown that this isotope localizes in regions of inflammation (156, 157). For example, ^{67}Ga will localize in the chest in disorders as diverse as pulmonary abscess, active tuberculosis, active sarcoidosis, silicosis, pleurisy, and bacterial pneumonia (158, 159). Although each condition varies in cause and histology, all are inflammatory disorders, and scan visualization gradually diminishes in intensity after appropriate therapy (156). Gallium-67 is used to detect and characterize the inflammation of idiopathic pulmonary fibrosis because it binds to neutrophils (probably in lysosomes) (157, 160), cells that are clearly found in the parenchyma in idiopathic pulmonary fibrosis.

Patients are scanned 48 to 72 h after the intravenous administration of 50 μCi of ^{67}Ga citrate/kg body weight. At the time of study, the tracer distributes primarily to liver, spleen, and skeletal tissues, with very little to normal lung (161,162). Sixty-seven percent of ^{67}Ga scans in patients with idiopathic pulmonary fibrosis showed increased pulmonary localization, whereas only 5% of control subjects showed an increase (163) (Figures 8*E* and *F*).

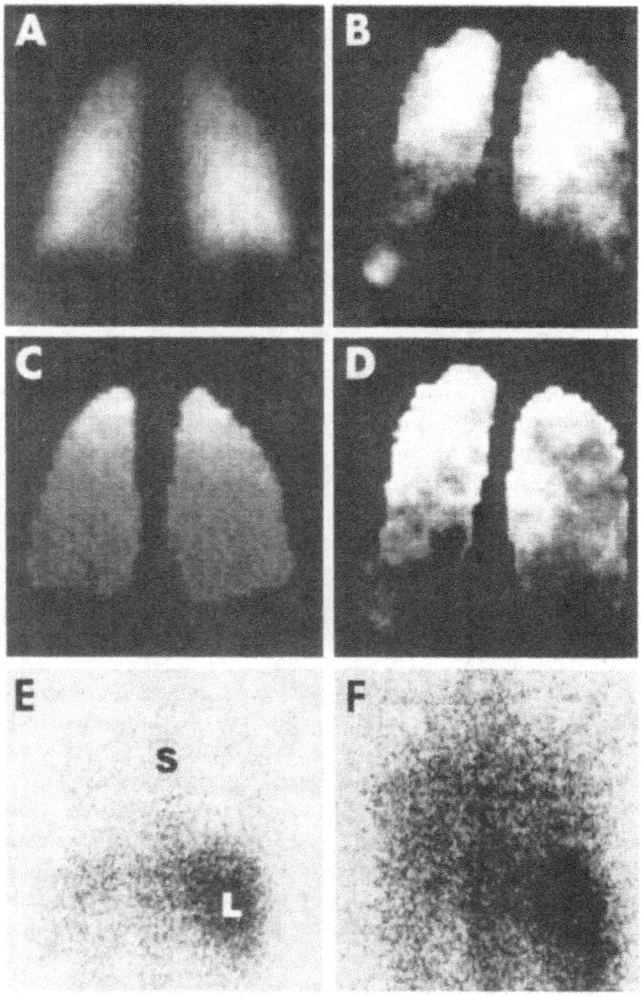

Figure 8. Dynamic ventilation, ventilation-perfusion, and gallium scans in a normal 57-year-old man (*A, C, E*) and a 48-year-old man with idiopathic pulmonary fibrosis (*B, D, F*). **A.** Normal dynamic ventilation; brighter regions indicate higher regional volume exchange per unit time. **B.** Idiopathic pulmonary fibrosis dynamic ventilation; patent but poorly ventilated basilar airspaces. **C.** Normal ventilation-perfusion ratio (V/Q) map; bright regions = high V/Q (relative dead space); gray = "good" V/Q match; dark = low V/Q (relative shunt). **D.** Same study as C but in idiopathic pulmonary fibrosis; there are patchy areas of high and low V/Q with fewer areas of "good" V/Q match compared with normal. **E.** Normal gallium scan; L= liver; S = spine; almost no gallium is taken up by normal parenchyma. **F.** Gallium scan in idiopathic pulmonary fibrosis showing prominent basilar tracer uptake, suggesting areas of active inflammation.

As a rule, interpretations of gallium scans are qualitative and include statements related to the presence and distribution of abnormal ^{67}Ga localization. It is difficult to quantitatively assess the degree of abnormality because of the wide spectrum of physiologic and technical influences on the ^{67}Ga image. However, by characterizing the percentage of lung involvement, the intensity of uptake, and the distribution of abnormalities, it is possible to rank the relative abnormality of gallium scans in idiopathic pulmonary fibrosis. Preliminary studies have shown that this quantitative assessment correlates well with the grading of alveolar and interstitial cellularity on open lung biopsy specimens of these patients. Thus the ^{67}Ga scan is a noninvasive, safe*, semiquantitative method of assessing the status of inflammation in idiopathic pulmonary fibrosis that may prove useful both in staging disease process and in evaluating the efficacy of treatment.

Bronchoalveolar Lavage in Idiopathic Pulmonary Fibrosis

Dr. Herbert Y. Reynolds†: One of the major limitations to understanding the pathogenesis of idiopathic pulmonary fibrosis is the inability to obtain samples of the same lung at different stages of the disease. However, the advent of the flexible fiberoptic bronchoscope and its adaptation to bronchoalveolar lavage has made it possible to evaluate repeatedly a representative sample of the fluid bathing the bronchoalveolar epithelial surface (165-167). We have adapted this method to study patients with idiopathic pulmonary fibrosis in order to [1] describe the cellular and protein components of their lower respiratory tract; [2] evaluate possible immune mechanisms that may contribute to the pathogenesis and continued activity of the disease; [3] determine if the therapy of idiopathic pulmonary fibrosis alters these components; and [4] correlate the cellular analysis of bronchoalveolar lavage fluid with the histologic findings.

We studied the bronchoalveolar lavage fluid in 19 of our 29 patients. To put these findings in perspective, we compared them to findings in seven patients with chronic hypersensitivity pneumonitis and 32 control subjects.

In all of these studies, the amount of lavage fluid retrieved varied from 31% to 48%. From the patients with idiopathic pulmonary fibrosis, an average of 18 million cells were recovered, with almost two times more cells found in fluid from untreated patients than treated patients. Interestingly, patients with idiopathic pulmonary fibrosis who did not smoke had more cells than those who did smoke; this is opposite to that found in control subjects (smokers normally have more than two times the cells of nonsmokers) (165). In general, patients with idiopathic pulmonary fibrosis had more cells recovered than those with chronic hypersensitivity pneumonitis, who in turn had more cells recovered than controls.

The variety in the types of cells recovered in lavage clearly distinguished the different local cellular responses of idiopathic pulmonary fibrosis and chronic hypersensitivity pneumonitis from each other and from controls (Table 6) (168). In general, patients with idiopathic pulmonary fibrosis had significant evidence of inflammation of the lower respiratory tract (an average of 33% neutrophils). The finding of these numbers of neutrophils in the lower respiratory tract was striking, since neutrophils in control lavage always represent less than 3% of the total cells. With treatment, perhaps secondary to corticosteroids, bronchoalveolar inflammation in idiopathic pulmonary fibrosis diminished (average neutrophils reduced to 14%, $P < 0.05$). Also striking was the invariable presence of eosinophils, a cell type almost never found in controls (165). In contrast to the reduction of lavage neutrophils with therapy, corticosteroids did not seem to influence the eosinophilic response in patients with idiopathic pulmonary fibrosis. Because these patients do not have a peripheral leukocytosis or eosinophilia, the findings suggest a local cellular response in the fluid bathing the bronchoalveolar epithelial surface. This is further strengthened by a comparison of the cells of patients with idiopathic pulmonary fibrosis to those of patients with chronic hypersensitivity pneumonitis. Lavage fluid of the latter group has an average of five times more lymphocytes than found in idiopathic pulmonary fibrosis, and an average of three times more lymphocytes than in controls.

The cell differential on bronchoalveolar lavage fluid in both groups of patients seems to correlate well with the histologic findings on open lung biopsy. Our findings corroborate those of Davis and co-workers (169), who have found cell analysis to be an accurate indicator of the alveolar cellular content in idiopathic pulmonary fibrosis. In addition, the lavage differential in idiopathic pulmonary fibrosis can predict which patients will show positive ^{67}Ga scans; those with more neutrophils tend to have more positive ^{67}Ga scans (163), as would be predicted from the evidence that ^{67}Ga is localized to areas of inflammation.

Quantitative determination of immunoglobulins (165-167) can also distinguish patients with idiopathic pulmonary fibrosis from control subjects and from patients with chronic hypersensitivity pneumonitis (Table 6). Compared with controls, both groups of patients have elevated IgG. Decreased IgE is seen only in patients with idiopathic pulmonary fibrosis, and IgM is found only in patients with chronic hypersensitivity pneumonitis. Therapy of idiopathic pulmonary fibrosis seems to reduce the bronchoalveolar fluid IgG levels, just as it reduces the neutrophil levels.

Not only are the IgG levels in lavage fluid from patients with idiopathic pulmonary fibrosis greater than those of controls, they are also more than two times higher than one would expect from transudation of serum alone*. Thus, the disease is probably associated with the local production of IgG or abnormalities in the mechanisms of lung IgG catabolism, or both. Part of the pathogenesis of idiopathic pulmonary fibrosis may be secondary to lung injury from locally produced IgG antibody in response to one or more as yet unidentified antigens. There is no evidence, however, of local complement use, since lavage fluid C4 and C6 levels were normal in idiopathic pulmonary fibrosis (Table 6).

These findings, together with the lack of elevated IgE or decreased complement, suggest that in this disorder the lung may act as a relatively independent immune organ; the immune reactions in this disease probably are not mediated by complement; and idiopathic pulmonary fibrosis is probably not an allergic disorder mediated by IgE (171, 172).

We have shown that limited bronchoalveolar lavage is an important tool for characterizing and understanding pulmonary disorders such as idiopathic pulmonary fibrosis.

* The total body dose of ^{67}Ga ordinarily amounts to less than 300 mrad/mCi of administered material (164).

† Chief, Pulmonary Section, Department of Medicine, Yale University School of Medicine, New Haven, Connecticut; formerly, Head, Section of Bacterial Diseases, Laboratory of Clinical Investigation, National Institute of Allergy and Infectious Diseases.

* The most rational basis for comparison of lavage proteins is to albumin, a protein synthesized external to lung that leaks across the alveolus and thus is representative of serum transudation (165-167, 170).

We have done this procedure in more than 150 patients with all forms of pulmonary disease. It is a simple extension of routine fiberoptic bronchoscopy and is well tolerated by patients. Analysis of the cell and protein content of the recovered lavage fluid is a direct attempt to evaluate those mechanisms that may contribute to the continued activity of the chronic lung disorders. These methods may also prove useful in following the response to specific therapy.

Biochemical Concepts and Overall Perspective of Idiopathic Pulmonary Fibrosis

Dr. Crystal: To begin to understand the biochemical basis of idiopathic pulmonary fibrosis, we must try to define the biochemical components of the deranged alveolar interstitium. Fibrosis is a histologic term that refers to the light microscopic assessment of an apparent excess of collagen, the macromolecule that is the major component of scar tissue. From studies of normal lung, we know that the alveolar interstitium contains at least two (and probably more) forms of collagen, distinguished from each other by their different amino acid sequences. The two major forms of collagen in the alveolar interstitium are termed collagen type I and collagen type III (173-179). Type I is the characteristic fibrillar collagen found in skin, bone, tendon, blood vessels, and lung. Type III is probably reticulin and is found in skin, blood vessels, intestine, and lung but not in bone or tendon*. In the normal human lung parenchyma, the ratio of type I to type III collagen is approximately 2:1 (178).

With light microscopy, the concentration of collagen in lung tissue from patients with idiopathic pulmonary fibrosis appears to be significantly greater than normal. This, however, is not the case, and studies of open lung biopsy specimens clearly show that collagen per unit dry weight is normal (143, 182, 183). There are several possible explanations for this: [1] the common light microscopy stains for collagen probably identify only fibrillar collagen. It is possible that the sum of fibrillar plus nonfibrillar interstitial collagen in idiopathic pulmonary fibrosis is normal, but there is a shift toward fibrillar collagen, thus giving the appearance of a relative increase in interstitial collagen; [2] collagen may be increased, but other lung components also increase in proportion, so that collagen per unit weight is constant; and [3] idiopathic pulmonary fibrosis is a disease of collagen rearrangement (more in some areas than others) rather than a total increase in fibrotic tissue. As we will see, all three still remain viable alternatives.

In other fibrotic disorders such as atherosclerosis, the ratio of type I to type III collagen increases (184). A recent study (178) of postmortem lung suggested that this is also true in idiopathic pulmonary fibrosis. Although type III collagen can form cross-banded fibers, it also exists in a loose fibril form. Thus, a change in the I/III ratio toward type I (but with the sum of I + III constant) might give the appearance of an increase in interstitial collagen when evaluated by light microscopy. Analagous to this hypothesis is the finding that tissues that are relatively compliant (fetal skin, lung, intestine, blood vessels) have a low type I/type III ratio (185); tissues with less compliance (adult skin, atherosclerotic blood vessel) have a higher ratio of type I to type III (184-186); and tissues that are very rigid (bone, tendon) have only type I and no type III (185). The lung in idiopathic pulmonary fibrosis is less compliant (*see* Figure 2), so a shift toward type I in this disease is certainly in concert with the concept that "stiffness" in lung is associated with more type I collagen.

Biochemical studies have not yet been done to verify that interstitial components other than collagen increase in idiopathic pulmonary fibrosis; however, one has only to look at the biopsy of a patient to appreciate the vast cellularity of the disease (Figures 3*B* and *D*). This is important because it suggests that this is a disease not only of collagen, but of many other components as well (143).

The most difficult hypothesis to approach biochemically is the possibility that the major collagen-related problem in idiopathic pulmonary fibrosis is a derangement of the connective tissue components of the normal alveolar

Table 6. Cells and Relative Concentrations of Proteins in Bronchoalveolar Lavage Fluid of Patients with Idiopathic Pulmonary Fibrosis and Chronic Hypersensitivity Pneumonitis Compared to Controls*†

	Controls§	Idiopathic Pulmonary Fibrosis‡		Chronic Hypersensitivity Pneumonitis‖
		Without Therapy	With Therapy	
Cells**				
Neutrophils	0-3	I (3+)††	I (2+)	I (1+)
Lymphocytes	8-18	N	N	I (4+)
Eosinophils	0	I (1+)	I (1+)	I (1+)
Alveolar macrophages	80-89	D (3+)	D (1+)	D (4+)
Proteins‡‡				
IgG, *mg/mg*	0.1-0.6	I (2+)	I (1+)	I (3+)
IgE, *ng/mg*	10-65	D (1+)	D (1+)	N
IgA, *mg/mg*	0.2-1.9	N	N	N
IgM, *mg/mg*	0	A	A	I (2+)
C4, $\times 10^{-3}$ *titer/mg*	0.5-3.0	N	N	N
C6, *titer/mg*	1-9	N	N	N

*Lavage was always carried out by positioning the bronchoscope in the lingula (B4 or B5) and infusing 100 ml of sterile saline (30- to 40-ml aliquots, immediately aspirated by suction).

† The quantitative data in this table were derived from Reynolds et al, *J Clin Invest*, in press.

‡ Nineteen patients with idiopathic pulmonary fibrosis (12 nonsmokers, seven smokers; seven receiving no therapy, 12 receiving a mean dose of 24.4 ± 4.0 mg daily of prednisone).

§ Controls consisted of 32 patients (age and sex matched to the patients with idiopathic pulmonary fibrosis; 11 nonsmokers, 21 smokers) with undiagnosed lesions limited to the right upper lobe; none had evidence of disease in the left lung.

‖ Seven patients with chronic hypersensitivity pneumonitis had a history of chronic intermittent respiratory and systemic symptoms related to their home or work environment; five had antibodies to thermophylic actinomycetes; granulomas in lung histopathology and reexposure to probable antigens helped confirm the diagnoses.

** Data presented as percentage of total cells.

†† I = increased compared with controls; N = normal and equal to controls; D = decreased compared with controls; A = absent; relative changes are indicated as 1 + to 4 +.

‡‡ Data presented relative to the lavage fluid albumin concentration (*See* text and references 165-168, 170).

* Type I collagen is the cross-banded material typically seen on electron micrographs; it is most of the material in the normal alveolar interstitium that stains blue with Masson trichrome. Most of the fine loosely bound fibrils on electron micrographs are type III collagen; this material is the silver staining "reticulin" seen by light microscopy (180, 181).

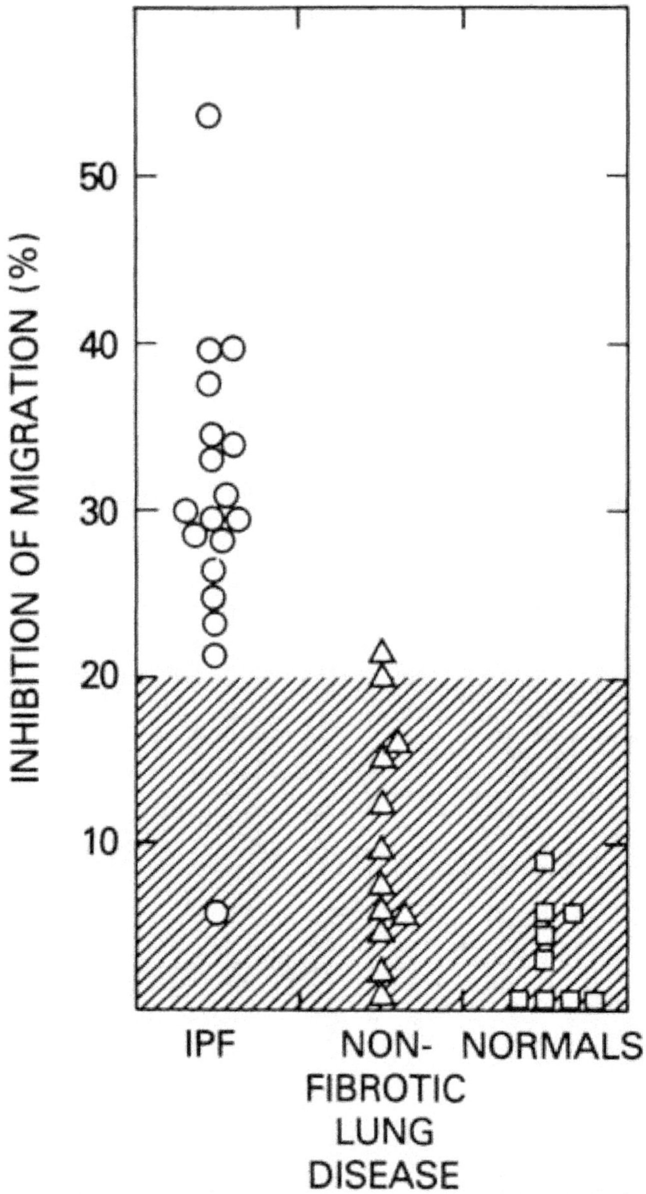

Figure 9. Collagen-induced production of migration inhibition factor by peripheral lymphocytes of patients with idiopathic pulmonary fibrosis. Lymphocytes were isolated from peripheral blood and exposed to 25 μg/ml of type I human lung collagen; production of migration inhibition factor was assayed using guinea pig peritoneal macrophages. Greater than 20% inhibition of migration was considered positive. Production of migration inhibition factor by lymphocytes of patients with idiopathic pulmonary fibrosis was completely obviated by exposing these lymphocytes to antihuman T-cell antiserum before incubation with the collagen antigen (187). Lymphocytes of patients with nonfibrotic lung disease seldom produce migration inhibition factor in response to collagen; lymphocytes of normal persons never do.

interstitium. We began by postulating that if collagen per unit weight was normal, perhaps it was turning over so rapidly that it would, by necessity, become deranged. To evaluate this, we quantitated the rate of collagen synthesis per cell in open lung biopsy specimens from our patients. However, in the eight biopsies evaluated thus far, the rate of collagen synthesis per cell (13.4 ± 2.6 μg of collagen/cell · h) is not significantly different from normal (15.9 ± 4.9 μg of collagen/cell · h) (143, 183). Thus, we have no evidence that collagen turns over more rapidly in idiopathic pulmonary fibrosis than normal.

As another, but much more indirect, approach to the question of derangement of the connective tissue in the idiopathic pulmonary fibrosis alveolar interstitium, we hypothesized that a derangement of collagen in the alveolar interstitium might result in the recognition of collagen as antigenic by the immune system. In studies in collaboration with Kravis and associates of the Navy Medical Research Institute (187), we showed that more than 95% of patients with idiopathic pulmonary fibrosis have circulating lymphocytes that produce lymphokines (migration inhibition factor) when exposed to type I collagen (Figure 9). In addition, these circulating lymphocytes will lyse collagen-coated erythrocytes. Studies with antihuman T-cell antiserum showed that these cell-mediated phenomena require viable T-cells to show these effects. These experiments indirectly suggest that collagen has become "non-self" in patients with idiopathic pulmonary fibrosis, a possible result of the anatomic derangement of the alveolar interstitium. These findings also suggest that a possible pathogenic mechanism in idiopathic pulmonary fibrosis is the continued injury to the alveolar interstitium by secretory products of cells such as macrophages that aggregate to sites of alveolar inflammation by collagen-induced cell-mediated immune phenomena.

However, the finding that collagen becomes antigenic to persons with idiopathic pulmonary fibrosis does not answer the question as to what triggers the disease. Perhaps clues to future studies lie in the historical information from patients with the disease, 25% to 40% of whom clearly relate that their disease began after a viral syndrome accompanied by chest symptoms. This, together with the reported familial clusterings of idiopathic pulmonary fibrosis (188-194), and our recent finding* of relative increases in HLA-12 and HLA-29 in patients with no family history of the disorder suggest that there may be predispositions to the disease, perhaps associated with cell surface antigens that could be altered by lung injury.

Regardless of the trigger of idiopathic pulmonary fibrosis, we now have several lines of evidence that strongly suggest that therapeutic intervention should be directed toward stopping the inflammatory and immune process, rather than toward stopping the fibrotic process.

1. Histologic observations clearly show that early aspects of the disease are highly cellular, with alveolar inflammation predominating. This concurs with the suggestion by Scadding and Hinson (18) that patients with "cellular" biopsies respond better to corticosteroids than those with late stages of fibrosis, and the suggestion by Carrington and co-workers (195) that patients with "desquamative interstitial pneumonitis" (that is, early idiopathic pulmonary fibrosis) also respond better to therapy.

2. The radiographic features of the disease suggest inflammation early in the course, fibrosis later.

3. The uptake of ^{67}Ga by 67% of these patients strongly suggests the lung parenchyma has areas of active neutrophilic inflammation.

* Fulmer JD, Spasovska M, Mittal K, et al: Unpublished.

4. Bronchoalveolar lavage in these patients shows elevated levels of neutrophils and IgG.

5. There is clear evidence of T-cell-mediated processes directed against collagen in this disease (187).

6. There is no evidence of increased amounts of collagen or increased rates of collagen synthesis in the lung parenchyma of patients with idiopathic pulmonary fibrosis (143, 182, 183).

Thus, we have an ongoing study to attempt to intervene in the abnormal inflammatory and immune processes in idiopathic pulmonary fibrosis (112). All patients are treated with standard levels of corticosteroids (prednisone daily dose: initially 1 mg/kg for 6 weeks, decreased by 0.05 mg /kg · week until 0.25 mg/kg is reached), and, in a double-blind fashion, 50% of the patients also receive azathioprine (daily dose: 2.5 mg/kg). These patients are being followed at 3-month intervals with routine studies and, more importantly, with exercise studies to follow the fibrotic process; bronchoalveolar lavage to follow inflammatory cells and IgG levels; ^{67}Ga scans to follow inflammation; ventilation-perfusion studies to follow the status of the capillary bed, cystic lesions, and small airways; and dynamic compliance, maximum expiratory flow-volume curves, and maximum flow-static recoil curves to follow the status of the small airways.

In summary, this multidisciplinary approach to evaluating the same set of patients with idiopathic pulmonary fibrosis has allowed us to make inroads into the pathogenesis, diagnosis, pathophysiology, and therapy of this disorder. Most importantly, it has enabled us to define idiopathic pulmonary fibrosis as a characteristic and specific disease entity. Rather than a clinical diagnosis of exclusion, idiopathic pulmonary fibrosis has a clear set of criteria that distinguish it from other disorders. It is a disease that has protean manifestations to those affected, and all indications are that if therapy is to be successful early diagnosis and treatment are essential.

ACKNOWLEDGMENTS: Received 3 September 1976; accepted 7 October 1976.

► Requests for reprints should be addressed to Ronald G. Crystal, M.D.; Chief, Pulmonary Branch, National Heart, Lung, and Blood Institute, National Institutes of Health; Bethesda, MD 20014.

References

1. Hamman L, Rich AR: Fulminating diffuse interstitial fibrosis of the lungs. *Trans Am Clin Climatol Assoc* 51:154-163, 1935
2. Hamman L, Rich AR: Acute diffuse interstitial fibrosis of the lungs. *Bull Johns Hopkins Hosp* 74:177-212, 1944
3. Rubin EH, Lubliner R: The Hamman-Rich syndrome: review of the literature and analysis of 15 cases. *Medicine* 36: 397-463, 1957
4. Mitchum WR, Brady BM: Differential diagnosis of fibrosing lung lesions. *Radiology* 68:36-47, 1957
5. Anderson AE Jr, Foraker AG: Morphological aspects of interstitial pulmonary fibrosis. *Arch Pathol* 70:79-93, 1960
6. Scadding JG: Chronic diffuse interstitial fibrosis of the lungs. *Br Med J* 1:443-450, 1960
7. Holland RAB: Physiologic dead space in the Hamman-Rich syndrome. Physiologic and clinical implications. *Am J Med* 28:61-68, 1960
8. Gross P: The concept of the Hamman-Rich syndrome. A critique. *Am Rev Respir Dis* 85:828-832, 1962
9. Nahmias BB, Churchwell AG, Bowles FN: Diffuse interstitial pulmonary fibrosis (Hamman-Rich syndrome). *Am J Med* 31:154-162, 1961
10. Doctor L, Snider GL: Diffuse interstitial pulmonary fibrosis associated with arthritis. With comments on the definition of rheumatoid lung disease. *Am Rev Respir Dis* 85:413-422, 1962
11. Muschenheim C: Some observations on the Hamman-Rich disease. *Am J Med Sci* 241:279-288, 1961
12. Herbert FA, Nahmias BB, Gaensler EA, et al: Pathophysiology of interstitial pulmonary fibrosis. Report of 19 cases and follow-up with corticosteroids. *Arch Intern Med* 110:628-648, 1962
13. Livingstone JL, Lewis JG, Reid L, et al: Diffuse interstitial pulmonary fibrosis. *Q J Med* 33:71-103, 1964
14. Stack BHR, Grant IWB, Irvine WJ, et al: Idiopathic diffuse interstitial lung disease. *Am Rev Respir Dis* 92:939-948, 1965
15. Liebow AA, Steer A, Billingsley JG: Desquamative interstitial pneumonia. *Am J Med* 39:369-404, 1965
16. Gaensler EA, Goff AM, Prowse CM: Desquamative interstitial pneumonia. *N Engl J Med* 274:113-128, 1966
17. Marks A: Diffuse interstitial pulmonary fibrosis. *Med Clin North Amer* 51:439-457, 1967
18. Scadding JG, Hinson KFW: Diffuse fibrosing alveolitis (diffuse interstitial fibrosis of the lungs). *Thorax* 22:291-304, 1967
19. Spencer H: Interstitial pneumonia. *Annu Rev Med* 18:423-442, 1967
20. Spencer H: Chronic interstitial pneumonia, in *The Lung*, edited by Liebow AA, Smith DE. Baltimore, Williams & Wilkins, 1968, pp. 134-150
21. Liebow AA: New concepts and entities in pulmonary disease, in *The Lung*, edited by Liebow AA, Smith DE. Baltimore, Williams & Wilkins, 1968, pp. 332-365
22. Liebow AA, Carrington CB: Alveolar diseases. The interstitial pneumonias, in *Frontiers of Pulmonary Radiology*, edited by Simon M. New York, Grune & Stratton, 1967, pp. 102-141
23. Parr LH: Hamman-Rich syndrome. Idiopathic pulmonary interstitial fibrosis of the lung. *J Natl Med Assoc* 61:8-12, 1969
24. Hinson KFW: Diffuse pulmonary fibrosis. *Hum Pathol* 1: 275-288, 1970
25. DeRemee RA, Harrison EG Jr, Anderson HA: The concept of classical interstitial pneumonitis-fibrosis (CIP-F) as a clinicopathologic syndrome. *Chest* 61:213-220, 1972
26. Stack HR, Choo-Kang YFJ, Heard BE: The prognosis of cryptogenic fibrosing alveolitis. *Thorax* 27:535-542, 1972
27. McCombs RP: Diseases due to immunologic reactions in the lungs. *N Engl J Med* 286:1186-1194, 1972
28. Fraire AE, Greenberg SD, O'Neal RM, et al: Diffuse interstitial fibrosis of the lung. *Am J Clin Pathol* 59:636-647, 1973
29. Patchefsky AS, Israel HL, Hoch WS, et al: Desquamative interstitial pneumonia: relationship to interstitial fibrosis. *Thorax* 28:680-693, 1973
30. Scadding JG: Diffuse pulmonary alveolar fibrosis. *Thorax* 29: 271-281, 1974
31. Dill J, Ghose T, Landrigan P, et al: Cryptogenic fibrosing alveolitis. *Chest* 67:411-416, 1975
32. Rankin J, Chester EH: Diffuse interstitial diseases of the lung as a cause of pulmonary insufficiency. The alveolar-capillary block syndrome, in *Textbook of Pulmonary Disease*, edited by Baum GL. Boston, Little, Brown and Co., 1974, pp. 609-645
33. Tukiainen P: Needle biopsy in diffuse lung manifestations. An analysis of 145 consecutive cases. *Scand J Respir Dis [Suppl]* 94:1-110, 1975
34. Liebow AA: Definition and classification of interstitial pneumonias in human pathology, in *Progress in Respiration Research, vol. 8. Alveolar Interstitium of the Lung. Pathological and Physiological Aspects*, edited by Basset F, Georges R. New York, Karger, 1975, pp. 1-33
35. Heard BE: Pathology of interstitial lung diseases, with particular reference to terminology, classification and trephine lung biopsy. *Chest* 69(suppl):252-253, 1976
36. Diamond I: The Hamman-Rich syndrome in childhood. *Pediatrics* 22:279-288, 1958
37. Weingärtner L: [Diffuse interstitial progressive pulmonary fibrosis in childhood.] (Germ.) *Dtsch Med Wochenschr* 90: 511-516, 1965
38. Austrian R, McClement JH, Renzetti AD Jr, et al: Clinical and physiologic features of some types of pulmonary diseases with impairment of alveolar-capillary diffusion. The syndrome of "alveolar-capillary block." *Am J Med* 11:667-685, 1951
39. Finley TN, Swenson EW, Comroe JH Jr: The cause of arterial hypoxemia at rest in patients with "alveolar-capillary block syndrome." *J Clin Invest* 41:618-622, 1962
40. Wagner PD, Dantzker DR, Dueck R, et al: Distribution of ventilation-perfusion ratios in patients with interstitial lung disease. *Chest* 69 (suppl):256-257, 1976
41. Cudkowicz L, Madoff IM, Abelmann WH: Rheumatoid lung

disease. A case report which includes respiratory function studies and a lung biopsy. *Br J Dis Chest* 55:35-40, 1961
42. Tomasi TB Jr, Fudenberg HH, Finby N: Possible relationship of rheumatoid factors and pulmonary disease. *Am J Med* 33:243-248, 1962
43. Talbot JA, Calkins E: Pulmonary involvement in rheumatoid arthritis. *JAMA* 189(12):911-913, 1964
44. Brannan HM, Good A, Divertie MB, et al: Pulmonary disease associated with rheumatoid arthritis. *JAMA* 189(12): 914-918, 1964
45. Patterson CD, Harville WE, Pierce JA: Rheumatoid lung disease. *Ann Intern Med* 62:685-697, 1965
46. Petty TL, Wilkins M: The five manifestations of rheumatoid lung. *Dis Chest* 49:75-82, 1966
47. Walker WC, Wright V: Pulmonary lesions and rheumatoid arthritis. *Medicine* 47:501-520, 1968
48. Scadding JG: The lungs in rheumatoid arthritis. *Proc R Soc Med* 62:227-238, 1969
49. Popper MS, Bogdonoff ML, Hughes RL: Interstitial rheumatoid lung disease. A reassessment and review of the literature. *Chest* 62:243-250, 1972
50. Frank ST, Weg JG, Harkleroad LE, et al: Pulmonary dysfunction in rheumatoid disease. *Chest* 63:27-34, 1973
51. Gordon DA, Stein JL, Broder I: The extra-articular features of rheumatoid arthritis. A systematic analysis of 127 cases. *Am J Med* 54:445-452, 1973
52. Ellman P, Cudkowicz L: Pulmonary manifestations in the diffuse collagen diseases. *Thorax* 9:46-57, 1954
53. Sullivan MA, Miller DK: Pulmonary manifestations in collagen disease. *Arch Intern Med* 110:769-787, 1962
54. Divertie MB: Lung involvement in the connective-tissue disorders. *Med Clin N Am* 48(4):1015-1030, 1964
55. Huang CT, Lyons HA: Comparison of pulmonary function in patients with systemic lupus erythematosus, scleroderma, and rheumatoid arthritis. *Am Rev Respir Dis* 93:865-875, 1966
56. Laitinen O, Salorinne Y, Poppius H: Respiratory function in systemic lupus erythematosus, scleroderma, and rheumatoid arthritis. *Ann Rheum Dis* 32:531-535, 1973
57. Spain DM, Thomas AG: The pulmonary manifestations of scleroderma. An anatomic-physiological correlation. *Ann Intern Med* 32:152-161, 1950
58. Adhikari PK, Bianchi FA, Boushy SF, et al: Pulmonary function in scleroderma. Its relation to changes in the chest roentgenogram and in the skin of the thorax. *Annu Rev Respir Dis* 86:823-831, 1963
59. Wilson RJ, Rodnan GP, Robin ED: An early pulmonary physiologic abnormality in progressive systemic sclerosis (diffuse scleroderma). *Am J Med* 36:361-369, 1964
60. Masi AT, D'Angelo WA: Epidemiology of fatal systemic sclerosis (diffuse scleroderma). A 15-year survey in Baltimore. *Ann Intern Med* 66:870-883, 1967
61. DeMuth GR, Furstenburg NA, Dabich L, et al: Pulmonary manifestations of progressive systemic sclerosis. *Am J Med Sci* 255:94-104, 1968
62. D'Angelo WA, Fries JF, Masi AT, et al: Pathologic observations in systemic sclerosis (scleroderma). A study of fifty-eight autopsy cases and fifty-eight matched controls. *Am J Med* 46:428-440, 1969
63. Medsger TA Jr, Masi AT, Rodnan GP, et al: Survival with systemic sclerosis (scleroderma). A life-table analysis of clinical and demographic factors in 309 patients. *Ann Intern Med* 75:369-376, 1971
64. Colp CR, Riker J, Williams MH Jr: Serial changes in scleroderma and idiopathic interstitial lung disease. *Arch Intern Med* 132:506-515, 1973
65. Grace WJ, Kennedy RJ, Formato A: Therapy of scleroderma and dermatomyositis. *NY State J Med* 63:140-144, 1963
66. Brundin A: Pulmonary fibrosis in scleroderma and dermatomyositis. *Scand J Respir Dis* 51:160-170, 1970
67. Goldfischer J, Rubin EH: Dermatomyositis with pulmonary lesions. *Ann Intern Med* 50:194-206, 1959
68. Medsger TA Jr, Robinson H, Masi AT: Factors affecting survivorship in polymyositis. *Arthritis Rheum* 14:249-258, 1971
69. Sandbank M, Grunebaum M, Katzenellenbogen I: Dermatomyositis associated with subacute pulmonary fibrosis. *Arch Dermatol* 94:432-435, 1966
70. Pearson CM: Polymyositis. *Annu Rev Med* 17:63-82, 1966
71. Weaver AL, Brundage BH, Nelson RA, et al: Pulmonary involvement in polymyositis: report of a case with response to corticosteroid therapy. *Arthritis Rheum* 11:765-773, 1968
72. Bohan A, Peter JB: Polymyositis and Dermatomyositis. *N Engl J Med* 292:344-347, 403-407, 1975
73. Thompson PL, Mackay IR: Fibrosing alveolitis and polymyositis. *Thorax* 25:504-507, 1970
74. Thompson JE: Lung involvement in polymyositis. *Med J Aust* 1:1332-1333, 1971
75. Webb DR, Currie GD: Pulmonary fibrosis masking polymyositis. *JAMA* 222:1146-1149, 1972
76. Camp AV, Lane DJ, Mowat AG: Dermatomyositis with parenchymal lung involvement. *Br Med J* 1:155-156, 1972
77. Olsen GN, Swenson EW: Polymyositis and interstitial lung disease. *Am Rev Respir Dis* 105:611-617, 1972
78. Frazier AR, Miller RD: Interstitial pneumonitis in association with polymyositis and dermatomyositis. *Chest* 65:403-407, 1974
79. Duncan PE, Griffin JP, Garcia A, et al: Fibrosing alveolitis in polymyositis. A review of histologically confirmed cases. *Am J Med* 57:621-626, 1974
80. Schwarz MI, Matthay RA, Sahn SA, et al: Interstitial lung disease in polymyositis and dermatomyositis: analysis of six cases and review of the literature. *Medicine* 55:89-104, 1976
81. Hoffbrand BI, Beck ER: "Unexplained" dyspnoea and shrinking lungs in systemic lupus erythematosus. *Br Med J* 1:1273-1277, 1965
82. Huang C, Hennigar GR, Lyons HA: Pulmonary dysfunction in systemic lupus erythematosus. *N Engl J Med* 272:288-293, 1965
83. Gold WM, Jennings DB: Pulmonary function in patients with systemic lupus erythematosus. *Am Rev Respir Dis* 93:556-567, 1966
84. Gross M, Esterly JR, Earle RH: Pulmonary alterations in systemic lupus erythematosus. *Am Rev Respir Dis* 105:572-577, 1972
85. Eisenberg H, Dubois EL, Sherwin RP, et al: Diffuse interstitial lung disease in systemic lupus erythematosus. *Ann Intern Med* 79:37-45, 1973
86. Mackay IR, Ritchie B: Diffuse fibrosing alveolitis (diffuse interstitial fibrosis of the lungs): two cases with autoimmune features. *Thorax* 20:200-205, 1965
87. Gottlieb AJ, Spiera H, Teirstein AS, et al: Serologic factors in idiopathic diffuse interstitial pulmonary fibrosis. *Am J Med* 39:405-410, 1965
88. Turner-Warwick M, Doniach D: Auto-antibody studies in interstitial pulmonary fibrosis. *Br Med J* 1:886-891, 1965
89. Hobbs JR, Turner-Warwick M: Assay of circulating immunoglobins in patients with fibrosing alveolitis. *Clin Exp Immunol* 2:645-652, 1967
90. Nagaya H, Buckley CE III, Sieker HO: Positive antinuclear factor in patients with unexplained pulmonary fibrosis. *Ann Intern Med* 70:1135-1145, 1969
91. Turner-Warwick M, Haslam P: Antibodies in some chronic fibrosing lung diseases. I. Non-organ-specific antibodies. *Clin Allergy* 1:83-95, 1971
92. Turner-Warwick M, Haslam P: Antibodies in some chronic fibrosing lung diseases. II. Immunofluorescent studies. *Clin Allergy* 1:209-219, 1971
93. Nagaya H, Sieker HO: Pathogenic mechanisms of interstitial pulmonary fibrosis in patients with serum antinuclear factor. A histologic and clinical correlation. *Am J Med* 52:51-62, 1972
94. DeHoratius RJ, Abruzzo JL, Williams RC Jr: Immunofluorescent and immunologic studies of rheumatoid lung. *Arch Intern Med* 129:441-446, 1972
95. Nagaya H, Elmore M, Ford CD: Idiopathic interstitial pulmonary fibrosis. An immune complex disease? *Am Rev Respir Dis* 107:826-830, 1973
96. Kang KY, Yagura T, Sera Y, et al: Antinuclear factor in pneumoconioses and idiopathic pulmonary fibrosis. *Med J Osaka Univ* 23:249-256, 1973
97. Turner-Warwick M: Immunologic aspects of systemic diseases of the lungs. *Proc R Soc Med* 67:541-547, 1974
98. Haslam P, Turner-Warwick M, Lukoszek A: Antinuclear antibody and lymphocyte responses to nuclear antigens in patients with lung disease. *Clin Exp Immunol* 20:379-395, 1975
99. Rodnan GP, McEwen C, Wallace SL, editors: *Primer on the Rheumatic Diseases, Seventh Edition.* New York, The Arthritis Foundation, 1973, pp. 1-152
100. Winkelmann RK: Classification and pathogenesis of scleroderma. *Mayo Clin Proc* 46:83-91, 1971
101. Snider GL: Case records of the Massachusetts General Hospital. *N Engl J Med* 293:136-143, 1975
102. Rose GA, Spenser H: Polyarteritis nodosa. *Q J Med* 26:43-81, 1957
103. Wolff SM, Fauci AS, Horn RG, et al: Wegener's granulomatosis. *Ann Intern Med* 81:513-525, 1974
104. Davies D: Ankylosing spondylitis and lung fibrosis. *Q J Med* 41:395-417, 1972

105. MENDLOWITZ M: Clubbing and hypertrophic osteoarthropathy. *Medicine* 21:269-306, 1942
106. CUDKOWICZ L, WRAITH DG: An evaluation of the clinical significance of clubbing in common lung disorders. *Br J Tuberc* 51:14-31, 1957
107. BALCERZAK SP, BROMBERG PA: Secondary polycythemia. *Semin Hematol* 12:353-382, 1975
108. TURNER-WARWICK M: Fibrosing alveolitis and chronic liver disease. *Q J Med* 37:133-149, 1968
109. HAMER J: Cause of low arterial oxygen saturation in pulmonary fibrosis. *Thorax* 19:507-514, 1964
110. MCCARTHY D, CHERNIACK RM: Regional ventilation-perfusion and hypoxia in cryptogenic fibrosing alveolitis. *Am Rev Respir Dis* 107:200-208, 1973
111. BACHOFEN H, SCHERRER M: Lung tissue resistance in diffuse interstitial pulmonary fibrosis. *J Clin Invest* 46:133-140, 1967
112. FULMER JD, ROBERTS WC, CRYSTAL RG: Diffuse fibrotic lung disease: a correlative study. *Chest* 69(suppl):263-265, 1975
113. JONES NL, MCHARDY GJR, NAIMARK A, et al: Physiological dead space and alveolar-arterial gas pressure differences during exercise. *Clin Sci* 31:19-29, 1966
114. WASSERMAN K, WHIPP BJ: Exercise physiology in health and disease. *Am Rev Respir Dis* 112:219-249, 1975
115. MACKLEM PT: New tests to assess lung function. *N Engl J Med* 293:339-342, 1975
116. MACKLEM PT, BECKLAKE MR: The relationship between the mechanical and diffusing properties of the lung in health and disease. *Am Rev Respir Dis* 87:47-56, 1963
117. BACHOFEN M, WEIBEL ER: Basic pattern of tissue repair in human lungs following unspecific injury. *Chest* 65 (suppl):14S-19S, 1974
118. KUHN C: The cells of the lung and their organelles, in *The Biochemical Basis of Pulmonary Function*, edited by CRYSTAL RG. New York, Dekker, Marcel, Inc., 1976, pp. 3-48
119. CLEMENTS JA, KING RJ: Composition of the surface active material, in *The Biochemical Basis of Pulmonary Function*, edited by CRYSTAL RG. New York, Dekker, Marcel, Inc., 1976, pp. 363-387
120. SHORTLAND JR, DARKE CS, CRANE WAJ: Electron microscopy of desquamative interstitial pneumonia. *Thorax* 24:192-208, 1969
121. BASSET F, SOLER P, BERNAUBIN JF, et al: Contribution of electron microscopy to the study of interstitial pneumonias, in *Progress in Respiration Research, vol. 8. Alveolar Interstitium of the Lung, International Symposium*, edited by BASSET F, GEORGES R. New York, Karger, 1975, pp. 45-58
122. FARR GH, HARLEY RA, HENNIGAR GR: Desquamative interstitial pneumonia. An electron microscopic study. *Am J Pathol* 60:347-354, 1970
123. BREWER BD, HEATH D, ASQUITH P: Electron microscopy of desquamative interstitial pneumonia. *J Path* 97:317-323, 1969
124. GLANCY DL, FRAZIER PD, ROBERTS WC: Pulmonary parenchymal cholesterol-ester granulomas in patients with pulmonary hypertension. *Am J Med* 45:198-210, 1968
125. DAVIES D, MACFARLANE A, DARKE CS, et al: Muscular hyperplasia ("cirrhosis") of the lung and bronchial dilations as features of chronic diffuse fibrosing alveolitis. *Thorax* 21:272-289, 1966
126. KAPANCI Y, ASSIMACOPOULOS A, IRLE C, et al: "Contractile interstitial cells" in pulmonary alveolar septa: a possible regulator of ventilation/perfusion ratio? Ultrastructural, immunofluorescence, and *in vitro* studies. *J Cell Biol* 60:375-392, 1974
127. SEAL RME, HAPKE EJ, THOMAS GO, et al: The pathology of the acute and chronic stages of farmer's lung. *Thorax* 23:469-489, 1968
128. RÜTTNER JR, SPYCHER MA, STICHER H: The detection of etiologic agents in interstitial pulmonary fibrosis. *Hum Pathol* 4:497-512, 1973
129. WINKELMANN RK, DITTO WB: Cutaneous and visceral syndromes of necrotizing or "allergic" angiitis: a study of 38 cases. *Medicine* 43:59-89, 1964
130. THEROS EG: The value of radiologic-pathologic correlation in the education of the radiologist. *Am J Roentgenol* 107:235-257, 1969
131. JOHNSON TH JR: Radiology and honeycomb lung disease. *Am J Roentgenol* 104:810-821, 1968
132. GENEREUX GP: The end-stage lung. *Radiology* 116:279-289, 1975
133. BENSON MK, HUGHES DT: Serial pulmonary function tests in fibrosing alveolitis. *Br J Dis Chest* 66:33-44, 1972
134. BROWN CH, TURNER-WARWICK M: The treatment of cryptogenic fibrosing alveolitis with immunosuppressant drugs. *Q J Med* 40:289-302, 1971
135. SCHLUETER DP, IMMEKUS J, STEAD WW: Relationship between maximal inspiratory pressure and total lung capacity (coefficient of retraction) in normal subjects and in patients with emphysema, asthma, and diffuse pulmonary infiltration. *Am Rev Respir Dis* 96:656-665, 1967
136. TURNER JM, MEAD J, WOHL ME: Elasticity of human lungs in relation to age. *J Appl Physiol* 25:664-671, 1968
137. MCFADDEN ER JR, LYONS HA: Airway resistance and uneven ventilation in bronchial asthma. *J Appl Physiol* 25:365-370, 1968
138. HILL DJ, LANDAU LI, PHELAN PD: Small airway disease in asymptomatic asthmatic adolescents. *Am Rev Respir Dis* 106: 873-880, 1972
139. HECKSCHER T, BASS H, ORIOL A, et al: Regional lung function in patients with bronchial asthma. *J Clin Invest* 47:1063-1070, 1968
140. WOOLCOCK AJ, VINCENT NJ, MACKLEM PT: Frequency dependence of compliance as a test for obstruction in the small airways. *J Clin Invest* 48:1097-1106, 1969
141. GELB AF, ZAMEL N: Simplified diagnosis of small-airway obstruction. *N Engl J Med* 288:395-398, 1973
142. MEAD J, TURNER JM, MACKLEM PT, et al: Significance of the relationship between lung recoil and maximum expiratory flow. *J Appl Physiol* 22:95-108, 1967
143. FULMER JD, CRYSTAL RG: The biochemical basis of pulmonary function, in *The Biochemical Basis of Pulmonary Function*, edited by CRYSTAL RG. New York, Dekker, Marcel, Inc., 1976, pp. 419-466
144. OSTROW D, CHERNIACK RM: Resistance to airflow in patients with diffuse interstitial lung disease. *Am Rev Respir Dis* 108: 205-210, 1973
145. MISHKIN FS, BRASHEAR RE: Pulmonary and systemic blood pressure responses to large doses of albumin microspheres. *J Nucl Med* 12:251-252, 1971
146. TAPLIN GV, MACDONALD NS: Radiochemistry of macroaggregated albumin and newer lung scanning agents. *Semin Nucl Med* 1:132-152, 1971
147. WAGNER HN JR, TOW DE, LOPEZ-MAJANO V, et al: Factors influencing regional pulmonary blood flow in man. *Scand J Respir Dis* 62(suppl):59-72, 1966
148. WAGNER HN JR, SABISTON DC, IIO M: The diagnosis of pulmonary embolism by radioisotope scanning (abstract). *J Nucl Med* 5:345-346, 1964
149. DUGARD A, NAIMARK A: Effect of hypoxia on distribution of pulmonary blood flow. *J Appl Physiol* 23:663-671, 1967
150. WAGNER HN JR: The use of radioisotope techniques for the evaluation of patients with pulmonary disease. *Am Rev Respir Dis* 113:203-218, 1976
151. FRIEDMAN WF, BRAUNWALD E: Alterations in regional pulmonary blood flow in mitral valve disease studied by radioisotope scanning. A simple nontraumatic technique for estimation of left atrial pressure. *Circulation* 34:363-376, 1966
152. LOKEN MK, WESTGATE HD: Evaluation of pulmonary function using xenon 133 and the scintillation camera. *Am J Roentgenol* 100:835-843, 1967
153. DE ROO MJK, GORIS M, VAN DER SCHUEREN G, et al: Computerized dynamic scintigraphy of the lungs. *Respiration* 26: 408-424, 1969
154. LOKEN MK, MEDINA JR, LILLEHEI JP, et al: Regional pulmonary function evaluation using Xenon 133, a scintillation camera, and computer. *Radiology* 93:1261-1266, 1969
155. MACINTYRE WJ, INKLEY SR, ROTH E, et al: Spatial recording of disappearance constants of xenon-133 wash out from the lung. *J Lab Clin Med* 76:701-712, 1970
156. JOHNSON G, JONES AE, (eds.): Atlas of Gallium-67 Scintigraphy. New York, Plenum Press, 1973
157. GELRUD LG, ARSENEAU JC, JOHNSTON GS: Gallium-67 localization in experimental and clinical abscesses (abstract). *Clin Res* 20:881, 1972
158. KINOSHITA F, USHIO T, MAEKAWA A, et al: Scintiscanning of pulmonary diseases with ^{67}Ga-citrate. *J Nucl Med* 15:227-233, 1974
159. SIEMSEN JK, GREBE SF, SARGENT EN, et al: Gallium-67 scintigraphy of pulmonary diseases as a complement to radiography. *Radiology* 118:371-375, 1976
160. SWARTZENDRUBER DC, NELSON B, HAYES RL: Gallium-67 localization in lysosomal-like granules of leukemic and nonleukemic murine tissues. *J Natl Cancer Inst* 46:941-952, 1971
161. NELSON B, HAYES RL, EDWARDS CL, et al: Distribution of gallium in human tissues after intravenous administration. *J Nucl Med* 13:92-100, 1972
162. LARSON SM, MILDER MS, JOHNSTON GS: Interpretation of the ^{67}Ga photoscan. *J Nucl Med* 14:208-214, 1973

163. Line BR, Fulmer JD, Jones AE, et al: [67]Gallium scanning in idiopathic pulmonary fibrosis: correlation with histopathology and broncho-alveolar lavage. *Am Rev Respir Dis* 113(4):244, 1976
164. Langhammer H, Glaubitt G, Grebe SF, et al: [67]Ga for tumor scanning. *J Nucl Med* 13:25-30, 1972
165. Reynolds HY, Newball HH: Analysis of proteins and respiratory cells obtained from human lungs by bronchial lavage. *J Lab Clin Med* 84:559-573, 1974
166. Reynolds HY, Atkinson JP, Newball HH, et al: Receptors for immunoglobulin and complement on human alveolar macrophages. *J Immunol* 114:1813-1819, 1975
167. Reynolds HY, Newball HH: Fluid and cellular milieu of the human respiratory tract, in *Immunologic and Infectious Reactions in the Lungs*, edited by Kirkpatrick CH, Reynolds HY. New York, Dekker, Marcel, Inc., 1976, pp. 3-27
168. Reynolds HY, Fulmer JD, Kazmierowski JA, et al: Analysis of broncho-alveolar fluid in patients with hypersensitivity pneumonitis (HP) (abstract). *Clin Res* 24:388A, 1976
169. Davis GS, Brody AR, Landis JH, et al: Quantitation of inflammatory activity in interstitial pneumonitis by bronchofiberscopic pulmonary lavage. *Chest* 69(suppl):254-255, 1976
170. Keimowitz RI: Immunoglobins in normal human tracheobronchial washings. *J Lab Clin Med* 63:54-59, 1964
171. McCombs RP: Diseases due to immunologic reactions in the lung. *N Engl J Med* 286:1186-1194, 1245-1252, 1972
172. Kaltreider HB: Expression of immune mechanisms in the lung. *Am Rev Respir Dis* 113:347-379, 1976
173. Bradley K, McConnell-Breul S, Crystal RG: Lung collagen heterogeneity. *Proc Natl Acad Sci USA* 71:2828-2832, 1974
174. Bradley K, McConnell-Breul S, Crystal RG: Collagen in the human lung. Quantitation of rates of synthesis and partial characterization of composition. *J Clin Invest* 55:543-550, 1975
175. Hance AJ, Crystal RG: The connective tissue of lung. *Am Rev Respir Dis* 112:657-711, 1975
176. Hance AJ, Bradley K, Crystal RG: Lung collagen heterogeneity. Synthesis of type I and type III collagen by rabbit and human lung cells in culture. *J Clin Invest* 57:102-111, 1976
177. Hance AJ, Crystal RG: Collagen, in *The Biochemical Basis of Pulmonary Function*, edited by Crystal RG. New York, Dekker, Marcel, Inc., 1976, pp. 215-271
178. Seyer JM, Hutcheson ET, Kang AH: Collagen polymorphism in idiopathic chronic pulmonary fibrosis. *J Clin Invest* 57:1498-1507, 1976
179. McLees BD, Schleiter G, Pinnell SR: Isolation of type III collagen from human adult parenchymal lung tissue. *Biochemistry*, in press
180. Gay S, Fietzek PP, Remberger K, et al: Liver cirrhosis: immunofluorescence and biochemical studies demonstate two types of collagen. *Klin Dtsch Med Wochenschr* 100: 205-207, 1975
181. Popper H: Hepatic fibrosis and collagen metabolism in the liver, in *Collagen Metabolism in the Liver*, edited by Popper H, Becker K. New York, Stratton Corp., 1975, pp. 1-14
182. Fulmer JD, Bienkowski RS, Cowan MJ, et al: Comparison of collagen concentration, distribution, and synthesis in fibrotic and normal lungs (abstract). *Clin Res* 24:384A, 1976
183. Hance AJ, Horwitz AL, Cowan MJ, et al: Biochemical approaches to the investigation of fibrotic lung disease. *Chest* 69(2)(suppl):257-261, 1976
184. McCullagh KA, Balian G: Collagen characterization and cell transformation in human atherosclerosis. *Nature* (Lond) 258:73-75, 1975
185. Epstein EH Jr, Munderloh NH: Isolation and characterization of CNBr peptides of human $[\alpha 1(III)]_3$ collagen and tissue distribution of $[\alpha 1(I)]_2\alpha 2$ and $[\alpha 1(III)]_3$ collagens. *J Biol Chem* 250:9304-9312, 1975
186. Epstein EH Jr: $[\alpha 1(III)]_3$ human skin collagen. Release by pepsin digestion and preponderance in fetal life. *J Biol Chem* 249:3225-3231, 1974
187. Kravis TC, Ahmed A, Brown TE, et al: Pathogenic mechanisms in pulmonary fibrosis: collagen induced migration inhibition factor production and cytotoxicity mediated by lymphocytes. *J Clin Invest*, 58:1223-1232, 1976
188. Hughes EW: Familial interstitial pulmonary fibrosis. *Thorax* 19:515-525, 1964
189. Bonanni PP, Frymoyer JW, Jacox RF: A family study of idiopathic pulmonary fibrosis. A possible dysproteinemic and genetically determined disease. *Am J Med* 39:411-421, 1965
190. Adelman AG, Chertkow G, Hayton RC: Familial fibrocystic pulmonary dysplasia: a detailed family study. *Can Med Assoc J* 95:603-610, 1966
191. Swaye P, Van Ordstrand HS, McCormack LJ, et al: Familial Hamman-Rich syndrome. Report of eight cases. *Dis Chest* 55: 7-12, 1969
192. Wagley PF: A new look at the Hamman-Rich syndrome. *Johns Hopkins Med J* 131:412-424, 1972
193. Solliday NH, Williams JA, Gaensler EA, et al: Familial chronic interstitial pneumonia. *Am Rev Respir Dis* 108:193-204, 1973
194. Davies BH, Tuddenham EGD: Familial pulmonary fibrosis associated with oculocutaneous albinism and platelet function defect. A new syndrome. *Q J Med* 45:219-232, 1976
195. Carrington CB, Gaensler EA, Coutu RE, et al: Usual and desquamative interstitial pneumonia. *Chest* 69(suppl):261-262, 1976

CONGENITAL OBSTRUCTIVE LESIONS INVOLVING THE MAJOR PULMONARY VEINS, LEFT ATRIUM, OR MITRAL VALVE: A Clinical, Laboratory, and Morphologic Survey

D. Luke Glancy, M.D., and William C. Roberts, M.D.

The clinical, laboratory, and morphologic features of congenitally obstructive lesions causing pulmonary venous hypertension are reviewed. These lesions are responsible for considerable infant mortality and morbidity, especially in the first weeks of life, are not infrequently encountered in older children, and are occasionally seen in adults. The presence of a malformation causing pulmonary venous hypertension often can be detected clinically, but precise anatomical and physiological diagnoses, usually necessary for optimal patient management, often can be made only by detailed laboratory study. Cardiac catheterization and angiocardiography remain the prime modes of accurate diagnosis in such patients, many of whom have other significant cardiovascular malformations, and echocardiography is an extremely useful adjunct, especially in patients with mitral valvular stenosis, hypoplasia, or atresia. The only definitive treatment in any of these patients is operative relief of the obstruction, and the chances of success depend not only on the skill of the surgeon, but also on the nature of the obstructing lesion, the types of associated malformations, and the precision with which these are defined preoperatively.

Key words: angiography, autopsy, cardiac catheterization, cardiac surgery, echocardiography, pulmonary venous hypertension

From the Cardiology Branch and the Section of Pathology, National Heart and Lung Institute, National Institutes of Health, Bethesda, Maryland 20014, and the Hôtel Dieu Hospital, New Orleans, Louisiana 70112

TABLE I. Congenitally Obstructive Lesions Causing Pulmonary Venous Hypertension

Pulmonary venous obstruction
With normal connection
With total or partial anomalous connection
Left atrial obstruction
Cor triatriatum
Supravalvular left atrial ring
Mitral valvular obstruction
Atresia
Hypoplasia
Stenosis

Pulmonary venous hypertension most commonly results from acquired lesions which interfere with left ventricular filling. The most common is left ventricular failure secondary to coronary or hypertensive heart disease or both. Another common one is rheumatic mitral stenosis. An infrequent but usually curable cause is obstruction to left ventricular filling from a left atrial mass (myxoma). In contrast to the frequency of the acquired lesions causing pulmonary venous hypertension, congenital causes are rare. This report focuses on the clinical, laboratory, and morphologic features of congenital lesions involving the pulmonary veins, left atrium, or mitral valve (Table I) that may produce pulmonary venous hypertension.

OBSTRUCTION OF THE MAJOR PULMONARY VEINS (Figs. 1–4)

Normal Connection

Pulmonary venous obstruction rarely occurs when all veins are normally connected. When this happens, however, the obstruction results from hypoplasia of a long segment of vein (1), from a discrete "diaphragm" (2, 3), or from *focal or diffuse intimal fibrosis* (4). One, several, or all of the pulmonary veins may be obstructed, and additional cardiovascular anomalies often coexist (2, 4–6). When most of the veins are involved, pulmonary arterial hypertension is the result and the clinical picture is virtually identical to that of cor triatriatum. Angiographic demonstration of the individual narrowings and failure to demonstrate an accessory chamber distinguish congenital pulmonary venous obstruction from cor triatriatum.

Narrowing of the major pulmonary veins and other obstructive lesions involving the left side of the heart must be distinguished from pulmonary veno-occlusive disease (Figs. 1 and 2), a condition only recently described (7), but characterized by severe narrowing of the lumens of the small intrapulmonary veins and venules. The patients, usually young males, present with features of severe pulmonary hypertension. The most common differential is primary or idiopathic pulmonary hypertension. The latter condition, however, most commonly involves young females rather than young males, and the pulmonary venous and pulmonary arterial wedge pressures are normal.

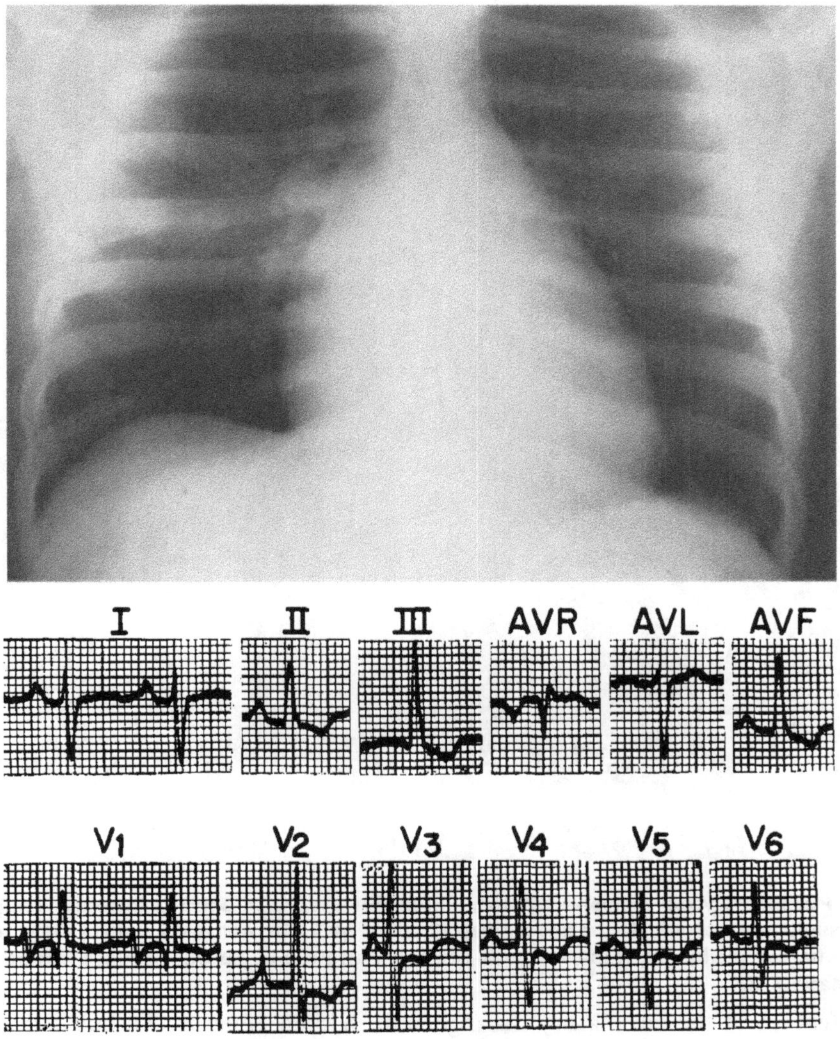

Fig. 1. Pulmonary veno-occlusive disease. Chest Roentgenogram and electrocardiogram, each taken 13 days before death, in a 17-yr old boy (A72-56) who was well (played competitive football) until 1 yr before death when symptoms and signs of congestive cardiac failure appeared. Catheterization 2 mo before death showed a pulmonary arterial wedge mean pressure of 17 with A waves of 20 and V waves of 14 mm Hg. Simultaneous pulmonary arterial and aortic pressures were 100/58 and 111/84 mm Hg, respectively. The right ventricular pressure was 100/14 and the left ventricular, 111/10 mm Hg. The pulmonary vascular resistance was 42 U/meter^2. Physical, radiographic, and electrocardiographic examinations showed evidence of right ventricular enlargement. He had precordial murmurs of tricuspid and pulmonic regurgitation. He died of progressive right-sided congestive cardiac failure.

Anomalous Connection

In patients with partial anomalous pulmonary venous connection, blood flow usually is unimpeded, but either the normally connected (Fig. 3) or the anomalously connected (8) veins may be obstructed. Usually, pulmonary venous obstruction is a

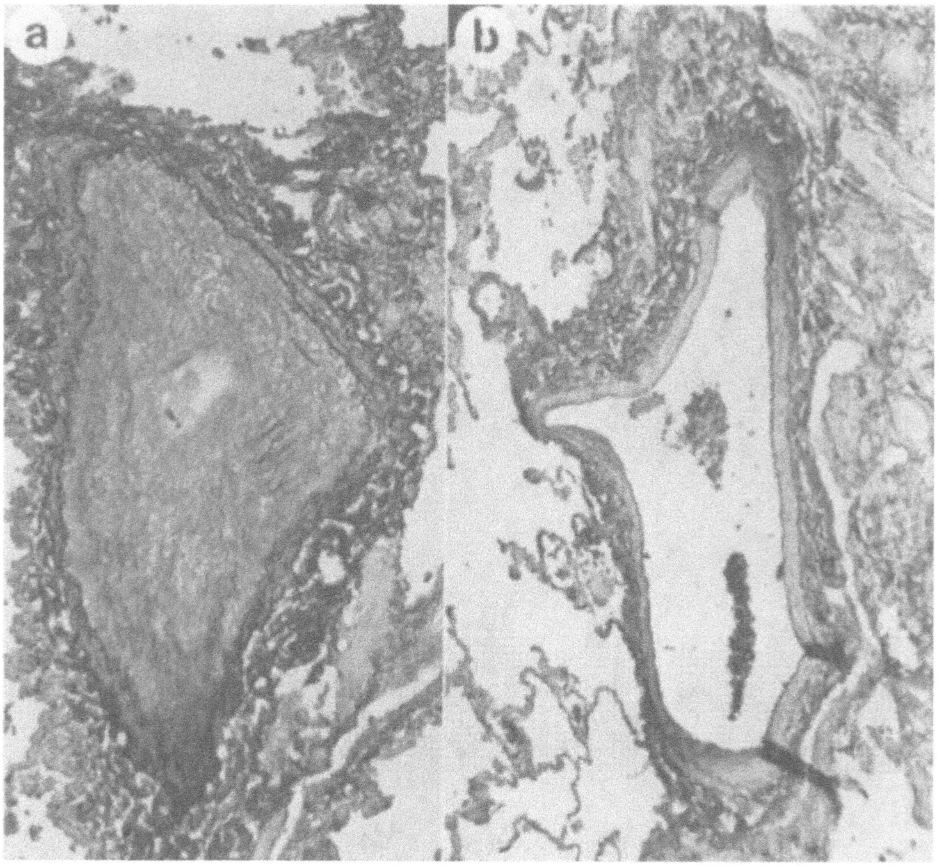

Fig. 2. Pulmonary veno-occlusive disease. Photomicrographs of small pulmonary venule (a) and of pulmonary artery (b) in the patient described in Fig. 1. The wall and lumen of the artery is normal whereas the lumen of the venule is severely narrowed by fibrous tissue. Elastic tissue stains; each × 63.

minor feature of the circulatory derangement in such patients (8), but it may be critically important (Fig. 3). In patients with total anomalous pulmonary venous connection (TAPVC) (Fig. 4), venous obstruction is rare when connection is to the coronary sinus or right atrium, is the rule when the connection is infradiaphragmatic, and often occurs when the connection is supracardiac (1, 5, 9–14). In the last situation, stenosis may result from fibrous intimal lesions, from compression of an anomalous vertical vein (Fig.4,left), or from both (1, 5, 12–14). When the anomalous connection is infradiaphragmatic to the portal vein or, less commonly, to the ductus venosus or inferior vena cava, several factors may contribute to the obstruction (5, 9, 11–13). The anomalous vein is long and often narrows progressively throughout its course. Focal stenosis also occurs, especially at the junction of the anomalous vein with an abdominal vein. In addition, the vein may be compressed as it descends through the diaphragm with the esophagus. Obstruction may be caused by a narrow ductus venosus when connection is to that structure. When connection is to the portal vein, progressive narrowing of the ductus venosus after birth causes an ever larger volume of pulmonary venous blood to traverse the hepatic sinusoids, and this resistance, in series with the others, undoubtedly contributes to the pulmonary venous hypertension.

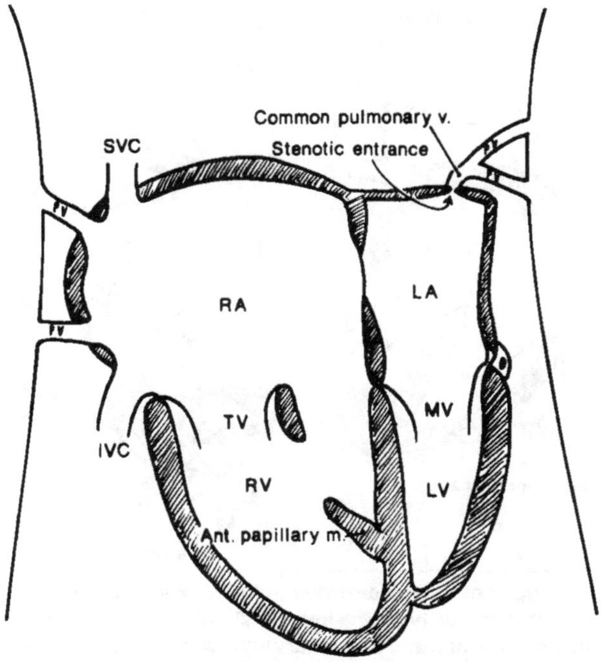

Fig. 3. Partial anomalous pulmonary venous connection in a 6-wk old girl (74A-28) who died of congestive cardiac failure, that first appeared during her 1st wk of life. She had no precordial murmurs. Chest Roentgenogram showed generalized cardiomegaly and increased pulmonary vascularity. Electrocardiogram showed right ventricular hypertrophy and right atrial enlargement.

At necropsy, the right side of the heart was much larger than the left as shown in the diagram. The two pulmonary veins (PV) from the right lung connected to the right atrium (RA). The two pulmonary veins from the left lung drained into a common pulmonary vein which in turn connected to the left atrium (LA). The entrance of the left common pulmonary vein (V) into the left atrium, however, was quite narrow (<2 mm dia). Although the anterior papillary muscle (m) of the right ventricle (RV) was quite hypertrophied, it did not appear to obstruct right ventricular outflow. MV = mitral valve; TV = tricuspid valve; LV = left ventricle; SVC = superior vena cava; IVC = inferior vena cava.

The heart in the above patient is similar from a functional standpoint to Lutembacher's syndrome. There was obstruction to inflow to the left ventricle (but proximal to the mitral valve, indeed proximal to the left atrium) and the drainage of the right pulmonary veins into the right atrium is equivalent to an atrial septal defect with left to right shunting. In both circumstances the obstructive lesion tends to increase the left to right shunt.

Atresia of the common pulmonary vein (5) in TAPVC is extremely rare. In this circumstance, the pulmonary veins join together behind the left atrium, but this confluence ends blindly. There are small communications with the systemic venous system through anastomoses of the pulmonary veins with bronchial veins, which in turn connect with mediastinal and esophageal veins.

Irrespective of whether the common pulmonary vein connects above or below the diaphragm or is atretic, the clinical features in these patients with TAPVC with obstruction are rather uniform (5, 9, 12, 14). Within a few days after birth, the infant, a boy in approximately 75% of cases, manifests cyanosis, increased sweating, and tachypnea. Respiratory distress is intensified during feeding, especially in infants with the infradiaphragmatic type of anomalous connection. In them, feeding may compress the common pulmonary vein in the esophageal hiatus. Weight gain is

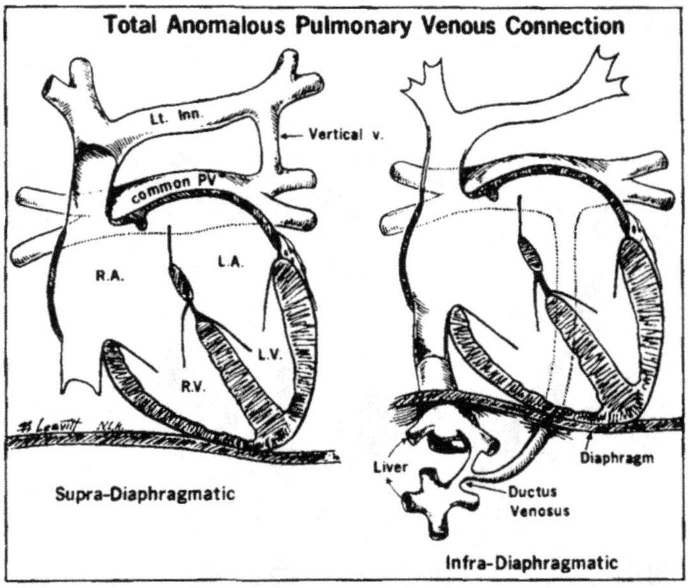

Fig. 4. Diagrams of two types of total anomalous pulmonary venous connection. On the left is the commonest supradiaphragmatic type: the individual pulmonary veins connect to a common pulmonary vein behind the left atrium and pulmonary venous blood is carried from there to the left innominate vein (Lt Inn) via an anomalous vertical vein. This vertical vein often is compressed between the left pulmonary artery and left main bronchus (so-called hemodynamic vice). On the right is the infradiaphragmatic type in which blood from the common pulmonary vein is carried by an anomalous vein through the esophageal hiatus to the portal vein, ductus venosus, or inferior vena cava. Venous obstruction is virtually always present in the infradiaphragmatic type (see text). LA = left atrium; LV = left ventricle; RA = right atrium; RV = right ventricle.

poor. Pulmonary rales occasionally are heard, and hepatomegaly is the rule. The second heart sound is widely split with a loud pulmonic component. Gallop rhythm due to the presence of third and/or fourth heart sounds is common. A systolic ejection murmur is heard along the left sternal edge in most infants, but it is usually soft and inconspicuous. A diastolic flow rumble may be heard. A continuous murmur is sometimes audible when the connection is to the left innominate vein and the vertical vein is compressed or, less often, when the connection is infradiaphragmatic. All of these signs, of course, may be difficult to detect in a severely ill newborn.

Right axis deviation and right ventricular hypertrophy of the systolic overload type are found on electrocardiogram, and right atrial enlargement usually is present by three months of age (12). Although the right-sided cardiac chambers are large at necropsy, overall heart size on chest X-ray usually is normal or only slightly increased. The lungs have the finely reticulated pattern of interstitial edema or the "ground glass" appearance of alveolar edema. In the newborn, this appearance together with the normal cardiac size strongly suggests the diagnosis of TAPVC with obstruction. When the connection is to the left innominate vein via an anomalous vertical vein, the cardiovascular silhouette characteristically has the so-called "snowman" appearance, but this is often difficult to recognize in the first months of life (12). While the echocardiogram of older patients with total anomalous pulmonary venous connection without obstruction typically shows the features of volume overload of the right ventricle, in the newborn with obstruction the echocardiogram may be normal (15). This normality is, of course, helpful in the differential diagnosis since it makes the hypoplastic left heart syndrome highly unlikely. When a common pulmonary vein lies behind the left atrium (Fig. 4, left) it may be detected echocardiographically (16) in some patients.

Diagnosis can be confirmed at catheterization by finding a markedly elevated pulmonary arterial wedge pressure, a normal left atrial pressure, a right to left shunt at atrial level, and a left to right shunt at superior or inferior vena caval level, depending on whether the anomalous connection is supra- or infracardiac. Pulmonary arterial pressure is higher than in TAPVC without obstruction and often is above systemic arterial pressure (9, 12). Pulmonary blood flow is much less in patients with obstruction than in those without, and gas exchange is hampered by pulmonary edema. Consequently, systemic arterial oxygen saturation is generally quite low. Systemic and pulmonary arterial saturations would be expected to be identical, but because of streaming often are different. On pulmonary arteriogram, the passage of contrast material through the lungs is markedly delayed (5, 9) and films taken up to 12 sec after injection may be needed. These usually, but not always, demonstrate the anomalous venous connection.

Without operation, prognosis in infants with TAPVC with obstruction is dismal; most die within 3 mo, and almost all within 12 mo after birth (9, 12). Operative anastomosis of the common pulmonary vein to the left atrium, with ligation of the vein forming the connection with the systemic venous system, is the only life-saving treatment.

COR TRIATRIATUM (Figs. 5–11)

In this rare anomaly [only 96 reported patients up to 1969 (17)], a fibromuscular septum divides the left atrium into two chambers: a posterior, rightward, and cephalad one (accessory or third chamber) receiving some, and usually all, of the pulmonary veins; and an anterior, leftward, and caudal one (true left atrium) emptying through the mitral valve (Fig. 5). The accessory chamber is believed to be a dilated common pulmonary vein that was not incorporated into the left atrium during embryonic life (5, 6, 17). The walls of both chambers and the partition dividing them contain cardiac muscle (Fig. 6), but at the junction site myocardium may be absent. The left atrial appendage always connects with the true left atrium, as does the foramen ovale. The remainder of the fossa ovalis, however, may be either above or below the left atrial partition, and thus it is possible for a catheter to pass from right atrium not only into true left atrium, but also into the accessory chamber either by the transseptal technique or through an atrial septal defect.

The size of the communication between the two left atrial chambers and the presence or absence of other cardiovascular anomalies are the primary determinants of the type and severity of the physiologic alterations in cor triatriatum (5, 18). The opening between the two left atrial chambers is usually single and less than 8 mm in maximal diameter (10, 17–19). Because forward flow occurs during systole as well as diastole, a smaller orifice can be tolerated than in mitral valve stenosis where flow occurs only during diastole (20, 21). Nevertheless, the opening is so small that death from pulmonary edema may occur before 6 mo of age (17, 19). On rare occasions, the communication between the accessory chamber and left atrium may be large enough that no obstruction to pulmonary venous return occurs; such was

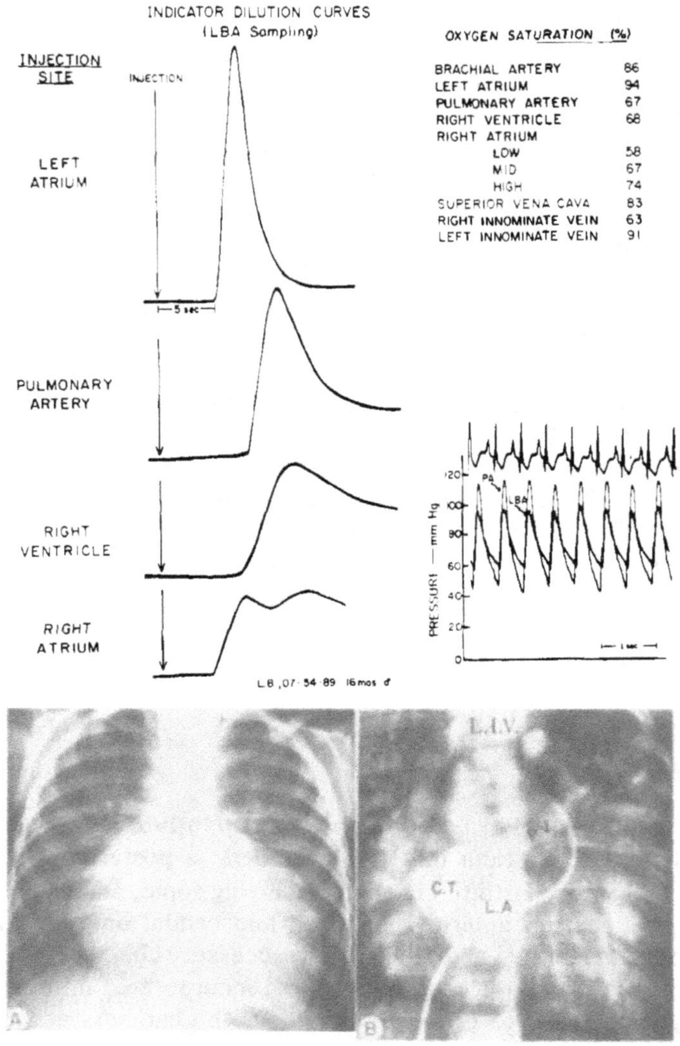

Fig. 5. Cor triatriatum in a 17-mo old boy (A67-226). He had been considered well except for frequent respiratory infections until age 9 mo when evidence of congestive cardiac failure appeared and cyanosis was noted during activity. At age 16 mo, examination disclosed rapid respirations, a grade 4/6 pansystolic murmur with a thrill along the left sternal edge and apex, and a grade 2/6 diastolic apical rumble. Electrocardiogram showed right axis deviation, right atrial enlargement, and right ventricular hypertrophy. Chest roentgenogram (A) showed massive cardiomegaly. Catheterization showed the following pressures in mm Hg: pulmonary artery (PA), 115/48; right ventricle, 115/8; right atrial mean, 13; true left atrial mean, 12; and brachial artery (LBA), 95/60. The indicator dilution curves established the presence of a right to left shunt at atrial level: dye appeared at the left brachial artery (LBA) earlier after right atrial injection than after injection into right ventricle or pulmonary artery. The elevated oxygen saturations in blood from left innominate vein and superior vena cava were the result of anomalous connection of the left upper lobe pulmonary vein. The depressed brachial arterial saturation was due to a right to left shunt at atrial level. On the late film of the pulmonary angiogram (B), the radiolucent line between the third chamber (CT) and the left atrium proper (LA) is the fibromuscular septum. The left pulmonary vein (PV) connects with the third chamber, and its upper lobe branch also connects with the left innominate vein (LIV) through an anomalous vertical vein. Operation was performed and the membrane separating the accessory left atrial chamber from the true left atrium was excised (Fig. 6). The child, however, could not be separated from cardiopulmonary bypass.

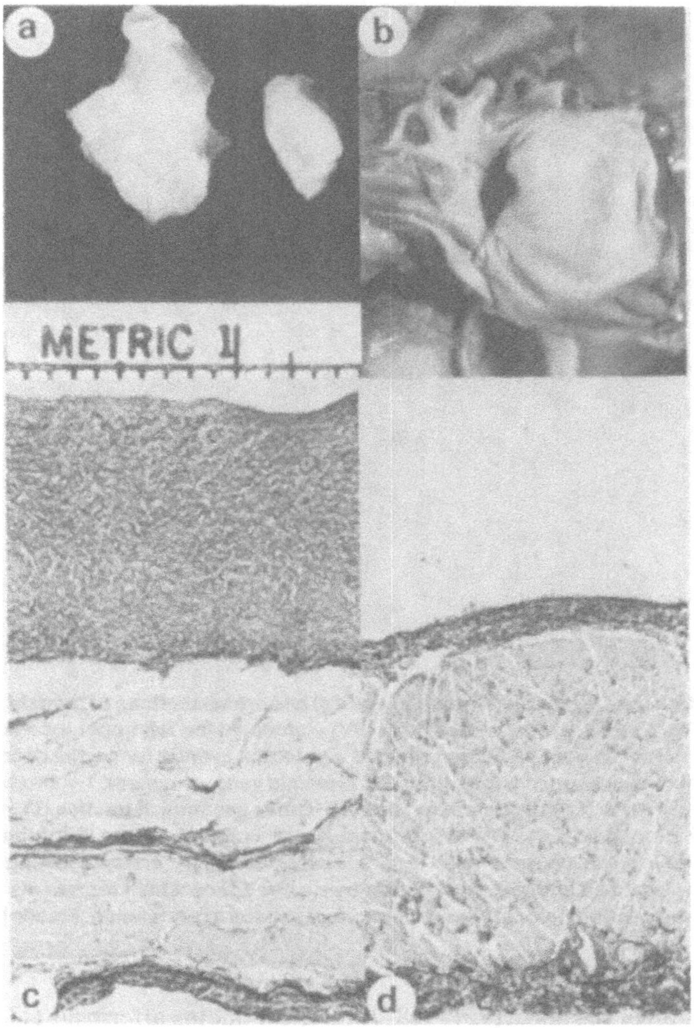

Fig. 6. Cor triatriatum. Resected "membrane" (a) and the opened accessory left atrial chamber (b) in the child described in Fig. 5. The amount of tissue resected was so small that the obstruction may not have been relieved. The endocardium of the accessory left atrium is quite thick (c) compared to the endocardium of the true left atrium (d). The higher the atrial pressure, the thicker the endocardium. Elastic tissue stains: each × 50 (c, d).

the case in McAllister's patient who never had cardiovascular symptoms and died at age 76 years during resection of a rectal carcinoma (22).

Although it may occur as an isolated anomaly, cor triatriatum often occurs in association with other cardiovascular malformations. Of these, partial anomalous pulmonary venous connection and atrial septal defect are the most common. Although various types of abnormal venous connections occur, often an anomalous vertical vein connects end to side both to a left upper lobe pulmonary vein and to the left innominate vein (10). This anatomic arrangement, found in two of our patients with anomalous veins, allows for some decompression of the accessory chamber, as well as of the involved segment of lung (Figs. 5–7). Ventricular septal defect (18,

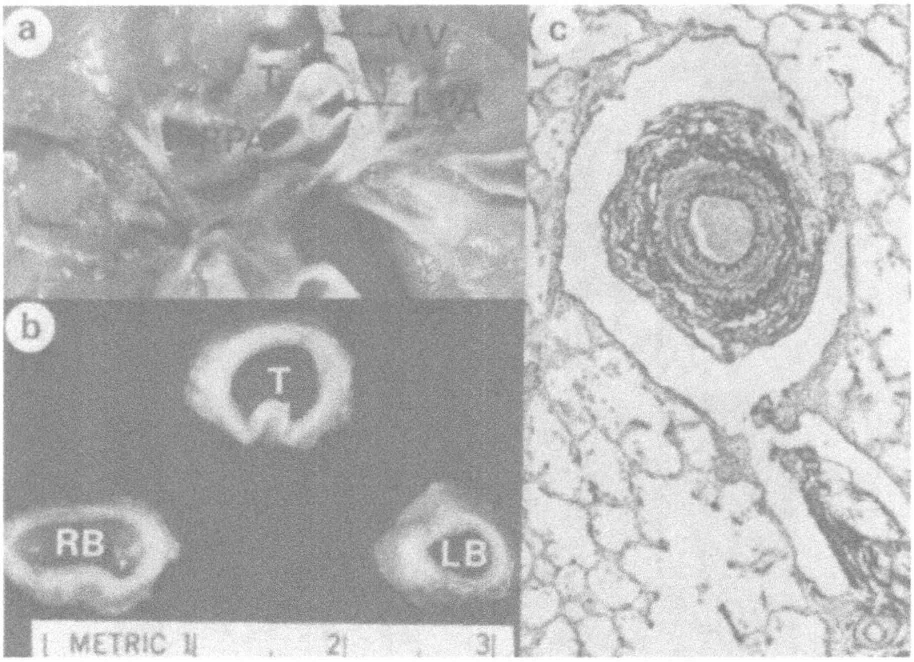

Fig. 7. Cor triatriatum. Pulmonary vessels (a and c) and cross-sections of bronchi (b) in the child described in Fig. 5 and 6. a, The vertical vein (VV) connected the left upper lobe pulmonary vein with the left innominate vein and thus provided a potential avenue for partial decompression of the high pressure accessory chamber into the systemic venous system. T = trachea; LPA = left pulmonary artery; RPA = right pulmonary artery. b, Cross sections of trachea (T), right bronchus (RB), and left bronchus (LB). The left bronchus was compressed by the high-pressure left pulmonary artery which coursed over it. c, A small pulmonary artery showing considerable medial hypertrophy. The artery is surrounded by a clear space which represents a very dilated lympathic channel, an indicator of severe pulmonary venous hypertension. Elastic tissue stain: × 48.

22), coarctation of the aorta (5, 17, 18, 22), patent ductus arteriosus (17, 18, 20, 22), persistent common atrioventricular canal (18), tetralogy of Fallot (17, 18, 23, 24), and TAPVC (22) are less common associated lesions, and other associated anomalies are extremely rare (10, 17, 18, 20).

When cor triatriatum is the only abnormality, the hemodynamic derangement is virtually identical to that of mitral stenosis. The pulmonary venous hypertension results in elevated pulmonary capillary pressures, pulmonary arterial hypertension, right ventriclar hypertrophy (Fig. 8), and right atrial enlargement. Pulmonary edema is common, and eventually right-sided cardiac failure occurs. Either partial anomalous pulmonary venous connection or an atrial septal defect between the accessory chamber and the right atrium may give rise to a left to right shunt, but pulmonary venous hypertension remains the dominant hemodynamic abnormality, just as in patients with combined mitral stenosis and partial anomalous pulmonary venous connection or a small atrial septal defect (25, 26). A right to left shunt may occur when a defect in atrial septum exists between right atrium and true left atrium (19) (Fig. 5). In a small number of patients, the fibromuscular septum in the left atrium is atretic. Under these circumstances pulmonary venous blood leaves the

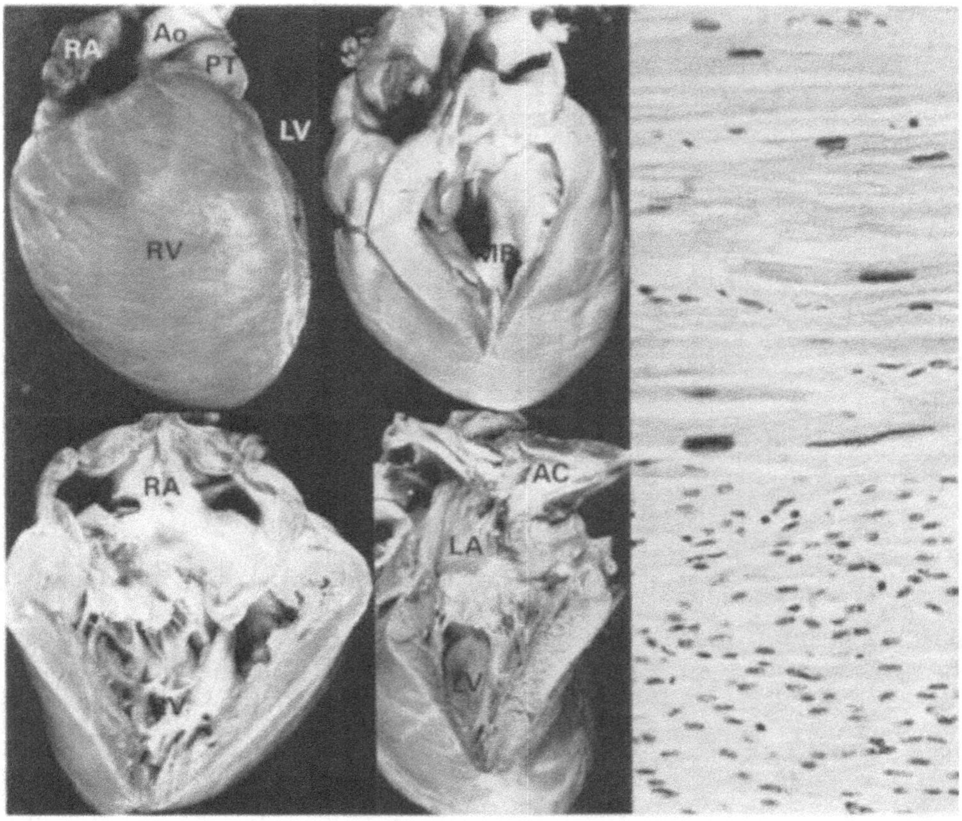

Fig. 8. Cor triatriatum. Gross (left) and microscopic (right) anatomy of the heart of the boy described in Figs. 5–7. The condition causes massive right ventricular hypertrophy because severe pulmonary hypertension is present from birth. Upper left, exterior view showing a huge right ventricle (RV) and a very small left ventricle (LV) in comparison. RA = right atrium; PT = pulmonary trunk; AO = aorta. Upper center, right ventricular outflow tract, pulmonic valve, and pulmonary trunk. The moderator band (MB) is enormously hypertrophied as is the entire right ventricular free wall. Lower left, opened right atrium, tricuspid valve, and right ventricular inflow tract, and lower center, opened accessory left atrium (AC), true left atrium (LA), mitral valve, and left ventricle (LV). (These photos were taken at the same magnification to show that the right ventricle is much bigger than the left ventricle.) Again, the thick endocardium of the accessory left atrium and the thin endocardium of the true left atrium are apparent. Actually, the endocardium of the right atrium is thicker than that of the true left atrium. The foramen ovale is valvular competent, but because, during life, pressure in right atrium exceeded that in true left atrium, the valve was open and a right to left shunt occurred (Fig. 5). Right, histologic sections (hematoxylin and eosin stains), photographed at the same magnification (× 232) show that the myocardial cells of the right ventricle (above) are enormously hypertrophied while those of the left ventricle (below) are normal.

accessory chamber either through an atrial septal defect or via a pulmonary vein which connects both with the accessory chamber and with a systemic vein. Blood reaches the true left atrium from right atrium through a patent foramen ovale or atrial septal defect. In such patients, the hemodynamic abnormality, and consequently the clinical picture, is virtually identical to that of TAPVC (19).

When the opening between the accessory chamber and true left atrium is extremely small, symptoms usually develop between ages 2 wk and 2 mo (5, 10, 19, 20,

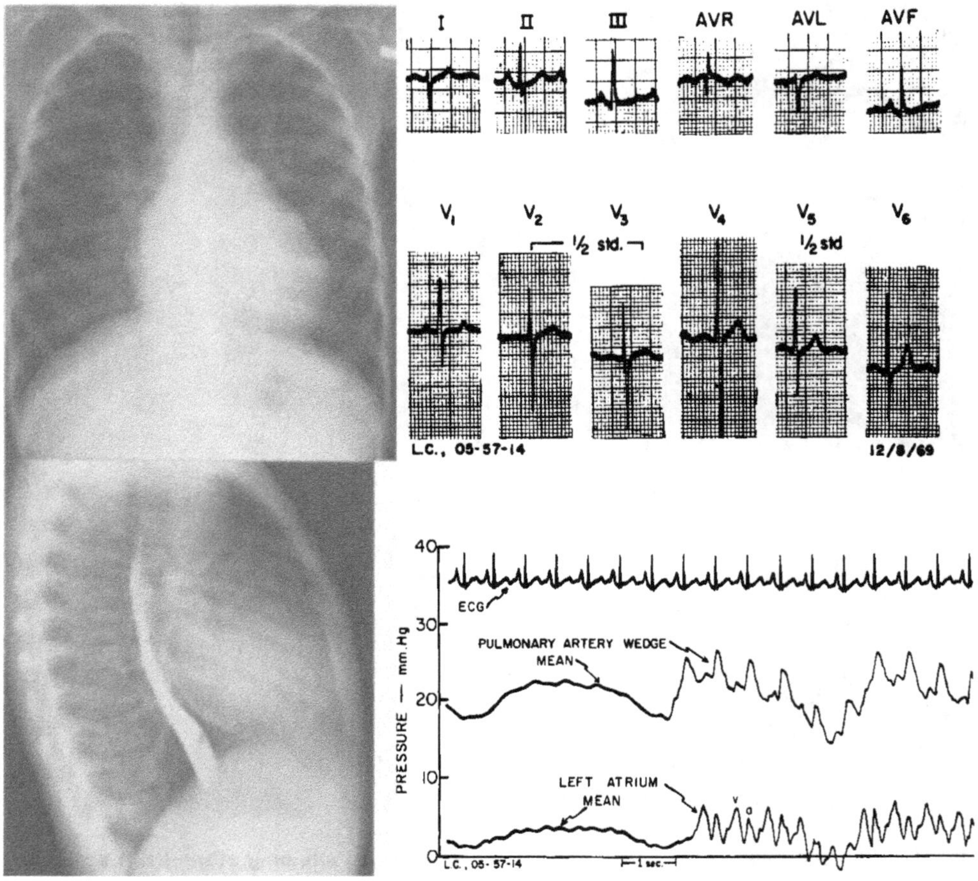

Fig. 9. Cor triatriatum in a 10-yr old girl, who for many years was believed to have primary pulmonary hypertension. The disproportionately prominent upper lobe vasculature and the "left atrial" enlargement on chest radiographs suggest, however, that the pulmonary arterial hypertension is secondary to pulmonary venous hypertension. Her electrocardiogram shows right axis deviation, right ventricular hypertrophy, and right atrial enlargement. At cardiac catheterization, pressure in left atrium was low normal while simultaneously measured pulmonary arterial wedge pressure was markedly elevated. After resection of the fibromuscular septum between accessory chamber and true left atrium, she was markedly improved.

27). The infant is irritable, feeds poorly, fails to gain weight, sweats excessively, coughs, breathes rapidly, and, episodically, may be cyanotic from pulmonary edema. In patients with less severe obstruction, symptoms often begin later in childhood or even during adult life. In them, effort and nocturnal dyspnea, orthopnea, and hemoptysis mimic mitral stenosis (19–21, 27). Occasionally, fatigue is the predominant symptom and, along with the findings of severe pulmonary arterial hypertension, prompts an erroneous diagnosis of primary pulmonary hypertension (Fig. 9).

Examination usually discloses a prominent A wave in the jugular pulse, reflecting an increase in resistance to right ventricular filling due to hypertrophy. Large V waves, hepatomegaly, and, in older patients, dependent edema indicate right ventricular failure, often accompanied by tricuspid regurgitation (10, 20). A prominent right ventricular lift usually is palpable parasternally and in the epigastrum (19, 20, 27). Basilar pulmonary rales may be heard (10). The pulmonic component of the second heart sound is loud (18) and often palpable. The second sound is either narrowly split or single (18–20, 27). A third heart sound may be heard (19), but there is no opening snap. Murmurs may be absent or systolic, diastolic, or continuous murmurs may occur. A systolic ejection murmur along the left sternal border is common (10, 18, 19). A pansystolic murmur at the lower sternal edge or apex is most often due to tricuspid regurgitation accompanying right ventricular failure (19, 20), but mitral valvular regurgitation also may occur (28). Because of the severe pulmonary arterial hypertension, pulmonic regurgitation with its high-pitched basal early diastolic murmur is common (18, 20, 29). Also occasionally heard along the left sternal border and at the apex is a low-pitched diastolic murmur, which presumably represents flow from the accessory chamber into the true left atrium (18, 19, 29). A continuous murmur may arise by the same mechanism since flow occurs throughout the cardiac cycle. In one of our patients (Fig. 9), a continuous murmur over the left upper chest was associated with anomalous connection of the left upper lobe pulmonary vein.

The electrocardiogram shows right axis deviation, marked right ventricular hypertrophy and P waves that suggest right (Fig. 9) or biatrial (Fig. 10) enlargement. Atrial fibrillation is uncommon (27, 29).

On chest radiographs, pulmonary venous distention (Figs. 9, 11) and interstitial edema (Fig. 11) are often seen; alveolar edema is less frequent. The pulmonary trunk and proximal pulmonary arteries are dilated. Overall heart size usually is only slightly to moderately increased (Figs. 9, 11), but occasionally the heart is huge (Fig. 5). The large right ventricle encroaches on the retrosternal space in the lateral film (Fig. 9). In addition, right atrial enlargement may be suggested by the prominent right border of the cardiac silhouette in both the posteroanterior and the left anterior oblique projections. Although it may be large (29), the "left atrium" usually is only mildly dilated (Fig. 9) or of normal size.

Although echocardiography can establish the diagnosis of cor triatriatum by demonstrating the septum between accessory chamber and true left atrium (30), a false negative diagnosis can be made if the plane of the septum is such that it does not reflect ultrasound waves back to the transducer (16). In addition, an echo of unknown origin frequently is seen in the left atrium of normal children (16), and it is a potential source of false positive diagnoses. Thus at the present time echocardiography is not a reliable means of diagnosing or excluding cor triatriatum.

At catheterization, pulmonary arterial pressure is elevated and often equals or exceeds systemic arterial pressure (Fig. 5). Pulmonary arterial wedge pressure also is markedly elevated (Fig. 9). In contrast, pressure is normal in the true left atrial chamber, which often can be entered via a patent foramen ovale, and this, of course, indicates that the obstruction is proximal to the mitral valve. When a patent foramen ovale cannot be crossed, the transseptal technique may be used to reach the true left atrium; occasionally, however, the accessory chamber is entered instead (19, 28) (Fig. 10). Because anomalous pulmonary venous connection and/or atrial septal defect coexist in many patients with cor triatriatum, an oxygen step-up may be found in the left innominate vein (Fig. 5), superior vena cava, or right atrium. When tetralogy of Fallot coexists, pulmonary arterial pressure is normal or only mildly increased, and consequently cor triatriatum has never been diagnosed before operation or necropsy in a patient with associated tetralogy of Fallot (24). The occurrence of a normal or slightly elevated, rather than a low pulmonary arterial pressure in a patient with tetralogy of Fallot should alert the physician to the

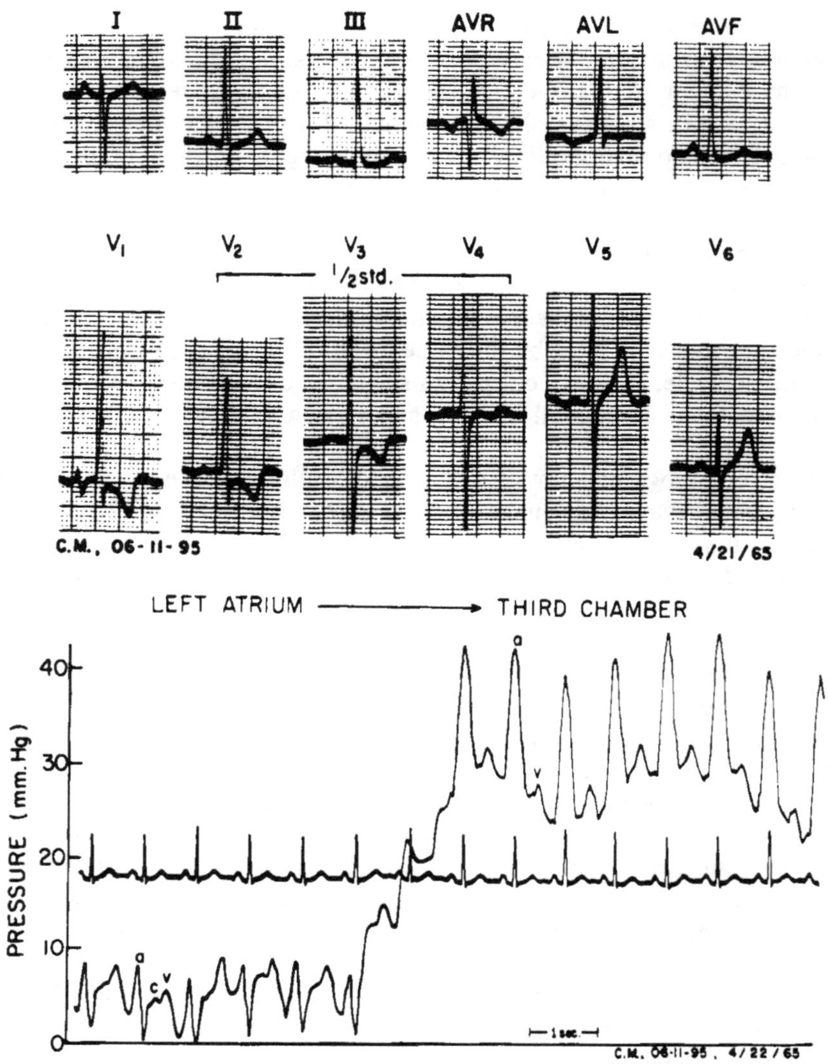

Fig. 10. Cortriatriatum in an 18-yr-old man. The electrocardiogram shows marked right axis deviation and right ventricular hypertrophy, and the P waves suggest biatrial enlargement. At cardiac catheterization, the third chamber was entered by the transseptal technique, and the catheter was then manipulated into true left atrium. The pressure tracing in the lower half of the figure was recorded as the catheter was withdrawn from left atrium, where pressure was normal, to the third chamber, where pressure was markedly elevated.

possibility of coexisting cor triatriatum. If in a patient with combined tetralogy and cor triatriatum, the ventricular septal defect is closed and the right ventricular outflow obstruction relieved without relieving the left-sided obstruction, the increased pulmony blood flow may produce pulmonary edema and death (23).

Pulmonary arteriography provides a definitive diagnosis when the fibromuscular septum separating the two left atrial chambers is visualized (29, 31) (Figs. 5, 11), and at present it is the only reliable way to distinguish cor triatriatum from obstruction of individual pulmonary veins preoperatively. Because the circulation time through the lungs is prolonged in cor triatriatum, films taken late after the injection often are

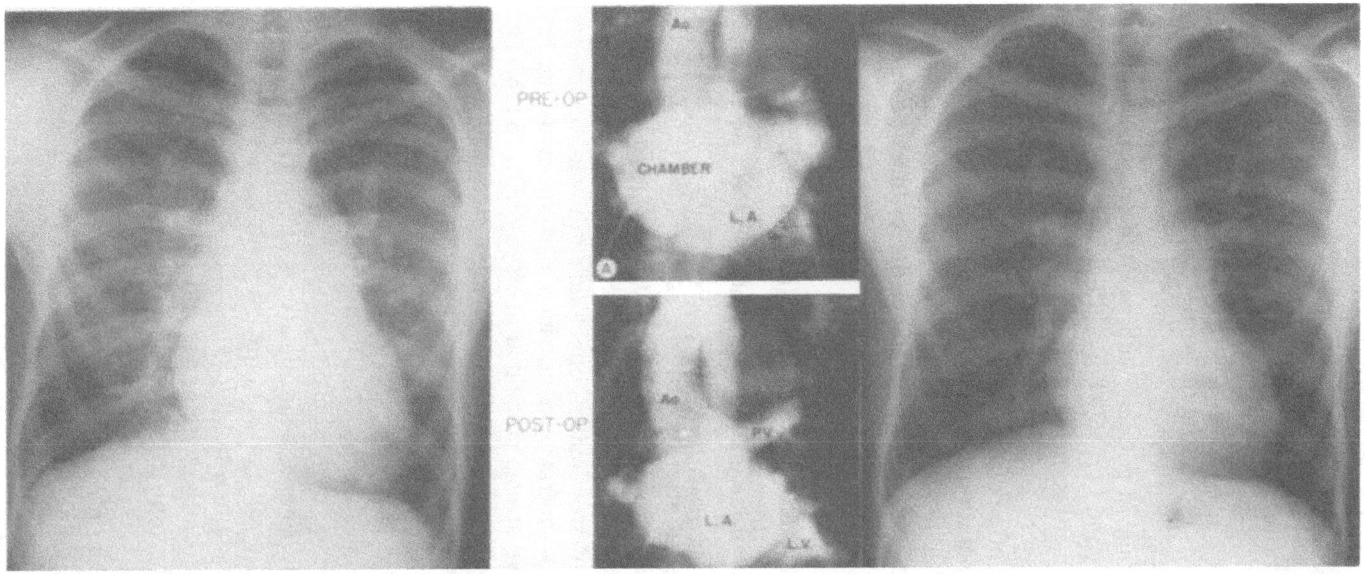

Fig. 11. Cor triatriatum. Radiography in the patient whose electrocardiogram and pressure tracings are shown in Fig. 10. The preoperative chest radiograph (left) shows slight cardiomegaly, a large pulmonary trunk, prominent upper lobe pulmonary vessels, and interstitial pulmonary edema with prominent B lines of Kerley (seen best at the right base). Postoperatively (right), heart size has decreased, and the features of pulmonary venous hypertension and interstitial edema have disappeared. The pulmonary trunk remains large. In both angiograms contrast material was injected through a transseptal catheter. Preoperatively, the third chamber is separated from the true left atrium (LA) by a fibromuscular septum that is seen as a radiolucency. Postoperatively, the radiolucency can no longer be seen. MV = mitral valve; PV = pulmonary vein; LV = left ventricle; Ao = aorta.

necessary if the left side of the heart is to be visualized. Unfortunately, even when these are obtained, the septum may not be seen because the true left atrium and the accessory chamber overlap. When the fibromuscular septum cannot be seen, a left atrial injection may be helpful in that the chamber visualized is much smaller than the left atrial chamber(s) seen after pulmonary arterial injection (27).

Prognosis in patients with cor triatriatum varies greatly depending on the size of the communication between the two left atria and on the presence or absence of additional anomalies. Among 76 patients with isolated cor triatriatum, 76% survived beyond 6 mo, 67% beyond 1 yr, 46% beyond 2 yr, and 20% beyond 20 yr (17).

The only definitive treatment is operative relief of the obstruction. Although the partition between the accessory and true left atrium has been incised during closed procedures, the results are often disappointing, and excision of the entire obstructing partition during open operation is preferred (18, 32). Results have been excellent in most older children and adults (Fig. 11). Rapidly improving methods for operating on critically ill infants should allow good results in the sick infant with cor triatriatum.

MITRAL VALVE ATRESIA AND HYPOPLASIA (Fig. 12–14)

Mitral atresia is never an isolated anomaly. In addition to a defect that virtually always is present in the atrial septum and is necessary for survival, there also is some abnormality of the great arteries or of the aortic valve or of the ventricular septum or of two of these three. Mitral atresia is most often seen in association with atresia of the aortic valve, and because aortic-valve atresia is common—indeed the most common cause of death from major congenital cardiovascular malformations during the 1st wk of life (33)—mitral valve atresia is also common (Fig. 12). Among 73 patients with aortic valve atresia studied at necropsy (33), 26 (36%) had mitral atresia. Of the remaining 47 patients with aortic valve atresia 44 had hypoplastic mitral valves. Except when ventricular septal defect occurs in association with aortic valve atresia, the mitral valve is always either atretic or extremely hypoplastic, and the left ventricular cavity is minute. In the infants with aortic atresia combined with mitral hypoplasia (Fig. 12, IB) the endocardium of the minute left ventricle is diffusely thickened by fibroelastic tissue that makes this small cavity inelastic and noncompliant. When the mitral valve is atretic rather than hypoplastic, in association with aortic valve atresia, the left ventricular cavity is even more hypoplastic, but its endocradium is not thickened (Fig. 12, IA). When mitral valve atresia or hypoplasia is associated with aortic valve atresia, only rarely (Fig. 12, IIA) is a defect present in the ventricular septum (33). Usually, the defect present in the atrial septum is in the form of a foramen ovale that is incompetent due to prolapse of its valve into the right atrium because of the much higher pressures in the left atrium. Presumably due to diminished blood flow through it during intrauterine life, the left atrium in mitral atresia is almost invariably quite small (10, 33). In addition, its endocardium is inordinately thick.

Less commonly, mitral valve atresia is associated with a nonatretic aortic valve (Fig. 13). When this circumstance exists, either a common ventricle or two well-developed ventricular cavities are present, and the great arteries may be transposed. Again, however, some type of defect must be present in the atrial septum.

The clinical manifestations of mitral atresia are variable and obviously depend to

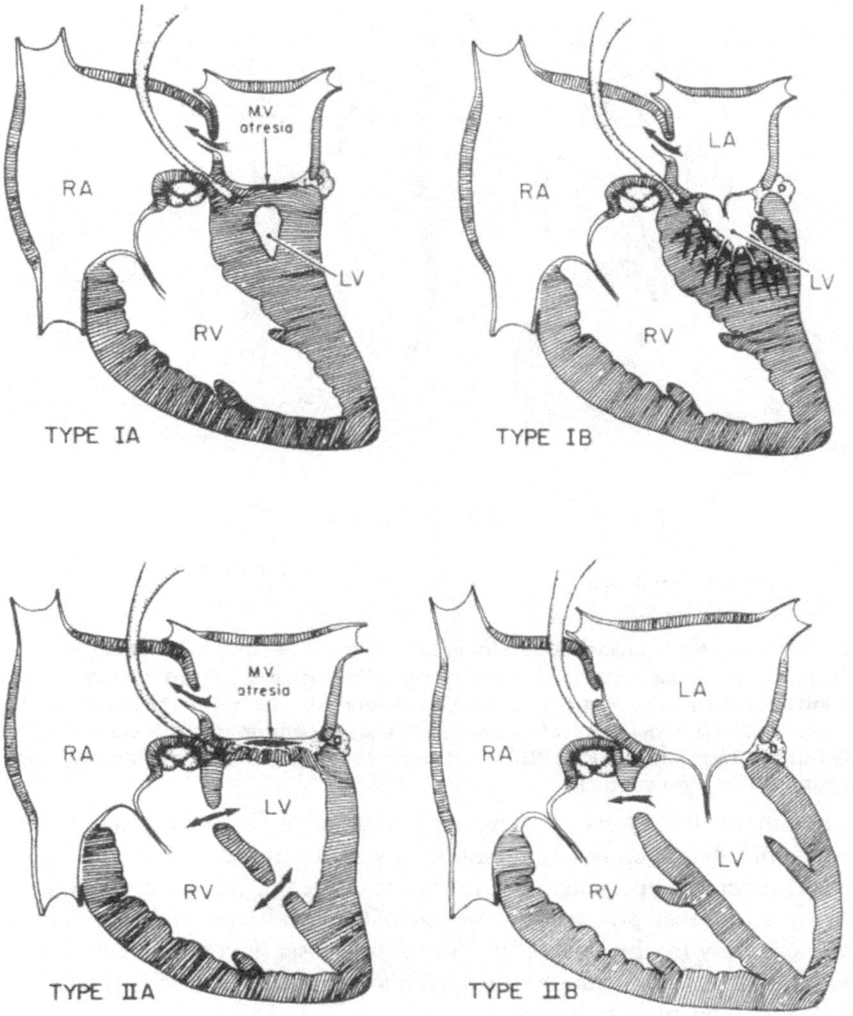

Fig. 12. The mitral valve in aortic valve atresia. Hearts with aortic valve atresia have been classified according to the morphology of the ventricular septum (VS) and of the mitral valve (MV) (33). Of 73 hearts examined, 25 (34%) were Type IA (intact VS, atretic MV); 44 (60%) were Type IB (intact VS, hypoplastic MV); 1 (1%) was Type IIA (VS defect, atretic MV); and 3 (4%) were Type IIB (VS defect, normal MV). Thus, the mitral valve is rarely normal in patients with aortic valve atresia, and a ventricular septal defect is a necessary condition for this normalcy. When the septum is intact, the mitral valve is always atretic or hypoplastic, and the left ventricular cavity is minute. In patients with mitral atresia all blood entering the left atrium (LA) must either cross the atrial septum, usually via a small opening produced by herniation of the valve of the fossa ovalis into the right atrium (RA), or rarely, when the foramen ovale has prematurely closed, be shunted to a systemic vein by a levoatriocardinal vein (5, 34). In patients with a hypoplastic mitral valve, left ventricular (LV) myocardial sinusoids provide additional pathways for the egress of blood which eventually reaches right atrium via the coronary sinus (33, 34). In all patients with aortic valve atresia, systemic and pulmonary venous returns are pumped by a large right ventricle (RV) to an equally large pulmonary trunk. All blood reaching the systemic arterial circuit does so via a large patent ductus arteriosus. (The left portion of Fig. 13 diagrams this in a patient whose aortic valve was severely hypoplastic rather than atretic.)

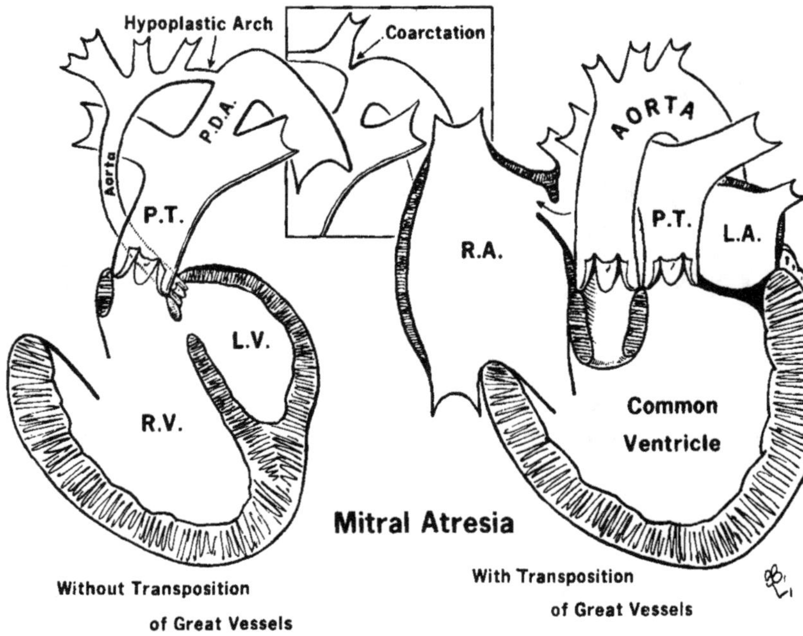

Fig. 13. Mitral atresia not associated with aortic valve atresia. In this circumstance, the aortic valve is usually either stenotic or severely hypoplastic (left) or a subaortic chamber is present (right), and the latter may be obstructive. The great arteries may or may not be transposed, and the ventricular septum is either absent (common ventricle) or perforated (ventricular septal defect). LA = left atrium; LV = left ventricle; PDA = patent ductus arteriosus; PT = pulmonary trunk; RA = right atrium; RV = right ventricle.

some extent on the types of associated anomalies. In most patients, a major hemodynamic derangement is pulmonary venous hypertension. The degree of pulmonary venous hypertension (but not the degree of pulmonary arterial hypertension) is determined primarily by the size of the atrial septal defect, which usually is small, or rarely by the size of an anomalous vessel (levoatriocardinal vein) that shunts blood from left atrium to the systemic venous system (5, 34) and is similar functionally to the anomalous vein described in Figs. 5 and 7. If the defect is small, the pulmonary venous pressures may be strikingly elevated. Since all pulmonary venous blood in mitral atresia must enter the right atrium, the hemodynamic abnormality is similar to that in TAPVC with obstruction. There exist under these circumstances both increased flow to the lungs and obstruction to flow from the lungs.

Like TAPVC with obstruction, mitral atresia with an obstructive atrial septum usually manifests itself clinically during the first days of extrauterine life, and the two conditions may be difficult to distinguish from one another. Respiratory distress is the most prominent feature. The infant feeds poorly, is irritable, and fails to gain weight. Because systemic arterial oxygen saturation is directly proportional to pulmonary blood flow and, consequently, inversely proportional to pulmonary resistance (35), infants with obstructive atrial septa tend to be more cyanotic than those with free communication between the two atria. Hepatomegaly is common. The right ventricle is prominent to palpation, and the pulmonic closure sound is generally loud. The high velocity jet of blood across the atrial septum may cause a continuous murmur (36), and murmurs due to other lesions may be heard.

The electrocardiogram often shows right atrial enlargement, right axis deviation, and marked right ventricular hypertrophy. On chest radiograph, the cardiac silhouette is often larger than in patients with TAPVC with obstruction. The pulmonary markings may suggest either venous hypertension or increased pulmonary arterial flow.

In most instances, mitral atresia or hypoplasia can be diagnosed accurately by echocardiography (15, 16, 30, 37, 38). The mitral valve echo is either absent or grossly distorted with an excursion that is less than normal. In the usual case in which mitral atresia or hypoplasia is associated with aortic atresia or hypoplasia, the right ventricular cavity is abnormally large; the left ventricular cavity is abnormally small or echocardiographically unidentifiable; and the aortic root is either unidentifiable or its diameter is greatly reduced. The severely hypoplastic left heart can usually be diagnosed with sufficient confidence by echocardiography that cardiac catheterization, which is hazardous in infants with these conditions, is unnecessary.

When a firm diagnosis cannot be established by echocardiography, definitive diagnosis is by cardiac catheterization and angiocardiography. A large oxygen step-up is detected in the right atrium, or in the left innominate vein in the rare event that the atrial septum has closed prematurely and a levoatriocardinal vein is present. The foramen ovale usually can be crossed, and any pressure gradient between the two atria (Fig. 14) will be detected by this means. Pressure in the pulmonary trunk is usually the same or slightly higher than in the descending aorta, which often can be entered via a patent ductus arteriosus. A left atrial angiogram showing that chamber to empty solely by way of an atrial septal defect is diagnostic. Usually diagnosis also can be made from the levophase of a pulmonary arterial injection and, occasionally, from a right atrial injection (Fig. 14). Aortography is the best means of diagnosing associated aortic atresia (35). The ascending aorta in this circumstance is hypoplastic and its only function is that of a common coronary artery.

Prognosis in mitral atresia or severe hypoplasia is dismal. Over 50% of the patients with atresia die within 1 mo of birth, usually within 1 wk if there is coexistent aortic atresia. In the presence of a normal left ventricular outflow tract and a ventricular septal defect, the patient may survive months (Fig. 14) or even years (36).

There is no definitive operative treatment. Severe hypoglycemia, which is common in these and other newborn infants with cardiac failure (39), can be prevented by continuous intravenous infusion of glucose. Atrial septostomy is of potential benefit. An occasional patient is improved by transthoracic atrial septostomy (Fig. 14), but several have died in the immediate postoperative period (35). In infants, balloon septostomy has the advantage of avoiding thoracotomy, but in some of them the left atrium may be too small to allow adequate inflation of the balloon. Occasionally the anatomic features in an individual patient with mitral atresia or hypoplasia are such that other types of operation may provide successful palliation (40).

SUPRAVALVULAR LEFT ATRIAL RING (Fig. 15–17)

In this malformation, a ridge of fibrous tissue extends partially or completely around the left atrial cavity just cephalad to, or at the level of, the mitral annulus.

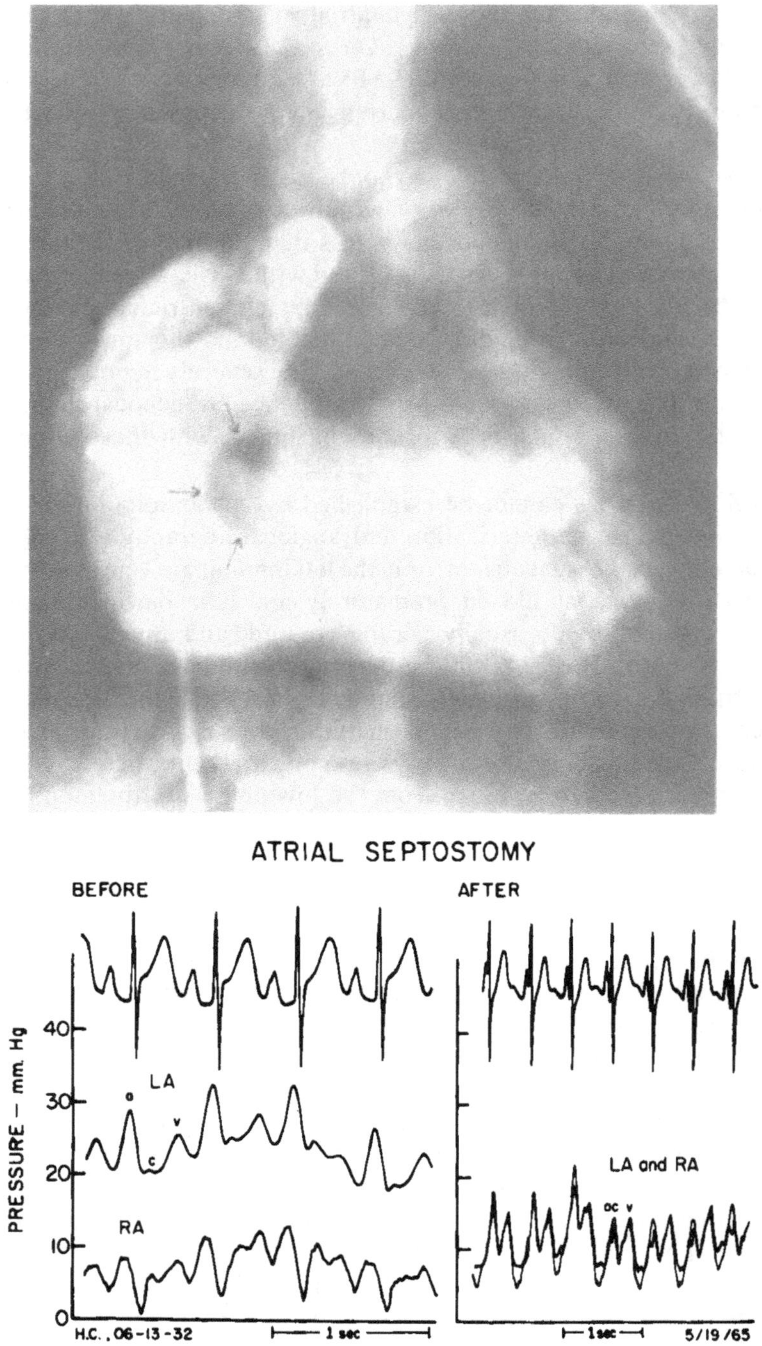

Fig. 14. **Mitral valve atresia in a 16-mo old boy with a large ventricular septal defect and a normal left ventricular outflow tract. In the preoperative right atrial angiogram (top) the herniated valve of the foramen ovale (arrows) is seen as a radiolucency in the middle of the opacified right atrium. Pressure tracings (bottom) recorded at operation (performed by Dr. A. G. Morrow) show a markedly elevated left atrial (LA) pressure and a large pressure gradient between LA and right atrium (RA) before atrial septostomy. After septostomy LA pressure is much lower and is virtually identical to that in RA. The patient also underwent pulmonary artery banding.**

The supravalvular ring may cause severe obstruction (Fig. 15), or be rudimentary and cause no hemodynamic disturbance (Fig. 16). Of 25 reported patients with this anomaly (41–45), only one has not had other cardiovascular malformations (45), and supravalvular left atrial ring usually forms part of the parachute mitral valve or single papillary muscle syndrome (Fig. 17).

When the supravalvular ring severely narrows the mitral orifice, the clinical features are those of mitral valvular stenosis, but the findings frequently are obscured in part by the associated lesions (42). The only bedside finding that might separate valvular from supravalvular mitral stenosis is an opening snap. Although found in a few patients with congenital valvular stenosis (Fig. 18), an opening snap has not been described in patients with supravalvular obstruction. Although, theoretically, supravalvular stenosis can be proved either by measuring left atrial pressure both above and below the ring (41) or by visualizing the ring echocardiographically (30, 45) or angiographically (45), the technical difficulties with each of these procedures in patients with this condition are formidable, and consequently the diagnosis is only rarely made before operation or necropsy. Echocardiography is of great value, of course, in determining the presence or absence of mitral valvular stenosis, which may be associated with or mimic supravalvular stenosis. Pulmonary arteriography is probably the best way to demonstrate the ring (45) but, as in cor triatriatum, the obstructing lesion may not be seen.

Treatment consists of operative excision of the ring as well as correction of the associated defects. When the supravalvular ring is the most important physiological malformation, excellent operative results may be obtained (41, 43, 45), but, in general, results have been poor, in large part because of the associated anomalies.

MITRAL STENOSIS (Figs. 18–27)

In contrast to rheumatic mitral stenosis, congenital mitral stenosis occurs with equal frequency in the two sexes. In congenital mitral stenosis, usually the entire mitral apparatus is malformed (46). The leaflets are thickened by fibrous tissue but calcific deposits are rare; the chordae tendineae are short, thick, fewer in number than usual, and those present are often fused resulting in diminished interchordal space. Most often, all chordae tendineae insert into a single papillary muscle producing the so-called parachute mitral valve (42, 44) (Figs. 15–17, 19, 21–23). Both papillary muscles may be present, however, and, in this circumstance when the leaflets insert directly onto the papillary muscles, an anomalous mitral arcade may result (47) (Fig. 27). With both of these malformations, mitral regurgitation may accompany stenosis and may even be the dominant hemodynamic abnormality (44, 51). Associated malformations are common (48–52), being present in 13 of our 16 patients with congenital mitral stenosis. In addition to the deformities commonly occurring in association with the parachute mitral valve (42), (Figs. 15, 17, 19, 21–22), valvular aortic stenosis, (Fig. 19, 27), valvular pulmonic stenosis (Figs. 23, 24), patent ductus arteriosis (Figs. 15, 20), and ventricular septal defect (Figs. 15, 19, 20, 25) also are common.

The degree of obstruction in congenital mitral stenosis is usually severe, and consequently symptoms appear early in life: before 1 mo of age in about one-third of patients and before 1 year in about three-fourths of them (48). Dyspnea, cough, difficulty feeding, frequent respiratory infections, and failure to thrive are usual.

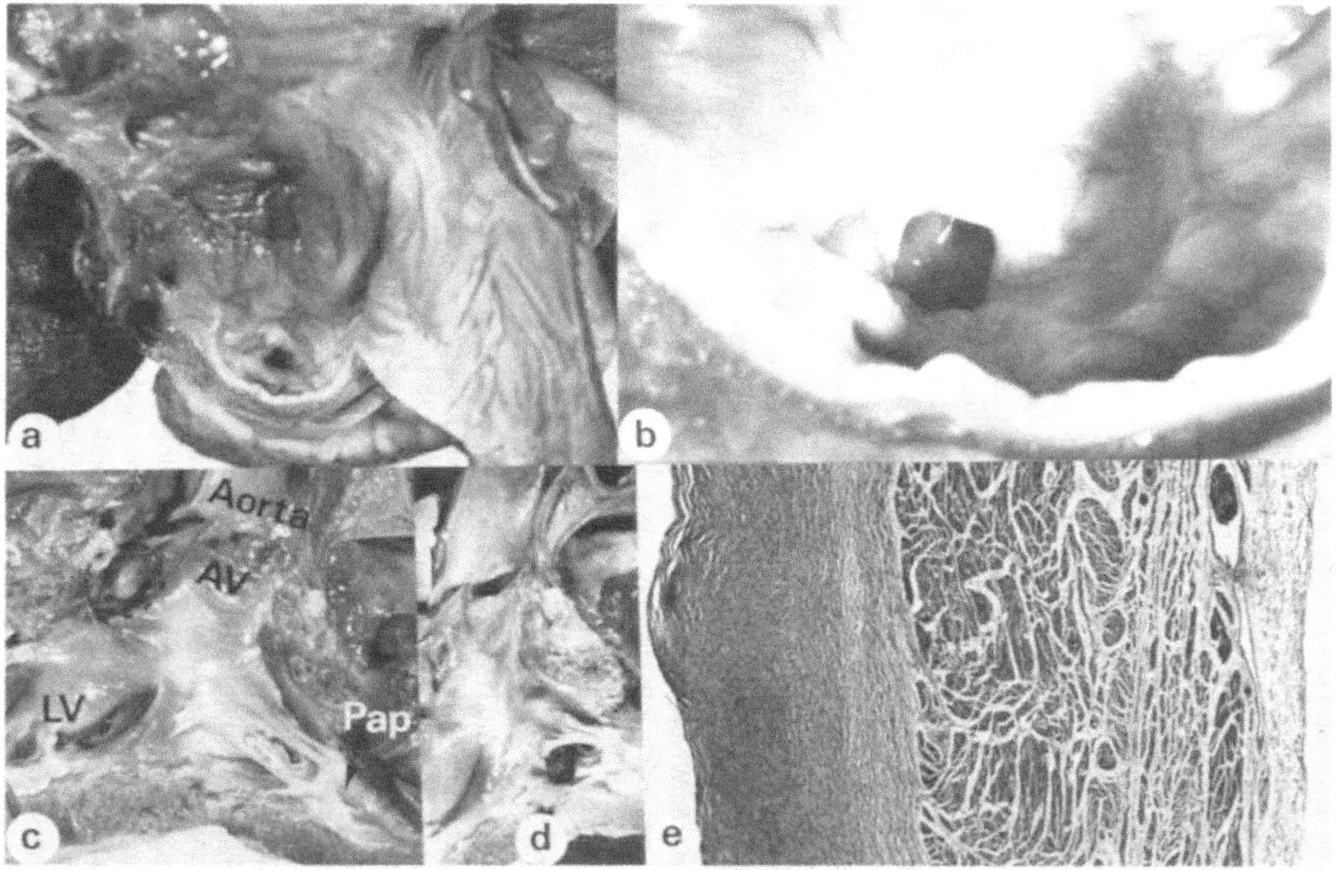

Fig. 15. Supravalvular mitral ring causing obstruction and associated with the parachute mitral valve syndrome in an infant (A69-264) who died of progressive congestive cardiac failure. a, Opened left atrium. The cavity is enormously dilated and the endocardium, enormously thickened (e). b, Close-up of the obstruction, located actually at, rather than just cephalad to the annulus. c, Opened left ventricle (LV) showing only one papillary muscle (pap) and a stenotic mitral orifice. A probe is placed through the mitral orifice in d. A ventricular septal defect (dashed circle) is located just caudal to the normal aortic valve (AV). In addition, coarctation of the aortic isthmus and patent ductus arteriosus were present. e, Photomicrograph of the thickened left atrial endocardium. Hematoxylin and eosin stain; × 18.

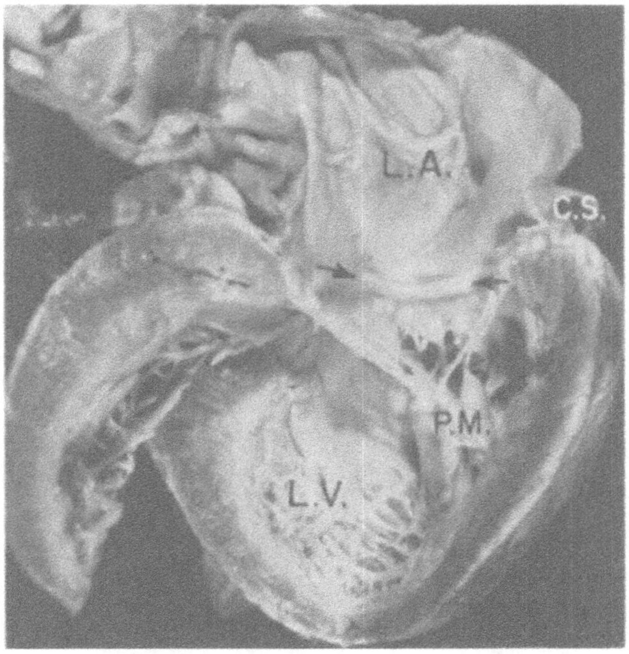

Fig. 16. Rudimentary supravalvular left atrial ring (arrows) of no hemodynamic consequence in the heart of a 6-yr-old girl. Parachute deformity of the mitral valve is present with all chordae tendineae inserting into a single left ventricular (LV) papillary muscle (PM). The interchordal spaces appear adequate, and the valve is not significantly stenotic. The patient also had a ventricular septal defect and right ventricular outflow obstruction due to an anomalous right ventricular muscle bundle. CS = coronary sinus which received a persistent left superior vena cava; LA = left atrium.

With episodes of pulmonary edema, the infant sweats excessively, is pale or even cyanotic, and may faint. Older children have exertional dyspnea, fatigue, and orthopnea. Dysphonia, due to compression of the recurrent laryngeal nerve by the hypertensive pulmonary trunk, and hemoptysis may occur, but each is rare.

In infants, the physical findings of mitral stenosis are often masked by those of associated anomalies; in older children without associated anomalies the findings are typical and usually easily demonstrated. The A wave in the jugular pulse is frequently prominent. The arterial pulse is normal. The precordium often bulges, and a right ventricular lift is palpable along the left sternal edge or in the epigastrum. The first heart sound is loud; the second sound is closely split, and the pulmonic component is loud and frequently palpable. An opening snap is heard occasionally (Fig. 18), but usually it is absent (35). An apical diastolic rumble, frequently accompanied by a thrill, is usually present in older children, and often has presystolic accentuation. A pansystolic murmur also may be present; it most often indicates mitral regurgitation but it also may be due to ventricular septal defect or to tricuspid regurgitation.

Under special circumstances other findings are present. Tachypnea and cyanosis occur with acute pulmonary edema or pneumonia. In addition, lower extremity cyanosis is noted when severe pulmonary arterial hypertension causes reversed flow through a patent ductus arteriosus. If pulmonary hypertension causes right ventricular failure, jugular venous distension, hepatomegaly, and edema may re-

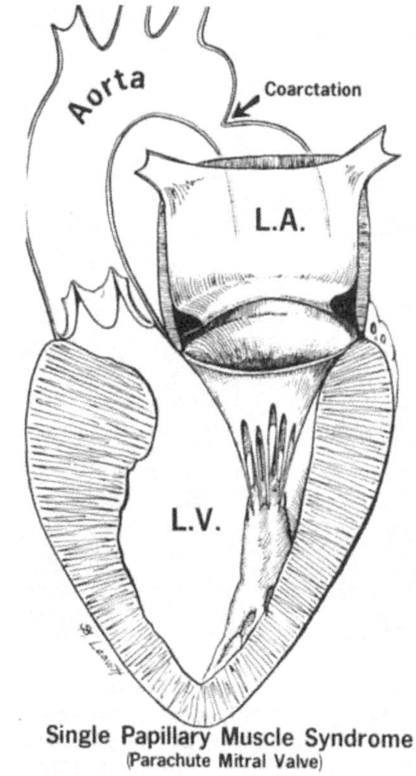

Fig. 17. Diagram demonstrating the major components of the parachute mitral valve syndrome: supravalvular mitral ring, single left ventricular papillary muscle, subaortic stenosis, bicuspid aortic valve, and coarctation of the aortic isthmus. All or virtually any combination of these malformations may occur in any one patient (42), and other anomalies may be present as well (44) (Figs. 15 and 16).

Fig. 18. Congenital mitral stenosis without associated anomalies. The electrocardiograms, taken at ages 2 and 10 yr, show right axis deviation of the QRS complex, right ventricular hypertrophy, and left atrial enlargement. The last two features are more striking in the 3/31/71 tracing. On the posteroanterior chest radiograph, a large left atrium and huge pulmonary trunk can be seen. The upper lobe vasculature and intersititial pulmonary markings are prominent. Striking right ventricular and left atrial enlargement are seen on the lateral film. The pressure tracings (lower left) show a large diastolic gradient between left atrium (LA) and left ventricle (LV) and a markedly elevated LA pressure. On the phonocardiogram (lower right) a loud first heart sound (S_1), prominent opening snap (OS), and long diastolic murmur (DM) with presystolic accentuation are recorded at the cardiac apex.

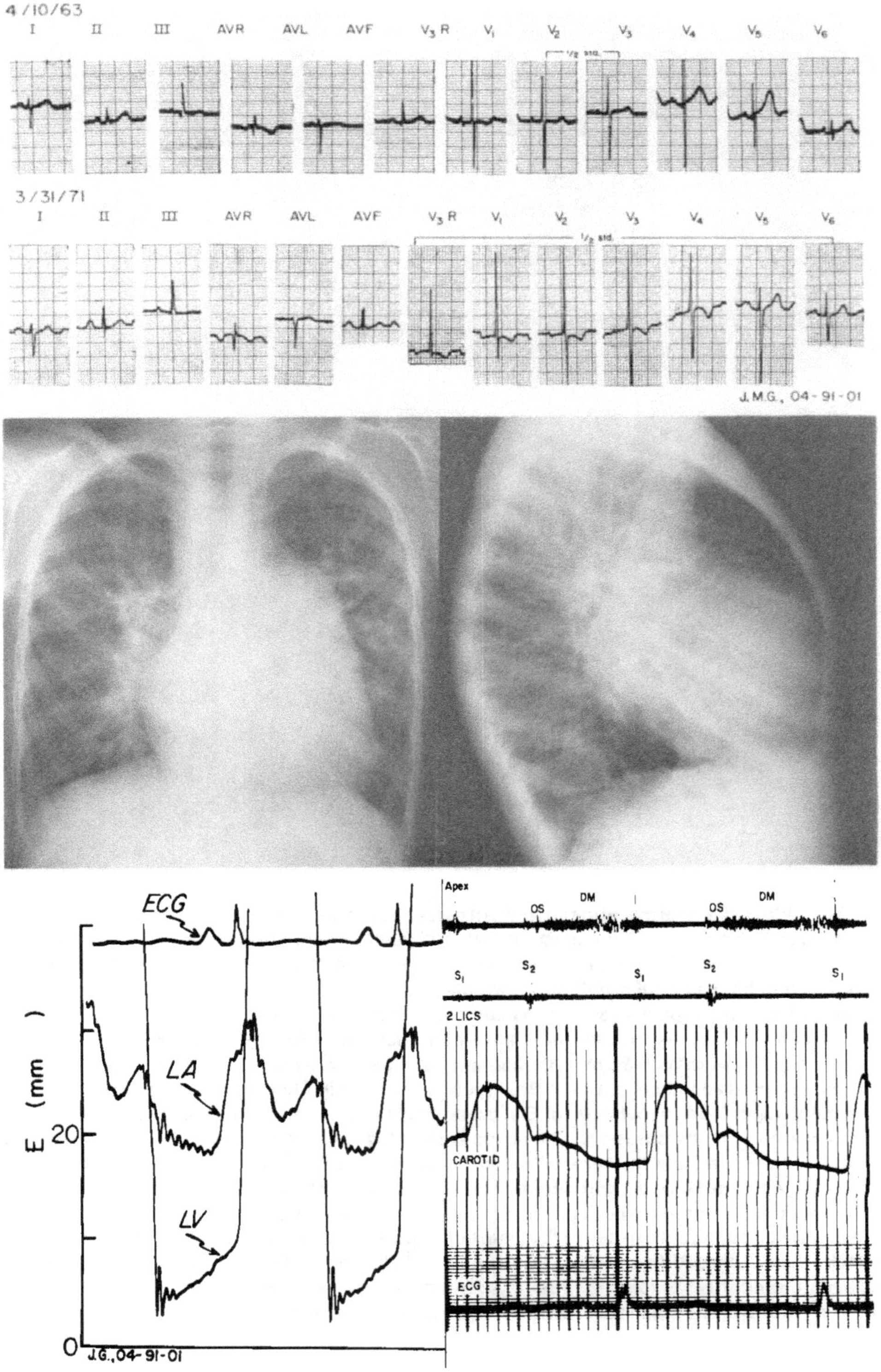
4/10/63
I
II
III
AVR
AVL
AVF
V3 R
V1
V2
V3
V4
V5
V6
1/2 std.
3/31/71
I
II
III
AVR
AVL
AVF
V3 R
V1
V2
V3
V4
V5
V6
1/2 std.
J.M.G., 04-91-01
ECG
LA
LV
E (mm)
20
0
J.G., 04-91-01
Apex
OS
DM
OS
DM
S1
S2
S1
S2
S1
2 LICS
CAROTID
ECG

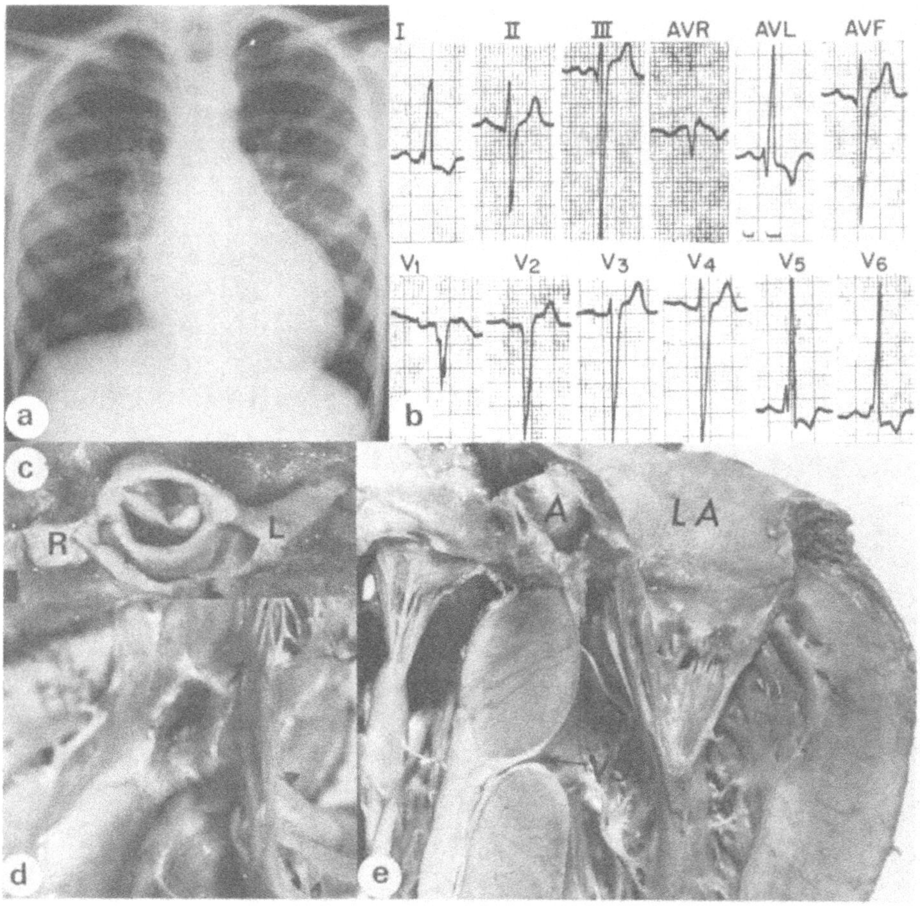

Fig. 19. Mild congenital mitral stenosis from parachute valve associated with discrete subaortic stenosis, bicuspid aortic valve, and spontaneous closure of ventricular septal defect in a 14-yr-old boy (71A-215) who had undergone resection of an aortic coarctation at age 5. His clinical features were those of left ventricular outflow obstruction, and no findings of mitral valve disease were audible. At age 13, the peak systolic pressure gradient between left ventricle and systemic artery was 80 mm Hg. Left ventricular end-diastolic and left atrial A-wave pressures (not recorded simultaneously) were both 30 mm Hg, and left atrial mean pressure was 27 mm Hg. He died of progressive cardiac failure. a, Chest Roentgenogram showing left ventricular enlargement and prominent upper lobe vasculature. b, Electrocardiogram showing marked left ventricular hypertrophy. c, Aortic valve from above. The cusps are located anteriorly and posteriorly. Both of them are mildly to moderately thickened. The aortic valve "annulus" and ascending aorta also are small. R = right and L = left coronary artery. d, View, from left ventricular body, of the discrete obstruction in the outflow tract. e, Longitudinal cut showing the parachute mitral valve. It has a funnel-shaped configuration due to the insertion of the leaflets and chordae into a single papillary muscle. Blood passed from left atrium (LA) into left ventricular cavity via the small spaces between the chordae tendineae. VSD = spontaneously closed ventricular septal defect; A = aortic valve cusps and small ascending aorta just above the discrete, fibrous, subaortic stenosis.

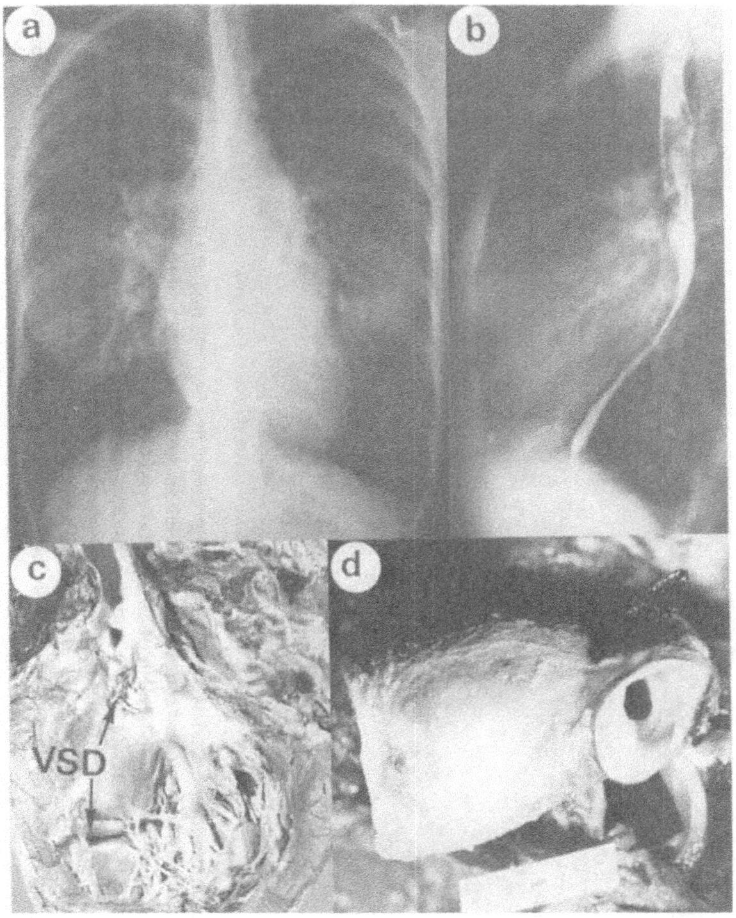

Fig. 20. Congenital mitral stenosis associated with ventricular septal defect, patent ductus arteriosus, and coarctation of aorta in a 25-yr-old, asymptomatic woman (A59-198). Examination disclosed an apical diastolic thrill, an opening snap, a loud S_1, and a grade 3/6 rumbling diastolic murmur over the apex. A grade 2/6 systolic ejection-type murmur also was heard along the left sternal edge. Pulmonic valve closure was loud. Electrocardiogram showed sinus rhythm and biventricular hypertrophy. Chest Roentgenograms (a, b) showed right ventricular and left atrial enlargement and enlarged pulmonary vessels centrally. The pressures in mm Hg were: pulmonary artery 104/60 (mean 82); left atrium, A 32, V 42, mean 35; left ventricle 122/4. The left atrial to left ventricular end-diastolic gradient was 20 mm Hg, and the cardiac output was normal. A transventricular mitral commissurotomy was performed but considerable mitral regurgitation was the consequence. The ventricular septal defect was closed by direct suture, and an unsuspected patent ductus arteriosus was ligated. She died 20 hr postoperatively after evidence of low cardiac output syndrome. c, Opened left ventricle, aortic valve, and aorta. There is more than one left ventricular papillary muscle, but they are not normally formed. The mitral leaflets are thickened but not calcified. Two ventricular septal defects (VSD) are present; the one just below the aortic valve was closed at operation. The aortic valve is congenitally bicuspid but functionally normal. d, Coarctation of aorta.

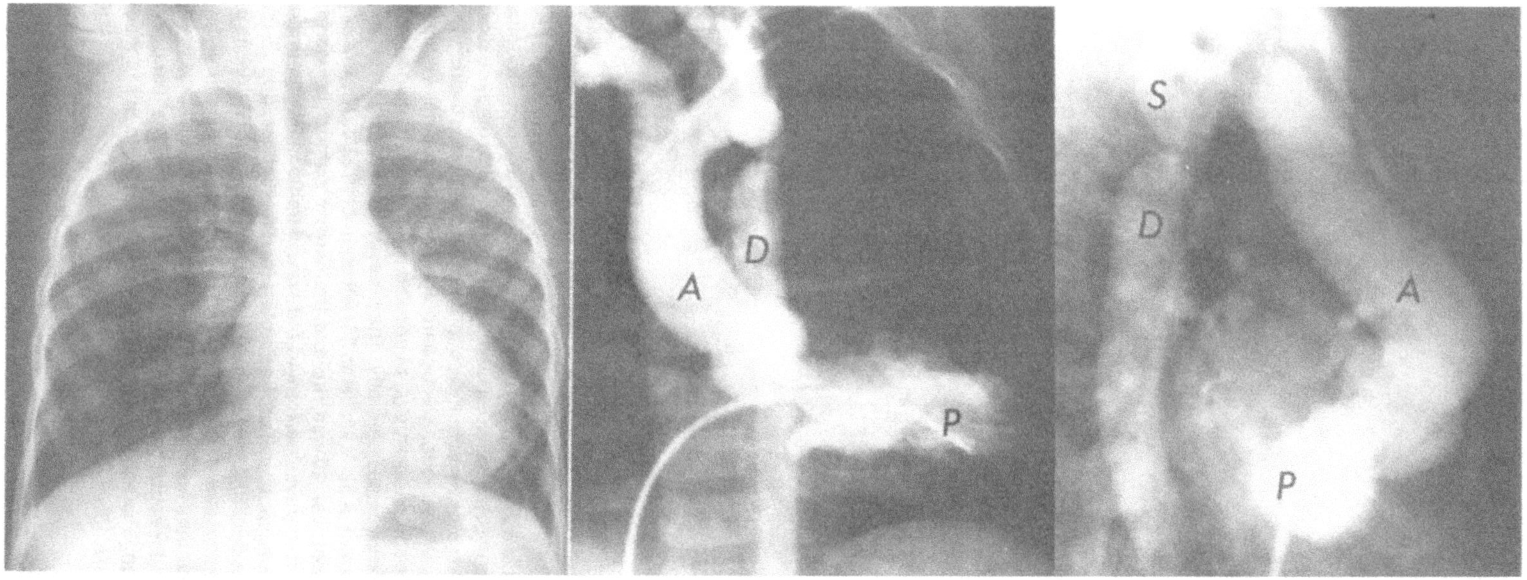

Fig. 21. Congenital mitral stenosis, subaortic stenosis, aortic coarctation, and a small atrial septal defect in a 5-yr-old boy. On the posteroanterior chest radiograph (left), the pulmonary vessels are more prominent in the upper than in the lower lobes, and left ventricular enlargement suggests other anomalies in addition to mitral stenosis. Catheterization revealed a 75 mm Hg peak systolic gradient between left ventricle and ascending aorta, a 25 mm Hg peak gradient (mean gradient = 10 mm Hg) between ascending and descending aorta, a 5 mm Hg mean diastolic gradient between left atrium and left ventricle, evidence of a small atrial septal defect or stretched foramen ovale with a small left to right shunt at atrial level (Qp/Qs = 1.2) and a large (10 mm Hg) pressure gradient between left and right atria, and a normal systemic cardiac index (3.6 L/min/M^2). Anteroposterior (middle) left ventriculogram shows a long area of subaortic narrowing. Mild poststenotic dilatation of the ascending aorta (A) is best seen on the lateral film (right). Typical aortic coarctation is seen just distal to the origin of the left subclavian artery (S). There is virtually no poststenotic dilatation of the descending aorta (D). Throughout systolic, shown here, and diastolic films in both projections, only one radiolucency compatible with left ventricular papillary muscle (P) is seen. This and the associated anomalies suggest that the patient has the parachute deformity of the mitral valve (42, 56).

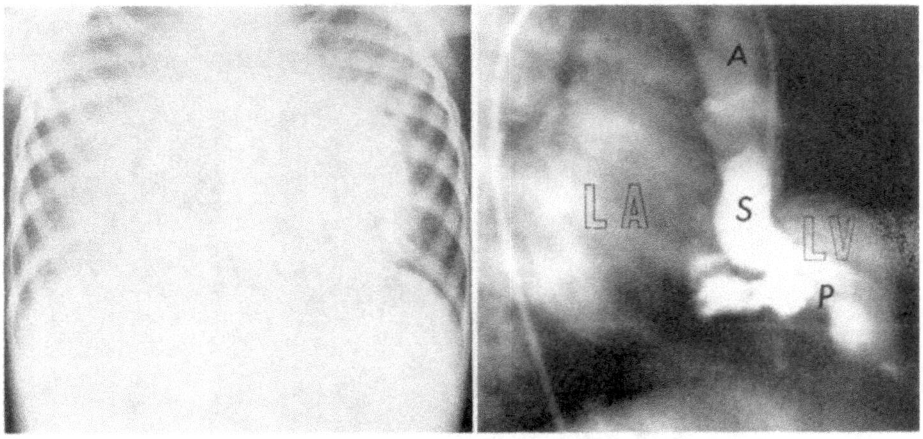

Fig. 22. Congenital mitral stenosis due to parachute deformity and associated with subvalvular aortic stenosis and pulmonic valvular stenosis (56). This 4-yr-old girl (A66-4) had congestive failure during her last 30 mo of life. Examination disclosed a continuous thrill at the apex and a systolic thrill in the suprasternal notch. A grade 3/6 systolic ejection murmur was heard over the pulmonic area, and a grade 4/6 holosystolic and grade 3/6 rumbling diastolic murmur were heard over the cardiac apex. Electrocardiogram showed right axis deviation, right atrial enlargement and right ventricular hypertrophy. Posteroanterior Roentgenogram (left) shows marked cardiomegaly and alveloar pulmonary edema. At cardiac catheterization, the pressures in mm Hg were: right ventricle, 142/6; pulmonary trunk 32/18; pulmonary arterial wedge M 19, A 25, V 24; left ventricular (LV) body, 168/15; LV outflow tract, 86/15; aorta, 86/42; and pulmonary arterial wedge–LV mean diastolic gradient, 9. The lateral angiogram (right), made following injection of contrast material into the LV, shows regurgitation through a thickened mitral valve into a markedly enlarged left atrium (LA). The single papillary muscle (P) appears as a radiolucency indenting the inferior margin of the LV cavity. A long subvalvular chamber (S) is present between the region of the LV outflow tract narrowing and the aortic valve. A = ascending aorta. At operation, the mitral valve was funnel shaped, and the leaflets inserted directly into a single papillary muscle. The mitral valve was excised and replaced with a caged disk prosthesis (Kay-Shiley type). Also, a pulmonic valvulotomy was performed. Hemodynamic measurements immediately postoperatively showed a reduction in the LV outflow gradient to 25 mm Hg and in the gradient across the pulmonic valve to 52 mm Hg. During the 42-hr postoperative period the child showed evidence of low cardiac output.

sult. Lower extremity pulses are delayed and of diminished amplitude when aortic coarctation coexists. An ejection click may occur in older children due to accompanying valvular aortic stenosis, pulmonic stenosis, or a dilated, hypertensive pulmonary artery. A continuous murmur may be caused by a high velocity jet through a stretched foramen ovale, or through a coexisting patent ductus arteriosus if pulmonary arterial pressure is less than systemic. An ejection-type systolic murmur may result from left or right ventricular outflow obstruction or, in the presence of severe pulmonary hypertension, from a ventricular septal defect or patent ductus arteriosus.

Chest radiographs (Figs. 18–22, 24, 25) show pulmonary congestion (Fig. 24) and, in older children, redistribution of flow with disproportionate prominence of the upper lobe veins (Figs. 18, 19, 21). In addition, interstitial (Figs. 18, 25) or alveolar (Fig. 22) edema may be present. Cardiomegaly is minimal to marked and, typically, there is enlargement of the left atrium, pulmonary trunk, right ventricle, and occasionally right atrium (Fig. 18). As with the physical findings, the radiographic signs are more typical in older children and may be modified by associated anomalies.

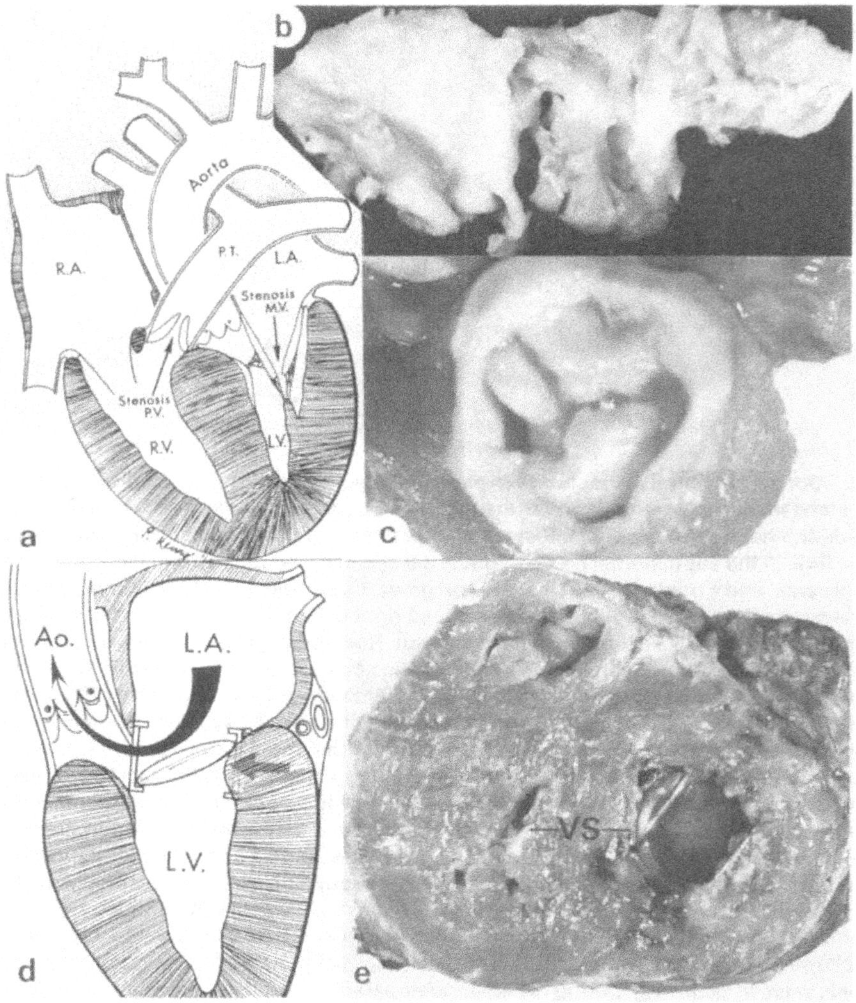

Fig. 23. Cardiac anatomic features in the patient whose Roentgenograms are shown in Fig. 22. a, Diagram summarizing the anatomic abnormalities. RA = right atrium; PV = pulmonic valve; PT = pulmonary trunk; RV = right ventricle; LA = left atrium; MV = mitral valve; LV = left ventricle. b, Excised mitral valve. The leaflets are diffusely thickened, the chordae tendineae are virtually absent, and only one papillary muscle is present. c, Stenotic pulmonic valve. d, Diagram showing an inadequate amount of space within the extremely hypertrophied left ventricle to accommodate the caged disk prosthesis. Myocardium from the left ventricular free wall bulged into the cage, preventing proper descent of the disk. Death resulted from prosthetic mitral stenosis. Ao = aorta. e, Transverse cut across the cardiac ventricles disclosing the impacted prosthesis which interferred with left atrial emptying. VS = ventricular septum.

The typical electrocardiogram (Fig. 18) shows right axis deviation, marked right ventricular hypertrophy, and abnormal P waves suggesting either left or right atrial enlargement or both. Atrial fibrillation (Fig. 25) is unusual. Left ventricular hypertrophy (Fig. 19) suggests an additional abnormality.

Echocardiography appears to be as useful in the diagnosis of congenital mitral stenosis as it is in acquired stenosis and the findings are similar (54). The E to F slope of the anterior mitral leaflet is reduced and there is a rough inverse correlation between the slope and the severity of the stenosis (54). Because other conditions may give rise to a reduced E to F slope and because some of these frequently coexist with congenital mitral stenosis, e.g., left ventricular outflow obstruction, analysis of posterior mitral leaflet motion will undoubtedly prove useful as it has in the diagnosis of acquired stenosis (55).

Cardiac catheterization is used to distinguish mitral stenosis from other causes of pulmonary venous hypertension when that is not possible by other means, to assess its severity, and to establish the presence or absence of additional anomalies. As in other congenital forms of pulmonary venous hypertension, pulmonary arterial and wedge pressures usually are moderately to markedly elevated. In addition, pressure in the left atrium, which can be entered through a patent foramen ovale or by the transseptal technique, also is elevated (Figs. 18, 24–26). This finding alone does not rule out cor triatriatum since, in that condition, the high pressure chamber may be entered with the transseptal catheter (Fig. 10). Manipulating the catheter into the left ventricle, however, and recording pressure during its withdrawal back to left atrium establish that the pressure gradient is at valvular level. In addition, any pressure gradient between left ventricle and systemic artery can be detected, and left to right shunts can be confirmed by oxygen series and/or indicator dilution curves. Because of the parabolic relation between flow across the valve and the pressure gradient, left to right shunts at ventricular or great artery level markedly accentuate the effects of mitral stenosis (Fig. 25).

A pulmonary arterial or left atrial angiogram demonstrates a large left atrium without the partition of cor triatriatum, usually shows a thickened mitral valve that domes into the left ventricle during diastole, and may detect additional anomalies. Left ventriculogram demonstrates mitral valvular anatomy (56), allows estimation of left ventricular cavity size and the amount of mitral regurgitation, and helps in assessing associated anomalies such as ventricular septal defect, left ventricular outflow obstruction, patent ductus arteriosus, and aortic coarctation (Figs. 21–22).

Congenital mitral stenosis must be distinguished from other causes of pulmonary venous hypertension, especially cor triatriatum. An opening snap is not encountered in patients with cor triatriatum, and an apical diastolic rumble with presystolic accentuation also strongly favors mitral stenosis. Cor triatriatum is suggested by a normal-sized left atrium on chest X ray, mitral stenosis by a greatly enlarged one. A slightly enlarged left atrium may occur in either condition. Echocardiography appears to be as accurate as cardiac catheterization and angiocardiography in diagnosing mitral stenosis and is more readily available and easier to employ. The invasive techniques may be required to assess severity and associated malformations. In older children isolated mitral stenosis is not likely to be overlooked or misdiagnosed, but in sick infants with additional anomalies it may not be suspected clinically and can be missed at catheterization unless looked for specifically (Fig. 24).

The prognosis in patients with congenital mitral stenosis generally is poor: at least 50% die during the 1st yr, and only 20% live 3 yr (48, 50). Prognosis is worse when other anomalies, especially aortic stenosis, coexist (48, 50). Occasional patients, however, live to adulthood despite congenital mitral stenosis and associated anomalies (Figs. 20, 25).

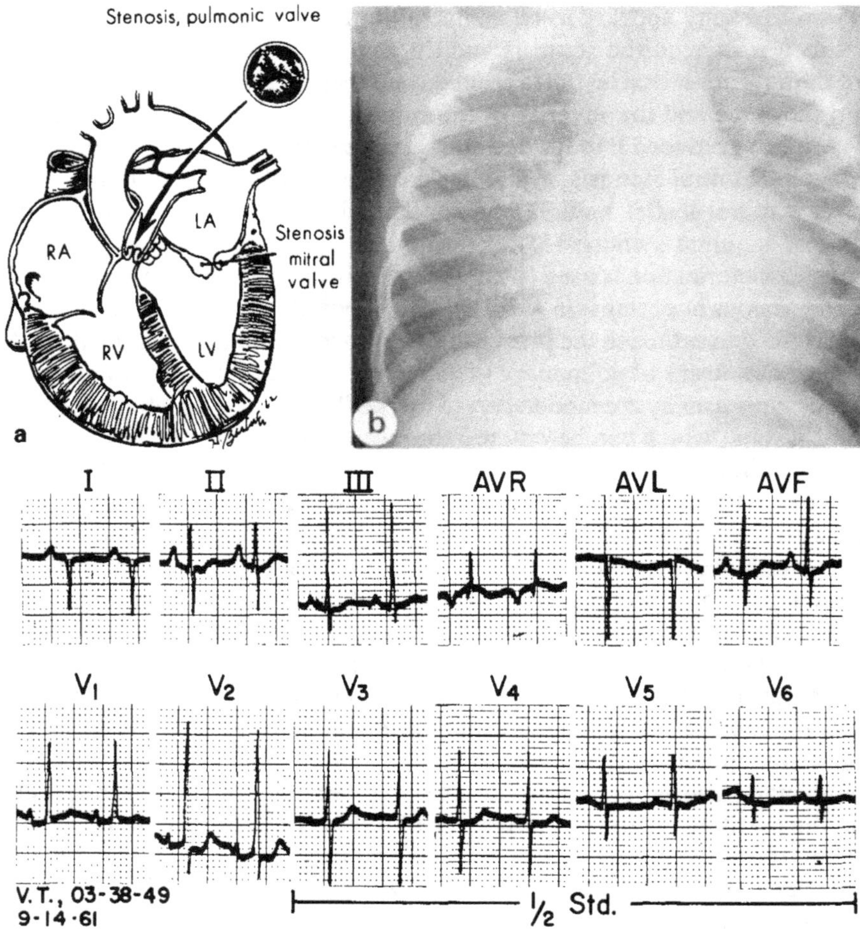

c

Fig. 24. Congenital mitral stenosis associated with valvular pulmonic stenosis in a 3-yr-old girl (A61-218). This child had frequent respiratory infections and evidence of right-sided congestive cardiac failure. A grade 4/6 ejection-type systolic murmur was audible over the pulmonic area, but an apical diastolic murmur was not heard. Chest Roentgenogram (b) showed cardiomegaly and pulmonary congestion. Electrocardiogram (c) showed right axis deviation, right ventricular (RV) hypertrophy, and atrial enlargement. At catheterization, neither pulmonary trunk nor the left ventricle could be entered; the left atrium was entered via a patent foramen ovale. The pressures in mm Hg were: right ventricle, 140/6 (g), left atrial A wave 38, V wave 30, mean 22 (f). The systolic pressure in the right ventricle (RV) was higher than that in the right brachial artery (RBA). Pullback from left atrium to right atrium showed a mean pressure drop from 20 to 7 mm Hg. Right ventricular angiogram disclosed a dome-shaped, thickened pulmonic valve. A closed pulmonic valvulotomy was performed, but following this procedure the pulmonary arterial systolic pressure was considerably elevated (70 mm Hg). The child died several hours after operation. At necropsy a thickened, severely stenotic mitral valve (MV) was found. The margins of the leaflets inserted directly into the papillary muscles (PM), and the endocardium of the left atrium (LA) was diffusely thickened (d). The pulmonic valve (PV) cusps also were thick (e). In this patient the pulmonary congestion and elevated left atrial pressure were unheeded clues to the presence of mitral stenosis. Failure to relieve this when the pulmonic stenosis was relieved resulted in pulmonary edema and death.

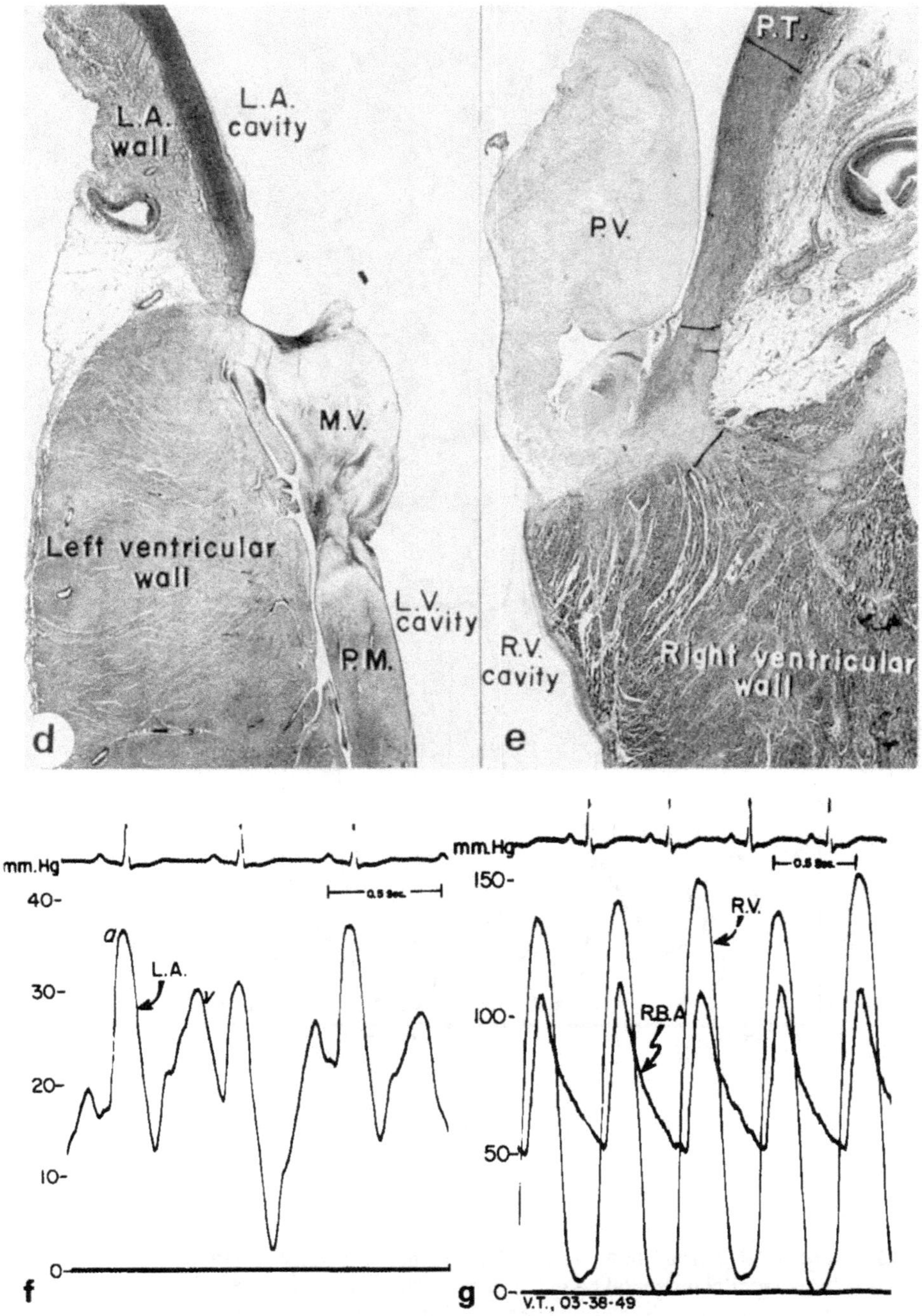

L.A. wall
L.A. cavity
M.V.
Left ventricular wall
L.V. cavity
P.M.
d
P.T.
P.V.
R.V. cavity
Right ventricular wall
e
mm.Hg
40-
30-
20-
10-
0-
a
L.A.
v
0.5 Sec.
f
mm.Hg
150-
100-
50-
0-
R.V.
R.B.A
0.5 Sec.
V.T., 03-38-49
g

24

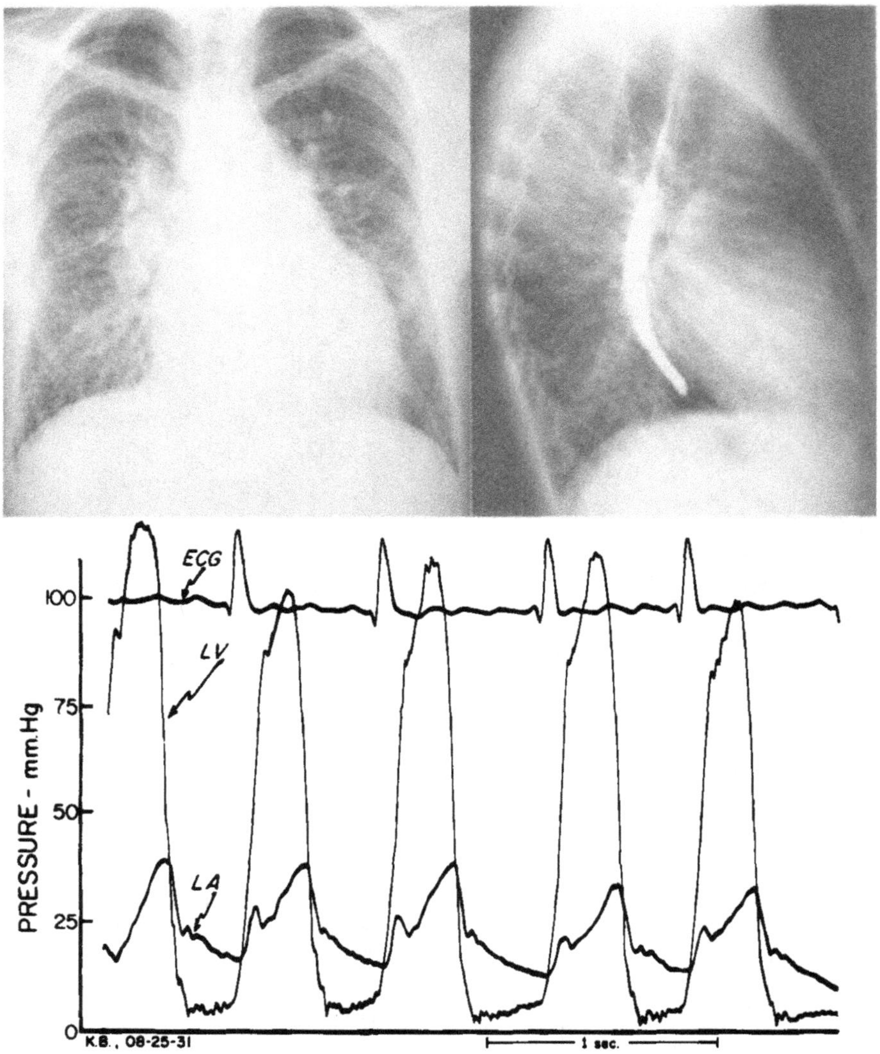

Fig. 25. Congenital "mitral" stenosis in a 26-yr-old man with corrected transposition of the great arteries, a large ventricular septal defect, and atrial fibrillation. The posteroanterior chest radiograph (upper left) shows moderate enlargement of the cardiac silhouette, a prominent pulmonary vasculature, and interstitial pulmonary edema. On the lateral radiograph (upper right), the barium-filled esophagus is displaced posteriorly by the enlarged left atrium. The pressure tracings (below) reveal a large diastolic gradient between left atrium (LA) and left ventricle (LV) and a markedly elevated LA pressure. The pressure gradient was in part due to increased forward flow across the mitral valve because of the left to right shunt, and at operation only mild mitral stenosis was found. The mitral valve was funnel shaped, had no chordal attachments at its free margin, and through the ventricular septal defect was in fibrous continuity with both the tricuspid and pulmonic valves.

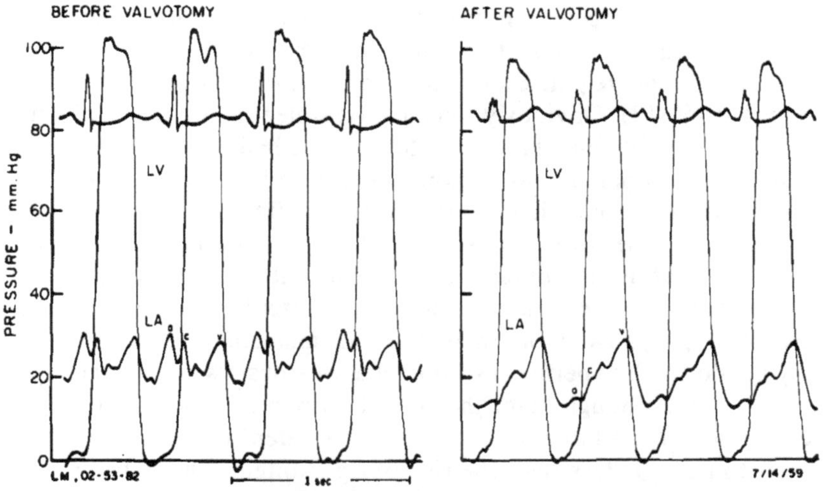

Fig. 26. **Congenital mitral stenosis: hemodynamic results of valvotomy in an 11-yr-old boy. Left atrial (LA) and left ventricular (LV) pressures were measured in the operating room before and after the procedure by Dr. A.G. Morrow. The diastolic pressure gradient between LA and LV was reduced by the procedure; LA mean pressure fell slightly; and the patient improved symptomatically. These hemodynamic results are not nearly as favorable, however, as those obtained in the majority of patients with rheumatic mitral stenosis (57).**

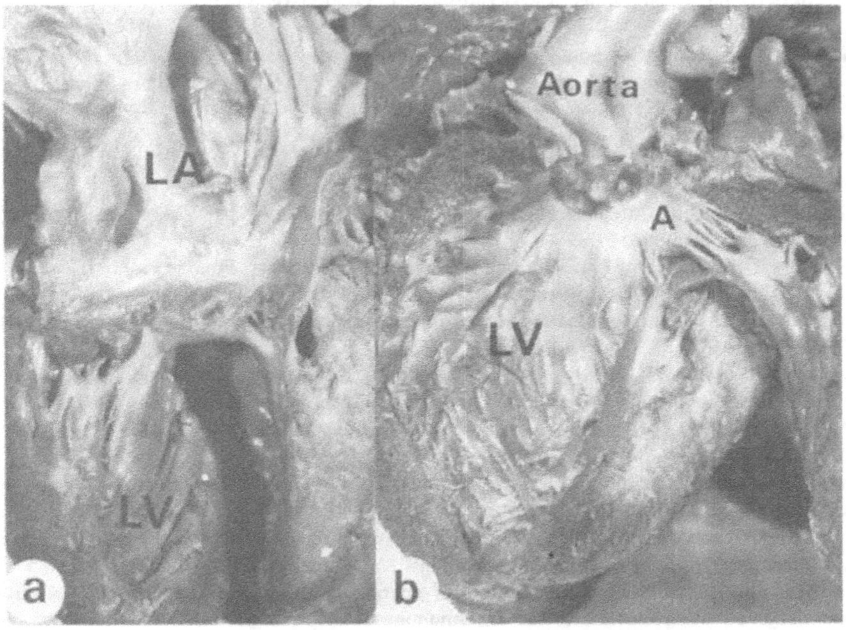

Fig. 27. **Arcade-type mitral valve probably causing both stenosis and regurgitation (51) in a 3-day old boy (A67-211) who clinically was believed to have "the hypoplastic left heart syndrome." a, Opened left atrium (LA), mitral valve, and left ventricle (LV). The mitral leaflets are mildly thickened and from the atrial aspect appear to insert virtually directly into the two papillary muscles. b, Opened left ventricle, aortic valve, and aorta. There are multiple nodular projections from each of the two aortic valve cusps and the valve "annulus" is small. These two lesions together resulted in valvular aortic stenosis. A = anterior mitral leaflet.**

Most patients with congenital mitral stenosis develop cardiac failure and need digitalis, diuretics, and a low sodium diet. In addition, they intermittently may require treatment for acute pulmonary edema and for a respiratory infection that so often precipitates it (53). Obviously, medical treatment is limited. Unfortunately, operative treatment of congenital mitral stenosis has had only partial success, and approximately 50% of patients undergoing operation for this condition have died (48, 52, 53). Although some relief of the stenosis is often possible with valvotomy (48, 49, 52) (Fig. 26), the severe deformity of the valve usually mitigates against a result as good as that usually obtained in patients with rheumatic disease (57). In older children valve replacement generally gives better hemodynamic results than valvotomy (46, 47, 52, 58–61), but in infants and small children the left ventricular cavity may be too small to permit insertion of a prosthesis with an adequate orifice size (Figs. 22, 23). Although high, the risk of correcting associated extracardiac anomalies, such as coarctation of the aorta or a patent ductus arteriosus that is shunting left to right, is less than the risk of operating on the mitral valve. Such correction may result in considerable clinical and hemodynamic improvement (49).

REFERENCES

1. Edwards JE: Congenital malformations of the heart and great vessels. J. Malformations of the thoracic veins. In, Pathology of the Heart and Blood Vessels, SE Gould, (Ed.). 3rd ed. Philadelphia, Charles C. Thomas, 1968.
2. Binet JP, Bouchard F, Langlois J, Chetochine F,Conso JF and Pottemain M: Unilateral congenital stenosis of the pulmonary veins: A very rare cause of pulmonary hypertension. J Thorac Cardiovasc Surg 63:397-402, 1972.
3. Snellen HA and Bruins C: Anomalies of venous return. In, Paediatric Cardiology, H Watson, (Ed.). St. Louis, The C.V. Mosby Company, 1968.
4. Shone JD, Amplatz K, Anderson RC, Adams P, Jr and Edwards JE: Congenital stenosis of individual pulmonary veins. Circulation 26:574-581, 1962.
5. Lucas RV, Jr, Anderson RC, Amplatz K, Adams P, Jr and Edwards JE: Congenital causes of pulmonary venous obstruction. Pediat Clin N Amer 10:781-836, 1963.
6. Edwards JE: Congenital stenosis of pulmonary veins. Pathologic and developmental considerations. Lab Invest 9:46-66, 1960.
7. Carrington CB and Liebow AA: Pulmonary veno-occlusive disease. Human Pathol 1:322-324, 1970.
8. Glancy, DL, Brauwald NS, O'Brien KP and Roberts WC: Scimitar syndrome associated with patent ductus arteriosus, aortic coarctation and irreversible pulmonary hypertension. Johns Hopkins Med J 123:297-304, 1968.
9. Hastreiter AR, Paul MH, Molthian ME and Miller RA: Total anomalous pulmonary venous connection with severe pulmonary venous obstruction: a clinical entity. Circulation 25:916-928, 1962.
10. Keith JD, Rowe RD and Vlad P: Heart Disease in Infancy and Childhood, 2nd edition, New York, The Macmillan Company, 1967.
11. Nakib A, Moller, JH, Kanjuh VI and Edwards JE: Anomalies of the puomonary veins. Amer J Cardiol 20:77-90, 1967.
12. Gathman GE and Nadas AS: Total anomalous pulmonary venous connection. Clinical and physiologic observations of 75 pediatric patients.. Circulation 42:143-154, 1970.
13. Elliot LP and Edwards JE: The problem of pulmonary venous obstruction in total anomalous pulmonary venous connection to the left innominate vein. Circulation 25:913-915, 1962.
14. Kauffman SL, Ores CN and Andersen DH: Two cases of total anomalous pulmonary venous return of the supracardiac type with stenosis simulating infradiaphragmatic drainage. Circulation 25:376-382, 1962.
15. Solinger RE: Ultrasound in congenital heart disease. In, Cardiac Ultrasound, R Gramiak and RC Waag, (Eds.). St. Louis, The C.V. Mosby Company, 1975.
16. Goldberg SJ, Allen HD and Sahn DJ: Pediatric and Adolescent Echocardiography. Chicago, Yearbook Medical Publishers, Inc. 1975.

17. Van Praagh R and Corsini I: Cor triatriatum: pathologic anatomy and a consideration of morphogenesis based on 13 postmortem cases and a study of normal development of the pulmonary vein and atrial septum in 83 human embryos. Am Heart J 78:379-405, 1969.
18. Marin-Garci J, Tandon R, Lucas RV, Jr and Edwards JE: Cor triatriatum: study of 20 cases. Amer J Cardiol 35:59-66, 1975.
19. Gasul, BM, Arcilla RA and Lev M: Heart Disease in Children. Philadelphia, J.B. Lippincott Co., 1966.
20. Perloff JK: The Clinical Recognition of Congenital Heart Disease. Philadelphia, W.B. Saunders Company, 1970.
21. McQuire LB, Nolan TB, Reeve R and Dammann JF, Jr: Cor triatriatum as a problem of adult heart disease. Circulation 31:263-272, 1965.
22. McAllister HA, Jr and Glancy DL: Unpublished observations on Armed Forces Institute of Pathology Collection.
23. Nagao GI, Daoud GI, McAdams AJ, Schwartz DC and Kaplan S: Cardiovascular anomalies associated with tetralogy of Fallot. Amer J Cardiol 20:206-215, 1967.
24. Danielson GK and Feldt RH: Successful repair of coexisting cor triatriatum and tetralogy of Fallot. J Thor Cardiovasc Surg 63:391-393, 1972.
25. Morrow AG, Oldham HN, Elkins RC and Braunwald E: Prosthetic replacement of the mitral valve. Preoperative and postoperative clinical hemodynamic assessments in 100 patients. Circulation 35:962-979, 1967.
26. Steinbrunn W, Cohn KE and Selzer A: Atrial septal defect associated with mitral stenosis. The Lutembacher syndrome revisited. Amer J Med 48:295-302, 1970.
27. Kaplan S: Cor triatriatum. In, Paediatric Cardiology, H. Watson, (Ed.). St. Louis, The C.V. Mosby Company, 1968.
28. Beller B, Childers R, Eckner F, Duchelle R, Ranniger K and Rabinowitz M: Cor triatriatum in the adult: complicated by mitral insufficiency and aortic dissection. Amer J Cardiol 19:749-754, 1967.
29. Miller GAH, Ongley PA, Anderson MW, Kincaid OW and Swan HJC: Cor triatriatum. Hemodynamic and angiographic diagnosis. Am Heart J 68:298-304, 1964.
30. Lundström N-R: Ultrasoundcardiographic studies of the mitral valve region in young infants with mitral atresia, mitral stenosis, hypoplasia of the left ventricle, and cor triatriatum. Circulation 45:324-334, 1972.
31. Ellis K, Griffiths SP, Jesse MJ and Jameson AG: Cor triatriatum. Angiocardiographic demonstration of the obstructing left atrial membrane. Amer J Roentgenol 92:669-675, 1964.
32. Jorgensen CR, Ferlic RM, Varco RL, Lillehei CW and Eliot RS: Cor triatriatum: Review of the surgical aspects with a follow-up report on the first patient successfully treated with surgery. Circulation 36:101-107, 1967.
33. Roberts WC, Perry LW, Chandra RS, Myers GE, Shapiro SR and Scott LP: Aortic valve atresia: a new classification based on necropsy study of 73 cases. Amer J Cardiol 37:753-756, 1976.
34. Beckman CB, Moller JH and Edwards JE: Alternate pathways to pulmonary venous flow in left-sided obstructive anomalies. Circulation 52:509-516, 1975.
35. Krovetz LJ, Rowe RD and Schiebler GL: Hemodynamics of aortic valve atresia. Circulation 42:953-959, 1970.
36. Ross J, Jr, Braunwald E, Mason DT and Morrow AG: Interatrial communication and left atrial hypertension. A cause of continuous murmur. Circulation 28:853-860, 1963.
37. Meyer RA and Kaplan S: Echocardiography in the diagnosis of hypoplasia of the left or right ventricles in the neonate. Circulation 46:55-64, 1972.
38. Godman MJ, Tham P and Langford Kidd BS: Echocardiography in the evaluation of the cyanotic newborn infant. Br Heart J 36:154-166, 1974.
39. Benzing G, III, Schubert W, Hug G and Kaplan S: Spontaneous hypoglycemia and acute congestive heart failure. Circulation 40:209-216, 1969.
40. Cayler GG, Smeloff EA and Miller GE, Jr: Surgical palliation of hypoplastic left side of the heart. N Engl J Med 282:780-783, 1970.
41. Lynch MF, Ryan NJ, Williams GR, Cayler GG, Richardson WR, Campbell GS and Taybi H: Preoperative diagnosis and surgical correction of supravalvular mitral stenosis and ventricular septal defect. Circulation 25:854-861, 1962.
42. Shone JD, Sellers RD, Anderson RC, Adams P Jr, Lillehei CW and Edwards JE: The developmental complex of "parachute mitral valve," supravalvular ring of left atrium, subaortic stenosis, and coarctation of aorta. Amer J Cardiol 11:714-725, 1963.

43. Anabtawi IN and Ellison RG: Congenital stenosing ring of the left atrioventricular canal (supravalvular mitral stenosis). J Thor Cardiovasc Surg 49:994-1005, 1965.
44. Glancy DL, Chang MY, Dorney ER and Roberts WC: Parachute mitral valve. Further observations and associated lesions. Amer J Cardiol 27:309-313, 1971.
45. Chung KJ, Manning JA, Lipchik EO, Gramiak R and Mahoney EB: Isolated supravalvular stenosing ring of left atrium: diagnosis before operation and successful surgical treatment. Chest 65:25-28, 1974.
46. Tank ES, Bernhard WF and Gross RE: Surgical anatomy of congenital mitral stenosis. Circulation 36 (Suppl II): II-246–II-247, 1967 (Abstr)
47. Castaneda AR, Anderson RC and Edwards JE: Congenital mitral stenosis resulting from anomalous arcade and obstructing papillary muscles. Report of correction by use of ball valve prosthesis. Amer J Cardiol 24:237-240, 1969.
48. Van der Horst RL and Hastreiter AR: Congenital mitral stenosis. Amer J Cardiol 20:773-783, 1967.
49. Easthope RN, Tawes RL, Jr, Bonham-Carter RE, Aberdeen E and Waterston DJ: Congenital mitral valve disease associated with coarctation of the aorta. A report of 39 cases. Am Heart J 77:743-754, 1969.
50. Vlad P: Mitral valve anomalies in children. Circulation 43:465-466, 1971.
51. Davachi F, Moller JH and Edwards JE: Diseases of the mitral valve in infancy. An anatomic analysis of 55 cases. Circulation 43:565-579, 1971.
52. Collins-Nakai RL, Rosenthal A, Castaneda AR and Nadas AS: Congenital mitral stenosis: course and effect of surgery on pulmonary vascular resistance. Circulation 52 (Suppl II): II-171, 1975 (Abstr.).
53. Daoud G, Kaplan S, Derrin EV, Dorst JP and Edwards FK: Congenital mitral stenosis. Circulation 27:185-196, 1963.
54. Lundström N-R: Echocardiography in the diagnosis of congenital mitral stenosis and in evaluation of the results of mitral valvotomy. Circulation 46:44-54, 1972.
55. Duchak JM, Jr, Chang S and Feigenbaum H: The posterior mitral valve echo and the echocardiographic diagnosis of mitral stenosis. Amer J Cardiol 29:628-632, 1972.
56. Simon AL, Friedman WF, Roberts WC: The angiographic features of a case of parachute mitral valve. Amer Heart J 77:809-813, 1969.
57. Mullin EM, Jr, Glancy DL, Higgs LM, Epstein SE and Morrow AG: Current results of operation for mitral stenosis: Clinical and hemodynamic assessments in 124 consecutive patients treated by closed commissurotomy, open commissurotomy, or valve replacement. Circulation 46:298-308, 1972.
58. Young D and Robinson G: Successful valve replacement in an infant with congenital mitral stenosis. N Engl J Med 270:660-664, 1964.
59. Prado S, Levy, M and Varco RL: Successful replacement of "parachute" mitral valve in a child. Circulation 32:130-133, 1965.
60. Terzaki AK, Leachman RD, Ali MK, Hallman GL and Cooley DA: Successful replacement of "parachute" mitral valve in a child. J. Thor Cardiovasc Surg 56:1-10, 1968.
61. Macartney FJ, Scott O, Ionescu MI and Deverall PB: Diagnosis and management of parachute mitral valve and supravalvar mitral ring. Br Heart J 36:641-652, 1974.

Small Airways in Idiopathic Pulmonary Fibrosis

COMPARISON OF MORPHOLOGIC AND PHYSIOLOGIC OBSERVATIONS

JACK D. FULMER, WILLIAM C. ROBERTS, EDWYNA R. VON GAL, and RONALD G. CRYSTAL

From the Pulmonary Branch and the Pathology Branch, National Heart, Lung, and Blood Institute, National Institutes of Health, Bethesda, Maryland 20014

ABSTRACT 18 patients with idiopathic pulmonary fibrosis were studied to determine if they had morphologic evidence of small airways disease and if physiologic testing could predict morphologic findings. In the presence of normal airway function by standard physiologic studies (forced expiratory volume in 1 s/forced vital capacity and airway resistance by plethysmography), dynamic compliance, maximum expiratory flow-volume curves, and maximum flow-static recoil curves were measured to detect physiologic alterations consistent with small airways abnormalities. These physiologic data were then compared with estimates of small airways diameter made in lung biopsy specimens.

94% (17 of 18) of the patients had peribronchiolar fibrosis or peribronchiolar inflammation or bronchiolitis. 67% (12 of 18) had an overall estimate of small airways diameter of "narrowed," whereas 33% (6 of 18) had airways that overall were "not narrowed." 59% (10 of 17) had frequency-dependent dynamic compliance, 50% (9 of 18) had abnormal maximum expiratory flow-volume curves, and 39% (7 of 18) had abnormal maximum flow-static recoil curves. Comparisons between morphologic and physiologic data revealed a significant correlation between the results of dynamic compliance and the overall estimate of small airways diameter ($P = 0.001$), and the results of maximum flow-volume curves and the overall estimate of small airways diameter ($P = 0.009$); there was no significant correlation between the results of maximum flow-static recoil curves and the overall estimate of small airways diameter ($P = 0.1$).

The results of this study suggest that: (*a*) idiopathic pulmonary fibrosis is a disease of small airways as well as alveoli; (*b*) dynamic compliance and the maximum expiratory flow-volume curve can predict the overall status of small airways diameter in idiopathic pulmonary fibrosis; and (*c*) whereas the maximum flow-static recoil curve predicts the overall estimate of small airways diameter in most patients with this disease, it is the least sensitive of these three monitors of small airways.

Reprint requests may be addressed to Dr. Fulmer, Room 6N260, Bldg. 10, National Institutes of Health, Bethesda, Md. 20014.

Received for publication 13 October 1976 and in revised form 11 April 1977.

INTRODUCTION

Idiopathic pulmonary fibrosis (IPF)[1] is a well-defined subgroup of the fibrotic lung disorders, characterized by distinct clinical, radiographic, physiologic, and morphologic features (1–16). These patients usually have exertional breathlessness, a diffuse interstitial infiltrate on chest X ray, decreased lung volumes, decreased diffusing capacity, and hypoxemia which worsens with exercise. Although the hypoxemia in IPF was initially thought to result from a diffusion barrier to oxygen (17), current data suggest that it mostly results from a ventilation-perfusion imbalance (18, 19).

In general, the most likely cause of hypoxemia secondary to a ventilation-perfusion imbalance is maldistribution of ventilation resulting either from airways disease or alterations in regional compliance or both. Because IPF has been considered to be a disease of alveoli and not of airways, maldistribution of ventilation in this disorder has previously been attributed to alterations in regional compliance (18). However, recent studies in disorders other than IPF (e.g. asthma)

[1] *Abbreviations used in this paper*: Cdyn, dynamic compliance; Cstat, static compliance; D_{LCO}, carbon dioxide diffusing capacity; $FEV_1\%$, forced expiratory volume in 1 s/forced vital capacity; FRC, functional residual capacity; IPF, idiopathic pulmonary fibrosis; MEFV, maximum expiratory flow volume; MFSR, maximum flow static recoil; P_L, transpulmonary pressure; Pst, static transpulmonary pressure; Raw, airway resistance; RV, residual volume; TLC, total lung capacity; VC, vital capacity; $\dot{V}_{max}$, maximum expiratory flow.

have demonstrated that hypoxemia can result from the maldistribution of ventilation due to narrowing of small (<2 mm) airways, an obstruction which is not detected by standard physiologic studies (20, 21).

In light of these newer concepts of small airways disease, the present study was designed to: (*a*) evaluate the morphology of small airways in IPF; (*b*) determine if patients with IPF have physiologic alterations consistent with small airways disease; and (*c*) attempt to correlate these morphologic and physiologic findings. To do so, we chose a group of patients with IPF who had normal airway function by standard physiologic studies and who had undergone lung biopsy within close proximity to a physiologic evaluation of small airways function. The results demonstrate that we must expand the concepts of IPF to consider it a disorder of small airways as well as alveoli.

METHODS

Patient population

Over an 18-mo period, 150 patients were referred to the Pulmonary Branch, National Heart, Lung, and Blood Institute for evaluation of interstitial lung disease. From this group, patients were determined to have IPF if they fit the following criteria (14–16).

Clinical. History of exertional breathlessness; no history of exposure to inorganic, organic, gaseous, physical, or pharmacologic agents known to cause pulmonary fibrosis; no history suggestive of an allergic pulmonary disorder; no history of chronic pulmonary infection; and no historical or physical evidence of left ventricular failure. All patients underwent fiberoptic bronchoscopy (B2F, Olympus Corporation of America, New Hyde Park, N. Y.) and were demonstrated to have normal airways within limits of the procedure.

Roentgenographic. The presence of a diffuse infiltrative pattern (reticular, reticulonodular, or ground glass) on a routine posterior-anterior chest film and no evidence of left ventricular disease.

Physiologic. Reduced lung volumes or reduced diffusing capacity or both; mild to moderate hypoxemia at rest which worsened with exercise, and a static volume-pressure curve consistent with fibrotic disease (see below for physiologic methods).

Morphologic. Lung biopsy showing varying degrees of alveolar septal fibrosis and inflammation with interstitial and intra-alveolar inflammatory cells (predominantly mononuclear cells, but often accompanied by neutrophils and eosinophils); no granuloma, no vasculitis, no evidence of inorganic material by polarized light microscopy, and negative cultures for bacteria and fungi.

Patients were included in the current study if they met all of the diagnostic criteria for IPF, and had no evidence of airways disease by standard criteria (forced expiratory volume in 1 s/forced vital capacity and airway resistance). In addition, they had to have had a recent lung biopsy demonstrating airways of <2 mm in diameter and be able to participate in measurement of at least two of three monitors of small airways (see below).

From the initial group of 150 patients, 50 had the diagnosis of IPF and 18 of these fit all of the criteria to be included in this study. Patients who were excluded from the study were done so largely because of failure to have a recent biopsy or because of advanced disease and inability to participate in physiologic studies. 15 had no evidence of a collagen vascular disease, two (M. C., V. J.) had rheumatoid arthritis, and one (O. N.) had an overlap connective tissue syndrome. Eight patients had open lung biopsy at our institution with physiologic testing performed within 2 wk before biopsy. The remaining 10 patients had lung biopsies performed at an outside institution with physiologic testing performed at our institution 3–18 mo (average 4 mo) after biopsy.

Airway morphology

Morphological observations were made by one of us (W. C. R.) without knowledge of the results of the physiological testing. All observations were made on surgical specimens fixed in formalin, processed in alcohols and xylene, imbedded in paraffin, sectioned at 6 μm intervals, and then stained with hematoxylin and eosin. Serial sections were evaluated whenever possible. Airways of 2-mm diameter or less which had nearly perpendicular cuts were selected for evaluation. Each biopsy contained an average of 7.7±0.7[2] airways which were suitable for study.

The following histologic features of small airways were noted if present: peribronchiolar fibrosis, peribronchiolar inflammation, and bronchiolitis. In addition, the diameters of small airways were graded as to whether they were normal, narrowed, or dilated by the following criteria: (*a*) comparing the diameter of the bronchiolar lumen to the diameter of the lumen of the accompanying pulmonary artery (the bronchiolar lumen should be as large or larger than the lumen of the artery); (*b*) comparing the diameter of the bronchiolar lumen in the biopsy to the bronchiolar lumen of noninflated normal lung with comparable sized bronchioles and pulmonary arteries; and (*c*) comparing the thickness of the bronchiolar wall to the thickness of the wall of comparably sized airways of noninflated normal lungs. Changes in pulmonary artery diameter associated with pulmonary hypertension were quantitated to adjust lumen diameter to a normal size and prevent over estimation of airway diameter. If an airway was normal or dilated, but on serial section was shown to be narrowed at some point, it was graded as narrowed.

To facilitate comparison of morphologic and physiologic studies, an overall estimate of the diameter of the small airways in each biopsy was made using the following criteria: if 60% or more airways in the biopsy were narrowed, airways diameter was considered "narrowed," independent of status of the other airways; if 70% or more of the airways in the biopsy were normal or dilated (i.e. 30% or less were narrowed), airways diameter was considered "not narrowed," independent of the status of the other airways. If 31–59% of the airways in the biopsy were narrowed, the morphologic data for that patient were not used for statistical comparison with the physiologic data.

Lung volumes, timed expiratory maneuver, and diffusing capacity

Lung volumes, timed expiratory maneuver and diffusing capacity were measured on a computerized lung analyzer (Warren E. Collins, Inc., Braintree, Mass.). Vital capacity (VC), forced vital capacity, forced expiratory volume in 1 s, and inspiratory capacity were done in the standing position. Functional residual capacity (FRC) was done in the sitting

[2] All data will be presented as mean±SEM.

position utilizing a closed circuit helium equilibration technique (22). Expiratory reserve volume was subtracted from FRC to obtain residual volume (RV) and VC was added to RV to obtain observed total lung capacity (TLC). Predicted values for VC, forced expiratory volume in 1 s, and forced expiratory volume in 1 s/forced vital capacity ($FEV_1\%$) were obtained from the data of Morris et al. (23). Predicted FRC and RV were obtained from the normals of Goldman and Becklake (24). Predicted TLC was obtained by adding predicted VC to predicted RV. The lower limit of lung volumes was considered to be −20% of the predicted value. The lower limit for $FEV_1\%$ was considered to be equal to the predicted $FEV_1\%$−5% (25).

Single-breath carbon monoxide diffusing capacity (D_{LCO}) was performed by the method of Ogilvie et al. (26). The program was modified so that alveolar volume was determined by a single-breath helium dilutional technique. Alveolar gas was quantitated after absorption of CO_2; gas concentrations were then adjusted by 6% for CO_2 removal (6% is the usual alveolar CO_2 concentration). The results were compared to the predicted values of Gaensler and Wright (27).

Airway resistance

Airway resistance (Raw) was determined by modification of the method of Dubois et al. (28) using a constant volume plethysmograph (Warren E. Collins, Inc.). Statham differential transducers (Pm 6 and 15, Gould, Inc., Oxnard, Calif.) were interfaced with carrier amplifiers (model 8805 B, Hewlett-Packard Co., Palo Alto, Calif.). Flow was measured with a heated number 3 Fleisch pneumotachograph (Medical Products, Blue Bell, Pa.). All transducers had a frequency response within ±5% up to 6 cycles/s. The Fleisch pneumotachograph was linear from 0.1–6 liters/s. Data were recorded on a storage oscilloscope (Tektronix, Inc., Beaverton, Oreg.) and either traced directly on cellulose paper or photographed. Raw was measured by the slope of where the loop crossed a flow of 1 liter/s. The resistance of the pneumotachograph, shutter assembly, and mouth piece (0.35 cm H_2O/liter per s) was subtracted from the total Raw. Normal Raw was considered to be ≷ 2.5 cm H_2O/liter per s (28).

Maximum expiratory flow-volume relationship

The relationship between maximum expiratory flow and volume (MEFV) was determined in the sitting position utilizing a wedge spirometer (570, Med-Science Electronics, Inc., St. Louis, Mo.) connected to a rapidly responding (1,500 in/s^2) XY recorder (model 7046A, Hewlett-Packard Co.). The apparatus was calibrated electronically and checked manually utilizing a 1-liter syringe (Warren E. Collins, Inc.) and a 0–10-liter/s flow meter (Vol-O-Flow, National Institute Laboratories Inc., Rockville, Md.). Calibration of flow was accomplished by incorporating a low resistance three-way valve (Warren E. Collins, Inc.) between a flow generator (vacuum cleaner) and flow meter and spirometer so that flow rate and time could be controlled; flow was linear from 0.1 to 10 liters/s.

A minimum of three MEFV curves were performed at each sitting and most patients had four to six curves done during their evaluation. The two most reproducible curves with the best flow rates and volumes within ±5% of VC (as quantitated by standard water spirometry) were accepted. Final MEFV curves were constructed from these data using the highest flow rates at all volumes.

The final MEFV data were analyzed by three methods: (*a*) with flow (liters/second) plotted against volume (observed VC); (*b*) with flow (liters/second) plotted against volume (percent observed TLC); and (*c*) with flow divided by observed TLC (liters/second per liter) plotted against volume (percent observed VC remaining). Because of the wide variation in lung volumes in the patient population, method *c* was found to be most useful; these data were compared to the normal values of Gelb et al. (29).

Static compliance, dynamic compliance, and isovolume pressure-flow curves

These data were obtained in the sitting position utilizing a wedge spirometer for quantitation of volume and flow rates. Transpulmonary pressure (P_L) was measured as the difference between mouth and esophageal pressure utilizing a Sanborn 268-B differential strain gauge and carrier preamplifier (Hewlett-Packard Co.). Volume, flow, and P_L signals were recorded on a Brush model 480, eight channel universal recorder (Gould, Inc.). The esophageal pressure signal was transmitted by a 10 cm, thin-walled, latex balloon (Young Rubber Co., Trenton, N.J.) positioned in the lower third of the esophagus by first passing it into the stomach and observing for a positive defection, then withdrawing the balloon approximately 10 cm so that the pressure signal was maximum and artifact free. Balloon volume was corrected by the methods of Milic-Emili et al. (30) or Lemen et al. (31); the latter technique was simpler and closely agrees with the former.

The wedge spirometer was calibrated electronically and checked manually utilizing a 1-liter syringe and a 0–10 liter/s flow meter. Using a sine wave generator, the frequency response of the spirometer was ±5% at 6 cycles/s and flow was linear from 0.1 to 10 liters/s. The Sanborn 268-B differential strain gauge was linear between 0–100 cm H_2O and had a frequency response which was ±5% at 6 cycles/s. Evaluation of phase lag between signals of flow, volume, and esophageal balloon pressure was performed by inserting the balloon inside the wedge spirometer and applying a sine wave (using a 500-ml pump) to the system. These signals were in phase (<5° shift) up to 3 cycles/s.

A constant volume history was assured by having the patient hyperventilate and then inspire to TLC three times (32). Static transpulmonary pressure (Pst) was measured at TLC and during deflation as the pressure difference between mouth and esophageal pressure with glottis open and flow being interrupted by a solenoid-operated shutter.

Static volume-pressure curves were constructed utilizing a mean of four deflation maneuvers with 12–14 points per maneuver. Volume was converted to body temperature and pressure saturated and required to be ±5% of VC (as recorded on standard spirometry). Because of the marked variability of Pst below 50% observed TLC, static volume-pressure curves were constructed from TLC to 50% observed TLC. Volume was expressed both as a percentage of observed and predicted TLC and compared to the predicted data of Turner et al. (32).

Data for generation of isovolume pressure-flow curves were obtained by having the patient exhale from TLC to RV at varying efforts from maximum flow to 0.5 liter/s. From simultaneously recorded flow, volume, and P_L data, isovolume pressure-flow curves were constructed at 70, 50, and 30% VC according to the method of Hyatt et al. (33).

Dynamic compliance (Cdyn) was measured by having the patient first hyperventilate, inspire to TLC three times, and then breathe at a constant tidal volume at increasing frequencies up to 100 breaths/min. Flow, volume, and P_L were simultaneously recorded while a constant resting end expiratory point and resting end inspiratory point were maintained by having the patient observe his breathing pattern (volume) on a time base oscilloscope. For each frequency, Cdyn was calculated by dividing the volume change by the change in pressure at points of zero flow over 10 or more breaths and averaging the results. Cdyn was expressed as a percentage of initial Cdyn (Cdyn/initial Cdyn) and plotted against respiratory frequency. A frequency dependent decrease in Cdyn/ initial Cdyn of > 20% was considered to be abnormal (34, 35).

To determine the effect of bronchodilators on Cdyn, these maneuvers were repeated immediately after 0.5 ml of 1% isoetherine was administered as an aerosol inhalant.

Maximum flow-static recoil relationship

The relationship between maximum flow and static recoil (MFSR) was determined by plotting maximum expiratory flow ($\dot{V}_{max}$; obtained from the MEFV curve from 80 to 50% observed TLC) against Pst (derived from the static volume-pressure curve) at the same lung volumes (36). These data were also plotted utilizing $\dot{V}_{max}$ and Pst expressed as percentage of predicted lung volume. Predicted MFSR curves were obtained by plotting $\dot{V}_{max}$ predicted by the data of Cherniack and Raber (37) against Pst at the same lung volume predicted by the data of Turner et al. (32). The prediction curves were grouped by age range from 25 to 45 yr and greater than 45 yr. These curves compare favorably to the normal curves of Mead et al. (36) and Ostrow and Cherniack. (38).

Statistical analysis of data

Three statistical methods were used for data analysis: Spearman rank correlation, two-tailed Student's *t*-test, and Fisher's exact test. To facilitate discussion of the analysis, the data were grouped as follows: "clinical data" include age, sex, duration of symptoms, smoking history, and drug therapy; "standard physiologic studies" include VC, FRC, TLC, RV/TLC, and D_{LCO}; "physiologic monitors of small airways" include Cdyn, MEFV curves, and MFSR curves; and "overall estimate of small airways diameter" refers to the rating ("narrowed" or "not narrowed") given to each biopsy as defined by the criteria listed above.

The choice of a statistical method for comparisons among clinical, physiologic, and morphologic data was dictated by the form of the data. Spearman rank correlation (39) was used when one variable was ranked and the other variable was ranked or continuous. The two-tailed Student's *t* test (40) was used when the mean values for a continuous variable could be determined for each of two ranked groups. Fisher's exact (41) test was used when both variables could be ranked in two categories and a contingency table could be constructed. In certain comparisons, more than one statistical comparison was used. A standard Pearson correlation was not used because it assumes a normal distribution for both variables and in all comparisons made at least one variable was ranked.

Utilizing these criteria, the following statistical comparisons were made:

(*a*) Spearman rank correlation of clinical data vs. overall estimate of small airways diameter; standard physiologic studies vs. overall estimate of small airways diameter; clinical data vs. physiologic monitors of small airways; and standard physiologic studies vs. physiologic monitors of small airways; (*b*) two-tailed Student's *t* test of standard physiologic studies vs. overall estimate of small airways diameter; and (*c*) Fisher's exact test of physiologic monitors of small airways vs. overall estimate of small airways diameter; and RV/TLC, MEFV curves and MFSR curves vs. Cdyn.

RESULTS

Clinical data. The 18 study patients ranged in age from 27 to 67 yr, 12 were male and 6 were female (Table I). Six patients never smoked; an additional three were light cigarette smokers (<10 pack yr) and one was a cigar smoker. The remaining eight patients were either moderate (10–25 pack yr) or heavy smokers (>25 pack yr) and none had a history of sputum production. The duration of symptoms (before study at National Institutes of Health) ranged from 0.5 to 10 yr, but was ≤ 2 yr in all but one patient (W. L.). Eight patients were taking prednisone at the time of evaluation; one was taking phenylbutazone, and none was taking sympathomimetic agents or xanthines.

Morphologic evaluation of small airways in IPF. A total of 138 small airways were suitable for evaluation in the lung biopsies of the 18 patients (Table II). The most frequently observed morphologic abnormality was peribronchiolar fibrosis, either alone or together with peribronchiolar inflammation and bronchiolitis (Fig. 1). No airway was seen with bronchiolitis alone. Only one patient (W. L. S.) had completely normal airways.

Each biopsy was graded an average of three times. Using the grading criteria for airway diameter, the mean intraobserver coefficient of variation was 9.1 ±0.2%; the mean interobserver error was 10%. Of the total airways evaluated, 19% were of normal diameter, 27% were dilated, and 54% were narrowed (Table II). The dominant histologic abnormality accompanying narrowed airways was peribronchiolar fibrosis with infolding and stenosis (Fig. 1 B); seen less frequently was peribronchiolar fibrosis or inflammation and bronchiolitis (Fig. 1 C). The presence of histologic abnormalities of small airways did not necessarily mean the airway would be narrowed; peribronchiolar inflammation and peribronchiolar fibrosis were associated with airways that were of normal diameter (Fig. 1 A) or dilated (Fig. 1 D).

Using the criteria listed in Methods, overall estimates of small airways diameter revealed that 12 of the 18 patients (67%) had "narrowed" airways (i.e. in these patients, 60% or more of the small airways evaluated were narrowed) and the remaining 6 patients (33%) had "not narrowed" airways (i.e. in these patients, 70% or more of the airways evaluated were normal or dilated).

Standard physiologic studies and routine monitors of airways. The lung volumes were variable in the 18 patients with IPF, but the mean predicted values were significantly reduced (Table III). Although patients with histologically proven IPF are generally considered to have reduced volumes, one (E. B.) had a TLC within the normal range. Likewise, although almost all of the patients had a reduced D_{LCO} (mean 52.7% predicted), one patient (B. T.) had a D_{LCO} within the normal range. Thus, all of the patients had either a reduced TLC or D_{LCO}, and 89% had both. The average RV/TLC was 31.8%; 10 patients had normal RV/TLC (<30% observed).

TABLE I
Clinical Data of 18 Patients with IPF

Patient	Age	Sex	Height	Weight	Smoking history*	Duration of symptoms	Drugs‡
	yr		*cm*	*kg*		*yr*	
E. B.	48	M	195	100	Heavy	1.5	None
M. C.	57	F	158	76	Nonsmoker	0.5	Phenylbutazone
R. C.	66	M	172	68	Nonsmoker	0.5	Prednisone
N. C.	27	M	174	53	Light	2.0	Prednisone
A. D.	67	M	164	65	Medium§	0.5	Prednisone
G. F.	51	M	183	76	Medium§	2.0	Prednisone
A. H.	26	F	178	62	Light§	2.0	None
W. H.	41	M	183	84	Light§	2.0	None
V. J.	27	F	162	48	Nonsmoker	0.5	None
W. L.	67	M	179	86	Heavy§	10.0	None
O. N.	27	F	171	63	Nonsmoker	1.5	Prednisone
P. R.	31	F	175	88	Medium	0.5	Prednisone
J. C. S.	61	M	172	77	Heavy§	1.5	None
W. E. S.	66	M	173	85	Cigars§	1.0	None
R. S.	52	M	186	66	Nonsmoker	2.0	Prednisone
J. K. S.	46	M	182	80	Medium§	2.0	Prednisone
W. L. S.	58	M	171	72	Medium§	1.0	None
B. T.	47	F	163	83	Nonsmoker	0.5	None
Mean±SEM	48.1±3.6		174.5±2.2	74.6±3.1		1.7±0.5	

* Light, <10 pack-yr; moderate, 10–25 pack-yr; heavy, >25 pack-yr.
‡ Only anti-inflammatory agents are listed; none of the patients was taking xanthines or sympathomimetics.
§ Stopped smoking >6 mo before study.

Routine monitors of airways ($FEV_1\%$, Raw) were normal in all patients tested. Four patients (G. F., W. L., J. K. S., R. S.) were unable to perform the necessary maneuvers to measure Raw because of marked resting breathlessness.

Volume-pressure relationship. Most patients exhibited increased elastic recoil at lung volumes above FRC with a shift of the volume-pressure curve downward and to the right when volume was expressed as a percentage of predicted TLC (Fig. 2). One patient (E. B.) had a borderline shift in the volume-pressure curve to the left of the predicted normal curve for his age. When volume was expressed as a percentage of measured TLC (Fig. 3), five patients (A. H., P. R., G. F., R. C., W. L.) had curves which were similar to normal except at high lung volumes.

Physiologic monitors of small airways. Cdyn, performed in 17 patients, was frequency independent in 7 and frequency dependent in 10 (Fig. 4). Three patients (G. F., P. R., and B. T.) exhibited Cdyn which was less frequency dependent after nebulized bronchodilators. In no case did the use of bronchodilators cause the Cdyn to become independent of frequency (data not shown).

Nine patients had abnormal MEFV curves with reduced flows at low lung volumes and nine had normal to increased flows at all lung volumes (Fig. 5). All three methods of analysis of the MEFV data (see Methods) give comparable results.

Seven patients had reduced flow rates for a given P_{st} with a shift of the MFSR curve to the right of the normal range. The remaining 11 patients had normal to increased flow rates for a given P_{st} (Fig. 6). Both methods of analysis (see Methods) gave comparable results.

Obtaining meaningful MEFV and MFSR curves depends upon achieving maximum flow. To verify that maximum flow was achieved in these studies, isovolume pressure-flow curves were constructed. 15 patients achieved maximum flow and effort independence at 50% VC (data not shown). The remaining three patients (M. C., G. F., W. E. S.) were not able to perform the necessary maneuvers to construct isovolume pressure-flow curves because of breathlessness and inability to perform sustained expiratory maneuvers at variable flow rates.

Comparison of clinical, physiologic, and morphologic studies. Of the 17 patients[3] whose clinical and physiologic data were used for statistical comparisons

[3] One patient (R. C.) was excluded from the statistical comparisons with the overall estimate of small airway diameter because the lung biopsy was a drill biopsy which contained only one airway.

TABLE II

Morphologic Evaluation of Small Airways in Lung Biopsy Specimens of 18 Patients with IPF

Patient	Biopsy site*	Number of airways examined	Histology‡			Small airway diameter			Overall estimate of small airway diameter§
			Peri-bronchiolar fibrosis	Peri-bronchiolar inflammation	Bronchiolitis	Normal	Dilated	Narrowed	
						Number (%)			
E. B.	LUL	6	+	0	0	2 (33)	0 (0)	4 (67)	Narrowed
M. C.	LLL	8	+	+	0	0 (0)	1 (13)	7 (87)	Narrowed
R. C.	RLL	1	0	+	0	0 (0)	0 (0)	1 (100)	Narrowed
N. C.	LLL	6	+	+	+	0 (0)	2 (33)	4 (67)	Narrowed
A. D.	LLL	11	+	0	0	1 (9)	7 (63)	3 (27)	Not narrowed
G. F.	LLL	2	+	0	0	0 (0)	0 (0)	2 (100)	Narrowed
A. H.	LUL	10	+	0	0	1 (10)	0 (0)	9 (90)	Narrowed
W. H.	LLL LUL	10	+	0	0	7 (70)	0 (0)	3 (30)	Not narrowed
V. J.	RLL	5	0	+	0	3 (60)	1 (20)	1 (20)	Not narrowed
W. L.	RLL	9	+	+	+	1 (11)	2 (22)	6 (67)	Narrowed
O. N.	LUL	9	0	+	0	1 (11)	6 (67)	2 (22)	Not narrowed
P. R.	LLL	7	+	+	+	2 (29)	0 (0)	5 (71)	Narrowed
J. C. S.	LLL	6	+	0	0	2 (33)	0 (0)	4 (67)	Narrowed
W. E. S.	RUL RLL RML	10	+	0	0	0 (0)	4 (40)	6 (60)	Narrowed
R. S.	RLL	10	+	0	0	1 (10)	2 (20)	7 (70)	Narrowed
J. K. S.	LLL	12	+	0	0	0 (0)	10 (83)	2 (17)	Not narrowed
W. L. S.	RLL	5	0	0	0	5 (100)	0 (0)	0 (0)	Not narrowed
B. T.	LLL	11	0	+	+	1 (9)	1 (9)	9 (82)	Narrowed
Total		138				27 (19)‖	36 (27)‖	75 (54)‖	

* LUL, left upper lobe; LLL, left lower lobe; RUL, right upper lobe; RML, right middle lobe; RLL, right lower lobe.

‡ +, present; 0, not present.

§ The overall estimate of small airway diameter was narrowed if ≥60% of the airways in the biopsy were narrowed, independent of the status (normal or dilated) of the other airways; the overall estimate of small airway diameter was not narrowed if ≤30% of the airways were narrowed, independent of the status (normal or dilated) of the other airways; if 31–59% of the airways were narrowed, the morphologic data was not used for statistical comparisons with the physiologic data. Patient R. C. had a needle biopsy with only one airway present; this data was not used for statistical comparisons.

‖ Percent total.

FIGURE 1 Examples of small airways in open lung biopsies of patients with IPF. A. Small airway of normal diameter in a 27-yr-old female (V. J.) demonstrating peribronchiolar inflammation (×130). B. Narrowed small airway in a 26-yr-old female (A. H.) demonstrating peribronchiolar fibrosis with infolding and stenosis (×220). C. Narrowed small airway in a 47-yr-old female (B. T.) demonstrating peribronchiolar inflammation and bronchiolitis (×130). D. Dilated small airway in a 67-yr-old male (A. D.) demonstrating peribronchiolar fibrosis (×80). All sections were stained with hematoxylin and eosin.

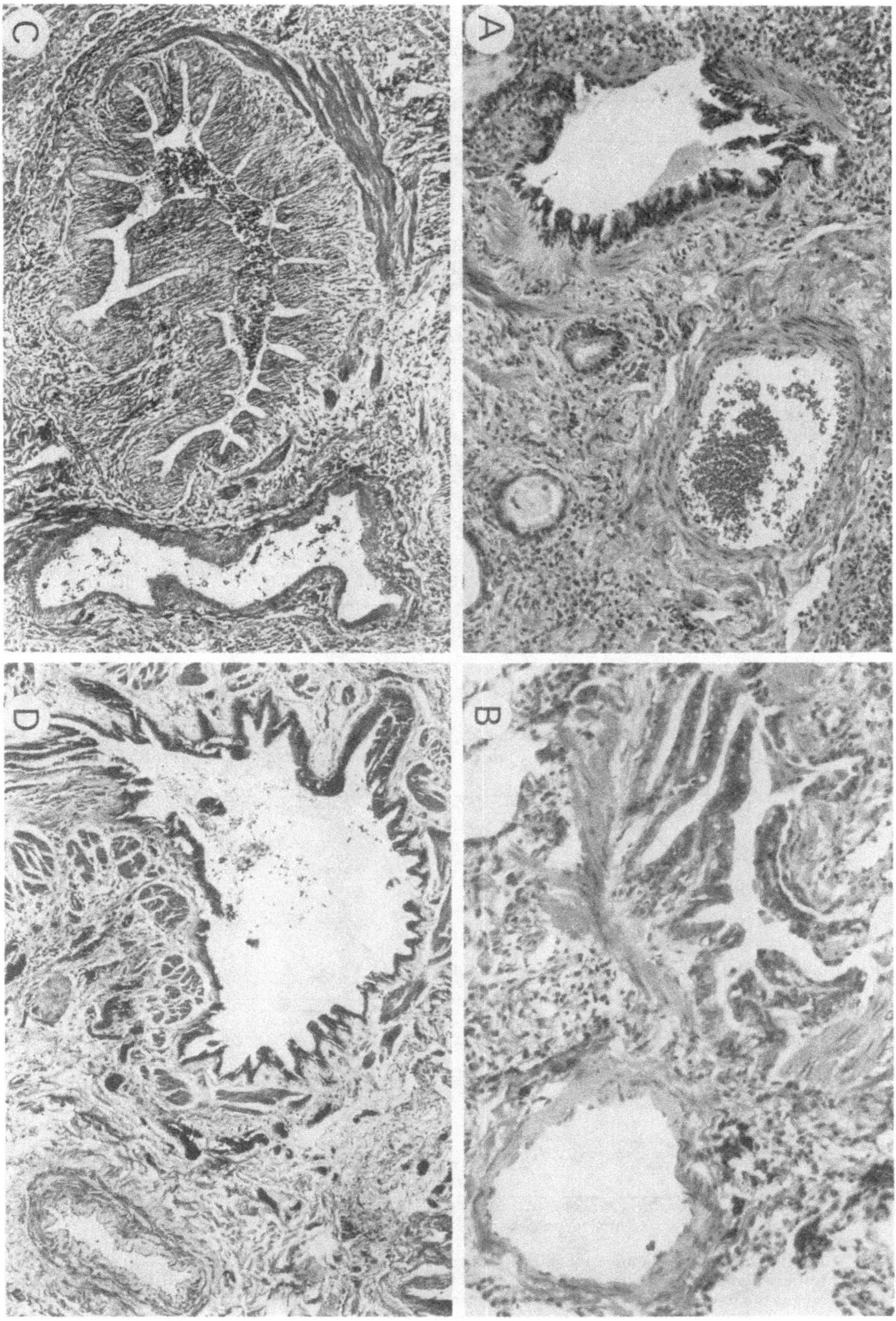
A
B
C
D

TABLE III
Standard Physiologic Studies of 18 Patients with IPF

Patient	VC		FRC		TLC		RV/TLC	Diffusing capacity*		FEV_1%		Raw
	Liters	% Predicted	Liters	% Predicted	Liters	% Predicted	% Observed	ml CO/mm Hg/min	% Predicted	% Observed	% Predicted	cm H_2O/liter/s
E. B.	4.84	83	3.53	73	7.17	86	31	16.3	48	72	96	1.16
M. C.	2.02	73	1.25	60	2.81	70	28	11.1	53	83	104	1.80
R. C.	2.98	71	2.14	60	4.17	64	28	8.9	42	78	109	2.38
N. C.	1.50	28	2.11	60	3.10	44	52	17.3	74	90	112	2.50
A. D.	2.19	59	1.85	63	3.52	61	37	11.8	49	86	122	1.60
G. F.	3.56	71	2.71	65	5.33	71	31	9.4	33	70	98	ND‡
A. H.	3.46	75	2.73	76	4.81	72	29	17.2	66	76	97	0.68
W. H.	2.85	50	1.93	43	3.66	46	25	12.6	52	83	113	0.99
V. J.	1.95	50	1.65	60	2.71	50	27	12.7	71	93	114	1.28
W. L.	2.90	65	2.43	61	4.35	62	33	7.0	31	74	109	ND‡
O. N.	1.86	45	1.73	54	2.62	43	29	9.5	57	98	125	2.12
P. R.	2.55	60	2.76	81	4.24	67	47	11.5	47	81	102	1.68
J. C. S.	2.34	55	1.42	55	4.02	74	41	12.7	57	77	109	1.50
W. E. S.	2.30	35	1.62	42	3.22	49	28	11.8	58	72	104	1.36
R. S.	1.41	33	1.49	34	2.57	33	29	5.0	25	96	120	ND‡
J. K. S.	3.42	65	2.91	85	4.70	68	27	8.3	30	91	123	ND‡
W. L. S.	3.32	78	1.91	53	4.32	67	24	14.8	60	32	114	0.82
B. T.	1.62	48	1.77	62	3.56	50	37	14.4	96	85	112	1.14
Mean	2.67	56.0	2.10	60.4	3.93	59.8	31.8	11.7	52.7	82.4	110.0	1.54
±SEM	±0.21	±3.7	±0.14	±2.9	±.27	±3.2	±1.7	±0.8	±4.2	±2.1	±2.1	±0.17

* Single-breath carbon monoxide diffusing capacity.
‡ ND, not done.

with the overall estimate of small airways diameter, 11 had "narrowed" airways and 6 had "not narrowed" airways. The overall estimate of small airway diameter did not correlate with age, sex, smoking history, duration of symptoms, drugs (on or off anti-inflammatory medications), lung volumes (VC, FRC, TLC), or diffusing capacity (Tables IV, V). There was, however, a significant association between RV/TLC and the over-

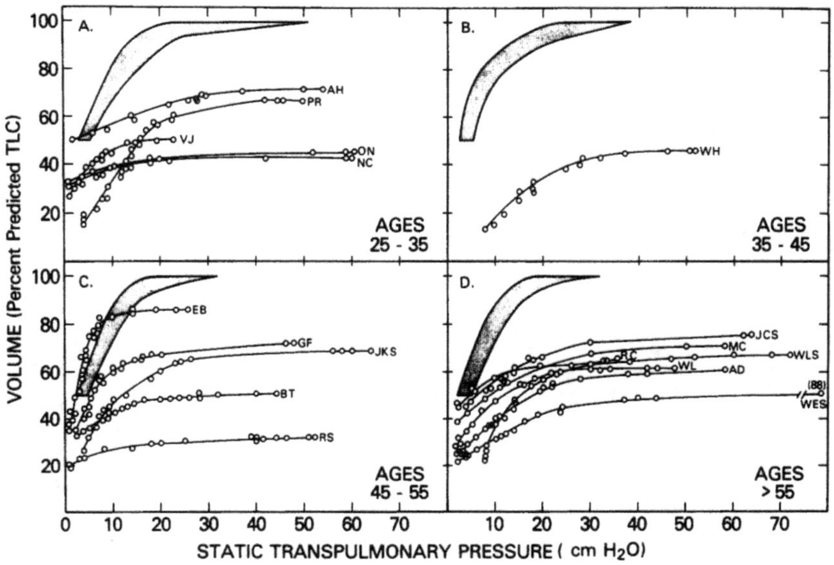

FIGURE 2 Static deflation volume-pressure curves for 18 patients with IPF grouped by age. Lung volume is expressed as percent predicted TLC. Pst is expressed in cm H_2O. Shaded area is the normal range established by Turner et al. (32).

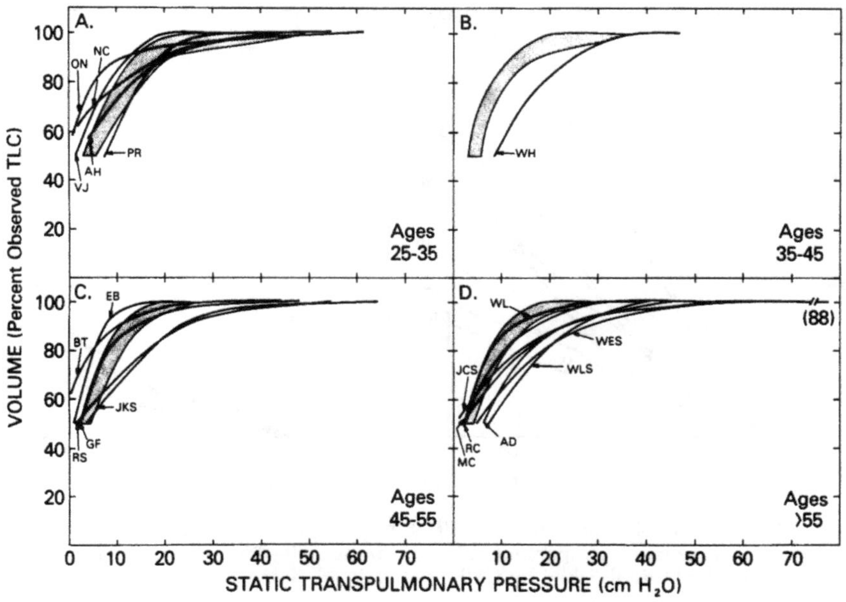

FIGURE 3 Static deflation volume-pressure curves for 18 patients with IPF grouped by age. Lung volume is expressed as percentage of observed (measured) TLC. Pst is expressed in cm H_2O. Shaded area is the normal range established by Turner et al. (32).

all estimate of small airways diameter whether the comparison was done by Spearman rank correlation ($P = 0.017$, Table IV) or Student's t test ($P = 0.046$, Table V). In general, patients with narrowed airways had elevated RV/TLC; in no case was an increased RV/TLC (>30% observed) associated with small airways whose overall status were not narrowed.

By entrance criteria for the study, all patients had normal $FEV_1\%$ and Raw, and thus there was no possible correlation between these monitors of large and

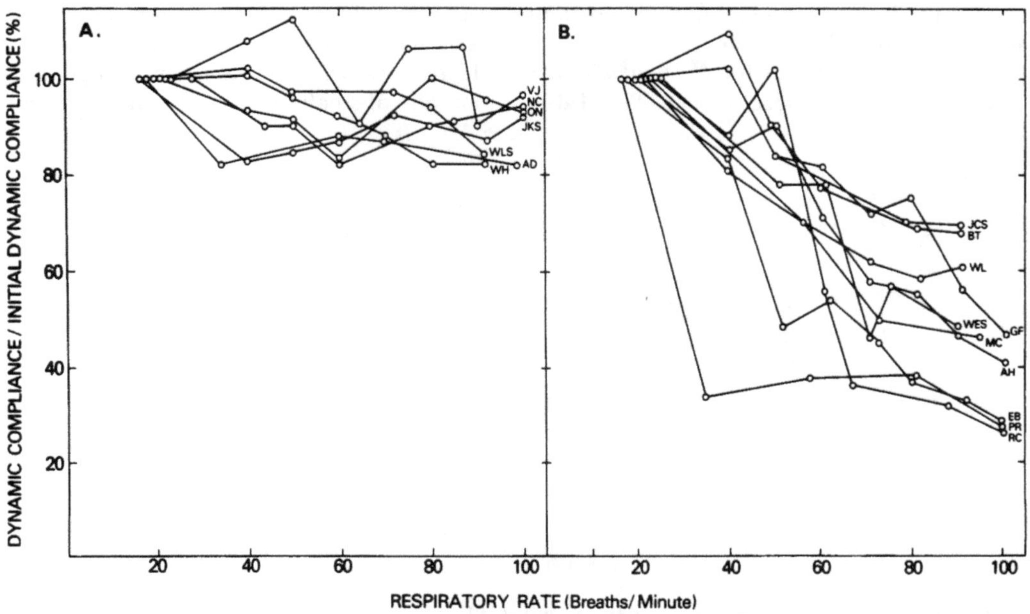

FIGURE 4 Cdyn in 17 patients with IPF expressed as a percentage of initial Cdyn. Respiratory rate is in breaths per minute. A. In seven patients Cdyn was independent of frequency. B. In 10 patients Cdyn was frequency dependent.

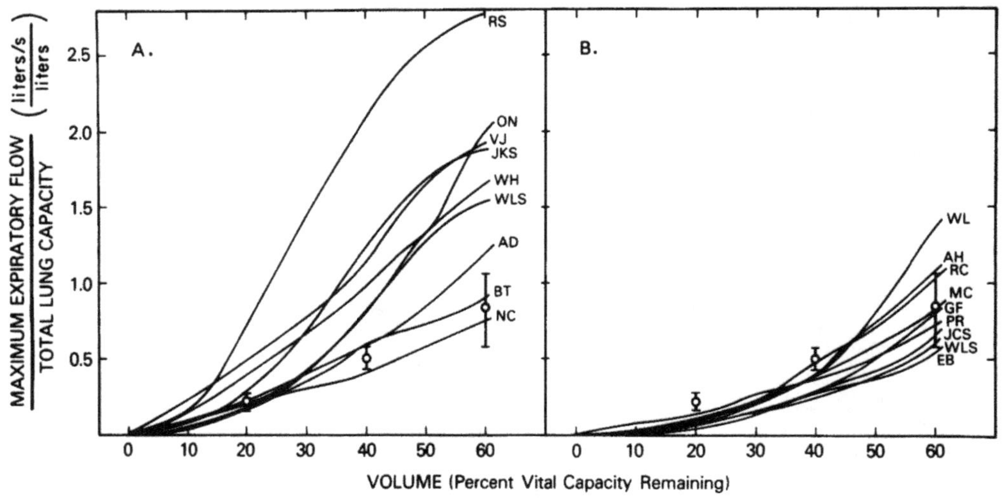

FIGURE 5 MEFV curves of 18 patients with IPF. Flow is expressed in liters per second/observed TLC; volume is expressed as percent VC remaining (60–0%). Open circles with error bars are the mean±SEM established by Gelb et al. (29).

medium airways and the morphologic evidence of narrowed small airways. In comparison, two of the physiologic tests of small airways function (Cdyn, MEFV curves) could predict the overall estimate of small airways diameter in open lung biopsy specimens.

Cdyn was the most sensitive predictor of the diameter of small airways ($P = 0.001$, Table VI); 9 of the 10 patients in whom airways were narrowed had frequency-dependent Cdyn and all 6 patients with not narrowed airways had normal Cdyn. Only one patient who had narrowed airways exhibited normal Cdyn; in no case was Cdyn frequency dependent in a patient who had airways of normal diameter.

The next most sensitive predictor of small airways diameter was the MEFV curve ($P = 0.009$, Table VI). 8 of the 11 patients in whom airways were narrowed had abnormal MEFV curves, whereas all 6 patients in whom airways were considered not narrowed had normal MEFV curves. However, three patients with narrowed small airways had normal MEFV curves. Like Cdyn, in no case was the MEFV curve abnormal in a patient who had airways that were considered not narrowed.

The third physiologic monitor of small airways, the MFSR relationship, was abnormal in 7 of the 11 patients with narrowed airways, and normal in all 6 patients with airways that were not narrowed (Table VI). However, four patients with narrowed airways had MFSR curves within the normal range. Like the other monitors of small airways, the MFSR curve was never

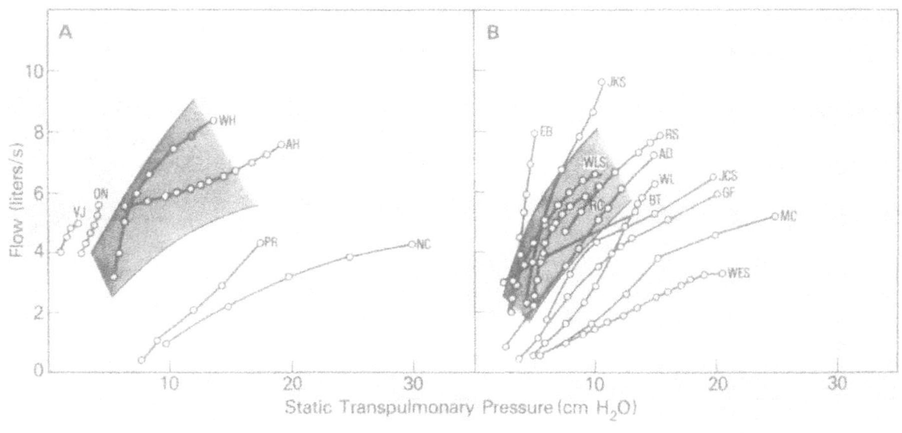

FIGURE 6 MRSR curves in 18 patients with IPF grouped by age. Flow is expressed in liters/second and Pst is expressed in cm H_2O. The shaded normal range is derived by plotting $\dot{V}_{max}$ predicted by the data of Cherniack and Raber (37) against Pst at the same lung volume predicted by the data of Turner et al. (32).

TABLE IV

Comparison of Clinical and Standard Physiologic Studies with the Overall Estimate of Small Airways Diameter of Patients with IPF

Comparison*	*r* value	*P* value
Clinical data‡ vs. overall estimate of small airways diameter§		
Age	0.139	0.601
Sex	0.030	0.904
Smoking history	−0.052	0.836
Duration of symptoms	0.144	0.588
Drugs	−0.044	0.862
Standard physiologic studies‖ vs. overall estimate of small airways diameter§		
VC	0.013	0.961
FRC	0.126	0.635
TLC	0.277	0.282
RV/TLC	0.568	0.017
Diffusing capacity	−0.050	0.842

* Comparison is by Spearman rank correlation.
‡ Data from Table I.
§ Data from Table II.
‖ Data from Table III.

TABLE V

Comparison of Standard Physiologic Studies between Groups of Patients with Overall Estimate of Small Airways that are Narrowed to Groups of Patients with Overall Estimate of Small Airways that Are Not Narrowed

Physiologic parameter	Mean value of physiologic parameter in each group of patients*: Those with airways that are narrowed‡	Those with airways that are not narrowed‡	*P* value§
VC	58.1	59.7	0.750
TLC	61.6	55.8	0.480
FRC	60.8	59.7	0.870
RV/TLC	35.5	28.2	0.046
Diffusing capacity	53.4	43.2	0.980

* Data from Table III; percent predicted values are used for all physiologic parameters except RV/TLC for which percent observed is used.
‡ Grouped according to the overall estimate of small airway diameter; see Table II.
§ Two-tailed Student's *t* test.

abnormal in a patient whose airways were considered not narrowed. Even so, the lack of a significant association between the MFSR curve and the overall estimate of small airways diameter suggested that the MFSR curve is not as sensitive as Cdyn or the MEFV curve in detecting narrowed small airways in patients with IPF.

There was no significant correlation between age, sex, smoking history, duration of symptoms, VC, FRC, RV/TLC, D_{LCO}, and the physiologic monitors of small airways (Table VII). However, there was a significant negative correlation between TLC and Cdyn and between TLC and the MEFV curves; patients with smaller total lung capacities tended to have normal Cdyn and normal MEFV curves, whereas those with larger total lung capacities tended to have frequency-dependent Cdyn and abnormal MEFV curves.

Although comparison of the physiologic data with the overall estimate of small airways diameter suggests that RV/TLC (Tables IV, V), Cdyn, and MEFV curves (Table VI) can predict narrowed small airways, only the results of the MEFV curves correlated with the results of Cdyn (the most sensitive predictor of the overall estimate of small airways diameter, Table VIII), suggesting a divergence in the physiologic functions monitored by some of these tests.

DISCUSSION

Although narrowing and stenosis of small airways were noted in the original description of IPF by Hamman and Rich (1), subsequent morphologic reports have largely concentrated on the alveoli and alveolar interstitium (3, 4, 8–10, 13); perhaps because the significance of small airways abnormalities in the pathophysiology of some chronic pulmonary disorders has only recently been recognized (42, 43). The data presented in this investigation indicate that morphologic and physiologic abnormalities of small airways are present

TABLE VI

Comparison between the Physiologic Monitors of Small Airways and the Overall Estimate of Small Airways Diameter in Patients with IPF

Physiologic study	Results*	Number of patients	Overall estimate of small airways diameter‡: Narrowed	Not narrowed	*P* value§
Cdyn	Normal	7	1	6	0.001
	Abnormal	9‖	9	0	
MEFV curve	Normal	9	3	6	0.009
	Abnormal	8‖	8	0	
MFSR curve	Normal	10‖	4	6	0.100
	Abnormal	7	7	0	

* Data from Figs. 4–6.
‡ Data from Table II.
§ Fisher's exact test.
‖ One patient (R. C.) was not included in the statistical analysis because the biopsy showed only one airway.

TABLE VII

Comparison of the Clinical Data and Standard Physiologic Studies with the Physiologic Monitors of Small Airways in Patients with IPF

	Physiologic monitors of small airways*					
	Cdyn		MEFV curve		MFSR	
	r value§	*P* value§	*r* value§	*P* value§	*r* value§	*P* value§
Clinical data‡						
Age	0.274	0.305	0.253	0.328	0.106	0.689
Sex	0.163	0.553	0.044	0.862	0.0635	0.803
Smoking history	0.042	0.870	0.250	0.665	0.219	0.598
Duration of symptoms	0.028	0.914	0.063	0.806	0.274	0.288
Standard physiologic studies‖						
VC	−0.3011	0.256	−0.047	0.055	−0.237	0.639
TLC	−0.5611	0.023	−0.663	0.004	−0.066	0.797
FRC	−0.261	0.332	0.289	0.259	−0.132	0.619
RV/TLC	−0.371	0.156	−0.266	0.303	−0.371	0.140
Diffusing capacity	−0.151	0.584	−0.217	0.592	−0.184	0.515

* Data from Figs. 4–6.
‡ Data from Table I.
§ Comparisons made using Spearman rank correlation.
‖ Data from Table III.

in IPF. The patients studied were representative of patients with IPF; the duration of symptoms and lung biopsy were typical of patients in mid-course (3–13). None had morphologic findings consistent with "end stage" lung (44).

Morphologic evaluation of small airways in IPF. Only one patient had completely normal airways; in the remainder, the majority of the small airways had peribronchiolar fibrosis or peribronchiolar inflammation or both; a smaller number of airways had coexisting bronchiolitis. Our data base does not allow for definitive conclusions as to whether these abnormalities are part of the same process that involves the alveolar interstitium; however, the localization of most of the airway pathology in the peribronchiolar tissue suggests that the inflammation and fibrosis of the small airways is secondary to the interstitial process. The dominant small airways abnormalities (peribronchiolar fibrosis, peribronchiolar inflammation, or both) were observed in all nonsmokers (M. C., R. C., V. J., O. N., R. S., B. T.) and all smokers (E. B., N. C., A. D., G. F., A. H., W. H., W. L., P. R., J. C. S., W. E. S., J. K. S.) except one (W. L. S.; Tables I, II). Thus, even though bronchiolar fibrosis and inflammation have been described in smokers (45–47), the lack of correlation of airway abnormalities and smoking history (Table IV, $P = 0.836$) suggests smoking was not the causative agent in these patients with IPF. In addition, there was no evidence that the airway abnormalities were secondary to intercurrent infection, because all bacterial, mycobacterial, fungal, and viral cultures of open lung biopsies done at our institution were negative.

TABLE VIII

Comparison of the Results of RV/TLC, MEFV Curve, and MFSR Curve with the Results of Cdyn in Patients with IPF

Physiologic study	Results	Number of patients	Cdyn* Normal	Cdyn* Abnormal	*P* value‡
RV/TLC*§	Normal	10	4	6	0.500
	Abnormal	7‖	2	5	
MEFV curve¶	Normal	8‖	7	1	0.001
	Abnormal	9	0	9	
MFSR curve**	Normal	10‖	6	4	0.310
	Abnormal	7	1	6	

* Data from Fig. 4.
‡ Fisher's exact test.
§ Data from Table III.
‖ One patient (R. S.) was excluded because he was unable to do Cdyn.
¶ Data from Fig. 5.
** Data from Fig. 6.

Some degree of bronchiolectasis was present in approximately one-fourth of all airways evaluated. Although there is no correlation between the morphologic assessment of the severity of disease and airway diameter, it is our impression that small airways in IPF progress through stages beginning with peribronchiolar inflammation leading to peribronchiolar fibrosis. With progressive fibrosis, it is probable that some airways stenose, whereas others become distorted and ectatic (44). However, this would be difficult to prove.

Even though almost all of the patients had morphologic abnormalities of small airways, these do not necessarily imply airways dysfunction. If intrinsic small airways abnormalities contribute significantly to airways dysfunction, the feature which should be compared to the physiologic studies is airway diameter (e.g. narrowed or not narrowed). 12 of the 18 patients had an overall estimate of small airways diameter of narrowed; the morphologic data, therefore, suggest that these patients have physiologic alterations consistent with obstruction of small airways.

It may be argued that biopsy specimens are not representative of the disease and that multiple samples, available only at autopsy, are necessary to fully evaluate IPF; or that biopsy specimens present special problems in the evaluation of airways diameter because it is not possible to "physiologically" inflate and fix an open lung biopsy as can be done with postmortem lung. However, it is critical that evaluation of small airways in IPF be done with biopsy (rather than postmortem) material because: (*a*) patients with IPF often die from a generalized pulmonary infection, a process which in itself may alter the morphology and diameter of small airways; (*b*) those who die without respiratory infection usually have "end-stage" lung, in which the disease is too far advanced to allow for rational morphologic analysis; and (*c*) to compare airway morphology with airway function (i.e. with physiologic studies), it is necessary to make the interval between the two as short as possible; a situation which is impossible when relying on postmortem lung.

Thus, to study small airway morphology in IPF in mid-course, it is mandatory that only biopsy material be used. To attempt to minimize errors in estimating airway diameter, detailed diameter grading was not attempted, only categories of narrowed, normal, or dilated were used. In addition, three independent criteria were used to estimate airway diameter; all done without knowledge of the physiologic data. Each method of diameter estimate gave similar results. In addition, to attempt to provide "representative" biopsies, the specimens were taken in areas appearing "average" on the chest roentgenogram.

Physiologic evaluation of small airways in IPF. None of the study patients had evidence of increased resistance to airflow by standard monitors of airway function ($FEV_1\%$, Raw). However, a significant number had abnormalities in physiologic tests considered to be monitors of small airways function. 59% had frequency-dependent Cydn (a decrease in Cdyn/initial Cdyn of greater than 20% with increasing respiratory rates). The remaining patients had normal Cdyn (a change of no more than 20% of Cdyn/initial Cdyn at increasing respiratory rates). In addition, 50% of the patients had abnormal MEFV curves and 39% had abnormal MEFV curves.

When the Cdyn data were plotted as percent of static compliance (Cstat) as described by Woolcock et al. (56), five of the seven patients (W. H., W. L. S., O. N., N. C., J. C. S.) with normal Cdyn (Fig. 3, group A.) had Cdyn/Cstat of $< 80\%$ at initial breathing frequencies (data not shown). This subgroup of patients did not, however, exhibit a progressive fall in Cdyn with increasing respiratory rates regardless of the method of analysis (Cdyn/initial Cdyn or Cdyn/Cstat). Four of these patients have been restudied at 3–6 mo intervals and exhibit identical reductions in Cdyn/Cstat at initial breathing frequencies without frequency dependence. Reduced Cdyn/Cstat at initial respiratory rates have been previously noted in fibrotic lung disease (49, 50). The reason for this is not clear, although alterations in surface forces which result in increased hysteresis are possible (49). In our patients, analysis of physiologic and morphologic data did not reveal significant differences between this subgroup of patients compared to those whose Cdyn/Cstat were $> 80\%$ at initial respiratory rates. The former did, however, tend to have more severe fibrosis.

Other physiologic studies have suggested that patients with IPF have small airways abnormalities. In a study of airway function in pulmonary fibrosis, Ostrow and Cherniack (38) included patients with "cryptogenic fibrosing alveolitis" whose physiologic features were similar to our patients. Like our study group, their patients had normal airway function by standard criteria, yet a significant number had physiologic evidence of increased resistance to airflow in small airways. A similar study by Yernalt et al. (49) also demonstrated that many of these patients have evidence of increased small airways resistance. In contrast, Schofield et al. (51) measured upstream conductance in patients with fibrotic lung disease (three with IPF), and found that these patients had normal upstream conductance. However, it is likely that those patients fall into the group of our patients (61%) that also had normal MFSR curves.

Recent studies have suggested that closing volume and closing capacity might be useful monitors of small airways in fibrotic lung disease (52, 53). In our group of 18 patients, we have performed more than 200 determinations of closing volume and closing capacity using the methods of Buist and Ross (54, 55). These tests were quite variable, even when performed on the same patient on consecutive days of the same hospitalization (data not shown). Thus, we do not find these to be useful in patients with IPF. Although closing volume and closing capacity may be useful for the detection of small airways abnormalities in patients with normal elastic recoil, they are less useful when recoil is increased as in patients with IPF. In addition, although the phase III data of the single breath nitrogen test was highly reproducible in these patients, there was no correlation between the slope of phase III (ΔN_2/liter) and any of the clinical, physiologic or morphologic parameters under study.

Comparison of clinical, physiologic, and morphologic data in IPF. Although it is generally accepted that MFSR curves can detect airflow obstruction in the presence of increased elastic recoil (48), it must be remembered that the use of Cdyn and MEFV curves as monitors of small airways function has been established only in the presence of normal lung resistance and normal elastic recoil (56–58). Inasmuch as patients with IPF have elevations of both (50, 59), it is possible that these physiologic abnormalities are secondary to alterations in regional compliance produced by the alveolar disease. To establish the valid use of these studies in IPF, it is necessary to demonstrate an association between these monitors of small airways function and the actual morphologic evidence of narrowed small airways.

The correlative data (Table VI) strongly suggest that Cdyn and MEFV curves detect, with a high degree of reliability, which patients with IPF have narrowed airways and which have not narrowed airways. These statistical comparisons are important because it could be argued that because both Cdyn and MEFV curves detect alterations in mechanical (resistance × compliance) time constants (56–58, 60), it is possible that abnormalities in these tests reflect abnormalities in regional compliance as well as airway resistance. However, if regional compliance abnormalities alone were responsible for making these tests abnormal in IPF, we would expect the results of Cdyn and MEFV curves to be randomly distributed, rather than yielding significant correlations with the morphologic estimates of small airways diameter. In addition, if volume pressure data are plotted with volume expressed as a percentage of measured TLC (Fig. 3) as Gibson and Pride have suggested (61), five patients who exhibited frequency-dependent Cdyn have curves which are similar to normals. This would suggest that there is uniform involvement of parenchyma and would favor the fact that frequency-dependent Cdyn is related to airways disease.

Even though 39% of the patients had abnormal MFSR curves, these data did not correlate with the morphologic assessment of airway narrowing ($P = 0.10$, Table VI). This lack of significant correlation occurred because although patients with not narrowed airways always had a normal MFSR curve, 4 of the 11 patients with narrowed airways also had normal MFSR studies. Thus, of the three physiologic methods (Cdyn, MEFV, MFSR) used in this study to test small airway function, the MFSR curve is the least sensitive. This may be due to the complexity of the volume-pressure curve in this disease, particularly at low lung volumes. Although almost all of our patients had increased elastic recoil near TLC, some had reduced recoil near FRC (Fig. 2 and 3). Similar volume-pressure curves were observed by Ostrow and Cherniack (38) and Yernalt et al. (49). The reduction in elastic recoil near FRC may result from a multitude of factors (e.g. rearrangements of connective tissue, increased tissue rigidity, destructive lesions), all of which may modify the usefulness of relying on measurement of upstream resistance as a monitor of small airways narrowing in IPF.

In comparison to Cdyn and MEFV curves, there were no significant associations among VC, FRC, and D_{LCO}, and the overall estimate of small airways diameter. Even though TLC correlated significantly with Cdyn and MEFV curves (Table VII), there was no correlation between TLC and overall estimate of small airways diameter. Thus, TLC cannot be used as a predictor of small airways disease in these patients. There was, however, a significant association between RV/TLC and airways diameter, suggesting that narrowing of small airways may account for the commonly observed increased RV/TLC seen in IPF (6, 7, 16). Although statistically significant, there was only a small difference in RV/TLC between patients grouped according to the estimate of airways diameter. Therefore, we do not believe that RV/TLC is a predictor of small airways diameter in IPF.

If we use frequency dependency of Cdyn as the best criterion for small airways dysfunction in IPF (Cdyn correlates best with the overall estimates of airway diameter, Table VI), it is interesting to note that results of MEFV curves correlate well with Cdyn, but the MFSR and RV/TLC results do not (Table VIII). These results are similar to that found by Martin et al. (62) and Gelb et al. (57) in evaluating these studies for use in patients with isolated small airways disease. Thus, Cdyn remains as the most sensitive and valid monitor of small airways disease, even in disorders as diverse as asthma (63) and IPF.

Inasmuch as age, sex, duration of symptoms, drugs, and smoking history could possibly modulate small airways disease, it was important to determine whether there were associations between these parameters and the morphologic assessment of small airways diameter or the physiologic monitors of small airways function. However, no significant correlates were found (Tables IV, V, VII).

Significance of small airways disease in IPF. The demonstration of morphologic and physiologic evidence of small airways abnormalities in IPF may have significant clinical implications. First, the detection of small airways dysfunction in IPF may be useful for staging this disease. Second, the hypoxemia may be, in part, secondary to ventilation-perfusion mismatching resulting from increased resistance to airflow in small airways. In our patient group, a small number of patients under therapy have demonstrated improvement of small airways function with lessening of hypoxemia with exercise. Thus, as suggested by Ostrow and Cherniack (38), small airways dysfunction may respond to therapeutic intervention which may significantly improve the level of oxygenation of patients with IPF.

ACKNOWLEDGMENTS

We thank Doctors Norton Elson and Byron McLees for their advice; Dr. David DeMetts for his help with the statistical analysis; Edwyna von Gal and Filippina Giacometti for their expert technical assistance; and Kirsten Cook and Nancy Wyne for their editorial assistance.

REFERENCES

1. Hamman, L., and A. R. Rich. 1944. Acute diffuse interstitial fibrosis of the lungs. *Bull. Johns Hopkins Hosp.* **74:** 177–212.
2. Rubin, E. H., and R. Lubliner. 1957. The Hamman-Rich syndrome: review of the literature and analysis of 15 cases. *Medicine (Baltimore).* **36:** 397–463.
3. Anderson, A. E., Jr., and A. G. Foraker. 1960. Morphological aspects of interstitial pulmonary fibrosis. *Arch. Pathol.* **70:** 79–93.
4. Scadding, J. G. 1960. Chronic diffuse interstitial fibrosis of the lungs. *Br. Med. J.* **1:** 443–450.
5. Herbert, F. A., B. B. Nahmias, E. A. Gaensler, and H. E. MacMahon. 1962. Pathophysiology of interstitial pulmonary fibrosis: report of 19 cases and follow-up with corticosteroids. *Arch. Intern. Med.* **110:** 628–648.
6. Livingstone, J. L., J. G. Lewis, L. Reid, and K. E. Jefferson. 1964. Diffuse interstitial pulmonary fibrosis: clinical, radiological, and pathological study based on 45 patients. *Q. J. Med.* **33:** 71–103.
7. Marks, A. 1967. Diffuse interstitial pulmonary fibrosis. *Med. Clin. North Am.* **51:** 439–457.
8. Scadding, J. G., and K. F. W. Hinson. 1967. Diffuse fibrosing alveolitis (diffuse interstitial fibrosis of the lungs): correlation of histology at biopsy with prognosis. *Thorax.* **22:** 291–304.
9. Liebow, A. A., and C. B. Carrington. 1967. Alveolar diseases: the interstitial pneumonias. *In* Frontiers of Pulmonary Radiology. M. Simon, E. J. Potchen, and M. LeMay, editors. Grune & Stratton, Inc., New York. 102–141.
10. Liebow, A. A. 1968. New concepts and entities in pulmonary disease. *In* The Lung. A. A. Liebow and D. E. Smith, editors. Williams and Wilkins, Baltimore. 332–365.
11. DeRemee, R. A., E. G. Harrison, Jr., and H. A. Andersen. 1972. The concept of classical interstitial pneumonitis-fibrosis (CIP-F) as a clinicopathologic syndrome. *Chest.* **61:** 213–220.
12. Stack, B. H. R., Y. F. J. Choo-Kang, and B. E. Heard. 1972. The prognosis of cryptogenic fibrosing alveolitis. *Thorax.* **27:** 535–542.
13. Scadding, J. G. 1974. Diffuse alveolar pulmonary fibrosis. *Thorax.* **29:** 271–281.
14. Kravis, T. C., A. Ahmed, T. E. Brown, J. D. Fulmer, and R. G. Crystal. 1976. Pathogenic mechanisms in pulmonary fibrosis: collagen-induced migration inhibition factor production and cytotoxicity mediated by lymphocytes. *J. Clin. Invest.* **58:** 1223–1232.
15. Reynolds, H. Y., J. D. Fulmer, J. A. Kazmierowski, W. C. Roberts, M. M. Frank, and R. G. Crystal. 1977. Analysis of cellular and protein content of broncho-alveolar lavage fluid from patients with idiopathic pulmonary fibrosis and chronic hypersensitivity pneumonitis. *J. Clin Invest.* **59:** 165–175.
16. Crystal, R. G., J. D. Fulmer, W. C. Roberts, M. L. Moss, B. R. Line, and H. Y. Reynolds. 1976. Idiopathic pulmonary fibrosis: clinical, histologic, radiographic, physiologic, scintigraphic, cytological, and biochemical aspects. *Ann. Intern. Med* **85:** 769–788.
17. Austrian, R., J. H. McClement, A. D. Renzetti, Jr., K. W. Donald, R. L. Riley, and A. Cournand. 1951. Clinical and physiologic features of some types of pulmonary diseases with impairment of alveolar-capillalry diffusion: the syndrome of "alveolar-capillary block." *Am. J. Med.* **11:** 667–685.
18. Finley, T. N., E. W. Swenson, and J. H. Comroe, Jr. 1962. The cause of arterial hypoxemia at rest in patients with "alveolar-capillary block syndrome." *J. Clin. Invest.* **41:** 618–622.
19. Wagner, P. D., D. R. Dantzker, R. Dueck, J. L. DePolo, K. Wasserman, and J. B. West. 1976. Distribution of ventilation-perfusion ratios in patients with interstitial lung disease. *Chest.* **69**(Suppl.): 256–257.
20. McFadden, E. R., Jr., and H. A. Lyons. 1968. Airway resistance and uneven ventilation in bronchial asthma. *J. Appl. Physiol.* **25:** 365–370.
21. Heckscher, T., H. Bass, A. Oriol, B. Rose, N. R. Anthonisen, and D. V. Bates. 1968. Regional lung function in patients with bronchial asthma. *J. Clin. Invest.* **47:** 1063–1070.
22. Meneely, G. R., and N. L. Kaltreider. 1949. The volume of the lung determined by helium dilution: description of method and comparison with other procedures. *J. Clin. Invest.* **28:** 129–139.
23. Morris, J. F., A. Koski, and L. C. Johnson. 1971. Spirometric standards for healthy nonsmoking adults. *Am. Rev. Respir. Dis.* **103:** 57–67.
24. Goldman, H. I., and M. R. Becklake. 1959. Respiratory function tests: normal values at medium altitudes and the predicition of normal results. *Am. Rev. Tuberc. Pulm. Dis.* **79:** 457–467.
25. Macdonald, J. B., T. J. Cole, and A. Seaton. 1975. Forced expiratory time—its reliability as a lung function test. *Thorax.* **30:** 554–559.
26. Ogilvie, C. M., R. E. Forster, W. S. Blakemore, and J. W. Morton. 1957. A standard breath holding technique for the clinical measurement of the diffusing capacity of the lung for carbon monoxide. *J. Clin. Invest.* **36:** 1–17.
27. Gaensler, E. A., and G. W. Wright. 1966. Evaluation of respiratory impairment. *Arch. Environ. Health* **12:** 146–189.
28. Dubois, A. B., S. Y. Botelho, and J. H. Comroe, Jr. 1956. A new method for measuring airway resistance in man using a body plethysmograph: values in normal subjects and in patients with respiratory disease. *J. Clin. Invest.* **35:** 327–335.
29. Gelb, A. F., W. M. Gold, R. R. Wright, H. R. Bruch, and J. A. Nadel. 1973. Physiologic diagnosis of subclinical emphysema. *Am. Rev. Respir. Dis.* **107:** 50–63.
30. Milic-Emili, J., J. Mead, J. M. Turner, and E. M. Glauser. 1964. Improved technique for estimating pleural pressure from esophageal balloons. *J. Appl. Physiol.* **19:** 207–211.
31. Lemen, R., M. Benson, and J. G. Jones. 1974. Absolute pressure measurements with hand-dipped and manufactured esophageal balloons. *J. Appl. Physiol.* **37:** 600–603.

32. Turner, J. M., J. Mead, and M. E. Wohl. 1968. Elasticity of human lungs in relation to age. *J. Appl. Physiol.* **25:** 664–671.
33. Hyatt, R. E., D. P. Schilder, and D. L. Fry. 1958. Relationship between maximum expiratory flow and the degree of lung inflation. *J. Appl. Physiol.* **13:** 331–336.
34. Seaton, Anthony, N. LeRoy Lapp, and W. K. C. Morgan. 1972. Lung mechanics and frequency dependence of compliance in coal miners. *J. Clin. Invest.* **51:** 1203–1211.
35. Blair, H. Thomas, S. B. Greenberg, P. M. Stevens, P. A. Bilunos, and R. B. Couch. 1976. Effects of rhinovirus infection on pulmonary function of healthy human volunteers. *Am. Rev. Respir. Dis.* **114:** 95–102.
36. Mead, J., J. M. Turner, P. T. Macklem, and J. B. Little. 1967. Significance of the relationship between lung recoil and maximum expiratory flow. *J. Appl. Physiol.* **22:** 95–108.
37. Cherniack, R. M., and M. B. Raber. 1972. Normal standards for ventilatory function using an automated wedge spirometer. *Am. Rev. Respir. Dis.* **106:** 38–46.
38. Ostrow, D., and R. M. Cherniack. 1973. Resistance to airflow in patients with diffuse interstitial lung disease. *Am. Rev. Respir. Dis.* **108:** 205–210.
39. Snedecor, G. W., and W. G. Cochran. 1967. Statistical Methods. Iowa State University Press, Ames, Iowa. 6th edition. 194.
40. Snedecor, G. W., and W. G. Cochran. 1967. Statistical Methods. Iowa State University Press, Ames, Iowa. 6th edition. 59–61.
41. Brownlee, K. A. 1960. Statistical Theory and Methodology in Science and Engineering. John Wiley & Sons, Inc., New York. 123–125.
42. Hogg, J. C., P. T. Macklem, and W. M. Thurlbeck. 1968. Site and nature of airway obstruction in chronic obstructive lung disease. *N. Engl. J. Med.* **278:** 1355–1360.
43. Despas, P. J., M. Leroux, and P. T. Macklem. 1972. Site of airway obstruction in asthma as determined by measuring maximal expiratory flow breathing air and a helium-oxygen mixture. *J. Clin. Invest.* **51:** 3235–3243.
44. Heppleston, A. G. 1956. The pathology of honeycomb lung. *Thorax.* **11:** 77–93.
45. Niewoehner, D. E., J. Kleinerman, and D. B. Rice. 1974. Pathological changes in the peripheral airways of young cigarette smokers. *N. Engl. J. Med.* **291:** 755–758.
46. Thurlbeck, W. M. 1973. Disease of small airways, with particular reference to lesions found in asymptomatic chronic bronchitis without emphysema. *Chest.* **63** (Suppl.): 70S–71S.
47. Zamel, N., J. Hogg, and A. Gelb. 1976. Mechanisms of maximal expiratory flow limitation in clinically unsuspected emphysema and obstruction of peripheral airways. *Am. Rev. Respir. Dis.* **113:** 337–345.
48. Macklem, P. T. 1975. Tests of lung mechanics. *N. Engl. J. Med.* **293:** 339–342.
49. Yernalt, J. C., M. DeJonghe, A. DeCoster, and M. Englert. 1975. Pulmonary mechanics in diffuse fibrosing alveolitis. *Bull. Physio-pathol. Respir.* **11:** 231–244.
50. Macklem, P. T., and M. R. Becklake. 1963. The relationship between the mechanical and diffusing properties of lung in health and disease. *Am. Rev. Respir. Dis.* **87:** 47–56.
51. Schofield, N. M., R. J. Davies, I. R. Cameron, and M. Green. 1976. Small airways in fibrosing alveolitis. *Am. Rev. Respir. Dis.* **113:** 729–735.
52. Levinson, R. S., L. F. Metzger, N. N. Stanley, J. S. Brody, and N. S. Cherniack. 1973. Airway function in interstitial disease. *Am. Rev. Respir. Dis.* **107:** 1105. (Abstr.)
53. Levinson, R. S., L. F. Metzger, N. N. Stanley, S. G. Kelsen, M. D. Altose, N. S. Cherniack, and J. S. Brody. 1977. Airway function in sarcoidosis. *Am. J. Med.* **62:** 51–59.
54. Buist, A. S., and B. B. Ross. 1973. Predicted values for closing volumes using a modified single breath nitrogen test. *Am. Rev. Respir. Dis.* **107:** 744–752.
55. Buist, A. Sonia. 1975. The single-breath nitrogen test. *N. Engl. J. Med.* **293:** 438–440.
56. Woolcock, A. J., N. J. Vincent, and P. T. Macklem. 1969. Frequency dependence of compliance as a test for obstruction of the small airways. *J. Clin. Invest.* **48:** 1097–1106.
57. Gelb, A. F., and N. Zamel. 1973. Simplified diagnosis of small-airway obstruction. *N. Engl. J. Med.* **288:** 395–398.
58. Gelb, A. F., and B. J. MacAnally. 1973. Early detection of obstructive lung disease by analysis of maximal expiratory flow-volume curve. *Chest.* **64:** 749–753.
59. Bachofen, H., and M. Scherrer. 1967. Lung tissue resistance in diffuse interstitial fibrosis. *J. Clin. Invest.* **46:** 133–140.
60. Otis, A. B., C. B. McKerrow, R. A. Bartlett, J. Mead, M. B. McIlroy, N. J. Selverstone, and E. P. Radford. 1956. Mechanical factors in distribution of pulmonary ventilation. *J. Appl. Physiol.* **8:** 427–443.
61. Gibson, A. J., and N. B. Pride. 1976. A reappraisal of lung mechanics in fibrosing alveolitis. *Chest.* **69**(Suppl.): 256.
62. Martin, R. R., D. Lindsay, P. Despas. D. Bruce, M. Leroux, N. R. Anthonisen, and P. T. Macklem. 1975. The early detection of airway obstruction. *Am. Rev. Respir. Dis.* **111:** 119–125.
63. Hill, D. J., L. I. Landu, and P. D. Phelan. 1972. Small airway disease in asymptomatic asthmatic adolescents. *Am. Rev. Respir. Dis.* **106:** 873–880.

Fibrosing Mediastinitis Causing Pulmonary Arterial Hypertension Without Pulmonary Venous Hypertension

Clinical and Necropsy Observations

ERNEST N. ARNETT, M.D.*
Bethesda, Maryland

JAMES M. BACOS, M.D.
ABE M. MACHER, M.D.†
H. BRANDIS MARSH, M.D.
Washington, D.C.

DANIEL D. SAVAGE, M.D., Ph.D.
JACK D. FULMER, M.D.
WILLIAM C. ROBERTS, M.D.
Bethesda, Maryland

Clinical and morphologic observations are described in two patients with severe pulmonary arterial hypertension without pulmonary venous hypertension from fibrosing mediastinitis. In one patient, both main pulmonary arteries and one major pulmonary vein were severely narrowed by dense fibrous tissue; in the second patient, only the right main pulmonary artery was severely narrowed. Both patients had normal intrapulmonary arteries and normal pulmonary parenchyma. Of nine previously described necropsy patients with pulmonary hypertension due to fibrosing mediastinitis, seven had severe narrowing of multiple large pulmonary veins and in six of them the pulmonary hypertension was entirely due to pulmonary venous obstruction. In one other patient, the pulmonary hypertension was due to obstruction of one main pulmonary artery and several large pulmonary veins. Each of these seven previously described patients had severe changes in the small intrapulmonary arteries. Of the other two previously described patients with pulmonary hypertension from fibrosing mediastinitis, one had severe narrowing of only the main right pulmonary artery, and the other, of both main pulmonary arteries. Thus, although pulmonary arterial hypertension in patients with fibrosing mediastinitis is usually due to obstruction of multiple large pulmonary veins and to severe secondary changes in small intrapulmonary arteries, fibrosing mediastinitis can cause severe pulmonary hypertension by obstructing the right or both main pulmonary arteries.

Fibrosing mediastinitis, an uncommon condition, is a rare cause of severe pulmonary hypertension. When occurring in patients with fibrosing mediastinitis, pulmonary hypertension usually is due to obstruction of multiple large pulmonary veins and to severe secondary narrowings of small intrapulmonary arteries. A rare cause of pulmonary hypertension in patients with fibrosing mediastinitis is extraluminal obstruction of major extrapulmonary pulmonary arteries. Recently, we studied two patients with severe pulmonary arterial hypertension without pulmonary venous hypertension secondary to obstruction of one or both main pulmonary arteries by fibrosing mediastinitis. Observations in them are described herein.

From the Pathology, Cardiology and Pulmonary Branches, National Heart, Lung and Blood Institute, National Institutes of Health, Bethesda, Maryland; and the Division of Cardiology, Department of Medicine, Washington Hospital Center, Washington, D.C. Requests for reprints should be addressed to Dr. William C. Roberts, Building 10A, Room 3E-30, National Institutes of Health, Bethesda, Maryland 20014. Manuscript accepted October 8, 1976.

* Present address: Department of Medicine, The Johns Hopkins Hospital, Baltimore, Maryland 21205.

† Present address: Laboratory of Clinical Investigation, National Institute of Allergy and Infectious Diseases, National Institutes of Health, Bethesda, Maryland 20014.

CASE REPORTS

Case 1. A 35 year old black woman, who was found to have a positive tuberculin skin test at age 14 years, was in good health until age 33 (25 months before death) when she coughed blood and for several days thereafter noted intermittent pleuritic chest pain. Chest roentgenogram showed an infiltrate in the upper lobe of the left lung, and fiberoptic bronchoscopy disclosed inflammation of the bronchus in the upper lobe of the left lung. Results of cytologic examination and cultures of bronchial washings were negative for tumor cells and for acid-fast organisms. Despite the negative cultures, the patient was treated with isoniazid for 18 months and with ethambutol for six months. She remained asymptomatic after the episode of hemoptysis until seven months before death when she noted the onset of exertional dyspnea which increased over the ensuing three months.

Four months before death, examination disclosed a precordial systolic murmur; an electrocardiogram showed right axis deviation and right ventricular hypertrophy. Chest roentgenograms showed mild cardiac enlargement, a "fibronodular" infiltrate in the upper lobe of the left lung and a pleural effusion in the right lung. Lung scan showed multiple perfusion defects and almost total lack of flow to the upper lobe of the right lung. Right-sided cardiac catheterization revealed the following pressures: mean pulmonary capillary wedge, 7 mm Hg; pulmonary artery, 85/25 mm Hg (mean 45 mm Hg); right ventricle 85/17 mm Hg and right atrium (mean) 17 mm Hg. Superior vena cavagram disclosed marked narrowing at the level of the carina. Pulmonary angiography revealed narrowed main right and left pulmonary arteries, and their branches at the hila of the lungs, with normal appearing intralung arteries. Examination 67 days before death disclosed her to be thin. The blood pressure was 120/90 mm Hg; pulse rate 110 beats/min, and respiratory rate 23 breaths/min. Percussion sound was dull, and auscultation disclosed egophony at the base of the right lung. A third heart sound was heard at the lower left sternal border. The first heart sound was normal, but the pulmonic component of the second heart sound was loud. A grade 3/6 holosystolic murmur which increased in intensity with inspiration was present at the lower left sternal border. The liver was enlarged and pulsatile, but no subcutaneous edema was present. An electrocardiogram (Figure 1) revealed right axis deviation and right ventricular hypertrophy. Chest roentgenograms (Figure 2) revealed cardiomegaly, a wide mediastinal shadow, an infiltrate in the upper lobe of the left lung, calcified right paratracheal lymph nodes and a pleural effusion in the right lung. The blood hematocrit value was 32 per cent; white blood cell count 9,800/mm^3 and erythrocyte sedimentation rate 24 mm in 1 hour. Tests for antinuclear factor, rheumatoid factor and lupus erythematosus cells yielded negative results. Histoplasma complement fixation test results were negative. Multiple cultures for acid-fast organisms in sputum, urine, bone marrow aspirate and pleural fluids were negative, and pleural biopsy specimens revealed no granulomas. Superior vena cavagram revealed discrete narrowing at the level of the innominate vein. Catheterization (nine days before death) disclosed the following pressures: peripheral right pulmonary artery, 10/0 mm Hg (mean 4 mm Hg) and pulmonary trunk, 70/11 mm Hg (mean 32 mm Hg). Pulmonary angiography disclosed no flow to the upper lobe of the right lung, severely diminished flow to the upper lobe of the left lung, and marked constriction of both right and left main pulmonary arteries at the hila.

Four days before death, thoracotomy disclosed extensive amounts of dense fibrous tissue in the mediastinum, surrounding both pulmonary arteries and the superior vena cava. The right pulmonary artery and the superior vena cava were dissected free: the main right pulmonary artery was widened with a Teflon® graft and the superior vena cava was widened with a pericardial patch. Postoperatively, the pressure in the pulmonary trunk and distal right pulmonary artery remained increased (60 to 70 mm Hg systolic). A chest roentgenogram, obtained 24 hours postoperatively, showed opacification of the entire upper lobe of the right lung; reexploration disclosed infarction of that lobe, and it was excised. The patient remained hypotensive, however, and she died three days later.

At necropsy (A76-223), dense fibrous tissue surrounded the great vessels, superior vena cava, major bronchi and lower trachea (Figures 3 and 4). The fibrous tissue caused marked narrowing of the lumens of the superior vena cava, both main right and left pulmonary arteries, and the lower left pulmonary vein (Figure 5). Although its grafted portion was widely patent (Figure 4), the main right pulmonary artery was still severely narrowed just distal to the distal attachment of the graft. The pericardial sac was free of excess fluid or fi-

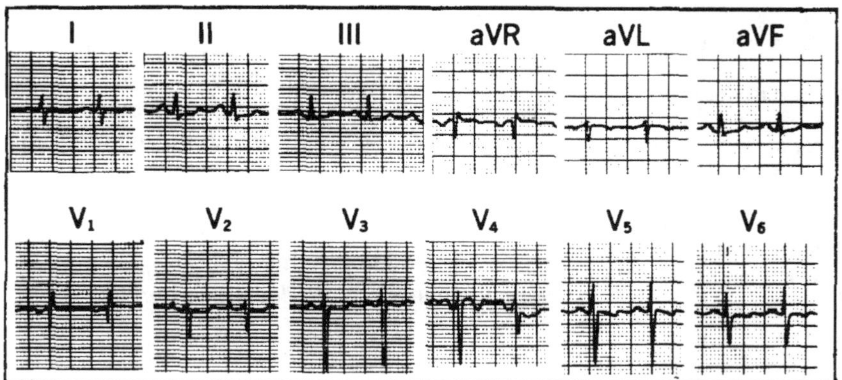

Figure 1. *Case 1. Electrocardiogram 67 days before death showing right axis deviation, right ventricular hypertrophy and incomplete right bundle branch block.*

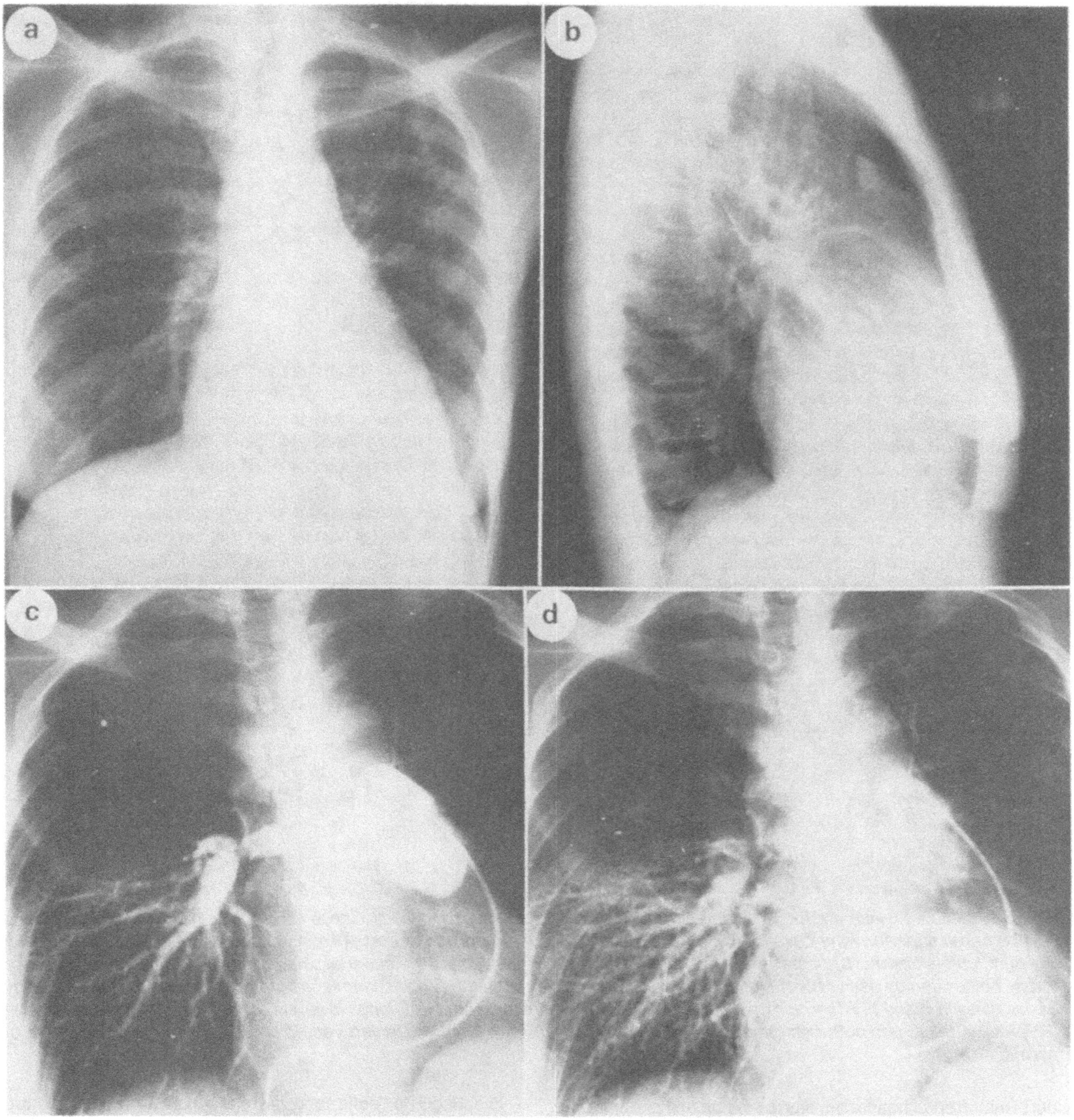

Figure 2. *Case 1.* ***a*** *and* ***b,*** *posteroanterior and lateral chest roentgenograms 67 days before death. The cardiac and mediastinal silhouettes are widened, the pulmonary trunk is prominent, and a coarse reticular infiltrate is present in the left upper lobe. A focal calcific deposit is present in the anterior mediastinum on the lateral film.* ***c*** *and* ***d,*** *pulmonary arteriograms nine days before death, 2.5 and 3.7 seconds, respectively, after injection of contrast material into the dilated pulmonary trunk. There is discrete narrowing of the main right pulmonary artery at the hilum and poststenotic dilatation of the branches to the right, middle and lower lobes. The arteries to the upper lobe of the right lung and to the entire left lung are totally obstructed.*

brous tissue. Histologic sections of the dense mediastinal tissue showed only a few scattered foci of mononuclear cells in addition to the scar. No granulomas were found in remnants of mediastinal lymph nodes, and no acid-fast bacilli or fungi were seen. The heart weighed 300 g; the wall of the right ventricle was hypertrophied, and both right-sided cardiac chambers were dilated (Figure 3). Histologic sections revealed focal interstitial scar and thromboembolic material in the lumen of a rare small muscular pulmonary artery in the upper lobe of the left lung.

Case 2. A 70 year old black woman was well until age 64 years when exertional dyspnea, dizziness, arthralgias of large joints, anorexia and weight loss were noted. Six months later,

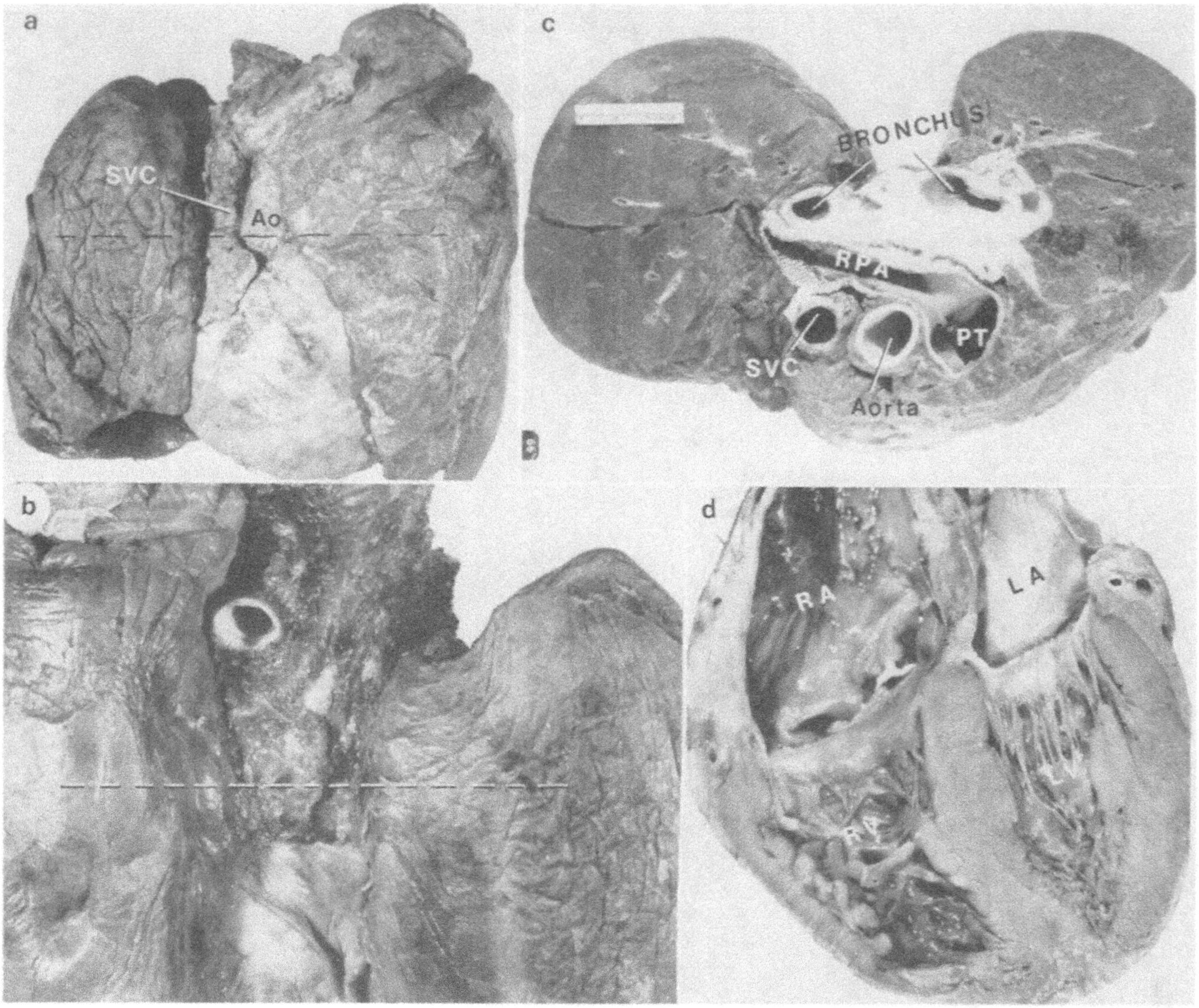

Figure 3. *Case 1. Heart and lungs.* ***a,*** *anterior view of the enblock heart and lungs. Dense fibrous tissue surrounds the cephalad portion of the superior vena cava (SVC), as well as the transverse portion of aorta (Ao) and its branches. The upper lobe of the right lung is absent.* ***b,*** *posterior view of the enblock heart and lungs. The superior and posterior mediastinal spaces are totally obliterated by dense fibrous tissue.* ***c,*** *transverse cut through the mediastinum and both lungs at the level indicated by dashed lines in* ***a*** *and* ***b.*** *PT = pulmonary trunk; RPA = right pulmonary artery.* ***d,*** *longitudinal cut of the heart. The right ventricular (RV) wall is thick, and both right ventricle and right atrium (RA) are dilated. The left ventricle (LV) and left atrium (LA) are of normal size.*

persistent frontal headache, blurred vision and photophobia of the right eye appeared. Examination revealed severe episcleritis and an enlarged tender right temporal artery. The hematocrit value was 32 per cent, erythrocyte sedimentation rate 38/mm in 1 hour, the results of the test for rheumatoid factor were weakly positive and of the tuberculin skin test negative. Chest roentgenogram and electrocardiogram disclosed no abnormalities. Biopsy of the right temporal artery revealed "atherosclerosis." Corticosteroid eye drops were prescribed. Prednisone therapy (60 mg/day) was started 65 months before death, marked symptomatic improvement followed, and seven months later administration of this drug was discontinued. Several months later, however, exertional dyspnea, dizziness and arthralgia recurred, and they were followed by cough, night sweats, exertional chest pain and dysphagia for solid foods. Examination 34 months before death disclosed a loud pulmonic component of the second sound and a systolic murmur which increased in intensity with inspiration and radiated into the right anterior precordium, right axilla and back. A chest roentgenogram showed marked enlargement of the cardiac silhouette, and an electrocardiogram showed right ventricular hypertrophy. Lung scan showed a large perfusion defect in the right lung, and pulmonary arteriography disclosed severe narrowing of the right main pulmonary artery and severely diminished flow to the right lung. The right-sided cardiac pressures were pulmonary artery wedge (mean) 8 mm Hg, a wave 8 mm Hg, v wave 12 mm Hg; pulmonary trunk 45/12 mm Hg (mean 23 mm Hg); right ventricle 45/8 mm Hg; and right atrium (mean) 7 mm Hg. The systolic pressure in the right pulmonary artery distal to

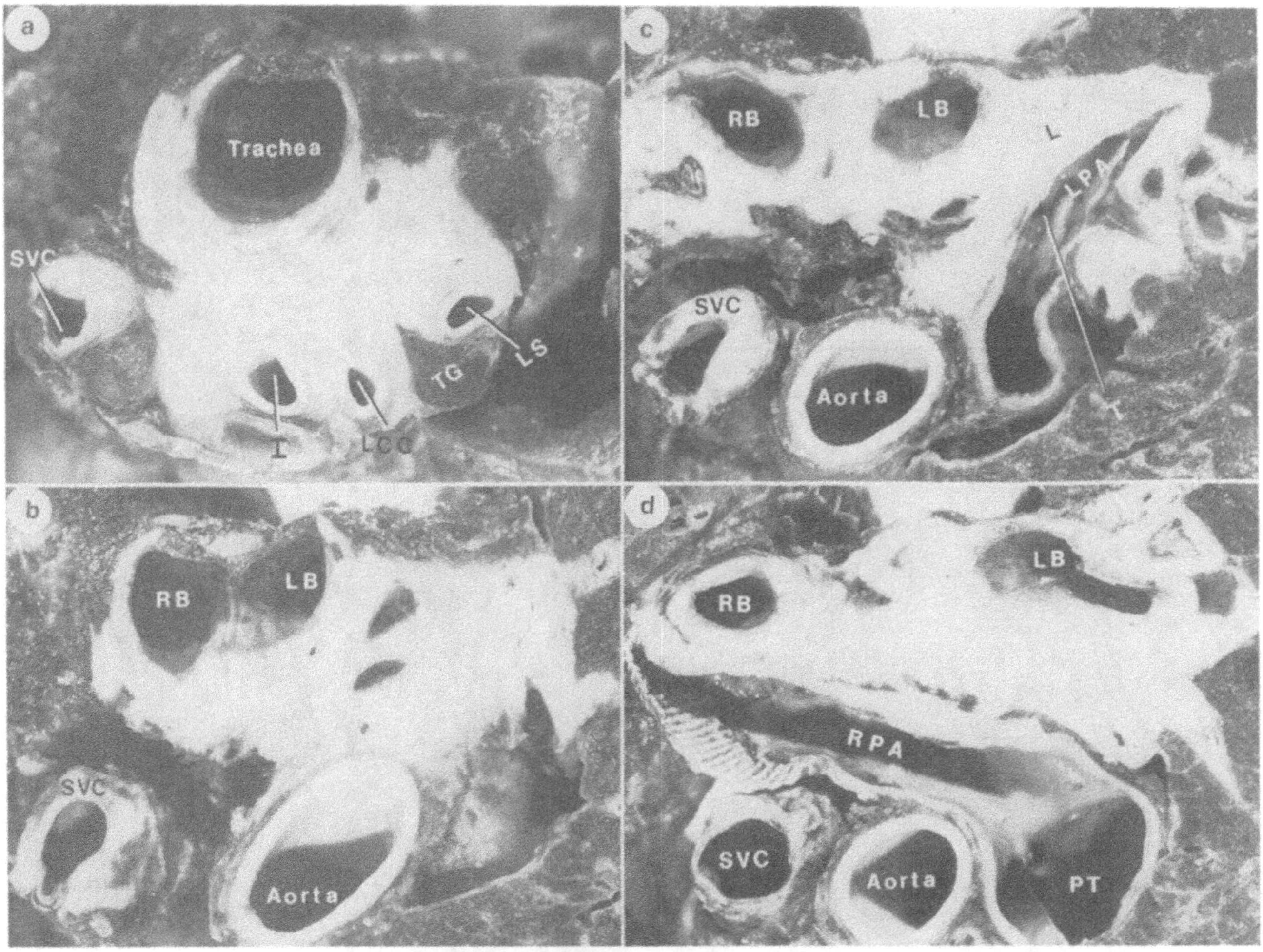

Figure 4. *Case 1. Transverse cuts through the mediastinum at successively more caudal levels.* ***a,*** *at the level of the innominate (I), left common carotid (LCC) and left subclavian (LS) arteries. Dense fibrous tissue (white) surrounds these structures and the trachea. The superior vena cava (SVC) is narrowed. TG = thymus gland.* ***b,*** *at level of the bifurcation of trachea into right (RB) and left bronchus (LB). The superior vena cava had been partially freed (at operation four days earlier) from the fibrous tissue.* ***c,*** *at level of left main pulmonary artery (LPA). The lumens of its major branches are totally compressed by the dense fibrous tissue and thrombus (T) is present in this artery.* ***d,*** *at level of right main pulmonary artery (RPA) and its grafted segment. Although the lumen of the proximal portion of this artery is patent, the branches to the middle and lower lobes remain markedly narrowed just beyond the graft. PT = pulmonary trunk.*

the narrowing was 22 mm Hg. Therapy with digoxin and furosemide was started.

Exertional dyspnea, orthopnea, dizziness and arthralgia associated with malaise and weight loss continued, however, and 28 months before death signs of superior vena caval obstruction appeared. A superior vena cavagram (Figure 6) disclosed severe narrowing at the level of the carina, and an 11 mm Hg gradient was measured between the cephalad portion of the superior vena cava and right atrium. A large pericardial effusion now was present. Results of histoplasma and coccidiodin complement fixation tests, and tests for antinuclear and rheumatoid factor were negative, but results of the tuberculin skin test were now strongly positive (42 mm). Pericardiocentesis yielded 500 ml of serosanguineous fluid with total protein 7 g/100 ml and mononuclear cells/ 10,000/mm^3; cultures of this fluid were negative for fungi and tuberculosis. Bronchoscopy yielded no abnormalities, but tomograms demonstrated an anterior mediastinal mass. Mediastinoscopy disclosed obliteration of the anterior mediastinal space by dense fibrous tissue. Consequently, 27 months before death, a saphenous vein was used to bypass the obstructed portion of superior vena cava. Biopsy specimens of the mediastinal mass revealed dense fibrous tissue with focal collections of mononuclear cells; of the parietal pericardium, diffuse chronic inflammation and fibrosis, and of mediastinal and scalene lymph nodes, reactive hyperplasia. Symptomatic improvement followed relief of the superior vena caval obstruction.

Pain in the right upper quadrant appeared intermittently beginning 12 months before death; one month before death, the patient had the abrupt onset of right upper quadrant pain and obstructive type jaundice. Laparotomy disclosed a dis-

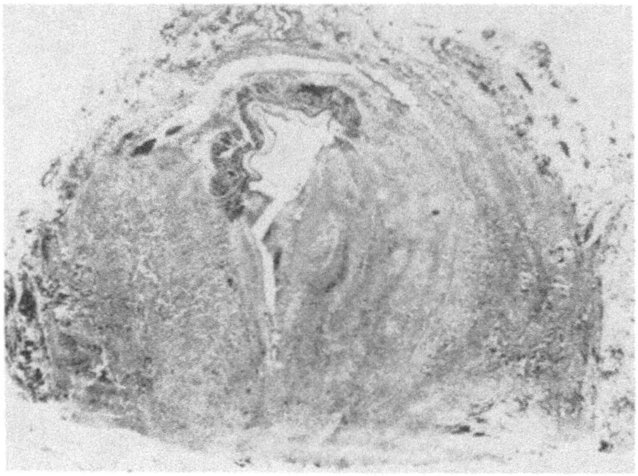

Figure 5. *Case 1. Histologic section of the left lower pulmonary vein. It is surrounded by dense fibrous tissue and its lumen is narrowed by extrinsic compression. Masson's trichrome stain; original magnification × 55.*

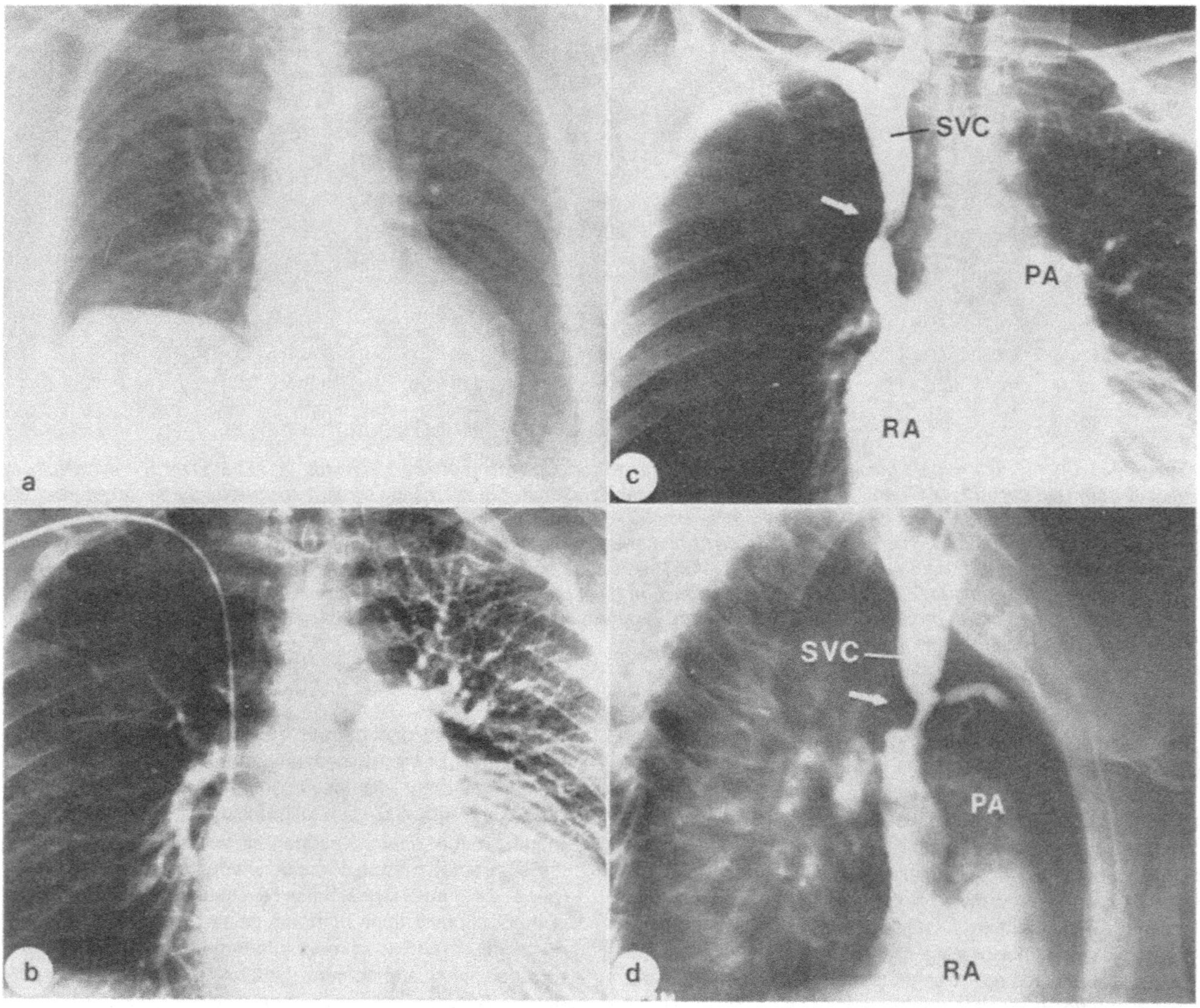

Figure 6. *Case 2.* ***a,*** *posteroanterior chest roentgenogram, and* ***b,*** *pulmonary angiogram 34 months before death. The cardiac silhouette is enlarged, and a large right pleural effusion is present. An arteriogram disclosed markedly diminished flow to the entire right lung with virtually no flow to the upper lobe. An area of discrete narrowing of the right pulmonary artery is present. A 23 mm Hg gradient was present across this area.* ***c*** *and* ***d,*** *superior vena cavagram 28 months before death. The lumen is severely narrowed at the level of the tracheal bifurcation (arrow). An 11 mm Hg gradient was measured across the narrowed segment.*

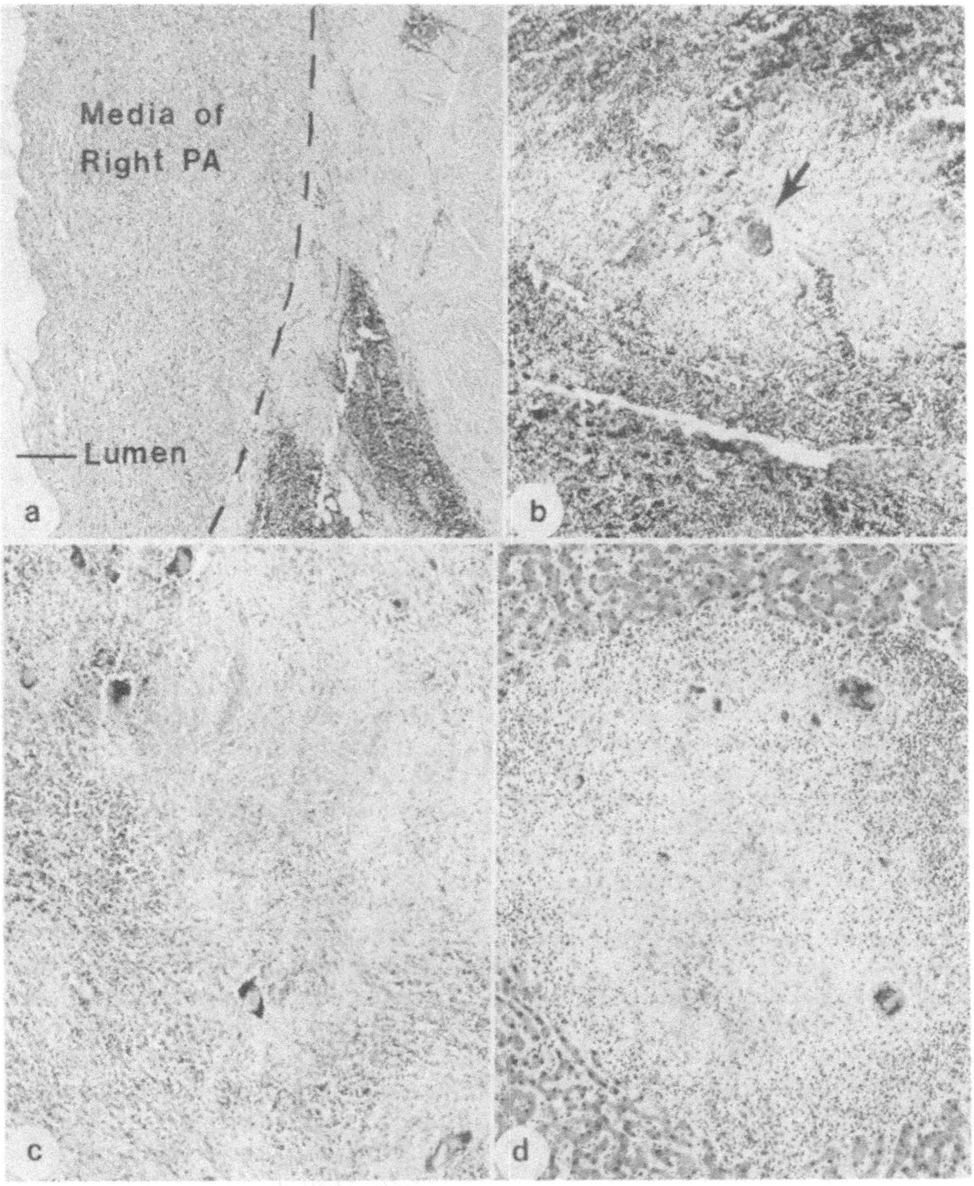

Figure 7. *Case 2.* ***a,*** *histologic section of the wall of the right pulmonary artery (PA) showing dense fibrous tissue with focal collections of mononuclear cells on its adventitial surface. The dense fibrous tissue encased the artery and caused marked narrowing of its lumen.* ***b,*** *histologic section of a mediastinal lymph node. A multinucleated giant cell (arrow) is present in an area of dense scar.* ***c,*** *histologic section of liver. A large caseating granuloma containing numerous giant cells is present.* ***d,*** *histologic section of a necrotic lymph node from the porta hepatis. Confluent granulomas with numerous giant cells and extensive central necrosis are present. Special stains revealed the presence of numerous acid-fast bacilli in these lymph nodes. Hematoxylin and eosin stains; original magnification × 54 (a), × 80 (b and c) and × 88 (d).*

tended gallbladder devoid of stones, and a hard fibrous mass surrounding and severely obstructing the common bile duct. Biopsy of the mass revealed only dense fibrous tissue with focal collections of chronic inflammatory cells. A cholecystojejunostomy was performed. Fifteen days postoperatively signs of thrombophlebitis in the lower extremities appeared, and heparin therapy was started. Two weeks later, the patient had the sudden onset of left-sided weakness followed by coma, and she died three days later.

At necropsy (WHC A74-343), the anterior and posterior mediastinal spaces were totally obliterated by dense fibrous tissue. The superior vena cava, ascending aorta, right and left main pulmonary arteries, major pulmonary veins and main stem bronchi were encased by fibrous tissue, and the lumens of the superior vena cava and right main pulmonary artery were severely narrowed by it. Although the lumen of the left main pulmonary artery was only slightly narrowed, the artery was totally inelastic due to the fibrous encasement. The pa-

TABLE I Observations in Previously Described Necropsy Patients with Pulmonary Hypertension Due to Fibrosing Mediastinitis (FM)

Source	Age (yr) and Sex	Cause of FM	ECG	PA Pressure (mm Hg) s/d (mean)	Obst. Main PA R	Obst. Main PA L	Obst. PV	PA Emboli	Narrowed Small PAs	IPF	Obst. SVC
Edwards, Burchell 1951 [18]	26,F	I	↓V	98/45	0	0	+	0	+	0	0
Davis, Andrus 1954 [19]	26,M	H	RVS	—	0	0	+	—	+	+	0
Bindelglass, Trubowitz 1958 [20]	25,M	I	RAD	—	0	0	+	0	+	0	0
Nelson et al. 1965 [21]	31,F	T	RVH	—	+	+	+	+	—	0	0
Clinicopathologic conference (JHHCPC 600747) 1966 [22]	42,F	H	RVS	82/45	0	0	+	0	+	+	0
Chesis, Dadey 1967 [23]	55, F	I	RAD P-pulm.	—	+	0	—	—	+	—	+
Nasser et al. 1967 [24]	21,F	I	RAD	50/22 (34)	0	0	+	—	+	0	0
Goodwin et al. 1972 [9]	27,F	H	RAD	—	+	0	+	+	+	0	+
Kittridge, Nash 1974 [25]	40,F	I	—	—	0	0	+	0	+	0	0

NOTE: H = histoplasmosis; I = idiopathic; IPF = idiopathic pulmonary fibrosis; L = left; Obst. = obstructed; PA = pulmonary artery; P-pulm. = P-pulmonale; PV = pulmonary vein; R = right; RAD = right axis deviation; RVH = right ventricular hypertrophy; RVS = right ventricular strain; SVC = superior vena cava; T = tuberculosis; V = voltage.

rietal pericardium was thickened and the pericardial space obliterated by numerous dense fibrous adhesions. The heart weighed 450 g; the walls of both ventricles were hypertrophied and the right-sided chambers were dilated. Histologic sections from mediastinum revealed dense hyalinized fibrous tissue with scattered foci of mononuclear cells (Figure 7). Several remnants of mediastinal lymph node contained granulomas with giant cells (Figure 7), but no acid-fast bacilli or fungi were found. Except for focal areas of intra-alveolar hemorrhage, the pulmonary parenchyma and intralung vessels were normal.

An extensive mass of dense fibrous tissue and enlarged lymph nodes was present in the porta hepatis, surrounding and compressing the bile duct. Histologically, it consisted of dense collagenous fibrous tissue, similar to that present in the mediastinum, surrounding regional lymph nodes which were virtually totally replaced by caseating granulomas containing numerous giant cells (Figure 7). Special stains disclosed acid-fast bacilli in the caseating granulomas. Caseating granulomas also were present in the liver (Figure 7), and in celiac and supraclavicular lymph nodes. Examination of histologic sections from several body organs, including the kidney, liver, heart, stomach, uterus, peripancreatic, periadrenal and perithyroidal fat, disclosed the presence of widespread segmental inflammation and fibrinoid necrosis of the walls of small- and medium-sized muscular arteries. Death resulted from a large subarachnoid hemorrhage.

COMMENTS

Although early reports [1,2] attributed it to syphilis, rheumatic fever or tuberculosis, fibrosing mediastinitis is now known to result most often from histoplasmosis [3–10]. Tuberculosis, however, remains a frequent cause [8,9,11,12]. The fibrosing mediastinitis in both our patients appears to have resulted from tuberculosis. In Case 1, the tuberculin skin test result was positive from childhood, the patient had an illness compatible with pulmonary tuberculosis two years before death and, although no acid-fast organisms were found at necropsy, she had received antituberculosis drugs during her last year. In Case 2, although the patient had polyarteritis nodosa, a condition which, on rare occasion, is associated with fibrosing mediastinitis [13], she also had untreated disseminated tuberculosis, which is the likely cause of her fibrosing mediastinitis.

Symptoms from fibrosing mediastinitis most often are due to obstruction of major systemic veins. Obstruction of the superior vena cava has been considered the hallmark of fibrosing mediastinitis [14–16]. Both our patients had obstructed superior vena cavae. The obstruction in Case 2 was operatively relieved 27 months before death [17].

Pulmonary hypertension from fibrosing mediastinitis is rare; it usually is due to obstruction of multiple major pulmonary veins and to secondary changes in the small intrapulmonary arteries. Among nine previously described necropsy patients (age range 21 to 42 years [average age 33 years]; seven women, three men) with fibrosing mediastinitis and pulmonary hypertension (Table I) [9,18–25], seven had obstruction of large pulmonary veins, the sole cause of the pulmonary hypertension in six. One other patient had pulmonary venous as well as pulmonary arterial obstruction. Each of these seven patients had severe secondary changes in the small intrapulmonary pulmonary arteries. Edwards and Burchell [18] in 1951 first described a patient with severe pulmonary arterial hypertension due to obstruction of three of four major pulmonary veins by fibrosing mediastinitis. In 1954, Davis and Andrus [19] described a similar patient whose initial clinical features strongly suggested mitral valve stenosis. Subsequently, additional patients with fibrosing mediastinitis were

TABLE II Causes of Pulmonary Hypertension in Patients with Fibrosing Mediastinitis

1. Obstruction of multiple large pulmonary veins
2. Obstruction of the right or both main pulmonary arteries
3. Associated pulmonary interstitial fibrosis with or without hypoxemia
4. Multiple occlusions of small intrapulmonary arteries by thromboembolic material
5. Combinations of these

described, and pulmonary hypertension due to pulmonary venous obstruction by fibrosing mediastinitis became well recognized [20].

Pulmonary hypertension in fibrosing mediastinitis may result from causes other than pulmonary venous obstruction (Table II). As illustrated by our two patients, obstruction of the main pulmonary arteries by fibrosing mediastinitis can cause pulmonary arterial hypertension in the absence of pulmonary venous hypertension. Both our patients had severe pulmonary arterial hypertension but normal pulmonary arterial wedge pressures. At necropsy, one (Case 1) had severe obstruction of both right and left main pulmonary arteries, partial obstruction of one major pulmonary vein and normal intrapulmonary arteries. A similar patient was described by Nelson et al. in 1965 [21]. In our Case 2, the right main pulmonary artery was severely narrowed, the left main pulmonary artery only mildly narrowed, none of the large pulmonary veins was obstructed and the intrapulmonary arteries of both lungs were normal.

Pulmonary hypertension has been shown, both clinically and experimentally to result from obstruction of only the right main pulmonary artery. Vogel and associates [26] ligated the right or left main pulmonary artery in 29 calves at sea level (17 calves) or at 5,280 feet above sea level (12 calves). At sea level, pulmonary hypertension developed in half the calves with right main pulmonary arterial ligation but in none with ligated left main pulmonary arteries. At the high altitude, however, ligation of the left main pulmonary artery also produced pulmonary hypertension. Cheris and Dadey [23] described a patient with fibrosing mediastinitis and pulmonary hypertension who had severe narrowing of only the right main pulmonary artery, and Cohn and associates [27] described a patient with isolated congenital stenosis of the right main pulmonary artery and severe pulmonary hypertension. Both patients had severe changes in the small intrapulmonary arteries. Why such changes were absent in the left lung in our Case 2 is unclear. It is clear, however, that fibrosing mediastinitis can cause pulmonary hypertension and cor pulmonale by obstructing only the right main pulmonary artery or both right and left main pulmonary arteries.

Another cause of pulmonary arterial hypertension in fibrosing mediastinitis is interstitial pulmonary fibrosis, which may be the consequence of fibrosing mediastinitis or due to the same condition which caused the fibrosing mediastinitis [28]. Two of the nine previously described necropsy patients with fibrosing mediastinitis and pulmonary hypertension also had considerable interstitial pulmonary fibrosis. How much the interstitial pulmonary fibrosis contributed to the pulmonary hypertension in them, however, is uncertain, because each also had obstruction of multiple large pulmonary veins.

Obstruction of multiple small intrapulmonary arteries by thromboembolic material also is a well known cause of pulmonary hypertension [29,30], and patients with fibrosing mediastinitis have an increased risk to thromboembolism. Superior vena caval constriction, the most frequent complication of fibrosing mediastinitis, is often accompanied by thrombosis of the residual lumen of the partially occluded vein. In 1903 Osler [31] described a patient with superior vena caval syndrome due to constriction of the superior vena cava by fibrosing mediastinitis, and the drawing of McCallum's autopsy findings show a thrombus in the residual lumen of the constricted vein. Among the nine previously described necropsy patients with fibrosing mediastinitis and pulmonary hypertension (Table I), two also had superior vena caval obstruction; at necropsy, two of the nine patients had thromboemboli in the lumens of multiple small intrapulmonary arteries.

Although patients with fibrosing mediastinitis with extensive changes in the small intrapulmonary arteries due to pulmonary venous obstruction or to thromboemboli and those with extensive interstitial pulmonary fibrosis are unlikely to benefit significantly from any form of therapy, patients with pulmonary hypertension due to obstruction of one or both main pulmonary arteries by fibrosing mediastinitis may be benefited by operative intervention unless the mediastinal fibrous tissue extends into the hilum of the lung as it did in our patient (Case 1).

REFERENCES

1. Knox LC: Chronic mediastinitis. Am J Med Sci 169: 807, 1925.
2. Keefer CS: Acute and chronic mediastinitis. A study of sixty cases. Arch Intern Med 62: 109, 1938.
3. Peabody JW Jr, Brown RB, Sullivan MB, et al.: Mediastinal granulomas. J Thorac Surg 35: 384, 1958.
4. Lull GF, Winn DF Jr: Chronic fibrous mediastinitis due to histoplasma capsulatum (histoplasmal mediastinitis). Report of three cases with different presenting symptoms. Radiology 73: 367, 1959.
5. Marshall RJ, Edmundowicz AC, Andrews CE: Chronic obstruction of the superior vena cava due to histoplasmosis.

A hemodynamic and angiographic correlation. Circulation 29: 604, 1964.
6. Clinicopathologic conference (JHH 664434). Bull Johns Hopkins Hosp 119: 288, 1966.
7. Hewlett TH, Steer A, Thomas DE: Progressive fibrosing mediastinitis. Ann Thorac Surg 2: 345, 1966.
8. Schowengerdt CG, Suyemoto R, Main FB: Granulomatous and fibrous mediastinitis: a review and analysis of 180 cases. J Thorac Cardiovasc Surg 57: 365, 1969.
9. Goodwin RA, Nickell JA, Des Prez RM: Mediastinal fibrosis complicating healed primary histoplasmosis and tuberculosis. Medicine (Baltimore) 51: 227, 1972.
10. Strimlan CV, Dines DE, Payne WS: Mediastinal granuloma. Mayo Clin Proc 50: 702, 1975.
11. Ferguson TB, Burford TH: Mediastinal granuloma. A 15-year experience. Ann Thorac Surg 1: 125, 1965.
12. McIntire FT, Sykes EM: Obstruction of the superior vena cava: a review of the literature and report of two personal cases. Ann Intern Med 30: 925, 1949.
13. Carton RW, Wong R: Multifocal fibrosclerosis manifested by vena caval obstruction and associated with vasculitis. Ann Intern Med 70: 81, 1969.
14. Erganian J, Wade LJ: Chronic fibrous mediastinitis with obstruction of the superior vena cava. J Thorac Surg 12: 275, 1943.
15. Hache L, Woolner LB, Bernatz PE: Idiopathic fibrous mediastinitis. Dis Chest 41: 9, 1962.
16. Miller RE, Sullivan FJ: Superior vena caval obstruction secondary to fibrosing mediastinitis. Ann Thorac Surg 15: 483, 1973.
17. Garcia J, Ramariz R, Bacos J, et al.: Technique of superior vena cava reconstruction in fibrosing mediastinitis. J Thorac Cardiovasc Surg 65: 547, 1973.
18. Edwards JE, Burchell HB: Multilobar pulmonary venous obstruction with pulmonary hypertension. "Protective" arterial lesions in the involved lobes. Arch Intern Med 87: 372, 1951.
19. Davis FW Jr, Andrus EC: Mitral stenosis in facsimile. N Engl J Med 251: 297, 1954.
20. Bindelglass IL, Trubowitz S: Pulmonary vein obstruction: an uncommon sequel to chronic fibrous mediastinitis. Ann Intern Med 48: 876, 1958.
21. Nelson WP, Lundberg GD, Dickerson RB: Pulmonary artery obstruction and cor pulmonale due to chronic fibrous mediastinitis. Am J Med 38: 279, 1965.
22. Clinicopathologic conference (JHH 600747). Bull Johns Hopkins Hosp 118: 73, 1966.
23. Cheris DN, Dadey JL: Fibrosing mediastinitis. An unusual cause for cor pulmonale. Am J Roentgenol Radium Ther Nucl Med 100: 328, 1967.
24. Nasser WK, Feigenbaum H, Fisch C: Clinical and hemodynamic diagnosis of pulmonary venous obstruction due to sclerosing mediastinitis. Am J Cardiol 20: 725, 1967.
25. Kittredge RD, Nash AD: The many facets of sclerosing fibrosis. Am J Roentgenol Radium Ther Nucl Med 122: 288, 1974.
26. Vogel JHK, McNamara DG, Hallman G, et al.: Effects of mild chronic hypoxia on the pulmonary circulation in calves with reactive pulmonary hypertension. Circ Res 21: 661, 1967.
27. Cohn LH, Sanders JH Jr, Collins JJ Jr: Surgical treatment of congenital unilateral pulmonary arterial stenosis with contralateral pulmonary hypertension. Am J Cardiol 38: 257, 1976.
28. Andrews EC: Five cases of an undescribed form of pulmonary interstitial fibrosis caused by obstruction of the pulmonary veins. Bull Johns Hopkins Hosp 100: 28, 1957.
29. Fowler NO, Black-Schaffer B, Scott RC, et al.: Idiopathic and thromboembolic pulmonary hypertension. Am J Med 40: 331, 1966.
30. Arnett EN, Battle WE, Russo JV, et al.: Intravenous injection of talc-containing drugs intended for oral use. A cause of pulmonary granulomatosis and pulmonary hypertension. Am J Med 60: 711, 1976.
31. Osler W: Obliteration of the superior vena cava. Bull Johns Hopkins Hosp 14: 169, 1903.

"Mitral Stenosis" Secondary to Combined "Massive" Mitral Anular Calcific Deposits and Small, Hypertrophied Left Ventricles

Hemodynamic Documentation in Four Patients

WILLIAM J. HAMMER, M.D.
Philadelphia, Pennsylvania

WILLIAM C. ROBERTS, M.D.
Bethesda, Maryland

ANTONIO C. deLEON, Jr., M.D.
Washington, D. C.

Certain observations are described in four elderly women with massive mitral anular calcific deposits, small thick-walled left ventricles and diastolic gradients between pulmonary artery wedge position (or left atrium) and left ventricle. All four patients had some degree of obstruction to left ventricular outflow. Examination at necropsy (two patients) or at operation (one patient) disclosed only focal fibrous thickening of the mitral leaflets without commissural or chordal fusion. By auscultation, none had mitral opening snaps, only two had loud first heart sounds and only one had a mitral diastolic rumble. Hemodynamic documentation of a diastolic gradient between pulmonary artery wedge position (or left atrium) and left ventricle in the presence of massive mitral anular calcific deposits and in the absence of diffuse disease of the mitral leaflets has not been demonstrated previously. The diastolic gradients are considered to result from the combination of the large mitral anular calcific deposits and the small, thick-walled, noncompliant left ventricles.

Although calcific deposits in the mitral anulus are extremely common [1], mainly in older persons, the hemodynamic consequences of these deposits are poorly understood. When the deposits are relatively small, i.e., not visible roentgenologically, it is unlikely that valvular dysfunction results. Large deposits, i.e., those visible during life by roentgenogram, of anular calcium, however, may be associated with mild to moderate degrees of mitral regurgitation but probably never severe regurgitation [1,2]. Although apical diastolic murmurs have been observed and stenosis of this valve suspected at necropsy in some patients with "massive" mitral anular calcific deposits [3], hemodynamic documentation of diastolic gradients between pulmonary artery wedge position (or left atrium) and left ventricle in patients with "massive" calcific deposits of the mitral anulus has not been reported. The present communication describes observations in four such patients.

From the Division of Cardiology, Department of Medicine, Georgetown University Medical Center, Washington, D.C.; and the Pathology Branch, National Heart, Lung and Blood Institute, National Institutes of Health, Bethesda, Maryland. This study was supported in part by the Benjamin May Memorial Fund. Requests for reprints should be addressed to Dr. Antonio C. deLeon, Jr., Division of Cardiology, Department of Medicine, Georgetown University Medical Center, 3800 Reservoir Road, N.W., Washington, D.C. 20007. Manuscript accepted June 22, 1977.

PATIENTS STUDIED AND METHODS

Certain clinical and hemodynamic observations in the four patients are presented in Table I. Three patients had angina pectoris and two had syncope. None had a history of acute rheumatic fever. The mean pressure gradients

TABLE I **Clinical and Hemodynamic Observations in the Four Patients Studied with Massive Calcific Deposits in the Mitral Anulus and Small Hypertrophied Left Ventricles**

Case No.	Age (yrs) and Sex	Rhythm	S_1	OS	S_3	S_4	Murmur (grade 0–6) of: MS	MR	AS	AR	HC	Hemodynamics (mm Hg): PA (s/d)	PAW a	PAW v	PAW m	LV (s/d)	SA s/d	PAW-LV mdg	Angiogram: LV-SA psg	MR (0–4)	AR (0–4)
1	70,F	Sinus	↑	0	+	+	0	2	5	0	0	46/22	34	46	30	268/4	115/60	15	153	1	1
2	70,F	Sinus	↑	0	+	+	1	0	2	2	0	45/22	33	28	22	179/22	170/90	15	9	1	1
3	74,F	Sinus	N	0	0	+	0	0	3	1	0	26/6	14*	6*	6*	210/5	120/80	8*	90	—	—
4	70,F	AF	Va		+	0	0	2	0	0	2	100/55	—	60	35	160/20†	95/60	21	65†	4	0

NOTE: A = a wave; AF = atrial fibrillation; AR = aortic regurgitation; AS = aortic stenosis; HC = hypertrophic cardiomyopathy; LV = left ventricle; m = mean; mdg = mean diastolic gradient; MR = mitral regurgitation; MS = mitral stenosis; N = normal; OS = opening snap; PAW = pulmonary arterial wedge; psg = peak systolic gradient; SA = systemic artery; S_1 = first heart sound; S_3 = ventricular diastolic gallop; S_4 = atrial diastolic gallop; s/d = peak systole/end diastole; v = v wave; Va = variable.

* Left atrial rather than pulmonary artery wedge pressure.

† On pullback from left ventricle to aorta the peak systolic pressure gradient was 120 mm Hg (LV body, 200/20; LV outflow, 80/20; aorta, 80/60 mm Hg).

between pulmonary arterial wedge position (left atrium in one patient) and left ventricle in the four patients ranged from 8 to 21 mm Hg (average 14.7 mm Hg) (Figures 1 and 2). In addition to these pressure gradients, all four patients also had left ventricular outflow tract obstruction: from valvular stenosis in three and from hypertrophic cardiomyopathy in one.

By auscultation, only one patient had an apical diastolic rumble, two had apical holosystolic murmurs consistent with mitral regurgitation, four had murmurs of aortic stenosis, and two of aortic regurgitation. By angiography, however, three had evidence of mitral regurgitation and two of aortic regurgitation. Of the three patients with sinus rhythm, the first heart sound was increased in intensity in one. Fourth hearth sounds were present in three patients, and third heart sounds in three patients. None had mitral opening snaps. All four had mitral anular calcific deposits large enough to be visible by routine chest roentgenogram; three also had calcific deposits in the aortic valve (Figure 3). The electrocardiogram showed normal sinus rhythm in three, atrial fibrillation in one, left ventricular hypertrophy in three, left atrial abnormality in two and right ventricular hypertrophy in none. Echocardiograms in two patients (Cases 1 and 2) disclosed large echoes in the region behind the posterior mitral leaflet. The E-F slope of the an-

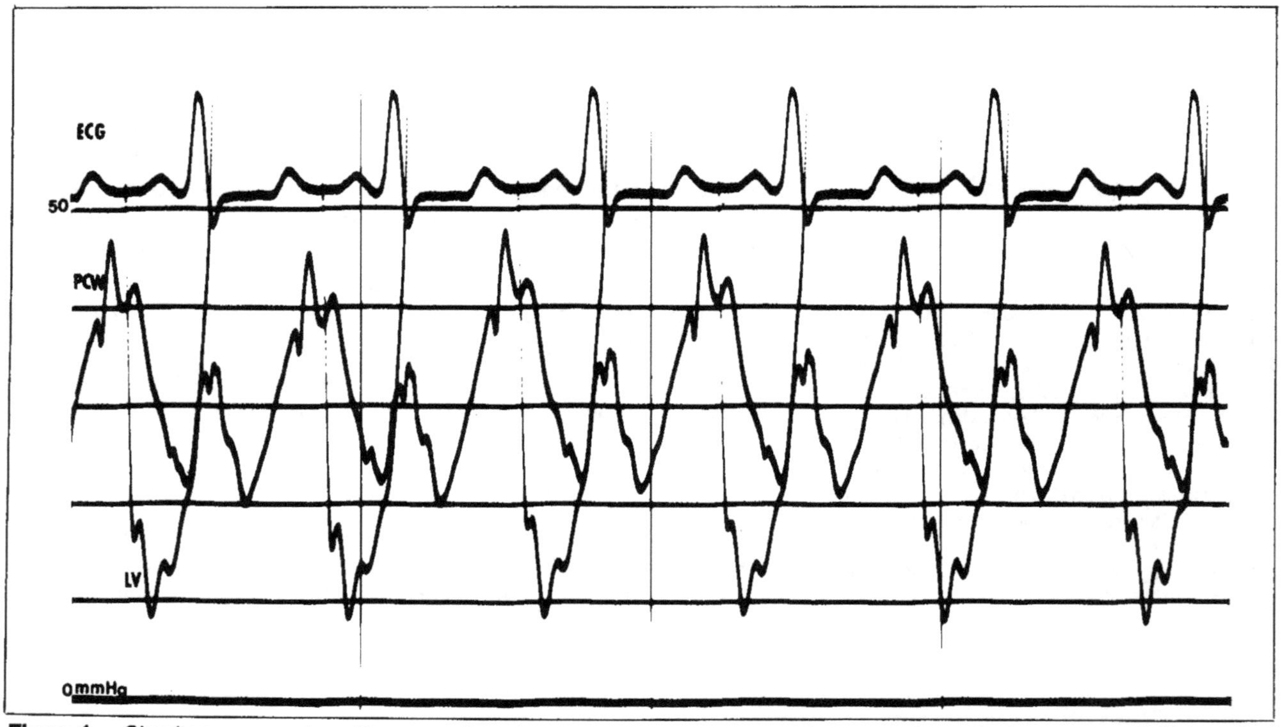

Figure 1. Simultaneous, equisensitive recording of pulmonary arterial wedge (PCW) and left ventricular pressures (LV) in patient (Case 2) demonstrating a sizable diastolic gradient.

terior mitral leaflet could not be satisfactorily demonstrated because of the large echoes from massive anular calcification.

Each of the two patients with significant valvular aortic stenosis underwent aortic valve replacement. The aortic valve was congenitally bicuspid in one (Case 1) (Figure 3) and three-cuspid without commissural fusion, the type most commonly seen in the elderly [1], in the other. The anterior mitral leaflet in both were freely mobile. One of these two patients died early, and necropsy confirmed the presence of massive mitral anular calcific deposits (Figure 3) and, other than focal aging changes, an otherwise normal mitral valve. Another patient (Case 3) died late after aortic valve replacement and necropsy was not performed. The third patient (Case 2) did not have surgery and is living. In none of the patients was a procedure performed on the mitral valve. One patient (Case 4) had hypertrophic cardiopathy and died of congestive cardiac failure. At necropsy, the mitral leaflets and chordae tendineae were quite mobile but focally thickened, and the amount of anular calcific deposits was large. In neither of the two necropsy patients was the chordae or commissures fused or the leaflets more than just focally thickened; in both, the calcific deposits were limited to the area behind the posterior mitral leaflets. In three patients, the left ventricular cavity appeared smaller than normal by left ventricular angiography (two patients) or by necropsy examination (two patients). The left ventricular cavity was judged "normal" by angiography in one patient (Case 2).

COMMENTS

Each of the four patients described in this report was a woman aged 70 years or older, each had "massive" deposits of calcium in the mitral anular region, each had diastolic gradients between pulmonary artery wedge position (of left atrium) and left ventricle, each had a relatively small left ventricular cavity and a hypertrophied left ventricular wall, and each had obstruction to left ventricular outflow. Other than focal fibrous thickening of the leaflets (the result of aging or hypertrophic cardiomyopathy, or both) disease of the mitral leaflets or chordae clearly was not the cause of the diastolic gradient. It is likely that the small and thick-walled left ventricles in association with the large mitral anular calcific deposits were responsible for the diastolic gradients. The small areas available for left ventricular inflow because of the left ventricular hypertrophy without dilatation were further compromised by the huge deposits of calcium behind the posterior mitral leaflets. That the small, thick-walled left ventricles did contribute to the diastolic gradients is supported by the lack of diastolic gradients in other patients with similarly large mitral anular calcific deposits and large left ventricular cavities (Figure 4). Although it is recognized that severe mitral regurgitation may further augment the degree of mitral stenosis, only one of the four patients (Case 4) had substantial mitral regurgitation by left ventricular angiography, one had none, and in two it was trivial. The unusually tall V waves and angiographically demonstrated 4+ mitral regurgitation in one patient (Case 4) indicated severe mitral regurgitation. The increased level of mean left atrial pressure caused by the mitral regurgitation may be a factor in the large (21 mm Hg)

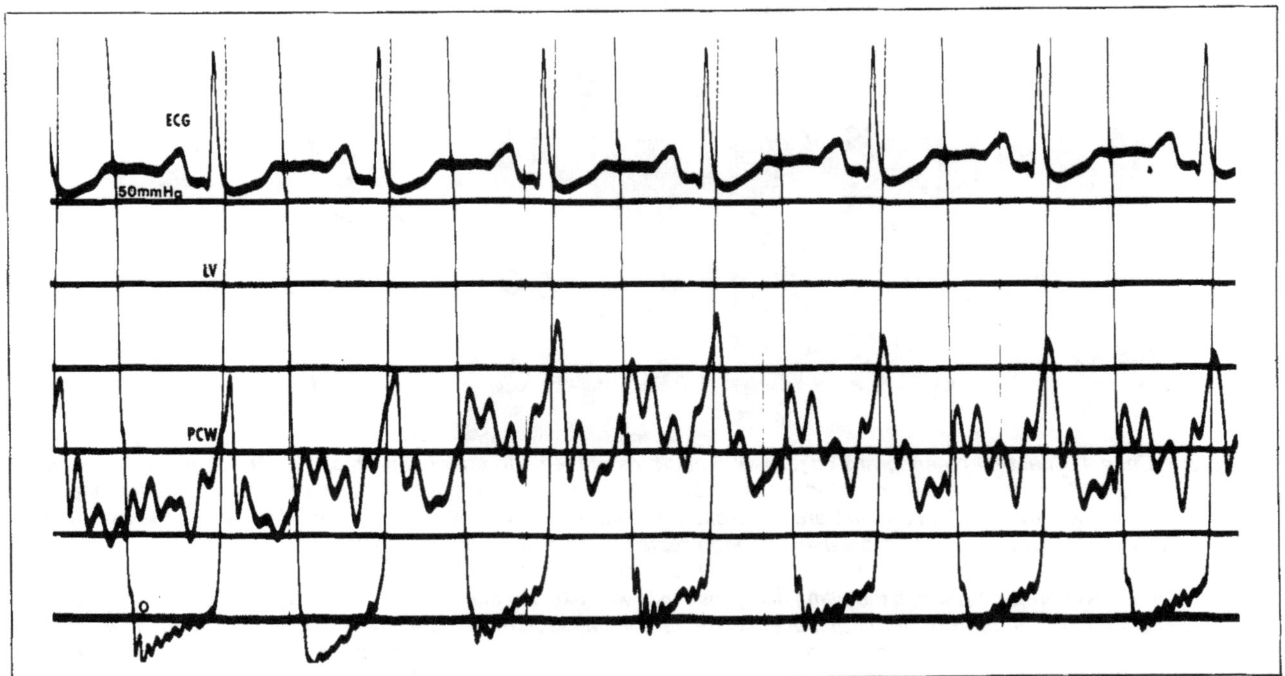

Figure 2. Simultaneous, equisensitive recording of pulmonary arterial wedge (PCW) and left ventricular pressures (LV) in patient (Case 1) demonstrating a diastolic gradient.

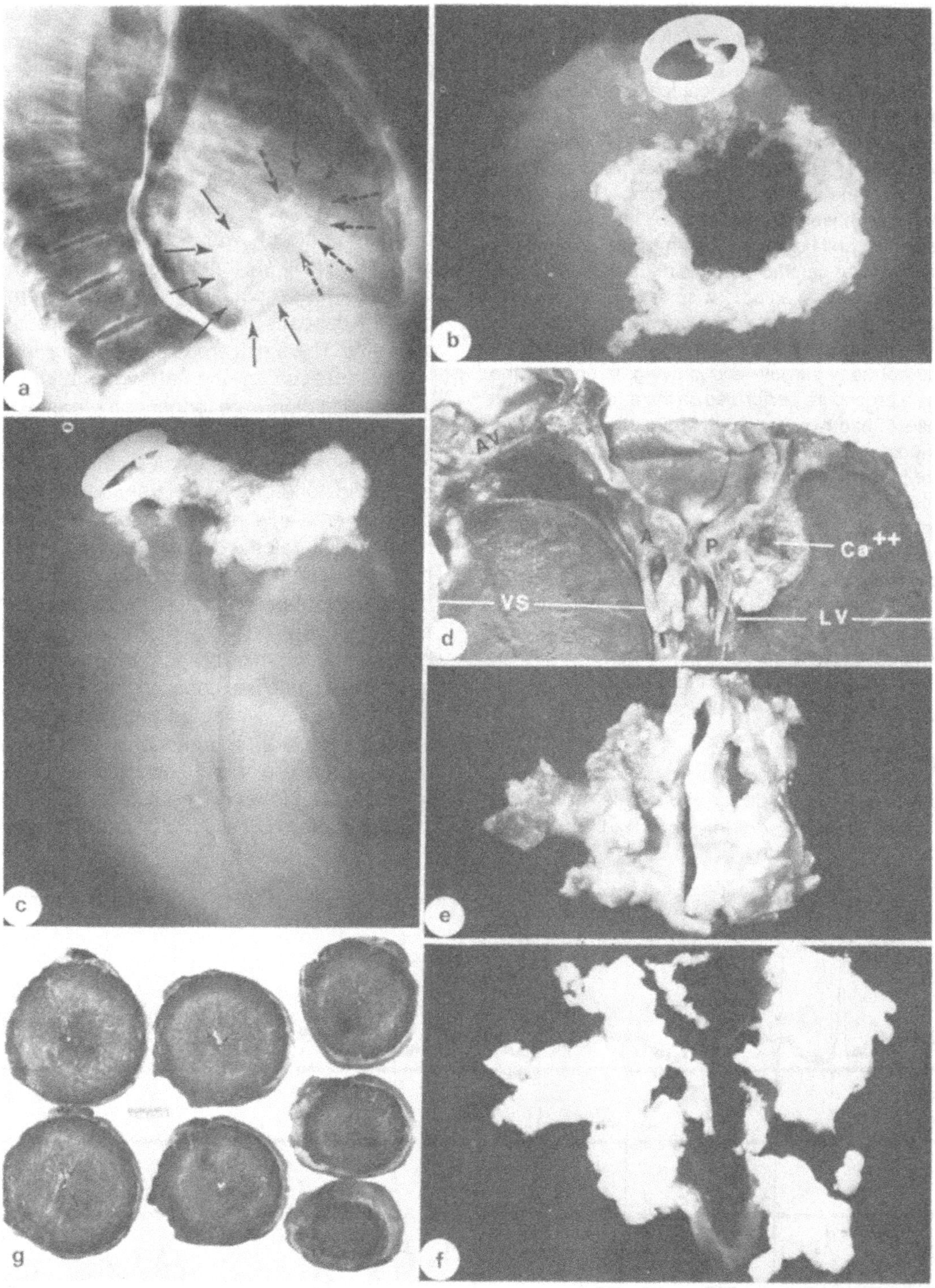

Figure 3. *Case 1. Chest roentgenogram (**a**), roentgenograms of the heart specimen (**b,c,f**) and photographs of the heart (**d,e,g**) in patient (Case 1). **a**, a u-shaped deposit of calcium in the mitral anular region (solid arrows) and another deposit of calcium in the aortic valve (dashed arrows) are apparent in this lateral view. **b**, this postmortem film shows the extent of the mitral anular calcific deposit. The aortic valve has been replaced by a Bjork-Shiley prosthesis. **c**, lateral view of the heart. The left ventricular cavity is minute. **d**, basal portion of left ventricle (LV) showing the anterior (A) and posterior (P) mitral leaflets and aortic valve (AV) area from which the tilting disc prosthesis was excised at necropsy. A large deposit of calcium is present behind, and attached to, the posterior mitral leaflet. VS = ventricular septum. **e**, operatively excised stenotic, bicuspid aortic valve. **f**, film of the excised aortic valve. **g**, transverse sections of the left ventricle (the right ventricular free wall was excised from these slices) showing a minute left ventricular cavity.*

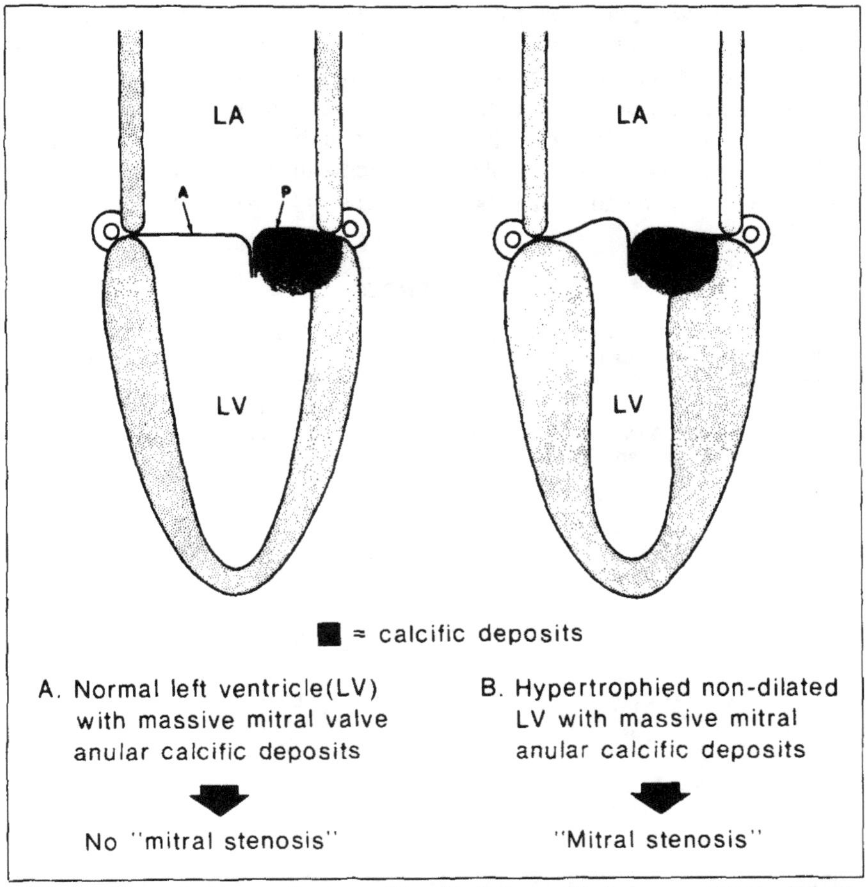

Figure 4. *Diagram showing the probable mechanism of the diastolic gradients in our patients. In both diagrams, the size of the mitral anular calcific deposits is similar and quite large. In **A** the left ventricular wall and cavity are normal. In **B** the left ventricular wall is considerably hypertrophied and the cavity is smaller than normal. The combination of the large calcific deposits in the mitral anulus in association with a small, thick-walled left ventricle is sufficient to produce a diastolic gradient whereas none results when the left ventricular cavity is enlarged and its wall thickness, normal.*

mean diastolic gradient in this case. However, it is unlikely that mitral regurgitation contributed in any significant degree to the mitral diastolic gradient in three of our four patients. The significant degree of pulmonary hypertension in this patient is in part due to the increased left atrial pressure, but abnormal pulmonary vascular resistance must also be a contributing factor. Pathologically, medial hypertrophy and intimal proliferation causing luminal narrowing of the smaller pulmonary arteries were present. The etiology of this could not be definitively determined.

The auscultatory findings in our four patients differed from the classic findings of rheumatic mitral stenosis [4]. Only two of the four patients had a loud first heart sound (S_1), none had a mitral opening snap, and only one had an apical diastolic rumble. The left ventricular outflow obstruction with resulting increase in left ventricular pressure, left ventricular hypertrophy and increased rate of left ventricular pressure (dp/dt), might explain the loud first heart sound in our two patients. The focal rather than diffuse nature of the mitral leaflet thickening may explain the absence of an opening snap in our patients. The consistent presence of rapid filling sounds (S4 and/or S3) presents an additional paradox in view of the mitral gradients. The presence of the diastolic filling sounds imply rapid blood flow into the left ventricle. One could postulate, therefore, that the degree of mitral valve obstruction was mild. Yet, in three of our patients, the measured mean resting mitral valve gradient was 15 and 21 mm Hg, suggesting severe obstruction. The mitral valves of the two patients examined at necropsy provide evidence that central rapid flow between the left atrium and left ventricle is possible. The additional presence of a small left ventricular cavity with stiff, relatively noncompliant left ventricular walls may explain the genesis of the diastolic filling sounds. It is certainly possible that the small left ventricular cavity in diastole and/or markedly diminished compliance of the left ventricular wall somehow plays a role in the genesis of the mitral diastolic pressure gradient. Rapid flow from the left atrium to the left ventricle is possible, but the volume of flow may be limited by the relatively small left ventricular cavity, resulting in lack of diastasis during the available diastolic filling period. This proposed mechanism can explain the paradox of rapid filling sound (S4 and/or S3) and presence of substantial pressure gradient across the mitral valve. Thus, because of a different mechanism for obstruction, its clinical presentation is different from that seen in rheumatic mitral stenosis. Massive mitral anular calcification represents a heretofore unemphasized cause of "obstruction" at the mitral valve level.

REFERENCES

1. Roberts WC, Perloff JK: Mitral valvular disease. A clinicopathologic survey of the conditions causing the mitral valve to function abnormally. Ann Intern Med 77: 939, 1972.
2. Perloff K, Roberts WC: The mitral apparatus. Functional anatomy of mitral regurgitation. Circulation 46: 227, 1972.
3. Korn D, DeSanctis RW, Sell S: Massive calcification of the mitral anulus. A clinicopathological study of fourteen cases. N Engl J Med 267: 900, 1962.
4. Reichek N, Shelburne JC, Perloff JK: Clinical aspects of rheumatic valvular disease. Prog Cardiovasc Dis 15: 491, 1973.

Calcific Deposits in Stenotic Mitral Valves

Extent and Relation to Age, Sex, Degree of Stenosis, Cardiac Rhythm, Previous Commissurotomy and Left Atrial Body Thrombus from Study of 164 Operatively-Excised Valves

ANTHONY S. LACHMAN, M.B., AND WILLIAM C. ROBERTS, M.D.

SUMMARY **The presence or absence and the extent of calcific deposits in excised stenotic mitral valves was determined by radiographs of the excised valve in 164 patients aged 26 to 72 years. The extent of the mitral calcific deposits was determined by the percent of the valvular circumference containing the deposits = grade 0 (14 patients); grade I = < 25% (43 patients); grade II = 25–50% (34 patients); grade III = 51–75% (39 patients); and grade IV = > 75% (34 patients). The amount of calcific deposits in the stenotic mitral valves correlated with sex and with the mean diastolic pressure gradient across the mitral valve ($P < 0.05$), but it did not correlate with the patient's age, cardiac rhythm, pulmonary arterial or pulmonary arterial wedge pressure, previous mitral commissurotomy, presence of thrombus in the body of left atrium or the presence of disease of one or more other cardiac valves.**

AMONG PATIENTS WITH MITRAL STENOSIS, we know that calcific deposits in the mitral leaflets are common, a higher percentage of men have the deposits in their stenotic valves than do women, the results of commissurotomy are less satisfactory in those with noncalcified compared to those with calcified mitral valves, and the presence of calcific deposits usually necessitates the performance of valve replacement. We do not know whether calcific deposits in stenotic mitral valves and age are correlated. Furthermore, the relationship between the presence of, or the degree of mitral calcific deposits and the degree of mitral stenosis or other clinical parameters has not been investigated. The present report, therefore, attempts to fill in these voids by summarizing observations in 164 patients in whom mitral valve replacement was performed because of mitral stenosis. Calcium in the excised valve was determined qualitatively and quantitatively by radiography of the excised valve itself. Previous studies have relied on the judgment of the surgeon at operation, or preoperative routine roentgenography, fluoroscopy, or tomography for identification and quantification of calcific deposits in stenotic mitral valves.

Materials and Methods

The patients included in this study were derived from review of photographs of mitral valves excised at the National Heart, Lung, and Blood Institute from 1963 through 1976. Photographs were taken routinely of all excised valves during this period. A total of 293 patients underwent mitral valve replacement for mitral stenosis during this period. Of this number, unsectioned stenotic mitral valves were available for re-examination in 164 patients and these 164 form the basis of this report. A radiograph was taken on each of these 164 operatively excised valves via a Field-Emission-Faxitron-X-ray unit at 35 KVP. The X-ray beam was directed more or less perpendicular to the valve orifice. The presence of and the amount of calcium was determined by examination of the single radiograph of each excised mitral valve. The amount of calcium in each valve was graded by the percent of circumference of the valve orifice occupied by calcium as follows: grade 0, no calcium; grade I, <25% of the circumference; grade II, 25–50%; grade III, 51–75%; and grade IV, >75%.

The degree of mitral stenosis and other clinical data were obtained from review of medical records. Mitral stenosis was confirmed by cardiac catheterization in all 164 patients. χ^2 tests were used on most of the two-way comparisons, and a distribution-free test for altered alternatives was used to compare the left atrial–left ventricular gradient to the degree of mitral valve calcium.

Results

The results are summarized in tables 1–5 and photographs of excised valves and radiographs of them are shown in figures 1–14. The 164 patients ranged in age from 26 to 72 years (median 51). The mean age of the 101 women was 52 years and for the 63 men, 48 years ($P < 0.05$). The amount of calcific deposits in the stenotic mitral valves did not correlate with age (table 1). Of the 91 patients with absent or light (grades 0, I, or II) calcific deposits, 41 (45%) were less than age 51 and 50 (55%) were greater than age 50; of the 73 patients with heavy (grades III or IV) calcific deposits, 37 (51%) were less than age 51 and 36 (49%) were greater than age 50. Of the total 164 patients, 78 (48%) were less than age 51 and 86 (52%) were greater than age 50.

The amount of calcific deposits in the stenotic mitral valves did correlate with sex (table 1). Of the 73 patients with heavy calcific deposits, 34 (47%) were men and 39 (53%) were women; of the 91 patients with absent or light calcific deposits, 29 (32%) were men, and 62 (68%) were women ($P < 0.05$). Of the 78 patients less than 51 years of age, 23 (61%) of the 38 men and 14 (35%) of the women had heavy calcific deposits ($P < 0.05$). Of the 15 patients less than age 41 with heavy calcific deposits, only 3 (20%) were women and 12 (80%) were men ($P < 0.05$). Of the 63 men, 20 (32%) had grade IV calcific deposits, and of the 101 women only 14 (14%) had similar sized deposits ($P < 0.05$). Furthermore, only 4 (6%) of the 63 men had no calcific deposits, whereas 10 (10%) of the 101 women had absent calcific deposits ($P < 0.05$).

From the Pathology Branch, National Heart, Lung, and Blood Institute, National Institutes of Health, Bethesda, Maryland.

Address for reprints: Dr. William C. Roberts, Building 10A, Room 3E-30, National Institutes of Health, Bethesda, Maryland 20014.

Received August 31, 1977; revision accepted October 31, 1977.

Table 1. *Calcific Deposits in Stenotic Mitral Valves: Amount of Calcium Related to Age and Sex*

Amount of Calcium	Ages (years) 25-40 M	25-40 F	41-50 M	41-50 F	51-60 M	51-60 F	61-75 M	61-75 F	Subtotals M	Subtotals F	Totals M + F
0	0	2	1	3	3	5	0	0	4	10	14 (8%)
I	3	7	4	6	5	11	1	6	13	30	43 (26%)
II	3	1	4	7	4	7	1	7	12	22	34 (21%)
III	3	3	5	8	4	9	2	5	14	25	39 (24%)
IV	9	0	6	3	4	7	1	4	20	14	34 (21%)
Totals	18	13	20	27	20	39	5	22	63	101	164 (100%)

Table 2. *Calcific Deposits in Stenotic Mitral Valves: Relation Between Valve Gradient and Sex*

Sex	Left atrial–Left ventricular mean diastolic gradient (mm Hg) < 7.5	7.5 - 15	> 15	Totals
Males	4 (7%)	38 (60%)	21 (33%)	63 (100%)
Females	19 (19%)	46 (45%)	36 (36%)	101 (100%)
Totals	23 (14%)	84 (51%)	57 (35%)	164 (100%)

Table 4. *Calcific Deposits in Stenotic Mitral Valves: Amount of Calcium Related to Cardiac Rhythm*

Amount of Calcium	Sinus Rhythm	Atrial Fibrillation	Total
0	4 (29%)	10 (71%)	14
I	11 (26%)	32 (74%)	43
II	5 (15%)	29 (85%)	34
III	6 (15%)	33 (85%)	39
IV	12 (35%)	22 (65%)	34
Totals	38 (23%)	126 (77%)	164

Table 3. *Calcific Deposits in Stenotic Mitral Valves: Amount of Calcium Related to Mitral Valve Gradient*

Amount of Calcium	Mean Diastolic Pressure Gradient (in mm Hg) Between Left Atrium and Left Ventricle < 7.5	7.5 - 15	> 15	Total
0	6	6	2	14
I	11	24	8	43
II	4	19	11	34
III	2	15	22	39
IV	0	20	14	34
Totals	23	84	57	164

Table 5. *Calcific Deposits in Stenotic Mitral Valves: Amount of Calcium Related Both to Left Atrial Body Thrombus and to Cardiac Rhythm*

Amount of Calcium	Left Atrial Thrombus	Sinus Rhythm	Atrial Fibrillation
0	1	0	1
I	4	1	3
II	7	1	6
III	7	0	7
IV	8	4	4
Totals	27	6	21

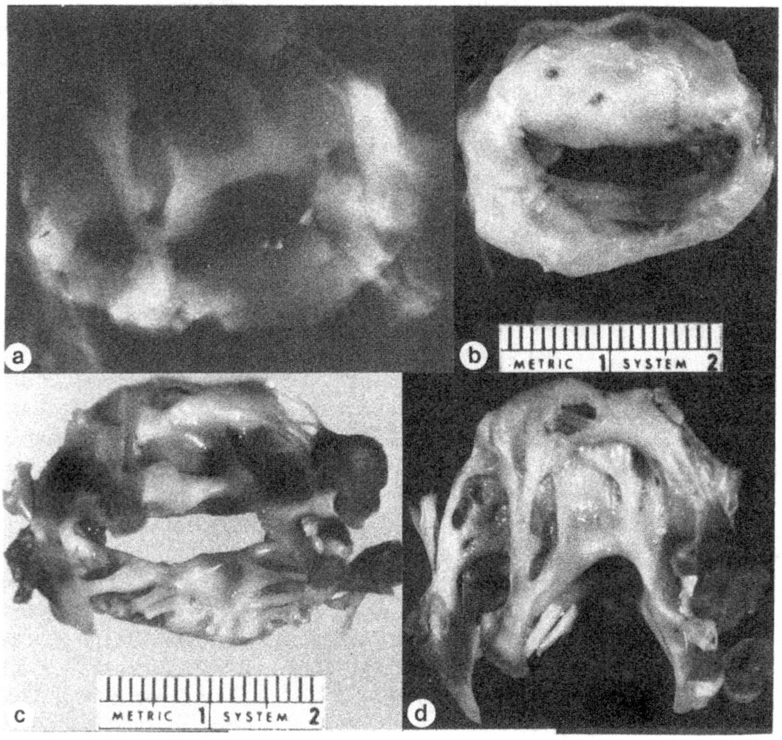

Figure 1. *Clinical data on each of the patients whose mitral valves are illustrated in this and the following figures are summarized in table 7.* a) *Radiograph.* b) *View from left atrium.* c *and* d) *View from left ventricle showing orifice in* c *and anterior leaflet and attached chordae tendineae in* d.

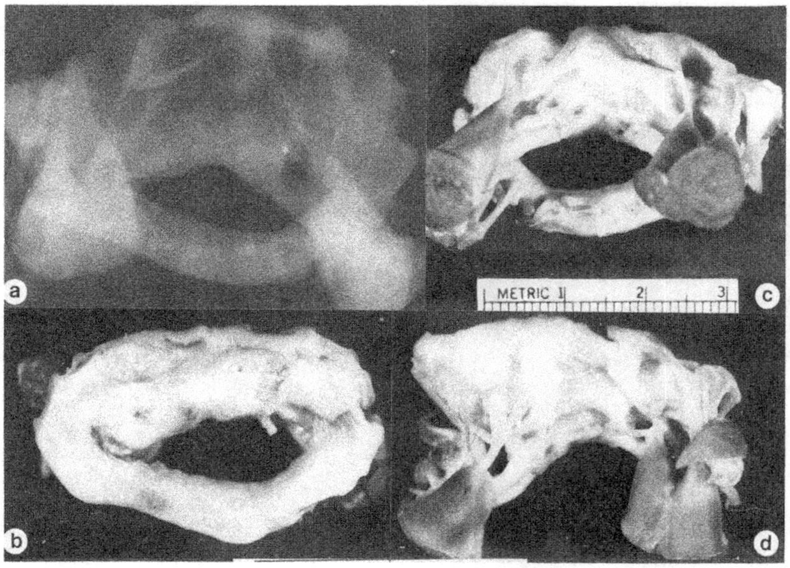

FIGURE 2. a) *Radiograph.* b) *View from left atrium.* c *and* d) *Views from left ventricle showing mitral orifice in* c *and anterior mitral leaflet in* d.

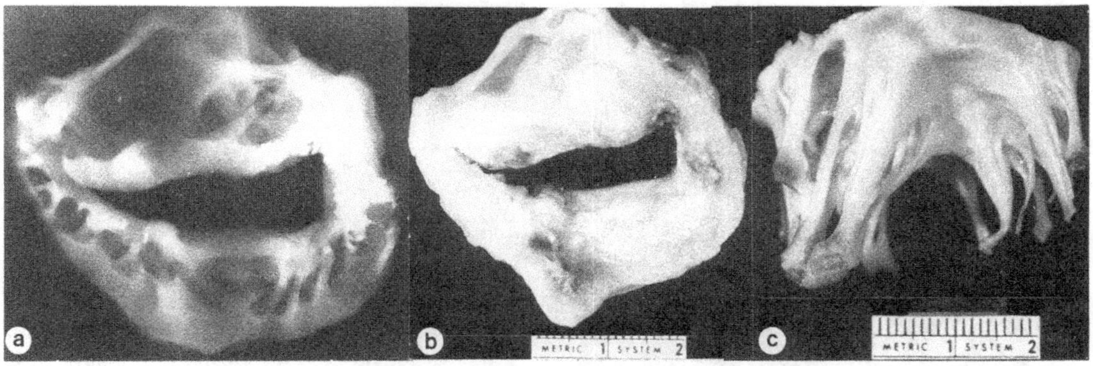

FIGURE 3. a) *Radiograph.* b) *View from left atrium.* c) *View of anterior leaflet from left ventricular aspect.*

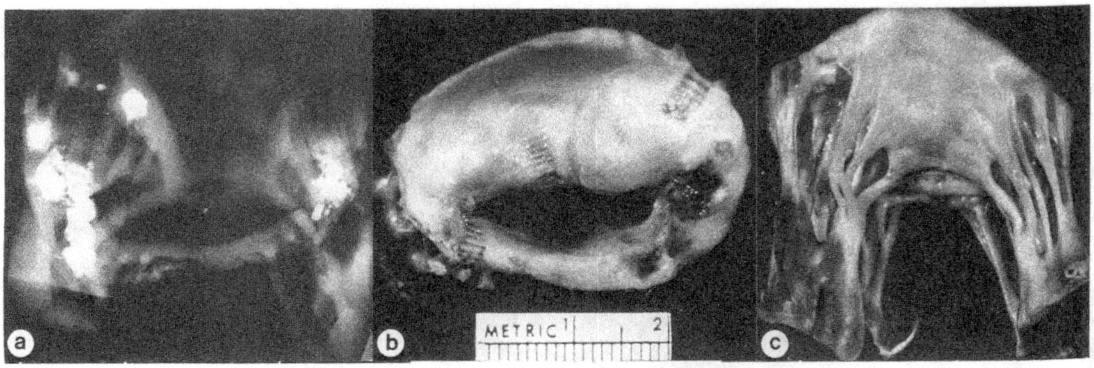

FIGURE 4. a) *Radiograph.* b) *View from left atrium.* c) *View of anterior leaflet from left ventricular aspect.*

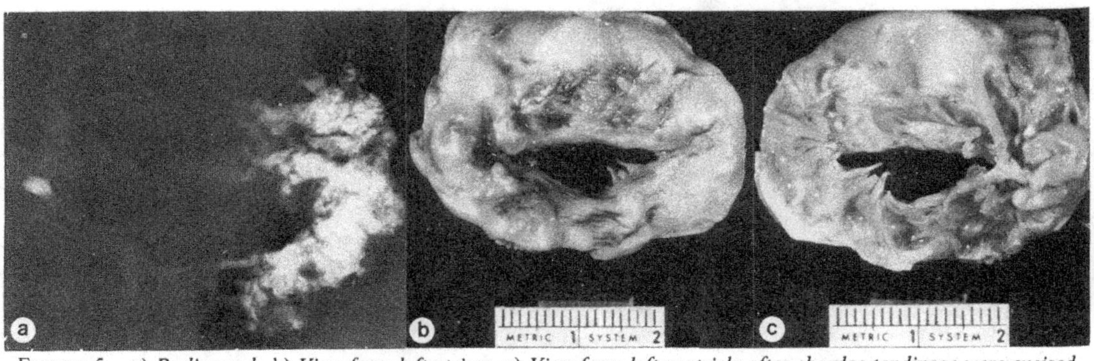

FIGURE 5. a) *Radiograph.* b) *View from left atrium.* c) *View from left ventricle after chordae tendineae were excised.*

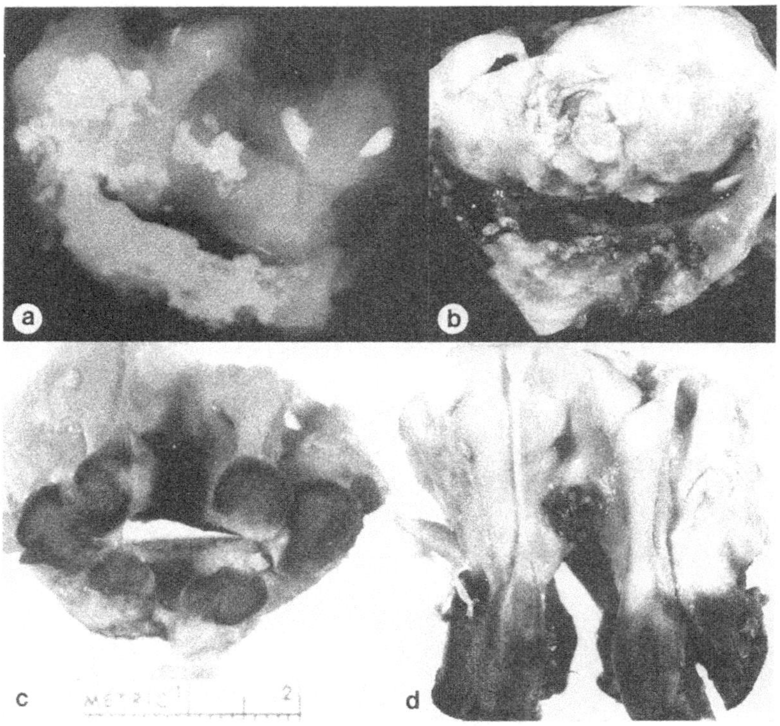

FIGURE 6. a) *Radiograph.* b) *View from left atrium.* c *and* d) *View of orifice* (c) *and anterior mitral leaflet* (d) *from left ventricular aspect.*

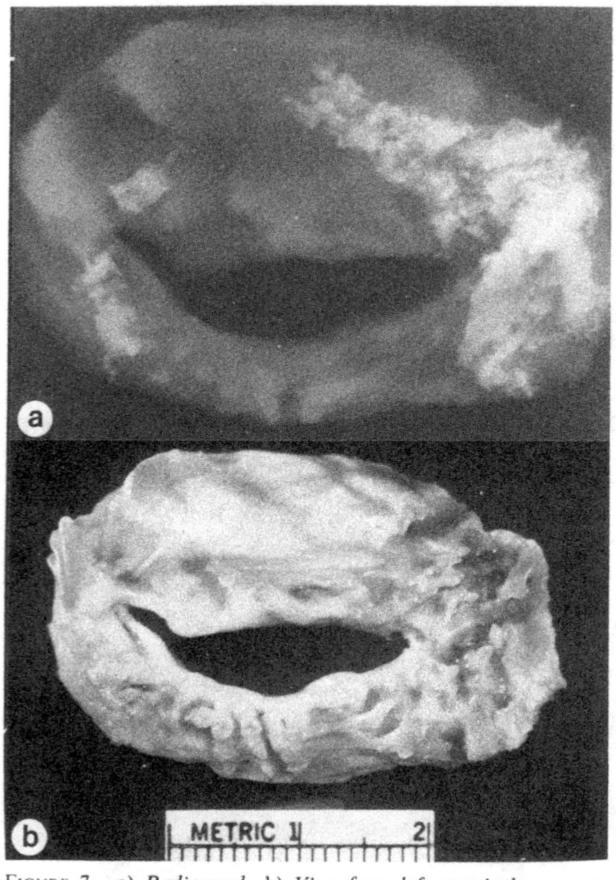

FIGURE 7. a) *Radiograph.* b) *View from left ventricular aspect after excision of the chordae tendineae.*

The *severity of the mitral stenosis* is summarized in tables 2 and 3 and in figure 15. The left atrial (or pulmonary arterial wedge) to left ventricular mean diastolic gradient in the 164 patients ranged from 4–30 mm Hg (avg 13.8 mm Hg). This gradient was identical in both men and women (13.8 mm Hg). Of the 164 patients, the gradients were greater than 15 in 57 (35%), between 7.5–15 in 84 (51%) and less than 7.5 in 23 (14%). The percent of men and women with gradients greater than 15 mm Hg was similar (33 and 36% respectively). Only four (6%) of the 63 men and 19 (19%) of the 101 women, however, had gradients less than 7.5 mm Hg ($P < 0.05$).

The degree of mitral stenosis did correlate with the amount of calcium present in the mitral leaflets (fig. 15). The left atrial to left ventricular mean diastolic gradient in the 57 patients with absent or grade I mitral calcific deposits averaged 10.7 mm Hg, whereas this gradient in the 73 patients with grade III or IV calcium averaged 16.4 mm Hg ($P < 0.01$) (fig. 15). This gradient in the 34 patients with grade II mitral calcium was midway between (13.5 mm Hg). Among the 57 patients with left atrial to left ventricular mean diastolic pressure gradients greater than 15 mm Hg, 36 (63%) had grade III or IV calcific deposits whereas only two (3%) had no calcific deposits ($P < 0.01$). Of the 23 patients with pressure gradients less than 7.5 mm Hg, only two (9%) had heavy (grade III or IV) calcific deposits, whereas 21 (91%) had absent or light (grades 0, I or II) calcific deposits ($P < 0.01$). Among the 84 patients with gradients between 7.5 and 15 mm Hg, 49 (58%) had absent or light and 35 (42%) had heavy calcific deposits.

Neither the pulmonary arterial systolic nor the pulmonary wedge mean pressures (144 patients) (left atrial mean

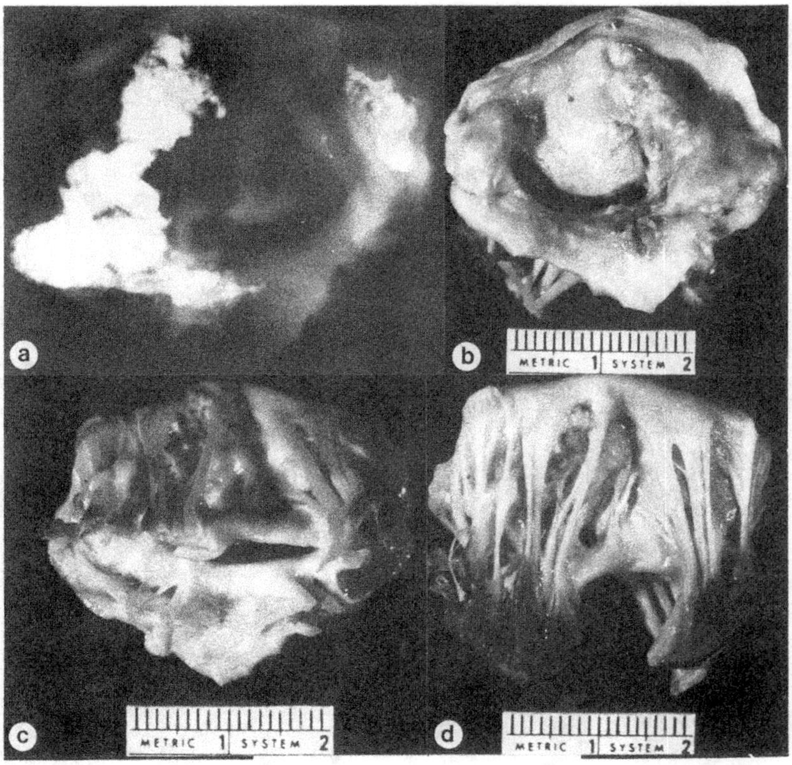

FIGURE 8. a) *Radiograph. Most of the calcific deposits are at and adjacent to the posteromedial commissure.* b) *View from left atrium.* c *and* d) *Views from left ventrical aspect showing the orifice* (c) *and anterior mitral leaflet* (d).

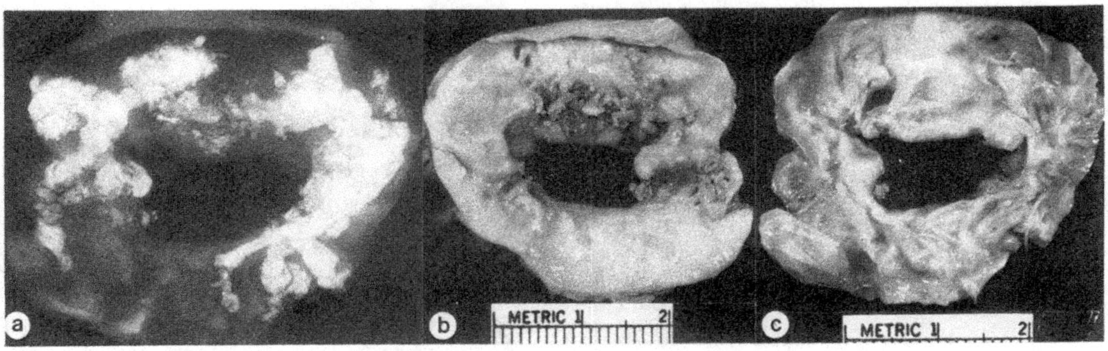

FIGURE 9. a) *Radiograph.* b) *View from left atrium.* c) *View from left ventricle.*

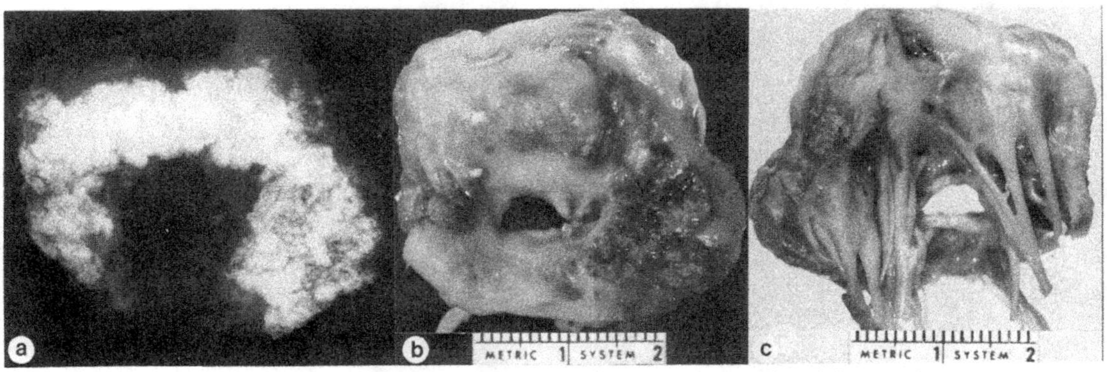

FIGURE 10. a) *Radiograph.* b) *View from left atrium.* c) *View from left ventricle.*

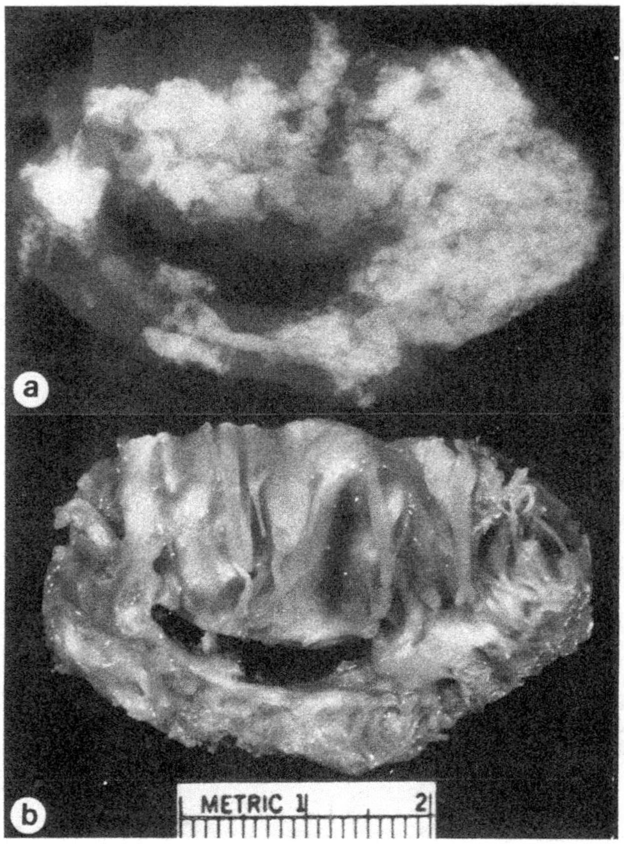

FIGURE 11. a) *Radiograph.* b) *View from left ventricle after excision of most chordae tendineae.*

pressure in 20 patients) correlated with the amount of mitral calcific deposits. Of the 162 patients with recorded pulmonary arterial systolic pressures, 50 (31%) were greater than 60 mm Hg, 54 (33%) were 45 to 60, 51 (32%) were 30 to 44, and only seven (4%) were normal (< 30 mm Hg). The pulmonary arterial wedge or left atrial mean pressures were greater than 25 mm Hg in 87 (53%) patients, between 12.5 and 25 mm Hg in 74 (45%) and less than 12.5 in four (3%) patients. The mitral valve area index decreased as the amount of the mitral calcific deposits increased.

Of the 164 patients before valve replacement, 38 (30%)

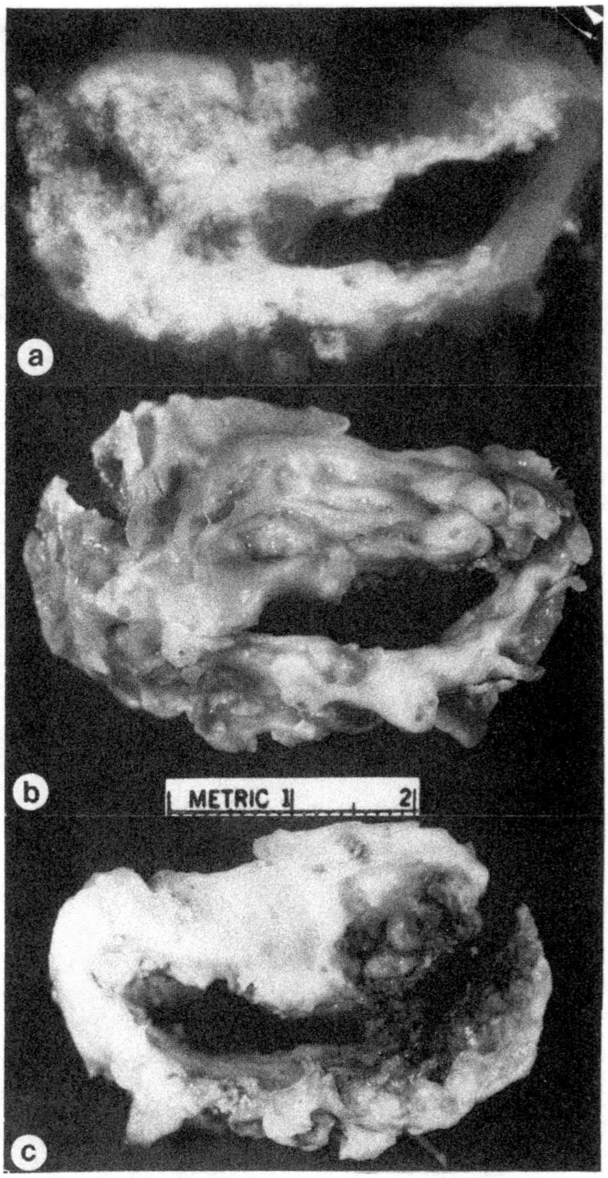

FIGURE 13. a) *Radiograph.* b) *View from left ventricle. The greatest amount of calcium is in the area of the posteromedial commissure.* c) *View from left atrial aspect.*

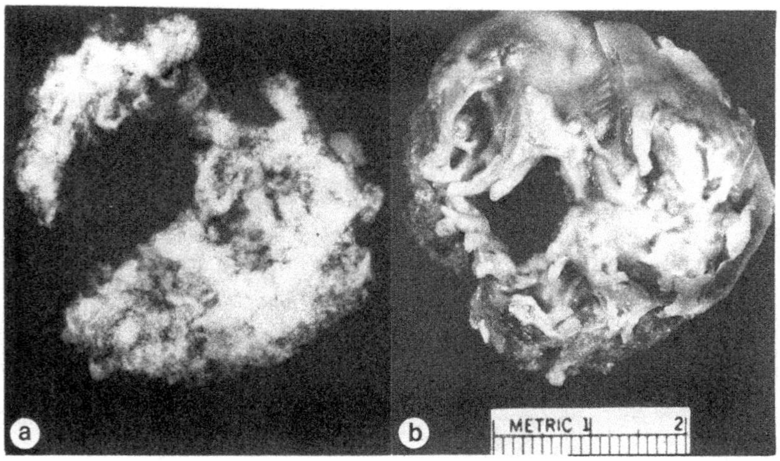

FIGURE 12. a) *Radiograph.* b) *View from left ventricular aspect after excision of most chordae tendineae.*

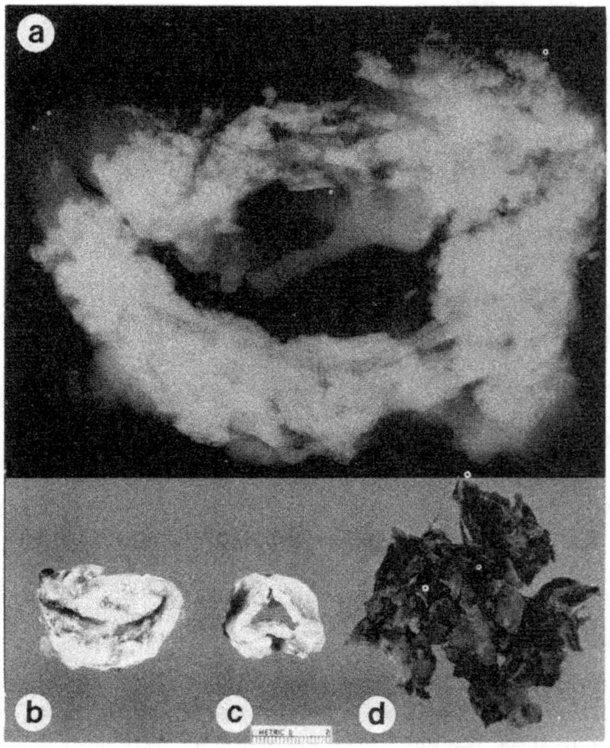

FIGURE 14. a) *Radiograph. Calcium extends around the entire 360° of the orifice.* b) *Mitral valve from left atrium.* c) *Excised, three-cuspid aortic valve with fusion of each of the 3 commissures.* d) *Thrombus excised from the body of left atrium.*

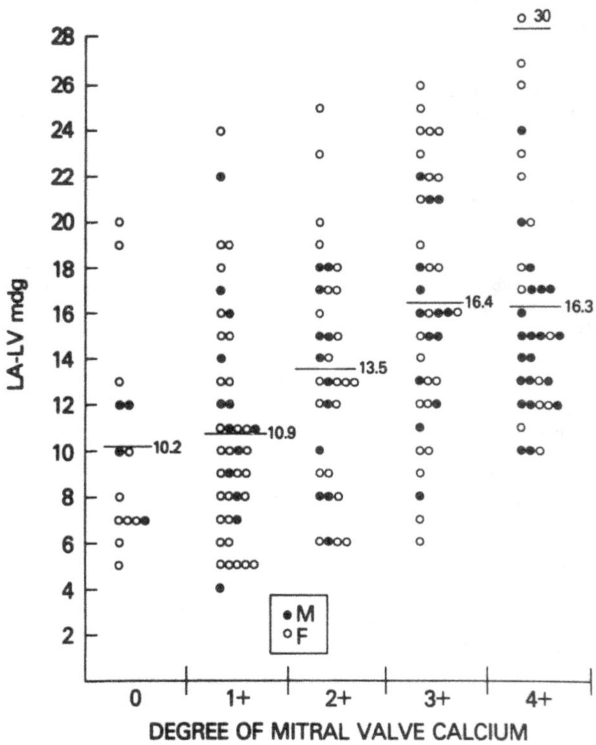

FIGURE 15. *Relation between left atrial (LA)-left ventricular (LV) mean diastolic gradient (mdg) and degree of mitral valve calcium.*

TABLE 6. *Calcific Deposits in Stenotic Mitral Valves: Amount of Calcium Related to Previous Mitral Commissurotomy (MC)*

Amount of Calcium	+ MC	O MC	Totals
0	6 (46%)	9 (64%)	14
I	18 (42%)	25 (58%)	43
II	11 (32%)	23 (68%)	34
III	14 (36%)	25 (64%)	39
IV	12 (35%)	22 (65%)	34
Totals	61 (37%)	103 (63%)	164

were in sinus rhythm and 126 (70%) were in chronic atrial fibrillation (table 4). The ages of the patients in sinus rhythm ranged from 33–68 years (avg. 47) and that of the 126 patients in atrial fibrillation, from 26–72 years (avg. 54) ($P < 0.05$). The rhythm, however, did not correlate with the amount of calcium in the stenotic mitral valves. Of the 126 patients in atrial fibrillation, 55 (44%) had heavy calcific deposits and of the 38 patients in sinus rhythm 18 (47%) had heavy calcific deposits.

The presence of *thrombus in the body of the left atrium* did not correlate with the amount of calcium in the stenotic mitral valves (table 5).

No relationship was found between the amount of mitral valve calcium and *previous mitral commissurotomy* (table 6). Of the 164 patients, 61 (37%) had mitral commissurotomy from 6 months to 19 years before mitral valve replacement.

No correlation was found between the amount of mitral calcium and the *presence of other cardiac valve lesions.* Of the 164 patients, 79 (48%) had isolated mitral stenosis with or without mitral regurgitation, and 85 (52%) patients had other valve lesions: aortic stenosis with or without aortic regurgitation in 47 patients (29%), pure aortic regurgitation in 30 (18%), and tricuspid stenosis with or without tricuspid regurgitation in 8 (5%). Pure tricuspid valve regurgitation was not included among the patients with associated valve lesions. In 59 (77%) of the 77 patients with associated aortic valve disease, aortic valve replacement also was carried out.

Comments

Clinical assessment of mitral calcific deposits has been made previously utilizing fluoroscopy, tomography, and angiocardiography.[1-3] While each could indicate the presence or absence of such deposits, these methods failed to quantify them. Radiography of the excised mitral valve allows accurate assessment of the amount of mitral calcific deposits. Wooley and associates[4] described the location and extent of such deposits in 23 patients with mitral stenosis, but they did not relate the morphologic changes to clinical or hemodynamic factors. Our method of expressing the degree of calcific deposits in this valve as a percentage of the valve orifice circumference provides a means of relating the morphological changes to the hemodynamic data.

The present study of 164 patients aged 26 to 72 years shows that the amount of calcific deposits in stenotic mitral valves correlated with *sex* and with the *mean diastolic pressure gradient* across the mitral valve, but not with the patient's age, cardiac rhythm, main pulmonary arterial or pulmonary arterial wedge pressure, previous mitral com-

TABLE 7. *Clinical Data in the 14 Patients Whose Mitral Valves Are Illustrated in Figures 1-14*

Fig. no.	Surgical number	MV Ca^{++} 1^+-4^+	Age (yrs.)	Sex	MVC in past	PAW-LV mdg (mm Hg)	PA Pressure (mm Hg) s/d	Rhythm SR	Rhythm AF	LV-SA psg (mm Hg)	LA Body Thr	MR (0-4^+) by LV cine
1	S73-5005	1^+	40	F	0	11	70/40	0	+	0	0	2^+
2	S67-686	1^+	40	F	+	13	50/18	0	+	0	0	3^+
3	S75-5138	2^+	41	F	0	7	32/14	0	+	0	0	3^+
4	S70-3120	2^+	55	F	0	9	28/12	0	+	0	0	2^+
5	S76-28	2^+	58	M	+	12	40/20	0	+	0	0	1^+
6	S71-3012	3^+	50	F	0	22	75/22	0	+	0	+	—
7	S67-4943	3^+	50	M	0	16	55/30	0	+	20	0	1^+
8	S76-52	3^+	50	F	0	16	60/30	0	+	0	+	1^+
9	S67-3587	4^+	45	F	0	24	110/52	+	0	0	0	1^+
10	S75-5128	4^+	33	M	0	15	120/60	+	0	0	0	3^+
11	S67-867	4^+	53	F	0	26	88/45	+	0	0	+	1^+
12	S70-3021	4^+	26	M	0	15	55/27	0	+	0	0	1^+
13	S66-4095	4^+	43	M	0	23	61/37	+	0	7	0	2^+
14	S70-3005	4^+	37	M	+	9	95/45	+	0	34	+	—

Abbreviations: AF = atrial fibrillation; Ca^{++} = calcium; F = female; Hg = mercury; M = male; mdg = mean diastolic gradient; mm = millimeters; MR = mitral regurgitation; MV = mitral valve; MVC = mitral valve commissurotomy; LA = left atrium; LV = left ventricle; PA = pulmonary artery; PAW = pulmonary artery wedge; psg = peak systolic gradient; SA = systemic artery; s/d = systolic/diastolic; SR = sinus rhythm; and Thr = thrombus.

missurotomy, presence of thrombus in the body of left atrium or the presence of disease in one or more other cardiac valves.

Men tend to have heavier calcific deposits in stenotic mitral valves and at an earlier age than do women with the same hemodynamic lesion. Over twice as many men had extremely heavy (grade IV) mitral calcific deposits than women, whereas the opposite occurred in the patients with no mitral calcific deposits. Olesen and associates,[2] from study by tomography, also demonstrated a much higher frequency of calcific deposits in stenotic mitral valves of men compared to women (nearly 3 to 1), but quantitation of the amount of calcium was not determined. Kitchin and Turner[3] determined the presence or absence of mitral calcific deposits by palpation at commissurotomy or by preoperative radiography, and they too found a higher incidence of mitral calcific deposits in men, and they also found an increased incidence of calcific deposits in stenotic mitral valves in their older patients. Neither of the latter two studies, however, attempted to quantitate the amount of calcific deposits in these stenotic mitral valves. We did not find heavier mitral calcific deposits in our older patients compared to the younger patients.

The mean diastolic pressure gradient across the mitral valve in our patients increased as the amount of calcium in this valve increased. This correlation has not been provided previously. A similar correlation regarding calcific deposits in stenotic *aortic* valves has been noted previously.[5]

Surprisingly, 12 (35%) of the 34 patients with the heaviest (grade IV) mitral calcific deposits had sinus rhythm. Of the 91 patients with absent or light (grade I and II) calcific deposits, 71 (78%) had atrial fibrillation.

Previous commissurotomy did not correlate with the extent of calcific deposits observed in the excised stenotic mitral valves. Indeed, the percent of patients in each of the five grades of mitral calcific deposits was similar. Thus, mitral valve commissurotomy does not appear to increase mitral valve calcific deposits and furthermore, an earlier mitral commissurotomy does not indicate that commissurotomy cannot be performed a second time. In retrospect, possibly several of the 24 patients in this analysis who had absent (6 patients) or only grade 1 (18 patients) mitral calcific deposits could have had another mitral commissurotomy rather than valve replacement during the second cardiotomy. None of the 18 patients with only grade I calcific deposits by radiography of the excised valve had calcific deposits by radiography (any method) before valve replacement.

Acknowledgments

This study was made possible because the mitral valves had been excised intact and because hemodynamic studies had been performed on all patients preoperatively. Therefore, we are enormously indebted to Dr. Andrew G. Morrow who has virtually always excised cardiac valves at operation *intact* and has stressed the importance of doing so to his associates. To Dr. Stephen E. Epstein and earlier to Dr. Eugene Braunwald and their colleagues we are grateful for free access to the hemodynamic information in their patients. Ms. Barbara E. Winterrowd and Filippina Giacometti provided technical assistance. The gross anatomy photographs were taken by Mr. L. Kenzie Edwards and James R. Banks, Jr. Mr. H. Robert Baird, Laboratory of Statistical and Mathematical Methodolology, Division of Computer Research and Technology, NIH, provided the statistical analyses.

References

1. Wynn A: Gross calcification of the mitral valve. Br Heart J **15:** 214, 1953
2. Olsen K, Dandoe E, Gudbjerg C: The higher incidence of valvular calcification in males than in females with mitral stenosis. Acta Medica Scand **177** (fasc. 1): 7, 1965
3. Kitchin A, Turner R: Calcification of the mitral valve. Results of valvotomy in 100 cases. Br Heart J **29:** 137, 1967
4. Wooley CF, Baba N, Kilman J, Rayna J: Thrombotic calcific mitral stenosis: Morphology of the calcific mitral valve. Circulation **49:** 1167, 1974
5. Glancy DL, Freed TA, O'Brien KP, Epstein SE: Calcium in the aortic valve. Roentgenologic and hemodynamic correlation in 148 patients. Ann Intern Med **71:** 245, 1969

Cells, Collagen and Idiopathic Pulmonary Fibrosis *

Ronald G. Crystal, Jack D. Fulmer, Bruce J. Baum, John Bernardo, Kathryn H. Bradley, Sally D. Bruel, Norton A. Elson, Gerald A. Fells, Victor J. Ferrans, James E. Gadek, Gary W. Hunninghake, Oichi Kawanami, Jeffrey A. Kelman, Bruce R. Line, John A. McDonald, Byron D. McLees, William C. Roberts, David M. Rosenberg, Paul Tolstoshev, Edwyna Von Gal and Steven E. Weinberger

Pulmonary Branch and Pathology Branch, National Heart, Lung, and Blood Institute, and Department of Nuclear Medicine, Clincial Center, National Institutes of Health, Bethesda, Maryland, USA

Abstract. Idiopathic pulmonary fibrosis (IPF) is a usually fatal disorder of lung with clearly defined clinical, roentgenographic, physiologic, morphologic, scintigraphic and bronchoalveolar lavage features. Current concepts of the pathogenesis of this disorder suggest a central role for a chronic alveolitis in causing changes in parenchymal cell populations and derangements in interstitial collagen. Of the many inflammatory and immune effector cells comprising the alveolitis of IPF, it is likely that the neutrophil is the most important mediator of parenchymal damage. To follow the status of lung neutrophils in patients with this disease, two methods have been utilized. Both gallium-67 scanning and bronchoalveolar lavage quantitate the extent of the alveolitis and can be used to stage and follow these patients. The treatment of IPF remains controversial, but it is likely that corticosteroids reduce the alveolitis and prolong the lifespan of these patients.

Key words: Lung - Cells - Collagen - Idiopathic pulmonary fibrosis - Alveolitis

---

Introduction

The interstitial lung diseases are chronic, diffuse, non-infectious, non-neoplastic disorders primarily affecting alveoli. In mid-course, these disorders are generally characterized roentgenographically by a nodular or reticular pattern, physiologically by decreased lung volumes and diffusing capacity, and morphologically by alveoli with altered cellular populations and deranged interstitial collagen. Because the deranged interstitial col-

* Presented at the 43rd Annual Meeting, American College of Chest Physicians, Las Vegas, Nevada, November 1977

lagen gives the alveolar septae a thickened, scarlike appearance when visualized by light microscopy, the term "interstitial fibrosis" is commonly used to describe this finding.

There are approximately 130 defined interstitial diseases, but the etiology can be identified in only about 30% of affected individuals [6]. The remaining 70% are categorized into specifically defined diseases, of which the most prevalent are idiopathic pulmonary fibrosis (IPF), chronic interstitial lung disease associated with the collagen-vascular disorders, and sarcoidosis. As an example of the current concepts of pathogenesis of the interstitial disorders, we will use IPF to demonstrate how alterations in alveolar cell populations can result in structural and functional abnormalities of gas-exchanging units.

Idiopathic Pulmonary Fibrosis

Because the etiology of IPF is unknown, and because lung biopsies from these patients do not have relatively unique morphologic features (e.g., granulomata), the diagnosis of IPF has often been considered "nonspecific" by pulmonary clinicians. However, as more information has accrued concerning these patients, it is apparent that IPF is a specific, independent disease entity, with clearly defined clinical, roentgenographic, physiologic, morphologic, scintigraphic and bronchoalveolar lavage features, including [4]:

1. Clinical. A history of breathlessness, particularly with exercise; no history suggesting a known etiology; no history or clinical evidence suggesting left ventricular failure or a defined collagen-vascular disease; no evidence of bronchitis; no history suggestive of hypersensitivity pneumonitis; and no exposure to inhalants or drugs known to cause interstitial lung disease;
2. Roentgenographic. A diffuse interstitial pattern on chest film; and no adenopathy;
3. Physiologic. Reduced total lung capacity or diffusing capacity; normal forced expiratory volume in 1 s/forced vital capacity; mild resting hypoxemia which worsens with exercise; and a deflation volume-pressure curve shifted downward and to the right;
4. Morphologic. Varying degrees of interstitial fibrosis; interstitial and intra-alveolar alveolitis[1] consisting predominantly of macrophages and lymphocytes but also including neutrophils and eosinophils; peribronchial inflammation and fibrosis; and no vasculitis, granulomata or significant refractile bodies by polarized light microscopy;
5. Scintigraphic. Diffuse uptake of gallium-67 in the lung parenchyma but not in lymph nodes; and
6. Bronchoalveolar lavage. Fluid recovered consisting of an increased proportion of polymorphonuclear leukocytes, normal lymphocyte subpopulations, and elevated levels of IgG.

[1] In reference to the interstitial lung disorders, "alveolitis" refers to the inflammatory and immune effector cells that accumulate within the interstitium and alveolar air spaces.

As the name implies, the process which incites the development of IPF is unknown, and all attempts to identify a responsible exogenous agent, such as a virus, have been unrewarding. Whatever the inciting process, the concept has arisen that genetic and host-acquired factors likely modulate susceptibility to IPF as well as the rate at which the disorder follows its characteristic pathogenic path.

In cases of early IPF that are biopsied, it is apparent that there is little, if any, fibrosis, but that the alveolar structures have two other distinguishing features (Fig. 1). First, there is a characteristic alveolitis, in which effector cells of the inflammatory and immune system accumulate within the alveolar interstitium and in the air spaces. Second, there are alterations in parenchymal cells, including changes in the proportions of epithelial, endothelial and interstitial cells that comprise the alveolus.

Although it is possible that some of the alveolitis and alterations in parenchymal cell populations are reversible, sequential biopsies have demonstrated that by the time IPF is in mid-course, the early changes have led to a progressive derangement of interstitial collagen (i.e., fibrosis) that is most likely irreversible once present (Fig. 2).

As this process continues, there are progressive alterations in the alveolar cellular and non-cellular structures such that the alveoli no longer can act as gas-exchanging units. As more and more alveoli follow this pathogenetic route, alveolar structures are no longer recognizable and are replaced by cystic spaces (Fig. 3). This late-stage IPF is termed "end-stage lung" and soon progresses to a state where the lung can no longer fulfill its function in gas exchange, and the patient dies.

It is clear from this discussion that three prominent features in the pathogenesis of IPF are: (1) a chronic alveolitis, (2) changes in parenchymal cell populations, and (3) a derangement in interstitial collagen (Fig. 4). Although it is useful to conceptualize each feature separately, it is important to understand that they are interdependent processes in which the cellular events within the alveolar structures lead to a progressive interstitial fibrosis and eventual destruction of the lung as a gas-exchanging organ. To understand how this may occur on a cellular level, it is first necessary to define the structure of the normal alveolus and how this structure is maintained.

The Normal Alveolus. The alveolus of the normal adult lung is comprised of four major parenchymal cells (epithelial type I, epithelial type II, capillary endothelial, interstitial mesenchymal) and two effector cell populations derived from the inflammatory and immune systems (alveolar macrophages, lymphocytes)[30]. The structural support for these cells is provided by the non-cellular connective tissue constituents of the alveolar interstitium, including collagen, elastic fibers, and proteoglycans [15, 17, 19]. Of these, collagen is the most abundant, comprising 15-20% of the alveolar dry weight and 60-70% of interstitial connective tissue. The other connective tissue components are critical to normal interstitial function, but as far as is known, they do not play an important role in the pathogenesis of IPF.

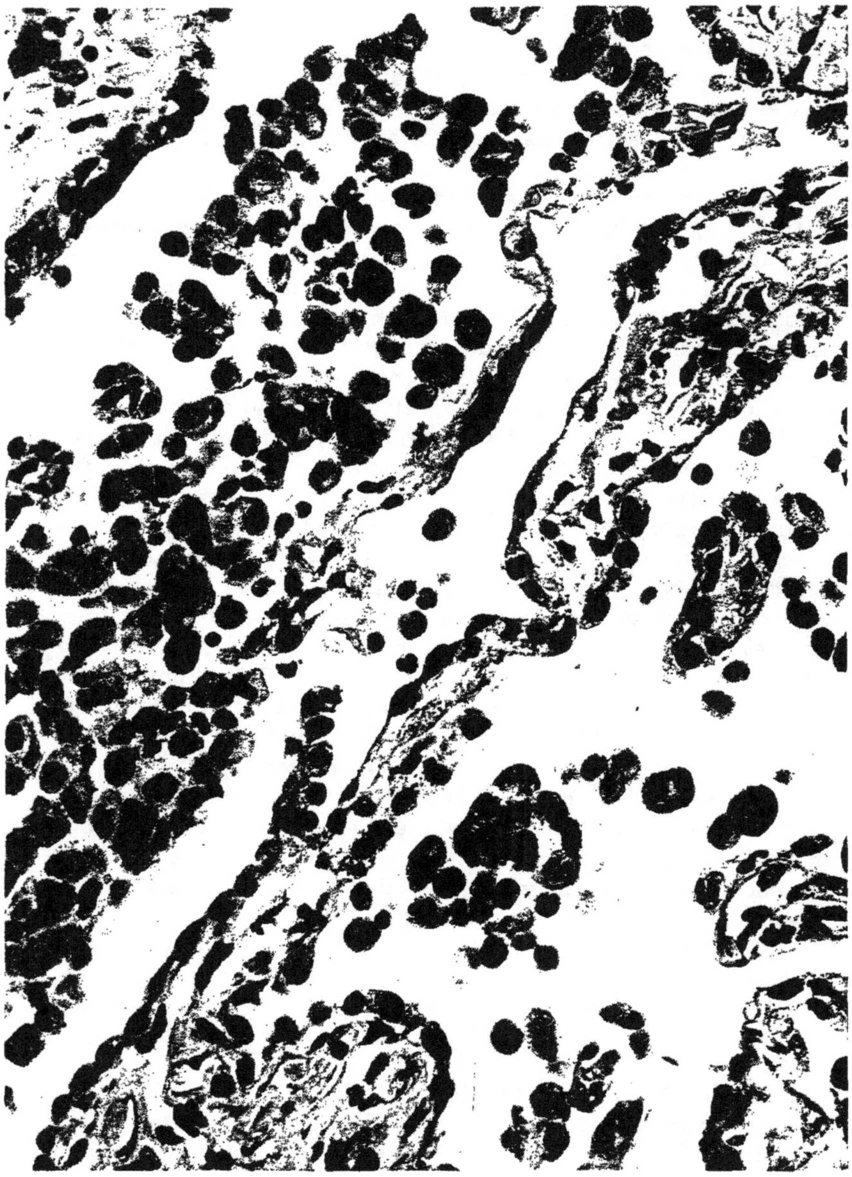

Fig. 1. Alveoli in lung biopsy specimen from patient with early IPF show minimal thickening but contain numerous inflammatory cells, including macrophages, polymorphonuclear leukocytes and lymphocytes. Hematoxylin and eosin stain, X 400.

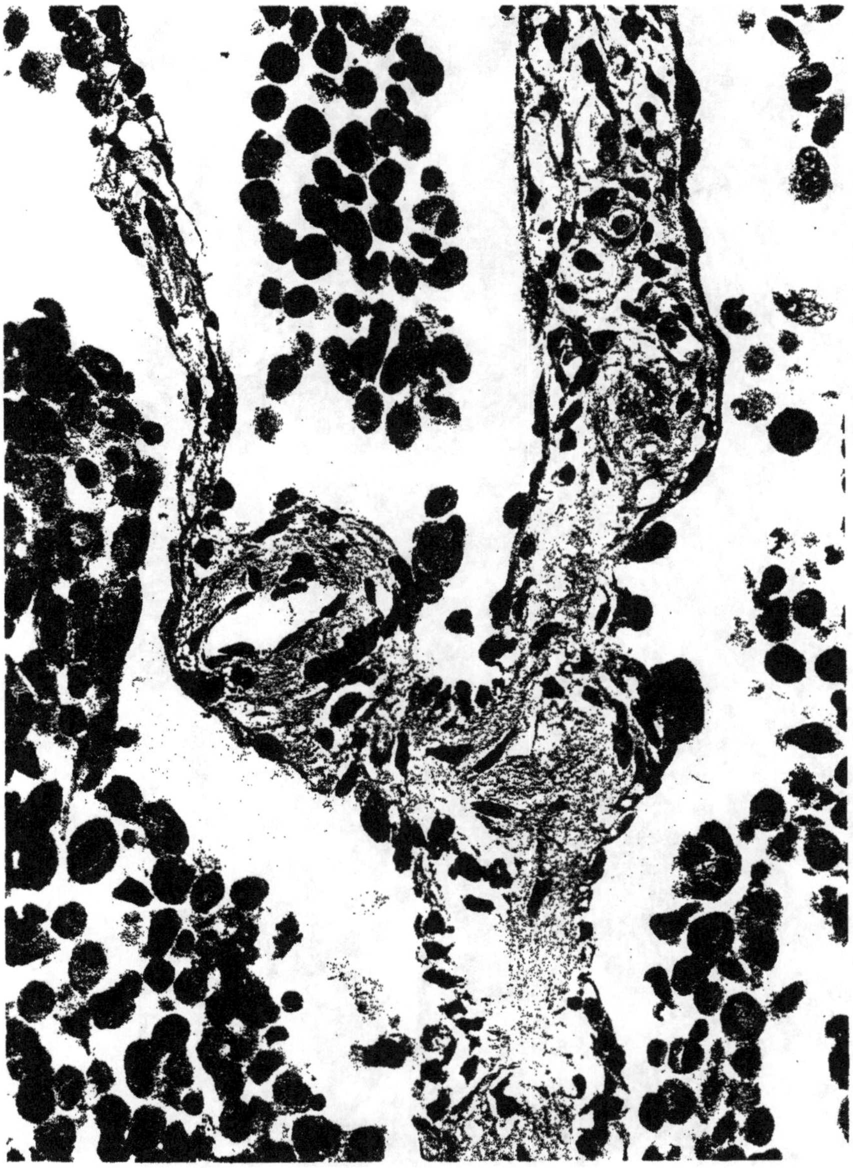

Fig. 2. Lung biopsy from patient with mid-course IPF showing inflammatory cells associated with marked thickening of the alveolar walls by fibrous connective tissue. Hematoxylin and eosin stain, X 400.

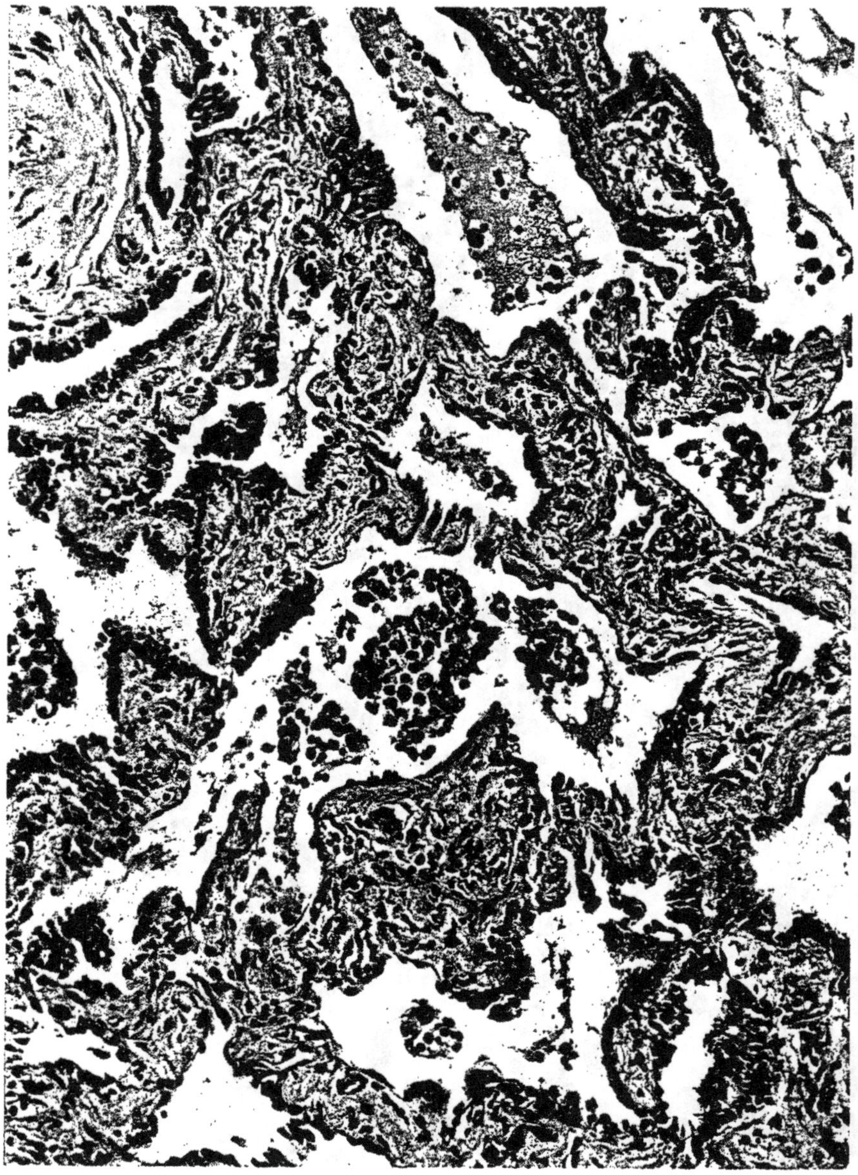

Fig. 3. Severely fibrotic, thickened and distorted alveolar walls in late IPF; cystic spaces that contain exudated material and numerous macrophages are evident. The epithelial cells vary in appearance; in some areas they are cuboidal and even multilayered. Hematoxylin and eosin stain, X 180.

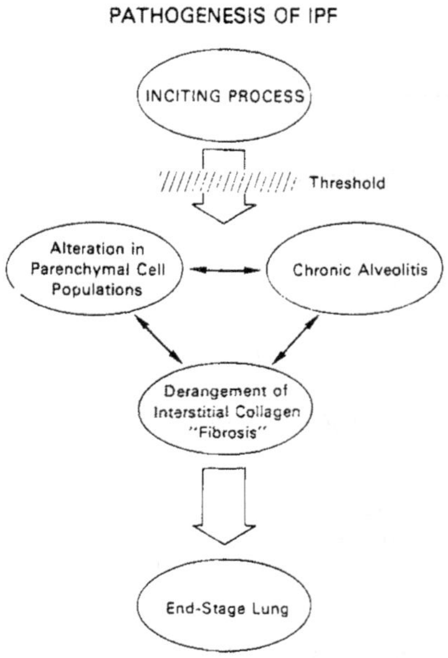

Fig. 4. Current concept of the pathogenesis of idiopathic pulmonary fibrosis (IPF). Although the inciting process has not been identified, it is likely that there exists a general threshold of alveolar injury above which characteristic pathogenic processes occur that result in IPF. See text for details.

The normal alveolar interstitium contains at least three types of collagen, each of which has a characteristic amino acid sequence [3, 15, 17]. Type I collagen (60-65% of the total) forms 500-1,000 μm banded fibers that usually run parallel to basement membrane. Most studies suggest that type I collagen is the most highly organized, least compliant form of interstitial collagen, and it plays a critical role in maintaining normal alveolar structure and function. Type III collagen (30-35% of the total) appears as 150-350 μm randomly dispersed fibrils that probably contribute to alveolar structure and function via their influence on the way in which type collagen forms fibers. The remaining collagen (< 5%) is that present in the basement membrane found beneath the alveolar epithelial and endothelial cells. The structure of alveolar basement membrane is not known, but from analogy to other basement membranes, it probably is composed of noncollagen glycoproteins together with collagens that are distinct from type I and type III. There is growing evidence that basement membrane collagens may differ depending on the cell responsible for synthesis, suggesting that the alveolar interstitium may include at least two types of basement membrane collagen (i.e., endothelial and epithelial). Alveolar basement membrane probably does not influence mechanical properties significantly, but it likely plays a critical role in directing the growth patterns of epithelial and endothelial cells following parenchymal injury.

Although it was originally thought that only mesenchymal, fibroblast-like cells could synthesize collagen, it is now known that a variety of differentiated cells are capable of this process [14, 15, 17]. Studies of individual cell types maintained in tissue culture suggest that most of the cells within the normal alveolar unit play an important role in production of the interstitial collagens (Table 1).

Table 1. Maintenance of interstitial collagen in normal lung and idiopathic

Cell type	Normal lung: Relative numbers	Normal lung: Role in the maintenance of interstitial collagen
Parenchymal cells		
Type I epithelial	8% of total parenchymal cells[a]	Probably synthesizes type I and III; ? synthesizes basement membrane
Type II epithelial	14% of total parenchymal cells	No known role
Capillary endothelial	39% of total parenchymal cells	Basement membrane synthesis[b]
Mesenchymal		
Fibroblast-like	39% of total parenchymal cells	Synthesizes types I and III collagen in a ratio of 10:1; secretes a collagenase that attacks collagens I and III at equal rates
Smooth muscle	Very rare	———
Inflammatory and immune effector cells		
Macrophage	80-90% of total effector cells	Produces collagenase which attacks types I and III collagen at an equal rate
Lymphocyte	10-20% of total effector cells; 70% T, 25%B	In collaboration with macrophages, probably suppresses collagen synthesis by fibroblasts [39]
Neutrophils	Very rare	———
Mast cells	Very rare	———
Eosinophils	Very rare	———

[a]Estimates are from rat lung [38].

[b]By analogy to endothelial cells derived from arteries and veins of sources other than lung [22].

pulmonary fibrosis

Idiophatic pulmonary fibrosis	
Relative numbers	Role in the derangement of interstitial collagen
Marked loss	
	Shifts in epithelial cell types probably affect the relative amounts and locations of interstitial collagen, but specific effects are unknown
Replacement of type I cells by a type II - like cell	
Decreased	Unknown
Increased	Predominant collagen-synthesizing cell of the IPF parenchyma; increased numbers probably play a critical role in the alterations of collagen found in IPF; unknown if differentiated state normal or altered in IPF
Increased	Synthesizes types I and III collagen and basement membrane[c]; likely alters relative collagen composition
Increased	IPF macrophages spontaneously secrete neutrophil chemotactic factor [11]
Increased	Proportions of T- and B - cells normal [24]; subpopulation produces MIF[d] in response to collagen [29]; may influence macrophages to secrete more collagenase[e];? loss of normal suppression of collagen synthesis
Increased	Collagenase attacks type I collagen selectively [20]; other neutral proteases destroy fibronectin [33]
Increased	Unknown
Increased	Unknown

[c] By analogy to smooth muscle cells derived from sources other than lung [32].

[d] MIF = Macrophage migration inhibiton factor.

[e] By analogy to studies of guinea pig cells in which activated lymphocytes induce peritoneal macrophages to secrete collagenase [37].

The synthesis of collagen, however, is only one side of the complex process involved in the maintenance of collagen in the normal lung. In the adult lung parenchyma, collagen is continually being synthesized, yet the amount of parenchymal collagen does not change [1, 2]. To provide this constancy, the normal parenchyma must have mechanisms to degrade collagen at the same rate at which it is produced. However, collagen is an unusual macromolecule in that only one class of enzymes, termed collagenases, is capable of degrading it under the physiologic conditions of the extracellular milieu. Thus, to maintain the normal alveolar interstitium, the cells of the alveolus must not only synthesize collagen, but they must also provide collagenase(s) to degrade it [18, 20, 21]. Although the production of collagenase is usually associated with cells of the inflammatory system (e.g., macrophages, neutrophils), tissue culture studies have demonstrated that parenchymal cells (e.g., mesenchymal cells) can also secrete a collagenase capable of attacking the major interstitial collagens [20, 40] (Table 1).

Cells, Collagen and IPF

The original light microscopic descriptions of IPF suggested that the "fibrosis" was simply an accumulation of interstitial collagen mediated by "activated" fibroblasts responding to "injury" [13, 36]. However, as more information has accrued using ultrastructural and biochemical techniques, it has become apparent that the "fibrosis" of IPF is much more complex and includes the following [5, 7, 26, 35]: (1) although the collagen is evenly distributed throughout the normal interstitium, in IPF there are localized accumulations such that some septa are markedly widened, whereas others are not (Fig. 2); (2) while the type I fibers of the normal interstitium (Fig. 5) are contained in sharply defined, relatively thin bundles running parallel to basement membrane, some fiber bundles in IPF are thickened, twisted, frayed and randomly oriented (Fig. 6); (3) on the average, the IPF interstitium contains relatively more type I and less type III collagen; and (4) basement membranes in the IPF lung are thickened, but in some areas they are thinned and occasionally disrupted, particularly on the epithelial surface.

This information, together with the knowledge that maintenance of interstitial collagen in the normal lung requires the balance of synthetic and degradative processes by a variety of cells, suggests that the "fibrosis" of IPF is not simply secondary to increased synthesis by "activated" fibroblasts. Rather the deranged collagen of the IPF interstitium must result from a number of processes involving multiple cell types in which the coordinated control of collagen synthesis and degradation is lost.

The key to understanding the pathogenesis of the fibrosis of IPF is the concept that this balance of collagen synthesis and degradation is upset through changes in the cells present in the alveolar structures. Most importantly, IPF is associated with significant alterations in all of the alveolar parenchymal cells (epithelial, endothelial and mesenchymal) as well as profound changes in the inflammatory and immune effector cells that are present within the alveolar structures.

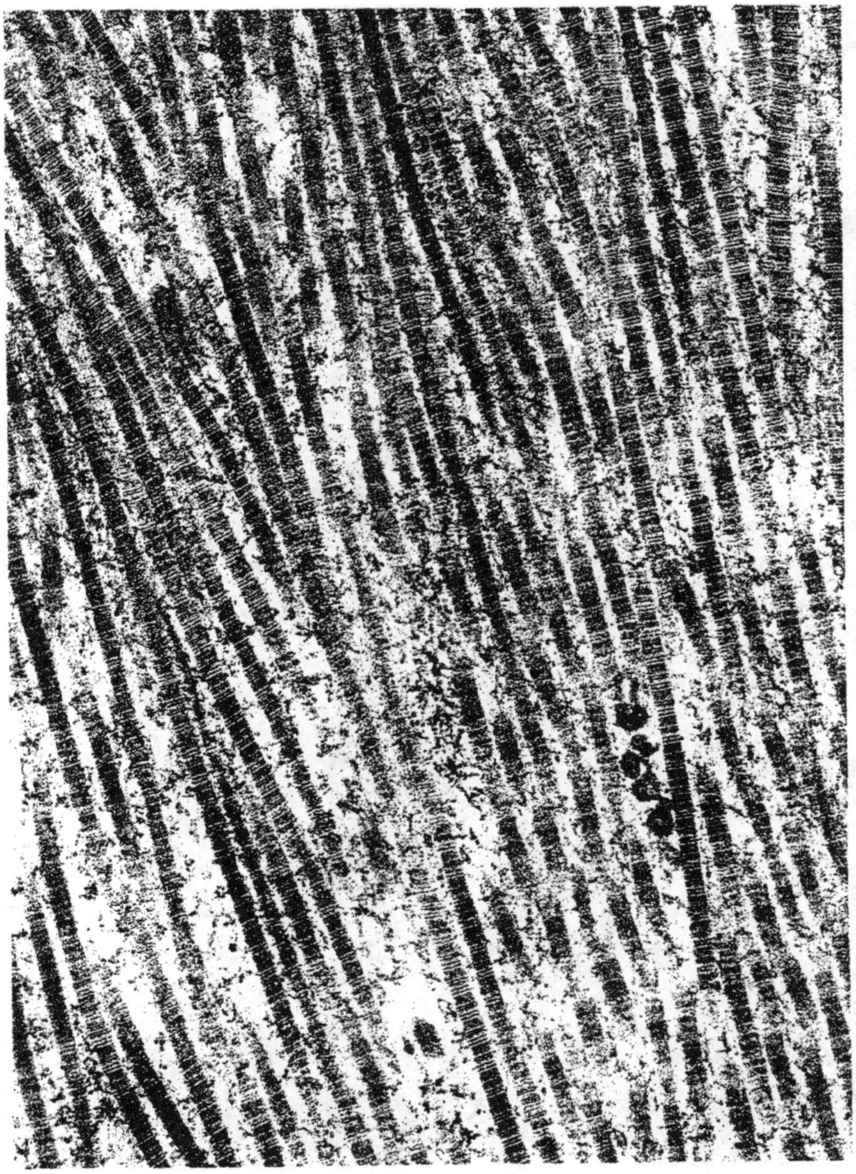

Fig. 5. Well-oriented interstitial collagen fibrils (presumed to be type I collagen) with typical periodic banding are associated with fine strands of material that probably represents proteoglycans. Pulmonary tissue removed from control patient (20-year-old woman) at the time of biopsy of metastatic (osteogenic sarcoma) pulmonary nodule. X 50, 000.

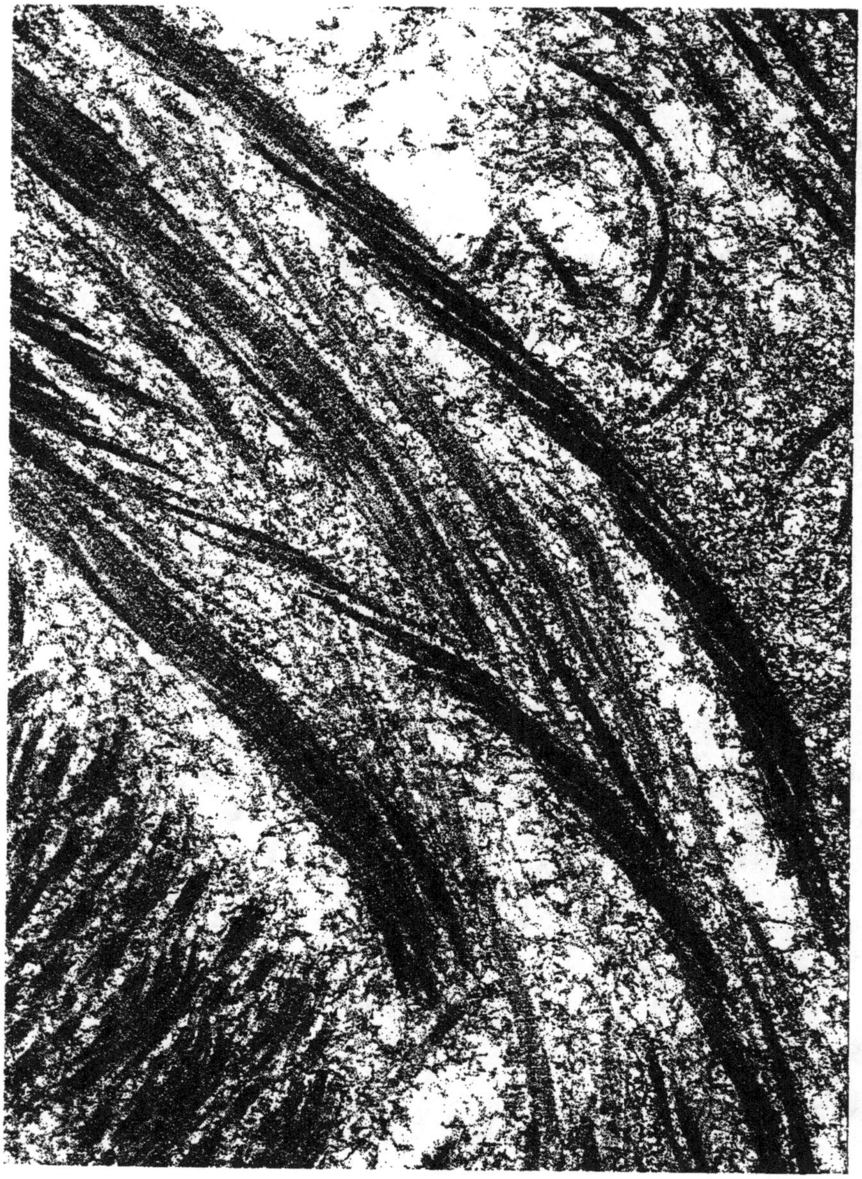

Fig. 6. Twisted, frayed, spiraling bundles of collagen (compare with normal collagen shown at same magnification in Fig. 5) are diversely oriented and are surrounded by abundant strands of material presumed to be proteoglycans. Tissue from same IPF patient as in light micrograph of Fig. 2. X 50,000.

Status of the Parenchymal Cell Populations in IPF. Although quantitative morphometric studies have not been carried out in lung biopsy specimens from patients with this disease, the general consensus is that the alveolar parenchymal cell populations in IPF in mid-course are modified in several ways, including [4]: (1) a marked decrease in the numbers of type I epithelial cells and a concomitant increase in the numbers of an epithelial cell that has many of the features of the fully differentiated type II epithelial cell (Figs. 7, 8); (2) a probable decrease in the total number of capillary endothelial cells; (3) an apparent increase in the total numbers of mesenchymal cells, including more fibroblast-like cells similar to those of the normal interstitium as well as the addition of clusters of smooth muscle cells (Figs. 7, 9); and (4) a striking derangement in the topologic associations between alveolar parenchymal cells and between these cells and the interstitial connective tissue matrix (Figs. 2, 3, 7, 9, 10).

In terms of the maintenance of collagen within the alveolar interstitium, such changes have multiple consequences (Table 1). Since the type I epithelial cell [8] and the endothelial cell [22] both synthesize collagen, the loss of these cells must have an effect on collagen homeostasis within the interstitium. In addition, since fibroblast-like mesenchymal cells synthesize collagen, the increased number of these cells is likely responsible for the localized accumulation of collagen in some alveolar septa [14, 16]. Although smooth muscle cells have not been cultured from the alveolar interstitium of patients with IPF, they have been isolated from other human sources, and they clearly synthesize types I and III collagen as well as basement membrane [32]. It is probable, therefore, that the clusters of smooth muscle cells within the IPF interstitium are responsible for at least some of the derangements of collagen found in this disorder.

The striking topologic derangement of the alveolar parenchymal cells in IPF is manifest in several ways [4, 26]: (1) cells are found in different locations, particularly the mesenchymal cells which are randomly distributed throughout the IPF interstitium; (2) cells are found piling up on one another (Fig. 3), most characteristically seen in the type II-like epithelial cells which replace the lost type I epithelial cells; (3) epithelial cell-basement membrane interactions are disturbed in IPF, as manifest by the partial separation of some epithelial cells from their basement membrane and by the presence of hemi-desmisomes attaching some epithelial cells to the underlying basement membrane (Fig. 10). In addition, anchoring fibrils attach the basement membrane to the underlying connective tissue (Fig. 10) [26]. One potential consequence of these topologic abnormalities is that parenchymal cells capable of collagen synthesis are found in the wrong locations and are oriented in the wrong directions. Although unproven, it is probable that this results in the deposition of collagen in improper locations and orientations, which are some of the characteristic findings in IPF.

The Chronic Alveolitis of IPF. The current concepts of pathogenesis of the fibrosis of IPF suggest two important roles for the effector cells of the inflammatory and immune systems that comprise the chronic alveolitis of the disease. First, a number of cells can alter collagen directly by secreting a collagenase and thus upsetting the relative balance between collagen synthesis and destruction within the interstitium. Second, the inflammatory and immune effector cells of the chronic alveolitis can

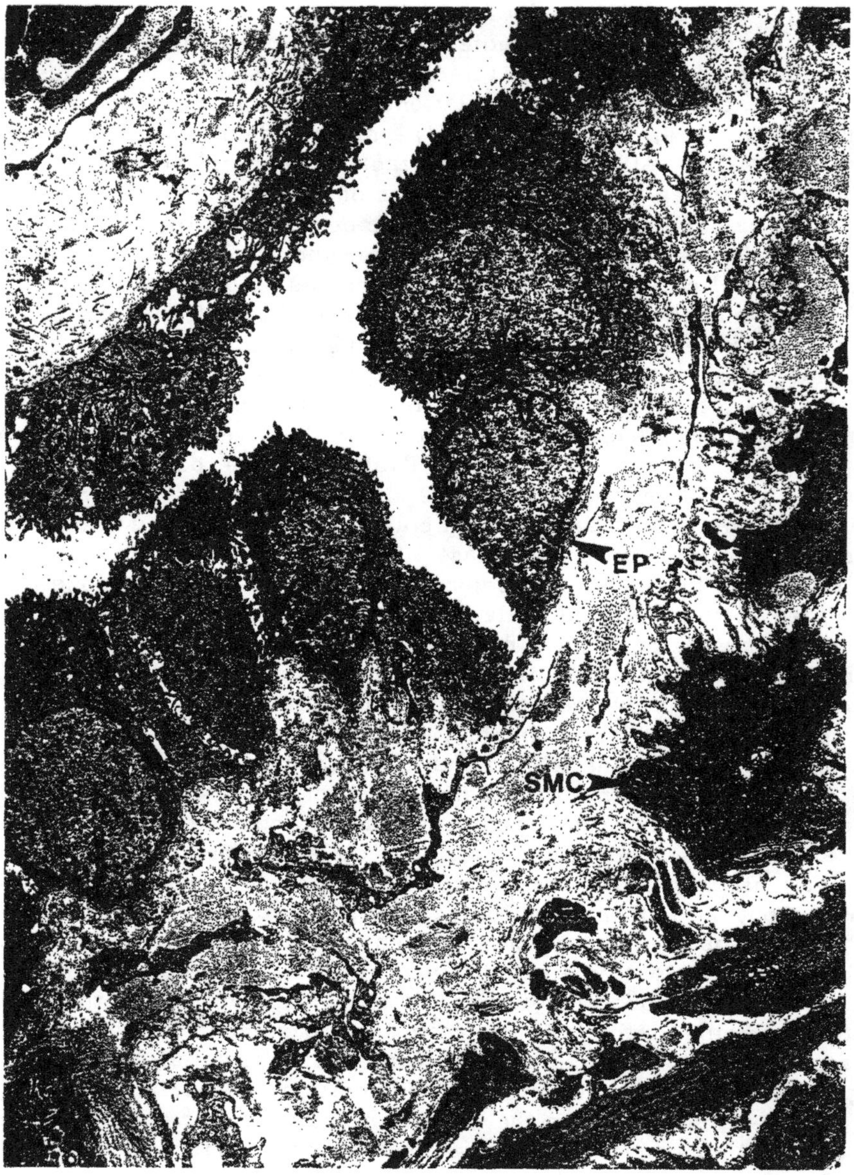

Fig. 7. Electron micrograph of alveolus in IPF. The alveolus is lined by cuboidal epithelial cells (EP), the luminal surfaces of which have numerous small cytoplasmic processes. Subjacent to the epithelium is a wide layer of dense, disordered fibrous connective tissue and a cluster of smooth muscle cells (SMC). X 5,480.

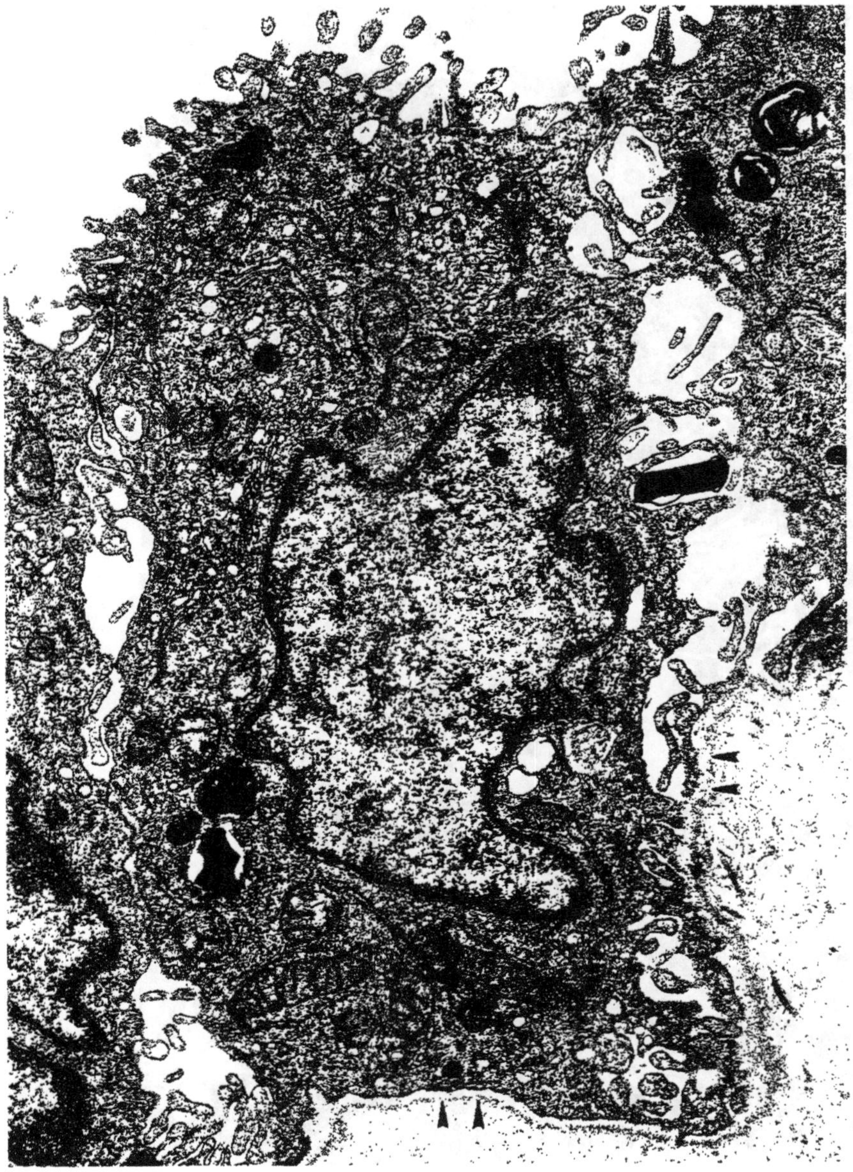

Fig. 8. View of cuboidal epithelial cells similar to those shown at low magnification in Fig. 7. The luminal surface is characterized by numerous short microvilli; the nucleus is idented, and the basement membrane (arrowheads) is prominent. The cytoplasm contains a well-developed Golgi complex, mitochondria, a few cisterns of rough-surfaced endoplasmic reticulum, and sparse numbers of lamellar bodies resembling those in normal type II alveolar epithelial cells. In contrast to normal alveolar epithelial cells, the cell in the center is loosely attached to its neighbors. X 18, 800.

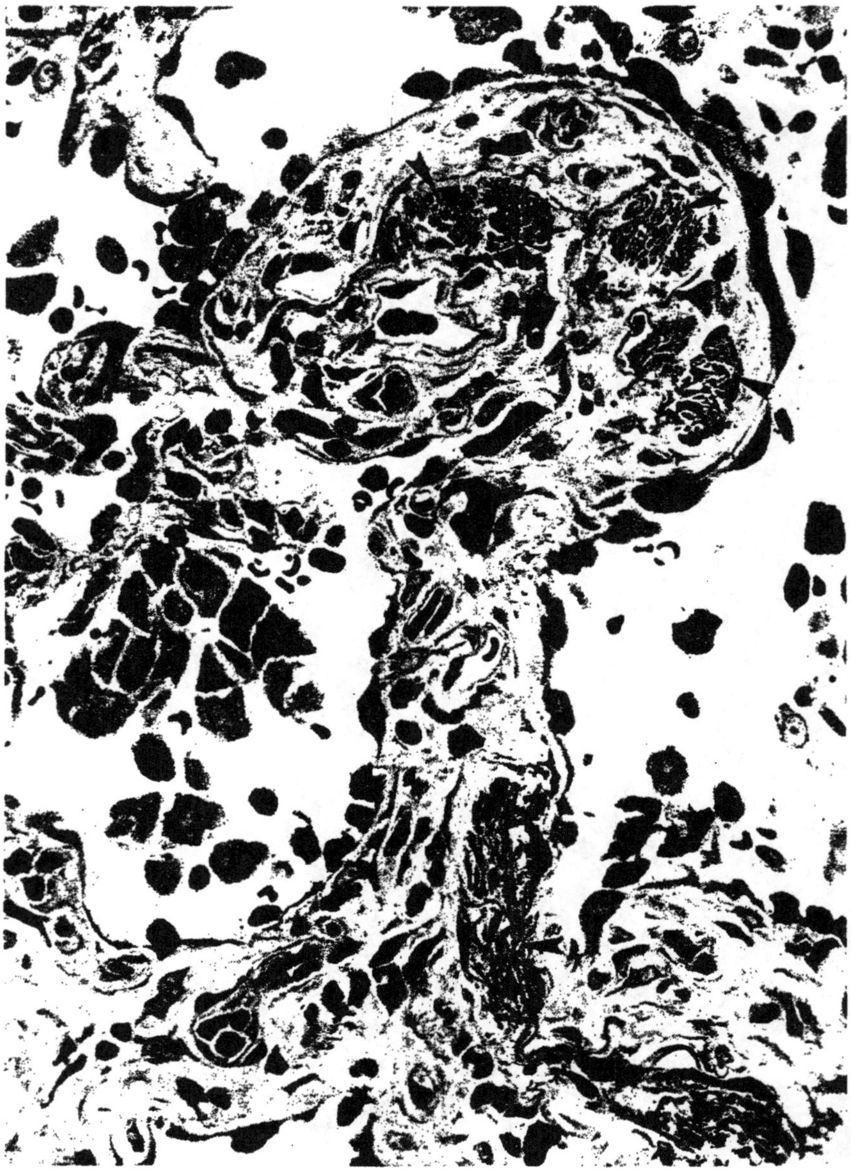

Fig. 9. Several clusters of smooth muscle cells (arrowheads) are present in widened, fibrotic pulmonary interstitium of patient with IPF. These smooth muscle cells are not related to blood vessels, from which they are clearly separated. The alveoli contain numerous macrophages and are lined by epithelial cells of various shapes. Half-micron-thick section of plastic-embedded tissue, alkaline toludine blue stain, X 1, 000.

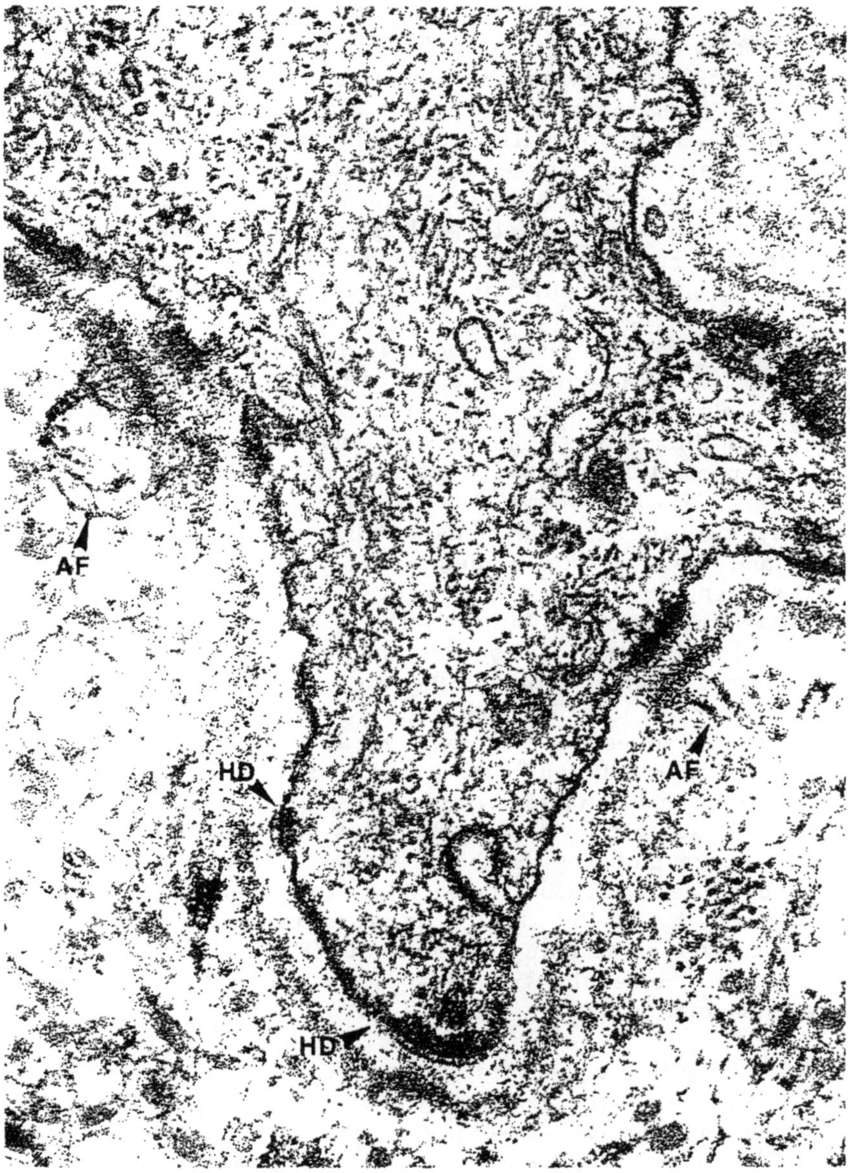

Fig. 10. Basal portion of cuboidal alveolar epithelial cell from patient with IPF shows abundant cytoplasmic filaments; several hemidesmosomes (HD) forming attachments between the plasma membrane and the basement membrane; anchoring fibrils (AF); and surrounding connective tissue containing collagen fibrils, connective tissue microfibrils and proteoglycan-like material. The anchoring fibrils [26] form arcs, the ends of which spread out fan-like and insert into the basement membrane; the banding pattern of anchoring fibrils differs from that of collagen fibrils. X 76,000.

alter collagen indirectly by affecting the parenchymal cells which normally synthesize and destroy collagen.

The effector cells that carry out these roles are present in the alveolar structures of the IPF lung in the following relative proportions: macrophages > lymphocytes and neutrophils > eosinophils and mast cells [4, 24, 34]. Although the relationship between these effector cells and the fibrosis of IPF has not been proven in all situations, convincing data have accumulated implicating certain dominant pathogenic processes. In many instances, the pathogenic process requires interdependence between different effector cells, but for convenience, we will discuss each cell separately.

Lymphocytes. The relative proportion of lymphocytes in the parenchyma of patients with IPF is normal, but since the number of inflammatory and immune effector cells is increased, the total number of lymphocytes (per alveolus) is also increased [4, 24, 34]. Although direct evaluation of the lymphocyte subpopulations in the IPF parenchyma has demonstrated that the proportions of T- and B-lymphocytes are normal, it is likely that at least certain lymphocyte subpopulations are different from those in normals. For example, there is some evidence that lymphocytes from patients with IPF recognize collagen as "non-self" and produce lymphokines such as macrophage migration inhibition factor (MIF) in response to it [29]. The mechanisms by which this occurs are not clear, but the T-lymphocyte is required in some fashion, since its removal completely obviates this phenomenon, at least in vitro.

Although completely untested, there are two additional roles that lymphocytes might play in relation to the fibrosis of IPF. First, there is evidence in guinea pigs that activated lymphocytes can "turn on" macrophages such that they secrete increased quantities of collagenase [37]. Second, evidence is accumulating that lymphocytes, in cooperation with monoclear phagocytic cells, produce factor(s) that suppress mesenchymal cell collagen synthesis by 30-40% [39]. Thus, it is theoretically possible that one fibrosis-related pathogenic mechanism in IPF is the loss of this suppressive effect and the resultant increased production of collagen by at least some mesenchymal cells.

Macrophages. As with lymphocytes, the relative proportion of macrophages in the IPF lung is not increased, but compared to normal lung, the total number of macrophages per alveolus is greatly elevated (Figs. 1-3, 9, 11) [4, 24, 34]. The reason why there are more macrophages present is not clear, but one possibility is that macrophages are induced to stay in affected alveoli by the influence of MIF produced by lymphocytes in the local area [29]. Since alveolar macrophages produce a collagenase capable of attacking types I and III collagen [20], one consequence of an increase in the numbers of macrophages per alveolus would be an imbalance in the maintenance of interstitial collagen toward collagen destruction. Further evidence that this might occur comes from the finding that 70% of patients with IPF have active collagenase in their lower respiratory tract while normals have none [28].

Recent evaluation of alveolar macrophages recovered from these patients suggests that the macrophage likely plays a critical role in the pathogenesis of IPF by recruiting neutrophils to the alveolar structures. This process is apparently mediated through the secretion by the macro-

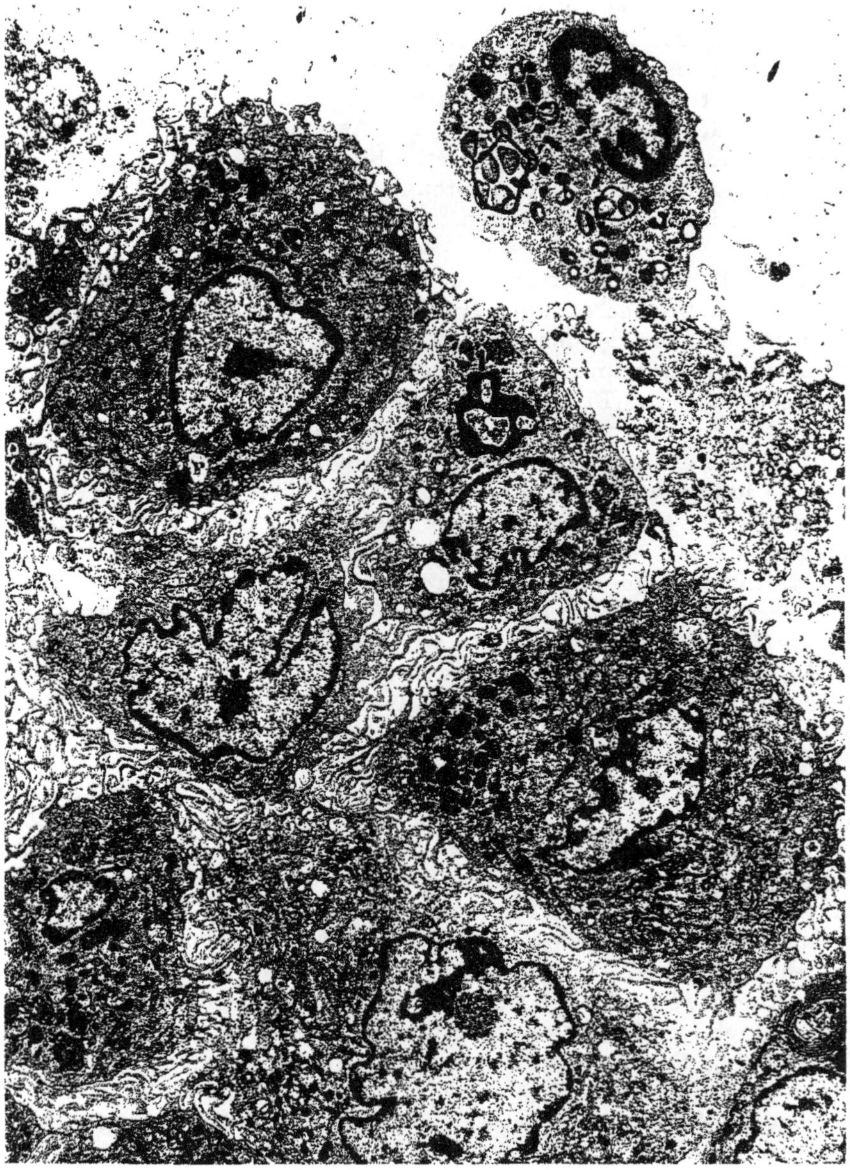

Fig. 11. View of cells in alveolar lumen in patient with IPF (compare with Figs. 1 and 2). The cell at upper right is an eosinophil leukocyte with typical cytoplasmic granules. The other cells are macrophages, characterized by marked irregularities of the contours of their plasma membranes (filopodia) and by their abundance of cytoplasmic dense bodies (lysosomes and residual bodies). X 5, 950.

phage of low-molecular-weight chemotactic factor which selectively attracts neutrophils [12, 23, 27]. Studies of IPF macrophages have shown that they are spontaneously secreting this neutrophil chemotactic factor, possibly mediated by the stimulation of immune complexes present in the lower respiratory tract of these patients [11]. As we will see, the recruitment of neutrophils to the alveoli is of particular importance, as the neutrophil is armed with a variety of proteases that can significantly influence the status of interstitial collagen.

P o l y m o r p h o n u c l e a r L e u k o c y t e s. Although eosinophils (Fig. 11) and mast cells are part of the chronic alveolitis of IPF, their role in the pathogenesis of the disease is unknown. In contrast, not only is there ample evidence that a significant number of neutrophils are present in the lung parenchyma of IPF patients (Fig. 12), but there is reason to believe the neutrophil may play an important role in the fibrosis of IPF.

There are two lines of evidence demonstrating a significant number of neutrophils in the lower respiratory tract of patients with IPF [24, 34]. First, analysis of cells recovered by bronchoalveolar lavage of these patients demonstrates that 10-20% of the cells recovered are neutrophils. Second, more definitive evidence comes from direct analysis of lung biopsies from these patients in which approximately 8% of the total inflammatory and immune effector cells recovered are neutrophils. Since these biopsies are sterile, and since they include rare airways relative to the number of alveoli, the neutrophils are undoubtedly part of the cells within the alveolar structures.

Unlike the macrophage, the neutrophil is a short-lived cell, suggesting neutrophil traffic in IPF from blood to alveoli must be large indeed. Since one consequence of neutrophil "death" is the release of proteolytic enzymes, it is likely that the presence of large numbers of neutrophils within the IPF parenchyma is associated with the release of relatively large quantities of collagenase, elastase and cathepsin-G, all of which are stored in neutrophil granules [25]. The consequences of having increased quantities of such enzymes within the interstitium are many, but two are particularly relevant to the disordered collagen that is part of the fibrosis of IPF. First, since neutrophil collagenase selectively attacks type I collagen over type III collagen [20], neutrophil collagenase may be responsible for some of the fraying of type I collagen seen on electron micrographs of the IPF interstitium. The finding that IPF patients have a collagenase in their lower respiratory tract active against type I collagen is consistent with this concept [28]. Second, there is recent evidence that fibronectin, a cell-surface macromolecule thought to be partially responsible for maintaining cell-cell and cell-connective tissue interactions, is particularly sensitive to destruction by neutrophil proteases such as elastase [33]. Thus, the presence of neutrophils in the IPF parenchyma may explain, in part, the mechanism by which parenchymal cells become topologically deranged in this disease, thus contributing to the disordering of collagen deposition that is so characteristic of the fibrosis of IPF.

The fact that IPF is a non-infectious disorder yet chronically associated with a significant number of neutrophils in the alveolar structures is so striking that IPF is now considered a chronic "neutrophil-accumulation" disorder of lung.

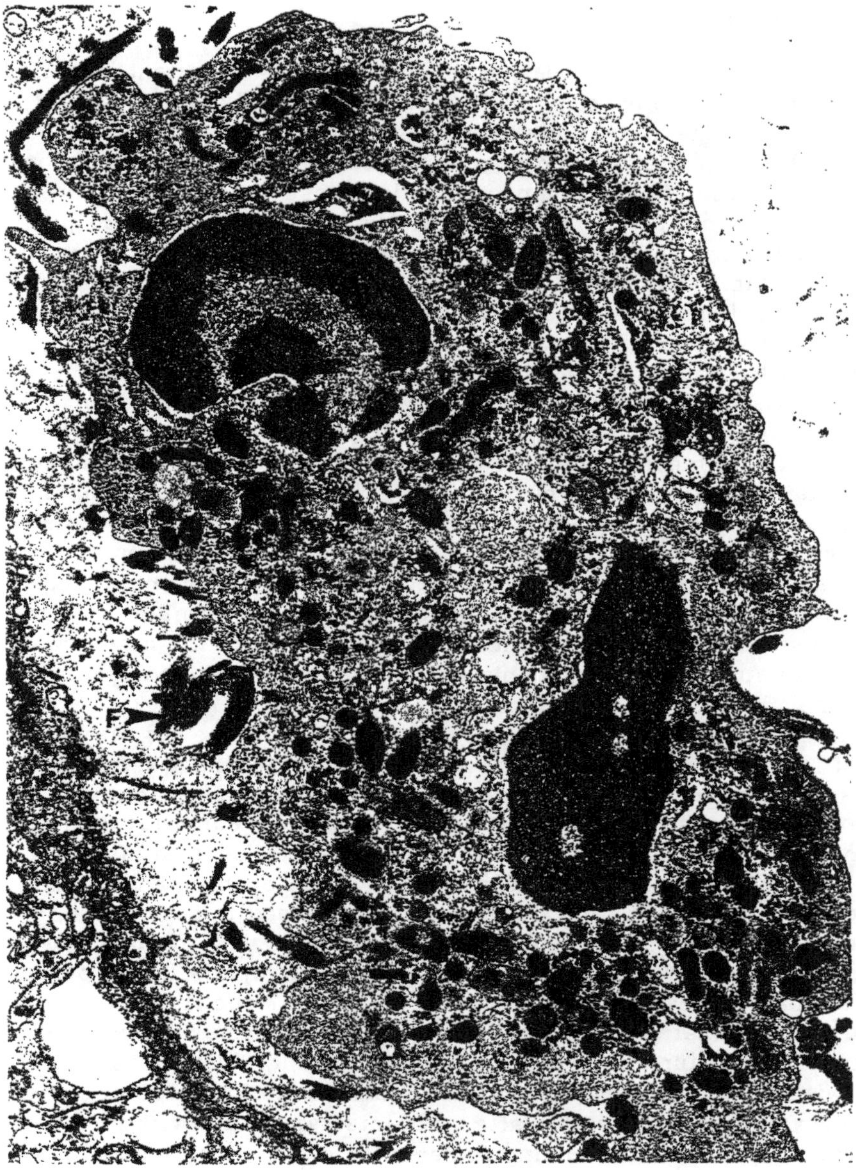

Fig. 12. Polymorphonuclear neutrophil leukocyte in fibrotic alveolar septum of patient with IPF is adjacent to collagen fibrils (upper right), strands of fibrin (F) and the basal portion of an alveolar epithelial cell (lower left). X 17, 600.

Clinical Considerations

It is clear from this discussion that, to stage and follow a patient with IPF, the clinician would like to have methods that independently and repeatedly assess the fibrosis, the alterations in parenchymal cells and the chronic alveolitis which are characteristic of this disease in mid-course. The open lung biopsy, of course, is one means of making these assessments, but biopsies are usually not performed sequentially, and it is difficult to quantitate the morphologic changes routinely. Although biopsy is currently the only method available to evaluate the alterations in parenchymal cells in IPF, recent methods have been developed to assess semiquantitatively the fibrosis and the alveolitis of this disease.

In a study of twenty-three patients with IPF in which the relative amount of fibrosis present in the biopsy was compared to a variety of physiologic monitors of the disease process, it became apparent that the results of traditional measurements such as volumes and diffusing capacity bore little relation to the degree of fibrosis [10]. In contrast, a number of parameters describing the deflation volume-pressure relationship of these patients (e.g., compliance at functional residual capacity, maximum transpulmonary pressure/total lung capacity), as well as parameters derived from steady-state exercise studies, did appear to correlate with the extent of fibrosis in each patient. Since exercise testing is the more routine of these two studies, it is probably the best available physiologic method to stage the fibrosis of IPF patients.

Two methods have been developed to stage and follow the degree of alveolitis of IPF, both of which are directly aimed at getting a semiquantitative measure of the number of neutrophils in the alveolar structures. The first is the analysis of the cells recovered by bronchoalveolar lavage [34]. As mentioned previously, the proportion of neutrophils found in lavage fluid closely parallels that found by direct analysis of open lung biopsies. The advantage of bronchoalveolar lavage is that it is easily performed, readily accepted by patients and carries little, if any, risk of morbidity if done carefully. Second, the relative number of neutrophils in the parenchyma of IPF patients can be assessed with gallium-67 rectilinear scans [31]. When conventional scanning methods are used, normal individuals do not accumulate gallium-67 in their lung parenchyma. In contrast, 70% of patients with IPF demonstrate significant quantities of this isotope within the parenchymal structures 48 h after administration. As with bronchoalveolar lavage, gallium-67 scanning is repeatable and carries little risk other than minor radiation exposure.

Therapy of IPF. The current concepts of the therapy of IPF involve attacking the disease in as early a stage as possible in the pathogenic process. Although it is theoretically attractive to think that at least some of the fibrosis of IPF could be prevented by agents that inhibit collagen synthesis, there is no agent available which will selectively provide this function in lung while sparing other organs [17]. Since collagen is the most abundant protein in the body, agents which inhibit collagen synthesis, secretion or maturation have significant "toxic" effects elsewhere, particularly in bone, where collagen is normally turning over at a rapid rate. Although some studies have suggested that such agents may be effective in experimental pulmonary fibrosis in animals [17], there is no evidence that these results can be directly transferred to the therapy of human disease.

More rational is the concept that IPF is vulnerable to attack by halting the chronic alveolits of the disorder. For several years, corticosteroids have been the mainstay of treatment of IPF [4, 6], and it is likely that their efficacy in slowing the progression of the disorder is through their anti-inflammatory properties. As evidence has accumulated that the alveolitis of IPF may also be mediated through immune mechanisms, clinicians have sought agents with broader anti-immune and anti-inflammatory actions than corticosteroids alone [6]. Although there are several anecdotal reports of the efficacy of immunosuppressive agents in IPF, there has only been one prospective double-blind study of corticosteroids alone vs. corticosteroids and azathioprine in the therapy of this disorder [9]. In the preliminary analysis of this data from twenty-seven patients followed over a one-year period, there was no additive effect of azathioprine in any of twenty-one parameters followed. This, together with the increased toxicity from an agent such as azathioprine, suggests that, at least for now, there is no proven role for immunosuppressive agents in the therapy of this disorder. In the Pulmonary Branch at the National Heart, Lung, and Blood Institute, we have several ongoing studies of other anti-inflammatory and anti-immune therapies in the treatment of these patients, but the results of these studies are not yet available.

References

1. Bradley, K., McConnell-Breul, S., Crystal, R. G.: Collagen in the human lung: Composition and quantitation of rates of synthesis. J. Clin. Invest. 55, 543-550 (1975)
2. Bradley, K. H., McConnell-Breul, S. D., Crystal, R. G.: Lung collagen composition and synthesis: Characterization and changes with age. J. Biol. Chem. 249, 2674-2683 (1974)
3. Bradley, K. H., McConnell-Breul, S. D., Crystal, R. G.: Lung collagen heterogeneity. Proc. Nat. Acad. Sci. 71, 2828-2832 (1974)
4. Crystal, R. G., Fulmer, J. D., Roberts, W. C., Moss, M. L., Line, B. R., Reynolds, H. Y.: Idiopathic pulmonary fibrosis: Clinical, histologic, radiographic, physiologic, scintigraphic, cytologic, and biochemical aspects. Ann. Int. Med. 85, 769-788 (1976)
5. Fulmer, J. D., Bienkowski, R. S., Cowan, M. J., Breul, S. D., Bradley, K. H., Ferrans, V. J., Roberts, W. C., Crystal, R. G.: Collagen concentration and rates of synthesis in idiopathic pulmonary fibrosis. (Unpublished ms.)
6. Fulmer, J. D., Crystal, R. G.: Interstitial Lung Disease. In: Current Pulmonology, vol. 1 (ed. D. H. Simmons), Pacific Palisades, California: Pinecliff Medical Publishing Company, 1978
7. Fulmer, J. D., Crystal, R. G.: The Biochemical Basis of Pulmonary Function. In: The Biochemical Basis of Pulmonary Function, pp. 419-466 (ed. R. G. Crystal). New York, Marcel Dekker, 1976
8. Fulmer, J., Elson, N., Bradley, K., Ferrans, V., Crystal, R. G.: Comparison of type-specific collagens synthesized by lung epithelial and mesenchymal cells. Clin. Res. 25, 416A (1977)

9. Fulmer, J., Elson, N., Von Gal, E., McLees, B., DeMets, D., Weinberger, S., Kelman, J., Crystal, R. G.: Treatment of idiopathic pulmonary fibrosis (IPF). Clin. Res. 26, 538A (1978)
10. Fulmer, J. D., Von Gal, E. R., Roberts, W. C., Crystal, R. G.: Morphologic-physiologic correlates of the severity of fibrosis in idiopathic pulmonary fibrosis. (Unpublished ms.)
11. Gadek, J., Hunninghake, G., Lawley, T., Kelman, J., Fulmer, J., Crystal, R. G.: Role of immune complexes in amplifying the alveolitis of idiopathic pulmonary fibrosis (IPF). Clin. Res. 26, 446A (1978)
12. Gadek, J., Hunninghake, G., Zimmerman, R., Crystal, R.: Mechanisms controlling release of neutrophil chemotactic factor by alveolar macrophages. Amer. Rev. Respir. Dis. 117 (Suppl.), 65 (1978)
13. Hamman, L., Rich, A. R.: Acute diffuse interstitial fibrosis of the lung. Bull. Johns Hopkins Hosp. 74, 177-212 (1944)
14. Hance, A. J., Bradley, K., Crystal, R. G.: Lung collagen heterogeneity. Synthesis of type I and type III collagen by rabbit and human lung cells in culture. J. Clin. Invest. 57, 102-111 (1976)
15. Hance, A. J., Crystal, R. G.: Collagen. In: The Biochemical Basis of Pulmonary Function, pp. 215-271 (ed. R. G. Crystal). New York, Marcel Dekker, 1976
16. Hance, A. J., Crystal, R. G.: Rigid control of the synthesis of collagen Types I and III by cells in culture. Nature 268, 152-154 (1977)
17. Hance, A. J., Crystal, R. G.: The connective tissue of lung. Amer. Rev. Respir. Dis. 112, 657-711 (1975)
18. Horwitz, A. L., Crystal, R. G.: Collagenase from rabbit pulmonary alveolar macrophages. Biochem. Biophys. Res. Commun. 69, 296-303 (1976)
19. Horwitz, A. L., Elson, N. A., Crystal, R. G.: Proteoglycans and Elastin. In: The Biochemical Basis of Pulmonary Function, pp. 273-311 (ed. R. G. Crystal). New York, Marcel Dekker, 1976
20. Horwitz, A. L., Hance, A. J., Crystal, R. G.: Granulocyte collagenase: Selective digestion of type I over type III collagen. Proc. Nat. Acad. Sci., 1977, 74, 897-901 (1977)
21. Horwitz, A. L., Kelman, J. A., Crystal, R. G.: Activation of alveolar macrophage collagenase by a neutral protease secreted by the same cell. Nature 264, 772-774 (1976)
22. Howard, B. V., Macarak, E. J., Gunson, D., Kefalides, N. A.: Characterization of the collagen synthesized by endothelial cells in culture. Proc. Nat. Acad. Sci. 73, 2361-2364 (1976)
23. Hunninghake, G. W., Gallin, J. I., Fauci, A. S.: Immunologic reactivity of the lung. The in vivo and in vitro generation of a neutrophil chemotactic factor by alveolar macrophages. Amer. Rev. Respir. Dis. 117, 15-23 (1978)
24. Hunninghake, G. W., Kelman, J. A., Gadek, J. E., Elson, N. A., Fulmer, J. D., Crystal, R. G.: Comparison of inflammatory and immune effector cell populations in lavage fluid and lung biopsies of patients with pulmonary fibrosis. Amer. Rev. Respir. Dis. 117 (Suppl.), 68 (1978)

25. Janoff, A.: At least three human neutrophil lysosomal proteases are capable of degrading joint connective tissue. Ann. New York Acad. Sci. 256, 402-408 (1975)
26. Kawanami, O., Ferrans, V. J., Roberts, W. C, Crystal, R. G., Fulmer, J. D.: Anchoring fibrils: A new connective tissue structure in fibrotic lung disease. Amer. J. Pathol. 92, 127-148 (1978)
27. Kazmierowski, J. A., Gallin, J. I., Reynolds, H. Y.: Mechanism for the inflammatory response in primate lungs. Demonstration and partial characterization of an alveolar macrophage-derived chemotactic factor with preferential activity for polymorphonuclear leukocytes. J. Clin. Invest. 59, 273-281 (1977)
28. Kelman, J., Weinberger, S., Fulmer, J., Reynolds, H., Crystal, R. G.: Connective tissue specific enzymes of bronchoalveolar fluid in idiopathic pulmonary fibrosis (IPF). Clin. Res. 25, 503A (1977)
29. Kravis, T. C., Ahmed, A., Brown, T. E., Fulmer, J. D., Crystal, R. G.: Pathogenic mechanisms in pulmonary fibrosis: Collagen induced migration inhibition factor production and cytotoxicity mediated by lymphocytes. J. Clin. Invest. 58, 1223-1232 (1976)
30. Kuhn, C.: The cells of the lung and their organelles. In: The Biochemical Basis of Pulmonary Function, pp. 3-48 (ed. R. G. Crystal). New York, Marcel Dekker, 1976
31. Line, B. R., Fulmer, J. D., Reynolds, H. Y., Roberts, W. C., Jones, A. E., Harris, E. K., Crystal, R. G.: Gallium-67 citrate scanning in the staging of idiopathic pulmonary fibrosis: Correlation with physiology, morphology and bronchoalveolar lavage. Amer. Rev. Respir. Dis. 118, 355-365 (1978)
32. Mayne, R., Vail, M. S., Miller, E. J.: Characterization of the collagen chains synthesized by cultured smooth muscle cells derived from rhesus monkey thoracic aorta. Biochemistry 17, 446-452 (1978)
33. McDonald, J., Baum, B., Rosenberg, D., Kelman, J., Senior, R., Crystal, R. G.: Fibronectin, the major cell surface protein of cultured human lung fibroblasts: Destruction of structure and biological activity by human neutrophil proteinases. Amer. Rev. Respir. Dis. 117 (Suppl.), 170 (1978)
34. Reynolds, H. Y., Fulmer, J. D., Kazmierowski, J. A., Roberts, W. C., Frank, M. M., Crystal, R. G.: Analysis of broncho-alveolar lavage fluid from patients with idiopathic pulmonary fibrosis and chronic hypersensitivity pneumonitis. J. Clin. Invest. 59, 165-175 (1977)
35. Seyer, J. M., Hutcheson, E. T., Kang, A. H.: Collagen polymorphism in idiopathic chronic pulmonary fibrosis. J. Clin. Invest. 57, 1498-1507 (1976)
36. Spencer, H.: Chronic interstitial pneumonia. In: The Lung, pp. 134-150, (ed. A. A. Liebow and D. E. Smith). Baltimore: Williams and Wilkins, 1968
37. Wahl, L. M., Wahl, S. M., Mergenhagen, S. E., Martin, G. R.: Collagenase production by lymphokine-activated macrophages. Science 187, 261-263 (1975)

38. Weibel, E. R., Gehr, P., Haies, D., Gil, J., Bachofen, M.: The cell population of the normal lung. In: Lung Cells in Disease, pp 3-16 (ed. A. Bouhuys). New York: North-Holland, 1976
39. Weinberger, S., Fells, G., Bradley, K., Hunninghake, G., Gadek, J., Crystal, R. G.: Mononuclear cell-fibroblast interactions in the synthesis of lung collagen. Amer. Rev. Respir. Dis. 117 (Suppl.), 84 (1978)
40. Werb, Z., Reynolds, J. J.: Purification and properties of a specific collagenase from rabbit synovial fibroblasts. Biochem. J. 151, 645-653 (1975)

Pulmonary Arteries in Congenital Heart Disease: A Structure-Function Analysis

Renu Virmani, M.D. and William C. Roberts, M.D.

For many years students of congenital heart disease were unable to explain the lack of survival patterns in patients with similar-sized, isolated communications between systemic and pulmonary circulations. Although in 1927 Moschcowitz[1] suggested that the explanation may be the result of pulmonary hypertension, hemodynamic and histologic studies during the past 30 years of the pulmonary vessels have helped enormously in explaining these differences. In 1935 Oscar Brenner in Birmingham, England, described histologic features of the normal pulmonary arteries and veins.[2] A year later Parker and Weiss,[3] at Boston City Hospital, described changes in the lungs and blood vessels in patients with mitral stenosis. Jesse Edwards, who also trained at Boston City Hospital in the late 1930s, began describing anatomic changes in the pulmonary vasculature in patients with congenital heart disease in the late 1940s; he too attributed the changes to the effects of pulmonary hypertension. Edwards, his colleagues, and many others described changes in a variety of congenital cardiac diseases,[4–45] and by 1958 a classification of the hypertensive pulmonary changes was formulated.[13] The recognition of the intimate association between the lung and the heart has been a major contribution to the understanding of congenital heart disease. Today it is well known that the state of the lung is the primary determinant of operability in a patient with a shunt. This chapter describes changes observed in the pulmonary vessels of adults with certain congenital cardiovascular malformations.

ANATOMIC CLASSIFICATION OF PULMONARY ARTERIAL HYPERTENSIVE CHANGES IN CONGENITAL HEART DISEASE

The anatomic classification of pulmonary hypertensive changes by Heath and Edwards[13] was based primarily on observations of patients with large ventricular septal defects, but it also was based on studies of a few patients with large patent ductus arteriosus and other defects associated with a free communication between the systemic and pulmonary circulations which causes *pulmonary hypertension from birth.** Their study also included a few patients with primary pulmonary hypertension.

The classification of Heath and Edwards is reproduced in Table 1. Although their classification of histologic changes observed in the pulmonary arteries in patients with

Table 1. Classification of hypertensive pulmonary vascular changes by Heath and Edwards in 1958.[13] (Reproduced with permission.)

	Change	Grade of hypertensive pulmonary vascular disease: 1	2	3	4	5	6
Type of intimal reaction	None	← None →					
	Cellular		←	—	Cellular —	—	→
	Fibrous and fibroelastic			←	Fibrous and fibroelastic —	—	→
	Plexiform lesion				←	Plexiform lesion —	→
State of media of arteries and arterioles	Hypertrophied	←	—	Hypertrophied —	—	—	→
	Some generalized dilatation			←	Some generalized dilatation —	—	→
	Local "dilatation lesions"*				←	Local "dilatation lesions"* —	→
	Pulmonary hemosiderosis†					← Pulmonary hemosiderosis†	→
	Necrotizing arteritis						← Necrotizing arteritis →

*Vein-like branches of hypertrophied muscular pulmonary arteries, angiomatoid lesion, and cavernous lesion

†Associated with distended, thin-walled, arterial vessels throughout the lung

pulmonary hypertension brought organization to a complex, previously unorganized subject, on re-evaluation, it is now apparent, 20 years later, that their classification has certain deficiencies. Considerable overlap exists between their grades 2 and 3, and between their grades 4 and 5. *Alveolar hemosiderosis* (grade 5) does not concern a pulmonary artery and is common in patients without pulmonary arterial hypertension. In our view, a classification of pulmonary arterial changes should not include changes in alveolar spaces (hemosiderosis). The grade 6 category implies that grades 1 through 5 are prerequisites, when, in actuality, necrotizing vasculitis may occur in the absence of grades 1 to 5. It seems to us that a classification of hypertensive changes in the pulmonary arteries should be applicable to all patients with pulmonary hypertension irrespective of cause and irrespective of whether the hypertension is congenital or acquired.

The classification of pulmonary arterial changes used herein is based entirely on the histologic alterations observed independent of etiology, time of appearance, and hemodynamic documentation of the pulmonary arterial pressure (Fig. 1). The major changes in the pulmonary arteries include: (1) *medial thickening* (MT), (2) *intimal thickening* (IT), and (3) *plexiform lesions* (PL). Only MT is grade I; MT and IT are grade II; and MT and IT with PL are grade III. We do not include arteritis (vasculitis), either necrotizing or non-necrotizing, in the grading system since pulmonary arteritis may occur in the absence of pulmonary hypertension.

Histologic Features of Normal Pulmonary Vessels

Much has been written on this subject.[1,9,13,25,45,–47] Table 2 summarizes some of the features of normal adult pulmonary vessels. The extrapulmonary arteries, i.e., the pulmonary trunk and right and left main pulmonary arteries, are *elastic* arteries. At birth the media of the pulmonary trunk consists of parallel elastic lamellae which are identical in number and configuration to those in the media of ascending aorta (Fig. 2). If the pulmonary arterial pressure falls to its normal level in the first few weeks of life, the thickness of the wall of the pulmonary trunk and its branches diminishes, and the number of elastic lamellae decrease; those which remain are disrupted (Fig. 2). In between the elastic fibers are smooth muscle cells and collagen fibrils. The integrity of the elastic pulmonary arteries in adults is dependent not on the disrupted elastic fibers

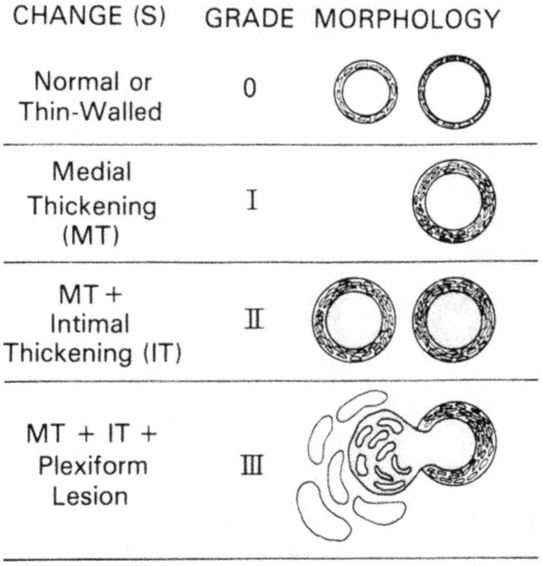

Figure 1. Types and grading of the morphologic pulmonary arterial changes in the patients studied (see text).

but on the integrity of the smooth muscle cells and collagen. The elastic pulmonary arteries extend into the lungs to the levels of the intrapulmonary cartilaginous bronchi.

The *muscular* pulmonary arteries begin, obviously, where the elastic arteries end. Although it contains occasional elastic and collagenous fibrils, the media consists predominantly of smooth muscle cells bordered by internal and external elastic membranes. The muscular arteries are adjacent to or associated with the terminal bronchioles, respiratory bronchioles, and alveolar ducts.

The pulmonary *arterioles* are branches of the muscular arteries. Except at their origin from the muscular arteries—where they have a thin muscular media between internal and external elastic membranes—the media is absent. An easily discernible elastic membrane covered by a single layer of endothelial cells borders the lumen. The arteriole divides into *capillaries* which course directly into the alveolar septa. The walls of the capillaries consist primarily of a single layer of endothelial cells covered by basement membrane. The capillary has a spiraling course within the alveolar septum rather than running parallel to the lining of the adjacent alveolus, as was originally believed.[3]

The capillaries drain into the pulmonary *venules* which are larger than, but virtually identical in structure to the capillaries: they consist of an endothelial layer covered by an elastic membrane. The *veins* have a thicker internal elastic membrane and are bordered by several irregularly arranged bundles of smooth muscle cells interspersed with collagenous fibrils and elastic fibrils.

The *bronchial arteries* are located within the walls of the bronchi, but otherwise are similar to the muscular pulmonary arteries. The *bronchial veins* also are in the bronchial walls and have thinner walls and larger lumens than the bronchial arteries. *Lymphatics* are present adjacent to pulmonary arteries and bronchi and in the interlobular septa and subpleural areas.

Histologic Features and Proposed Causes of Abnormal Pulmonary Arteries

Medial Thickening

This applies to an increase in the thickness of the media, either in the wall of the pulmonary artery or in the proximal portion of the pulmonary arteriole. Whether this

Table 2. Histologic features of normal pulmonary vessels in adults

		Media			*Lumen Diameter*	*Internal*	*External*	
	External Diameter	*Elastic Fibers (0–4)*	*SM Cells (0–4)*	*Collagen (0–4)*	*÷ Wall Thickness*	*Elastic Membrane*	*Elastic Membrane*	*Adventitia (0–4)*
Extrapulmonary Arteries								
Pulmonary trunk	1.6 cm.	+ + + +	+ +	+		+	+	+
Right main PA	1.3 cm.	+ + + +	+ +	+		+	+	+
Left main PA	1.3 cm.	+ + + +	+ +	+		+	+	+
Intrapulmonary Vessels								
Elastic arteries	>1000μ	+ + +	+ +	+	10	+	+	+
Muscular arteries	100–1000μ	+	+ + + +	+	4	+	+	+
Arterioles	<100μ	0	0*	0	6	+	0	+ +
Capillaries	<10μ	0	0	0		0**	0	0
Venules	10–100μ	0	0	0		+	0	+ +
Veins	>100μ	+ +	+	+ +	4	+	0	+ + +
Bronchial arteries	100–300μ	+	+ + + +	+	4	+	±	+
Bronchial veins		0	+	+	2	+	0	+
Lymphatic channels		0	0	0		0***	0	0

*A thin muscular media is present in its most proximal portion
**Endothelial layer plus basement membranes
***Actually an endothelial lining rather than an internal elastic membrane
SM = smooth muscle

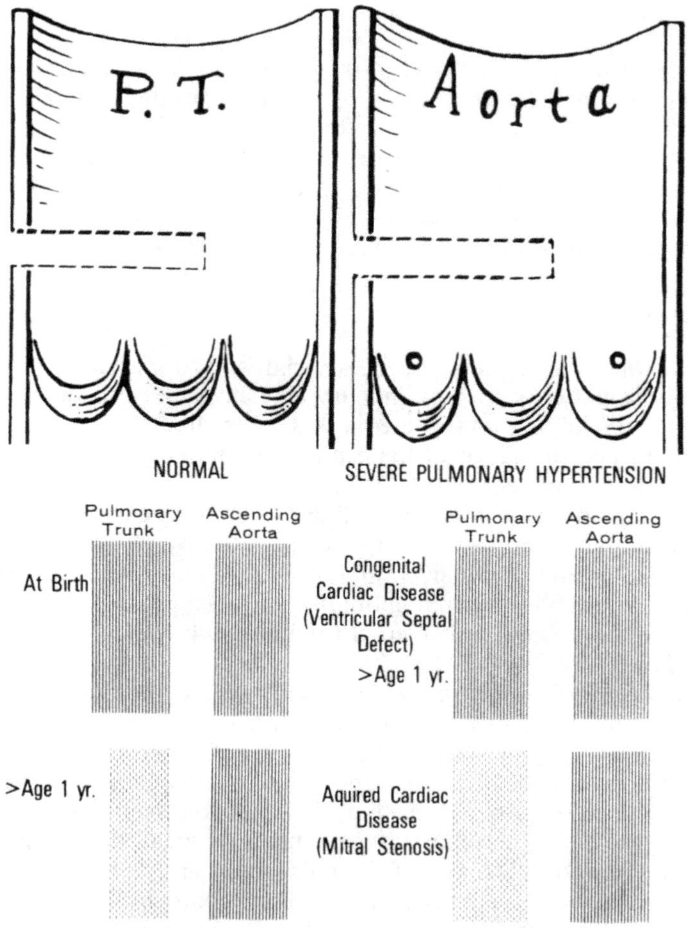

Figure 2. Configuration of elastic fibers in the pulmonary trunk at birth, after 1 year of age, with pulmonary hypertension from birth (VSD), and with an acquired condition (mitral stenosis). The sketch (top) shows the sites in the pulmonary trunk (P.T.) and aorta at which the sections for histologic examination were taken. At birth the configuration of the elastic fibers in both the pulmonary trunk and ascending aorta are identical and wall thicknesses are similar. Normally, after a year of age the number of elastic fibers in the pulmonary trunk diminishes considerably to reach an "adult configuration," and the thickness of the wall also diminishes. If a large VSD or aorticopulmonary defect is present from birth, both the configuration of the elastic fibers and wall thickness of the pulmonary trunk remains similar to that of the ascending aorta ("fetal configuration"). If pulmonary hypertension is acquired later in life, however, as in mitral stenosis, the configuration of the elastic fibers of the pulmonary trunk remains like that of the normal adult but wall thickness increases. The information on the configuration of elastic fibers in the pulmonary trunk is based on original work by Heath and associates.[69]

occurs entirely from hypertrophy of smooth muscle cells or whether both hypertrophy and hyperplasia cause the thickening is unclear.

Intimal Thickening

There are two types of intimal thickening—cellular and acellular. In the cellular variety the proliferated intima consists primarily of strap cells with collagen in between. The strap cells appear to be primarily smooth muscle cells. The acellular variety consists mostly of dense fibrous tissue (collagen) with minimal smooth muscle cells or none at all.

Plexiform Lesion

This is an aneurysmal or glomus-like structure which emerges at a right angle from a muscular pulmonary artery. The beginning of the right-angle branch is usually apparent; from there it rapidly dilates into a plexus of channels, the walls of which consist primarily of fibrous tissue covered by endothelial cells. The plexiform structure ends by giving off thin-walled channels, which probably are dilated arterioles; these branch quickly into alveolar septal capillaries. When these thin-walled channels are considerably dilated they are sometimes called *dilatation lesions*.

Proposed Causes

Medial thickening is a response of the arterial wall to increased pressure and therefore occurs only in patients with pulmonary arterial hypertension. As mentioned earlier, whether the thickening of the media is a consequence of hypertrophy alone, of hypertrophy and hyperplasia, or of hyperplasia alone, is unclear. Medial thickening is never simply a normal consequence of aging.

Intimal thickening, be it cellular or acellular, is not necessarily the consequence of pulmonary arterial hypertension, but it is accelerated by elevation of pulmonary arterial pressure. Cellular and acellular intimal proliferation is observed commonly in older persons, most of whom have normal pulmonary arterial pressures.[47] The occurrence of intimal thickening combined with medial thickening, however, is indicative of pulmonary hypertension.

Plexiform lesions occur only in patients with severe pulmonary hypertension, although some patients with severe pulmonary hypertension do not have them. These lesions can occur in patients with large left-to-right shunts or primary pulmonary hypertension, but do not occur in patients with severe pulmonary hypertension secondary only to left-sided cardiac disease (i.e., mitral stenosis). Plexiform lesions do not occur if the cause of the pulmonary hypertension is located distal to the pulmonary capillary level, or, stated differently, if the pulmonary arterial hypertension is the consequence of pulmonary venous hypertension. For plexiform lesions to occur the cause of the hypertension must orginate at the capillary or precapillary level.[48]

The exact cause of plexiform lesions is unknown. Serial sections of lung at sites of plexiform lesions generally show extreme narrowing or almost total obstruction of the lumen of the muscular pulmonary artery distal to the origin of the small muscular pulmonary artery or arteriole which is the site of the lesions.[25] Kanjuh and colleagues[30] have speculated that the plexiform lesion is a consequence of a *jet lesion* caused by blood rapidly changing its course because of the distal obstruction of the relatively large muscular pulmonary artery distal to the site of the plexiform lesion. Thus, the plexiform lesion might act as a dissipater of the extremely high pulmonary arterial pressure.

Other proposed causes of plexiform lesions are that they represent *sites of anastomoses of pulmonary arteries and veins*[49–52] or that they are a *congenital malformation*.[53,54] The latter theory appears particularly unlikely because plexiform lesions have never been observed in the lungs at birth. The earliest these pulmonary lesions have been observed is 2 months of age;[24,30,55,56] they are rare, however, under the age of 5 years. Another proposal is that the plexiform lesions represent *sites of thrombosis which have subsequently recanalized*.[57,58] Recently, Wagenvoort[45] proposed that plexiform lesions represent sites of necrotizing arteritis and, therefore, *represent healing of a necrotizing inflammatory process*. The arteritis weakens the arterial wall which becomes focally aneurysmal. Fibrin and platelets are deposited in the aneurysm and organization of the resulting thrombus produces multiluminal channels lined by endothelial cells.

We believe that plexiform lesions may represent aneurysms formed at sites of *congenitally underdeveloped or weak media* (analagous to the formation of intracerebral berry aneurysms in systemic hypertension) and that the aneurysm is filled by thrombus which organizes into multiple minute vascular channels. Distal to the weak or thin media, the lumen of the muscular artery is obliterated.

NECROPSY OBSERVATIONS OF PATIENTS OVER AGE 15 YEARS WITH CONGENITAL HEART DISEASE

To secure information on the lungs of adults with congenital cardiovascular anomalies, we reviewed clinical records accessioned in the Pathology Branch of the National Heart, Lung, and Blood Institute of the National Institutes of Health, often re-examining the heart itself and histologic sections of lung. All patients over age 15 with major anomalies of the heart and great vessels associated with a communication between pulmonary and systemic circulations were examined. A few cases were eliminated because histologic sections of lung were not available; a total of 87 patients were analyzed. At least five blocks of lung portions (all larger than 2 by 2 cm.) had been processed in alcohol and xylene and embedded in paraffin from each patient. At least one section of lung from these paraffin blocks was stained by hematoxylin and eosin, and at least one additional section from each paraffin block was stained for elastic fibers by either the Van Gieson or the Movat method. The status of the intrapulmonary pulmonary arteries was determined by histologic examination of each of the stained sections of lung, and the presence or absence of medial thickening, intimal thickening, plexiform lesions, and luminal thrombus was recorded. The presence and frequency of cholesterol-ester granulomas were also recorded.

Operated and Unoperated Patients

Certain clinical and morphologic observations in the 87 study patients are summarized in Tables 3–14. The 87 patients ranged in age from 16 to 83 (mean 34); 47 (54 percent) were women and 40 (46 percent) were men. One or more cardiovascular operations had been performed in 65 patients (75 percent), and observations in this group are summarized in Table 3. The other 22 patients (25 percent) never had a cardiovascular operation, and observations in this group are summarized in Table 4. The 22 unoperated patients ranged in age from 16 to 33 (mean 36), and the 65 operated patients were between 16 and 64 years old (mean 33). In Tables 3 and 4 the patients are grouped by the type of congenital cardiovascular malformation present. Patients with multiple nonobligatory anomalies—those who presumably represent more than a single embryologic defect—are grouped together under the term "complex anomaly;" observations in them are summarized in Table 5.

Patients with Abnormal Pulmonary Arteries

Medial thickening with or without intimal thickening or plexiform lesions was observed in the intrapulmonary pulmonary arteries by examination of lung sections of 44 (50 percent) of the 87 patients. The abnormalities consisted entirely of medial thickening in 6 patients (14 percent), medial and intimal thickening in 25 patients (57 percent), and medial and intimal thickening with plexiform lesions in 13 patients (29 percent). In addition, fibrin or fibrin-platelet thrombi were observed in the lumen of one or more small pulmonary arteries in 31 patients: 12 (39 percent) had neither medial nor intimal thickening, nor plexiform lesions; one or more of these three lesions were present in 19 (61 percent).

Table 3. Observations in 65 necropsy patients with various congenital cardiovascular malformations and one or more cardiovascular operations

Malformation: Sex of Patients/Age Range/Mean Age	*PA Systolic Pressure, mm. Hg*					*Shunts*			*Pulmonary Arterial Changes*				
	<30	*30–60*	*61–90*	*>90*	*U*	*L→R*	*R→L*	*Both*	*None*	*MT only*	*MT + IT*	*PL*	*T*
ASD													
Fossa ovale: 8F/43–64/61	1	4	2	1	0	8	0	0	4	1	3	0	4
Partial AV canal: 5F/21–54/38	1	3	0	0	1	4	0	1	2	1	2	0	2
Sinus venosus: 1M/37	1	0	0	0	0	1	0	0	1	0	0	0	0
VSD: 4F, 2M/16–54/29	0	1	4	1	0	4	1	1	1	2	2	1	2
Patent ductus arteriosus: 2F, 5M/16–44/30	0	0	1	6	0	5	2	0	0	0	1	6	1
VSD + PS (TOF): 5F, 10M/16–53/29	9	0	0	0	6	1	11	3	14	0	0	1	5
VSD + PV atresia: 1F/22	0	0	0	0	1	0	0	1	1	0	0	0	1
Complete transposition + VSD													
With PS: 3F/21–59/32 Without PS: 0	1	0	0	0	2	0	2	1	3	0	0	0	0
Corrected transposition + VSD: 1M/38	0	0	1	0	0	0	0	1	0	0	1	0	1
Double outlet right ventricle: 1F/24	0	1	0	0	0	1	0	0	0	0	1	0	0
Ebstein's anomaly + ASD: 1F, 1M/20–31/25	1	0	0	0	1	0	1	1	0	0	2	0	1
PS with intact VS + ASD: 3F/28–43/36	2	0	0	0	1	0	3	0	3	0	0	0	1
Tricuspid atresia: 1M/27	0	0	0	0	1	0	1	0	1	0	0	0	0
Parachute MV syndrome: 1F/24	0	0	0	1	0	1	0	0	0	0	1	0	0
Complex anomaly: 5F, 5M/16–39/27*	4	0	1	1	4	2	3	5	7	0	2	1	2
TOTALS: 39F, 26M/16–64/33	20	9	9	10	17	27	24	14	37	4	15	9	20

*See Table 5 for additional information on these cases.

ASD = atrial septal defect; AV = atrioventricular; F = female; IT = intimal thickening; L = left; M = male; MT = medial thickening; MV = mitral valve; PA = pulmonary artery; PL = plexiform lesions + MT + IT; PS = pulmonic stenosis; PV = pulmonic valve; R = right; T = thrombi; TOF = tetralogy of Fallot; U = unknown; VS = ventricular septum; VSD = ventricular septal defect.

Table 4. Observations in 22 unoperated necropsy patients with various congenital cardiovascular malformations*

Malformation: Sex of Patients/ Age Range/Mean Age	*PA Systolic Pressure, mm. Hg*					*Shunts*			*Pulmonary Arterial Changes*				
	<30	*30–60*	*61–90*	*>90*	*U*	*L→R*	*R→L*	*Both*	*None*	*MT only*	*MT + IT*	*PL*	*T*
ASD													
Fossa ovale: 5F, 2M/29–83/55	0	1	1	1	4	6	0	1	3	1	2	1	4
Partial AV canal: 0													
Sinus venosus: 1M/58	0	0	0	1†	0	1	0	0	0	0	1	0	1
VSD: 2M/16–37/27	1	0	0	0	1	2	0	0	1	0	1	0	0
PDA: 3F/17–34/21	0	0	0	2	1	0	1	2	0	1	0	2	1
VSD + PS (TOF): 1M/22	0	0	0	0	1	0	1	0	1	0	0	0	1
VSD + PV atresia: 1M/28	0	0	0	0	1	0	0	1	1	0	0	0	0
Complete transposition + VSD													
With PS: 0													
Without PS: 1F, 1M/21–39/30	0	0	0	0	2	1	0	1	0	0	2	0	1
Complex anomaly: 5M, /20–41/26**	0	1	0	1	3	2	2	1	0	0	4	1	3
TOTALS: 9F, 13M/16–83/36	1	2	1	5	13	12	4	6	6	2	10	4	11

*Abbreviations listed in Table 3.

**See Table 5 for additional information on these cases.

†This patient died of carcinoma of the lung; some of this elevation probably is the result of the severe pulmonary cancer.

Table 5. Observations in 15 necropsy patients with complex anomalies*

Patient Age	*Malformation*				*PA Pressure*	*SA Pressure*	*Shunt*		*SA* O_2		*Pulmonary Arterial Changes*				
(years)/Sex	*PS*	*VSD*	*ASD*	*Other*	*mm. Hg (s/d)*	*mm. Hg (s/d)*	*L→R*	*R→L*	*Sat., %*	*OP*	*None*	*MT only*	*MT + IT*	*PL*	*T*
WITHOUT RIGHT VENTRICULAR OUTFLOW OBSTRUCTION															
31/F	0	+	0	CS→LA	75/25	130/75	+	0	81	+	0	0	+	0	+
39/M	0	+	0	COA	105/54	152/64	+	+	87	+	0	0	0	+	0
41/M	0	+	0	PDA + CT + IAA		120/70	0	+		0	0	0	0	+	0
21/M	0	+	0	DORV + CT	92/48	104/64	+	0	90	0	0	0	+	0	0
21/M	0	+	0	DORV + CT		102/64	+	0	90	0	0	0	+	0	0
WITH RIGHT VENTRICULAR OUTFLOW OBSTRUCTION															
33/M	+	0	+	AS		80/62	+	+	81	+	+	0	0	0	0
19/M	+	0	+	RPV→RA	18/9	144/78	+	+	97	+	+	0	0	0	0
20/M	+	0	+	AV canal		180/100	0	+		0	0	0	+	0	+
25/F	+	+	+	AS		100/65	0	+	61	+	+	0	0	0	+
38/F	+	+	0	CT		125/48	0	+	62	+	0	0	+	0	0
17/M	+**	+	+	DORV, CT	20/12	90/60	+	0	93	+	+	0	0	0	0
22/F	+**	+	0	SV	15/6	100/65	+	+	81	+	+	0	0	0	0
16/M	+**	+	0	SV + CT		100/75	+	+	51	+	+	0	0	0	0
25/M	+	0	+	TAPVC	55/20	110/50	+	+	72	0	0	0	+	0	0
17/M	+**	0	+	TAPVC	20/8	95/60	0	+	92	+	+	0	0	0	+

*Last category in Tables 3 and 4.

**Subvalvular

AS = aortic stenosis; ASD = atrial septal defect; AV = atrioventricular; COA = coarctation of aorta; CS = coronary sinus; CT = corrected transposition; DORV = double outlet right ventricle; F = female; IT = intimal thickening; L = left; LA = left atrium; M = male; MT = medial thickening; OP = cardiovascular operation; PA = pulmonary artery; PDA = patent ductus arteriosus; PL = plexiform lesion + MT + IT; PS = pulmonic stenosis; R = right; RA = right atrium; RPV = right pulmonic vein; RV = right ventricle; SA = systemic artery; Sat. = saturation; s/d = systolic/diastolic; SV = single ventricle; T = thrombi; TAPVC = total anomalous pulmonary venous connection; VSD = ventricular septal defect.

Pulmonary Arterial Systolic Pressure and Shunt Direction

Of the 57 patients in whom pulmonary arterial pressures were recorded, the systolic pressure was ≤ 30 mm. Hg in 21 (37 percent); 30 to 60 mm. Hg in 11 (19 percent); 61 to 90 mm. Hg in 10 (18 percent); and > 90 mm. Hg in 15 (26 percent). All 87 patients had one or more communications between systemic and pulmonary circulations and were comprised as follows: (1) 39 patients with left-to-right shunt only (Tables 6 through 8); (2) 28 patients with right-to-left shunt only (Tables 6, 7, and 9); and (3) 20 patients with both left-to-right and right-to-left shunts (Tables 6, 7, and 9). Right ventricular outflow obstruction occurred in 36 (41 percent) of the 87 patients, including 18 of the 57 patients in whom pulmonary arterial systolic pressures were recorded. Pulmonary arterial systolic pressures were ≤ 30 mm. Hg in 5 (13 percent) of the 39 patients without right ventricular outflow obstruction, and in 16 (89 percent) of the 18 patients with obstruction. Conversely, the pulmonary arterial systolic pressure was elevated (>30 mm. Hg) in 34 (87 percent) of 39 patients without right ventricular outflow obstruction and in 2 (11 percent) of the 18 patients with obstruction (Tables 6, 8, and 9).

Anatomic Features of the Pulmonary Vessels

Figures 3 to 13 illustrate some of the anatomic features observed in the pulmonary vessels of the study patients.

Left-to-Right Shunts

Of these 39 patients, the pulmonary arterial pressure had been recorded in 31: 4 patients (13 percent) had only medial thickening; 13 patients (42 percent) had medial and intimal thickening; 3 patients (10 percent) had medial and intimal thickening with plexiform lesions; and 11 patients (35 percent) had none of these changes. The pulmonary arterial systolic pressures in the 11 patients ranged from 20 to 63 mm. Hg (mean 36 mm. Hg): in 5 it was ≤ 30 mm. Hg. In the 4 patients with medial thickening only, this pressure ranged from 58 to 80 mm. Hg (mean 70 mm. Hg). In the 13 patients with medial and intimal thickening, pressures ranged from 37 to 118 mm. Hg (mean 81 mm. Hg). In the 3 patients with plexiform lesions, pulmonary arterial systolic pressure was 120 mm. Hg in 2 and 136 mm. Hg in the other.

Right-to-Left Shunts

Of these 13 patients, 9 had pulmonary arterial systolic pressures ≤ 30 mm. Hg (mean 15 mm. Hg) from right ventricular outflow obstruction, and none of them had morphologic changes in the pulmonary arteries. The 4 other patients who had no right ventricular outflow obstruction had pulmonary arterial systolic pressures ranging from 98 to 132 mm. Hg (mean 114 mm. Hg) and all had plexiform lesions in the pulmonary arteries.

Both Left-to-Right and Right-to-Left Shunts

Of these 13 patients, 6 had right ventricular outflow obstruction and 7 did not. There were no morphologic changes in the pulmonary arteries in 6 patients whose pressures ranged from 15 to 20 mm. Hg (mean 15 mm. Hg); 4 had medial and intimal thickening and their pressures ranged from 22 to 83 mm. Hg (mean 55 mm. Hg). The 3 patients with plexiform lesions had pressures of 108, 110 and 138 mm. Hg.

Table 6. Observations in 87 necropsy patients over age 15 with congenital cardiovascular malformations

Direction of Shunt	*Totals*	*L→R*	*R→L*	*Both*	*L→R*	*R→L*	*Both*	*Pulmonary Arterial Changes*				
								None	*MT only*	*MT + IT*	*PL*	*T*
No. Patients	87	3	22	11	36	6	9	43	6	25	13	31
RV Outflow Obst.		3	22	11	0	0	0					
PA systolic Pressure (mm. Hg.)												
≤30	21	2	9	5	3	0	2	20	0	1	0	5
31–60	11	0	0	1	9	0	1	5	1	5	0	2
61–90	10	1	0	0	8	0	1	1	3	6	0	5
>90	15	0	0	0	8	4	3	0	0	5	10	7
Unknown (U)	30	0	13	5	8	2	2	17	2	8	3	12
Morphologic changes in PAs												
None	43	3	19	10	10	0	1					
MI alone	6	0	0	0	6	0	0					
MT + IT	25	0	2	1	17	1	4					
PL	13	0	1	0	3	5	4					
Thrombi	31	1	8	2	13	2	5					

IT = intimal thickening; L = left; MT = medical thickening; obst = obstruction; PA = pulmonary artery; PL = plexiform lesions + MT + IT; R = right; RV = right ventricle; T = thrombi

Table 7. Observations in 36 necropsy patients over age 15 with right ventricular outflow or inflow obstruction

Malformation: Sex of Patients/ Age Range/Mean Age	*PA Systolic Pressures (mm. Hg)*					*OP*	*SA O_2 Sat. (%)*	*Pulmonary Arterial Changes*						
	<30	*31–60*	*61–90*	*>90*	*U*			*None*	*H*	*IT only*	*MT only*	*MT + IT*	*ARL*	*T*
LEFT-TO-RIGHT SHUNT ONLY														
VSD + PS(TOF): 1M/22	1	0	0	0	0	1	92	1	0	0	0	0	0	1
VSD + RVOTO: 1F/25	0	0	1	0	0	1	91	1	0	0	0	0	0	0
Complex anomaly: 1M/17	1	0	0	0	0	1	93	0	1	0	0	0	0	0
RIGHT-TO-LEFT SHUNT ONLY														
VSD + PS(TOF): 5F, 7M/17–36/27	5	0	0	0	7	11	9(82)	2	7	6	0	1(PL)	5	5
CT + PS + VSD + DORV: 1F/55	1	0	0	0	0	1		0	1	1	0	0	0	0
CT + PS + VSD + ASD: 1M/21	0	0	0	0	1	1		0	1	1	0	0	0	0
TVA + ASD: 1M/27	0	0	0	0	1	1	83	0	0	1	0	0	0	0
PS + IVS + ASD: 3F/28–43/36	2	0	0	0	1	3	2(75)	1	3	1	0	0	0	1
Complex anomaly: 2F, 2M/17–38/34	1	0	0	0	3	3	3(72)	1	1	2	0	2	0	3
BOTH LEFT-TO-RIGHT AND RIGHT-TO-LEFT SHUNTS														
VSD + PS(TOF): 3M/16–53/37	3	0	0	0	0	3	3(81)	0	1	2	0	0	2	0
VSD + PVA: 1F, 1M/22–28/25	0	0	0	0	2	1	2(67)	0	0	2	0	0	1	1
CT + VSD + PS: 1M/21	0	0	0	0	1	1	71	0	0	1	0	0	1	1
Complex anomaly: 1F, 4M/16–33/23	2	1	0	0	2	4	4(83)	1	1	2	0	1	0	0

ARL = Arnold Rich lesions; ASD = atrial septal defect; CT = corrected transposition; DORV = double outlet right ventricle; F = female; H = hypoplastic; IT = intimal thickening; M = male; MT = medial thickening; OP = cardiovascular operation; PA = pulmonary artery; PL = plexiform lesions + MT and IT; PS = pulmonic stenosis; PVA = pulmonic valve atresia; RVTO = right ventricular outflow tract obstruction; SA = systemic artery; Sat. = saturation; T = thrombus; TOF = tetralogy of Fallot; TVA = tricuspid valve atresia; U = unknown; IVS = intact ventricular septum; VSD = ventricular septal defect.

Table 8. Clinical and morphologic observations in 36 necropsy patients over age 15 with CHD, L-R shunts, and no right ventricular outflow or inflow obstruction

Malformation Sex of Patients/ Age Range/Mean Age	*PA Systolic Pressure (mm. Hg)*				*U*	*OP*	*Pulmonary Arterial Changes*				
	<30	*31–60*	*61–90*	*>90*			*None*	*MT only*	*MT + IT*	*PL*	*T*
ASD											
Fossa ovale: 13F, 1M/43–83/57	1	5	3	1	4	8	7	2	5	0	7
Partial AV canal: 4M/21–54/39	0	3	0	0	1	4	1	1	2	0	2
Sinus venosus: 2M/37–58/48	1	0	0	1	0	1	1	0	1	0	1
VSD: 2F, 3M/16–54/28	1	0	3	0	1	4	1	2	2	0	1
PDA: 1F, 4M/16–44/28	0	0	1	4	0	5	0	1	1	3	0
Complete transposition with VSD: 1F/39	0	0	0	0	1	0	0	0	1	0	0
DORV: 1F/24	0	1	0	0	0	1	0	0	1	0	0
Parachute MV syndromes: 1F/24	0	0	0	1	0	1	0	0	1	0	0
Complex anomaly: IF, 2M/21–31/26	0	0	1	1	1	1	0	0	3	0	2
TOTALS: 20F, 16M/16–83/42	3	9	8	8	8	27	10	6	17	3	13

Abbreviations as in Tables 3, 5, and 6.

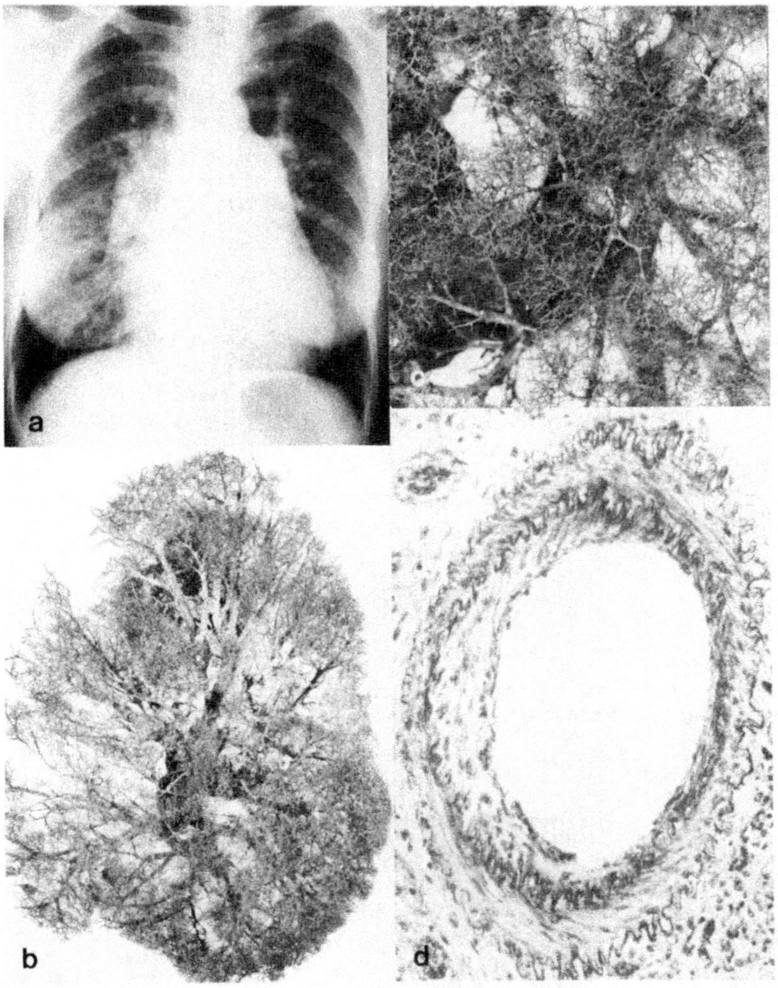

Figure 3. Atrial septal defect in a 45-year-old woman who died 11 days after operative closure. Preoperative pulmonary arterial pressure was 40/14 mm. Hg; left-to-right shunt was 2.8 to 1; and pulmonary to systemic resistance was 0.17 to 1. *a*, Radiograph immediately before operation. *b*, Mold of pulmonary arteries in one lung. *c*, Close-up of wide-open arteries. *d*, Typical muscular pulmonary artery showing mild medial and intimal thickening. (Movat stain, x 252; reduced 30%.)

Table 9. Clinical and morphologic observations in 15 necropsy patients over age 15 with CHD and R-L shunts only or both R-L and L-R shunts, without right ventricular outflow or inflow obstruction

	F	*M*	*ASD*	*VSD*	*PDA*	*Other*	*PA Systolic Pressure mm. Hg*	*OP*	*PA Lesions*
						RIGHT-TO-LEFT SHUNT ONLY			
17	+	0	0	0	+	0	120	0	PL,T
20	+	0	+	0	0	Ebstein's + LSVC	U	+	MT + IT
25	+	0	0	+	0	0	98	+	PL
33	0	+	0	+	+	0	106	+	PL,T
40	+	0	0	0	+	0	132	+	PL
41	0	+	0	+	+	IAA + CT	U	0	PL
						BOTH RIGHT-TO-LEFT AND LEFT-TO-RIGHT SHUNTS			
16	+	0	0	+	0	0	60	+	MT + IT,T
21	+	0	0	+	+	0	138	0	PL,T
21	0	+	+	+	0	Comp T	U	0	MT + IT
24	+	0	0	0	+	0	U	0	PL
29	+	0	+	0	0	0	110	0	PL,T
31	0	+	+	0	0	Ebstein's	22	+	MT + IT,T
38	0	+	0	+	0	CT	83	+	MT + IT,T
39	0	+	0	+	0	COA	108	+	PL
40	+	0	+	0	0	TAPVC	20	+	O

Abbreviations as in Table 5 and 6; EA = Ebstein's anomaly.

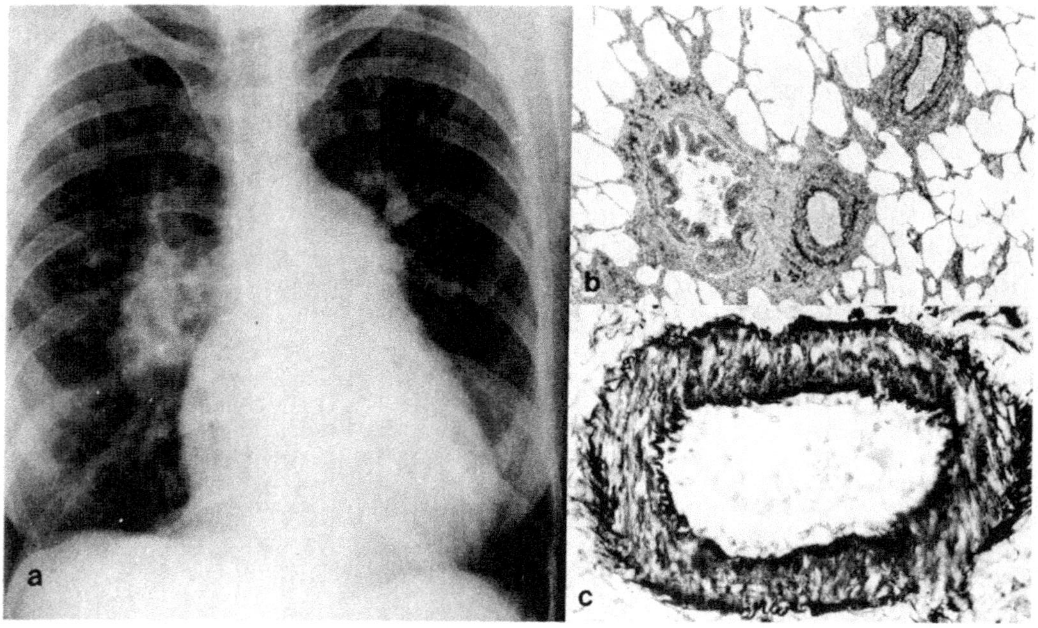

Figure 4. Atrial septal defect in a 50-year-old woman who died 11 days after operative closure of the defect. Preoperative pulmonary arterial pressure was 95/30 mm. Hg; the shunt was entirely left-to-right. *a*, Radiograph immediately before operation. *b*, Two muscular pulmonary arteries with thickened media (x 60). *c*, Close-up (x 330) of one of the two muscular pulmonary arteries shown in *b*. (Movat stains; reduced 30%.)

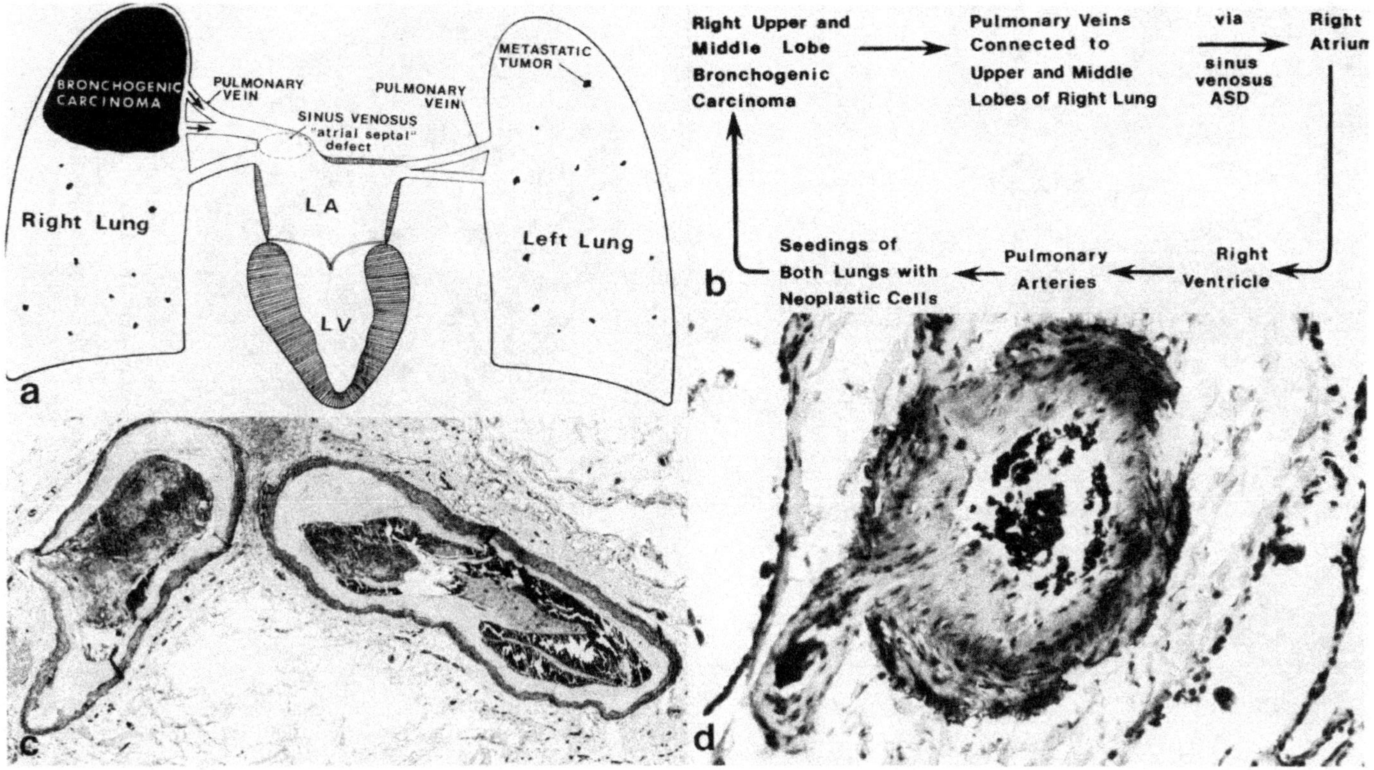

Figure 5. Sinus venosus type ASD with anomalous pulmonary venous return from the right lung associated with bronchogenic carcinoma in a 58-year-old man. Three years before he died his pulmonary arterial pressure was 100/22 mm. Hg and left-to-right shunt was 1.5 to 1. *a,* Diagram of the heart and lungs. LA = left atrium; LV = left ventricle. *b,* Path of metastatic spread of the tumor in both lungs. *c,* Large pulmonary arteries with thickened intima and antemortem blood clot (x 85). *d,* Typical muscular artery and branching arteriole with thickened media and intima (x 220). (Movat stains; reduced 12%.)

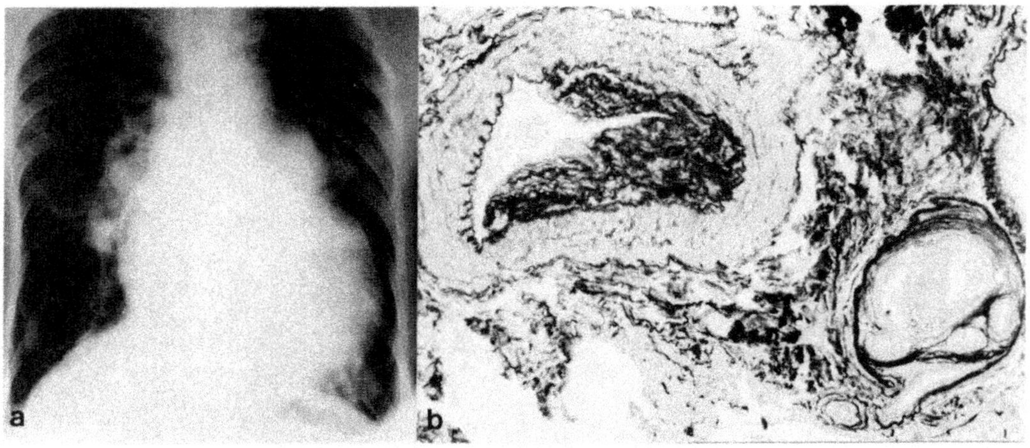

Figure 6. Patent ductus arterosus in a 36-year-old man who died during attempted closure of the calcified ductus. Preoperative pulmonary arterial pressure was equal to systemic arterial pressure (136/96 mm. Hg). The shunt was entirely left to right. *a,* Radiograph immediately before operation. *b,* Muscular pulmonary artery showing marked medial and intimal thickening and a plexiform lesion. (Elastic van Gieson stain; x 220; reduced 30%.)

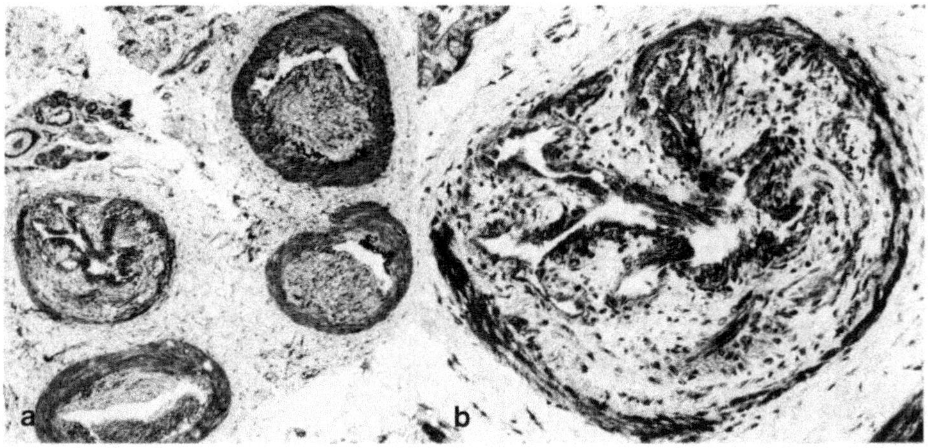

Figure 7. Patent ductus arteriosus in a 40-year-old woman who died during attempted operative closure. Simultaneous pulmonary arterial and femoral arterial pressures were 110/58 (mean 80) and 128/46 mm. Hg (mean 80), respectively. The shunt was right-to-left, femoral arterial oxygen saturation was 70 percent, and blood hematocrit was 46 percent. *a,* Muscular pulmonary arteries with thickened media and intima and narrowed lumens (x 80). *b,* Plexiform lesions (x 240). (Movat stains; reduced 30%.)

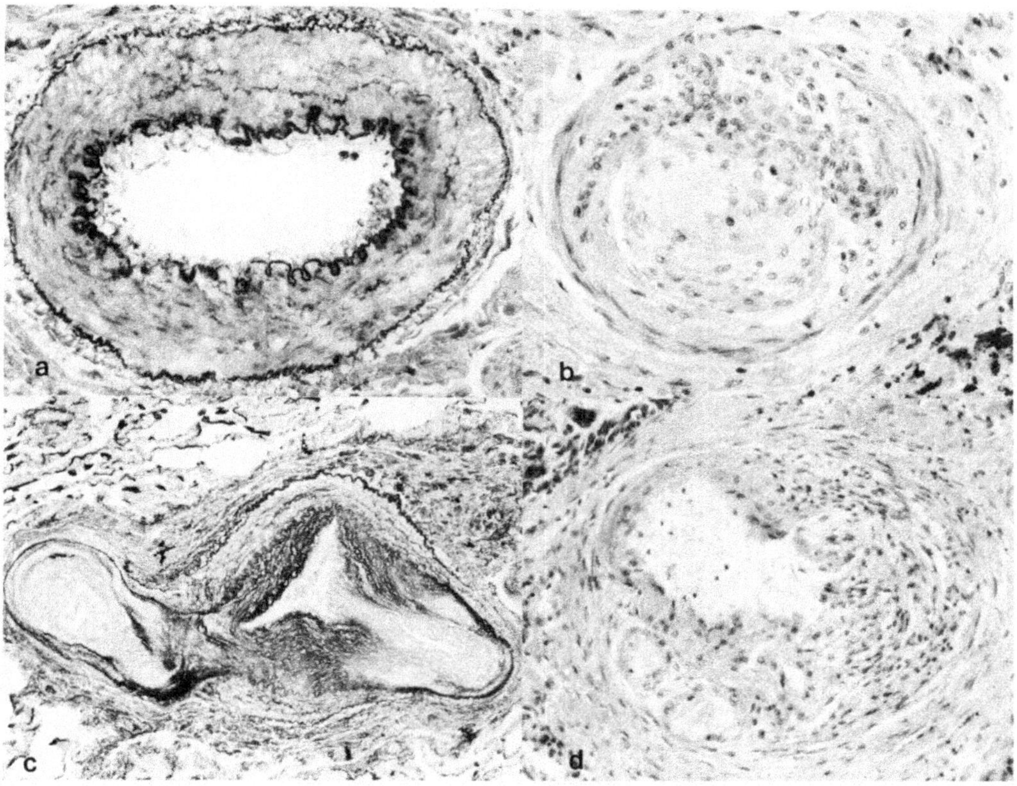

Figure 8. Combined PDA and discrete subaortic stenosis in a 17-year-old boy. Peak systolic pressure gradient between left ventricle and brachial artery was 78 mm. Hg. Pulmonary arterial pressure was 128/70 mm. Hg and the shunt was entirely left-to-right. Muscular pulmonary arteries (*a* through *d*) shows severe medial hypertrophy and luminal narrowing by intimal thickening. *c*, *d*, Plexiform lesions. (Elastic Van Gieson stains: x 255 (*a*) and x 65 (*c*); hematoxylin and eosin stains: x375 (*b*) and x 240 (*d*); reduced 34%.)

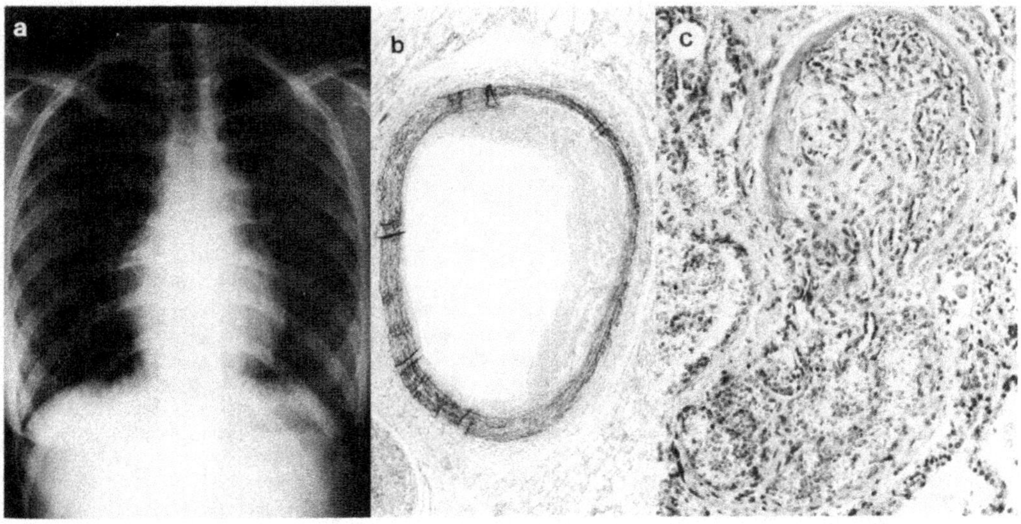

Figure 9. Combined PDA and VSD in a 21-year-old woman who died soon after catheterization. The pulmonary and systemic arterial pressures were both 138/86 mm. Hg (mean 107). The shunt through the ductus was mainly right-to-left and the shunt through the VSD was minute. Oxygen saturation was 89 percent in the brachial artery and 75 percent in the femoral artery; blood hematocrit was 66 percent. *a*, Chest radiograph. *b*, Intrapulmonary elastic artery (x 27). *c*, Plexiform lesion (x 225). (Hematoxylin and eosin stains; reduced 40%.)

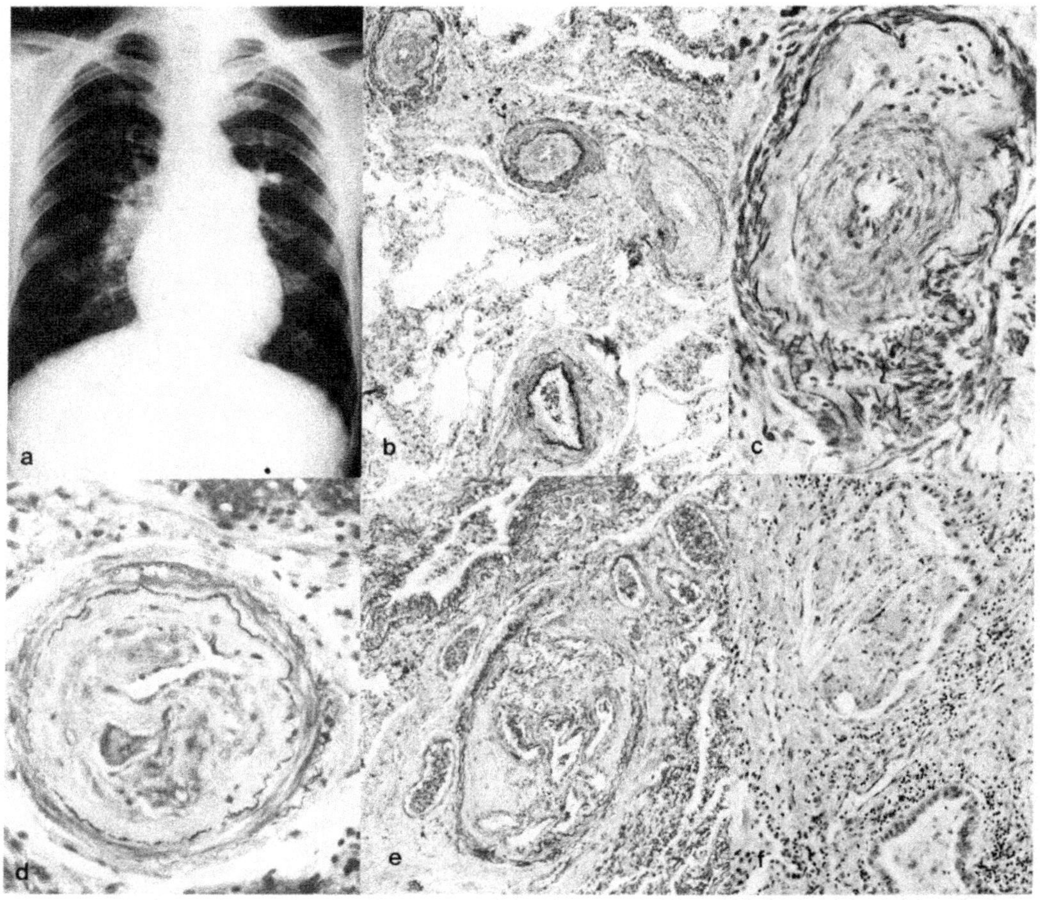

Figure 10. Combined PDA and VSD in a 33-year-old man who died during attempted operative closure of the ductus. Simultaneous pulmonary and femoral arterial pressures were 106/64 and 132/52 mm. Hg, respectively. The femoral and brachial arterial oxygen saturations were 69 and 80 percent, respectively. Blood hematocrit was 54 percent but severe iron deficiency anemia was present. The shunt at the ductus was primarily right-to-left and no shunt was detected at the ventricular level. *a,* Chest radiograph immediately before operation. *b, c, d,* Severe medial and intimal thickening with luminal narrowing (x 95, x 380, x 385, respectively). *e,* Plexiform lesions (x 130). *f,* Cholesterol-ester granuloma (x 160). (Movat stains: *b, c, d, e;* hematoxylin and eosin stain: *f;* reduced 42%.)

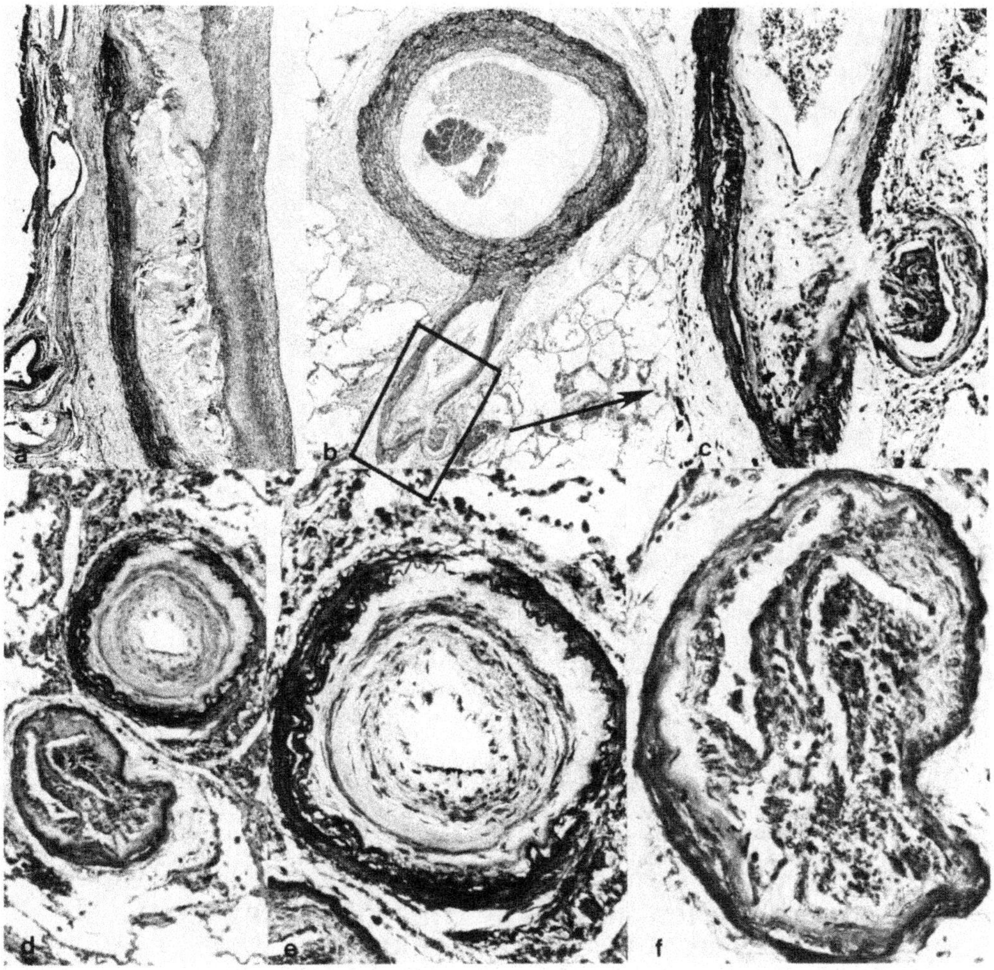

Figure 11. Combined VSD and coarctation of aorta in a 39-year-old man who died 24 hours after operative closure of the defect. Simultaneous pulmonary arterial and aortic pressures were 131/76 (mean 93) and 144/84 (mean 100) mm. Hg, respectively. Left brachial arterial oxygen saturation was 87 percent, blood hematocrit was 54 percent, and the shunt was bidirectional, but predominantly left-to-right. The pulmonary arteries had thick media, thick intima, narrowed lumens, and plexiform lesions. *a,* Intrapulmonary elastic artery (media stains black) with a huge atherosclerotic plaque (x 40). *b,* Large pulmonary artery with a muscular branch which has an obliterated lumen (x 60). *c,* Close-up of the area in brackets shown in *b* (x 155). This is a plexiform lesion. *d,* Muscular pulmonary artery (x 130). *e,* Close-up of artery shown in *d* (x 248). *f,* Close-up of plexiform lesion shown in *d* (x 330). (Movat stains; reduced 40%.)

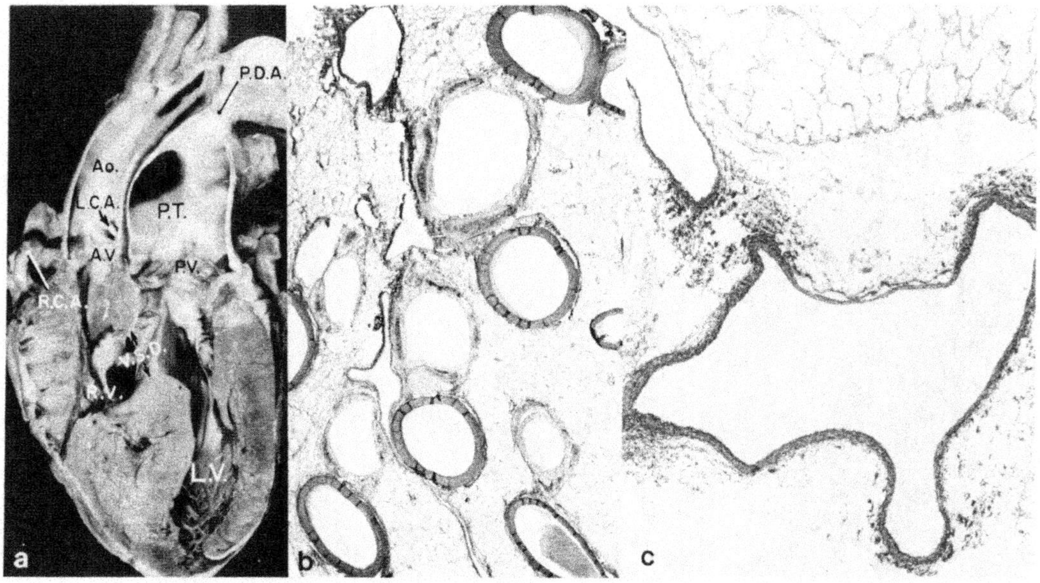

Figure 12. Ventricular septal defect and PDA associated with the Taussig-Bing malformation in a 39-year-old woman described in detail elsewhere.[70] Pulmonary arterial pressure was 91/58 mm. Hg; brachial arterial pressure, 93/56 mm. Hg. Blood hematocrit was 75 percent; systemic arterial oxygen saturation, 47 percent. *a,* Longitudinal view of heart showing the pulmonary trunk (P.T.) and pulmonic valve (P.V.) overriding a large ventricular septal defect (V.S.D.). The aorta (A.) arises anteriorly and from the right ventricle (R.V.). The patent ductus arteriosus (P.D.A.) is large. L.V. = left ventricle; L.C.A. = ostium of left coronary artery; R.C.A. = right coronary artery. *b,* Greatly dilated pulmonary arteries near hilum of one lung (x 5). Media is thickened but intima is normal or only minimally thickened. The pulmonary arteries in this patient were everywhere wide open and dilated. *c,* Dilated pulmonary veins (x 40). Despite the balanced pulmonary and systemic arterial pressures maintained over many years the anatomic pulmonary arterial changes were mild. (Elastic Van Gieson and Movat stains; reduced 33%.)

MORPHOLOGIC CHANGES IN THE PULMONARY ARTERIES: THE EFFECTS OF PULMONARY ARTERIAL SYSTOLIC PRESSURE, DIRECTION AND LOCATION OF SHUNT, AND PATIENT AGE

The observations described above and presented in detail in Tables 3 through 14 indicate that the crucial determinant of anatomic change in the muscular pulmonary arteries of patients over age 15 with congenital cardiac disease is the *level of the pulmonary arterial pressure.* These observations in our 57 necropsy patients in whom pulmonary arterial pressures were recorded are summarized in Fig. 14. Of the 26 patients without morphologic pulmonary arterial changes, the average pulmonary arterial systolic pressure was 25 mm. Hg (range 9 to 63 mm. Hg) and only 6 patients had pressures > 30 mm. Hg. In contrast, of the 10 patients with plexiform lesions, the average pulmonary arterial systolic pressure was 119 mm. Hg (range 98 to 138 mm. Hg; $p < .01$). The 21 patients with medial thickening only or medial and intimal thickening had similar average pulmonary arterial systolic pressures (70 and 75 mm. Hg, respectively). The average pulmonary arterial systolic pressure in the patients with medial thickening with or without intimal thickening was significantly ($p < .01$) different than the pressures of patients without morphologic pulmonary arterial changes and patients with plexiform lesions (Fig. 14).

The *direction of the intravascular shunt* appeared to have only indirect effect on the pulmonary arteries. As shown in Figures 14 through 16, 15 of the 26 patients without structural pulmonary arterial abnormalities (average pulmonary arterial systolic pres-

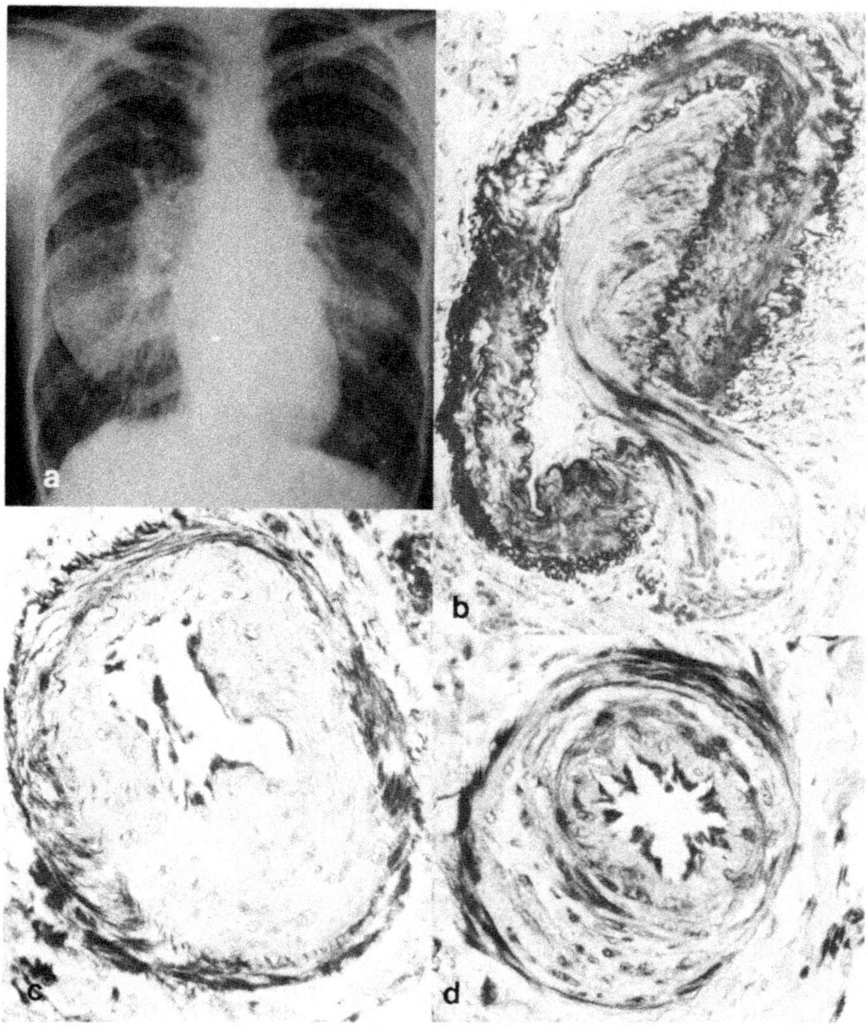

Figure 13. Congenital mitral stenosis, VSD, PDA, and coarctation of aorta in a 25-year-old asymptomatic woman.[71] Pulmonary arterial pressure was 104/60 mm. Hg (mean 82); left ventricular pressure, 122/4 mm. Hg. Left atrial to left ventricular end-diastolic gradient was 20 mm. Hg and cardiac output was normal. *a*, Preoperative chest radiograph. A mitral commissurotomy was performed but considerable mitral regurgitation resulted; the VSD was closed by direct suture, and an unsuspected ductus was ligated. The patient died 20 hours after operation. *b* (x 220), *c* (x 330), *d* (x 435), Pulmonary arteries show severe intimal and medial thickening with luminal narrowing, and pulmonary venous and alveolar septal and space lesions are typical of mitral stenosis.[72–75] (Movat stains; reduced 25%.)

sure = 15 mm. Hg) had right-to-left or bidirectional shunts and 7 of the 10 patients with plexiform lesions (average pulmonary arterial systolic pressure = 116 mm. Hg) (Fig. 15) also had right-to-left or bidirectional shunts. Thus, the pressure and not the direction of the shunt determines anatomic pulmonary arterial changes in these patients. As shown in Figure 16, patients with left-to-right shunts only, also had all degrees of anatomic change in the muscular pulmonary arteries, again demonstrating that structural changes in these patients depend on the pulmonary arterial pressure.

The anatomic changes in the muscular pulmonary arteries were only secondarily dependent on the *location of the shunt* in the heart or great arteries. Among our 40 patients with isolated atrial septal defect (ASD) or ventricular septal defect (VSD) or

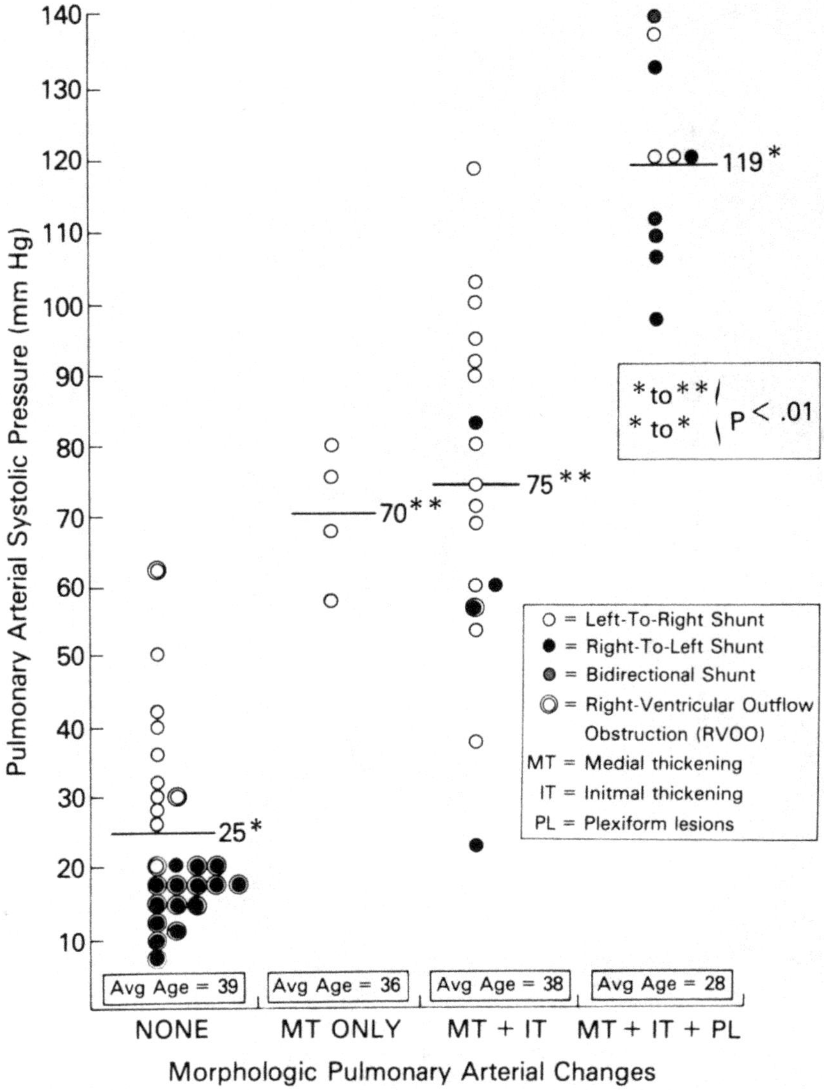

Figure 14. Morphologic pulmonary arterial changes, pulmonary arterial systolic pressure, and direction of shunt in 57 necropsy patients over age 15 with congenital heart disease. In 26 patients the media of the pulmonary arterial wall was normal or thinner than normal, in 4 there was medial thickening only, in 17 there was both medial and intimal thickening, and in 10 there was medial and intimal thickening with plexiform lesions. The average pulmonary arterial systolic pressure in the patients with medial thickening with or without intimal thickening was significantly ($p < .01$) different from the average pressure in patients without any morphologic changes and from the average pressure in those with plexiform lesions.

patent ductus arteriosus (PDA) (Tables 3 and 4), 33 had pulmonary arterial pressures recorded at catheterization. As shown in Figures 17 and 18, the anatomic changes in the muscular pulmonary arteries in these 33 patients depended not on the location of the shunt but on the pressure in the pulmonary artery. Of course, the location of the communication played a major role in determining the pulmonary arterial pressure. Generally, the closer the shunt is to the pulmonary circulation the greater the pulmonary arterial pressure. Thus, the average pulmonary arterial systolic pressure in our patients was highest (118 mm. Hg) (Fig. 17) in the 9 patients with PDA, lowest (58 mm.

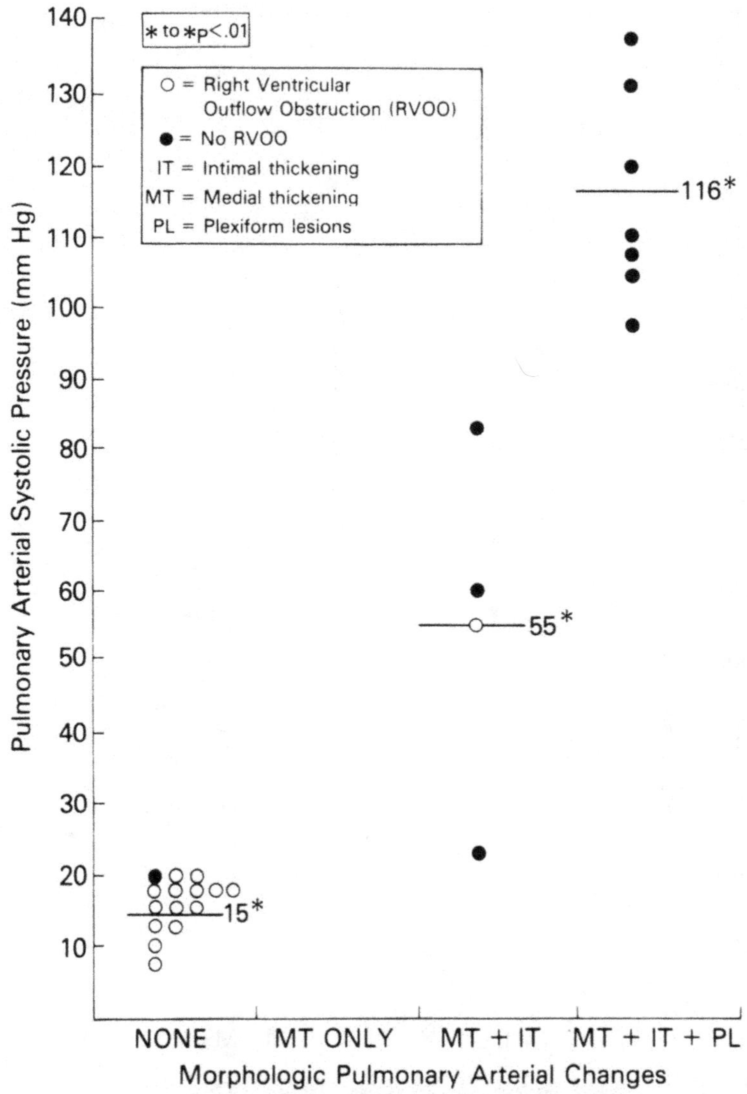

Figure 15. Morphologic pulmonary arterial changes and pulmonary arterial systolic pressure in 26 necropsy patients over age 15 with right-to-left or bidirectional shunts. In 15 patients the media of the pulmonary arteries was normal or thinner than normal; 4 patients had both medial and intimal thickening; 7 patients had both medial and intimal thickening with plexiform lesions. The average pulmonary arterial systolic pressure increased significantly as morphologic pulmonary arterial changes worsened.

Hg) in the 17 patients with ASD, and intermediate (68 mm. Hg) in the 7 patients with isolated VSD. Surprisingly, no significant difference in average pulmonary arterial systolic pressure was observed between the 17 patients with isolated ASD and the 7 patients with isolated VSD (Fig. 17). The average pulmonary arterial systolic pressure in the 9 patients with isolated PDA was nearly twice that of the patients with either ASD or VSD, and this difference was highly significant ($p < .001$).

Plexiform lesions were observed in 1 of the 17 patients with ASD, in 1 of the 7 with VSD, and in 7 of the 9 with PDA. All 9 patients with plexiform lesions had pulmonary arterial systolic pressures > 90 mm. Hg.

Age was not an important determinant of anatomic changes in the muscular pulmo-

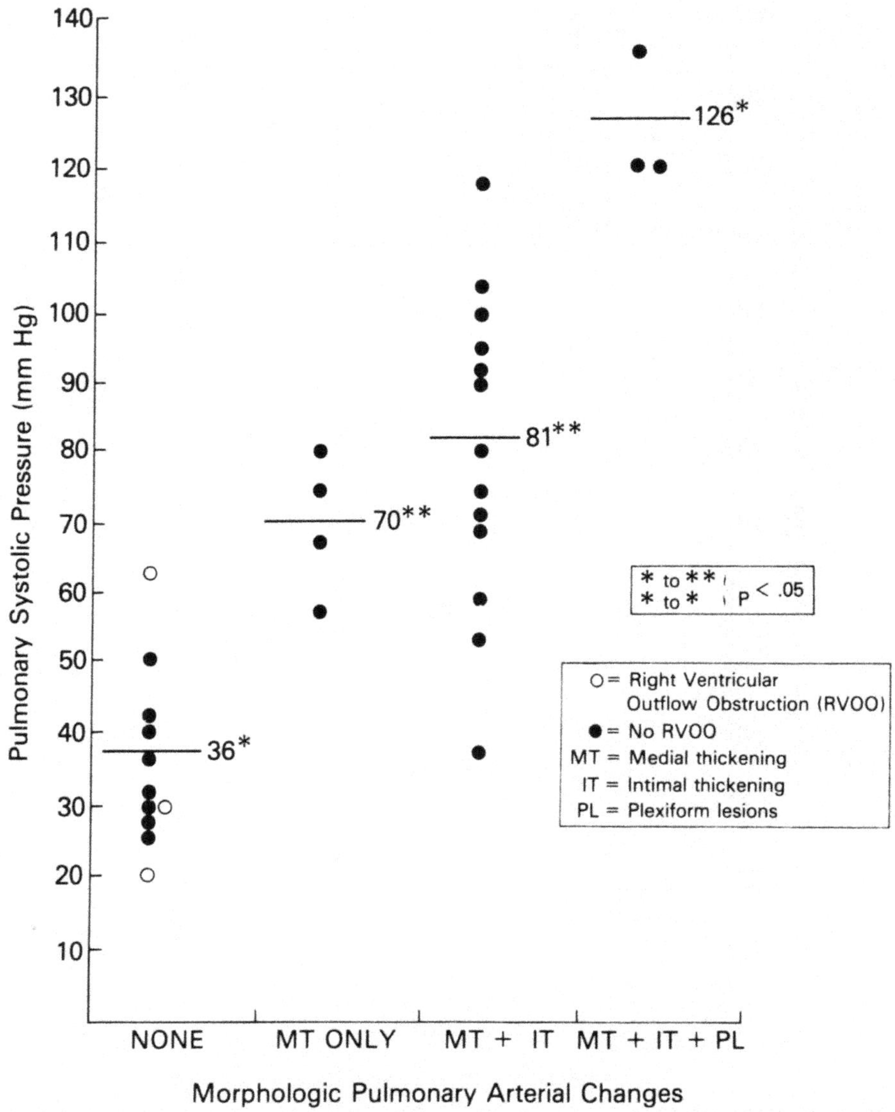

Figure 16. Morphologic pulmonary arterial changes and pulmonary arterial systolic pressure in 31 necropsy patients over age 15 with only left-to-right shunts. In 11 patients the media of the pulmonary arteries was normal or thinner than normal; 4 patients had only medial thickening; 13 patients had both medial and intimal thickening; 3 patients had both medial and intimal thickening with plexiform lesions. The average pulmonary arterial systolic pressure in the patients with medial thickening with or without intimal thickening was significantly ($p < .05$) different from the average pressure in patients without morphologic changes and from the average pressure in those with plexiform changes.

nary arteries (Fig. 19). Among the 40 patients with isolated ASD or VSD or PDA, the group with ASD was oldest (mean 51 years) and yet they had the least severe pulmonary arterial anatomic changes. Furthermore, the patients with VSD and PDA were younger and had the same mean age (28 years); yet, the anatomic pulmonary arterial changes were far worse among the patients with PDA ($p < .001$). The lack of severe morphologic pulmonary arterial changes in the patients with ASD appears to explain the much longer survival among these patients than among those with either isolated VSD or PDA (Fig. 19).

Observations of Other Investigators

Although several investigators have described previously the effect of pressure, direction and location of shunt, and age on the anatomic changes in the pulmonary arteries, the only previous study which allows direct comparison to ours is the one by Heath and associates.[14] Among their 40 patients with isolated ASD or VSD or PDA, 23 were over 15 years of age (range 17 to 55; mean 32) and pulmonary arterial systolic pressures were available in all patients. Figures 20 to 22 show our plotting of their observations in 23 patients in the same way we plotted our own observations (Figs. 17

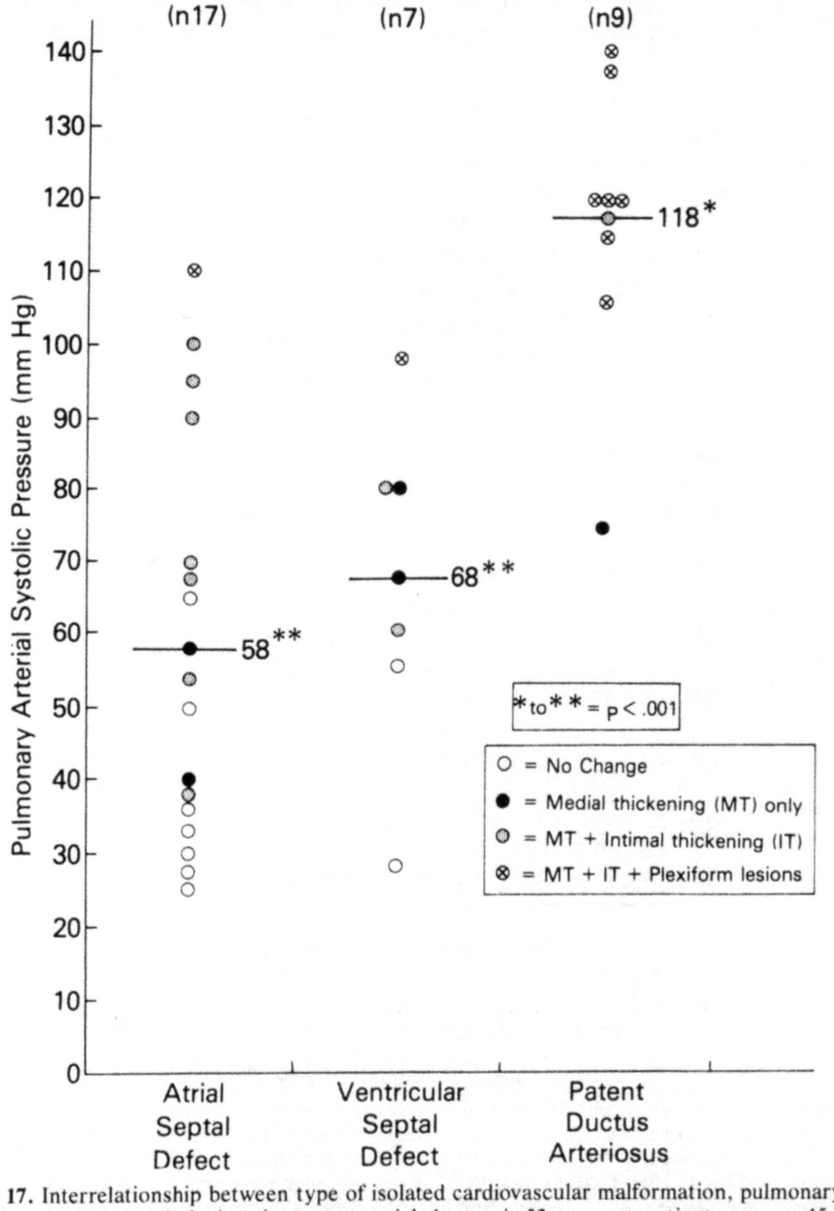

Figure 17. Interrelationship between type of isolated cardiovascular malformation, pulmonary arterial systolic pressure, and morphologic pulmonary arterial changes in 33 necropsy patients over age 15. There was no significant difference in the average systolic pressures in patients with ASD and VSD, but both these averages were significantly ($p < .001$) different from the average pressure in patients with PDA.

through 19). As shown in Figure 21, the pulmonary arterial systolic pressures were significantly ($p < .01$) lower in the patients in whom the morphologic pulmonary arterial changes consisted only of medial thickening. Surprisingly, in contrast to our patients, no significant differences in these average pressures were observed between the patients with medial and intimal thickening and the patients with plexiform lesions. Furthermore, the average systolic pressure in their patients with isolated ASD was only slightly lower—although significantly ($p < 0.01$)—than the average pressures in their patients with either VSD or PDA (Fig. 20).

As in our patients, their patients with ASD were significantly older than their patients with either VSD or PDA, even though their pulmonary arterial systolic pressures were significantly lower. As pointed out by Heath and associates,[14] however, in patients with

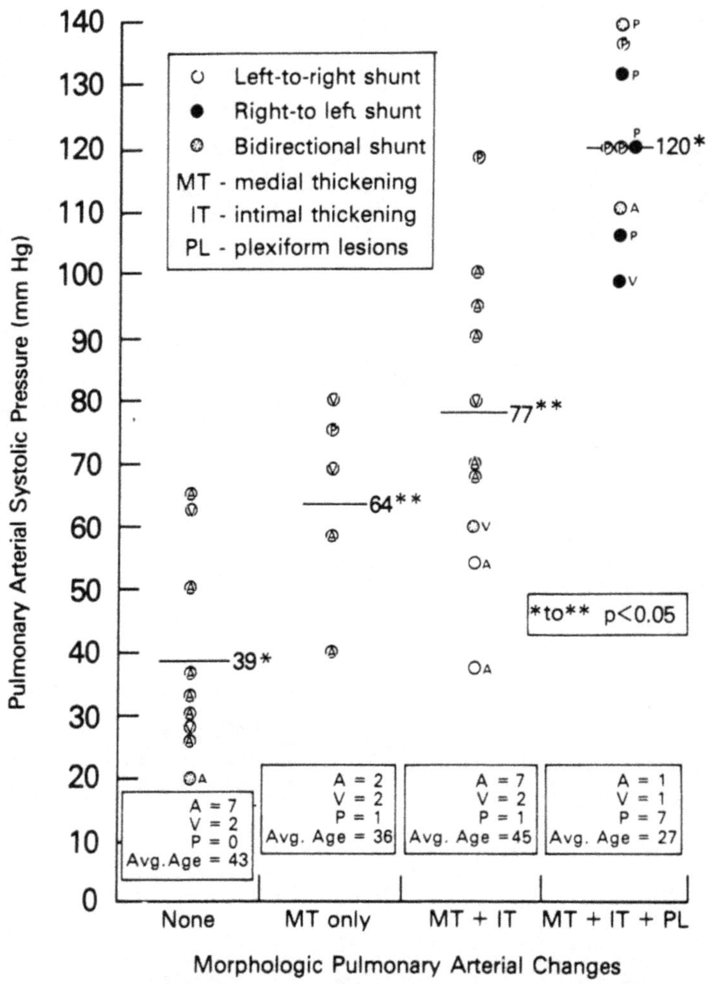

Figure 18. Morphologic pulmonary arterial changes, pulmonary arterial systolic pressure, and shunt direction in 33 necropsy patients over age 15 with isolated ASD or VSD or PDA. The pulmonary arteries were normal in 9 patients; 5 had medial thickening only; 10 had both medial and intimal thickening; 9 had both medial and intimal thickening with plexiform lesions. The average pulmonary arterial systolic pressures in the patients with medial thickening with or without intimal thickening was significantly ($p<.05$) different from average pressure in patients without morphologic changes and from the average pressure in those with plexiform changes.

large VSD or PDA the systemic pressure is freely propagated into the pulmonary circulation from birth. Hence, the age of the patient is synonymous with the duration of the pulmonary arterial hypertension. As seen in Figure 22, there was an inverse correlation with the morphologic pulmonary arterial changes and the average age of their patients. In patients with medial thickening only, the average age was 37; in the group with medial and intimal thickening, the average age was 34; and in their patients with plexiform lesions the average age was 29. A similar trend occurred in our patients (Fig. 18).

The direction of the shunt, as shown in Figure 21, played a role in causing the morphologic pulmonary arterial changes in that their patients with bidirectional or only right-to-left shunts had higher pulmonary arterial systolic pressures than those with only left-to-right shunts.

Thus, the study by Heath and associates[14] showed no significant pulmonary arterial systolic pressure differences between patients with plexiform lesions and those with both medial and intimal thickening (Fig. 21). Our study, in contrast, showed a significant difference in pulmonary arterial systolic pressure between these two anatomic groups (Fig. 18). Their study showed a clear difference in pulmonary arterial systolic pressure in the patients with only medial thickening compared to those with both medial and intimal thickening and those with plexiform lesions (Fig. 21). Our study (Fig. 18), in contrast, showed no significant difference in the patients with medial thickening only as compared to those with both medial and intimal thickening.

When comparing pulmonary arterial systolic pressures to the location of the shunt, there was no significant difference in pulmonary pressures in their patients with VSD and PDA; there was a significant difference between the pressures of these two groups and pressures of patients with ASD (Fig. 20). In contrast, our study showed a highly significant difference between average pulmonary systolic pressure in patients with PDA and in those with VSD, but no significant difference between patients with ASD and in those with VSD (Fig. 17).

The results of our study were similar to that of Heath and associates[14] in regard to age (Figs. 19 and 22) and direction of the shunt.

How might the differences in the results of the two studies be explained? First, the patients were different. We studied only necropsy patients and many histologic sections from each patient. How many, if any, of their patients were studied at necropsy is not stated. It appears likely that the lung tissue in most of their patients was obtained at biopsy at the time of cardiac operation. Second, the investigators were different and judgments of morphologic changes possibly were different. Third, the numbers of patients in each study were relatively small so that differences may have been magnified. Fourth, their study excluded patients without anatomic changes in the pulmonary arteries whereas ours did not. Nevertheless, when we exclude our patients without anatomic pulmonary arterial changes, the differences between the two studies persist.

Wagenvoort and associates[33,40,41] studied lung tissue biopsied at the time of thoracotomy in patients with various congenital cardiovascular malformations. They also have shown that the primary cause of anatomic pulmonary arterial changes is elevation of the pulmonary arterial pressure, and that the magnitude of pulmonary flow is not, in itself, a determinant of these anatomic changes. This group did find, however, that the location of the shunt was an important factor in determining the extent of the anatomic pulmonary arterial changes. Of 77 lung samples studied from patients with isolated ASD (mean age, 22 years), medial thickening occurred in only 22 (29 percent), intimal thickening occurred in only 14 (18 percent), and none had plexiform lesions. In contrast, of 44 patients with isolated VSD (mean age, 9 years) and of 74 with isolated PDA (mean age, 9 years), 44 (34 percent) had medial thickening, 36 (28 percent) had intimal thickening, and only 2 (2 percent) had plexiform lesions. Severe intimal thicken-

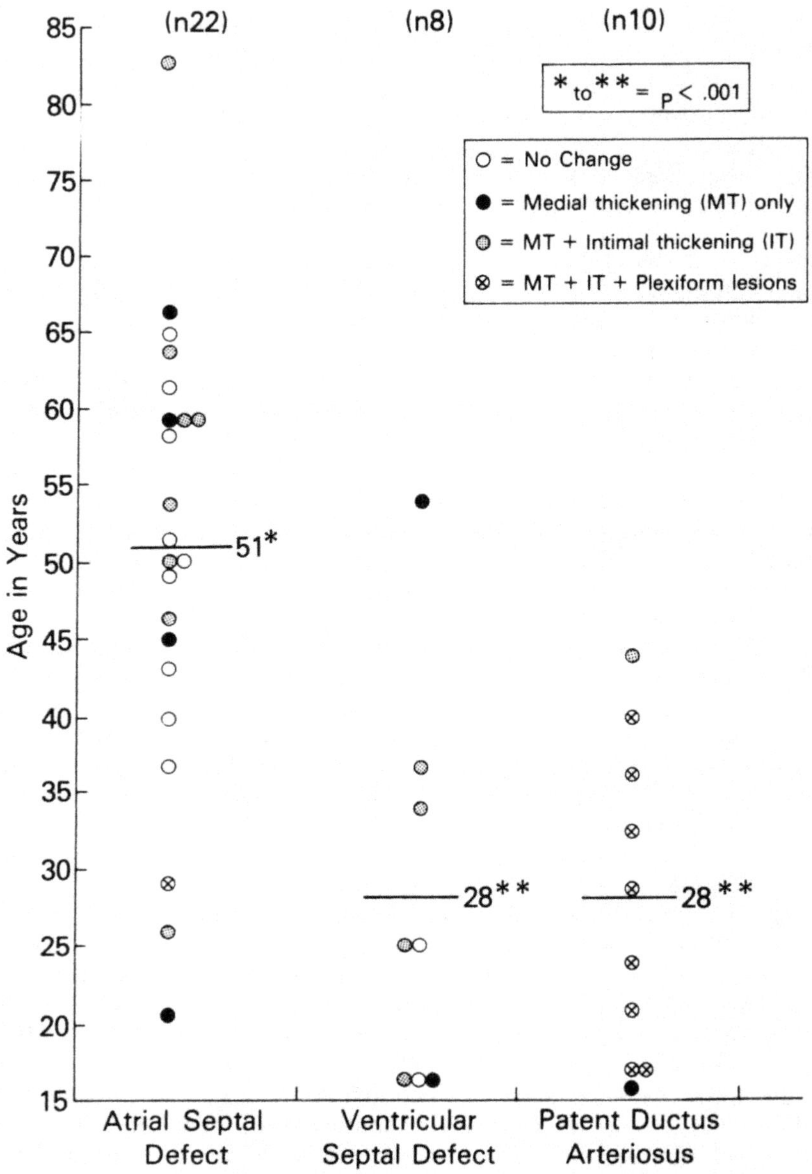

Figure 19. Interrelationship between type of isolated congenital cardiovascular malformation (ASD, n = 22; VSD, n = 8; PDA, n = 10) and morphologic pulmonary arterial changes in 40 necropsy patients over age 15. The average ages of patients with VSD and PDA are significantly ($p < .001$) different than the average age of patients with ASD.

ing was not observed in any patient with ASD or PDA but it occurred in 12 (27 percent) of the 44 patients with VSD.

The Wagenvoort study emphasized that the pulmonary vessels of their patients with ASD (much younger than ours and Heath's) did not differ significantly from those of his "control subjects." Among Wagenvoort's 105 patients with left-to-right shunts and pulmonary atrial systolic pressures greater than 60 mm. Hg, all had medial thickening and 74 (70 percent) had intimal thickening. In contrast, of his 45 patients with only right-to-left or bidirectional shunts, all had medial thickening and 44 (98 percent) had

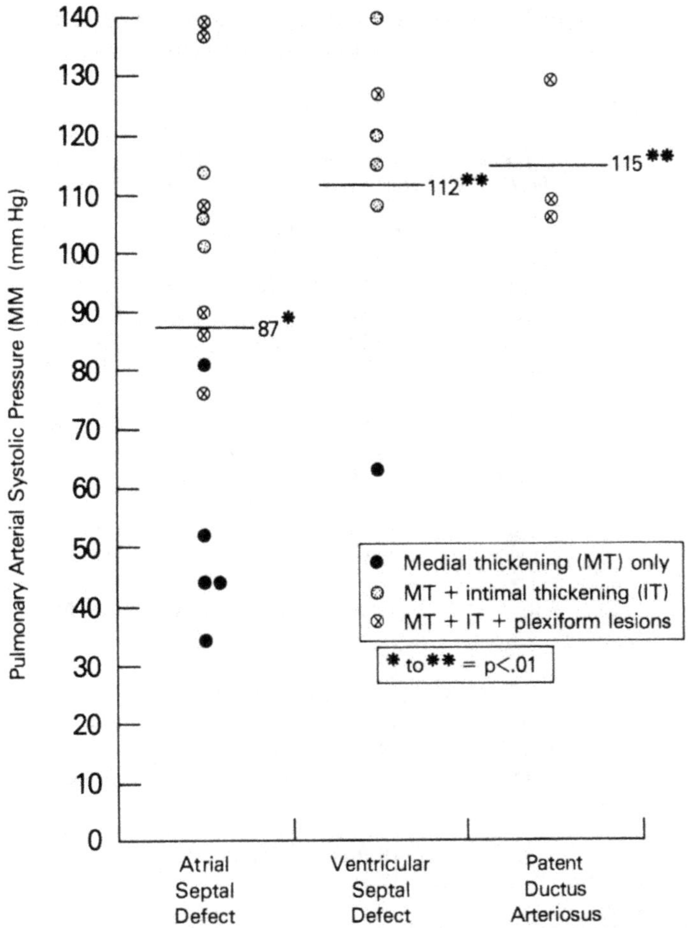

Figure 20. Data from Heath and associates[14] showing interrelationship between type of isolated congenital cardiovascular malformation (ASD, n = 14; VSD, n = 6; PDA, n = 3), pulmonary artery systolic pressure, and morphologic pulmonary arterial changes in 23 patients over age 15. There was no significant difference between the average pulmonary arterial systolic pressures in patients with VSD and in patients with PDA, but pressures in these two groups were significantly ($p < .01$) different from those in the patients with ASD.

intimal thickening. Plexiform lesions were not described in any of these 150 patients but, again, they were much younger than our patients.

SIGNIFICANCE OF PLEXIFORM LESIONS IN PATIENTS WITH PRIMARY PULMONARY HYPERTENSION

Plexiform lesions in the lung are indicative of severe pulmonary arterial hypertension which is almost always irreversible. Of our 87 patients, 13 (15 percent) had plexiform lesions: they occurred in 12 (23 percent) of the 51 patients without and in 1 (3 percent) of the 36 patients with right ventricular outflow or inflow obstruction (Table 10). The latter patient, however, developed plexiform lesions after operative creation of a large end-to-side communication between aorta and right main pulmonary artery. The pulmonary arterial systolic pressures were known in 11 of our 13 patients with plexiform lesions and in each this pressure was greater than 90 mm. Hg (mean 118 mm. Hg). Of the 13 patients with lesions, 12 had either VSD or PDA and only one had isolated ASD; they were between 17 and 41 years old (mean 28).

Table 10. Observations in 18 necropsy patients over age 15 with CHD, pulmonary arterial systolic pressures >90 mm. Hg, and no right ventricular outflow or inflow obstruction

Patient Age, Sex Malformation	PA Pressure (mm. Hg, s/d)	SA Pressure (mm. Hg, s/d)	Shunt	SA O_2 Sat. (%)	Cardiac Operation	Interval (days) OP to Death
WITH PLEXIFORM LESIONS						
29 F/ASD, RPV→SVC	110/60	110/60	both		none	
25 F/VSD	98/62	104/66	R-L	88	VSD closed	1
33 M/VSD, PDA	106/64	136/68	R-L	61	PDA closed	0
21 F/VSD, PDA	138/86	140/88	both	89	none	
39 M/VSD, COA	108/54	152/64	both	87	VSD closed	1
41 M/VSD, PDA, IAA +CT		120/70	none	*	none	
40 F/PDA	132/64	128/68	R-L	70	PDA closed	0
24 F/PDA		128/70	none	*	none	
28 M/PDA	120/60	120/60	L-R	96	PDA closed	1
17 F/PDA	120/65	110/60	R-L	*	none	
36 M/PDA	136/96	136/96	L-R	95	PDA closed	0
17 M/PDA, SS	120/65	122/65	L-R	97	PDA closed; SS resectioned	1
19 F/TOF	105/—	108/78	R-L	70	right PA-DA anastomosis	14 yrs.
WITHOUT PLEXIFORM LESIONS						
50 F/ASD	95/30	105/80	L-R	96	ASD closed	11
58 M/ASD	100/22	140/90	L-R		none	
44 F/PDA	118/52	150/70	L-R	92**	PDA closed	7
24 F/VSD, PDA, MS +COA	104/60	118/70	L-R		PDA and VSD closed; MVC	1
21 M/VSD, DORV +CT	92/48	102/64	L-R	90	none	0

*Central cyanosis present.
**Right brachial artery; 89 percent in femoral artery.
Abbreviations as in Tables 5 and 6; DA = descending aorta; IAA = interrupted aortic arch; MVC = mitral valve commissurotomy; MS = mitral stenosis; SS = subaortic stenosis; SVC = superior vena cava.

Heath and associates[14] described plexiform lesions in 10 (43 percent) of their 23 patients over 15 years of age with isolated ASD or VSD or PDA (Fig. 21). In their 10 patients with plexiform lesions the pulmonary arterial systolic pressures ranged from 76 to 139 mm. Hg (mean 111 mm. Hg), and in 8 of the 10 this pressure was 90 mm. Hg or greater. These lesions were observed in 6 (43 percent) of their 14 patients with ASD, in 1 (17 percent) of 6 with VSD, and all of the 3 with PDA. Among our patients, in contrast, plexiform lesions were seen in 1 (6 percent) of 17 with ASD, in 1 (14 percent) of 7 with VSD, and in 7 (78 percent) of 9 with PDA. Except for the patients with ASD, the frequency of plexiform lesions in our patients was similar to that observed in the patients studied by Heath and associates.[14]

Plexiform lesions are observed in highest frequency not in patients with congenital cardiovascular malformations but in patients with primary or idiopathic pulmonary hypertension. Observations in 16 necropsy patients with this condition are summarized in Table 11. Fourteen (87 percent) of these 16 patients had plexiform lesions in the lungs; in 13, pulmonary arterial systolic pressures ranged from 60 to 192 mm. Hg (mean 117 mm. Hg). In 11 of these 13 patients this pressure was greater than 90 mm. Hg. In the 2 patients without plexiform lesions, pulmonary arterial systolic pressures were 49 and 101 mm. Hg.

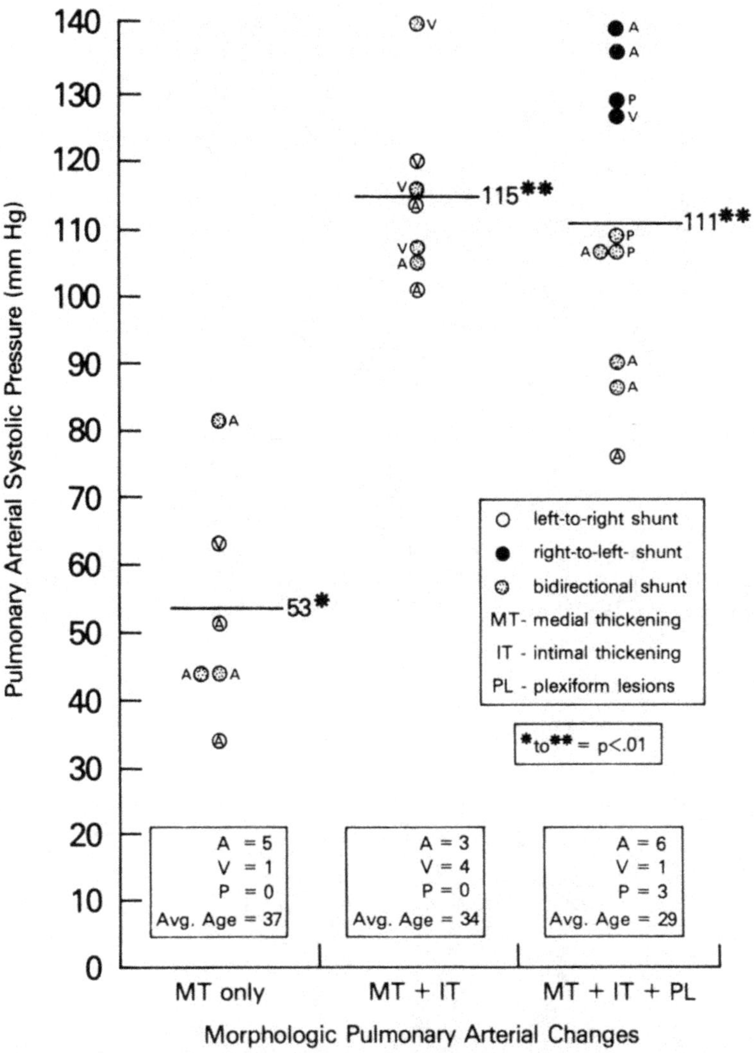

Figure 21. Data from Health and associates[14] showing interrelationship between morphologic pulmonary arterial changes, pulmonary arterial systolic pressure, and direction of shunt in 23 patients over age 15 with isolated ASD or VSD or PDA. Medial thickening only occurred in 6 patients; 7 had medial and intimal thickening; 10 had both medial and intimal thickening with plexiform lesions. The average pulmonary arterial systolic pressures in the patients with medial and intimal thickening were not significantly different from those of patients who had medial and intimal thickening with plexiform lesions. Pressures in both of these groups were significantly ($p < .01$) different from pressures in patients with only medial thickening.

Of the 10 patients with primary pulmonary hypertension with plexiform lesions and known pulmonary arterial pressures reported by Walcott and associates,[59] the pulmonary arterial systolic pressures ranged from 76 to 168 mm. Hg (mean 99 mm. Hg) and in only 2 patients was this pressure less than 90 mm. Hg.

Wagenvoort and Wagenvoort[60] summarized pulmonary morphologic observations in 110 patients (age range, infancy to 69 years; mean 23) with primary pulmonary hypertension, and 77 (70 percent) had plexiform lesions. Of their 110 patients, however, only 70 were 16 years of age or older and of the remaining 39 patients, many were infants and young children. Had these authors included only patients over age 15 their frequency of plexiform lesions almost certainly would have been higher.

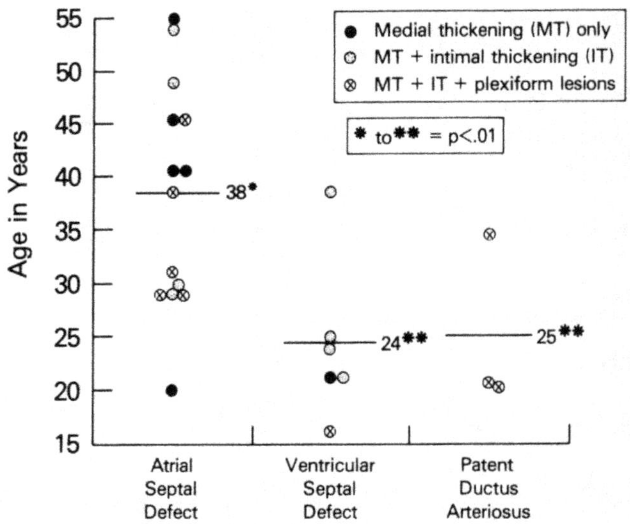

Figure 22. Data from Heath and associates[14] showing interrelationship between type of isolated congenital cardiovascular malformation (ASD, n = 14; VSD, n = 6; PDA, n = 3), age, and morphologic pulmonary arterial changes in 23 patients over age 15. The patients with VSD and PDA were significantly ($p < .01$) younger than those with ASD.

Table 11. Observations in 16 necropsy patients with primary pulmonary hypertension

Patient Age, Sex	*Duration of Symptoms (months)*	*Pressures (mm. Hg)* *PA (s/d)*	*SA (s/d)*	*CI (ml./min./m.^{2})*	*SA O_2* Sat. (%)	*Heart Weight* (gm.)	*PL*	*CEF-PT*
8 F*	24	190/100	90/55			160	+	A + F
17 F*	24	192/5	138/90	2.1	91	340	+	F
18 M	1	135/90	92/68	1.9	66	440	+	A
22 M**	36	88/54	100/60	1.5	86		+	A
25 F	30	92/39	130/78	2.0	98	460	+	A
25 F	54	122/49	122/80	2.7		360	+	A
25 F**	24	91/41	104/67	2.0	95		+	A
25 F	48	112/41	109/70	2.5			+	
28 M	24	108/58	127/80	3.2	92	630	+	A
29 F*	60	120/40	110/80	1.5	91	320	+	A
35 F*	84	101/38	108/72		86	400	0	A
38 M	144	138/88	138/88		↓†	880	+	F
39 F*	30	49/30	96/73		81†	390	0	A
39 F*	6	60/45	112/85			360	+	A
43 M	4	70/30	115/72	2.5		500	+	
56 M**	24		110/80				+	

*Death during or shortly after cardiac catheterization.
**Father-son-daughter relationship reported in detail elsewhere.[76]
†Right-to-left shunt via patent foramen ovale.
CEF-PT = configuration of elastic fibers of pulmonary trunk (A = adult; F = fetal); CI = cardiac index; PA = pulmonary artery; PL = plexiform lesion; SA = systemic artery; Sat. = saturation; s/d = systole diastole.

SIGNIFICANCE OF PULMONARY PARENCHYMAL CHOLESTEROL-ESTER GRANULOMAS

Among our 87 necropsy patients with various congenital cardiovascular malformations, 8 (11 percent) had pulmonary parenchymal cholesterol-ester granulomas (Table 12, Fig. 23). The cause of these granulomas is uncertain, but most patients who have them also have pulmonary hypertension.[61] We observed 13 necropsy patients with cholesterol-ester pulmonary granulomas (Table 12); 11 had pulmonary arterial systolic pressures recorded and these ranged from 50 to 138 mm. Hg (mean 108 mm. Hg). The other 2 patients had pulmonic stenosis and probably normal or only mildly elevated pulmonary arterial pressures.

PULMONARY ARTERIAL *HYPO*TENSION

To this point we have discussed changes in pulmonary arteries primarily in patients with pulmonary *hyper*tension. Now we focus on patients with pulmonary arterial *hypo*tension. The media of the pulmonary arteries in patients with chronic pulmonary hypertension is usually thicker than normal; the reverse is true in patients with chronic pulmonary hypotension in whom the media is thinner than normal. In addition, the lumens of these arteries, as well as those of the capillaries and pulmonary veins, are dilated.[45] The medial thinning and the luminal widening appears to be a consequence of the decreased pulmonary arterial pressure and not a consequence of decreased pulmonary arterial flow because these findings are present both in patients with isolated pulmonic stenosis (normal pulmonary flow) and in patients with pulmonic stenosis associated with VSD and right-to-left shunt (diminished pulmonary flow) (Figs. 24 and 25).

Table 12. Observations in 13 necropsy patients over age 15 with cholesterol-ester granulomas

Patient		*Pressure (mm. Hg)*			*Anatomic*
Age, Sex	*Diagnosis*	*PA (s/d)*	*SA (s/d)*	*Shunt*	*Grade of PA Changes*
29 F	ASD	110/60	110/60	both	III
33 M	VSD + PDA	106/60	136/68	R-L	III
21 F	VSD + PDA	138/86	140/88	both	III
38 M	VSD + CT	83/20	102/65	both	II
24 F	VSD + DORV	60/12	80/48	L-R	II
38 F	ASD + PS			R-L	0
24 F	VSD + PDA + MS + COA	104/60	118/70	L-R	II
25 F*	VSD + PS + AS		100/65	R-L	0
25 F	PPH	122/49	122/80	0	III
25 F	PPH	91/41	104/67	0	III
17 F	PPH	192/5**	138/90	0	III
38 M	PPH	138/88	138/88	0	III
39 F	PPH	50/30	96/73	L-R	II

*Patient also had pulmonary tuberculosis.

**Right ventricular pressure; pulmonary artery not entered.

AS = aortic stenosis; ASD = atrial septal defect; COA = coarctation of aorta; CT = corrected transposition; DORV = double outlet right ventricle; MS = mitral stenosis; PDA = patent ductus arteriosus; PPH = primary pulmonary hypertension; PS = pulmonic stenosis; PA = pulmonary artery; SA = systemic artery; s/d = systole/diastole; VSD = ventricular septal defect.

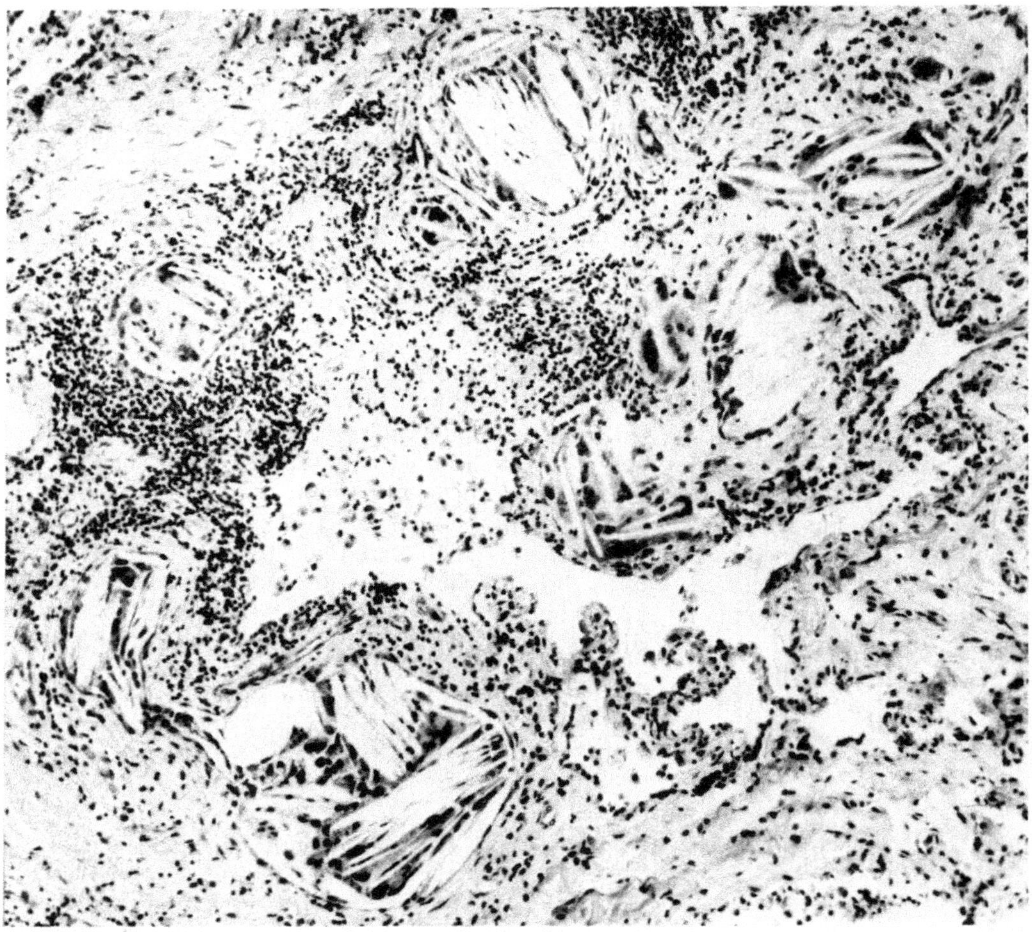

Figure 23. Multiple cholesterol-ester granulomas in the pulmonary parenchyma of a 38-year-old woman with VSD and corrected transposition. She had severe pulmonary hypertension (83/20 mm. Hg). Brachial arterial pressure was 102/65 mm. Hg and the left-to-right shunt was 2.1:1. (Hematoxylin and eosin stain, x 82; reduced 30%.)

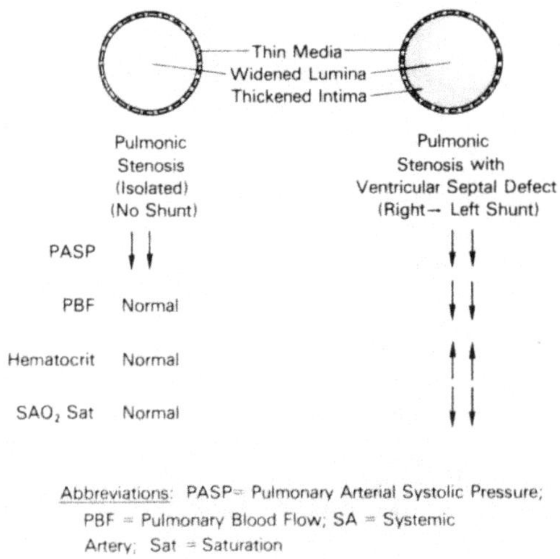

Figure 24. Diagram showing appearance of the pulmonary arteries in patients with pulmonary *hypo*tension. Patients with pulmonic stenosis have thinned media and wide lumina. If isolated, there is usually no thickening of the intima, but if pulmonic stenosis is combined with VSD the intima is usually thickened.

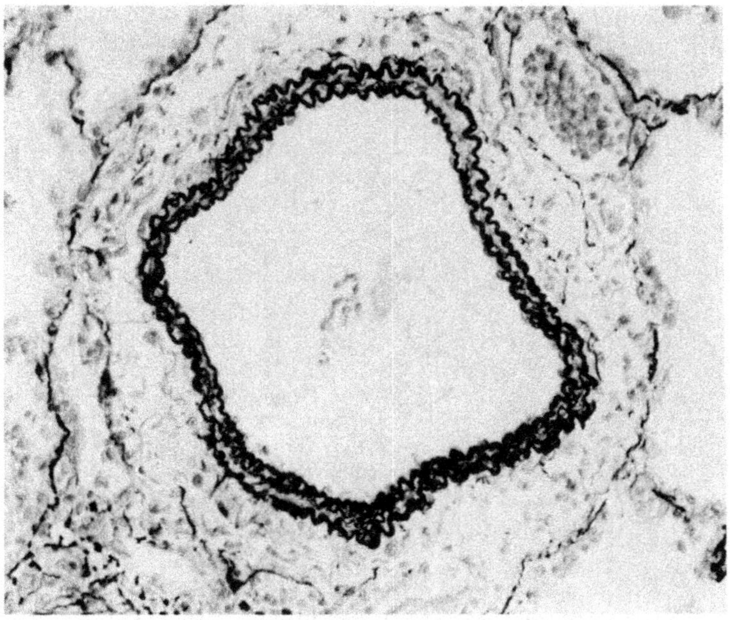

Figure 25. Pulmonic stenosis with ASD and anomalous drainage of the right pulmonary veins into the right atrium in a 19-year-old man who died three days after closure of the defect, pulmonic valvulotomy, and rerouting of the anomalous pulmonary veins. Preoperatively, pulmonary arterial pressure was 18/9 mm. Hg (mean 15), right ventricular pressure was 78/6 mm. Hg, brachial arterial pressure was 144/84 mm. Hg (mean 100), pulmonary to systemic flow ratio was 1.6 to 1, and systemic arterial oxygen saturation was 97 percent. Pulmonary arteries in this patient had thin medial walls and no intimal thickening, changes typical of pulmonary *hypo*tension. (Elastic van Gieson stain, x 272)

Another finding in some patients with pulmonary hypotension caused by congenital cardiovascular malformations is intimal fibrinous and fibrous changes. These intimal lesions were described intially by Arnold Rich[4] and are illustrated in Figure 26. Although pulmonary hypotension accompanies these lesions, it does not appear to be their cause. Evidence for this conclusion is provided by the fact that these lesions are rare in patients with pulmonic stenosis unassociated with communications between systemic and pulmonary circulations, but they are common in patients with pulmonic stenosis associated with VSD and right-to-left shunts (Table 13). The cause for the intimal lesions, therefore, must be related to the decreased pulmonary blood flow and associated polycythemia. It is also possible that "sludging" of blood flowing through the pulmonary vascular bed plays a role. Our observations in necropsy patients over age 15 with pulmonic stenosis are summarized in Table 13.

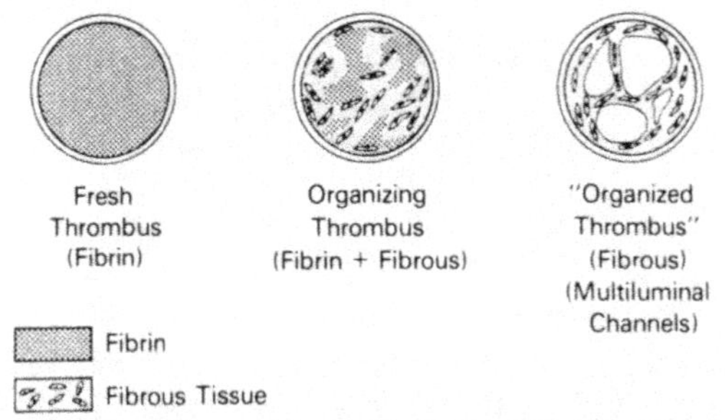

Figure 26. Diagram of Arnold Rich lesions occurring in patients with pulmonary hypotension and inadequate pulmonary blood flow.

Table 13. Observations in 9 necropsy patients over age 15 with pulmonic stenosis associated with either patent foramen ovale or ventricular septal defect

Patient Age, Sex	*Pressures (mm. Hg, s/d)*			*SA O₂*	*Blood*		*Interval (days)*	*PAs*		
Associated Defect	*PA*	*RV*	*SA*	*Sat. (%)*	*Hct. (%)*	*OP*	*OP to Death*	*M*	*I*	*AR*
28 F/PFO	9/4	170/4	123/70	67	61	PV	4	↓	nl	0
38 F/PFO						PV	60	↓	nl	0
43 F/PFO	13/8	172/12	130/70	83	65	PV	0	↓	↑	+
35 F/VSD	20/10	88/6		87	54	BT	21	↓	nl	0
22 M/VSD		145/9	148/105	88	71	0		↓	nl	0
53 M/VSD	17/8	95/8	110/65	77	69	TC	1	nl	↑	+
30 M/VSD	20/10	124/11	116/73	72	76	TC	45	↓	↑	+
23/M/VSD	12/4	112/4	131/85	68	72	TC	0	↓	↑	0
55 M/VSD	15/7	135/7	125/71	71	65	BT	6	↓	↑	0

AR = Arnold Rich lesions; Art = arterial; BT = Blalock-Taussig; Hct. = hematocrit; I = intima; nl = normal; M = media; OP = Cardiovascular operation; PA = pulmonary artery; PFO = patent foramen ovale; PV = pulmonic valvulotomy; RV = right ventricle; SA = systemic artery; Sat. = saturation; TC = total correction; ↓ = thinner than normal; ↑ = thickened; VSD = ventricular septal defect

Operative Creation of Systemic-to-Pulmonary Arterial Communications in Patients with Pulmonary Hypotension

Although development of pulmonary arterial hypertension is a recognized complication of operative creation of pulmonary-to-systemic arterial anastomoses,[62–66] the actual occurrence of pulmonary hypertension is uncommon. Therefore, anatomic pulmonary arterial changes indicative of pulmonary hypertension are also uncommon (Figs. 27 through 30).

Table 14 summarizes our observations in 10 necropsy patients over 15 years of age in whom pulmonary-to-systemic shunts had been created operatively between 3 and 23 years (mean 14) before death because of inadequate pulmonary blood flow. Nine patients had tetralogy of Fallot and one combined pulmonic stenosis and ASD. Surprisingly, 9 of the 10 patients showed neither pulmonary arterial medial or intimal thickening; 5 showed media of normal thickness and 4 had media thinner than normal. The one patient (Table 14) who did have medial and intimal thickening also had plexiform lesions. This patient, reported elsewhere,[65] was the only one of the 10 patients who had a Potts[67] operation rather than a Blalock-Taussig[68] anastomosis. The anastomosis in her was an end-to-side connection between right pulmonary artery and aorta. The right lung consequently developed systemic pressures and plexiform lesions (Fig. 29).

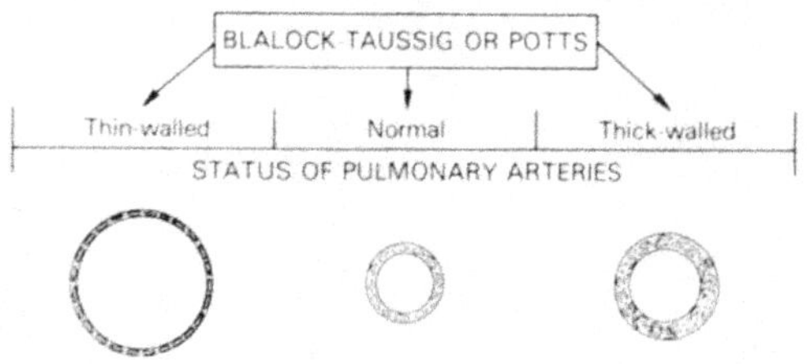

Figure 27. Diagram illustrating the effect of operative creation of systemic to pulmonary arterial communications on pulmonary arteries of patients with pulmonary *hypo*tension. The media of the pulmonary arteries may remain thin-walled and dilated (left), may increase to normal thickness (center), or may develop abnormally thickened media.

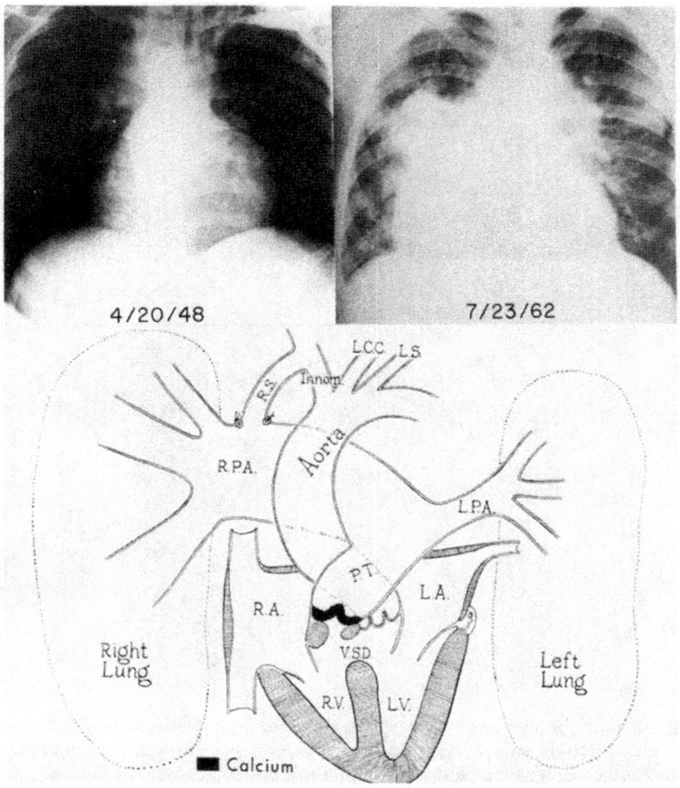

Figure 28. Tetralogy of Fallot in a 35-year-old man described in detail elsewhere.[65] By age 16 he was severely cyanotic and clubbed. Hemoglobin was 19.5 gm./100 ml. Chest radiograph (4/20/48) disclosed decreased pulmonary vascularity, and a subclavian-to-pulmonary arterial anastomosis was performed. Postoperatively, exercise tolerance improved and cyanosis had disappeared. At age 26 he had the first of many episodes of rapid heart action; three years later a chest radiograph (7/23/62) showed aneurysmal dilatation of the right pulmonary artery; systemic blood pressure was 150/25 mm. Hg. The patient died at age 35 of progressive right- and-left-sided congestive heart failure. Shortly before death the hematocrit was 44 percent.

The diagram of the heart and lungs at necropsy shows total obstruction of the pulmonic valve, ventricular septal defect (VSD), severely dilated pulmonary trunk (PT) and right main pulmonary artery (RPA), and widely patent right subclavian (RS) artery and anastomosis. LCC = left common carotid artery; LS = left subclavian artery; LPA = left pulmonary artery; LA = left atrium; LV = left ventricle; RA = right atrium; RV = right ventricle. Histologically, there was neither medial nor intimal thickening of the pulmonary arteries of either lung.

It is now well appreciated that pulmonary hypertension and anatomic pulmonary arterial changes of pulmonary hypertension are far more likely to develop after Potts than after Blalock-Taussig anastomoses. The various changes which may develop after creation of pulmonary to systemic anastomoses in patients with previous pulmonary hypotension are shown diagrammatically in Figure 30.

SUMMARY

Our three-grade anatomic classification of pulmonary arterial changes for patients with pulmonary arterial hypertension is a modification of the classification of Heath and Edwards. Our new classification consists of medial thickening only, grade I; medial and intimal thickening, grade II; and both medial and intimal thickening plus plexiform lesions, grade III. These anatomic changes in the pulmonary arteries result entirely

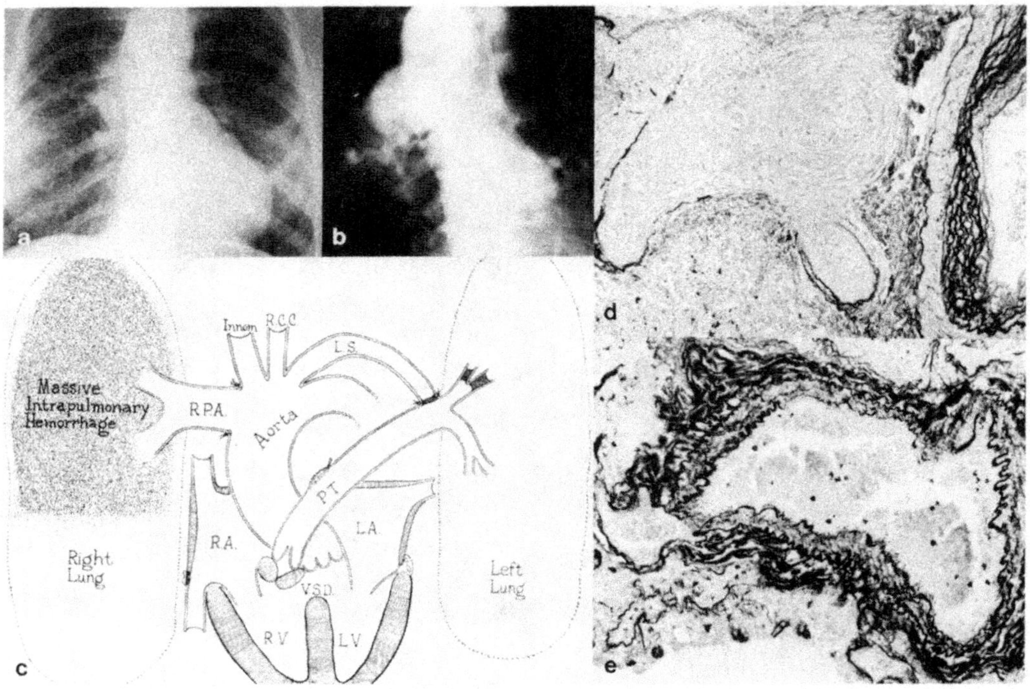

Figure 29. Tetralogy of Fallot in a 19-year-old woman described in detail elsewhere.[65] A left subclavian to left pulmonary arterial anastomosis was performed at age 3. There was little improvement, however, and an end-to-side anastomosis between aorta and right main pulmonary artery was performed two years later. She was nearly asymptomatic thereafter until age 11, when exercise tolerance diminished and cyanosis returned. At age 18 hematocrit was 80 percent. *a*, Chest radiograph shows right-aortic arch, decreased vascularity in the left lung, and increased vascular markings in the central portions of the right lung. The pulmonary trunk could not be entered by catheter from the right ventricle. Simultaneous right ventricular, femoral arterial, and right main pulmonary arterial systolic pressures were equal (108 mm. Hg). Oxygen saturation in the femoral artery was 70 percent. *b*, At right ventricular angiography all contrast material was ejected into the aorta and the lumens of the intrapulmonary branches of the right main pulmonary artery were severely narrowed. The left subclavian artery was occluded just proximal to its connection to the left main pulmonary artery. No contrast material entered the pulmonary trunk, left main pulmonary artery, or left lung. Because of systemic pressure in the right pulmonary arteries and absent blood flow to the left lung, the patient was considered inoperable. At age 19 she died suddenly of massive intrapulmonary hemorrhage. *c*, Diagram of findings in heart and lungs at necropsy (abbreviations in Figure 28). *d*, A portion of wall of a right pulmonary artery. Arising from it (but not connected in this section) is a plexiform lesion. *e*, Left pulmonary artery is normal. (Elastic van Gieson stain, x 160; reduced 41%.)

from pulmonary hypertension. Intimal thickening without medial thickening, however, is observed in older persons, and, in itself, is not a consequence of pulmonary hypertension.

Observations in our 87 necropsy patients over age 15 with major congenital cardiovascular malformations indicate that the changes in the pulmonary arteries are directly related to the level of pulmonary arterial pressure. Direction of the shunt, location of the shunt, and age of the patient were important only by their effect on the pulmonary arterial pressure. The patients with patent ductus arteriosus had the most severe changes in the pulmonary arteries and the highest average pulmonary arterial pressures.

Although not *all* patients with pulmonary arterial systolic pressures >90 mm. Hg had them, plexiform lesions were only observed in patients in whom the pulmonary arterial systemic pressure was >90 mm. Hg. Plexiform lesions indicate the irreversible nature

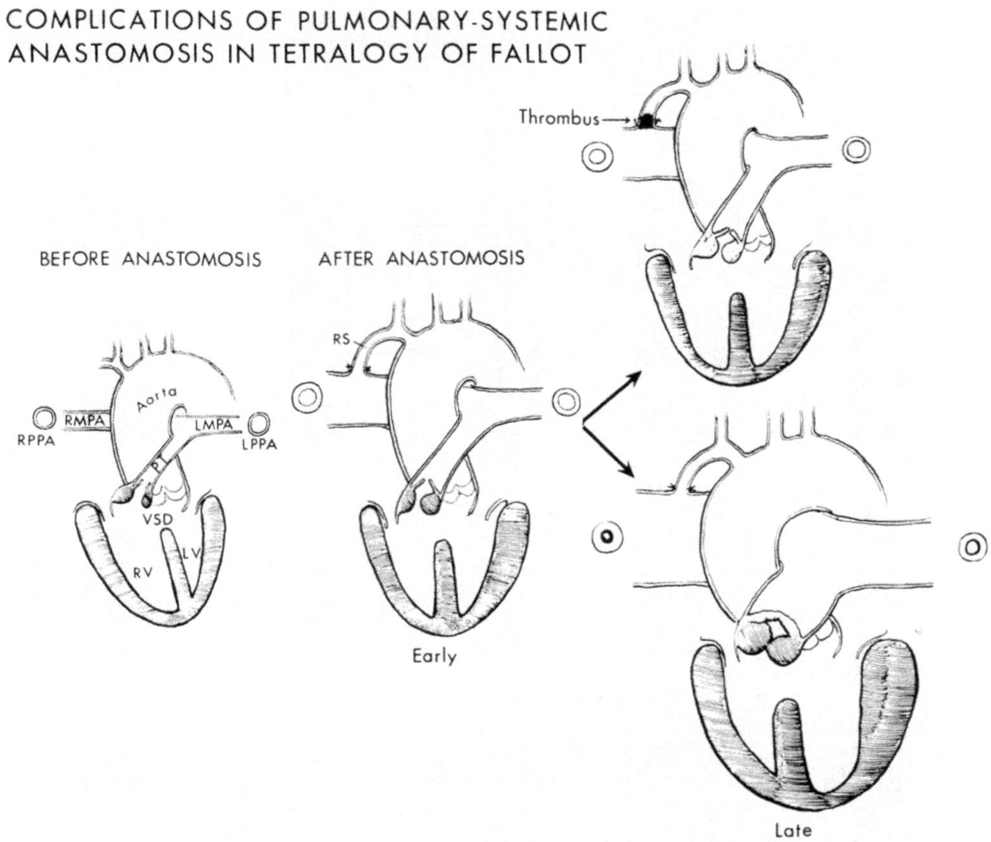

Figure 30. Diagram illustrating complications of pulmonary-systemic anastomosis in patients with tetralogy of Fallot. After anastomosis the early changes are related to the beneficial effects of increased blood flow to the lungs. With the shunt wide open, blood flow through the right ventricular outflow tract decreases and the amount of blood shunted from the right ventricular body to the left ventricle in diastole increases. As a result of the increased blood flow and pressure, the major pulmonary arteries widen and their wall thicknesses increase. Late complications include occlusion of the shunt and of the pulmonic valve or right ventricular infundibulum. LV = left ventricle; LPPA and RPPA = left and right peripheral pulmonary arteries; LMPA and RMPA = left and right main pulmonary arteries; RS = right subclavian artery; RV = right ventricle; VSD = ventricular septal defect.

of pulmonary hypertension and are more frequent in patients with primary pulmonary hypertension than in patients with congenital cardiovascular malformations.

The cause of plexiform lesions is unknown. We believe they are aneurysmal dilatations at sites of congenitally weak and/or thin walls of muscular pulmonary arteries. Distal to the weak or thin media the lumen of the muscular artery is obliterated. The aneurysmal protrusion is filled with thrombus which organizes into multiluminal channels.

Cholesterol-ester granulomas in the lungs usually indicate the presence of pulmonary hypertension; their cause is also uncertain.

In patients with pulmonary *hypo*tension (isolated pulmonic stenosis) and in patients with pulmonic stenosis and ventricular septal defect (tetralogy of Fallot), the media of the pulmonary arteries is thinner than normal and the lumens are larger than normal. Intimal thickening is usually seen in patients with tetralogy of Fallot even though the media is not thickened.

Surgical creation of systemic-to-pulmonary arterial anastomoses may cause the pul-

Table 14. Observations in 10 necropsy patients over age 15 with cyanotic CHD: Pulmonary vascular changes in patients having operatively created systemic to pulmonary arterial shunts for inadequate pulmonary blood flow (or severe systemic arterial desaturation)

Patient Age, Sex	*Anomalies*	*SA* O_2 Sat. (%)*	*RV Pressure (mm. Hg, s/d) PRE–PO*	*PA Pressure (mm. Hg, s/d) PRE–PO*	*SA Pressure (mm. Hg, s/d) PRE–PO*	*Type Operative Shunt Created*	*Direction of PO Shunt R→L*	*L→R*	*Interval (yrs) OP-Shunt to Death*	*Cause of Death/ Status of Operative Shunt*	*Morphologic Pulmonic Arterial Changes*
19 F	PS, VSD	70	NA–105/6	NA–108/78**	NA–108/78	(1)LSA→LPA (2)Ao→RPA	+	+	16 14	bleeding, lung/(1)C; (2)O	(1)H, (2)PL
35 M	PS, VSD		172/18–NA	20/10–NA	108/85–150/25	RSA→RPA	+	+	19	CHF/O	H, T
36 M	PS, VSD		NA	NA	NA–104/63	Ao→LPA			20	reoperation	H, T
24 F	PS, VSD	89	NA–40/0	NA–14/4	NA–90/70	(1)RSA→RPA (2)RSA→RPA	+	0	18 23	reoperation/O↓↓	H
27 M	PS, VSD		NA	NA	NA	LSA→LPA	+	0	9	CHF/(1) + (2)O↓↓↓	H
21 M	PS, VSD, ASD, CT		NA	NA	NA–120/80	LSA→LPA	+	0	11	polycythemia/O↓↓↓	none
21 M	PS, VSD, CT	71	125/0–NA	NA	NA–125/80	(1)LSA→LPA (2)RSA→RPA	+	+	6 3	reoperation/(1)C, (2)O↓	(1)T, (2)none
33 M	PS, ASD	81	NA–130/10	NA	NA–80/55†	LSA→LPA	+	+	20	reoperation/O	none
27 M	PS,VSD,ASD, TA	88	NA	NA	NA–112/66	LSA→LPA	+	+	20	reoperation/O	none
22 F	PS,VSD	72	145/0–154/13	15/0–NA	120/65–196/75	LSA→LPA	+	0	8	reoperation C	none

*Last year of life
**Right pulmonary artery
†Left brachial artery: right femoral artery = 98/58

ASD = atrial septal defect; C = closed; CHF = congestive heart failure; CT = complete transposition; H = hypoplastic; LPA = left main pulmonary artery; LSA = left subclavian artery; NA = data not available; OP = cardiovascular operation; O = open; PA = pulmonary artery; PL = plexiform lesion + medial hypertrophy + intimal proliferation; PO = postoperative; PRE = preoperative; PS = pulmonic or subpulmonic stenosis; RPA = right pulmonary artery; RSA = right subclavian artery; RV = right ventricle; T = thrombi containing fibrin; TA = tricuspid atresia; SA = systemic artery; Sat. = saturation; s/d = systolic/diastolic; VSD = ventricular septal defect.

monary arterial media to thicken to normal widths or even to widths thicker than normal, but the development of pulmonary hypertension after such operations is infrequent.

REFERENCES

1. Moschcowitz, E.: *Hypertension of the pulmonary circulation; its causes, dynamics and relation to other circulatory states.* Am. J. Med. Sci. 174:388,1927.
2. Brenner, O.: *Pathology of the vessels of the pulmonary circulation.* Arch. Intern. Med. 56:211,1935.
3. Parker, F., and Weiss, S.: *The nature and significance of the structural changes in the lungs in mitral stenosis.* Am. J. Pathol. 12:573,1936.
4. Rich, A. R.: *A hitherto unrecognized tendency to the development of widespread pulmonary vascular obstruction in patients with congenital pulmonary stenosis (tetralogy of Fallot).* Bull. Johns Hopkins Hosp. 82:389,1948.
5. Edwards, J. E., Douglas, J. M., Burchell, H. B., et al.: *Pathology of the intrapulmonary arteries and arterioles in coarctation of the aorta associated with patent ductus arteriosus.* Am. Heart J. 38:208,1949.
6. Civin, W. H., and Edwards, J. E.: *Pathology of the pulmonary vascular tree. I. A comparison of the intrapulmonary arteries in the Eisenmenger complex and in stenosis of ostium infundibuli associated with biventricular origin of the aorta.* Circulation 21:545,1950.
7. Heath, D., and Witaker, W.: *The pulmonary vessels in patent ductus arteriosus.* J. Pathol. Bacteriol. 70:285,1955.
8. Brewer, D. B.: *Fibrous occlusion and anastomosis of the pulmonary vessels in a case of pulmonary hypertension associated with patent ductus arteriosus.* J. Pathol. Bacteriol. 70:299,1955.
9. Dammann, J. F., and Ferencz, C.: *The significance of the pulmonary vascular bed in congenital heart disease. I. Normal lungs, II. Malformations of the heart in which there is pulmonary stenosis.* Am. Heart J. 52:7,1956.
10. Dammann, J. F., Jr., and Ferencz, C.: *The significance of the pulmonary vascular bed in congenital heart disease. III. Defects between the ventricles or great vessels in which both increased pressure and blood flow may act upon the lungs and in which there is a common ejectile force.* Am. Heart J. 52:210,1956.
11. Edwards, J. E.: *Functional pathology of the pulmonary vascular tree in congenital cardiac disease.* Circulation 15:164,1957.
12. Heath, D., Dushane, J. W., Wood, E. H., et al.: *The etiology of pulmonary thrombosis in cyanotic congenital heart disease with pulmonary stenosis.* Thorax 13:213,1958.
13. Heath, D., and Edwards, J. E.: *The pathology of hypertensive pulmonary vascular disease. A description of six grades of structural changes in the pulmonary arteries with special reference to congenital cardiac defects.* Circulation 18:533,1958.
14. Heath, D., Helmholz, H. F., Burchell, H. B., et al.: *Graded pulmonary vascular changes and hemodynamic findings in cases of atrial and ventricular septal defect and patent ductus arteriosus.* Circulation 18:1155,1958.
15. Heath, D., Helmholz, H. F., Burchell, H. B., et al.: *Relation between structural changes in the small pulmonary arteries and the immediate reversibility of pulmonary hypertension following closure of ventricular and atrial septal defects.* Circulation 18:1167,1958.
16. Wagenvoort, C. A.: *The morphology of certain vascular lesions in pulmonary hypertension.* J. Pathol. Bacteriol. 78:503,1959.
17. Ferencz, C.: *The pulmonary vascular bed in tetralogy of Fallot. I. Changes associated with pulmonic stenosis.* Bull. Johns Hopkins Hosp. 106:81,1960.
18. Ferencz, C.: *The pulmonary vascular bed in tetralogy of Fallot. II. Changes following a systemic-pulmonary arterial anastomosis.* Bull. Johns Hopkins Hosp. 106:100,1960.
19. Heath, D.: *Pathology of the pulmonary vessels.* Br. J. Dis. Chest 54:182,1960.
20. Wagenvoort, C. A., Dushane, J. W., and Edwards, J. E.: *Hypertensive pulmonary arterial lesions as a result of anastomosis of systemic and pulmonary circulations.* Mayo Clin. Proc. 35:186,1960.
21. Naeye, R. L.: *Perinatal changes in the pulmonary vascular bed with stenosis and atresia of the pulmonic valve.* Am. Heart J. 61:586,1961.
22. Wagenvoort, C. A., Neufeld, H. N., Dushane, J. W., et al.: *The pulmonary arterial tree in ventricular septal defect. A quantitative study of anatomic features in fetuses, infants, and children.* Circulation 23:740,1961.
23. Wagenvoort, C. A., and Edwards, J. E.: *The pulmonary arterial tree in pulmonic atresia.* Arch. Pathol. 71:646,1961.

24. WAGENVOORT, C. A.: *Pulmonary arteries in infants with ventricular septal defect.* Med. Thorac. 19:354,1962.

25. HARRIS, P., AND HEATH, D.: *The Human Pulmonary Circulation. Its Forms and Function in Health and Disease.* E & S Livingstone, Ltd., Edinburgh and London, 1962.

26. THOMAS, M. A.: *Pulmonary vascular changes in pulmonary stenosis with and without ventricular septal defect.* Br. Heart J. 26:655,1964.

27. FERENCZ, C.: *Pulmonary vascular changes in tetralogy of Fallot.* Dis. Chest 46:664,1964.

28. WAGENVOORT, C. A., HEATH, D., AND EDWARDS, J. E.: *The Pathology of the Pulmonary Vasculature.* Charles C Thomas, Springfield, Ill., 1964.

29. THOMAS, M. A.: *Pulmonary vascular changes in pulmonary stenosis with and without ventricular septal defect.* Br. Heart J. 26:655,1964.

30. KANJUH, V. I., SELLERS, R. D., AND EDWARDS, J. E.: *Pulmonary vascular plexiform lesion.* Arch. Pathol. 78:513,1964.

31. FERENCZ, C.: *Transposition of the great vessels; pathophysiologic consideration based upon a study of the lungs.* Circulation 33:232,1966.

32. ANDERSON, R. A., LEVY, A. M., NAEYE, R. L., ET AL.: *Rapidly progressive pulmonary vascular obstructive disease. Association with ventricular septal defects during early childhood.* Am. J. Cardiol. 19:854,1967.

33. WAGENVOORT, C. A., NAUTA, J., VAN DER SCHAAR, P. J., ET AL.: *Effect of flow and pressure on pulmonary vessels. A semiquantitative study based on lung biopsies.* Circulation 35:1028,1967.

34. WAGENVOORT, C. A., NAUTA, J., VAN DER SCHAAR, P. J., ET AL.: *Vascular changes in pulmonic stenosis and tetralogy of Fallot studied in lung biopsies.* Circulation 36:924,1967.

35. WAGENVOORT, C. A., NAUTA, J., VAN DER SCHAAR, P. J., ET AL.: *The pulmonary vasculature in complete transposition of the great vessels judged from lung biopsies.* Circulation 38:746,1968.

36. VILES, P. H., ONGLEY, P. A., AND TITUS, J. L.: *The spectrum of pulmonary vascular disease in transposition of the great arteries.* Circulation 40:31,1969.

37. WAGENVOORT, C. A.: *Hypertensive pulmonary vascular disease complicating congenital heart disease: A review.* Cardiovasc. Clin. 5:43,1973.

38. HISLOP, A., AND REID, L.: *Stuctural changes in the pulmonary arteries and veins in tetralogy of Fallot.* Br. Heart J. 35:1178,1973.

39. NEWFELD, E. A., PAUL, M. H., MUSTER, A. J., ET AL.: *Pulmonary vascular disease in complete transposition of the great arteries: A study of 200 patients.* Am. J. Cardiol. 34:75,1974.

40. WAGENVOORT, C. A.: *Classification of pulmonary vascular lesions in congenital and acquired heart disease.* Adv. Cardiol. 11:48,1974.

41. WAGENVOORT, C. A., AND WAGENVOORT, N.: *Pathology of the Eisenmenger syndrome and primary pulmonary hypertension.* Adv. Cardiol. 11:123,1974.

42. HOFFMEISTER, H. -E., APITZ, J., AND BACKMANN, R.: *The correlation between pulmonary hypertension and histological findings of the pulmonary vessels in congenital heart disease.* Thoraxchir. Vask. Chir. 23:436,1975.

43. BESSINGER, F. B., BLIEDEN, L. C., AND EDWARDS, J. E.: *Hypertensive pulmonary vascular disease associated with patent ductus arteriosus. Primary or secondary?* Circulation 52:157,1975.

44. NEWFELD, E. A., SHER, M., PAUL, M. H., ET AL.: *Pulmonary vascular disease in complete atrioventricular canal defect.* Am. J. Cardiol. 39:721,1977.

45. WAGENVOORT, C. A., AND WAGENVOORT, N.: *Pathology of Pulmonary Hypertension.* John Wiley & Sons, New York, 1977.

46. CIVIN, W. H., AND EDWARDS, J. E.: *The postnatal structural changes in the intrapulmonary arteries and arterioles.* Arch. Pathol. 51:192,1951.

47. WAGENVOORT, C. A., AND WAGENVOORT, N.: *Age changes in muscular pulmonary arteries.* Arch. Pathol. 79:524,1965.

48. ROBERTS, W. C., AND FREDRICKSON, D. S.: *Gaucher's disease of the lung causing severe pulmonary hypertension with associated acute recurrent pericarditis.* Circulation 35:783,1967.

49. SPENCER, H.: *Primary pulmonary hypertension and related vascular changes in the lungs.* J. Pathol. Bacteriol. 62:75,1950.

50. GORDON, A. J., DONOSO, E., KUHN, C. L. A., ET AL.: *Patent ductus arteriosus with reversal of flow.* N. Engl. J. Med. 251:923,1954.

51. HUFNER, R. F., AND MCNICOL, C. A.: *The pathologic physiology of microscopic pulmonary vascular shunts.* AMA Arch. Pathol. 65:554,1958.

52. ROSSALL, R. E., AND THOMPSON, H.: *Formation of new vascular channels in the lungs of a patient with secondary pulmonary hypertension.* J. Pathol. Bacteriol. 76:593,1958.

53. PLANT, A.: *Hemangioendothelioma of the lung. Report of two cases.* Arch. Pathol. 29:517,1940.

54. MOSCHCOWITZ, E., RUBIN, E., AND STRAUSS, L.: *Hypertension of the pulmonary circulation due to congenital glomoid obstruction of the pulmonary arteries.* Am. J. Pathol. 39:75,1961.

55. CROSS, K. R., AND KOBAYASHI, C. K.: *Primary pulmonary vascular sclerosis: Report of case.* Am. J. Clin. Pathol. 17:155,1947.

56. HRUBAN, Z., AND HUMPHREYS, E. M.: *Congenital anomalies associated with pulmonary hypertension in an infant.* Arch. Pathol. 70:766,1960.

57. NAEYE, R. L., AND VENNART, G. P.: *Structure and significance of pulmonary plexiform structures.* Am. J. Pathol. 36:593,1960.

58. KAPANCI, Y.: *Hypertensive pulmonary vascular disease. Endothelial hyperplasia and its relations to intravascular fibrin precipitation.* Am. J. Pathol. 48:665,1965.

59. WALCOTT, G., BURCHELL, H. B., AND BROWN, A. L.: *Primary pulmonary hypertension.* Am. J. Med. 49:70,1970.

60. WAGENVOORT, C. A., AND WAGENVOORT, N.: *Primary pulmonary hypertension. A patholytic study of the lung vessels in 156 clinically diagnosed cases.* Circulation 42:1163,1970.

61. GLANCY, D. L., FRAZIER, P. D., AND ROBERTS, W. C.: *Pulmonary parenchymal cholesterol-ester granulomas in patients with pulmonary hypertension.* Am. J. Med. 45:198,1968.

62. ROSS, R. S., TAUSSIG, H. B., AND EVANS, M. H.: *Late hemodynamic complications of anastomotic surgery for the treatment of the tetralogy of Fallot.* Circulation 18:553,1958.

63. PAUL, M. H., MILLER, R. A., AND POTTS, W. J.: *Long-term results of aortic-pulmonary anastomosis for tetralogy of Fallot: An analysis of the first 100 cases eleven to thirteen years after operation.* Circulation 23:525,1961.

64. MCCAGG, C. J., ROSS, R. S., AND BRAUNWALD, E.: *The development of elevated pulmonary vascular resistance in man following increased pulmonary blood flow from systemic pulmonary anastomoses.* Am. J. Med. 33:201,1962.

65. ROBERTS, W. C., FRIESINGER, G. C., COHEN, L. S., ET AL.: *Acquired pulmonic atresia. Total obstruction to right ventricular outflow after systemic to pulmonary arterial anastomoses for cyanotic congenital cardiac disease.* Am. J. Cardiol. 24:335,1969.

66. NEWFELD, E. A., WALDMAN, J. D., PAUL, M. H., ET AL.: *Pulmonary vascular disease after systemic-pulmonary arterial shunt operations.* Am. J. Cardiol. 39:715,1977.

67. POTTS, W. J., SMITH, S., AND GIBSON, S.: *Anastomosis of the aorta to a pulmonary artery. Certain types in congenital heart disease.* JAMA 132:627,1946.

68. BLALOCK, A., AND TAUSSIG, H. B.: *Surgical treatment of malformations of the heart in which there is a pulmonary stenosis or pulmonary atresia.* JAMA 128:189,1945.

69. HEATH, D., DUSHANE, J. W., WOOD, E. H., ET AL.: *The structure of the pulmonary trunk at different ages and in cases of pulmonary hypertension and pulmonary stenosis.* J. Pathol. Bacteriol. 77:443,1959.

70. PERLOFF, J. K., URSCHELL, C. W., ROBERTS, W. C., ET AL.: *Aneurysmal dilatation of the coronary arteries in cyanotic congenital cardiac disease.* Am. J. Med. 45:802,1968.

71. GLANCY, D. L., AND ROBERTS, W. C.: *Congenital obstructive lesions involving the major pulmonary veins, left atrium, or mitral valve: A clinical, laboratory, and morphologic survey.* Cathet. Cardiovasc. Diagn. 2:215,1976.

72. PARKER, F., JR., AND WEISS, S.: *The nature and significance of the structural changes in the lungs in mitral stenosis.* Am. J. Pathol. 12:573,1936.

73. HEATH, D., AND WHITAKER, W.: *The pulmonary vessels in mitral stenosis.* J. Pathol. Bacteriol. 70:291,1955.

74. ABER, C. P., CAMPBELL, J. A., AND MEECHAM, J.: *Arterial patterns in mitral stenosis.* Br. Heart J. 25:109,1963.

75. TANDON, H. D., AND KASTURI, J.: *Pulmonary vascular changes associated with isolated mitral stenosis in India.* Br. Heart J. 37:26,1975.

76. KINGDON, H. S., COHEN, L. S., ROBERTS, W. C., ET AL.: *Familial occurrence of primary pulmonary hypertension.* Arch. Intern. Med. 118:422,1966.

Mitral valve *commissurotomy* versus *replacement*

Considerations based on examination of operatively excised stenotic mitral valves

William C. Roberts, M.D.
Anthony S. Lachman, M.B., F.C.P. (S.A.)
Bethesda, Md.

Recently, we studied 164 operatively-excised stenotic mitral valves and by radiography of the excised valve quantitated the amount of calcific deposits in them.[1] Of the 164 stenotic valves, 14 had absent and 43 had minimal calcific deposits by x-ray of the excised valve. Of these 57 patients with absent or minimal calcific deposits, 37 had moderate to severe mitral regurgitation, and, therefore, clearly deserved mitral valve replacement. The remaining 20 had absent or minimal mitral regurgitation, absent or minimal calcific deposits, and mitral valve replacement, nevertheless, was carried out. This report focuses on these latter 20 patients to ask if mitral valve replacement was preferable to mitral valve commissurotomy.

Patients studied

Of the 20 patients, 19 underwent mitral valve replacement from 1970 to 1976 and one in 1967. The mitral valve operations on these 20 patients during the 8 years were done by five different surgeons (see Acknowledgment). Certain clinical and morphologic features in the 20 patients are summarized in Table I and morphologic and radiographic features of the excised mitral valves are illustrated in Figs. 1 to 5. A radiograph was taken of each of the excised mitral valves via a Field-Emission-Faxitron x-ray unit at 35 KVP. No calcific deposits were present in the excised valve in five patients and in the other 15, calcific deposits were trace, minimal, or mild and in no patient were they visible before operation by routine chest roentgenogram or by fluoroscopy.

The 20 patients ranged in age from 36 to 62 years (average, 52 years); 12 (60 per cent) were women and eight were men. Cardiac catheterization was carried out during the 2 months before mitral valve replacement in all 20 patients (Table I). The mean diastolic pressure gradients between pulmonary artery wedge and left ventricle ranged from 5 to 21 mm. Hg (average, 11.5 mm. Hg). The pulmonary arterial systolic pressures (19 patients) ranged from 32 to 75 mm. Hg (average, 50 mm. Hg). The mean pulmonary arterial wedge pressures ranged from 15 to 35 mm. Hg (average, 25 mm. Hg). In eight patients, a systolic pressure gradient was present between left ventricle and systemic artery and it ranged from 10 to 95 mm. Hg (average, 50 mm. Hg). The cardiac index ranged from 1.2 to 3.6 L./min./M.^{2} (average, 2.09 L./min./M.^{2}). Left ventricular angiography in 19 patients indicated minimal (1+/4+) mitral regurgitation in 16 patients and no regurgitation in three patients. The one patient (No. 10, Table I) in whom left ventricular angiography was not performed had no precordial systolic murmur. Injection of contrast material into the aortic "root" in 18 patients indicated various degrees of aortic regurgitation in 14.

In addition to mitral valve replacement, the aortic valve was replaced in 12 (60 per cent) of the 20 patients and the tricuspid valve, in four (20 per cent), three of whom also had aortic valve replacement. The average mean diastolic pressure gradient between pulmonary arterial wedge posi-

From the Pathology Branch, National Heart, Lung, and Blood Institute, National Institutes of Health, Bethesda, Md.

Received for publication June 2, 1978.

Accepted for publication July 14, 1978.

Reprint requests to: Dr. William C. Roberts, Building 10A, Room 3E30, National Institutes of Health, Bethesda, Md. 20014.

Table I. Clinical and hemodynamic data in the 20 patients analyzed

	Surgical Number	Age (yrs)	Sex	Interval MVC to MVR (yrs)	PAW-LV mdg* (mm. Hg)	PA* (s/d) (mm. Hg)	CI* (L./min. /M.²)	MR by LV cine* (0-4+)	MV Ca⁺⁺ by x-ray of excised valve (0+ 4+)	LV-SA PSG* (mm. Hg)	AR by AA cine* (0-4+)	AVR	TVR	Fig. No.
No previous mitral-valve commissurotomy														
1	67-3005	36	M	–	8	32/10	1.7	1+	1+	26	2+	+	0	–
2	70-3094	47	M	–	11	50/20	1.8	1+	1+	0	2+	+	0	–
3	70-3127	44	F	–	15	45/32	1.7	1+	1+	10	3+	+	+	–
4	72-4096	57	F	–	5	34/18	2.0	0	0	40	4+	+	0	–
5	73-5085	60	M	–	17	–	1.5	1+	1+	0	3+	+	0	–
6	74-5139	48	M	–	12	50/20	3.1	0	1+	50	3+	+	0	–
7	75-5067	52	F	–	21	60/30	2.3	1+	0	90	2+	+	+	–
8	75-5106	58	M	–	10	70/40	3.6	1+	0	0	0	0	0	1
9	76-28	58	M		12	40/20	2.3	1+	1+	0	0	0	0	–
Previous mitral-valve commissurotomy														
10	71-3125	59	F	17 & 14	11**	36/18	1.7	–***	1+	0	–	0	0	2
11	71-3136	62	F	15	11	48/23	2.6	1+	1+	0	1+	0	0	3
12	71-3144	61	F	19	10	70/35	3.4	1+	1+	0	1+	0	0	4
13	72-5003	64	F	10	15	75/35	1.2	0	1+	0	1+	0	0	–
14	73-5032	57	F	12	8	55/25	2.3	1+	1+	0	0	0	0	–
15	73-5071	49	M	18	10	50/20	2.2	1+	1+	95	2+	+	0	–
16	74-5047	47	M	2	14	45/24	2.5	1+	1+	0	2+	+	0	–
17	74-5156	36	F	8	7	40/20	1.0	1+	0	75	–	+	+	5
18	75-5162	43	F	15 & 8	10	55/25	1.7	1+	1+	0	0	0	+	
19	76-95	51	F	6	16	55/28	2.0	1+	1+	10	2+	+	0	–
20	76-99	42	F	4	7	32/15	1.2	1+	0	0	3+	+	0	–

*At cardiac catheterization performed during the 2 months before mitral valve replacement.

**Left atrial pressure.

***A precordial systolic murmur was absent.

Abbreviations: AA = ascending aorta; AR = aortic regurgitation; AVR = aortic valve replacement; CI = cardiac index; F = female; LA = left atrial; LV = left ventricular; M = male; mdg = mean diastolic gradient; MR = mitral regurgitation; MV = mitral valve; MVC = mitral valve commissurotomy; MVR = mitral valve replacement; PA = pulmonary arterial; PAW = pulmonary arterial wedge; PSG = peak systolic gradient; SA = systemic arterial; s/d = systolic/diastolic; TVR = tricuspid valve replacement.

tion and left ventricle in the patients who underwent aortic valve replacement was 11.9 mm. Hg, and in those in whom this valve was not replaced, it was 10.9 mm. Hg.

Of the 20 patients, 11 had had mitral commissurotomy from 2 to 19 years (average, 12 years) previously. Two patients (No. 10 and No. 18, Table I) had had two previous commissurotomies. The pulmonary arterial wedge to left ventricular mean diastolic pressure gradients in these 11 patients ranged from 7 to 16 mm. Hg (average, 10.8 mm. Hg), whereas this gradient in the nine patients without previous commissurotomy ranged from 5 to 21 mm. Hg (average, 12.3 mm. Hg).

Thrombus was found in the body of left atrium at the time of valve replacement in two patients (No. 10 and No. 18, Table I).

Comments

The absence of significant calcific deposits (as determined by radiography of the excised valve) and the absence of significant mitral regurgitation (as determined by left ventricular angiography) in the operatively-excised stenotic mitral valves described above raises the question as to whether mitral valve replacement in these 20 patients was preferable to commissurotomy. To answer this question the stenotic mitral valves in patients having only commissurotomy would have to be studied morphologically and radiographically in the same manner as the valves which were excised and replaced. Obviously, the non-excised valve cannot be examined in the same manner as the excised valve. Nevertheless, the ideal valve for mitral commissurotomy in the past has been considered to be the stenotic one

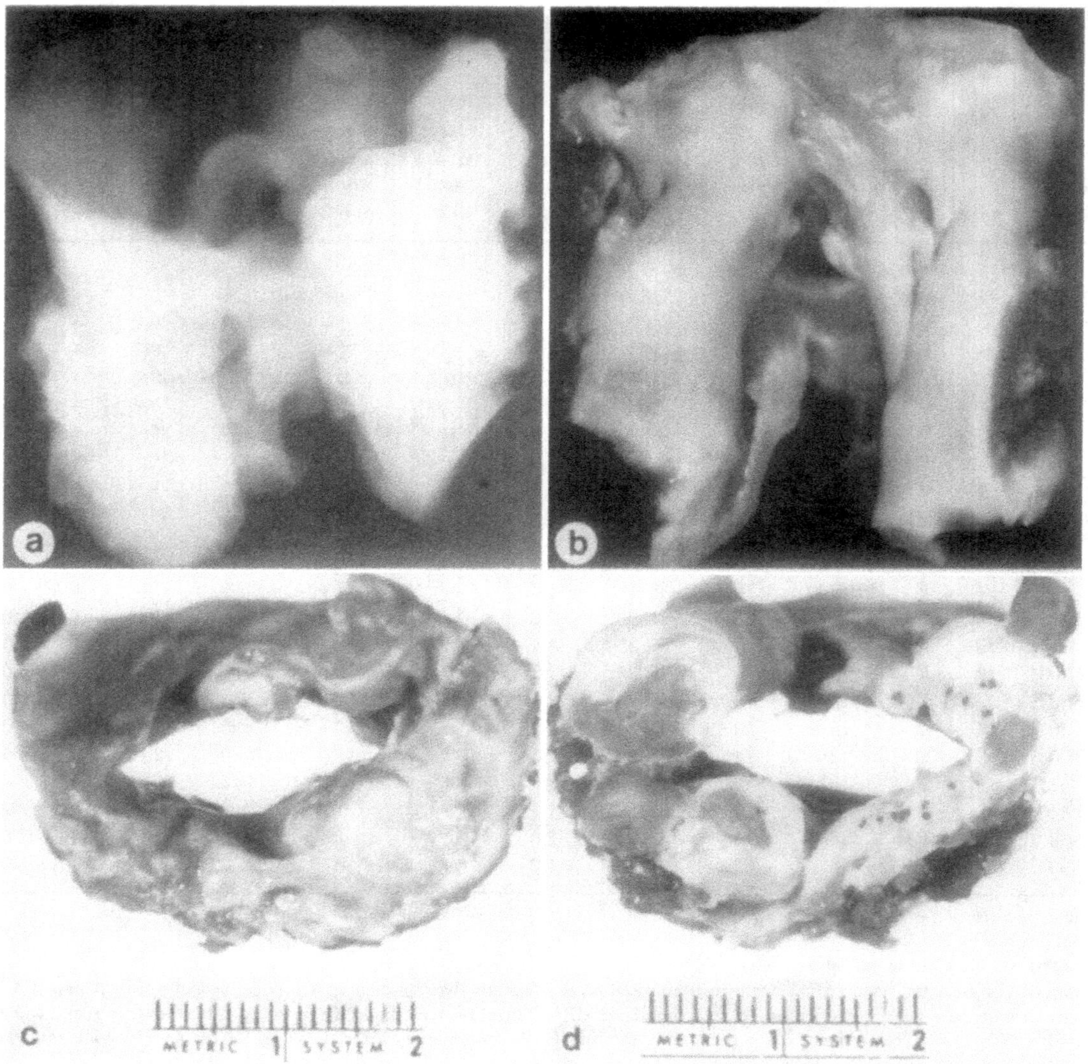

Fig. 1, a through d. Case No. 8 (Table I). *a,* Radiograph showing no calcific deposits. *b,* View of anterior leaflet and papillary muscles from left ventricle. The papillary muscles are covered by thick fibrous tissue. *c,* View from left atrium. *d,* View of orifice from left ventricle again showing the thick fibrous tissue overlying the papillary muscles.

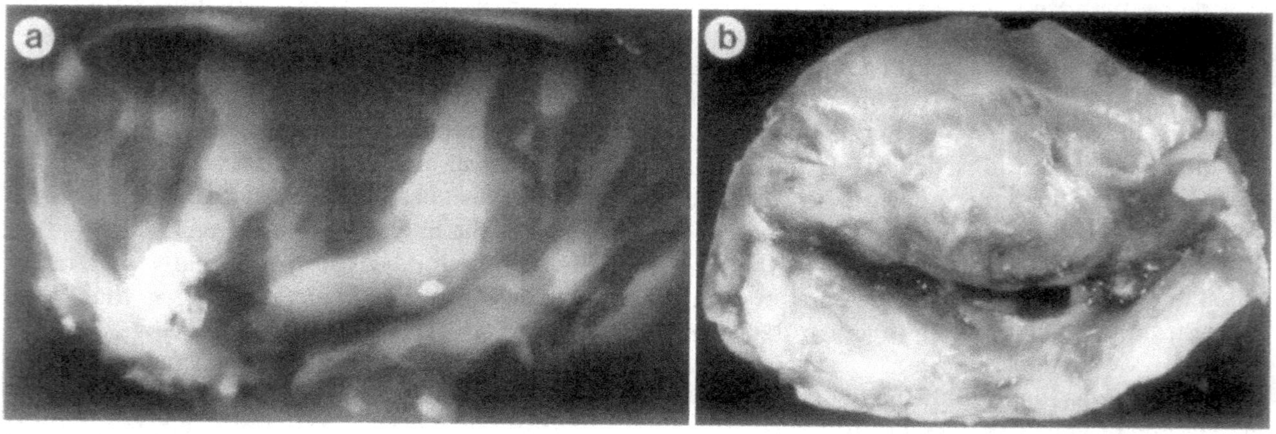

Fig. 2, a and b. Case No. 10 (Table I). *a,* Radiograph showing two calcific deposits. *b,* View from left atrium.

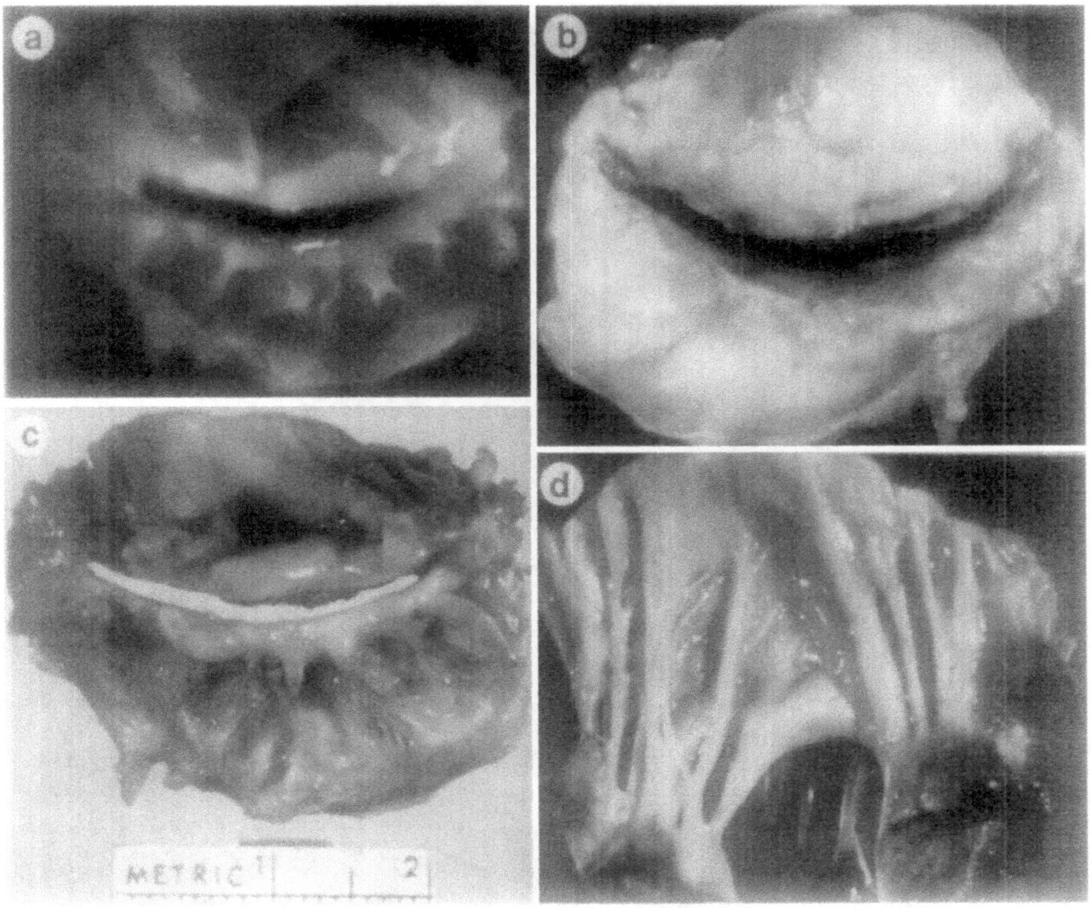

Fig. 3, a through d. Case No. 11 (Table I). *a,* Radiograph showing three minute calcific deposits. *b,* View from left atrium. *c,* View from left ventricle after excision of the chordae tendineae. *d,* View of anterior leaflet from left ventricle.

which is free of calcific deposits, free of significant mitral regurgitation, and mobile.[2-10] The excised mitral valves in the 20 patients analyzed here were free of calcific deposits by preoperative examination, and none had significant mitral regurgitation by preoperative evaluation. Mobility of the mitral valve at the time of valve replacement was described in the operative note in six of the 20 patients and in each mobility was limited, particularly so in four patients. Small calcific deposits in the mitral leaflets, however, were noted at operation in 10 patients; in three others, calcific deposits were noted to be absent, and in the remaining seven patients no mention was made in the operative note regarding their presence or absence. Radiography, however, of the excised valve disclosed no calcific deposits in five patients and minimal deposits in 15. In two of the patients stated to have calcific deposits in the mitral valve at operation, radiography of the excised valve disclosed no calcific deposits, indicating that palpation and visual inspection is not always accurate with respect to calcific deposits.

It seems likely that all 20 patients analyzed here would have been acceptable candidates for mitral commissurotomy alone in the pre-valve replacement era. Why then was mitral valve replacement rather than commissurotomy carried out? One factor certainly was the fact *that one or more other valves were replaced.* Thirteen of the 20 patients also underwent replacement of the aortic or tricuspid valve or both. Under these circumstances, mitral replacement may be advisable rather than risk possible significant regurgitation or incomplete relief of the stenosis by mitral commissurotomy.

Another consideration was the fact that *cardiopulmonary bypass was utilized* in each patient. This procedure obviously allows visual

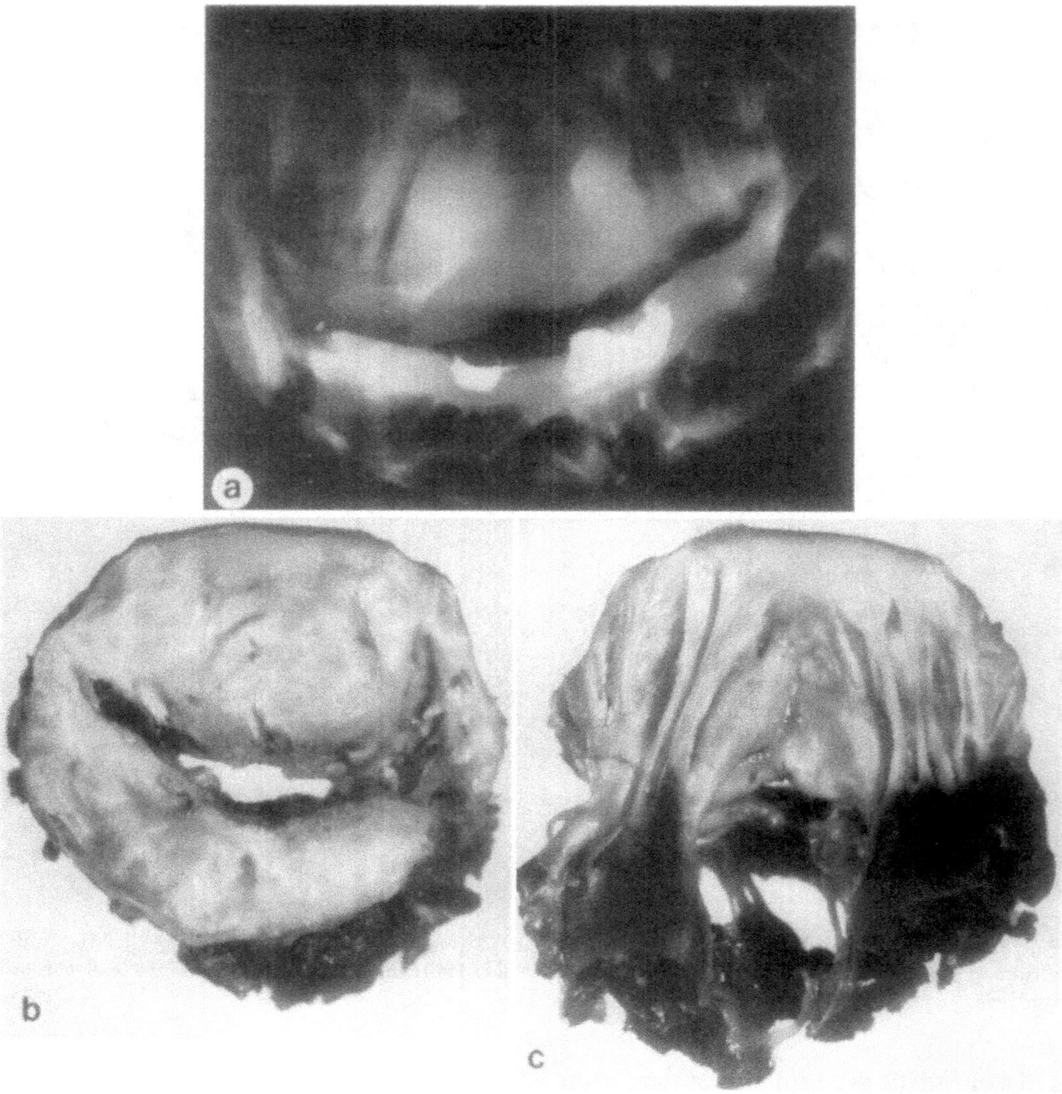

Fig. 4, a through c. Case No. 12 (Table I). *a*, Radiograph. *b*, View from left atrium. *c*, View of anterior leaflet and papillary muscles from left ventricle.

inspection of the valve, something not possible when commissurotomy was done as a "closed" procedure. We suspect that the visually inspected stenotic mitral valve is more frightening to the observer than is the stenotic valve which is only palpated. Thus, visual inspection alone, particularly when valve replacement is a reasonable and uncriticized option, may push the surgeon in some patients toward replacement rather than simple commissurotomy.

Another factor was *relatively little experience of some surgeons with mitral commissurotomy*, particularly as an open procedure, compared to valve replacement. Of the 20 study patients, 17 were operated upon by surgeons less than 40 years of age when the operation was done. The younger surgeons have had less experience with the commissurotomy procedure than with valve replacement, and consequently may feel more comfortable with the latter procedure.

Another factor was *displeasure with the attempted commissurotomy*. Three patients (No. 3, No. 4, and No. 6, Table I) had open mitral commissurotomy attempted but the surgeon was not satisfied with his results and valve replacement, therefore, was done.

And finally, *previous mitral valve commissurotomy* probably contributed to the decision. Eleven of the 20 patients had had at least one previous mitral commissurotomy. Examination of the

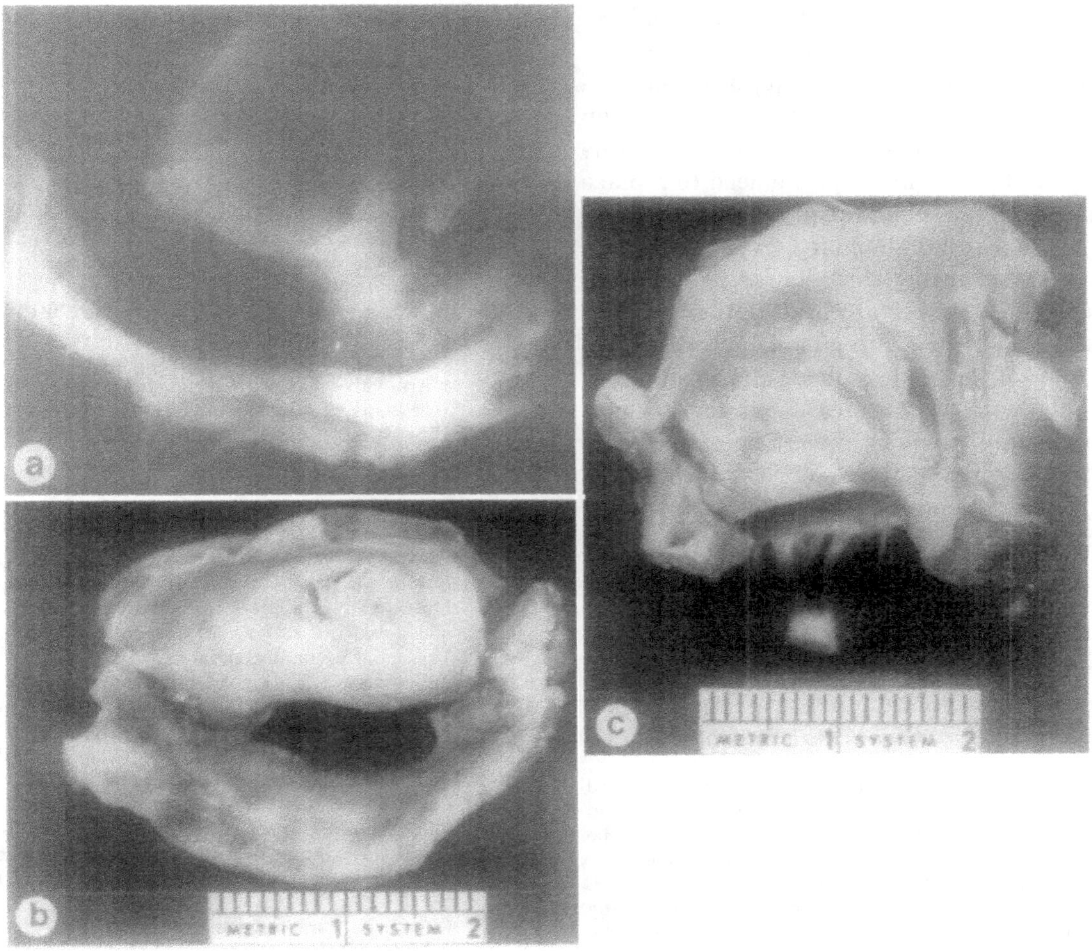

Fig. 5, a through **c**. Case No. 17 (Table I). *a*, Radiograph showing no calcific deposits. *b*, View from left atrium. *c*, View of anterior leaflet from left ventricle.

excised mitral valve in several of these 11 patients, however, showed no anatomic residua of the previous commissurotomy. Therefore, as is already recognized,[11] a mitral valve which has had one previous commissurotomy and later becomes severely stenotic again can, nevertheless, have another commissurotomy so long as calcific deposits are absent and mitral regurgitation is absent or is minimal.

Thus as emphasized recently by Spencer[12] "... the relative frequency of mitral valve reconstruction (i.e., commissurotomy) versus replacement will vary not only with the *experience* and *attitude* of the surgeon but with the *type of valve pathology seen* ... a surgeon experienced and enthusiastic about reconstruction might perform commissurotomy in 95 per cent of cases if patients are referred for operation with relatively early disease, while a similar surgeon might find it necessary to perform replacement in over 30 per cent of cases if patients are referred only with far advanced disease and extensive calcification."[12] Nevertheless, the definition of "advanced disease" appears to be changing, but as yet there is insufficient information to know whether this apparent change will prove to be beneficial or detrimental to the patient.

Summary

Among 164 patients who underwent mitral valve replacement because of mitral stenosis (with or without mitral regurgitation) and had radiographs taken of their operatively excised mitral valves, 20 had absent or minimal calcific deposits in the excised valves and absent or minimal mitral regurgitation as determined, except for one patient, by left ventricular angiography preoperatively. This report focuses on these 20 patients to ask if mitral valve replacement was preferable to mitral valve commissurotomy. Although in the pre-valve replacement era, all 20 patients almost surely would have been considered good candidates for mitral commissurotomy, other factors, namely, the need to replace one or more other cardiac valves (13 patients), the utilization of cardiopulmonary bypass allowing visual inspection rather than simple palpation of the diseased mitral valve (all 20 patients), relatively little experience with mitral commissurotomy in four of the five surgeons (17 patients), displeasure with attempted commissurotomy (three patients), previous mitral commissurotomy (11 patients), and incorrect identification of mitral calcific deposits (two patients), each contributed in one or more patients to the final decision of replacement versus commissurotomy. Even though mitral commissurotomy has been in use for 30 years, the mere alternative of valve replacement may have altered somewhat the definition of the stenotic mitral valve previously considered ideal for mitral commissurotomy.

The authors are indebted to the five surgeons who operated on the 20 patients analyzed in this report. These surgeons and the number of patients operated on by them were the following: Charles L. McIntosh (7), Lawrence L. Michaelis (7), Andrew G. Morrow (3), Robert L. Reis (2), and Edward B. Stinson (1). We thank Dr. Andrew G. Morrow for reviewing the manuscript, and Dr. Stephen E. Epstein for free use of the hemodynamic data in the study patients.

REFERENCES

1. Lachman, A. S., and Roberts, W. C.: Calcific deposits in stenotic mitral valves. Extent and relationship to age, sex, degree of stenosis, cardiac rhythm, previous commissurotomy and left atrial body thrombus from study of 164 operatively-excised valves, Circulation **57**:808, 1978.
2. Ellis, L. B., and Harken, D. E.: Closed valvuloplasty for mitral stenosis. A twelve-year follow-up study of 1571 patients, N. Engl. J. Med. **270**:643, 1964.
3. Morrow, A. G., Harrison, D. C., Ross, J., Jr., Braunwald, N. S., Clark, W. D., and Ross, R. S.: The surgical management of mitral valve disease: A symposium on diagnostic methods, operative techniques and results. Combined Clinical Staff Conference at the National Institutes of Health, Ann. Intern. Med. **60**:1073, 1964.
4. Ellis, F. H., Jr., Callahan, J. A., McGoon, D. C., and Kirklin, J. W.: Results of open operation for acquired mitral-valve disease, N. Engl. J. Med. **272**:869, 1965.
5. Hoeksema, T. D., Wallace, R. B., and Kirklin, J. W.: Closed mitral commissurotomy. Recent results in 291 cases, Am. J. Cardiol. **17**:825, 1966.
6. Dahl, J. C., Winchell, P., and Borden, C. W.: Mitral stenosis. A long-term postoperative follow-up, Arch. Intern. Med. **119**:92, 1967.
7. Glenn, W. W., Goodyear, A. V., Stansel, H. C., Jr., Calabrese, C., and Hume, H.: Mitral valvulotomy. II. Operative results after closed valvulotomy: A report of 500 cases, Am. J. Surg. **117**:493, 1969.
8. Higgs, L. M., Glancy, D. L., O'Brien, K. P., Epstein, S. E., and Morrow, A. G.: Mitral restenosis: An uncommon cause of recurrent symptoms following mitral commissurotomy, Am. J. Cardiol. **26**:34, 1970.
9. Keith, T. A., and Fowler, N. O.: Closed mitral commissurotomy. Complications and their effect on survival, Chest **61**:24, 1972.
10. Nanda, N. C., Gramiak, R., Shah, P. M., and DeWeese, J. A.: Mitral commissurotomy versus replacement. Preoperative evaluation by echocardiography, Circulation **51**:263, 1975.
11. Fraser, K., and Sugden, B. A.: Second closed mitral valvotomy for recurrent mitral stenosis, Thorax **32**:759, 1977.
12. Spencer, F. C.: A plea for early, open mitral commissurotomy, AM. HEART J. **95**:668, 1978.

Small Airways and Interstitial Pulmonary Disease

The concept of disease of the small airways was introduced in 1968 by Hogg and associates.[1] These workers defined the site and nature of obstruction of the airways in chronic obstructive pulmonary disease (COPD) at the small airways. Morphologically, small (less than 2 mm) airways were narrowed or obliterated by inflammation, mucus, or fibrosis. The concept of two components to disease of the small airways was introduced by them, *ie*, a reversible component due to acute inflammation or mucous plugging and an irreversible component due to fibrosis, distortion, and narrowing or obliteration of small airways. These findings suggested that disease of the small airways may be one of the earliest changes in COPD, and current data strongly support that suggestion.[2-4] The role of small airway disease in the eventual development of COPD, particularly emphysema, is unclear;[3,4] however, it is likely that small airway disease contributes to trapping of air and mechanical disruption of alveolar septae[4] and to the development of a distal chronic alveolitis. Once this last process has been initiated, the release of macrophagic or neutrophilic proteases may result in degradation of elastin and subsequent emphysema.[5]

In contrast to its occurrence in COPD, disease of the small airways was not considered to be a part of interstitial pulmonary disease until recently. Although grouped together because of common clinical, roentgenographic, physiologic, and morphologic features, interstitial pulmonary diseases are heterogeneous and have a variety of causes.[6] Just as COPD is characterized by an obstructive ventilatory defect with normal or increased pulmonary volumes, interstitial pulmonary disease has classically been characterized by a restrictive defect (reduced pulmonary volumes and compliance) without evidence of obstruction to airflow.[6] Because interstitial pulmonary disease is characterized morphologically by fibrosis of the supporting tissues of lung, primarily alveolar interstitium,[6] the concept of a restrictive ventilatory defect in this disorder is easy to accept. However, recent physiologic and morphologic observations indicate that disease of the small airways is not limited to COPD and that many of the morphologic and pathophysiologic features of COPD may be evident in interstitial pulmonary disease.

Although narrowing of small airways in acute idiopathic pulmonary fibrosis was mentioned by Hamman and Rich[7] in their original communication, only recently has emphasis been placed on small airways in interstitial pulmonary disease. Except for the "bronchiolitis obliterans interstitial pneumonia" described by Liebow and Carrington,[8] most reports have concentrated on alveolar pathologic abnormalities. The suggestion that functional alterations in interstitial pulmonary disease were consistent with small airway disease was made in 1973 by Ostrow and Cherniack[9] and subsequently by Yernalt et al.[10] Both groups found that some patients with interstitial pulmonary disease had evidence of increased resistance to airflow in small airways. In a study of 29 patients with idiopathic pulmonary fibrosis we[11] found small airways to be narrowed in 20 patients (70 percent). A detailed physiologic-morphologic correlative study of 18 of these 29 patients was made by obtaining pulmonary tissue and performing detailed testing of pulmonary function in the same patients.[12] Seventeen (94 percent) had peribronchiolar fibrosis or inflammation or bronchiolitis, and 12 (71 percent) of these 17 had narrowed small airways.[12] Furthermore, a good correlation was seen between the finding of narrowed small airways in the specimens from biopsy and two physiologic studies considered to be useful detectors of small-airway disease, *ie*, dynamic compliance and maximum expiratory flow-volume curves. Our study demonstrated that idiopathic pulmonary fibrosis is a disease that can involve small airways and that physiologic studies can define the function of small airways in this disease. Subsequent studies have shown that other diseases with pulmonary morphologic changes that can be indistinguishable from idiopathic pulmonary fibrosis (interstitial pulmonary disease associated with specific collagen vascular diseases and essential mixed cryoglobulinemia) may also have physiologic alterations consistent with disease of the small airways.[13-15]

Granulomatous interstitial pulmonary disease may also involve small airways. Young and associates[16] in 1967 demonstrated such an involvement by graulomata in patients with sarcoidosis. Although these workers noted no evidence of obstruction to airflow on simple spirometric testing, this publication preceded our current concepts of the relative insensitivity of this test to mild degrees of obstruction to airflow. Subsequent studies have shown that granulomata can involve small airways and that patients with sarcoidosis can have physiologic alterations consistent with disease of the small airways.[17-20]

At least three occupational or environmental interstitial diseases (hypersensitivity pneumonitis, asbestosis, and coal dust disease) have been shown to have physiologic alterations consistent with disease of the small airways.[21-23] A bronchiolo-alveolitis, the characteristic morphologic finding of hypersensitivity pneumonitis, is the morphologic equivalent of such functional abnormalities.[24] Similarly, the early morphologic change of coal dust disease is the coal macula which involves the small airways.[23]

Although many studies have now demonstrated its occurrence in interstitial pulmonary disease, small airway disease is not always present,[25-27] which suggests that several factors must determine its occurrence. These factors might include severity of the disease process, chronicity of the disease, susceptibility of the host, and certain environmental factors.[6,12,26,27] The functional significance of disease of the small airways is also variable. While it is likely that small airway disease is the earliest functional alteration in COPD, the significance of small airway disease in interstitial pulmonary disease is speculative. It is likely that disease of the small airways contributes to the ventilation-perfusion mismatching in interstitial pulmonary disease and hence to the hypoxemia of this disease.[6,12] In addition, small airway disease may be partly responsible for alterations in pulmonary recoil and pulmonary volumes[4] for example, trapping of air may mask the effects of alveolar fibrosis. Perhaps this is why pulmonary volumes correlate poorly or not at all with the severity of fibrosis in interstitial pulmonary fibrosis and in many of the inorganic dust diseases.[28,29] Disease of the small airways may also contribute to the development of chronic obstruction of airflow in interstitial pulmonary disease. Indeed, it is well documented but poorly recognized that some patients with interstitial pulmonary disease progress to show a pattern of chronic obstruction of airflow. The most notable example is chronic sarcoidosis, in which there may be functional evidence of chronic obstruction of airflow with an increased residual volume and normal or near normal total lung capacity.[30,31] Roentgenographically, there are dense areas of fibrosis with coexisting cystic lesions and hyperinflation.[31] Similarly, chronic obstruction of airflow may be present in patients with chronic hypersensitivity pneumonitis,[32] some of the inorganic dust diseases,[33] and chronic histiocytosis X of lung.[34] Although there are scant data on the mechanism of obstruction of airflow in these forms of interstitial pulmonary disease, both intrinsic narrowing of small airways and loss of elastic recoil probably contribute to the obstruction.[6,18]

In this issue (see page 473), McCarthy and associates describe two patients with idiopathic pulmonary fibrosis which rapidly progressed to COPD. Both patients initially had restrictive ventilatory defects (with normal timed spirometric data), but, in addition, both had evidence of increased resistance to airflow in small airways. Pulmonary biopsies in each showed an active alveolitis and either an obliterative bronchiolitis or endobronchiolar fibrosis. Both patients were treated with corticosteroids and improved initially. Six to 12 months later, both had physiologic, clinical, and radiographic findings typical of COPD. Pressure-flow studies indicated that a reduction in flow during maximum expiration was due mainly to reduced elastic recoil and increased dynamic compression. These data would be consistent with emphysema.[35] The report of McCarthy et al and the data cited in this editorial strongly support the concept that there are distinctive similarities between the interstitial and obstructive pulmonary diseases. The report by McCarthy et al also raises questions on the possibility of acute interstitial injury as a cause for COPD. It is well documented that acute bronchiolar injury can lead to COPD, for example, that resulting from acute inhalation of smoke.[36] Could an acute viral alveolitis and bronchiolitis or subclinical idiopathic pulmonary fibrosis do the same? Current data suggest that lobar emphysema is associated with acute viral pneumonias.[37] Certainly, influenza can be associated with physiologic alterations consistent with disease of the small airways.[38] This type of injury in the susceptible person may lead to classic COPD or to chronic obstructive disease of the small airways, as described by Macklem and colleagues.[39] Recently, Miller et al[40] suggested that sarcoidosis may cause diffuse bullous emphysema.

The report by McCarthy and associates also raises important therapeutic questions. Whereas Ostrow and Cherniack[9] and we[12] observed improvement in the physiologic abnormalities of small airways on treatment with corticosteroids, the two patients of McCarthy et al developed obstructive pulmonary disease despite corticosteroid treatment. This suggests that most small airways were irreversibly damaged, perhaps with fibrosis. Could agents that interfere with collagen synthesis, secretion, or cross-linking have altered the disease process? Of even greater importance is the question of the overall significance of small airway disease in interstitial pulmonary disease. Clearly, we should be actively investigating mechanisms of alveolar and bronchiolar injury and repair in both the "interstitial" and "obstructive" pulmonary diseases. The functional distinction between these two classes of diseases becomes less distinct as our knowledge of them increases.

*Jack D. Fulmer, M.D., F.C.C.P.**
Birmingham, Ala
*and William C. Roberts, M.D., F.C.C.P.***
Bethesda, Md

*Veterans Administration Medical Center and Department of Medicine, University of Alabama.
**Pathology Branch, National Heart, Lung, and Blood Institute.
Reprint requests: Dr. Fulmer, Department of Medicine (Pulmonary), University of Alabama Medical Center, Birmingham 35294

References

1 Hogg JC, Macklem PT, Thurlbeck WM. Site and nature of airway obstruction in chronic obstructive lung disease. N Engl J Med 1968; 278:1355-60.
2 Cosio M, Ghezzo H, Hogg JC, et al. The relations between structural changes in small airways and pulmonary function tests. N Engl J Med 1977; 298:1277-81.
3 Thurlbeck WM. Changes in lung structure. In: Macklem PT, Permutt S, eds. The lung in the transition between health and disease. New York: Marcel Dekker, Inc, 1979:17-41.
4 Macklem PT. Changes in lung mechanics: pressure-volume and pressure-flow relations. In: Macklem PT, Permutt S, eds. The lung in the transition between health and disease. New York: Marcel Dekker, Inc, 1979:53-71.
5 Kuhn C, Senior RM. The role of elastases in the development of emphysema. Lung 1978; 155:185-97.
6 Fulmer JD, Crystal RG. Interstitial lung diseases. In Simmons DE, ed. Current pulmonology. Boston: Houghton Mifflin Professional Publishers, 1979; 1:1-65.
7 Hamman L, Rich AR. Acute diffuse interstitial fibrosis of the lungs. Bull Johns Hopkins Hosp 1944; 74:177-212.
8 Liebow AA, Carrington CB. Alveolar diseases: the interstitial pneumonias. In: Simon M, Potchen EJ, LeMay M, eds. Frontiers of Pulmonary Radiology. New York: Grune and Stratton, Inc, 1967: 102-41.
9 Ostrow D, Cherniack RM. Resistance to airflow in patients with diffuse interstitial lung disease. Am Rev Respir Dis 1973; 108:205-10.
10 Yernalt JC, Dejoinghe M, DeCoster A, et al. Pulmonary mechanics in diffuse fibrosing alveolitis. Bull Physiopathol Respir 1975; 11:231-44.
11 Roberts WC. Histologic observations in idiopathic pulmonary fibrosis. (pp 773-776). In: Crystal RG (moderator). Idiopathic pulmonary fibrosis: clinical, histologic, radiographic, physiologic, scintigraphic, cytologic, and biochemical aspects. Ann Intern Med 1976; 85:769-88.
12 Fulmer JD, Roberts WC, Von gal ER, et al. Small airways in idiopathic pulmonary fibrosis: comparison of morphologic and physiologic observations. J Clin Invest 1977; 60:595-610.
13 Guttadauria M, Ellman H, Emmanuel G, et al. Pulmonary function in scleroderma. Arthritis Rheumatism 1977; 20:1071-9.
14 Wohlgelernter D, Loke J, Matthay RA, et al. Systemic and discoid lupus erythematosis: analysis of pulmonary function. Yale J Biol Med 1978; 51:157-64.
15 Bombardieri S, Paoletti P, Ferri C, et al. Lung involvement in essential mixed cryoglobulinemia. Am J Med 1979; 66:748-55.
16 Young RC Jr, Carr C, Shelton TG, et al. Sarcoidosis: relationship between changes in lung structure and function. Am Rev Respir Dis 1967; 95:224-38.
17 Young RC Jr, Headings VE, Bose S, et al. Alpha-1 antitrypsin levels in sarcoidosis: relationship to disease activity. Chest 1973; 64:39-45.
18 Kaneko K, Sharma OP. Airway obstruction in pulmonary sarcoidosis. Bull Eur Physiopathol Respir 1977; 13:231-40.
19 Levinson RS, Metzger LF, Stanley NN, et al. Airway function in sarcoidosis. Am J Med 1977; 62:51-9.
20 Carrington CB, Gaensler EA, Mikus JP, et al. Structure and function in sarcoidosis. NY Acad Sci 1976; 278: 265-83.
21 Allen DH, Williams GV, Woolcock AJ. Bird breeders' hypersensitivity pneumonitis: progress studies of lung function after cessation of exposure to the provoking antigen. Am Rev Respir Dis 1976; 114:555-66.
22 Jodoin G, Gibbs GW, Macklem PT, et al. Early effects of asbestos exposure on lung function. Am Rev Respir Dis 1971; 104:525-35.
23 Seaton A, Lapp NL, Morgan WKC. Lung mechanics and frequency dependence of compliance in coal miners. J Clin Invest 1972; 51:1203-11.
24 Seal RME, Hapke EJ, Thomas GO, et al. The pathology of the acute and chronic stages of farmers lung. Thorax 1968; 23:469-89.
25 Schofield NM, Davies RJ, Cameron IR, et al. Small airways in fibrosing alveolitis. Am Rev Respir Dis 1976; 113:729-35.
26 DeTroyer A, Yernalt JC, Dierekx P, et al. Lung and airways mechanics in early pulmonary sarcoidosis. Bull Eur Physiopathol Respir 1978; 14:299-310.
27 Bjerke RD, Tashkin DP, Clements DJ, et al. Small airways in progressive systemic sclerosis. Am J Med 1979; 66:201-9.
28 Fulmer JD, Roberts WC, Von Gal ER, et al. Morphologic-physiologic correlates of the severity of fibrosis and degree of cellularity in idiopathic pulmonary fibrosis. J Clin Invest 1979; 63:665-76.
29 Gaensler EA, Carrington CB, Coutu RE, et al. Radiographic physiologic-pathologic correlates in interstitial pneumonias. Prog Respir Res 1975; 8:223-41.
30 Miller A, Teirstein AS, Jackler I, et al. Airway function in chronic pulmonary sarcoidosis with fibrosis. Am Rev Respir Dis 1974; 109:179-89.
31 DeRemee RA, Andersen HA. Sarcoidosis: a correlation of dyspnea with radiographic stage and pulmonary function changes. Mayo Clin Proc 1974; 49:742-5.
32 Braun SR, doPico GA, Tsiatis A, et al. Farmer's lung

disease: long-term clinical and physiologic outcome. Am Rev Respir Dis 1979; 119:185-91.

33 Morgan WKC, Seaton A. Occupational lung diseases. Philadelphia: WB Saunders Co, 1975: 132-4, 174-92.

34 Basset F, Corrin B, Spence H, et al. Pulmonary histiocytosis X. Am Rev Respir Dis 1978; 118:811-20.

35 Leaver DG, Tattersfield AE, Pride NB. Contributions of loss of lung recoil and of enhanced airways collapsibility to the airflow obstruction of chronic bronchitis and emphysema. J Clin Invest 1973; 52:2117-34.

36 Kirkpatrick MB, Bass JB. Severe obstructive lung disease after smoke inhalation. Chest 1979; 76:108-10.

37 Fraser RG, Paré JAP. Diagnosis of diseases of the chest. Philadelphia: WB Saunders Co, 1979; 3:1431.

38 Little JW, Hall WJ, Douglas RG, et al. Amantadine effect on peripheral airways abnormalities in influenza. Ann Intern Med 1976; 85:177-82.

39 Macklem PT, Thurlbeck WM, Fraser RG. Chronic obstructive disease of small airways. Ann Intern Med 1971; 74:167-77.

40 Miller A, Teirstein AS, Chuang MT. The sequence of physiologic changes in pulmonary sarcoidosis: correlation with radiographic stages and response to therapy. Mt Sinai J Med 1977; 44:852-65.

Self-Induced Pulmonary Granulomatosis*

A Consequence of Intravenous Injection of Drugs Intended for Oral Use

Bruce F. Waller, M.D.; William J. Brownlee, M.D.; and William C. Roberts, M.D., F.C.C.P.

Dr. William C. Roberts: Herein we will discuss pulmonary and cardiac findings in a girl who injected into her systemic veins dissolved drugs originally intended for oral use. Dr. Brownlee will describe the patient.

Dr. William J. Brownlee: An 18-year-old white woman began injecting heroin intravenously at the age of 15 years, about 30 months before her death.

*From the Pathology Branch, National Heart, Lung, and Blood Institute, National Institutes of Health, Bethesda, Md, and the District of Columbia Medical Examiner's Office, Washington, DC.
Reprint requests: Dr. Roberts, National Institutes of Health, Bldg 10A, Room 3E30, Bethesda 20205

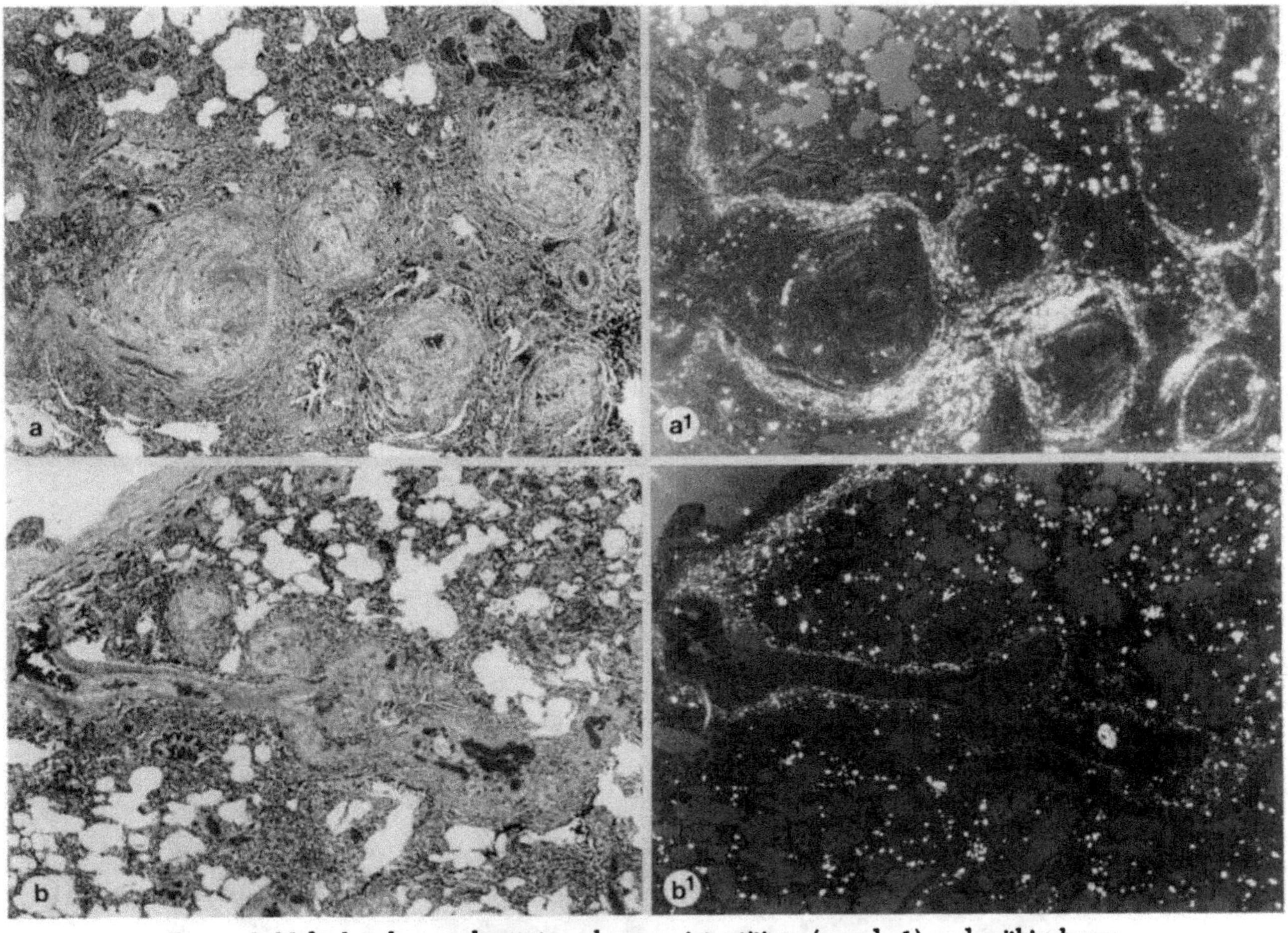

FIGURE 1. Multiple talc granulomas in pulmonary interstitium (*a* and a^1) and within lumen of pulmonary artery (*b* and b^1). Polarized sections (a^1 and b^1) are from the same areas shown in *a* and *b*, respectively. Refractile material, for most part, represents talc (hematoxylin-eosin, original magnifications × 60 [*a* and a^1] and × 22 [*b* and b^1]).

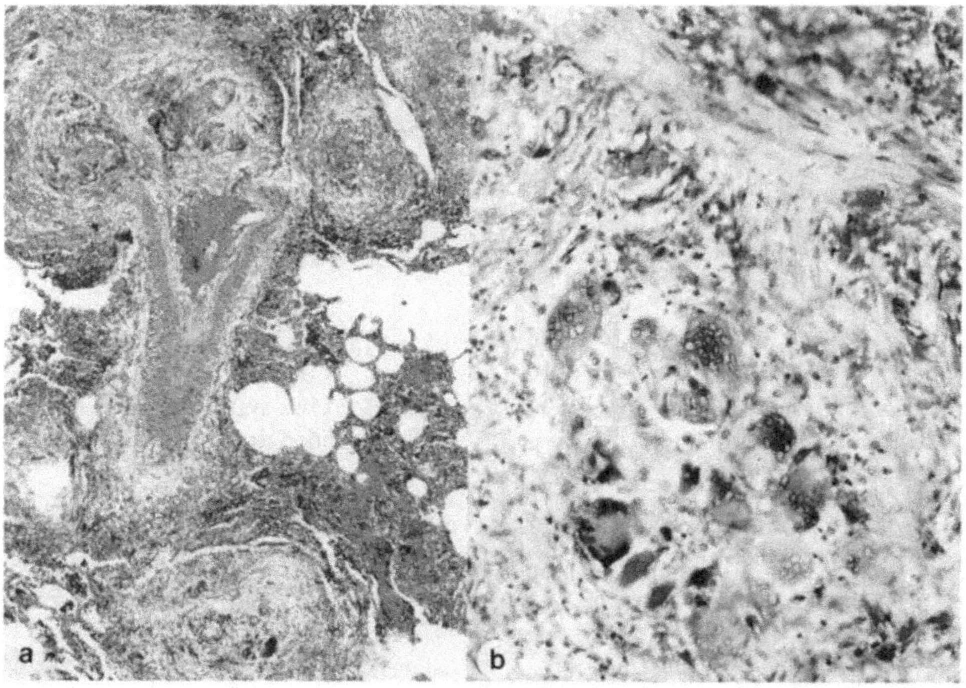

FIGURE 2. Talc granulomas located within pulmonary artery (*a*) and close-up of large granuloma adjacent to pulmonary artery (*b*) (hematoxylin-eosin, original magnifications × 100 [*a*] and × 220 [*b*]).

About six months later, she began injecting regularly into her systemic veins various other drugs, including methylphenidate (Ritalin), after dissolving them in liquids. She noted periodic wheezing and exertional dyspnea about 12 months before death, and these symptoms gradually progressed thereafter. The patient died suddenly at home after an episode of severe dyspnea. She had never sought medical care.

At necropsy, the surfaces of both lungs appeared normal; but on sectioning, multiple small (about 1 to 2 mm) relatively firm lesions were present throughout all lobes. Histologically, these little nodules were granulomas containing refractile material typical of talc (Fig 1 and 2). The alveolar septa contained similar refractile material and also numerous inflammatory cells (Fig 3). In addition, the media and intima of many pulmonary arteries

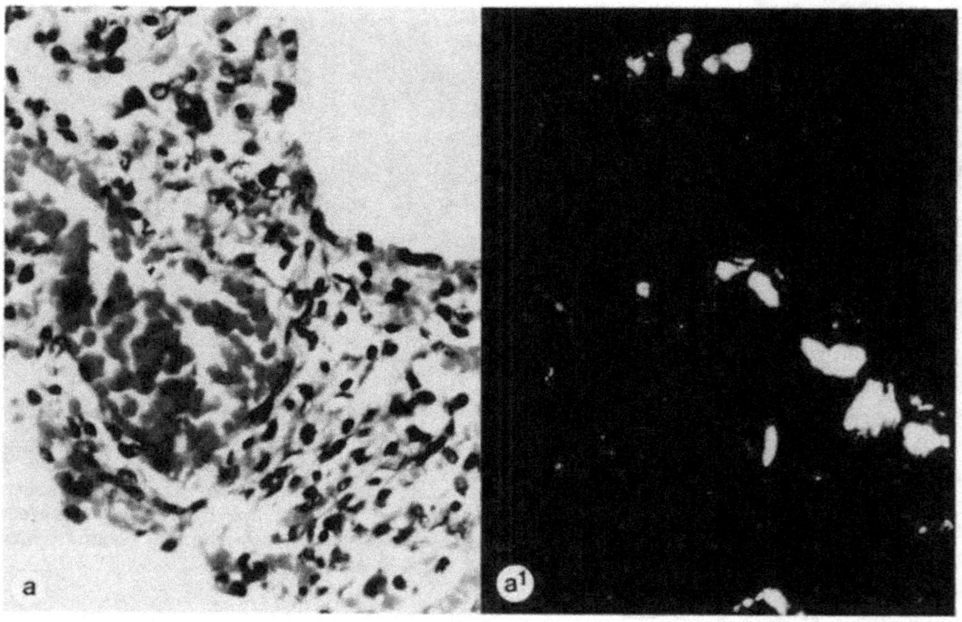

FIGURE 3. Alveolar septum containing many mononuclear inflammatory cells producing "active-appearing" alveolitis (*a*). Same section polarized is shown (*b*). Lumina of septal capillaries contain birefringent particles typical of talc (*b*) (hematoxylin-eosin, original magnification × 500).

were thickened, and many small pulmonary arteries were totally obstructed by talc-containing granulomas (Fig 2). The heart, which weighed 440 gm, was typical of that observed in cor pulmonale; both the right atrial and right ventricular cavities were dilated, and their walls were quite thickened; the tricuspid valvular anulus was dilated.

Dr. Roberts: This girl obviously died from self-induced pulmonary granulomatosis, causing morphologic evidence of severe pulmonary hypertension. Because it holds the components of the pill together, talc is present in virtually all tablets; and, consequently, if tablets of nearly any variety are dissolved in a fluid and injected into systemic veins, rather than swallowed, pulmonary talc granulomas are the expected consequence. If few talc granulomas form, no functional consequence ensues. If numerous talc granulomas develop, the consequence is either obstruction of the lumina of many pulmonary arteries, producing pulmonary hypertension and cor pulmonale or interstitial pulmonary fibrosis or both. Although nearly all contain talc, the tablets most commonly used for intravenous injection after crushing and dissolving are methylphenidate (Ritalin) (as in our patient), methadone, tripalennamine (Pyribenzamine), propoxyphene hydrochloride (Darvon), phenmetrazine (Preludin), and amphetamines.

Dr. Waller, would you summarize the findings in previously reported necropsies of patients with pulmonary talc granulomatosis?

Dr. Bruce F. Waller: From 1950 to June 1979, at least 16 necropsies of patients with pulmonary talc granulomas from intravenous injection of dissolved tablets were reported (Table 1).[1-12] All patients were known to have repeatedly injected intravenously drugs intended for oral use for periods ranging from 2 to 20 years (average, ten years). In each patient, foreign material consistent with talc was present in the pulmonary granulomas. The 16 patients ranged in age from 22 to 52 years (average, 31 years); 13 were men, and three were women. In all 16 patients the granulomas were present in both pulmonary interstitium and in the lumina of the

Table 1—***Data from 16 Necropsies of Patients with Pulmonary Talc Granulomas from Intravenous Injection of Dissolved Tablets***

Reference	Patient's Sex and Age (yr)	Duration of Addiction, yr*			Pulmonary Granuloma**		Alveolitis†				Pulmonary Arteries‡			Weight of Heart, gm	RV Wall >5 mm§
		IV	Oral	Total	PA	I	Leu	PC	Lym	AH	MT	IT	PL		
Spain[1]	M, . . .	. . .	. . .	. . .	+	++	−	−	−	−	0	0	0	. . .	+
Wendt et al[2]	F, 32	← 2→		2	++	+	+	−	+	+	+	+	+	720	+
Burton et al[3]	M, 25	. . .	. . .	. . .	+	++	−	−	−	+	0	0	0	400	+
Butz[4]	M, 29	. . .	. . .	. . .	++	+	+	−	+	+	+	+	+	375	+
Hahn et al[5]	M, 30	. . .	. . .	. . .	+	++	−	−	−	−	0	0	0	. . .	−
Hahn et al[5]	F, 28	. . .	. . .	. . .	+	++	−	−	−	−	0	0	+	. . .	−
Bainborough and Jerico[6]	M, 35	. . .	. . .	. . .	+	++	−	−	−	−	0	0	0	. . .	+
Douglas et al[7]	M, 52	←30→		30	+	++	−	−	−	−	0	0	0	. . .	+
	F, 28	←10→		10	+	++	−	−	−	−	0	0	0	. . .	−
	M, 42	← 5→		5	+	+	−	−	−	−	+	+	+	. . .	−
Lewman[8]	M, 30	← 7→		7	++	+	−	−	−	−	+	+	+	400	+
Groth et al[9]	M, 40	5	?	5	+	++	−	−	+	−	−	−	−	. . .	+
Genereux and Emson[10]	M, 52	←25→		25	+	++	−	−	−	−	0	0	0	. . .	+
	M, 32	←"Many"→		. . .	+	++	−	−	+	−	0	0	0	. . .	0
Arnett et al[11]	M, 22	← 7→		7	++	+	−	−	−	−	+	+	+	550	+
Paré et al[12]	M, 25	5	1.5	6.5	+	++	−	−	−	−	−	−	−	. . .	−

*IV, intravenous.
**PA, pulmonary arteries; and I, interstitium.
†Leu, leukocytes; PC, plasma cells; Lym, lymphocytes; and AH, alveolar hemorrhage.
‡MT, medial thickening; IT, intimal thickening; and PL, plexiform lesion.
§RV, right ventricular.

pulmonary arteries. In 11 patients the interstitium appeared to be the predominant location; in four, the pulmonary arteries were the predominant location; and in one patient, it was not mentioned. The interstitial location led to pulmonary interstitial fibrosis, and the arterial location led to pulmonary arterial narrowing with changes consistent with pulmonary hypertension. The patients who had been taking dissolved tablets intravenously the longest tended to have the talc granulomas located primarily in the pulmonary interstitium, and those with the shortest duration of addiction tended to have the granulomas predominantly in the lumina of the pulmonary arteries. Morphologic evidence (right ventricular hypertrophy or pulmonary arterial changes or both) of pulmonary arterial hypertension was present in 13 of the 16 patients. In addition to the 16 necropsies, at least 13 living patients[1,5,11,13,14] have been reported to have talc granulomas in pulmonary biopsies. Of them, seven had pulmonary arterial changes indicative of pulmonary hypertension. Thus, of 29 previous reports of cases of pulmonary talc granulomas, 20 had morphologic evidence of pulmonary hypertension, and six had plexiform lesions indicating that the pulmonary hypertension was severe.[15]

Dr. Roberts: Dr. Waller, what does the roentgenogram of the chest disclose in patients with pulmonary talc granulomatosis?

Dr. Waller: The roentgenographic changes appear, to some extent at least to be dependent on the stage of the process at which the patient is examined. When the pulmonary granulomas are few in number, the pulmonary parenchyma is normal by radiographic examination. When the pulmonary granulomas are widespread and fatal, the pulmonary parenchyma by roentgenographic examination may still be normal.[4,12,16] Thus, a normal roentgenogram of the chest does not rule out the presence of extensive pulmonary talc granulomatosis. In a study of 17 living patients who administered intravenously at least 2,500 to 50,000 dissolved tablets of methadone during periods ranging from one to nine years, ten patients had normal and seven had abnormal chest roentgenograms.[12] The abnormalities consisted of widespread nodules measuring 1 mm or less in diameter (seven patients) and diminished pulmonary volumes (two patients). Surprisingly, pulmonary infarcts appear to be infrequent, despite the frequent total obliteration of the lumina of many pulmonary arteries. Of course, the patients with pulmonary hypertension may have dilated pulmonary trunks and right ventricular and right atrial cavities. The electrocardiogram in the latter patients also may provide evidence of right ventricular hypertrophy and right atrial abnormality.

Dr. Roberts: Dr. Waller, what alterations in pulmonary function occur in patients with pulmonary talc granulomatosis?

Dr. Waller: Relatively few reported necropsies of cases of fatal pulmonary granulomatosis were from patients who had pulmonary function tests during life, and most patients with pulmonary function tests have not had the pulmonary granulomatosis confirmed anatomically (biopsy or necropsy). Nevertheless, several patients who took dissolved tablets intravenously for long periods have undergone tests of pulmonary function.[12,14] The major functional abnormality is a slowed diffusion of air from the alveolar spaces to the alveolar capillaries (decreased diffusing capacity). A second abnormality described is an increased period of time to expel a certain amount of pulmonary air (diminished forced expiratory volume in one second and diminished midexpiratory flow rate). These latter disturbances may result in an increased pulmonary volume (*ie*, hyperinflation). Whether or not this diminished expiratory flow rate and increased residual pulmonary volume are the result of the pulmonary granulomatosis or whether they are the result of associated cigarette smoking, which is extremely common in the drug addicts, is unclear. Surprisingly, despite the extensive distribution of the pulmonary talc granulomas, systemic arterial hypoxia is usually absent; or at least, cyanosis, except terminally, is uncommon. *Dyspnea* is the usual symptom resulting from the pulmonary talc granulomatosis. Again, clinical evidences of pulmonary infarcts are not reported.

Dr. Roberts: I have a few comments regarding pulmonary morphologic findings in patients with talc granulomatosis. As shown in Figure 1, numerous birefringent particles may be present throughout the pulmonary parenchyma. These birefringent particles are more numerous in alveolar septa not containing granulomas than in the granulomas *per se*. The alveolar septa usually contain many mononuclear inflammatory cells, producing a very "active"-appearing diffuse *alveolitis* as a consequence of the talc granulomatosis (Fig 3). The inflammatory cells generally consist of lymphocytes, plasma cells, and eosinophils; or at least, this was the finding in our patient. In our patient, large numbers of plasma cells and eosinophils were present in many alveolar septa. The alveolitis is consistent with the pulmonary functional abnormality of slowed perfusion of air from alveolar space to alveolar capillary. There has been

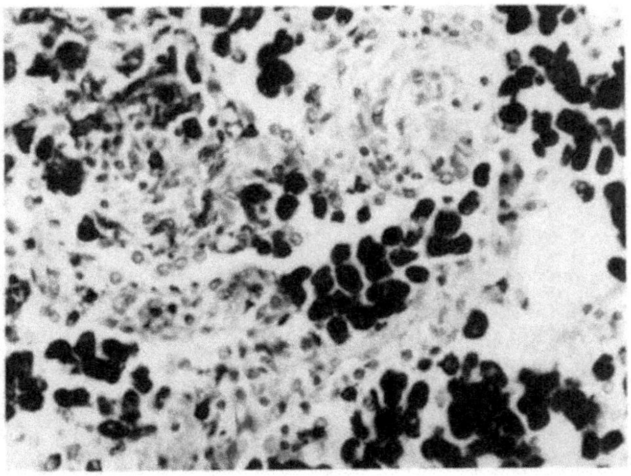

FIGURE 4. Hemosiderin-laden macrophages located within alveolar spaces (Mallory's stain for iron, original magnification × 400).

very little comment regarding alveolitis in previous reports on pulmonary talc granulomatosis. Another infrequently mentioned abnormality in the lungs of these patients is the presence of hemosiderin-laden macrophages within the alveolar spaces. We interpret this abnormality, which was quite extensive in our patient, as resulting from a rupture of the membranes of alveolar capillaries, allowing extravasation of erythrocytes and other blood products into the alveolar spaces (Fig 4). Thus, it might be possible to find hemosiderin or iron deposits in the pulmonary expectorates; however, talc spicules or granulomas are infrequent in the alveolar spaces.

I have one final comment regarding diagnosis. Some patients with pulmonary talc granulomatosis initially have evidence of severe pulmonary hypertension. A male patient with pulmonary talcosis, who was previously studied by us,[11] was initially diagnosed as having primary or idiopathic pulmonary hypertension. The finding of evidence of severe pulmonary hypertension in a man should arouse suspicion of the possibility of pulmonary talc granulomatosis as the cause of the pulmonary hypertension, because most patients with primary pulmonary hypertension are women, and most patients with pulmonary talc granulomatosis are men.

REFERENCES

1 Spain DM: Patterns of pulmonary fibrosis as related to pulmonary function. Ann Intern Med 33:1150-1163, 1950

2 Wendt VE, Puro HE, Shapiro J, et al: Angiothrombotic pulmonary hypertension in addicts: "Blue velvet" addiction. JAMA 188:755-757, 1964

3 Burton JF, Zawadzki ES, Wetherell HR, et al: Mainliners and blue velvet. J Forensic Sci 10:466-472, 1965

4 Butz WC: Pulmonary arteriole foreign body granulomata associated with angiomatoids resulting from the intravenous injection of oral medications, e.g., propxyphene hydrochloride (Davron®). J Forensic Sci 14:317-325, 1969

5 Hahn HH, Schweid AL, Beaty HN: Complications of injecting dissolved methylphenidate tablets. Arch Intern Med 123:656-659, 1969

6 Bainborough AR, Jerico KWF: Cor pulmonale secondary to talc granulomata in the lungs of a drug addict. Can Med Assoc J 103:1297-1298, 1970

7 Douglas FG, Kafilmont KJ, Patt NL: Foreign particle embolism in drug addicts. Ann Intern Med 75:865-872, 1971

8 Lewman LV: Fatal pulmonary hypertension from intravenous injection of methylphenidate (Ritalin) tablets. Hum Pathol 3:67-70, 1972

9 Groth DH, Mackay GR, Crable JV, et al: Intravenous injection of talc in a narcotics addict. Arch Pathol 94:171-178, 1972

10 Genereux GP, Emson HE: Talc granulomatosis and angiothrombotic pulmonary hypertension in drug addicts. J Can Assoc Radiol 25:87-93, 1974

11 Arnett EN, Battle WE, Russe JV, et al: Intravenous infection of talc-containing drugs intended for oral use: A cause of pulmonary granulomatosis and pulmonary hypertension. Am J Med 60:711-717, 1976

12 Paré JAP, Fraser RG, Hogg JC, et al: Pulmonary "mainline" granulomatosis; Talcosis of intravenous methadone abuse. Medicine 58:229-239, 1979

13 Szwed JJ: Pulmonary angiothrombosis caused by "blue velvet" addiction. Ann Intern Med 73:771-774, 1970

14 Robertson CH, Reynolds J, Wilson JE III: Pulmonary hypertension and foreign body granulomatosis, in intravenous drug abusers: Documentation by cardiac catheterization and lung biopsy. Ann J Med 61:657-663, 1976

15 Virmani R, Roberts WC: Pulmonary arteries in congenital heart disease: A structure-function analysis. Cardiovasc Clin 10:455-499, 1979

16 Hopkins GB, Taylor DG: Pulmonary talc granulomatosis. Ann Rev Respir Dis 101:101-108, 1970

Pulmonary Sarcoidosis: A Disease Characterized and Perpetuated by Activated Lung T-Lymphocytes

Moderator: RONALD G. CRYSTAL, M.D. *Discussants:* WILLIAM C. ROBERTS, M.D.; GARY W. HUNNINGHAKE, M.D.; JAMES E. GADEK, M.D.; JACK D. FULMER, M.D.; and BRUCE R. LINE, M.D.; Bethesda, Maryland

The alveolitis of pulmonary sarcoidosis is characterized by an intense, mononuclear cell infiltrate that probably precedes granuloma formation. Pathogenic mechanisms underlying pulmonary sarcoidosis can be shown by study of the mononuclear cells composing the alveolitis. Bronchoalveolar lavage has shown that the sarcoid lung is characterized by increased numbers of "activated" T-lymphocytes within the alveolar structures. In contrast to normal control cells, the lung T-lymphocytes of patients with sarcoid release the mediator, monocyte chemotactic factor, that probably contributes to the pathogenesis of sarcoidosis by recruiting blood monocytes to the lung, thus providing cellular building blocks for granuloma formation. Conventional monitors of the activity of pulmonary sarcoidosis, such as blood studies, pulmonary function testing, and chest roentgenograms, show little relation to the intensity of the T-lymphocyte alveolitis as assessed by bronchoalveolar lavage or by histopathologic studies. In contrast, quantification of lavage T-lymphocyte populations and ^{67}Ga scintigraphy of the chest provide a sensitive and specific means of assessing the activity of the alveolitis in pulmonary sarcoidosis and may provide a rational basis for therapy.

DR. RONALD G. CRYSTAL (Chief, Pulmonary Branch, National Heart, Lung, and Blood Institute): Sarcoidosis is a multisystem disease of undetermined cause characterized by the presence of noncaseating granulomas in many organs (1-6). Although the cause is unknown and the morphologic findings nonspecific, the combination of clinical, roentgenographic, histologic, and physiologic findings are so characteristic that in modern clinical practice the diagnosis of sarcoidosis is usually unambiguous (6-11). Sarcoidosis has been described in most tissues of the body, but for most patients lung involvement has the most serious consequences. At least 90% of all patients have pulmonary manifestations (1, 3-6, 12-14). Of these, 20% to 25% will have permanent loss of lung function, and 5% to 10% will die from the disease (1, 3, 4, 14-18).

The presence of granulomas in the alveolar structures in pulmonary sarcoidosis has long been considered histologic evidence that there are heightened cellular immune processes. However, many studies have documented a nonspecific depression of cellular immunity in this disorder. For example, most patients with active sarcoidosis have anergy to skin tests (12, 19, 20), impairment of the in-vitro proliferative response of blood mononuclear cells to antigens and mitogens (21-23), and a peripheral blood T-lymphocytopenia (24-28).

One explanation for this apparent paradox is that studies of uninvolved tissues such as skin and blood do not reflect the ongoing immune processes at the site of granuloma formation. The development of methods to directly evaluate the inflammatory and immune effector systems within the human lung has led to remarkable insights into the pathogenesis of this disease. Specifically, by 1978 it had become obvious that pulmonary sarcoidosis is characterized and perpetuated by increased numbers of activated T-lymphocytes within the alveolar structures (28-34).

To show the importance and ramifications of lung T-lymphocytes in this disease, we have used a study population of 45 persons with biopsy proven pulmonary sarcoidosis. Included were 20 males and 25 females, with an average age of 37 ± 5 years (all data are presented as the mean ± SE). By conventional clinical criteria, 19 were classified as having "active" disease.

First, we will define the disease morphologically, stressing the temporal sequence of the histologic findings. Second, we will detail the types, numbers, and function of lung inflammatory and immune effector cells, emphasizing the critical role of lung T-lymphocytes. Third, we will evaluate the tests available for staging sarcoidosis in terms of the sensitivity and specificity of these methods in staging the activity of the disease within the alveolar structures. Finally, we will review the therapy of pulmonary sarcoidosis, emphasizing the importance of using measures of inflammatory and immune activity within the lung as criteria for making decisions.

Morphologic Aspects

Dr. William C. Roberts (Chief, Pathology Branch, National Heart, Lung, and Blood Institute): The characteristic morphologic feature of pulmonary sarcoidosis is the presence of multiple noncaseating granulomas in the lung (Figure 1, *upper left*). The granulomas are always present in the alveolar septa (Figure 1, *upper right*) and usually in the walls of bronchi, pulmonary arteries, and veins (Figure 1, *lower left* and *right*) (1-3, 7, 35, 36).

COMPOSITION OF THE SARCOID GRANULOMA

The sarcoid granuloma is usually sharply circumscribed. Its central follicle consists of tightly packed cells,

▸ An edited transcription of a Combined Clinical Staff Conference at the Clinical Center, Bethesda, Maryland, 29 June 1978, by the National Institutes of Health, U.S. Department of Health, Education, and Welfare.

▸ Authors who wish to cite a section of the conference and specifically indicate its author can use this example for the form of reference:
ROBERTS WC. Morphologic aspects of pulmonary sarcoidosis, pp. 73-6. In: CRYSTAL RG, moderator. Pulmonary sarcoidosis: a disease characterized and perpetuated by activated lung T-lymphocytes. *Ann Intern Med.* 1981;**94**:73-94.

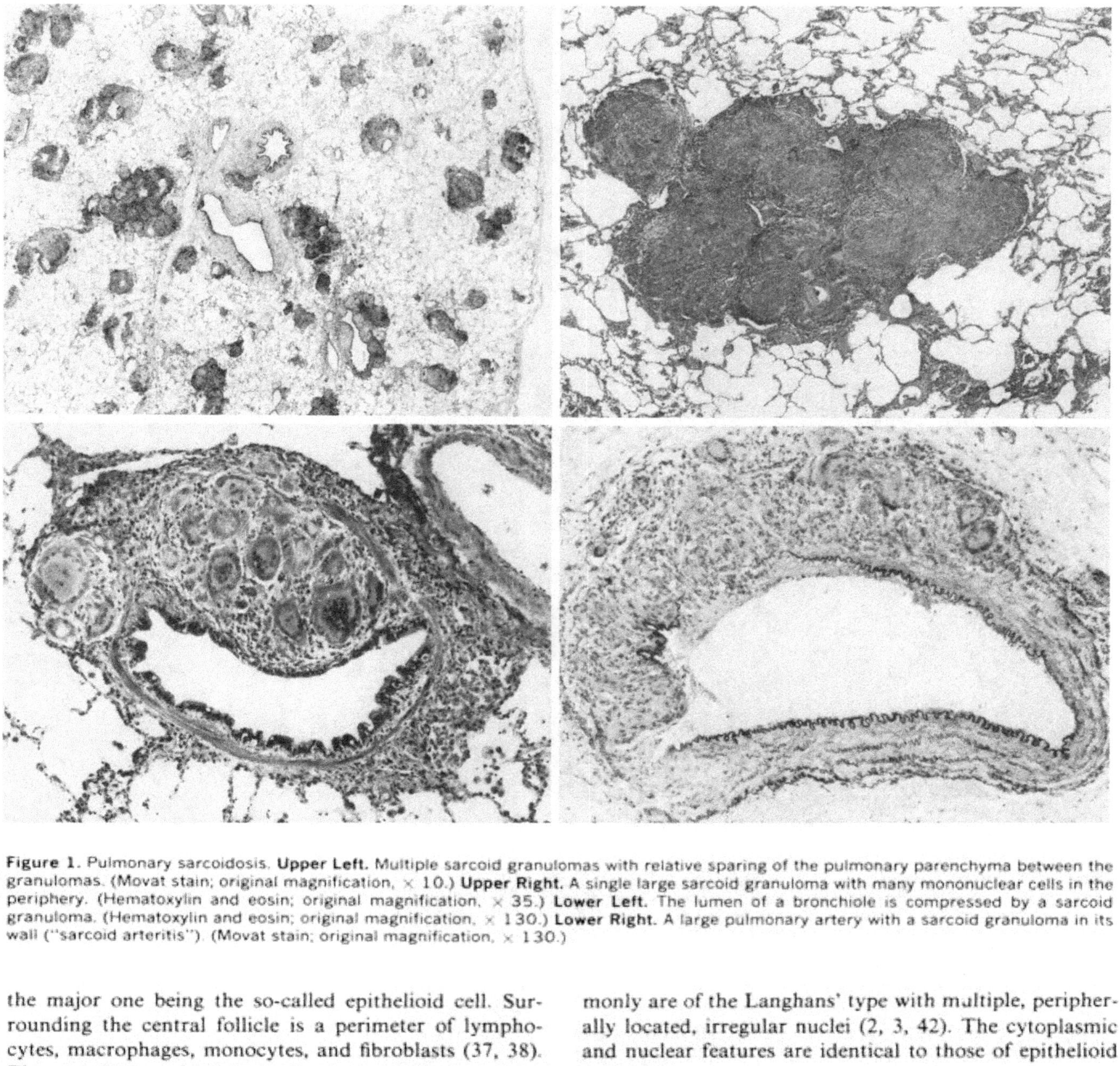

Figure 1. Pulmonary sarcoidosis. **Upper Left.** Multiple sarcoid granulomas with relative sparing of the pulmonary parenchyma between the granulomas. (Movat stain; original magnification, × 10.) **Upper Right.** A single large sarcoid granuloma with many mononuclear cells in the periphery. (Hematoxylin and eosin; original magnification, × 35.) **Lower Left.** The lumen of a bronchiole is compressed by a sarcoid granuloma. (Hematoxylin and eosin; original magnification, × 130.) **Lower Right.** A large pulmonary artery with a sarcoid granuloma in its wall ("sarcoid arteritis"). (Movat stain; original magnification, × 130.)

the major one being the so-called epithelioid cell. Surrounding the central follicle is a perimeter of lymphocytes, macrophages, monocytes, and fibroblasts (37, 38). The sarcoid granuloma is similar in appearance to those in all other types of granulomatous disease with the exception of tuberculosis (1-6).

Epithelioid cells occupy the body of the follicle as nodular collections of tightly packed cells. The term *epithelioid* was originally used because the size and arrangement of the cells were similar to the cells of epithelium; the epithelioid cell is now known, however, to be derived from the mononuclear-phagocyte system (39). Because epithelioid cells do have abundant cytoplasmic organelles, it has been suggested that they have secretory capabilities (40-42). Several populations of epithelioid cells have been described, but these "subclasses" are now believed to represent stages in the development of one cell type (6, 42-44).

Multinucleated giant cells, often up to 150 μm in diameter, are frequently found among the epithelioid cells within the granuloma follicle. The giant cells most commonly are of the Langhans' type with multiple, peripherally located, irregular nuclei (2, 3, 42). The cytoplasmic and nuclear features are identical to those of epithelioid cells (37).

The macrophages within the follicle are 10 to 25 μm in diameter and have numerous cytoplasmic processes that interdigitate with those of adjacent cells. The nuclei are indented and contain finely dispersed chromatin. The macrophages are rich in cytoplasmic organelles; but like epithelioid cells, the macrophages have a paucity of phagosomes or phagolysosomes, suggesting that they are not actively involved in phagocytosis (37). However, the macrophages within the granulomas do have numerous electron-dense lysosomes, suggesting that they are secretory cells (45).

The monocytes of the sarcoid follicle have a smoother surface then the macrophages (37). The nuclei are dark, and the cytoplasm has fewer organelles then the macrophage or epithelioid cell. Many of the lymphocytes of the follicle have the morphologic features of *activated* lymphocytes (37, 42, 43, 46). They are larger than the usual

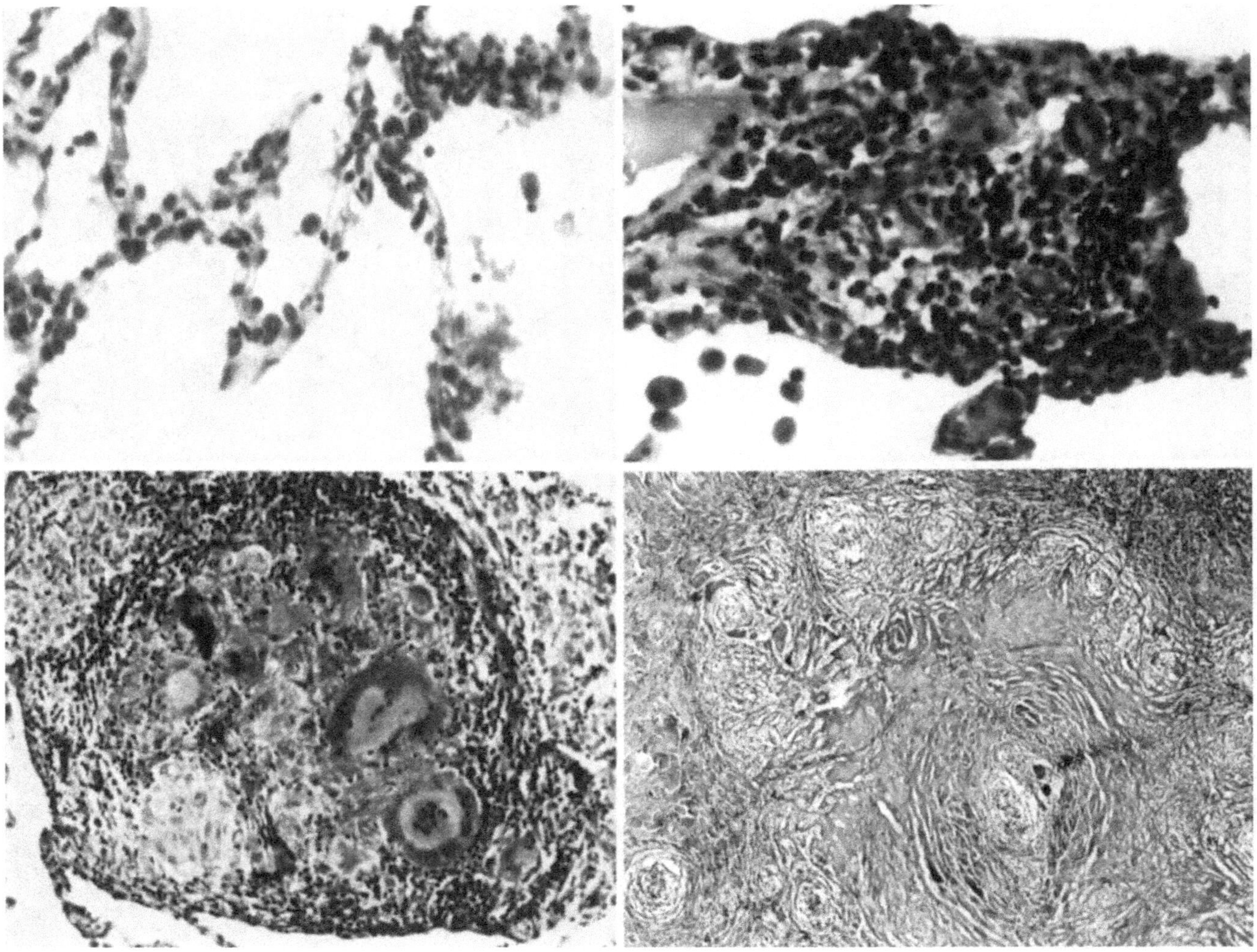

Figure 2. Stages of pulmonary sarcoidosis. **Upper Left.** Alveolar septae with increased numbers of mononuclear cells ("sarcoid alveolitis") Hematoxylin and eosin; original magnification, × 500.) **Upper Right.** Larger collection of mononuclear cells with few epithelioid cells and one giant cell in an alveolar septum. (Hematoxylin and eosin; original magnification, × 500.) **Lower Left.** A well-developed sarcoid granuloma with many giant cells and mononuclear cells only in the periphery. (Hematoxylin and eosin; original magnification, × 220.) **Lower Right.** The final stage in the organization of a sarcoid granuloma. The granulomas now consist mainly of relatively dense fibrous tissue, and only an occasional giant or epithelioid cell remains. (Hematoxylin and eosin; original magnification, × 55.)

lymphocyte and contain an irregular nucleus, often with centrioles; the cytoplasm contains large numbers of mitochrondria, dense granules, ribosomes, and rough endoplasmic reticulum.

The extracellular material within and surrounding the central follicle is classically described as *amorphous hyaline material* or *reticulin* (2). Although it has been suggested that some of this material was "para-amyloid" (47), electron microscopy has shown that it is mostly ground substance with interspersed fibers of various diameters (48). The exact nature of the latter is unknown. It has been described as amyloid or fibrin-like, but is more likely one or more types of collagen.

When involving alveolar septa, the sarcoid granuloma distorts the interstitium by its physical bulk and, thus, probably causes derangements in air-blood relations (37, 49). The presence of granulomas, however, does not seem to affect structures composing the so-called alveolar-capillary membrane; measurements of the pathway between air and blood in the sarcoid lung have shown it to be normal or, at most, slightly increased (50).

ALVEOLITIS OF SARCOIDOSIS; EVOLUTION OF DISEASE

Whereas early reports described the granuloma of sarcoid as being monotonously uniform (suggesting they begin at the same time) (51), it is now clear that the lesions of pulmonary sarcoidosis can originate at different times (5, 6). Moreover, although the granulomas are the morphologic hallmarks of pulmonary sarcoidosis, the alveolar structures in this disease also are characterized by accumulations of inflammatory and immune-effector cells within the interstitium and alveolus (5, 36, 52). Commonly referred to as the *alveolitis* of sarcoidosis, these inflammatory and immune effector cell accumulations consist of monocytes, macrophages, and lymphocytes that are present in approximately equal numbers. In most patients, the majority of effector cells are found within the interstitium rather than the alveolar air spaces (36, 52).

Although the diagnosis of sarcoidosis cannot be made without the presence of granulomas, there is increasing evidence that the alveolitis of sarcoidosis precedes the formation of the granulomas (Figure 2) (34, 36, 52-55). The extensive studies by Rosen and associates (52) have shown that early, developing granulomas are composed of a loose collection of inflammatory and immune effector cells in which monocytes, macrophages, and lymphocytes predominate over epithelioid cells. As the granuloma matures, numbers of epithelioid cells increase and numbers of monocytes, macrophages, and lymphocytes decrease (37, 52, 56). In patients with extensive alveolitis, few granulomas are present, but in patients with numerous granulomas, the alveolitis is minimal or absent, further supporting the concept that the alveolitis precedes the granulomas (52). At least part of the alveolitis of sarcoidosis is derived from circulating inflammatory and immune effector cells; Soler and Bassett (37) have presented morphologic evidence that blood monocytes pass from capillaries to the interstitium in this disease.

The fate of the sarcoid granuloma has been well documented morphologically. Although it can appear *fresh* from months to years, the granuloma ultimately either resolves leaving few or no morphologic changes or it undergoes progressive fibrosis (1, 5, 6, 57). The fibrosis begins as a rim of collagen around the granuloma and proceeds in a centripetal fashion until the entire structure is replaced by fibrous tissue (1, 2, 37, 53, 56). It is likely, although unproven, that the collagen composing the fibrous tissue originates from the fibroblasts in the periphery of the granuloma (37). As the lesion "matures," fibroblasts proliferate in the periphery of the granuloma (56). In older granulomas, peripheral fibroblasts are extensive, and the inflammatory and immune effector cells in the periphery of the granuloma disappear (56). As the fibrosis proceeds inward, capillaries in the region are trapped and disappear (37, 55).

In about 20% of patients with sarcoidosis, there is progression to interstitial fibrosis, distortion, and replacement of the pulmonary architecture (58, 59). These progressive lesions are associated with increased amounts of collagen fibers within the interstitium, obliteration of capillaries, and destruction of architecture by inflammatory and immune effector cells, granulomas, and fibroblasts (37). Eventually, the normal alveolar architecture disappears, resulting in cystic spaces interspersed with bands of connective tissue producing the so-called *end-stage*.

Thus, on morphologic grounds, pulmonary sarcoidosis appears to begin as a mononuclear alveolitis that proceeds to a multinucleated, giant cell granulomatous disease. Thereafter, two alternatives are available: The granulomas resolve leaving relatively normal lung (80% of patients), or progressive fibrosis ensues producing end-stage lung. In either case, the process takes place in various alveolar structures at different times and progresses at different rates.

Characterization of the Alveolitis of Sarcoidosis

Dr. Gary W. Hunninghake (Senior Investigator, Pulmonary Branch, National Heart, Lung, and Blood Institute): Pulmonary sarcoidosis is characterized by the presence of granulomas in the lung parenchyma (5, 6, 60). However, as we have just seen, the earliest lesion of this disease is an alveolitis, a diffuse infiltration of the lung parenchyma by mononuclear cells (36, 52-54). We may conceive, therefore, of the sequence of events in the development of pulmonary sarcoidosis as follows. A stimulus, at present not defined, results in an accumulation of mononuclear cells in the lung parenchyma (that is, the alveolitis). The alveolitis either resolves spontaneously or leads to the formation of granulomas. The presence of granulomas is usually associated with at least some degree of alteration of interstitial connective tissue and epithelial, endothelial, and mesenchymal cells that compose the normal alveolar structures. Although whether it is the alveolitis or granulomas, or both, that mediate these alterations is unclear, it is evident that in some cases the derangement of the alveolar structure is progressive, leading to interstitial fibrosis and the eventual end-stage of alveolar-capillary units.

The sequence of events outlined above does not take place in all of the alveolar structures at the same time or at the same rate. Rather, small groups of units are affected at different times and progress through the phases of alveolitis to granulomas, fibrosis, and cellular derangement to end-stage at different rates. Also, the disease within each group of alveoli may halt, resolve, or progress, making the overall picture a montage of alveolar-capillary units in various stages of inflammation and derangement. Thus, a patient with sarcoidosis will have some alveoli that are normal, some with alveolitis, and others with various mixtures of alveolitis, granuloma, fibrosis, and alterations of parenchymal cells. Over a time, the number of units in each phase will probably change, giving an overall picture of either no lung disease, stable lung disease, or progressive lung disease.

On the basis of these observations, it is clear that characterization and quantification of the alveolitis of sarcoidosis is an important means of defining the pathogenesis as well as the activity and prognosis of the disease.

TECHNIQUE

The inflammatory and immune effector cells forming the alveolitis of sarcoidosis can be recovered from the alveolar structures by a technique termed *bronchoalveolar lavage* (28, 32-34, 61-64). With this method, the effector cells within the lower respiratory tract are obtained by placing a fiberoptic bronchoscope in a distal airway, instilling 1 dL of sterile saline in five 20-mL aliquots, and recovering the lavage fluid by suction. With this technique, from 10 to 30 $\times$ 10^6 effector cells can be recovered; with the immunologic methods now available, this is sufficient to permit detailed characterization of the type, number, and state of activation of the cells that are present. Also, because bronchoalveolar lavage is rapid and safe, the procedure can be used to contrast the effector cell populations of the lungs of sarcoidosis patients with those of normal persons and of persons with other lung disorders and can be used to evaluate the effector cell populations of the same patient over a period of time.

One area of concern in using bronchoalveolar lavage to evaluate the inflammatory and immune effector cell populations in the lower respiratory tract is the possibility that the cells recovered by lavage do not accurately reflect the true alveolitis of the disease. However, studies comparing the effector cells in open lung biopsies of patients to the effector cells recovered by lavage have shown that the cells recovered by lavage accurately reflect the ongoing inflammatory and immune processes within the lower respiratory tract (31, 33, 65). In addition, the inflammatory and immune effector cells obtained by lavage of one segment of the lung appear to be representative of the alveolitis of the sarcoid lung as a whole (66). Although it is not known how many alveolar-capillary units are washed out during the lavage procedure, it is apparent that enough alveoli are sampled so that the local differences from one group of alveolar-capillary units to another are averaged out in the lavage specimen.

The current methods of handling the lavage fluid and characterizing and quantifying the recovered cells have been detailed in a recent review (33). The cell populations are usually quantified as a percentage of the total bronchoalveolar cells. Quantifying the absolute numbers of these cells is not very meaningful, because the yield of cells may be influenced by multiple factors such as the placement of the bronchoscope or the relative "stickiness" of the cells to the alveolar epithelial surface.

GENERAL CHARACTERISTICS OF THE ALVEOLITIS OF SARCOIDOSIS

Evaluation of the inflammatory and immune effector cell populations recovered from the lungs of patients with sarcoidosis shows that the alveolitis of this disease contrasts sharply with the effector cell populations of normal lung and is markedly different than the alveolitis of most other interstitial disorders (28, 32-34, 63-71).

The effector cells present in the alveolar structures of normal nonsmokers consist of more than 90% alveolar macrophages, less than 10% lymphocytes, and less than 1% polymorphonuclear leukocytes (28, 32, 33, 64). In contrast, sarcoidosis is characterized by a marked increase in the proportions of lymphocytes in the lower respiratory tract (28, 31-34, 63-71). On the average, our study population had 33% ± 6% lymphocytes in their lavage fluid compared to less than 10% for normal nonsmokers and smokers. In our sarcoidosis patients with clinical criteria associated with active disease (such as fever, weight loss, erythema nodosum, progressive deterioration of lung function) the proportion of lung lymphocytes was 55% ± 8%, almost twofold higher than that of the group average.

Most other interstitial disorders are associated with normal proportions of lymphocytes in the alveolar structures. Other than sarcoidosis, the only lung disorders know to be associated with increased proportions of lymphocytes in lavage fluid are hypersensitivity pneumonitis (62), tuberculosis (33, 72), and lymphoma involving the lung parenchyma (33). As more lung disorders are evaluated by bronchoalveolar lavage, this list is likely to grow; from the pattern emerging, it will probably include most granulomatous lung diseases in addition to lymphocyte-derived malignancies involving lung parenchyma (33).

In addition to lymphocytes, the remainder of the effector cells characterizing the alveolitis of sarcoidosis are monocytes and macrophages (5, 6, 28, 31-34, 36, 52-54, 61-71); as in normal persons, nonsmoking patients with sarcoidosis have less than 1% neutrophils in their lower respiratory tract (28-34, 64, 65). With the technology presently available, it is not possible to distinguish between the small young macrophage and the blood monocyte that has recently migrated to the alveolar structures; hence the terms *macrophages* or *mononuclear phagocytes* are used interchangeably when this population of cells in bronchoalveolar lavage fluid analyses is discussed. Although the proportions of these cells are lower in lavage fluid recovered from patients with sarcoidosis as compared to those in normal persons, it is important to emphasize that the total number of inflammatory and immune effector cells in the sarcoid lung is many times that in the normal lung. Thus, in terms of total numbers, the alveolitis of sarcoidosis is characterized not only by increased numbers of lymphocytes but also by increased numbers of mononuclear phagocytes.

From these studies, it is apparent that bronchoalveolar lavage analysis yields a picture of the alveolitis of pulmonary sarcoidosis similar to that of the open lung biopsy: Sarcoidosis is a disease characterized by the accumulation of large numbers of lymphocytes, monocytes, and macrophages within the alveolar structures.

CHARACTERIZATION AND QUANTIFICATION OF LYMPHOCYTE SUBTYPES

Estimates of the relative numbers of lymphocyte subtypes in the lower respiratory tract can be expressed either as a percentage of the total lymphocytes present or as a percentage of total inflammatory and immune effector cells present. Both methods are valuable, as they give somewhat different insights into the importance of the various cells as components of the inflammatory and immune effector cell populations of the lower respiratory tract. Whereas expressing the numbers of lymphocyte subtypes as a percentage of total lymphocytes present gives an estimate of relative shifts in lymphocyte subpopulations, expressing the numbers of lymphocyte subtypes as a percentage of total alveolar effector cells gives an estimate of the overall intensity of each lymphocyte component of the pulmonary inflammatory and immune process.

In normal persons, the percentage of lung lymphocytes that is T-lymphocytes varies from 65% to 80%; this is also the case for interstitial disorders such as idiopathic pulmonary fibrosis, the collagen-vascular disorders, and histiocytosis-X (28, 32, 33, 64). In marked contrast, our study population with sarcoidosis, unselected for disease activity, had an average of 90% ± 4% of all lung lymphocytes as T-lymphocytes. In fact, T-lymphocytes represented more than 80% (the high normal value) of all lung lymphocytes in 91% of the persons in the study population, in spite of the fact that these patients were unselected in terms of any clinical, roentgenographic, or physiologic criteria. Of the patients with less than 80% T-lymphocytes, none had any evidence of lung disease at

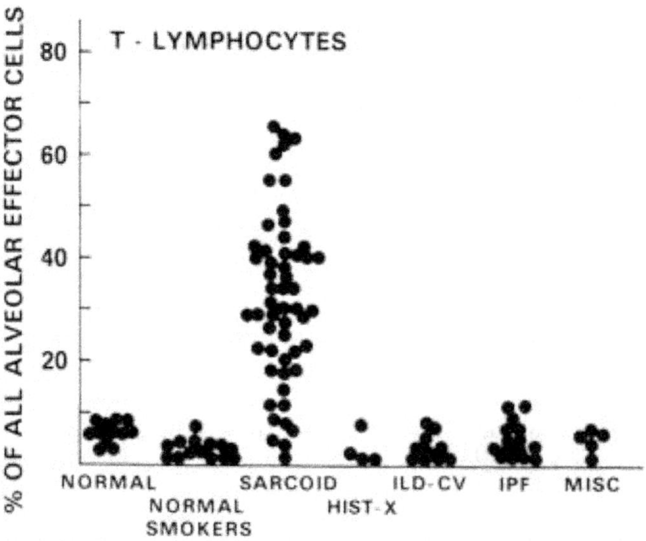

Figure 3. Proportion of all inflammatory and immune effector cells in the alveolar structures that are T-lymphocytes in normal persons and in persons with various chronic lung disorders, including untreated patients with sarcoidosis. The lung effector cells were recovered by bronchoalveolar lavage. For normal persons (nonsmokers and smokers), T-lymphocytes represent less than 8% of all effector cells present. Hist-X = histiocytosis-X; ILD-CV = interstitial lung disease associated with collagen vascular disease (included are patients with rheumatoid arthritis, progressive systemic sclerosis, systemic lupus erythematosus, and mixed connective tissue disease); IPF = idiopathic pulmonary fibrosis; Misc = various miscellaneous lung disorders (included are patients with familial pulmonary fibrosis, Kartagener's syndrome, inorganic dust disease, squamous cell carcinoma, and cystic fibrosis).

the time of evaluation. Thus, pulmonary sarcoidosis is a disease characterized by shifts in the proportions of lung lymphocytes toward more T-lymphocytes (28-34, 65).

That patients with pulmonary sarcoidosis have increased proportions of T-lymphocytes in their alveolar structures is even more remarkable when compared to the findings in their peripheral blood. Although these persons have large amounts of T-lymphocytes in lung, they simultaneously have peripheral blood T-lymphocytopenia (23-34), suggesting that observations of cellular immune processes in blood may give a false view of what is actually occurring in lung. In comparison to persons with sarcoidosis, normal persons have the same proportions of T-lymphocytes in lung and blood as do patients with idiopathic pulmonary fibrosis, interstitial lung disease associated with collagen-vascular disease, and histiocytosis-X (28, 32, 33).

When the numbers of T-lymphocytes in the sarcoid lung are expressed as a proportion of the total inflammatory and immune effector cells present, it becomes apparent that this disease is characterized not only by shifts in the proportions of lung lymphocytes that are T-lymphocytes but also by an intense T-lymphocyte alveolitis. Whereas in normal persons, T-lymphocytes account for less than 8% of all inflammatory and immune effector cells within the alveolar structures, in persons with sarcoidosis, T-lymphocytes represent 31% ± 8% of the effector cells present (Figure 3). By comparison, in most other interstitial disorders, less than 8% of all effector cells present in the lower respiratory tract are T-lymphocytes (28-33). This increased proportion of T-lymphocytes in the sarcoid lung becomes even more impressive when one considers that although normal persons have approximately 25×10^9 effector cells in their lower respiratory tract (73), morphologic observations of biopsies of patients with sarcoidosis with active alveolitis suggest that there are probably five to 20 times more effector cells within their alveolar structures (5, 6, 36, 52-54, 60). It is apparent, therefore, that in absolute numbers T-lymphocytes are tremendously increased within the alveolar structures of the sarcoid lung.

Although the proportions of lung lymphocytes that are T-lymphocytes are increased in the sarcoid lung, the proportions of lung lymphocytes that are B-lymphocytes are significantly reduced (28, 32, 33). In contrast, the proportions of lymphocytes that are B-lymphocytes are increased in the blood of sarcoid patients compared to their own lungs and to the blood of normal persons. Because the sarcoid lung is characterized by an overall increase in total lymphocytes, it is likely that the total number of B-lymphocytes is increased within the sarcoid lung even though the proportion of these cells is reduced. Even so, the total number of T-lymphocytes is still far in excess; on the average, the sarcoid lung has 20 to 25 times more T-lymphocytes than B-lymphocytes (28-33). In comparison, the normal lung has only seven to 10 times more T-lymphocytes than B-lymphocytes (28-33).

If, as suggested above, lung T-lymphocytes are actively involved in the pathogenesis of pulmonary sarcoidosis, many of these lung T-lymphocytes are probably in a state of relative activation and thus function as effector T-lymphocytes. In support of this concept are the findings that in parallel with the marked increase in the numbers of T-lymphocytes in the sarcoid lung, there are also increases in numbers of various subtypes of T-lymphocytes in the alveolar structures of these patients (28-34). Most importantly, persons with sarcoidosis have increased proportions of lung T-lymphocytes that form rosettes with sheep erythrocytes at 37 °C, a subset of T-lymphocytes well known to be in a relative state of activation (Figure 4) (28, 32, 33, 74, 75). Additional evidence of increased numbers of activated T-lymphocytes in the lungs of sarcoid patients comes from the observation that these patients have increased numbers of T-lymphocytes that have receptors for the crystallizable fragment (Fc) portion of IgG (so-called Tγ cells) (28, 32, 33). Although the exact role of Tγ cells in the pathogenesis of sarcoidosis is unknown, several studies have shown that increased numbers of this subset of T-lymphocytes are present when a population of T-lymphocytes has been activated in some manner (76-78).

As pointed out by other investigators, there are increased proportions of T-lymphocytes forming rosettes with sheep erythrocytes at 37 °C (79) and Tγ cells (80) in the blood of patients with sarcoid compared to blood of normals. Although this was also true in our study population, the proportion and total numbers of these T-lymphocyte subtypes in blood were far less than those found in lung, further suggesting that analysis of blood does not give a true picture of the character and magnitude of the immune processes within the lung.

Further evidence of the presence of increased numbers of activated T-lymphocytes in the sarcoid lung comes from studies of the relative proportions of these cells undergoing spontaneous transformation. In this regard, unstimulated, highly purified T-lymphocytes isolated from the lungs of patients with sarcoidosis spontaneously incorporate three- to fourfold greater amounts of [^{3}H]thymidine than do equal numbers of lung T-lymphocytes from normal persons (HUNNINGHAKE GW, CRYSTAL RG. Unpublished observations). In addition, as will be discussed by Dr. Gadek, lung T-lymphocytes from patients with sarcoidosis spontaneously release a variety of lymphokines whereas lung T-lymphocytes from normal persons do not (28, 33, 34).

Thus, it is clear that the alveolitis of sarcoidosis is characterized by increased numbers of lymphocytes, monocytes, and macrophages. Whereas the effector role of the monocytes and macrophages in the sarcoid lung has not been evaluated, it is apparent that this disease is distinguished by large numbers of activated T-lymphocytes within the alveolar structures. Furthermore, these activated T-lymphocytes probably play a major role in the pathogenesis of the disease. Because the activity of the alveolitis can be accurately gauged by analysis of the cell populations in bronchoalveolar lavage fluid, this technique should prove useful in staging patients with sarcoidosis and following their response to therapy.

Maintenance of the Alveolitis of Sarcoidosis

Dr. James E. Gadek (Senior Investigator, Pulmonary Branch, National Heart, Lung, and Blood Institute): Although the initiating stimulus for sarcoidosis is unknown, increasingly there are clues as to how the sarcoid granuloma is formed and maintained. As discussed by Drs. Roberts and Hunninghake, the appearance of granuloma is preceded by an accumulation of monocytes, macrophages, and lymphocytes, particularly T-lymphocytes, within the alveolar structures. I will outline the importance of all these cell types in forming and maintaining granuloma within the lower respiratory tract.

IMPORTANCE OF MONONUCLEAR PHAGOCYTES

Monocytes and alveolar macrophages are part of the *mononuclear phagocyte* system, a term applied to a specific class of phagocytic cells derived from monoblasts within the bone marrow (39, 81-83). The mononuclear phagocyte system forms a continuum of cells that progressively mature from precursor marrow cells to blood monocytes and finally to macrophages. In addition, the evidence is overwhelming that epithelioid cells and giant cells are derived from monocytes and macrophages (53, 54, 83-88). Thus, in pulmonary sarcoidosis, granuloma formation is conceived as a coalescence and maturation of mononuclear phagocytes that are in the alveolar structures. Consequently, although mononuclear phagocytes have a variety of effector functions that may be relevant to the pathogenesis of sarcoidosis (64, 68, 83, 89-98), one critical role of these cells in this disease is to serve as a building block for granuloma formation.

Because granulomas are dynamic structures, there is a need for the constant replenishment of mononuclear phagocytes as epithelioid cells and giant cells either die or move out of granuloma (85, 88). This constant requirement for a monocyte and macrophage pool in the formation of new granuloma and maintenance of established granuloma suggests processes that maintain the mononuclear phagocyte series of cells within the alveolar structures are relevant to the pathogenesis of sarcoidosis.

There are two mechanisms that could serve to replenish the monocyte and macrophage pool within the lung: Monocytes and macrophages within the alveolar structures could proliferate locally, or monocytes could be recruited to the lung from the blood monocyte pool, or both could occur. There are several reasons to think that the second mechanism is more important in pulmonary sarcoidosis. First, although monocytes and macrophages in the lower respiratory tract have the capacity to proliferate (99, 100), large numbers of monocytes and macrophages would have to be constantly dividing to maintain the monocyte series within the sarcoid lung (82). However, evaluation of biopsies of sarcoid lung rarely shows these cells in mitosis (2, 3, 36, 37). Second, studies with experimental models of granuloma formation have shown that most cells composing granuloma are derived from the circulating pool of blood monocytes (45, 53, 68, 83-88). Consistent with this concept, biopsies of patients with sarcoidosis show monocytes migrating from capillaries to the alveolar interstitium (37).

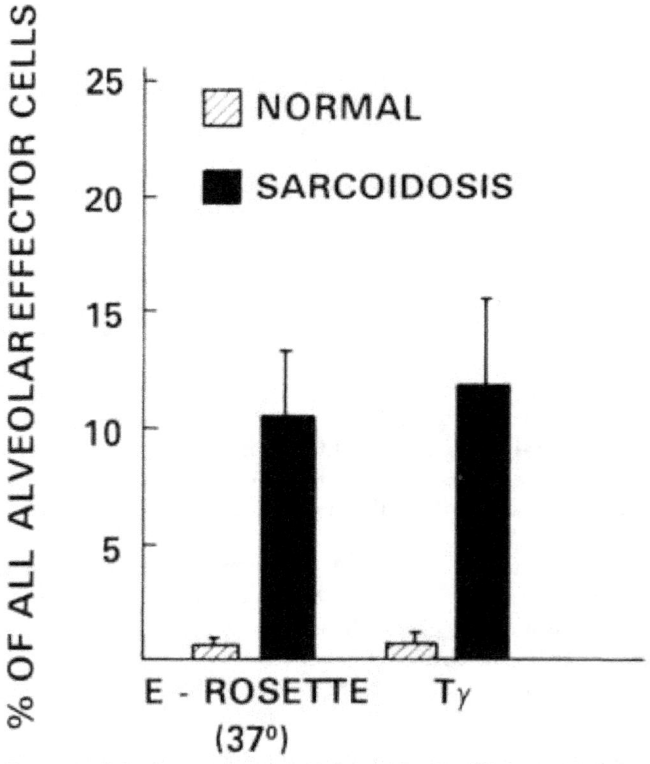

Figure 4. Subtypes of T-lymphocytes in the lungs of patients with sarcoidosis. Two subtypes of T-lymphocytes were evaluated, those forming rosettes with sheep erythrocytes at 37 °C (*E-Rosette, 37 °*) and those with receptors for the Fc portion of IgG (*Tγ*). The data are presented as the proportions of all inflammatory and immune effector cells represented as each T-lymphocyte subtype. The normal study population consisted of eight persons and the sarcoid population, of nine. The error bars represent SEM.

Table 1. Role of Lung T-Lymphocytes in Recruiting Blood Monocytes to the Lung in Patients With Pulmonary Sarcoidosis*

Mediator	Function	Normal Persons†		Patients with Sarcoid†	
		Blood	Lung	Blood	Lung
Monocyte chemotactic factor‡	Recruitment of circulating monocytes to the site of mediator release	0	0	1+	4+
Leukocyte inhibitory factor§	Inhibition of polymorphonuclear leukocyte migration	0	0	1+	4+

* Production of soluble mediators of inflammatory cell migration by lung and blood T-lymphocytes of normal persons and patients with pulmonary sarcoidosis.
† Lung and blood T-lymphocytes were incubated for 48 h. at 37 °C and the supernatants evaluated for the production of monocyte chemotactic factor and leukocyte inhibitory factor. The relative amounts of the factors produced are expressed on an arbitrary scale of 0 (none) to 4+ (maximum, equivalent to mitogen-stimulated T-lymphocytes) (28, 34).
‡ Quantified using purified blood monocytes as target cells in a modified Boyden chemotaxis assay (34).
§ Quantified using unfractionated blood leukocytes as target cells in a chemotaxis under agarose assay (28).

MONOCYTE RECRUITMENT TO THE SARCOID LUNG: ROLE OF T-LYMPHOCYTES

The process of recruitment of leukocytes from one compartment to another is known as chemotaxis (101). Chemotactic stimuli are generally protein or lipid and are referred to as "chemotactic factors." A vast array of such factors has been described, some derived from serum and others produced directly by cells (102-115). In addition, a number of chemotactic inhibitors have been characterized (116-121), and thus the process of chemotaxis must be considered as a balance between the attractive nature of chemotactic factors and the restraining influence of chemotactic inhibitors. Whereas some of these processes are directed toward all leukocytes, others affect one cell type more than others allowing for the expression of specificity in cell migrations. This concept is important because neutrophils are rarely found in the sarcoid lung, suggesting that blood monocytes are recruited to the sarcoid lung, and blood neutrophils are excluded.

Chemotactic factors are conventionally evaluated in vitro by the use of chemotactic chambers in which the target cells and putative chemotactic stimuli are separated by a membrane of calibrated pore size. In such a system, chemotactic activity is usually quantitated as the number of target cells moving through the membrane toward the stimulus per unit time (122). To evaluate the role played by lung inflammatory and immune effector cells in recruiting blood monocytes, unstimulated lung T-lymphocytes obtained from sarcoid patients by bronchoalveolar lavage were cultured for 48 hours, after which the supernatants of these cells were evaluated for chemotactic activity using blood monocytes as target cells (34).

Such studies convincingly demonstrate that T-lymphocytes comprising the alveolitis of sarcoidosis are spontaneously elaborating a specific factor (monocyte chemotactic factor) that attracts blood monocytes (34) (Table 1). In contrast, T-lymphocytes present in normal alveolar structures have no influence on the migration of blood monocytes. Monocyte chemotactic factor has a molecular mass of 10 to 15 000 daltons and is probably a protein (110). Whereas T-lymphocytes from the normal lung can be induced to elaborate monocyte chemotactic factor (for example, by stimulation with a mitogen such as concanavalin A), the T-lymphocytes obtained from the lungs of sarcoid patients are spontaneously secreting it (34). This finding is consistent with the concept that increased numbers of T-lymphocytes found in the sarcoid lung are activated.

In addition, comparison of T-lymphocytes from lung and blood of sarcoid patients demonstrates that lung T-lymphocytes spontaneously secrete larger amounts of monocyte chemotactic factor than blood T-lymphocytes of the same person (Table 1). The difference between lung and blood is striking; sarcoid lung T-lymphocytes produce an average of 25 times more of this chemotactic factor per cell than do sarcoid blood T-lymphocytes (34). This observation, together with the finding that the sarcoid lung contains large numbers of T-lymphocytes, suggests that concentrations of this chemotactic factor are higher in lung than in blood. Thus, a gradient of monocyte chemotactic factor between lung and blood of these patients is likely, resulting in the chronic accumulation of blood monocytes within the alveolar structures. In light of this observation, it is not difficult to understand how the pool of mononuclear phagocytes may be maintained within the sarcoid lung, providing a continuous source of basic building blocks for granuloma formation.

Although the elaboration of monocyte chemotactic factor by sarcoid lung T-lymphocytes explains the attraction of blood monocytes to the lung in this disease, it does not explain why monocytes, and not polymorphonuclear leukocytes, are recruited. When neutrophils are used as the target cell, chemotactic chamber studies show that monocyte chemotactic factor attracts neutrophils as well as monocytes (123). Thus, we have to look elsewhere to explain the specificity of the recruitment of monocytes in this disease.

One clue comes from analysis of other products elaborated by activated T-lymphocytes. Along with monocyte chemotactic factor, lung T-lymphocytes from sarcoid patients also spontaneously produced leukocyte inhibitory factor (28), a 68 000-dalton product that prevents the migration of polymorphonuclear leukocytes, but not monocytes (119) (Table 1). In addition, patients with sarcoidosis have elevated levels of serum lysozyme (68), an enzyme that inhibits the migration of neutrophils (124). In sarcoidosis, therefore, blood leukocytes are probably under a number of attractive and inhibitory stimuli, the net result of which is to recruit monocytes, but no neutrophils, to the alveolar structures.

Various studies have shown that blood monocytes of sarcoid patients are in a relative state of activation compared to blood monocytes of normal persons. Monocytes of sarcoid patients have increased numbers of IgG-Fc and C3 receptors (125), show increased spreading (126), and contain more lysozyme (68, 127), β-galactosidase (128), and angiotensin-converting enzyme (68, 129-131), all of which are considered criteria for mononuclear phagocyte activation (68). Although the mechanism of monocyte activation in sarcoidosis is undoubtedly complex and involves a variety of processes, T-lymphocytes probably play a role. In this regard, products elaborated by activated T-lymphocytes are known to be able to stimulate blood monocytes as well as attract them (132). The results of monocyte activation are probably important in helping the monocyte negotiate tissue barriers in its migration from capillary lumen to alveolar interstitium and in preparing the monocyte for its role in granuloma formation. In addition, that lung T-lymphocytes from sarcoid patients also spontaneously elaborate macrophage migration inhibitory factor (HUNNINGHAKE GW, GADEK JE, CRYSTAL RG. Unpublished observations) may provide a mechanism for the immobilization of the monocyte once it arrives within the alveolar structures. Although the relative state of cells composing sarcoid granuloma has not yet been studied, evidence from other forms of granuloma, such as that found in tuberculosis and schistosomasis, suggests that monocytes, macrophages, and epithelioid cells forming granuloma are in a relative state of activation (68, 83-88).

In addition to locally produced T-lymphocyte products, numerous inhibitory factors have been found in serum of patients with sarcoidosis. Although these circulating inhibitory factors probably play an important role in the cutaneous anergy of sarcoidosis, their presence does not seem to be related to disease activity in the lung (133-141). Thus, their role, if any, in the recruitment of blood monocytes to the sarcoid lung is unclear.

In summary, quantitative analysis of the alveolitis of sarcoidosis has shown that it is made up of monocytes, macrophages, and lymphocytes, including large numbers of activated T-lymphocytes. Analysis of the products elaborated by T-lymphocytes composing the alveolitis of sarcoidosis shows that these cells produce factors whose net effect is to attract blood monocytes specifically. Although these observations are relevant only to a part of the pathogenesis of sarcoidosis, they explain how one important cellular constituent of the sarcoid alveolitis is maintained.

Skin Testing, Blood Studies, and Bronchoalveolar Lavage to Assess Activity

Dr. Ronald G. Crystal: Traditionally, the activity of pulmonary sarcoidosis has been assessed with a number of loosely defined clinical criteria such as the presence or absence of weight loss, fatigue, weakness, malaise, fever, erythema nodosum, dry cough, progressive dyspnea, and worsening exercise intolerance (1, 3-5, 7, 12-16, 35). However, true activity of pulmonary sarcoid can be defined only in terms of the actual disease process in the lung. Because the alveolitis of sarcoidosis clearly precedes, and probably causes, the anatomic derangements of the alveolar structures that are characteristic of this disease, assessments of disease activity must take into account the number, type, and functional state of the inflammatory and immune effector cells in the lower respiratory tract. Thus, in view of our previous discussions, monitors of disease activity should assess the status of lung T-lymphocytes, lung mononuclear phagocytes, or both.

Table 2. Skin Test and Blood Studies Suggested in the Literature as Means to Assess the Activity of Pulmonary Sarcoidosis

Test	References
Skin testing	
Evaluation of anergy to a variety of antigens	1, 3-5, 12, 19-23, 143-149
Rebuck skin window	170
Evaluation of circulating mononuclear cells	
Number of lymphocytes	24, 25, 146, 150-151
Number of T-lymphocytes	24-27, 145, 149, 151, 152
Number of activated T-lymphocytes	70, 79, 80, 153
Response of lymphocytes to mitogens and antigens	21-23, 35, 145, 146, 154, 155
Response of lymphocytes to mixed lymphocyte cultures	143
Generation of killer cells	143
Spontaneous production of migration inhibition factor	146
Mediation of antibody dependent cellular cytotoxicity	152
Quantitation of serologic variables	
Immune complexes	156-159
Antibodies against infectious agents	160
Serum inhibitors of sheep erythrocyte binding to normal T-lymphocytes	137-139
IgG levels	149
Presence of autoantibodies	149
Anti T-lymphocyte antibodies	161
Lysozyme	7, 162-166, 180
Angiotensin-converting enzyme	7, 11, 131, 166-178, 180

SKIN TESTS AND BLOOD STUDIES

The mechanisms causing the anergic state in sarcoidosis are not well understood but probably involve circulating "factor(s)" that suppress the normal response of circulating inflammatory and immune effector cells to intradermal antigens (*see* Table 2). However, although anergy is a classic finding in pulmonary sarcoidosis (1, 3-5, 12, 19, 20, 133-143), there is no evidence that the anergic state reflects a concomitant high-intensity alveolitis or that normal skin test responses are characteristic of patients with low-intensity alveolitis (143-149). Likewise, although the numbers and function of blood mononuclear cells may have a broad correlation with disease activity, there is little evidence suggesting that such measurements accurately gauge the quantity and activity of the alveolitis of the sarcoid lung (23-29, 150-155).

The same reservations exist for most serologic tests proposed as monitors of disease activity. For example,

Table 3. Comparison of Proportions of T-Lymphocytes in Lavage Cell Differential with Biopsy Assessment of the Intensity of Alveolitis of Sarcoidosis Patients

Biopsy Assessment*	Percentages of T-Lymphocytes in the Lavage Cell Differential†	
	(≤28)	(>28)
Low-intensity alveolitis	6‡	0
High-intensity alveolitis	2	12‡

* Lung biopsies (approximately 1 cm by 1 cm, hemotoxylin and eosin stain), divided in a blinded fashion, were placed into a low- or high-intensity alveolitis group using criteria based on the number of mononuclear cells infiltrating the gas exchange exchange units (36).

† Patients were divided into two groups: those in whom lavage T-lymphocytes represented ≤28% of all inflammatory and immune effector cells present (low-intensity alveolitis) and those in whom T-lymphocutes represented >28% effector cells present (high-intensity alveolitis).

‡ The groupings of low-intensity alveolitis with ≤28% lavage T-lymphocytes and the high-intensity alveolitis with >28% lavage T-lymphocytes was significant at the $p < 0.01$ level.

there is no evidence that circulating immune complexes or various types of antibodies found in the serum of sarcoid patients are related to the inflammatory and immune processes within their lungs (156-161). However, two serologic variables, lysozyme and angiotensin-converting enzyme, should be considered because in theory, serum levels of these enzymes are linked to the class of phagocytic cells composing the alveolitis of sarcoidosis (11, 68, 162-180).

Lysozyme is an enzyme produced and secreted by many different cell types including cells of the mononuclear phagocytic series. In vitro, activated mononuclear phagocytes have an increased content of lysozyme and secrete more lysozyme into the culture medium (179). Thus, when the observation was made that patients with sarcoidosis frequently had increased levels of serum lysozyme, it was suggested that such measurements might reflect the activity of mononuclear phagocytes in these persons (68, 127, 163, 180). Several studies seem to support this concept. Blood monocytes of sarcoid patients secrete increased amounts of lysozyme compared to controls, monocyte lysozyme secretory rates correlate with the patient's lysozyme levels, and alveolar macrophages of these patients have more lysozyme activity than normal macrophages (68, 127).

Angiotensin-converting enzyme is generally regarded as a product of endothelial cells, where it acts to convert serum angiotensin I to angiotensin II and metabolizes bradykinin (181). However, when it was discovered that patients with sarcoidosis had increased serum levels of angiotensin-converting enzymes (168, 170), attention was directed toward the mechanism of this finding. Alveolar capillary endothelial cells seemed unlikely to be the source, because many chronic lung diseases are associated with injury to the alveolar capillary bed, yet increased angiotensin-converting enzyme levels are much commoner in sarcoidosis (11, 171). It was soon ascertained, however, that angiotensin-converting enzyme was present in lymph nodes, higher levels were present in nodes containing sarcoid granuloma (165), cells of the mononuclear phagocyte series contained and secreted angiotensin-converting enzyme (68, 128), and alveolar macrophages from sarcoid patients contained increased levels of this enzyme (68, 131). Thus, the concept evolved that cells of the mononuclear phagocyte series were the source of increased angiotensin-converting enzyme levels in sarcoidosis, and it was proposed that serum angiotensin-converting enzyme levels might reflect the inflammatory and immune processes in the lung parenchyma.

Unfortunately, in spite of the strong theoretical basis for the use of serum lysozyme and angiotensin-converting enzyme levels to gauge the activity of pulmonary sarcoidosis, there is conflicting evidence on the use of these variables in actually staging patients. Wheras some investigators have found that serum lysozyme and angiotensin-converting enzyme levels roughly correlate with disease activity (defined by symptoms or chest film) (11, 68, 131, 164, 166, 167, 169, 171-174), others have found either little or no correlation (168, 177) or have found that more patients with chronic disease than with acute disease have elevated levels (175). In addition, there have been no clinical studies showing a correlation of serum angiotensin-converting enzyme or lysozyme levels with the intensity of the alveolitis of sarcoidosis. In fact, there is direct evidence suggesting there is no correlation; quantitation of angiotensin-converting enzyme levels in lung parenchyma of sarcoid patients has shown them to be no different from those in normal persons (130, 131). Further confusing the picture is the observation that elevated serum angiotensin-converting enzyme levels also have been found in persons with disorders not involving the lungs, such as degenerative arthritis (171), cirrhosis (171), and granulomatous hepatitis (68, 169), suggesting that the quantity of this enzyme in the serum reflects a contribution from many organs. Because sarcoidosis is a systemic disease, the serum angiotensin-converting enzyme level probably reflects disease activity in many organs and has no specificity for disease activity within the alveolar structures.

In view of the above considerations, although it is clear that activated mononuclear phagocytes produce increased amounts of lysozyme and angiotensin converting enzyme, and that these cells are important components of the alveolitis of sarcoidosis, there is little evidence at present that these serum enzyme levels reflect the intensity of the alveolitis.

BRONCHOALVEOLAR LAVAGE

In contrast to the variables listed in Table 2, several lines of evidence support the concept that bronchoalveolar lavage is a useful clinical tool to sequentially measure the intensity of the inflammatory and immune processes within the alveolar structures of patients with pulmonary sarcoidosis.

1. As Dr. Hunninghake has discussed, bronchoalveolar lavage can be used to characterize the type and state of activation of the cells present within the alveolar structures (33). Although this method samples only cells on the epithelial surface of the lower respiratory tract, comparisons with analyses of effector cells in open lung biop-

sy specimens have shown that lavage analyses yield a representative average of the relative proportions of the various inflammatory and immune effector cells present throughout the alveolar structures (33, 65).

2. Even though lavage analyses are usually expressed in proportional terms (for example, proportion of all inflammatory and immune effector cells that are T-lymphocytes), comparison of lavage data with histologic data showed that for patients with pulmonary sarcoidosis, lavage analyses not only characterize the type of cells present but also estimate the overall intensity of the alveolitis (Table 3). To show this, we compared the proportions of T-lymphocytes recovered by lavage of a group of patients with sarcoidosis with a histologic estimate of the intensity of the alveolitis made by open lung biopsy. The biopsies, taken within 1 month of the lavage, were divided into two groups: those showing a high-intensity alveolitis (that is large numbers of mononuclear cells with the alveolar structures) and those showing a low-intensity alveolitis (that is, small numbers of mononuclear cells within the alveolar structures). Likewise, the lavage analyses were divided into two groups: those in which T-lymphocytes accounted for more than 28% of all cells recovered and those in which T-lymphocytes made up less than 28% of the effector cells present. Comparisons of these groupings showed a significant correlation between large numbers of mononuclear cells present in the biopsies and large proportions of T-lymphocytes recovered by lavage (65).

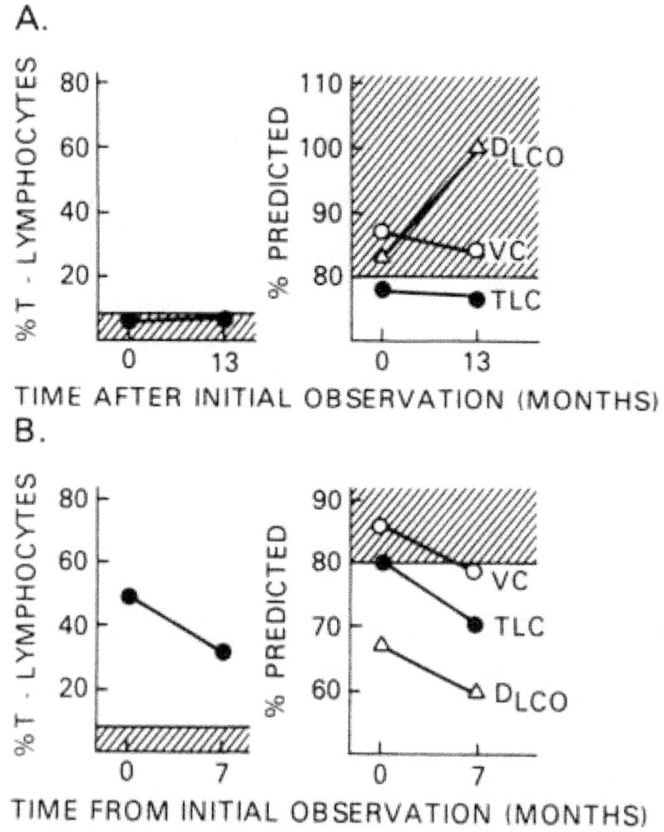

Figure 5. Prognostic use of bronchoalveolar lavage to evaluate the T-lymphocyte component of the alveolitis of pulmonary sarcoidosis. **A.** An untreated 22-year-old woman with pulmonary sarcoidosis seen over 13 months. During this period the alveolitis remained at a low level, and the pulmonary function variables remained stable or improved. **B.** An untreated 25-year-old woman with pulmonary sarcoidosis had a high-intensity alveolitis when first evaluated. After 7 months the alveolitis remained active, and all lung function variables had deteriorated. In both examples, the T-lymphocyte data are presented as the proportion of all lung effector cells that were T-lymphocytes, whereas the pulmonary function data are given in percent of predicted values. Shaded areas represent normal ranges. VC = vital capacity; TLC = total lung capacity; and D_{LCO} = single breath diffusing capacity (predicted based on alveolar volume and hemoglobin).

3. In our laboratories, bronchoalveolar lavage has been carried out in over 500 persons; it is associated with minimal discomfort, little morbidity, and no mortality (33). To ensure patient safety, however, it is important not to do lavage in patients with a forced expiratory volume in 1 s of less than 0.8 L. In addition, if inflammatory airway disease is present, lavage analyses must be interpreted cautiously, as it is difficult to estimate the relative contributions of bronchi and alveoli to the recovered cells.

4. Repeat lavage analyses over time show that in persons with pulmonary sarcoidosis in whom the proportion of T-lymphocytes remains low, there is little if any change in lung function over the same period (Figure 5A) (71). In contrast, for untreated patients in whom the proportion of lung T-lymphocytes remains high, lung function deteriorates (Figure 5B).

Such data support the concept that the alveolitis of sarcoidosis is a predecessor and cause of the anatomical derangements characteristic of sarcoidosis and that lavage is a useful monitor of the activity of the sarcoid alveolitis.

Roentgenograms and Physiologic Studies to Assess Activity

Dr. Jack D. Fulmer (Chief, Clinical Service, Pulmonary Branch, National Heart, Lung, and Blood Institute): The most commonly used monitors of pulmonary sarcoidosis are the chest roentgenogram and pulmonary function studies. Inherent in the use of these tests is the assumption that they help to stage the patient, that is, establish the extent and activity of the disease process, the prognosis, and the need for and efficacy of therapy. We will describe, therefore, the roentgenographic and physiologic findings in sarcoidosis and examine the available data concerning the sensitivity and specificity of these tests as monitors of disease activity. Also, because active pulmonary sarcoidosis is characterized by increased numbers of activated T-lymphocytes within the alveolar structures, we will evaluate the usefulness of the chest roentgenogram and common pulmonary function tests as detectors of the T-lymphocyte component of the alveolitis of this disease.

CHEST ROENTGENOGRAMS

The roentgenographic findings in pulmonary sarcoidosis have been well defined, and various classifications have been developed (12, 182-194). However, by international convention, the chest roentgenograms of patients with sarcoidosis are grouped according to the following scheme (12, 186): stage O, normal; stage I, bilateral hilar adenopathy; stage II, hilar adenopathy and diffuse parenchymal changes; and stage III, diffuse pulmonary infiltrates without hilar adenopathy. In this classification, the parenchymal changes most commonly described are fine or coarse nodules or a fluffy, cottonwood appearance; films with fibrotic changes, cysts, and bullae are usually assigned to stage III (12, 186). The proponents of this classification scheme view stages I through III as the roentgenographic manifestations of disease progression (186, 188). A worldwide review of 3676 patients with sarcoidosis showed that at the initial presentation to a physician, 8% had stage O roentgenograms, 51% had stage I, 29% had stage II, and 12% had stage III (186).

Although this international staging scheme is widely used in epidemiologic studies, most investigators believe that it often gives a false impression of the extent and activity of the disease process. Importantly, comparative morphologic-radiographic studies have shown that alveolitis and granulomas are present in the lung parenchyma of persons with stage I roentgenograms (5, 36, 195-198), even though the lung fields appear normal on the roentgenogram. In addition, although stage III roentgenograms are usually found only in those persons with progressive disease, it cannot be assumed that roentgenographic stages I and II always precede stage III (5).

To evaluate the usefulness of the classic roentgenographic staging in detecting the alveolitis in sarcoidosis, we categorized our study population into roentgenographic stages O to III and compared theses stages to estimates of the intensity of the alveolitis made from the lung biopsy. Consistent with the concept that the classic roentgenogram does not yield specific information concerning the activity of pulmonary sarcoidosis, no association was found between the roentgenographic stage and the quantitation of inflammatory and immune effector cells seen in the biopsy (33, 65). Further, comparison of the classic roentgenographic stages to the proportion of the T-lymphocytes recovered by bronchoalveolar lavage also showed no correlation.

In an attempt to escape the rigidity of the classic roentgenographic staging system, many investigators choose to simply describe the pattern seen; the most commonly described parenchymal patterns are reticulonodular, acinar, and fibrotic (189-192). Occasional patients also have large nodular lesions that simulate pulmonary metastasis, and cavitary lesions are sometimes found (184, 189, 193, 194). Although reticulonodular, acinar, and fibrotic patterns are widely recognized as manifestations of sarcoidosis, like the classic roentgenographic stages, their usefulness in staging the disease is unclear. It is generally accepted that the acinar and reticulonodular patterns precede the fibrotic pattern (189, 199, 200), but most evidence suggests that the chest film cannot be used to predict the morphologic findings (5, 36, 195, 201). Closely packed mononuclear cells within the alveolar air spaces have been suggested as the cause of the acinar pattern in sarcoidosis (191, 192), but there is also evidence that it is brought about by interstitial granulomas compressing the air spaces (190, 191). Attempts to correlate the alveolitis of sarcoidosis with these various roentgenographic presentations of sarcoidosis have failed. Evaluation of our study population also shows that there is little relation between the reticulonodular, acinar, and fibrotic patterns and the extent of alveolitis estimated by lung biopsy. Patients with acinar or nodular patterns generally had alveolitis and those with a coarse reticular pattern generally did not, but there was a great deal of overlap between groups. Likewise, no relationship could be found between the roentgenographic pattern and the proportion of bronchoalveolar lavage cells that were T-lymphocytes (33).

PHYSIOLOGIC TESTING

The usual physiologic findings in a patient with pulmonary sarcoidosis are characteristic of those of other patients with interstitial lung disease (3, 8, 189, 202-207). Lung volumes are reduced as are the diffusing capacity and lung compliance (202, 208-215). In addition, airway obstruction is a frequent physiologic finding in patients with sarcoidosis and seems to be unrelated to smoking history or the presence of bronchitis (8, 205, 206, 211, 215-223). Although many patients with sarcoidosis have a normal resting arterial oxygen tension, the resting alveolar-arterial oxygen gradient is often widened. In mild sarcoidosis, the arterial Po_2 may not change with exercise, but in persons with moderate and severe disease, increasing workloads cause the arterial oxygen tension to fall and the alveolar-arterial oxygen gradient to widen (8, 224-226).

Part of the problem in defining the functional consequences of sarcoidosis is that instead of using morphologic data as the standard for classifying patients, most investigators analyze the functional derangements from the perspective of the patient's roentgenographic stage (224). However, even though those with extensive roentgenographic changes usually have severe functional disturbances and those with minimal radiographic findings usually have few functional abnormalities (214), chest film and pulmonary function tests clearly have only a rough correlation to each other. A few studies have suggested that there is progressive impairment of pulmonary function with progressive roentgenographic changes (that is, stage I to III) (207), but for the majority of patients with sarcoidosis, most investigators have found little association between the chest film and physiologic tests (205, 211, 224, 227).

Functional testing is clearly more sensitive, however, to the disease process than the chest film. Many studies have shown examples of patients with stage I sarcoidosis who have abnormal diffusing capacity (189, 202, 207, 211, 224, 226). However, pulmonary function testing can be normal in the presence of parenchymal involvement (226, 227). Likewise, pulmonary function tests can be markedly abnormal but with the patient having little awareness of the functional derangement (228, 229).

As might be expected, some pulmonary function tests are more sensitive than others to this disease process. Measurements of lung volume are generally less sensitive than diffusing capacity, which in turn is less sensitive than gas exchange studies (particularly with exercise) (226, 227).

In our study population, comparison of the lung biopsy to the vital capacity, total lung capacity, diffusing capaci-

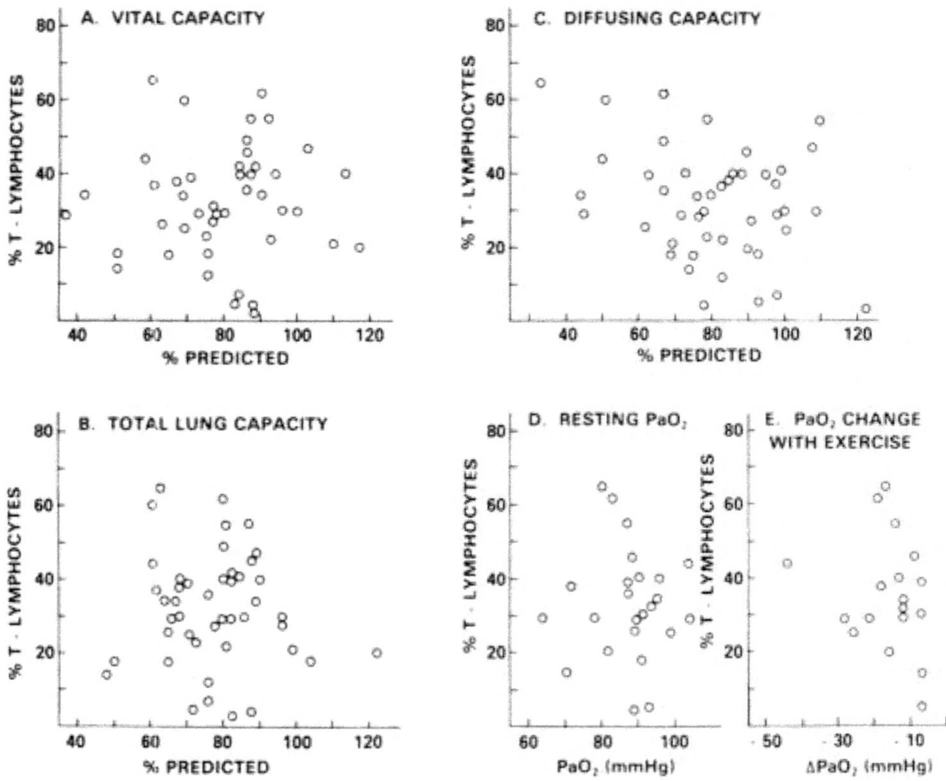

Figure 6. Evaluation of the ability of various pulmonary function variables to monitor the extent of the T-lymphocyte component of the alveolitis of sarcoidosis. The proportion of all lung effector cells that were T-lymphocytes (*% T-lymphocytes*) are compared to the percent predicted values for the following: **A.** Vital capacity. **B.** Total lung capacity. **C.** Single breath diffusing capacity (predicted based on alveolar volume and hemoglobin). **D.** Resting arterial oxygen tension. **E.** Change in arterial oxygen tension with exercise (PaO_2 [exercise]; PaO_2 [rest]).

ty, and resting exercising gas exchange data suggests that those studies are abnormal in the presence of alveolitis but cannot predict the extent of parenchymal inflammation. In addition, comparison of the proportion of T-lymphocytes in the lower respiratory tract to these variables showed that the magnitude of the functional abnormality has no relationship to the magnitude of the T-lymphocyte component of the alveolitis (Figure 6).

In summary, although radiographic and functional tests are useful to estimate the extent of disease within the alveolar structures, they cannot distinguish between alveolitis and anatomic derangement. Because the pathogenesis of the disease appears to be closely associated with the magnitude and characteristics of the alveolitis, we do not rely on roentgenographic and pulmonary function tests alone to make prognostic and therapeutic decisions in this disease (71).

Gallium Scanning to Assess Activity

Dr. Bruce R. Line (Senior Investigator, Department of Nuclear Medicine, Clinical Center and Laboratory of Applied Studies, Division of Computer Research and Technology): Gallium-67 (^{67}Ga) is a cyclotron-produced radionuclide with a half-life of 78 hours. This isotope was first used clinically to detect neoplastic disease (230-235). Soon thereafter, it was recognized that ^{67}Ga would also concentrate in sites of acute and chronic inflammation (231, 232, 235, 236). This property of ^{67}Ga is now widely used in the scintigraphic assessment of occult inflammation (237-245). It is thus natural to consider ^{67}Ga scanning as a noninvasive means of assessing the intensity of the alveolitis of sarcoidosis.

Gallium-67 scans are technically simple to do, cause no patient discomfort, and are associated with low radiation exposures (246, 247). The localization of ^{67}Ga in the region from the head to the pelvis is assessed from anterior and posterior rectilinear scans obtained 48 to 72 hours after intravenous administration of ^{67}Ga citrate (35 to 50 μCi/kg). Normal lung tissue does not exceed the uptake of the nonspecific body background. Tissues that show significant physiologic uptake include the skeleton (spine, sternum, pelvis), the liver, and the spleen (Figure 7A) (248). To estimate the quality of ^{67}Ga taken up by lung alveolar tissues and minimize the effects of body structure and interpretive subjectivity, a semiquantitative "^{67}Ga-index" was devised (Figure 7) (249).

Abnormal gallium uptake in the lung is found in various pulmonary disorders with different pathogenesis and by itself is not diagnostic for any particular disease. Most categories of active interstitial lung disease have been associated with positive gallium scans (8). In some of these disorders, such as untreated idiopathic pulmonary fibrosis (249) and sarcoidosis (236, 242, 250, 251), positive gallium scans are the rule. In others, such as histiocytosis-X (Line BR, Fulmer JD, Crystal RG. Unpublished observations), pulmonary uptake of ^{67}Ga is only occasionally observed. The reason for this wide range in sensitivity of the gallium scan is not clear but is probably associated with the type, intensity, and duration of the alveolitis of each disease.

GALLIUM SCANNING IN PULMONARY SARCOIDOSIS

A spectrum of ^{67}Ga uptake patterns can be found in the lungs of patients with sarcoidosis (Figure 7B to D). Diffuse mid- and lower lung zone parenchymal uptake are frequent, but focal or patchy localizations may be

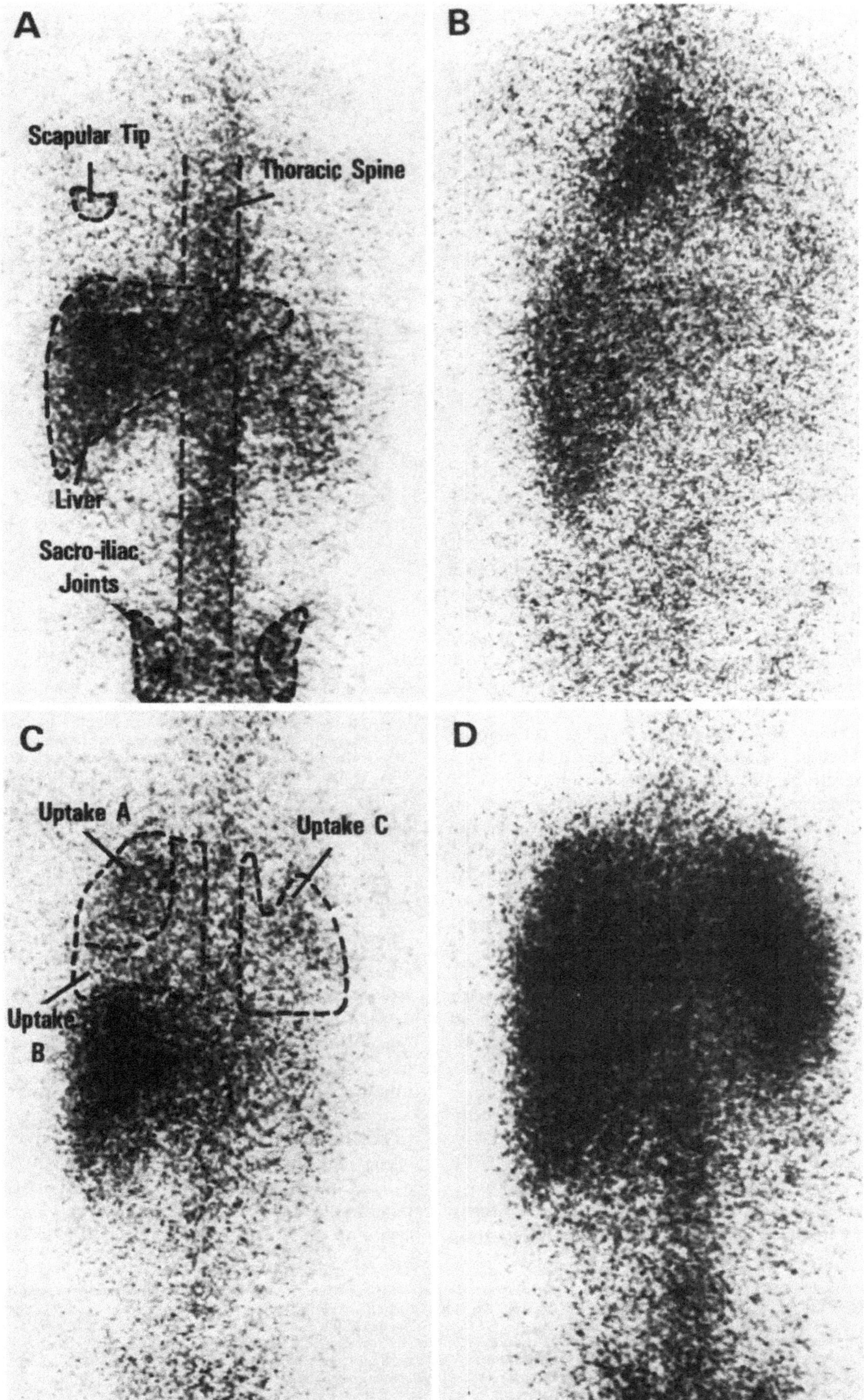

Figure 7. For Legend, see facing page.

present in any lung zone.

Although ^{67}Ga uptake is seen in other thoracic structures other than the lung parenchyma (such as hilar and paratracheal nodes), such uptake is not indicative of alveolitis and therefore not included in the computation of the parenchymal gallium uptake (249).

SIGNIFICANCE OF POSITIVE GALLIUM SCANS

The uptake of gallium in the lungs of patients with sarcoidosis is not associated with age, sex, smoking history, or duration of symptoms. In addition, there is no relation between the level of ^{67}Ga uptake and the functional status of the lung as assessed by lung volumes, by diffusing capacity, or by arterial blood gases at rest or with exercise.

To evaluate the usefulness of ^{67}Ga scans as an indicator of the alveolitis of sarcoidosis, we correlated ^{67}Ga-index estimates of pulmonary ^{67}Ga uptake with assessments of parenchymal inflammation by bronchoalveolar lavage. In the studies to date, there is a significant association of gallium uptake and the proportion of lung effector cells that are lymphocytes but an even stronger association of gallium uptake with the proportion of effector cells that were T-lymphocytes (unpublished observations). Because T-lymphocytes are important in the alveolitis of sarcoidosis, this evidence suggests that gallium uptake reflects the intensity of the T-lymphocyte component of the alveolitis. Consistent with the concept that T-lymphocytes may be responsible for ^{67}Ga uptake in sarcoidosis, Mertz and associates (252) showed in vitro that ^{67}Ga binds to the plasma membrane of lymphocytes. Further, the uptake was doubled when the lymphocytes were activated with phytohemagglutinin.

Further evidence for the usefulness of ^{67}Ga scans in assessing the alveolitis of sarcoidosis comes from the studies in Niden and associates (253) who showed good agreement between ^{67}Ga uptake and the presence of active inflammation in lung tissue obtained by biopsy. In addition, several studies have shown that parenchymal ^{67}Ga uptake is reduced when there is clinical remission of the disease (242, 250-252).

The spectrum of ^{67}Ga index in untreated patients with sarcoidosis (Figure 8) shows uptake scored from 10 to 340 units with indexes in more than two/thirds of patients above the normal limit of 50 units. Scans of untreated patients with sarcoid, compared to untreated patients with idiopathic pulmonary fibrosis, are generally more intense (Figure 8).

EXTRATHORACIC GALLIUM SCANNING

Although most interest in ^{67}Ga scanning in sarcoidosis has centered on the ^{67}Ga uptake by thoracic structures,

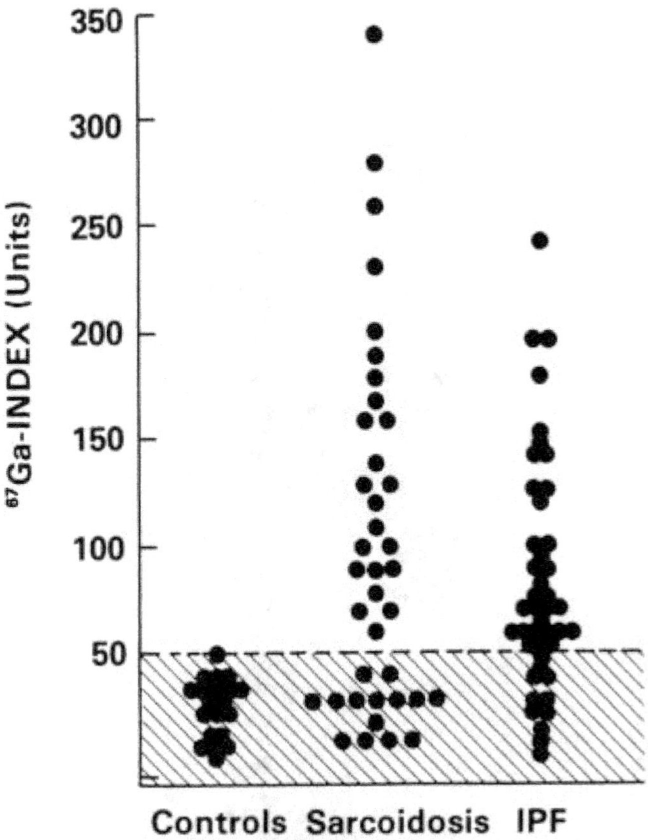

Figure 8. Distribution of ^{67}Ga index in control patients and in untreated patients with sarcoidosis and idiopathic pulmonary fibrosis (*IPF*). All control scans show ^{67}Ga index values below 50 ^{67}Ga index units. Sixty-three percent of the untreated patients with sarcoidosis show ^{67}Ga index values greater than 50 index units. In contrast, 74% of the untreated patients with idiopathic pulmonary fibrosis have ^{67}Ga index values greater than 50 index units (249). As a group, untreated patients with sarcoidosis show greater gallium lung uptake than do untreated patients with idiopathic pulmonary fibrosis. Shaded area represents normal range.

gallium often localizes in extrathoracic tissues in this disease (Figures 9 and 10). As in the lung, ^{67}Ga uptake in extrathoracic structures is probably associated with increased proportions of T-lymphocytes. For example, the left iliac crest localization in the patient shown in Figure 10 was associated with larger than normal numbers of T-lymphocytes in the bone marrow of that region. In comparison, the iliac crest on the right did not take up gallium and has normal proportions of T-lymphocytes (28).

In summary, although not diagnostically specific, the ^{67}Ga scan can be used to repetitively characterize the severity and anatomic location of regions of alveolitis and can provide a longitudinal assessment of the degree of inflammation in the whole parenchyma. Gallium-67 scanning is available, noninvasive, and involves low radi-

Figure 7. Examples of ^{67}Ga index computation in a normal person and in three patients with pulmonary sarcoidosis; the method used to quantitate the ^{67}Ga index is as outlined in reference 249. **A.** Normal scan in a 36-year-old man showing physiologic ^{67}Ga uptake in skeletal tissues (scapular tips, spine, pelvis, sacroiliac joints), liver, and spleen. Localization in the pulmonary parenchyma is similar to background (estimated from uptake in abdominal region below kidneys). Gallium-67 index = 10 index units. **B.** Scan of 45-year-old woman with pulmonary sarcoidosis showing right paratracheal and bilateral hilar nodal uptake and mild lower lung zone ^{67}Ga uptake (intensity = 1, area = 30%, equivalent to a ^{67}Ga index of 30 units. **C.** Scan of a 42-year-old man with pulmonary sarcoidosis. Three regions show uptake greater than the background area. Region A (intensity = 2, area = 20%, index = 40 units), region B (intensity = 1 area = 20%, index = 20 units), and region C (intensity = 1, area = 30%, index = 30 units) are summed to give a total ^{67}Ga index of 90 units. **D.** Diffuse high intensity ^{67}Ga uptake in a 36-year-old man with pulmonary sarcoidosis. The ^{67}Ga index is equivalent to 340 units.

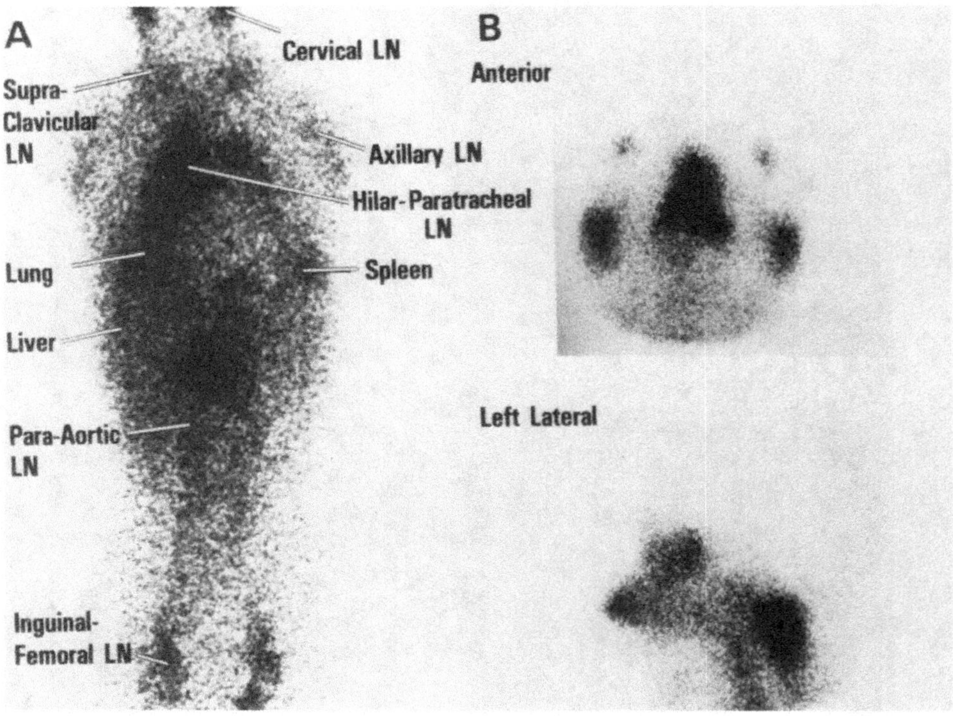

Figure 9. Extrathoracic ^{67}Ga localization in sarcoidosis. **A.** Sarcoidosis in 32-year-old woman. Gallium localization is noted in cervical, supraclavicular, axillary, mediastinal, para-aortic, inguinal, and femoral lymph nodes (*LN*) and in pulmonary parenchyma at base of right lung. **B.** Nasopharyngeal and parotid gland uptake of ^{67}Ga in 24-year-old man with sarcoidosis. There was clinical evidence of sarcoidosis of the nasopharynx but not of the parotids.

ation exposures. It should prove useful in staging patients with sarcoidosis and in following their response to therapy.

Treatment of Pulmonary Sarcoidosis

Dr. Ronald G. Crystal: Although the cause of pulmonary sarcoidosis is unknown, the disease clearly is characterized and perpetuated by activated T-lymphocytes within the alveolar structures. This is probably only part of the picture. For example, an important effector role will probably be found for mononuclear phagocytes in the lung other than simply as building blocks for granuloma formation. However, the knowledge that activated lung T-lymphocytes play a central role in the pathogenesis of this disease permits a rational assessment of therapeutic strategies.

CORTICOSTEROID THERAPY

Corticosteroids are the principal therapy against sarcoidosis. During the past 25 years, the following concepts have emerged (1, 3, 5, 7, 13, 15, 16, 35, 215, 254-261): [1] Corticosteroids generally improve symptoms, may or may not improve roentgenographic abnormalities, and variably improve lung function. [2] To be effective, corticosteroids must be given early and for at least 3 to 6 months. When they are withdrawn, relapses are frequent. Although long-term corticosteroid therapy seems to benefit most patients, the conditions of a small proportion will still deteriorate. [3] If low doses are used for maintenance therapy (for example, prednisone $\leq$ 0.25 mg/kg of body weight a day), complications are infrequent and mild.

Most of these observations are consistent with the concept that corticosteroids suppress the alveolitis of sarcoidosis but have little direct influence on the anatomic derangements of the alveolar structures that occurred before the institution of therapy. In humans, corticosteroids impair T-lymphocyte proliferation (262-264) and T-cell effector functions (265-266). They may affect the distribution of immune effector cells, including the proportioning of T-lymphocytes between blood and various organs (267, 268). These agents also have a profound effect on the capacity of mononuclear phagocytes to respond to mediators produced by T-lymphocytes (269). Thus it is reasonable to hypothesize that when corticosteroids are given in appropriate doses to patients with pulmonary sarcoidosis, they should prevent T-lymphocyte-mediated recruitment of blood monocytes to the lung and thus inhibit granuloma formation. Also, because granulomas are dynamic structures (85, 88), the reduction in recruitment of blood monocytes probably will cause a reduction in the number and size of existing granulomas.

Because both the alveolitis and granulomas impair lung function, therapy with corticosteroids should improve lung function by reducing the intensity of the alveolitis and reducing the lung burden of granuloma. In addition, by suppressing the alveolitis, corticosteroids prevent future derangements of the alveolar structures. However, there is no evidence that corticosteroids can improve interstitial fibrosis or alterations in lung parenchymal cells once present, that is, a deranged alveolus cannot be rebuilt and is lost forever as a gas-exchanging unit (270, 271).

Generally, studies evaluating the efficacy of corticosteriods in pulmonary sarcoidosis have relied on one or more of the following criteria as evidence for a beneficial therapeutic effect: a reduction in symptoms related to the lungs, particularly dyspnea; improvement in the chest roentgenogram; and improvement in functional tests such as lung volumes, diffusing capacity, and arterial

Figure 10 Left. Extrathoracic uptake in left posterior iliac crest of a 63-year-old man. There is also diffuse parenchymal ^{67}Ga uptake with right apical prominence and mediastinal-bilateral hilar node involvement. Right. Biopsy of left posterior iliac crest of the patient in left-hand panel showing noncaseating granulomas consistent with sarcoidosis.

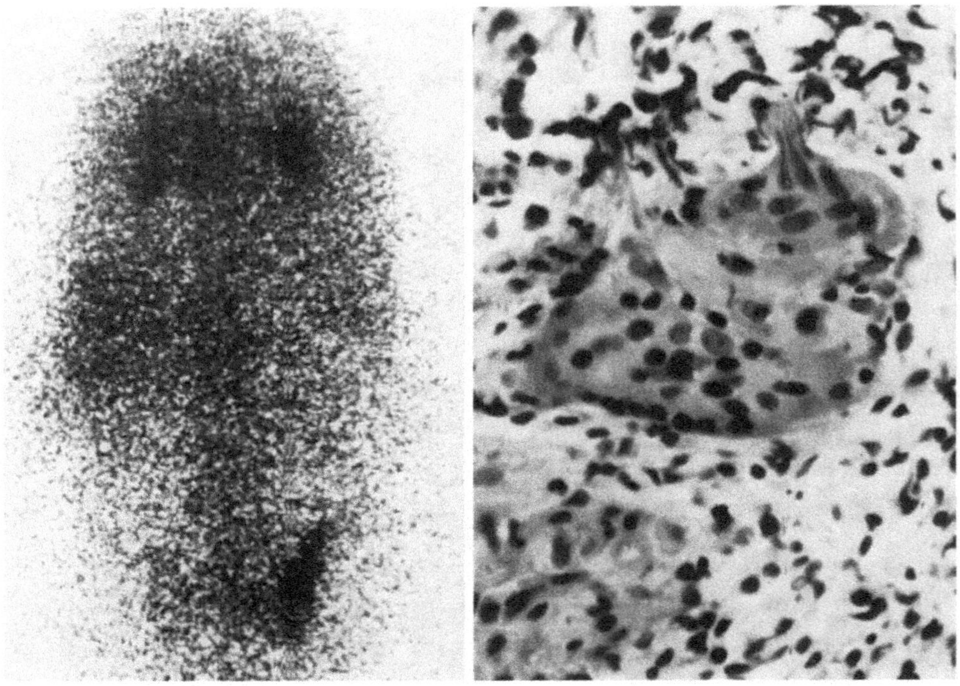

blood gases at rest and during exercise. However, in view of our previous discussions, the difficulty assessing the efficacy of corticosteroids using these variables is understandable. Corticosteroids act on the alveolitis, not the derangements of the alveolar structures, yet there have been no studies comparing pulmonary symptoms to the intensity of the alveolitis or the anatomic derangements of the alveolar structures; the chest roentgenogram cannot clearly distinguish between alveolitis and anatomic derangement and is relatively insensitive to the presence of alveolitis; and because functional tests probably detect alveolitis as well as granulomas, fibrosis, and other derangements of the alveolar structures, they cannot be used to follow change in the alveolitis. Thus, even if corticosteroids were to effectively reduce the proportion of T-lymphocytes within the lung of a person with sarcoidosis, this beneficial effect may not be detected by the conventional monitors of the disease process. Because both alveolitis and anatomic derangements seem to influence radiographic and functional tests, an improvement in the alveolitis may be masked by a stabilized, but abnormal, anatomic arrangement of the alveolar structures.

THERAPY OF SARCOIDOSIS: OTHER AGENTS

Besides corticosteroids, chloroquine (272), D-penacillamine (273), spironolactone (274), allopurinol (275), levamisole (276), heparin (277), and phenylbutazone (278) have also been used in the therapy of sarcoidosis. Except for chloroquine, none have been evaluated by controlled trials, and the results with chloroquine are equivocal (272). In view of the current concepts of the disease, there is little theoretical basis for the use of any of these agents. Cytotoxic agents such as chlorambucil (279), azathioprine (280), and methotrexate (279) have also been used, but only in a few patients. No controls were used, the patients were mostly those with advanced disease, and the effect of these drugs on the alveolitis was not evaluated. Thus, although such drugs might suppress lung T-lymphocytes, at this time they cannot be considered as tested therapies for this disease.

FUTURE APPROACHES

The observations that T-lymphocytes play an important role in the pathogenesis of pulmonary sarcoidosis and that the alveolitis of this disease precedes anatomic derangements in the alveolar structures suggest that monitors of lung T-lymphocyte number may provide a convenient and logical guide to therapy decisions and the assessment of new treatment protocols.

ACKNOWLEDGMENTS: The authors thank Drs. Gordon Head and Andrew Dwyer of the Radiology Department, Clinical Center, National Institutes of Health, for assistance in classifying the chest radiographs; Charlotte Kenton of the National Library of Medicine for invaluable help in searching the extensive sarcoidosis literature; and Mrs. Lou West and Mrs. Ellen Wright for excellent editorial assistance.

▶ Requests for reprints should be addressed to Ronald G. Crystal, M.D.; Building 10, Room 6D06, National Institutes of Health; Bethesda, MD 20205.

References

1. Scadding JG. *Sarcoidosis.* London: Eyre and Spottiswoode Ltd.; 1967.
2. Spencer H. *Pathology of the Lung.* New York: Pergammon Press; 1977.
3. Crofton J, Douglas A. *Respiratory Disease.* Oxford: Blackwell Scientific Publications; 1975.
4. Fraser RG, Pare JAP. *Diagnosis of Diseases of the Chest.* Philadelphia: W. B. Saunders Co.; 1979.
5. Mitchell DN, Scadding JG. Sarcoidosis. *Am Rev Respir Dis.* 1974;**110**:774-802.
6. Mitchell DN, Scadding JG, Heard BE, et al. Sarcoidosis: histopathological definition and clinical diagnosis. *J Clin Pathol.* 1977;**30**:395-408.
7. Israel H. Sarcoidosis. In: Simmons DH, ed. *Current Pulmonology.* Vol. 1. Boston: Houghton Mifflin; 1979:163-82.
8. Fulmer JD, Crystal RG. Interstitial lung disease. In: Simmons DH, ed. *Current Pulmonology.* Vol. 1. Boston: Houghton Mifflin; 1979:1-65.
9. Kent DC, Houk VN, Elliott RC, Sokolowski JW Jr, Baker JH,

Sorensen K. The definitive evaluation of sarcoidosis. *Am Rev Respir Dis.* 1970;**101**:721-7.

10. Koerner SK, Sakowitz AJ, Appelman RI, Becker NH, Schoenbaum SW. Transbronchial lung biopsy for the diagnosis of sarcoidosis. *N Engl J Med.* 1975;**293**:268-70.
11. Lieberman J, Nosal A, Schlessner L, Sastre-Foken A. Serum angiotensin-converting enzyme for diagnosis and therapeutic evaluation of sarcoidosis. *Am Rev Respir Dis.* 1979;**120**:329-35.
12. Siltzbach LE, James DG, Neville E, et al. Course and prognosis of sarcoidosis around the world. *Am J Med.* 1974;**57**:847-52.
13. James DG, Neville E, Siltzbach LE, et al. A worldwide survey of sarcoid. In: Siltzbach LE, ed. Seventh International Conference on Sarcoidosis. *Ann NY Acad Sci.* 1976;**278**:321-34.
14. Mayock RL, Bertrand P, Morrison CE, Scott JH. Manifestations of sarcoidosis: analysis of 145 patients with a review of 9 series selected from the literature. *Am J Med.* 1963;**35**:67-89.
15. Israel HL. Prognosis of sarcoidosis. *Ann Intern Med.* 1970;**73**:1038-9.
16. Sones M, Israel HL. Course and prognosis of sarcoidosis. *Am J Med.* 1960;**28**:84-93.
17. Bacharach T. Sarcoidosis: a clinical review of 111 cases. *Am Rev Respir Dis.* 1961;**84**:12-6.
18. Longcope WT, Freiman DG. A study of sarcoidosis. *Medicine (Baltimore).* 1952;**31**:1-132.
19. Geraint-James D. Immunology of sarcoidosis. *Lancet.* 1966;**2**:633-4.
20. Sones M, Israel HC. Altered immunologic reactions in sarcoidosis.
21. Hirschorn K, Schreibman RR, Bach FH et al. *In vitro* studies of lymphocytes from patients with sarcoidosis and lymphoproliferative diseases. *Lancet.* 1964;**2**:842-3.
22. Sharma OP, James DG, Fox RA. A correlation of *in vitro* delayed type hypersensitivity and *in vitro* lymphocyte transformation in sarcoidosis. *Chest.* 1971;**60**:35-7.
23. Kataria YP, Sagone AL, LoBuglio AF, et al. *In vitro* observations on sarcoid lymphocytes and their correlation with cutaneous anergy and clinical severity of disease. *Am Rev Respir Dis.* 1973;**108**:767-76.
24. Hedfors E, Holm G, Petterson E. Lymphocyte subpopulations in sarcoidosis. *Clin Exp Immunol.* 1974;**17**:219-26.
25. Daniele RP, Rowlands DT Jr. Lymphocyte subpopulations in sarcoidosis: correlation with disease activity and duration. *Ann Intern Med.* 1976;**85**:593-600.
26. Ramachandar K, Douglas SD, Siltzbach LE, et al. Peripheral blood lymphocyte subpopulations in sarcoidosis. *Cell Immunol.* 1975;**16**:422-6.
27. Sorensen SF, Hardt F, Veien NF. Estimation of lymphocyte subpopulations in peripheral blood of patients with sarcoidosis. *Scand J Immunol.* 1976;**5**:117-22.
28. Hunninghake GW, Fulmer JD, Young RC Jr, Gadek JE, Crystal RG. Localization of the immune response in sarcoidosis. *Am Rev Respir Dis.* 1979;**120**:49-57.
29. Hunninghake G, Kelman J, Weinberger S, Young R, Fulmer J, Crystal RG. Lung lymphocyte subpopulations in sarcoidosis. *Clin Res.* 1978;**26**:448A. Abstract.
30. Hunninghake GW, Kelman JA, Gadek JE, Elson NA, Fulmer JD, Crystal RG. Comparison of inflammatory and immune effector cell populations in lavage fluid and lung biopsies of patients with pulmonary fibrosis. *Am Rev Respir Dis.* 1978;**177** (suppl): 68. Abstract.
31. Hunninghake G, Gadek J, Weinberger S, et al. Comparison of the alveolitis of sarcoidosis and idiopathic pulmonary fibrosis. *Chest.* 1979;**75S**:266S-67S.
32. Hunninghake GW, Fulmer JD, Young RC, Crystal RG. Comparison of lung and blood lymphocyte subpopulations in pulmonary sarcoidosis. In: Williams, WJ, Davies, BH, eds. *Proceedings of the 8th International Conference on Sarcoidosis and Other Granulomatous Disease.* London: Alpha Omega Publishing, Ltd.; 1980:426-35.
33. Hunninghake GW, Gadek JE, Kawanami O, Ferrans VJ, Crystal RG. Inflammatory and immune processes in the human lung in health and disease: evaluation by bronchoalveolar lavage. *Am J Pathol.* 1979;**97**:149-206.
34. Hunninghake GW, Gadek JE, Young RC Jr, Kawanami O, Ferrans VJ, Crystal RG. Mechanisms of granuloma formation in pulmonary sarcoidosis by T-lymphocytes within the lung. *N Engl J Med.* 1980;**302**:594-8.
35. Siltzbach LE. Sarcoidosis. In: Fishman AP, ed. *Pulmonary Diseases and Disorders.* New York: McGraw-Hill; 1980:899-908.
36. Carrington CB, Gaensler EA, Milsus JP, et al. Structure and function in sarcoidosis. *Ann NY Acad Sci.* 1976;**278**:265-82.
37. Soler P, Basset F. Morphology and distribution of the cells of a sarcoid granuloma: ultrastructural study of serial sections. *Ann NY Acad Sci.* 1976;**278**:147-60.
38. Soler P, Bernaudin JF, Basset F, Basset G. Epithelioid cell and sarcoid-like granuloma: a review of human and experimental material. *Mt Sinai J Med.* 1977;**44**:767-71.
39. Van Furth R. Origin and kinetics of monocytes and macrophages. *Semin Hematol.* 1970;**7**:125-41.
40. James EM, Williams WJ. Fine structure and histochemistry of epithelioid cells in sarcoidosis. *Thorax.* 1974;**29**:115-20.
41. Wanstrup J, Christensen HE. Sarcoidosis: I. Ultrastructural investigations on epithelioid cell granulomas. *Acta Pathol Microbiol Scand.* 1966;**66**:169-85.
42. Jones-Williams W, Erazmus DA, Valerie-James EM, Davies T. The fine structure of sarcoid and tuberculous granulomas. *Postgrad Med J.* 1970;**46**:496-500.
43. Fuse Y, Hiragi Y. The fine structures of sarcoidal and Kveim granulomas. In: Iwai K, Hasodo Y, eds. *Proceedings of the VI International Conference on Sarcoidosis.* Baltimore: University Park Press; 1974;269-75.
44. Fukushiro R, Hirone T, Eryn Y. Ultrastructural and cytochemical observations on sarcoid granulomas. In: Levinsky L, Macholda F, eds. *Fifth International Conference on Sarcoidosis.* Prague: Universita Karlova; 1971:276-9.
45. Carr I, Norris P. The fine structure of human machrophage granules in sarcoidosis. *J Pathol.* 1977;**122**:29-32.
46. Biberfield P. Morphogenesis in blood lymphocytes stimulated with phytohaemagglutinin (PITA): a light and electron microscopic study. *Acta Pathol Microbiol Scand [A].* **223** (suppl):1-70.
47. Teilum G. Allergic hyperglobulinosis and hyalinosis (paraamyloidosis) in the reticulo-endothelial system in Boecks sarcoid and other conditions: a morphologic immunity reaction. *Am J Pathol.* 1948;**24**:389-407.
48. Kalifat SR, Bouteille M, Belarue J. Changes in connective tissue in sarcoid granuloma: hyalin, paraamyloid and fibrinoid: electron microscopic study of 11 cases. *Virchows Arch Abt B Zellpath.* 1969;**3**:348-58.
49. Weinberger SE, Crystal RG. Reactions of the interstitial space to injury. In: Fishman AP, ed. *Pulmonary Diseases and Disorders.* New York: McGraw-Hill; 1980;640-7.
50. Divertie MB, Cassan SM, Brown AL. Ultrastructural morphometry of blood-air barrier in pulmonary sarcoidosis. *Chest.* 1976;**69**:154-7.
51. Pinner M. Noncaseating tuberculosis. *Am Rev Tuberc.* 1938;**37**:690-728.
52. Rosen Y, Athanassiades TJ, Moon S, et al. Nongranulomatous interstitial pneumonitis in sarcoidosis: relationship to the development of epithelioid granulomas. *Chest.* 1978;**74**:122-5.
53. Takahashi M. Histopathology of sarcoidosis and its immunological basis. *Acta Pathol Jpn.* 1970;**20**:171-82.
54. Teilum G. Morphogenesis and development of sarcoid lesions: similarities to the group of collagenosis. *Acta Med Scand.* 1964;**425** (suppl):14-8.
55. Judd PA, Finnegan P, Curran RC. Pulmonary sarcoidosis: a clinicopathologic study. *J Pathol.* 1975;**115**:191-8.
56. Cain H, Kraus B. Asteroid bodies: derivatives of the cytosphere. *Virchows Arch [Cell Pathol].* 1977;**26**:119-32.
57. Obel AL, Löfgren S. Pathogenesis of hyaline formation in sarcoidosis lymph nodes. *Acta Med Scand.* 1964;**425**(suppl):27-30.
58. DiBenedetto RJ, Ribaudo C. Bronchopulmonary sarcoidosis. *Am Rev Respir Dis.* 1966;**94**:952-5.
59. Scadding JG. The late stages of pulmonary sarcoidosis. *Postgrad Med J.* 1970;**46**:530-6.
60. Boros OL. Granulomatous inflammations. *Prog Allergy.* 1978;**24**:183-267.
61. Reynolds HY, Newball HH. Analysis of proteins and respiratory cells obtained from human lungs by bronchial lavage. *J Lab Clin Med.* 1974;**84**:559-73.
62. Reynolds HY, Fulmer JD Kazmierowski JA, Roberts WC, Frank MM, Crystal RG. Analysis of bronchoalveolar lavage fluid from patients with idiopathic pulmonary fibrosis and chronic hypersensitivity pneumonitis. *J Clin Invest.* 1977;**59**:165-75.
63. Weinberger SE, Kelman JA, Elson NA, et al. Bronchoalveolar lavage in interstitial lung disease. *Ann Intern Med.* 1978;**89**:459-66.
64. Hunninghake GW, Gadek JE, Szapiel SV, et al. The human alveolar macrophage. In: Harris CC, Trump BF, Stoner GD, eds. *Cultured Human Cells and Tissues in Bio-Medical Research.* New York: Academic Press; 1980. *(Methods and Perspectives in Cell Biology,* Vol. 1).
65. Hunninghake GW, Kawanami O, Ferrans VI, et al. Characterization of the inflammatory and immune effector cells in lung parenchyma of patients with interstitial lung disease. *Am Rev Respir Dis.* In press.
66. Yeager J, Williams MC, Beekman JF, Bayly TC, Beaman BL, Hawley RJ. Sarcoidosis: analysis of cells obtained by bronchial lavage. *Am Rev Respir Dis.* 1977;**116**:951-5.
67. Reynolds HY. The importance of lymphocytes in pulmonary health and disease. *Lung.* 1978;**155**:225-42.
68. Gee JB, Godel PT, Zorn SK, et al. Sarcoidosis and mononuclear

phagocytes. *Lung.* 1978;**155:**243-53.

69. DANEL C, ARNOUX A, MARSAC J, et al. Cellular data from bronchoalveolar lavages in various interstitial diseases. *Bull Europ Physiopath Respir.* 1979;**15:**42P-43P.
70. ROSSMAN MD, DANIELE RP, DAUBER JH. Bronchoalveolar lymphocytes in sarcoidosis. *Am Rev Respir Dis.* 1979;**119:**795.
71. KEOGH B, HUNNINGHAKE G, LINE B, et al. Therapeutic decisions in sarcoidosis: prospective evaluation of the effect of corticosteroids on lavage lymphocytes and [67] gallium scans. *Clin Res.* 1979;**27:**400A. Abstract.
72. CLOT J, ANDARY M, BONSEQUET J, GODART P, MICHEL FB. Lous populations lymphocytaires des iquides de lavage bronchoalveolaire. *Bull Europ Physiopath Respir.* 1979;**15:**27P-28P.
73. BARRY BE, CRAPO JD, GEHR P, BACHOFEN M, WEIBEL ER. Population characteristics of the cells in normal human lung. *Am Rev Respir Dis.* 1979;**119:**287A. Abstract.
74. WYBRAN JM, CARR C, FUDENBERT HH. The human-rosette forming cell as a marker of a population of thymus-derived cells. *J Clin Invest.* 1972;**51:**2537-43.
75. KATOH AK, CHAROENSIRI S. The formation of stable E-rosettes by human T-lymphocytes activated by phytohemagglutinin. *J Immunol.* 1977;**118:**2291-2.
76. FERRANRINI M, MORRETTA L, ABILE R, DURANTE ML. Receptors for IgG molecules on human lymphocytes forming spontaneous rosettes with sheep red cells. *Eur J Immunol.* 1975;**5:**70-2.
77. KRAMMER PH, HUDSON C, SPRENT J. Fc receptor, Ia-antigens, and immuno-globulin on normal and activated mouse T-lymphocytes. *J Exp Med.* 1975;**142:**1403-14.
78. FRIDMAN WH, FRADELIZI D, GUIMEZANES A, PLATES C, LECLERC JC. The role of the Fc receptor (FcR) on thymus-derived lymphocytes. II. Presence of FcR on suppressor cells and direct involvement in suppression. *Eur J Immunol.* 1977;**8:**549-54.
79. ROSSMAN MD, DAUBER JH, DANIELE RP. Elevation of stable (37°) E-rosettes in sarcoidosis. *Am Rev Respir Dis.* (suppl:73)1977:111.
80. KATZ P, HAYNES BF, FAUCI AS. Alteration of T-lymphocyte subpopulations in sarcoidosis. *Clin Immunol Immunopathol.* 1978;**10:**350-4.
81. HOCKING WG, GOLDE DW. The pulmonary-alveolar macrophage. *N Engl J Med.* 1979;**301:**580-7.
82. BLUSSE VAN OUD ALBLAS A, VAN FURTH R. Origin, kinetics, and characteristics of pulmonary macrophages in the normal steady state. *J Exp Med.* 1979;**149:**1504-18.
83. CARR I. *The Macrophage.* London: Academic Press, Inc.; 1973:80-5.
84. ADAMS DO. The structure of mononuclear phagocytes differentiating *in vivo. Am J Pathol.* 1974;**76:**17-39.
85. SPECTOR WG. The dynamics of granulomas and the significance of epithelioid cells. *Pathologie-Biologie.* 1975;**6:**437-9.
86. BLACK MM, EPSTEIN WL. Formation of multinucleate giant cells in organized epithelioid cell granulomas. *Am J Pathol.* 1974;**74:**262-74.
87. SUTTON JS, WEISS L. Transformation of monocytes in tissue culture into macrophages, epithelioid cells, and multinucleated giant cells: an electron microscope study. *J Cell Biol.* 1966;**28:**303-32.
88. MARIANO M, SPECTOR WG. The formation and properties of macrophage polykaryous (inflammatory giant cells). *J Pathol.* 1974;**113:**1-19.
89. JOHNSTON RB JR, GODZIK CA, COHN ZA. Increased superoxide anion production by immunologically activated and chemically elicited macrophages. *J Exp Med.* 1978;**148:**115-27.
90. DRATH DB, KARNOVSKY ML, HUBER GL. Hydroxyl radical formation in phagocytic cells of the rat. *Am J Physiol.* 1979;**46:**136-40.
91. WERB Z, GORDON S. Secretion of a specific collagenase by stimulated macrophages. *J Exp Med.* 1975;**142:**346-60.
92. HOROWITZ AL, KELMAN JA, CRYSTAL RG. Activation of alveolar macrophage collagenase by a neutral protease secreted by the same cell. *Nature.* 1976;**264:**772-4.
93. JANOFF A, ROSENBERG R, GLADSTON M. Elastase-like esteroprotease activity in human and rabbit alveolar macrophage granules. *Proc Soc Exp Biol Med.* 1971;**136:**1054-8.
94. POLVERINI PF, COTRAN RS, GIMBROME MA, UNANUE ER. Activated macrophages induce vascular proliferation. *Nature.* 1977;**269:**804-6.
95. ROSENTHAL AS, LIPSKY PE, SHEVACH EM. Macrophage-lymphocyte interaction and antigen recognition. *Fed Proc.* 1975;**34:**1743-8.
96. UNANUE ER. Secretory function of mononuclear phagocytes. *Am J Pathol.* 1976;**83:**396-417.
97. EVANS R, ALEXANDER P. Mechanisms of extracellular killing of nucleated mammalian cells by macrophages. In: NELSON DS, ed. *Immunobiology of the Macrophage.* New York: Academic Press; 1976:535-76.
98. WARD PA, UNANUE ER, GORALNICK SJ, SCHREINER GF. Chemotaxis of rat lymphocytes. *J Immunol.* 1977;**119:**416-421.
99. GOLDE DW, BYERS LD, FINLEY TN. Proliferative capacity of the human alveolar macrophage. *Nature.* 1974;**247:**373-5.
100. ADAMSON IYR, BOWDEN DH. Role of monocytes and interstitial cells in the generation of alveolar macrophages. *Fed Proc.* 1979;**38:**1205.
101. BOYDEN S. The chemotactic effect of mixtures of antibody and antigen on polymorphonuclear leukocytes. *J Exp Med.* 1962;**115:**453-66.
102. KAZMIEROWSKI JA, GALLIN JI, REYNOLDS HY. Mechanisms for the inflammatory response in primate lungs: demonstration and partial characterization of an alveolar macrophage-derived chemotactic factor with preferential activity for polymorphonuclear leukocytes. *J Clin Invest.* 1977;**59:**273-81.
103. HUNNINGHAKE GW, GALLIN JI, FAUCI AS. Immunologic reactivity of the lung. The *in vivo* and *in vitro* generation of a neutrophil chemotactic factor by alveolar macrophages. *Am Rev Respir Dis.* 1978;**117:**15-23.
104. HUNNINGHAKE GW, GADEK JE, CRYSTAL RG. Human alveolar macrophage chemotactic factor for neutrophils: stimuli and partial characterization. *J Clin Invest.* In press.
105. MERRILL WW, NAEGEL GP, MATTHAY RA, REYNOLDS HY. Alveolar macrophage-derived chemotactic factor: kinetics of *in vitro* production and partial characterization. *J Clin Invest.* 1980;**65:**268-76.
106. GADEK JE, HUNNINGHAKE GW, ZIMMERMAN RL, CRYSTAL RG. Regulation of release of the alveolar macrophage-derived chemotactic factor. *Am Rev Respir Dis.* 1980;**121:**823-33.
107. GALLIN JI, QUIE PG. *Leukocyte Chemotaxis: Methods, Physiology, and Clinical Implications.* New York: Raven Press; 1978:1-429.
108. WARD PA, REMOLD HG, DAVID JR. Leukotactic factor produced by sensitized lymphocytes. *Science.* 1969;**163:**1079-81.
109. SNYDERMAN R, ALTMAN LC, HAUSMAN MS, et al. Human mononuclear leukocyte chemotaxis: a quantitative assay for humoral and cellular chemotactic factors. *J Immunol.* 1972;**108:**857-60.
110. ALTMAN LC, SNYDERMAN R, OPPENHEIM JJ, et al. A human mononuclear leukocyte chemotactic factor: characterization, specificity and kinetics of production by homologous leukocytes. *J Immunol.* 1973;**110:**801-10.
111. KAY AB, STECHSCHULTE DJ, AUSTEN KF. An eosinophilic leukocyte chemotactic factor of anaphylaxis. *J Exp Med.* 1971;**133:**602-19.
112. ZIGMOND SH, HIRSCH JG. Leukocyte locomotion and chemotaxis: new methods for evaluation and demonstration of cell-derived chemotactic factor. *J Exp Med.* 1973;**137:**387-410.
113. GOETZL EJ, WOODS JM, GORMAN RR. Stimulation of human eosinophil and neutrophil polymorphonuclear leukocyte chemotaxis and random migration by 12-L-hydroxy-5,8,10,14-eicosatetraenoic acid. *J Clin Invest.* 1977;**59:**179-83.
114. SOBEL JD, GALLIN JI. Polymorphonuclear leukocyte and monocyte chemoattractants produced by human fibroblasts. *J Clin Invest.* 1979;**63:**609-18.
115. KAPLAN AP, GOETZL EJ, AUSTEN KF. The fibrinolytic pathway of human plasma. II. The generation of chemotactic activity by activation of plasminogen proactivator. *J Clin Invest.* 1973;**52:**2591-5.
116. BERENBERG JL, WARD PA. Chemotactic factor inactivator in normal human serum. *J Clin Invest.* 1973;**52:**1200-6.
117. GOETZL EJ, ROCKLIN RE. Amplification of the activity of human leukocyte inhibitory factor (LIF) by the generatipn of a low molecular weight inhibitor of PMN leukocyte chemotaxis. *J Immuno.* 1978;**121:**891-6.
118. TILL G, WARD PA. Two distinct chemotactic factor inactivators in human serum. *J Immunol.* 1975;**114:**843-7.
119. ROCKLIN RE. Products of activated lymphocytes: leukocyte inhibitory factor (LIF) distinct from migration inhibitory factor (MIF). *J Immunol.* 1974;**112:**1461-6.
120. GOETZL EJ. Plasma and cell-derived inhibitors of human neutrophil chemotaxis. *Ann NY Acad Sci.* 1975;**256:**210-21.
121. WRIGHT DG, GALLIN JI. Modulation of the inflammatory response by products released from human polymorphonuclear leukocytes during phagocytosis: generation and inactivation of the chemotactic factor C5a. *Inflammation.* 1975;**1:**23-39.
122. CATES KL, RAY CA QUIE PG. Modified Boyden chamber method of measuring polymorphonuclear leukocyte chemotaxis. In: GALLIN JI, QUIE PG, eds. *Leukocyte Chemotaxis: Methods, Physiology, and Clinical Applications.* New York: Raven Press; 1978:67-72.
123. ALTMAN LC. Chemotactic lymphokines. In: GALLIN JI, QUIE PG, eds. *Leukocyte Chemotaxis: Methods, Physiology, and Clinical Implications.* New York: Raven Press; 1978:267-88.
124. GORDON LI, DOUGLAS SD, KAY NE, YAMADA O, OSSERMAN EF, JACOB HS. Modulation of neutrophil function by lysozyme: potential feedback system of inflammation. *J Clin Invest.* 1979;**64:**226-32.
125. DOUGLAS SE, DOUGHADAY CC, SCHMIDT ME, SILTZBACH LE. Kinetics of monocyte receptor activity for immunoproteins in patients with sarcoidosis. *Ann NY Acad Sci.* 1976;**278:**190-6.
126. DOUGLAS SE. Human monocyte spreading *in vitro*: inducers and effects on Fc and C3 receptors. *Cell Immunol.* 1976;**21:**344-9.
127. HIMAN LM, STEVENS CA, MATTHAY RA, REYNOLDS HY, GEE JBL. Lysozyme and angiotensin convertase activity in human alveolar macrophages: the effects of cigarette smoking and pulmonary sarcoidosis.

Am Rev Respir Dis. 1978;**117**(Part 2):67. Abstract.

128. Shima K, Tamiya J, Tsuda T, Tokuomi H. Lysosomal enzyme activation of monocytes in sarcoid patients and activation factor in their sera. In: *Proceedings of the 8th International Conference on Sarcoidosis;* Cardiff, Wales, UK. 1978:9.
129. Friedland J, Setton C, Silverstein E. Induction of angiotensin converting enzyme in human monocytes in culture. *Biochem Biophys Res Comm.* 1979;**83**:843-9.
130. Silverstein E, Friedland J, Lyons HA, et al. Markedly elevated angiotensin converting enzyme in lymph nodes containing non-necrotizing granulomas in sarcoidosis. *Proc Nat Acad Sci USA.* 1976;**73**:2137-41.
131. Silverstein E, Friedland J, Lyons HA, et al. Elevation of angiotensin-converting enzyme in granulomatous lymph nodes and serum in sarcoidosis: clinical and possible pathogenic significance. *Ann NY Acad Sci.* 1976;**278**:498-513.
132. David JR, Remold HG. Macrophage activation by lymphocyte mediators and studies on the interaction of macrophages and lymphocytes. In: Nelson DS, ed. *Immunobiology of the Macrophage.* New York: Academic Press, 1976;401-27.
133. Gordon LI, Doublas SE, Kay NE, Osserman EF, Jacob HD. Modulation of neutrophil function by lysozyme: a macrophage secretory product. In: Williams WJ, Davies BH, eds. *Proceedings of the 8th International Conference on Sarcoidosis and Other Granulomatous Disease.* London: Alpha Omega Publishing, Ltd; 1980:76-83.
134. Maderazo EG, Ward PA, Woronick CL, Kubik J, DeGraff AC Jr. Leukotactic dysfunction in sarcoidosis. *Ann Intern Med.* 1976;**84**:414-9.
135. Campbell PB. Defective monocyte leukotaxis in sarcoidosis: possible relationship to a plasma factor. *Am Rev Respir Dis.* 1977;**116**:251-9.
136. Yoshida T, Siltzback LE, Masih N, Cohen S. Serum-migration inhibitory activity in patients with sarcoidosis. *Clin Immunol Immunopathol.* 1979;**13**:39-46.
137. Shima K, Ikeda S, Horiuchi S, Tokuomo H. Lysosomal enzyme activity of monocytes and activation factors in the sera of sarcoidosis patients. In: Williams WJ, Davies BH, eds. *Proceedings of the 8th International Conference on Sarcoidosis and Other Granulomatous Disease,* London: Alpha Omega Publishing, Ltd; 1980:89-98.
138. Semenzato G, Ciorani A, Colombatti M, Amadori G, Gasparotto G. Inhibitors of T-cell immune function in sarcoidosis. In: Williams WJ, Davies BH, eds. *Proceedings of the 8th International Conference on Sarcoidosis and Other Granulomatous Disease.* London: Alpha Omega Publishing, Ltd.; 1980:466-71.
139. Davies BH, Jones KP, Evans P, Jones-Williams W. Thymic lymphocyte responses in sarcoidosis: effect of sera and levamisole. In: Williams WJ, Davies BH, eds. *Proceedings of the 8th International Conference on Sarcoidosis and Other Granulomatous Disease.* London: Alpha Omega Publishing, Ltd.; 1980:477-84.
140. Horsmanheimo A, Horsmanheimo M, Fudenberg HH, Siltzback LE, McKee KT. Kveins test reactivity with leukocyte migration in agarose and lymphocyte transformation tests. In: Williams WJ, Davies BH, eds. *Proceedings of the 8th International Conference on Sarcoidosis and Other Granulomatous Disease.* London: Alpha Omega Publishing, Ltd.; 1980:186-90.
141. Mangi RJ, Dwyer JM, Kantor FS. The effect of plasma upon lymphocyte responses *in vitro:* demonstration of a humoral inhibitor in patients with sarcoidosis. *Clin Exp Immunol.* 1974;**18**:519-28.
142. Drutz DJ, Cline MJ. Intermittent neutrophil-monocyte bactericidal defects in a patient with sarcoidosis. *Am Rev Respir Dis.* 1975;**112**:387-92.
143. Broom BC, Maclaurin BP. Sarcoidosis: correlation of delayed hypersensitivity, MLC reactivity and lymphocytotoxicity with disease activity. *Clin Exp Immunol.* 1973;**15**:355-64.
144. Friou GJ. Delayed cutaneous hypersensitivity in sarcoidosis. *J Clin Invest.* 1952;**31**:630.
145. Horsmanheimo M. Correlation of tuberculin-induced lymphocyte transformation with skin test reactivity and with clinical manifestations of sarcoidosis. *Cell Immunol.* 1974;**10**:329-37.
146. Kataria YP, LoBuglio AF, Bromberg PA. Sarcoid lymphocytes: spontaneous transformation and release of macrophage migration inhibition activity. *Am Rev Respir Dis.* 1976;**113**:315-23.
147. Selroos O, Niemisto M. Tuberculin sensitivity in active and cured sarcoidosis in Finland. In: Iwai K, Hosoda Y, eds. *Proceedings of the VI International Conference on Sarcoidosis,* Baltimore: University Park Press; 1974;248-52.
148. Sones M, Israel HL. Altered immunologic reactions in sarcoidosis. *Ann Intern Med.* 1954;**40**:260-8.
149. Veien NK, Hardt F, Bendixen G, et al. Immunological studies in sarcoidosis: a comparison of disease activity and various immunologic parameters. *Ann NY Acad Sci.* 1976;**278**:47-51.
150. Hoffbrand BI. Occurrence and significance of lymphopenia in sarcoidosis. *Am Rev Respir Dis.* 1968;**98**:107-10.
151. Sorensen SF, Hardt F, Veien NK. Estimation of lymphocyte subpopulations in the peripheral blood of patients with sarcoidosis. *Scand J Immunol.* 1976;**5**:1117-22.
152. Kalden JR, Peter HH, Lohmann E, Schedel J, Diehl V, Valke D. Estimation of T- and K-cell activity in the peripheral blood of sarcoidosis patients. *Ann NY Acad Sci.* 1976;**278**:52-68.
153. Hsu CCS, Wu SJY, Celic L, Weaver LJ, Solliday N. Increased proportion of active sheep erythrocyte rosette-forming lymphocytes and plasma rosette enhancement in sarcoidosis. *Am Rev Respir Dis.* 1979;**119**:383-9.
154. Goldstein RA, Janicki BW, Mirro J, Foellmer JW. Cell-mediated immune responses in sarcoidosis. *Am Rev Respir Dis.* 1978;**117**:55-62.
155. Siltzbach LE, Glade PR, Hirshant Y, Vieira LOBD, Celikoglu IS, Hirschhorn K. In vitro stimulation of peripheral lymphocytes in sarcoidosis. In: Levinsky L, Macholda F. *Fifth International Conference on Sarcoidosis.* Prague: University Karlova; 1971:217-20.
156. Daniele RP, McMillan LJ, Dauber JH, Rossman MD. Immune complexes in sarcoidosis: a correlation with activity and duration of disease. *Chest.* 1978;**74**:261-4.
157. Gupta RC, Kueppers F, DeRemee RA, et al. Pulmonary and extrapulmonary sarcoidosis in relation to circulating immune complexes: a quantification of immune complexes by two radioimmunoassays. *Am Rev Respir Dis.* 1977;**116**:261-6.
158. Hedfors E, Norberg R. Evidence for circulating immune complexes in sarcoidosis. *Clin Exp Immunol.* 1974;**16**:493-6.
159. Verrier-Jones J, Cumming RH, Asplin CM. Evidence for circulating immune complexes in erythema nodosum and early sarcoidosis. *Ann NY Acad Sci.* 1976;**278**:212-9.
160. Kueppers F, DeRemee RE. Search for a specific antibody in sera from patients with sarcoidosis. *Ann NY Acad Sci.* 1976;**278**:220-4.
161. Daniele RP, Rowlands DT. Antibodies to T cells in sarcoidosis. *Ann NY Acad Sci.* 1976;**278**:88-100.
162. Klockars M, Selroos O. Immunohistochemical demonstration of lysozyme in the lymph nodes and Kveim reaction papules in sarcoidosis. *Acta Pathol Microbiol Scand.* 1977;**85A**:169-73.
163. Pascual RS, Gee JBL, Finch SC. Usefulness of serum lysozyme measurement in diagnosis and evaluation of sarcoidosis. *N Engl J Med.* 1973;**289**:1074-6.
164. Selroos O, Klockars M. Serum lysozyme in sarcoidosis. Evaluation of its usefulness in determination of disease activity. *Scand J Respir Dis.* 1977;**58**:110-6.
165. Silverstein E, Friedland J, Ackerman T. Elevation of granulomatous lymph node and serum lysozyme in sarcoidosis and correlation with angiotensin-converting enzyme. *Am J Clin Pathol.* 1977;**68**:219-24.
166. Siltzback LE, Krakoff L, Dorph D, Tierstein AS. Elevated levels of serum angiotensin-converting enzyme (ACE) and lysozyme (L) levels in sarcoidosis. In: Williams WJ, Davies BH, eds. *Proceedings of the 8th International Conference on Sarcoidosis and Other Granulomatous Disease.* London: Alpha Omega Publishing, Ltd.; 1980:298-302.
167. Ashutosh K, Keighley JFH. Diagnostic value of serum angiotensin converting enzyme activity in lung disease. *Thorax.* 1976;**31**:552-7.
168. Fanburg BL, Schoenberger MD, Bachus B, Snider GL. Elevated serum angiotensin I converting enzyme in sarcoidosis. *Am Rev Respir Dis.* 1976;**114**:525-8.
169. Ferlitsch A, Kohout J, Kummer F, Legenstein E, Muller MM. Angiotensin converting enzyme in the diagnosis of sarcoidosis. In: Williams WJ, Davies BH, eds. *Proceedings of the 8th International Conference on Sarcoidosis and Other Granulomatous Disease.* London: Alpha Omega Publishing, Ltd.; 1980:22.
170. Lieberman J. Elevation of serum angiotensin-converting-enzyme (ACE) level in sarcoidosis. *Am J Med.* 1975;**59**:365-72.
171. Lieberman J. The specificity and nature of serum angiotensin-converting-enzyme (serum ACE) elevations in sarcoidosis. *Ann NY Acad Sci.* 1976;**278**:488-97.
172. Lieberman J, Kaneshiro W, Weisser K, et al. Update on serum ACE: angiotensin converting enzyme assays for diagnosis and therapeutic evaluation in sarcoidosis. In: Williams WJ, Davies BH, eds. *Proceedings of the 8th International Conference on Sarcoidosis and Other Granulomatous Disease.* London: Alpha Omega Publishing, Ltd.; 1980:320-7.
173. Rohrbach MS, Dereme RA. Serum angiotensin converting enzyme activity in sarcoidosis as measured by a simple radiochemical assay. *Am Rev Respir Dis.* 1979;**119**:761-7.
174. Sandron D, Lecossier D, Moreun F, Basset G, Battesti JP. Comparison between two methods of determining serum angiotensin converting enzyme in sarcoidosis and other pulmonary diseases. In: Williams WJ, Davies BH, eds. *Proceedings of the 8th International Conference on Sarcoidosis and Other Granulomatous Disease.* London: Alpha Omega Publishing, Ltd.; 1980; 317-9.
175. Abboy R, Kanada DJ, Sharma OP. Serum angiotensin converting

enzyme in sarcoidosis. In: Williams WJ, Davies BH, eds. *Proceedings of the 8th International Conference on Sarcoidosis and Other Granulomatous Disease.* London: Alpha Omega Publishing; 1980:273-6.

176. Simonowitz LJ, Solliday N, Celic L, Cugell E. Serial measurements of angiotensin converting enzyme and diffusing capacity in sarcoidosis. *Am Rev Respir Dis.* 1977;**115**(suppl):164. Abstract.
177. Studdy P, Bird R, Geraint JD, Sherberb S. Serum angiotensin converting enzyme (SACE) in sarcoidosis and other granulomatous disorders. In: Williams WJ, Davies BH, eds. *Proceedings of the 8th International Conference on Sarcoidosis and Other Granulomatous Disease.* London: Alpha Omega Publishing, Ltd.; 1980:259-65.
178. Ueda E, Hishimurak, Hawada K, et al. Serum angiotensin-converting enzyme activity in patients with sarcoidosis. *Jpn J Thorac Dis.* 1976;**14:**736-42.
179. Nelson DS. *Immunobiology of the Macrophage.* New York: Academic Press; 1976.
180. Pascual RS, Perille PE, Gee JBL, Finch SC. Serum and urine lysozyme in sarcoidosis. In: Osserman E, Cenfield R, Beychok S, eds. *Lysozyme.* New York: Academic Press; 1974:391.
181. Ng KKF, Vane JR. Fate of angiotensin I in the circulation. *Nature (London).* 1968;**218:**144-50.
182. Renzi G, Dutton RE. Pulmonary function in diffuse sarcoidosis. *Respiration.* 1973;**31:**124-31.
183. James DG, Carstairs LS, Trowell J, Sharma OP. Treatment of sarcoidosis: report of a controlled therapeutic trial. *Lancet.* 1967;**2:**526-8.
184. Kirks DR, McCormick VD, Greenspan RH. Pulmonary sarcoidosis: roentgenologic analysis of 150 patients. *Am J Roentgenol Radium Therap Nucl Med.* 1973;**117:**777-8.
185. James DG. Diagnosis and treatment of sarcoidosis. *Br Med J.* 1956;**2:**900-04.
186. James DG, Neville E, Siltzbach LE, et al. A worldwide view of sarcoidosis. *Ann NY Acad Sci.* 1976;**278:**321-34.
187. DeRemee RA, Andersen HA. Sarcoidosis: a correlation of dyspnea with roentgenographic stage and pulmonary function changes. *Mayo Clin Proc.* 1974;**49:**742-5.
188. Freundlich IM, Libshitz HI, Glassman LM, Israel HL. Sarcoidosis: typical and atypical thoracic manifestations and complications. *Clin Radiol.* 1970;**21:**376-83.
189. Fraser RG, Pare JAP. *Diagnosis of Diseases of the Chest.* Philadelphia: W.B. Saunders; 1979:1659-90.
190. Felson B. *Chest Roentgenology.* Philadelphia: W.B. Saunders; 1973:302.
191. Rabinowitz JG, Ulreich S, Soriano C. The usual unusual manifestations of sarcoidosis and the "hilar haze"—a new diagnostic aid. *Am J Roentgenol Rad Therap Nucl Med.* 1974;**120:**821-39.
192. Shigematsu N, Emori K, Matsuba K, Harada S, Takahahi T. Clinico-pathologic characteristics of pulmonary acinar sarcoidosis. *Chest.* 1978;**73:**186-8.
193. Felson B. Uncommon roentgen patterns of pulmonary sarcoidosis. *Dis Chest.* 1958;**34:**357-67.
194. Sharma OP, Hewlett R, Gordonson J. Nodular sarcoidosis: an unusual radiographic appearance. *Chest.* 1973;**64:**189-92.
195. Kirks DR, McCormick VD, Greenspan RH. Pulmonary sarcoidosis: roentgenologic analysis of 150 patients. *Am J Roentgenol.* 1973;**117:**777-86.
196. Young RC, Titus-Dillon PY, Schneider ML, Shelton TG, Hackney RL, Harden KA. Sarcoidosis in Washington, D.C.: clinical observations in 105 black patients. In: Levinsky DL, Macholda F, eds. *Fifth International Conference on Sarcoidosis.* Prague: Universita Karlova; 1971:513-20.
197. Rosen Y, Amorosa JK, Moon S, Cohen J, Lyons HA. Occurrence of lung granulomas in patients with stage I sarcoidosis. *Am J Roentgenol.* 1977;**129:**1083-85.
198. Epler GR, McLoud TC, Gaensler ER, Mickus JP, Carrington CB. Normal chest roentgenograms in chronic diffuse infiltrative lung disease. *N Engl J Med.* 1978;**298:**934-9.
199. McCort JJ, Pare JAP. Pulmonary fibrosis and cor pulmonale in sarcoidosis. *Radiology.* 1954;**62:**496-504.
200. Scadding JG. Prognosis of intrathoracic sarcoidosis. *Br Med J.* 1961;**2:**1165-72.
201. Mikhail JR, Drury RA, Mitchell DN. Evaluation of the clinical and histological features of paratracheal and hilar gland enlargement. *Postgrad Med J.* 1970;**46:**515-8.
202. Boushy SF, Kurtzman RS, Martin ND, Lewis BM. The course of pulmonary function in sarcoidosis. *Ann Intern Med.* 1965;**62:**939-55.
203. Berg GR. Pulmonary function in sarcoidosis. *N Engl J Med.* 1968;**278:**1019. Letter.
204. O'Brien LE, Forsman PJ, Wiltse HE. Early onset sarcoidosis with pulmonary function abnormalities. *Chest.* 1974;**65:**472-4.
205. Renzi G, Dutton RE. Pulmonary function in diffuse sarcoidosis. *Respiration.* 1974;**31:**124-36.
206. Colp C, Park SS, Williams MH Jr. Pulmonary function follow-up to 120 patients with sarcoidosis. *Ann NY Acad Sci.* 1976;**278:**301-07.
207. Miller A, Chuang M, Teirstein AS, Siltzbach LE. Pulmonary function in stage I and II pulmonary sarcoidosis. *Ann NY Acad Sci.* 1976;**278:**292-300.
208. Hamer NA. Changes in the components of the diffusing capacity in pulmonary sarcoidosis. *Thorax.* 1963;**18:**275-87.
209. Saumon G, Georges R, Loiseau A, Turiaf J. Membrane diffusing capacity and pulmonary capillary blood volume in pulmonary sarcoidosis. *Ann NY Acad Sci.* 1976;**278:**284-91.
210. Sellers RD, Siebens AA. The effects of sarcoidosis on pulmonary function with particular reference to changes in pulmonary compliance. *Am Rev Respir Dis.* 1965;**91:**660-4.
211. Ting GY, Williams MH Jr. Mechanics of breathing in sarcoidosis of the lung. *JAMA.* 1965;**192:**619-24.
212. Harden KA, Young RC Jr, Carr C, Laurey JR. Oxygen cost of breathing. II. Studies in patients with sarcoidosis. *Am Rev Respir Dis.* 1968;**97:**1127-30.
213. Snider GL, Doctor LR. The mechanics of ventilation in sarcoidosis. *Am Rev Respir Dis.* 1964;**89:**897-908.
214. Tabiri G, Arndt H, Behrend H, Dombrowski H. Lung volumes, compliance and diffusing capacity in advanced pulmonary sarcoidosis. In: Levinsky DL, Macholda F, eds. *Fifth International Conference on Sarcoidosis.* Prague: Universita Karlova; 1971:442-6.
215. Young RL, Harkleroad CE, Lordon RE, Weg JG. Pulmonary sarcoidosis: a prospective evaluation of glucocorticoid therapy. *Ann Intern Med.* 1970;**73:**207-12.
216. Kaneko K, Sharma OP. Airway obstruction in pulmonary sarcoidosis. *Bull Eur Physiopathol Respir.* 1977;**13:**231-40.
217. Rizzato G, Brambilla I, Bertoli L, Conti F, Merlin R, Mantaro O. Impaired airway function and pulmonary hemodynamics in sarcoidosis. In: Williams WJ, Davies BH, eds. *Proceedings of the 8th International Conference on Sarcoidosis and Other Granulomatous Disease.* London: Alpha Omega Publishing, Ltd.; 1980:349-60.
218. Sahetya GK, Covy WB, Facen HK, Hassan S, Kumar B, Young RC. Pulmonary sarcoidosis: a significant cause of chronic airway obstruction. In: Williams WJ, Davies, BH, eds. *Proceedings of the 8th International Conference on Sarcoidosis and Other Granulomatous Disease.* London: Alpha Omega Publishing, Ltd.; 1980:361-7.
219. Miller A, Teirstein AS, Jackler I, Chuang M, Siltzbach LE. Airway function in chronic pulmonary sarcoidosis with fibrosis. *Am Rev Respir Dis.* 1974;**109:**179-89.
220. Tammeling GJ, de Vries K, Sluiter HJ, et al. Obstructive lung disease in pulmonary sarcoidosis. *Acta Med Scand.* 1964;**176**(suppl):275-77.
221. Levinson RS, Metzger LF, Stanley NN, et al. Airway function in sarcoidosis. *Am J Med.* 1977;**62:**51-9.
222. Radwan L, Grebska E, Koziorowski A. Small airway function in pulmonary sarcoidosis. *Scand J Respir Dis.* 1978;**59:**37-43.
223. Sharma OP. Airway obstruction in sarcoidosis. *Chest.* 1978;**73:**6-7. Editorial.
224. Bates DV, Macklem PT, Christie RV. Pulmonary sarcoidosis, In: *Respiratory Function in Disease.* Philadelphia: W.B. Saunders Co.; 1971:287-9.
225. Staneck V, Widimsky J, Navratil M, Daum S, Levinsky L. The pulmonary gas exchange during exercise in patients with pulmonary fibrosis. *Scand J Respir Dis.* 1967;**48:**11-2.
226. Sears MR. Pulmonary gas transfer and alveolar-oxygen differences in sarcoidosis. In: Williams WJ, Davies BH, eds. *Proceedings of the 8th International Conference on Sarcoidosis and Other Granulomatous Disease.* London: Alpha Omega Publishing, Ltd.; 1980:343-8.
227. Colp C. Sarcoidosis: course and treatment. *Med Clin N Am.* 1977;**61:**1267-78.
228. Young RC Jr, Carr C, Shelton TG, et al. Sarcoidosis: relationship between changes in lung structure and function. *Am Rev Respir Dis.* 1967;**95:**224-38.
229. Young RL, Lordon RE, Krumholz RA, Harkleroad LE, Branam GE, Weg JG. Pulmonary sarcoidosis. I. Pathophysiologic correlations. *Am Rev Respir Dis.* 1968;**97:**997-1008.
230. Edwards CL, Hayes RL. Tumor scanning with ^{67}Ga citrate. *J Nucl Med.* 1969;**10:**103-5.
231. Lavender PJ, Lowe J, Barker JR, Burn JI, Chaudhri MA. Gallium-67 citrate scanning in neoplastic and inflammatory lesions. *Br J Radiol.* 1971;**44:**361-6.
232. Kanno I. Diagnostic evaluation of ^{67}Ga scanning of lung cancer and other diseases. *Radiology.* 1971;**101:**355-62.
233. Hisasi T, Nakayama Y. Clinical evaluation of ^{67}Ga citrate scanning. *J Nucl Med.* 1972;**13:**196-201.
234. van der Schoot JB, Groen AS, de Jons J. Gallium-67 scintigraphy in lung diseases. *Thorax.* 1972;**27:**543-6.
235. Teates CD, Bray ST, Williamson BR. Tumor detection with ^{67}Ga citrate: a literature survey (1970-1978). *Clin Nucl Med.* 1978;**3:**456-60.
236. Dise-Peterson H, Heckscher T, Hertz M. ^{67}Ga-scintigraphy in

nonmalignant lung diseases. *Scand J Respir Dis.* 1972;**53**:314-31.
237. Littenberg RL, Taketa RM, Alazraki NP, Halpern SE, Ashburn WL. Gallium-67 for localization of septic lesions. *Ann Intern Med.* 1973;**79**:403-6.
238. Israel HL, Atkinson GW. Sarcoidosis: basics of respiratory disease. *Am Thoracic Soc.* 1978;**7**:1-6.
239. Silberstein EB. Gallium detection of inflammation. *Ann Intern Med.* 1974;**80**:774. Letter.
240. Teates CD, Hunger JG. Gallium scanning as a screening test for inflammatory lesions. *Radiology.* 1975;**116**:383-7.
241. Kumar B, Coleman RE, Alderson PO. Gallium citrate Ga-67 imaging in patients with suspected inflammatory processes. *Arch Surg.* 1975;**110**:1237-42.
242. Siemsen JK, Grebe SF, Sargent EN, Wentz D. Gallium-67 scintigraphy of pulmonary diseases as a complement to radiography. *Radiology.* 1976;**118**:371-5.
243. Vallieres BJ, Johnston GS, Jones AE, Line BR. Gallium-67 citrate scintigraphy: II. Clinical aspects. *Union Med Can.* 1977;**106**:1382-91.
244. Staab EV, McCartney WH. Role of gallium-67 in inflammatory disease. *Semin Nucl Med.* 1978;**8**:219-34.
245. Myerson PJ, Myerson DA, Spencer RP. Anatomic correlations in radiogallium imaging of the peritoneum and retroperitoneum. *Semin Nucl Med.* 1979;**9**:66-70.
246. Lanshammer H, Glaubitt G, Grebe SF, et al. Gallium-67 for tumor scanning. *J Nucl Med.* 1972;**13**:25-30.
247. Nelson B, Hayes RL, Edwards CL, et al. Distribution of gallium in human tissues after intravenous administration. *J Nucl Med.* 1972;**13**:92-100.
248. Larson SM, Milder MS, Johnston GS. Interpretation of the ^{67}Ga photoscan. *J Nucl Med.* 1973;**14**:208-14.
249. Line BR, Fulmer JD, Reynolds HY, et al. Gallium-67 citrate scanning in the staging of idiopathic pulmonary fibrosis: correlation with physiologic and morphologic features and bronchoalveolar lavage. *Am Rev Respir Dis.* 1978;**118**:355-65.
250. Siemsen JK, Grebe SF, Waxman AD. The use of gallium-67 in pulmonary disorders. *Semin Nucl Med.* 1978;**8**:235-49.
251. Heshiki A, Schatz SL, McKusick KA, Bowersox DW, Soin JS, Wagner HN. Gallium-67 citrate scanning in patients with pulmonary sarcoidosis. *Am J Roentgenol Radium Ther Nucl Med.* 1974;**122**:744-9.
252. Mertz T, Malmud L, McKusick KA, Wagner HN. Mechanisms of ^{67}Ga association with lymphocytes. *Cancer Res.* 1974;**34**:2495-9.
253. Niden AH, Mishkin FS, Khurana ML. ^{67}Gallium citrate lung scans in interstitial lung disease. *Chest.* 1976;**69**:266-8.
254. Stone DJ, Schwartz A, Feltman JA, Lovelock FJ. Pulmonary function in sarcoidosis: results with cortisone therapy. *Am J Med.* 1953;**15**:468-78.
255. Israel HL, Sones M, Harrell D. Cortisone treatment of sarcoidosis: experience with thirty-six cases. *JAMA.* 1954;**156**:461-8.
256. Smellie H, Apthorp GH, Marshall R. The effect of corticosteroid treatment on pulmonary function in sarcoidosis. *Thorax.* 1960;**16**:87-90.
257. Sharma OP, Colp C, Williams MH. Course of pulmonary sarcoidosis with and without corticosteroid therapy as determined by pulmonary function studies. *Am J Med.* 1966;**41**:541-51.
258. Siltzbach LE. Sarcoidosis: clinical features and management. *Med Clin N Am.* 1967;**51**:483-502.
259. American Thoracic Society Medical Section of the National Tuberculosis and Respiratory Disease Association: Treatment of sarcoidosis. *Am Rev Respir Dis.* 1971;**103**:433-4.
260. Israel HL, Fouts DW, Beggs RA. A controlled trial of prednisone treatment of sarcoidosis. *Am Rev Respir Dis.* 1973;**107**:609-14.
261. Johns CJ, Zachary JB, Ball WC. A ten-year study of corticosteroid treatment of pulmonary sarcoidosis. *Hopkins Med J.* 1974;**134**:271-83.
262. Hedfors E. Influence of steroid treatment on lymphocyte response in sarcoidosis. *Clin Immunol Immunopathol.* 1975;**4**:96-100.
263. Balow JE, Hurley DL, Fauci AS. Immuno-suppressive effects of glucocorticoids: differential effects of acute vs. chronic administration on cell-mediated immunity. *J Immunol.* 1975;**114**:1072-6.
264. Fauci AS, Dale DC, Balow JE. Glucocorticosteroid therapy: mechanisms of action and clinical considerations. *Ann Intern Med.* 1976;**84**:304-15.
265. Rosenau W, Moon HD. The inhibitory effect of hydrocortisone on lysis of homologous cells by lymphocytes in vitro. *J Immunol.* 1962;**89**:422-6.
266. Stavey L, Cohen IR, Feldman M. The effect of hydrocortisone on lymphocyte-mediated cytolysis. *Cell Immunol.* 1973;**7**:302-12.
267. Fauci AS. Corticosteroids and circulating lymphocytes. *Transplant Proc.* 1975;**7**:37-40.
268. Haynes BF, Fauci AS. The differential effect of in vivo hydrocortisone on the kinetics of subpopulations of human peripheral blood thymus-derived lymphocytes. *J Clin Invest.* 1978;**61**:703-7.
269. Balow JE, Rosenthal AS. Glucocorticoid suppression of macrophage migration inhibitory factor. *J Exp Med.* 1973;**137**:1031-41.
270. Crystal RG, Fulmer JD, Baum B, et al. Cells, collagen and idiopathic pulmonary fibrosis. *Lung.* 1978;**155**:199-224.
271. Vracko R. Significance of basal lamina for regeneration of injured lung. *Virchows Arch [Pathol Anat].* 1972;**355**:264-74.
272. British Tuberculosis Association: Chloroquine in the treatment of sarcoidosis. *Tubercle.* 1967;**48**:257-72.
273. Breyne H. Experiences with immunological therapy of sarcoidosis over 13 years. *Z Erkrank Atm Org.* 1977;**149**:160-3.
274. Wandett-Freerksen E. Aldactone in the treatment of sarcoidosis of the lungs. *Z Erkrank Atm Org.* 1977;**149**:156-9.
275. Rosof BM. Allopurinol for sarcoid. *N Engl J Med.* 1964;**294**:447. Letter.
276. Rosenthal M, Trabert U, Müller W, Müller S, Wurm K. Levamisole in sarcoidosis. *N Engl J Med.* 1974;**294**:112-3.
277. Hedfors E. Possible role for anticoagulant treatment in sarcoidosis. *Mt Sinai J Med.* 1977;**44**:745-7.
278. Geraint-James D, Carstairs LS, Trowell J, Sharma OP. Treatment of sarcoidosis: report of a controlled therapeutic trial. *Lancet.* 1967:526-8.
279. Israel HL. Effects of chlorambucil and methotrexate in sarcoidosis. In: Levinsky L, Mackolda F, eds. *Fifth International Conference on Sarcoidosis.* Prague: Universita Karlova; 1971:632-4.
280. Sharma O, Hughes DTD, Geraint-James D, Naish P. Immunosuppressive therapy with azathioprine in sarcoidosis. In: Levinsky L, Macholda F, eds. *Fifth International Conference on Sarcoidosis.* Prague: Universita Karlova; 1971:635-7.

Characterization of the Inflammatory and Immune Effector Cells in the Lung Parenchyma of Patients with Interstitial Lung Disease[1,2]

GARY W. HUNNINGHAKE, OICHI KAWANAMI, VICTOR J. FERRANS, ROSCOE C. YOUNG, JR., WILLIAM C. ROBERTS, and RONALD G. CRYSTAL

SUMMARY The pathogenesis of the interstitial lung disorders is intimately related to the number, type, and state of activation of inflammatory and immune effector cells (the alveolitis) within the alveolar structures. To directly characterize the type and status of the cells comprising the alveolitis of various interstitial lung disorders, a method was developed to isolate inflammatory and immune effector cells from open lung biopsies of patients with idiopathic pulmonary fibrosis (n = 9) and sarcoidosis (n = 6). The cells isolated from these biopsies were compared with effector cells obtained from normal lung (n = 3). The effector cell populations in normal lung contained alveolar macrophages (84 ± 17%), lymphocytes (16 ± 4%), and rare polymorphonuclear leukocytes (<1%); of the lymphocytes present, 73 ± 4% were T-lymphocytes, 7 ± 2% were "activated" T-lymphocytes, and 9 ± 2% were B-lymphocytes. In contrast, a characteristic feature of the alveolitis of idiopathic pulmonary fibrosis was the presence of increased proportions of polymorphonuclear leukocytes, primarily neutrophils (18 ± 4%); the percentages of lymphocytes and various lymphocyte subpopulations were similar to those found in the normal lung. By comparison, the alveolitis of sarcoidosis was characterized by the presence of increased proportions of lymphocytes (57 ± 7%), T-lymphocytes (91 ± 5%), and "activated" T-lymphocytes (19 ± 4%); neutrophils were rarely found in the lung of nonsmoking patients with sarcoidosis. The proportions of various inflammatory and immune effector cells isolated from the lung of normal subjects as well as from biopsies of patients with idiopathic pulmonary fibrosis and sarcoidosis were similar to those cell populations that were present in the respective bronchoalveolar lavage fluids. Thus, the alveolitis of the interstitial lung diseases can be directly characterized by the types of inflammatory and immune effector cells present within the lung parenchyma. In addition, the cells recovered by bronchoalveolar lavage accurately reflect the alveolitis of these disorders.
AM REV RESPIR DIS 1981; 123:407-412

Introduction

The interstitial lung diseases are a heterogeneous group of disorders characterized by a chronic accumulation of increased numbers of inflammatory and immune effector cells within the alveolar structures (the "alveolitis"), a derangement of interstitial collagen (the "fibrosis"), alterations in lung parenchymal cells, and a progressive disordering of alveolar-capillary units (1-13). Although the fibrosis of interstitial disease likely plays an important role in disordering alveolar-capillary units, the current concepts of the pathogenesis of these disorders suggest that the alveolitis occurs early in the disease process and likely mediates both the fibrosis and the alterations in lung parenchymal cells (5, 10-14). Thus, to understand the pathogenesis of the different interstitial diseases, it was first necessary to define the type and function of the cells comprising the alveolitis that is characteristic of each disorder.

The classic approach to evaluate the alveolitis of interstitial disease has been to biopsy the lung parenchyma and, using conventional histologic methods, to describe qualitatively the inflammatory and immune effector cells that have accumulated within the alveolar structures (1-13). However, although such methods are useful to determine the degree of the cellular infiltrate, the integrity of the alveolar structures, and the amount of fibrosis, they yield little information as to the type and function of the cells comprising the alveolitis.

A newer approach to evaluate the alveolitis of interstitial disease has been the use of the fiberoptic bronchoscope to lavage the lower respiratory tract of these patients to obtain inflammatory and immune effector cells that are lining the epithelial surface of the lung parenchyma (5, 11-13, 15-22). This technique holds great promise, because, for the first time, it permits detailed morphologic surface marker, and functional evaluation of the inflammatory and immune effector cells involved in various chronic lung diseases. In addition, bronchoalveolar lavage is a safe, easily repeatable procedure that can be used to follow the status of the alveolitis of interstitial disease and its response to therapy (11-13, 15-21).

Although the formation derived from bronchoalveolar lavage of patient with interstitial disease is consistent with the theoretical concepts of the pathogenesis of these disorders, it has not been demonstrated that the inflammatory and immune effector cells collected by lavage are truly representative of the effector cells within the alveolar structures. The present study, therefore, was designed to study directly the inflammatory and immune effector cells that comprise the alveolitis of these disorders by isolating these cells from biopsies of lung parenchyma of patients with interstitial disease and comparing these cells with the cell populations obtained by bronchoalveolar lavage of the same patients. Two diverse disorders, sarcoidosis and idiopathic pulmonary fibrosis, were chosen for study, because they likely represent diseases whose pathogenesis is me-

(Received in original form January 31, 1980 and in revised form December 10, 1980)

[1] From the Pulmonary Branch and Pathology Branch, National Heart, Lung and Blood Institute, National Institutes of Health, Bethesda, MD 20205, and the Pulmonary Division, Department of Medicine, Howard University, Washington, DC 20001.

[2] Requests for reprints should be addressed to Gary W. Hunninghake, M.D., Building 10, Room 6D06 National Heart, Lung and Blood Institute, Bethesda, MD 20205.

diated through markedly different inflammatory and immune effector cells (1–21). For comparison, similar studies were carried out using lung biopsies from normal lung obtained from patients who underwent thoracotomy and biopsy of what turned out to be nonmalignant, noninfectious localized pulmonary lesions.

Methods

Study population: normal control subjects. Fiberoptic bronchoscopy was performed on 6 nonsmoking normal volunteers (2 men and 4 women with a mean ± SE age of 28 ± 6yr). The pulmonary function tests and chest roentgenograms of all 6 subjects were within normal limits, and none of the subjects were taking medication. Open lung biopsies were not performed on these 6 volunteers.

Normal lung parenchyma was obtained from patients who underwent thoracotomy for removal of solitary lung nodules. The nodule and a portion of the surrounding parenchyma were examined histologically and the remaining parenchyma was used for isolation of inflammatory and immune effector cells, as described subsequently. Data were used from only those patients fulfilling he following criteria: (*1*) nonsmoking, (*2*) normal pulmonary function tests and normal chest roentgenograms (except for the solitary nodules), and (*3*) nodules that proved to be noninfectious and nonmalignant and surrounding parenchyma that was normal by histologic examination. Three patients fulfilled all of these criteria. There were 2 men and 1 woman with a mean age of 42 ± 8 yr.

Study population: patients with idiopathic pulmonary fibrosis. A diagnosis of idiopathic pulmonary fibrosis (IPF) was made in 9 nonsmoking patients (5 men and 4 women with a mean age of 46 ± 8 yr) by established criteria (5, 10, 11, 13). All patients were in mid-course of their disease and none were taking medication. As a group, the patients with IPF had the following functional abnormalities: vital capacity, 71 ± 14% predicted; total lung capacity, 65 ± 9% predicted; single breath diffusing capacity, 58 ± 7% predicted, forced expiratory volume in one second/forced vital capacity, 96 ± 8% predicted; resting Pa_{O_2}, 77 ± 7 mm Hg; Pa_{O_2} at maximal steady-state exercise, 56 ± 12 mm Hg. All 9 patients underwent open lung biopsy and fiberoptic bronchoscopy with lavage.

Study population: patients with sarcoidosis. A diagnosis of sarcoidosis was established in 6 patients using the following criteria (10–13, 21): (*1*) an open lung biopsy demonstrating noncaseating epithelioid granulomata with giant cell formation in the lung parenchyma and coexisting morphologic features compatible with sarcoidosis; (*2*) a compatible clinical picture without evidence of mycobacterial, fungal, or parasitic infection; (*3*) no history of exposure to inorganic or organic material known to cause granulomatous lung disease; (*4*) a positive reaction to a Kveim-Siltzbach skin test (materials for the Kveim-Siltzbach skin test were kindly provided by Dr. L. Siltzbach). All patients had active sarcoidosis with lung parenchymal and hilar node involvement. None was taking medication. As a group, these patients had the following functional abnormalities: vital capacity, 74 ± 9% predicted; total lung capacity, 77 ± 7% predicted; single breath diffusing capacity, 62 ± 14% predicted; forced expiratory volume in one second/forced vital capacity, 101 ± 8% predicted; resting Pa_{O_2}, 87 ± 9 mm Hg; Pa_{O_2} at maximal steady-state exercise, 74 ± 12 mm Hg. All 6 patients underwent open lung biopsy and fiberoptic bronchoscopy with lavage.

Bronchoalveolar lavage. Patients and normal subjects were premedicated intravenously with valium (2 to 10 mg) and intramuscularly with atropine (0.8 mg). After local anesthesia with 2% lidocaine spray, examination of the airways was carried out with a flexible fiberoptic bronchoscope (Model BF-B2; Olympus Corporation of America, New Hyde Park, NY). The tip of the bronchoscope was then wedged in B4 or B5 in the left lung. Lavage was carried out with 100 ml of sterile saline in 5 20-ml aliquots with immediate vacuum aspiration after each aliquot. Immediately after lavage, the fluid was filtered through several layers of surgical gauze and the volume was measured. The cells were separated from the lavage fluid by centrifugation (500 *g* for 5 min) and resuspended in Hanks' balanced salt solution (HBSS) without Ca^{++} or Mg^{++}. The cells were then evaluated for total number (Model FN, Coulter Electronics, Hialeah, FL), viability (trypan blue dye exclusion), and differential count (Wright-Giemsa stained cytocentrifuge preparation, Cytospin®, Shandon Southern Instruments, Sewickley, PA). Macrophages were distinguished from lymphocytes by nonspecific esterase stains (11). The bronchoalveolar lavage cells (in HBSS) were then subjected to Hypaque-Ficoll density (1.077 to 1.080 g/ml) centrifugation (23), and the purified mononuclear cells were suspended in HBSS at a concentration of 4×10^6 cells/ml.

Lung biopsy. All lung biopsy specimens were immediately placed in sterile heparanized 0.9% saline (100 units/ml) at 4° C and portions removed for histologic examination and culture. The remaining tissue was then used to obtain inflammatory and immune effector cell populations by first teasing the parenchyma in HBSS in a petri dish. The resulting material was filtered through several layers of sterile surgical gauze to obtain a single cell suspension. Mononuclear cells were then isolated from these cell suspensions by Hypaque-Ficoll density centrifugation (23) and resuspended in HBSS at a concentration of 4×10^6 cells/ml. A small aliquot of the original cell suspension, the mononuclear cell band from the Hypaque-Ficoll gradient, and the cells going to the bottom of the Hypaque-Ficoll gradient were used to make a cytocentrifuge smear for cell differential, as described previously. Evaluation of these cell differentials demonstrated that, in addition to inflammatory and immune effector cells, additional lung cells were also present in the unfractionated biopsy cell suspensions. These cells were distinguished from lymphocytes and alveolar macrophages by their morphologic features, their inability to phagocytize, their lack of cell surface markers, and their density on Hypaque-Ficoll (these cells went to the bottom along with polymorphonuclear leukocytes). For these reasons, these cells were not considered to be inflammatory and immune effector cells, and they were not considered during subsequent analyses. Only polymorphonuclear leukocytes, macrophages, and lymphocytes were included in the cell differentials; in all biopsies, these cells comprised more than 75% of the cells isolated.

Identification of lymphocyte subpopulations. Identical methods were used to identify lymphocyte subpopulations in the post-Hypaque-Ficoll mononuclear cell suspensions from lavage fluid and the lung biopsies (11, 20). The viability of the cell suspensions was more than 95% in all cases. To exclude phagocytic cells from quantitation of lymphocyte subpopulations, neutral red dye was added to the mononuclear cell suspensions before the rosetting procedure used to identify lymphocyte subpopulations. "Total lymphocytes" were arbitrarily identified as all cells not taking up the red dye. The use of the dye did not affect the percentages of lymphocytes forming rosettes in any of the testing procedures subsequently described.

The T-lymphocytes were identfied by their ability to form spontaneous rosettes at 4° C with neuraminidase-treated sheep red blood cells (SRBC) (24) and B-lymphocytes by the presence of surface immunoglobulin using a fluorescein conjugated $F(ab')_2$ goat antihuman immunoglobulin reagent (Cappel Laboratory, Cochranville, PA) (25). Both tests were performed as previously described (11, 21).

"Activated" T-lymphocytes, defined as a subset of T-lymphocytes capable of forming rosettes with SRBC (not neuraminidase-treated) at 37° C, were identified by combining 0.25 ml of the mononuclear cell suspension (4×10^6 cells/ml in HBSS) with 0.25 ml of 0.5 SRBC and incubating at 37° C for 5 min (26–28). The cells were then pelleted (100 *g* for 5 min at 37° C), incubated (at 37° C for 15 min), and the rosette-forming cells enumerated as previously described (11, 21).

Analysis of data. All data were presented as mean ± SE of the mean; comparisons between values were made using the two-tailed *t* test.

Results

Bronchoalveolar lavage was performed without difficulty in each of the patients and in each of the normal volunteers. Visualization of the tracheobronchial tree prior to lavage demonstrated normal airways in all of the subjects, with no evidence of bronchitis. There was no significant difference in the total fluid recovered from the normal or the patient groups ($p > 0.2$, all comparisons). The recovered fluid was sterile in all cases, except for rare oral flora.

The biopsies of normal lung were characterized by thin alveolar septums and pleura, and the alveolar walls formed a fine, fishnet pattern. Within the interstitium and the alveoli there were a few mononuclear cells, primarily alveolar macrophages. Polymorphonuclear leukocytes were rarely found in the alveolar structures of the normal lung (data not shown).

The biopsies of the IPF lung were characterized by thickened interstitial areas and a derangement of the structure of alveolar-capillary units. In addition to alveolar macrophages/monocytes, increased numbers of polymorphonuclear leukocytes and lymphocytes were also present both within the interstitium and on the epithelial surface of the alveoli. Granulomata were not present within the lung in these patients (data not shown).

The biopsies of sarcoid lung were also characterized by thickened interstitial areas and a derangement of alveolar-capillary units. In contrast to the IPF lung, the inflammatory and immune effector cells present within the interstitium and alveoli of the sarcoid lung were comprised primarily of lymphocytes and monocytes/macrophages. Polymorphonuclear leukocytes were only rarely found in the lung in nonsmoking patients with this disorder. The lung lesions of sarcoidosis were always associated with the presence of granulomata within the lung parenchyma (data not shown).

The unfractionated single cell suspensions isolated from normal lung biopsies contained alveolar macrophages, small numbers of lymphocytes, and a variety of lung parenchymal cells; polymorphonuclear leukocytes were not present. After Hypaque-Ficoll centrifugation, the lung parenchymal cells pelleted to the bottom of the gradient and the macrophages and lymphocytes remained at the top of the gradient (data not shown).

In contrast to normal lung, the unfractionated single cell suspensions from the IPF lung were characterized by the presence of polymorphonuclear leukocytes in addition to macrophages, small numbers of lymphocytes, and lung parenchymal cells. After Hypaque-Ficoll centrifugation, the polymorphonuclear leukocytes and the lung parenchymal cells pelleted to the bottom of the gradient and the macrophages and lymphocytes remained at the top of the gradient (data not shown).

Compared with those from both normal and IPF lung, the unfractionated single cell suspensions from the sarcoid lung were characterized by the presence of large numbers of both lymphocytes and alveolar macrophages together with small numbers of eosinophils, basophils, and lung parenchymal cells; neutrophils were not present in these cell suspensions. After Hypaque-Ficoll centrifugation, the lung parenchymal cells, eosinophils, and basophils pelleted to the bottom of the gradient and the macrophages and lymphocytes remained at the top of the gradient (data not shown).

Comparison of the inflammatory and immune effector cells in lavage fluid and the lung biopsies. The cell yield per standard 100-ml bronchoalveolar lavage was $14 \pm 5 \times 10^6$ cells in normal subjects, $22 \pm 6 \times 10^6$ cells in patients with IPF, and $66 \pm 8 \times 10^6$ cells in patients with sarcoidosis (table 1).

An average of $7 \pm 3 \times 10^6$ inflammatory and immune effector cells/cm^3 of tissue were obtained from normal lung, $11 \pm 5 \times 10^6$ cells/cm^3 of lung tissue from patients with IPF, and $44 \pm 13 \times 10^6$ cells/cm^3 of lung tissue from patients with sarcoidosis (table 1). Sufficient numbers of cells were obtained from all biopsies to characterize the inflammatory and immune effector cells that were present in the lung tissues. This technique appeared to isolate almost all inflammatory and immune effector cells from the biopsies since histologic analysis of the parenchymal tissue that remained after teasing the specimens revealed only a rare macrophage, lymphocyte, or neutrophil (data not shown). Using the total number of red blood cells recovered in the biopsies as a reference, the percentages of blood-derived mononuclear cells were calculated; in all cases it was < 3%.

In the normal lung, the percentages of lymphocytes were 7 ± 1% in lavage fluid and 16 ± 4% in the unfractionated cell suspensions from the lung biopsies ($p < 0.01$) (figure 1). Polymorphonuclear leukocytes were rarely present in either lavage fluid or in the cell suspensions from the lung biopsies. Macrophages comprised the rest of the cell differential in both the lavage and biopsy cell suspensions. The other lung cells present in the unfractionated cell suspensions that were not considered inflammatory and immune effector cells were not included in the cell differentials.

In the IPF lung, the percentages of lymphocytes were 5 ± 3% in lavage fluid and 14 ± 5% in the unfractionated biopsy cell suspensions (figure 2). The percentages of these cells in lavage fluid and the lung biopsies were not significantly different from those in lavage fluid and lung biopsies of normal lung ($p > 0.2$, each comparison). In contrast to the normal lung, there was a marked increase in the percentages of polymorphonuclear leukocytes, primarily neutrophils but including eosinophils, in both lavage fluid and in

TABLE 1

ABSOLUTE NUMBER OF INFLAMMATORY AND IMMUNE EFFECTOR CELLS RECOVERED FROM OPEN LUNG BIOPSIES AND BRONCHOALVEOLAR LAVAGE FLUID OF PATIENTS WITH SARCOIDOSIS AND IPF AND NORMAL CONTROL SUBJECTS

	Cell Yield ($\times 10^{-6}$)	
Patient Groups	Biopsy*	Lavage Fluid†
Sarcoidosis	44 ± 13‡	66 ± 8
IPF	11 ± 5	22 ± 6
Normal subjects	7 ± 3§	14 ± 5‖

* Cell yield per cm^3 of lung tissue.
† Cell yield per standard 100 ml lavage.
‡ Mean ± SEM.
§ Includes normal lung from 3 patients with solitary lung nodules; *see* Methods.
‖ Includes 6 normal volunteers; *see* Methods.

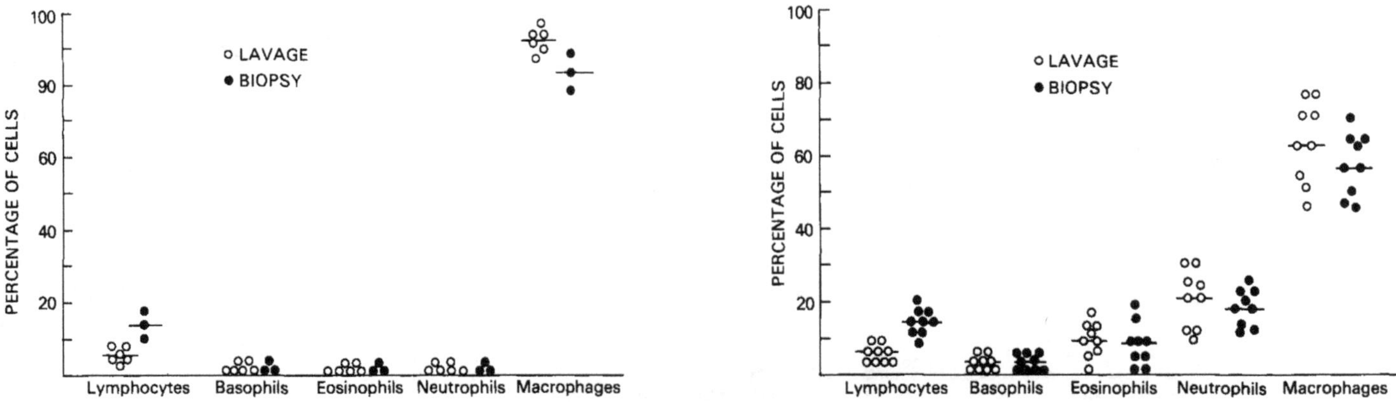

Fig. 1. (*left*) Inflammatory and immune effector cells obtained from bronchoalveolar lavage and open lung biopsies of normal lung. The percentage of cells is on the ordinate, and various cell types including macrophages, lymphocytes, basophils, eosinophils, and neutrophils are indicated on the abscissa. The data represent the mean ± SEM of cells from bronchoalveolar lavage of 6 normal subjects and cells from biopsies of 3 normal subjects. Fig. 2. (*right*) Inflammatory and immune effector cells obtained from bronchoalveolar lavage and open lung biopsies of patients with idiopathic pulmonary fibrosis. The percentage of cells is on the ordinate, and various cell types including macrophages, lymphocytes, basophils, eosinophils, and neutrophils are indicated on the abscissa. The data represent the cells from bronchoalveolar lavage and open lung biopsies of 9 patients with IPF.

the lung biopsies of patients with IPF ($p < 0.01$, each comparison). There was no significant difference in the percentages of either neutrophils or eosinophils in lavage fluid of patients with IPF compared with the IPF biopsy cell suspensions ($p > 0.2$, each comparison). Macrophages comprised the rest of the cell differentials in both the lavage and biopsy cell suspensions.

In the sarcoid lung, there was a marked increase in the percentages of lymphocytes in both lavage fluid and lung biopsies, compared with both control subjects and patients with IPF ($p < 0.01$, all comparisons) (figure 3). There was no significant difference in the percentages of lymphocytes in lavage fluid compared with the biopsy cell suspensions in patients with sarcoidosis (48 ± 12% versus 57 ± 7%, respectively, $p > 0.2$). In addition, there were no significant numbers of neutrophils in the lung of these patients. However, 2 to 3% basophils and eosinophils were routinely present in both lavage fluid and the biopsy cell suspensions. Macrophages comprised the rest of the cell differential in both the lavage and biopsy cell suspensions.

Comparisons of lymphocyte subpopulations in lavage fluid and the biopsy cell suspensions. In normal subjects, the percentages of T-lymphocytes, "activated" T-lymphocytes, and B-lymphocytes were similar in cell suspensions from lavage fluid and from lung parenchyma ($p > 0.2$). In addition, in patients with IPF or with sarcoidosis there also were no differences in the proportions of each of these lymphocyte subpopulations in cell suspensions isolated from lavage fluid compared with those isolated from lung parenchyma ($p > 0.2$, each comparison). Thus, the lymphocytes in lavage fluid reflected those present in the lung parenchyma in normal subjects as well as in patients with IPF or sarcoidosis (figure 4).

There were no significant differences in the percentages of T-lymphocytes, "activated" T-lymphocytes, or B-lymphocytes between control subjects and patients with IPF in either the lavage cell suspensions or the post-Hypaque-Ficoll biopsy cell suspensions ($p > 0.2$, all comparisons). In patients with sarcoidosis, however, the percentages of T-lymphocytes and "activated" T-lymphocytes were significantly increased in both lavage fluid and in the lung biopsies, compared with both the normal and the IPF lung ($p < 0.01$, all comparisons). In contrast, the percentages of B-lymphocytes were significantly decreased in both lavage fluid and lung biopsies of patients with sarcoidosis, compared with the normal and IPF lung ($p < 0.01$, all comparisons). Although the percentages of B-lymphocytes were decreased in the lung of patients with sarcoidosis, it is likely that the absolute numbers of these cells as well as the T-lymphocytes were actually increased because of the marked increase in the total number of lymphocytes that were present in the lungs of these patients.

Discussion

From histologic studies, it has been known for some time that the cell populations of the alveolar structures of the human lung include significant numbers of inflammatory and immune effector cells (1–14). The present study demonstrated that these effector cells can be isolated directly from lung biopsies in numbers adequate to characterize them. By comparing the effector cell populations present in biopsies of normal, IPF, and sarcoid lung, it has become apparent that the inflammatory and immune effector cells present in the IPF and the sarcoid lung are markedly different from those in normal lung and from each other. In addition, these studies have also shown that the proportions of effector cells recovered by bronchoalveolar lavage of patients with IPF or sarcoidosis closely resemble the proportions of effector cells actually present within the alveolar structures of the lungs of these patients. This observation, together with the study which demonstrated that samples of lavage fluid obtained from different sites within the lung contain a similar composition of cell types (18) validates the concept that bronchoalveolar lavage is a useful technique by which to characterize the alveolitis of these disorders.

Effector cells in the normal lung. Consistent with histologic studies, most of the inflammatory and immune effector cells isolated directly from normal lung were alveolar macrophages; a smaller proportion were lymphocytes. The lymphocytes present were primarily T-lymphocytes; most of these cells were not activated. The B-lymphocytes were also present, but in much smaller numbers than the T-lymphocytes. In normal lung, polymorphonuclear leukocytes were rarely found.

Lavage of the normal lung yielded

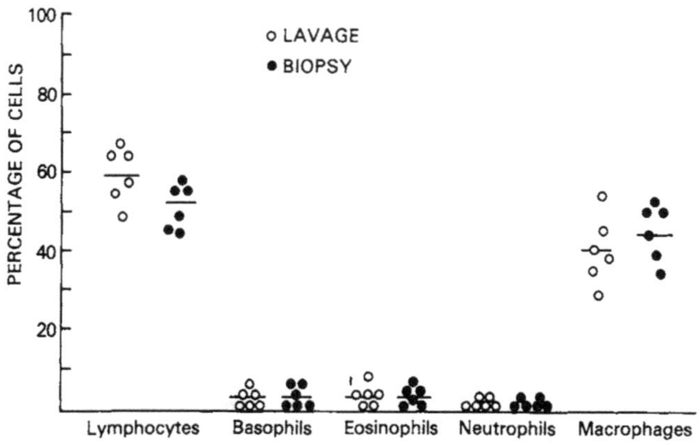

Fig. 3. Inflammatory and immune effector cells obtained from bronchoalveolar lavage and open lung biopsies of patients with pulmonary sarcoidosis. The percentage of cells is on the ordinate, and various cell types including macrophages, lymphocytes, basophils, eosinophils, and neutrophils are indicated on the abscissa. The data represent the cells from bronchoalveolar lavage and open lung biopsies of 6 patients with sarcoidosis.

similar results. The only significant difference between the effector cells recovered from the biopsies of normal lung and the lavage of normal lung was that a relatively larger proportion of lymphocytes were present in the parenchyma than was reflected by lavage analysis. This observation was consistent with animal studies (29) and histologic observations (30) of human lung showing that, in normal lung parenchyma, the majority of lymphocytes are in the interstitium, not in the alveolar air spaces. However, analysis of the lymphocytes present in lavage did accurately reflect the distribution of lymphocyte subtypes in the alveolar structures (figure 4).

Effector cells in the IPF lung. In contrast to the normal lung, the effector cells isolated from biopsies of patients with IPF were characterized by the presence of large proportions of neutrophils. The proportions and subtypes of lymphocytes, however, closely resembled those of normal lung.

Analysis of effector cells recovered by bronchoalveolar lavage of the same IPF patients revealed similar results. This is particularly important in relation to the neutrophils found in lavage of these patients (10, 11, 13, 17–21). Although patients with IPF do not as a rule have bronchitis, lavage samples containing neutrophils must be interpreted in the context that clinically occult inflammatory airway disease might be present, and thus the neutrophils might be airway, rather than alveolar, derived. However, the fact that the proportions of neutrophils recovered from IPF parenchymal biopsies were similar to those in lavage strongly supported the concept that bronchoalveolar lavage of these patients yields a valid assessment of the character and intensity of the alveolitis that is present.

Effector cells in the sarcoid lung. The inflammatory and immune effector cells associated with the alveolitis of sarcoidosis were characterized by much larger proportions of lymphocytes than were found in either the normal or the IPF lung. Not only were there increased proportions of lymphocytes in the sarcoid lung, but more of these lymphocytes were T-lymphocytes and more of these T-lymphocytes were "activated." In addition, the alveolitis of sarcoid lung was further distinguished by the absence of neutrophils from the alveolar structures of these patients.

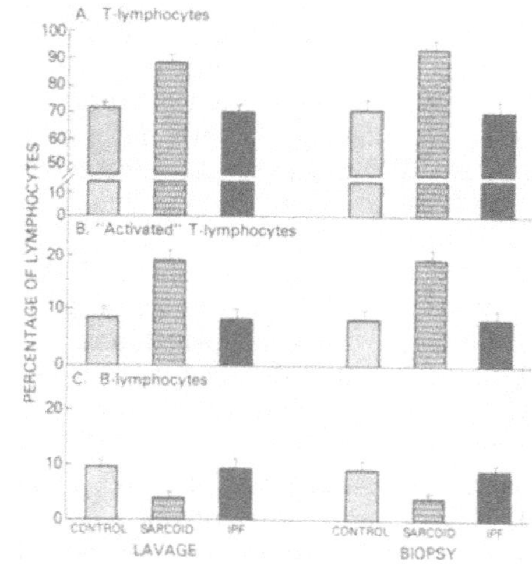

Fig. 4. Lymphocyte subpopulations in bronchoalveolar lavage fluid and open lung biopsies of patients with normal lung and patients with IPF and sarcoidosis. The percentage of lymphocytes is on the ordinate and the source of cells is indicated on the abscissa. A. percentage of T-lymphocytes; B. percentage of "activated" T-lymphocytes; C. percentage of B-lymphocytes. The lavage data represent the mean ± SEM of cells obtained from 6 normal subjects, 9 patients with IPF, and 6 patients with sarcoidosis; and the biopsy data represent cells obtained from 3 normal subjects, 9 patients with IPF, and 6 patients with sarcoidosis.

When the alveolitis of sarcoidosis was characterized by lavage techniques, it was found to consist of increased proportions of activated T-lymphocytes (10–13, 19–21, 31–35), similar to what was found on direct analysis of the biopsy specimens. Thus, as in IPF, lavage is a valid means to assess the alveolitis of sarcoidosis.

The present study demonstrated that adequate numbers of effector cells can be isolated directly from biopsies of normal subjects and patients with common forms of interstitial lung disease. These techniques should be generally applicable to the evaluation of other interstitial disorders and permit a validation of lavage assessments of the alveolitis of each disease. In addition, the numbers of effector cells recovered from the biopsies are sufficient to permit detailed characterizations of the types and functions of various subpopulations of effector cells comprising the alveolitis of these disorders. This should prove useful in helping to understand the pathogenesis of the interstitial lung diseases, and also in staging the intensity of the alveolitis of individual patients. The latter is critical in terms of making rational therapy decisions in these disorders.

References

1. Spencer H. Interstitial pneumonia. Annu Rev Med 1967; 18:423–42.

2. Scadding JG, Hinson KFW. Diffuse fibrosing alveolitis (diffuse interstitial fibrosis of the lungs): correlation with histology at biopsy with prognosis. Thorax 1967; 22:291–304.

3. Hinson KFW. Diffuse pulmonary fibrosis. Hum Pathol 1970; 1:275–88.

4. Scadding JG. Diffuse pulmonary alveolar fibrosis. Thorax 1974; 29:271–81.

5. Crystal RG, Fulmer JD, Roberts WC, Moss ML, Line BR, Reynolds HY. Idiopathic pulmonary fibrosis: clinical, histologic, radiographic, physiologic, scintigraphic, cytologic and biochemical aspects. Ann Intern Med 1976;85: 769–88.

6. Fulmer JD, Crystal RG. The biochemical basis of pulmonary function. In: Crystal RG, ed, The Biochemical Basis of Pulmonary Function. New York: Marcel Dekker, 1976:419–66.

7. Weinburger SE, Crystal RG. Reactions of the interstitial space to injury. In: Fishman AP, ed, Textbook of pulmonary diseases. New York: McGraw-Hill, 1979:640–47.

8. Basset F, Soler P, Bernandin JF. Contribu-

tion of electron microscopy to the study of interstitial pneumonias. Prog Respir Dis 1975; 8:45–58.

9. Brody AR, Craighead JE. Interstitial association of cells lining air spaces in human pulmonary fibrosis. Virchows Arch [Pathol Anat] 1976; 372:39–49.

10. Fulmer JD, Crystal RG. Interstitial lung disease. In: Simmons DH, ed, Current pneumonology. Boston: Houghton Mifflin, 1979:1–65.

11. Hunninghake GW, Gadek JE, Kawanami O, Ferrans VJ, Crystal RG. Inflammatory and immune processes in the human lung in health and disease: evaluation by bronchoalveolar lavage. Am J Pathol 1979; 97:149–206.

12. Crystal RG, Roberts WC, Hunninghake GW, Gadek JE, Fulmer JD, Line BR. Pulmonary sarcoidosis: a disease characterized and perpetuated by activated lung T-lymphocytes. Ann Intern Med (in press).

13. Crystal RG, Ferrans VJ, Gadek JE, Fulmer JD. Line BR, Hunninghake GW. Interstitial lung disease: current concepts of pathogenesis, staging, and therapy. Am J Med (in press).

14. Rosen Y, Athanassiades TJ, Moon S, Lyons HA. Nongranulomatous interstitial pneumonitis in sarcoidosis. Relationship to development of epithelioid granulomas. Chest 1978; 74:122–5.

15. Finley TN, Swenson EW, Curran WS, Huber GL, Todman AJ. Bronchopulmonary lavage in normal subjects and patients with obstructive lung disease. Ann Intern Med 1967; 66:651–8.

16. Reynolds HY, Newball HH. Analysis of proteins and respiratory cells obtained from human lungs by bronchial lavage. J Lab Clin Med 1974; 84:559–73.

17. Reynolds HY, Fulmer JD, Kazmierowski JA, Roberts WC, Frank MM, Crystal RG. Analysis of bronchoalveolar lavage fluid from patients with idopathic pulmonary fibrosis and chronic hypersensitivity pneumonitis. J Clin Invest 1977; 59:165–75.

18. Weinberger SE, Kelman JA, Elson NA, *et al.* Broncholalveolar lavage in interstitial lung disease. Ann Intern Med 1978; 89:459–66.

19. Hunninghake GW, Fulmer JD, Young RC, Crystal RG. Comparison of lung and blood lymphocyte subpopulations in pulmonary sarcoidosis. In: Eighth International Congress on Sarcoidosis and Other Granulomatous Diseases 1980 (in press).

20. Hunninghake GW, Gadek JE, Szapiel SV, *et al.* The human alveolar macrophage. In: Harris CC, Trump BF, Stoner GD, eds, Methods and perspectives in cell biology: cultured human cells and tissues in biomedical research. New York: Academic Press, 1980 (in press).

21. Hunninghake GW, Fulmer JD, Young RC, Gadek JE, Crystal RG. Localization of the immune response in sarcoidosis. Am Rev Respir Dis 1979; 120:49–57.

22. Daniele RP, Altrose MD, Rowlands DT. Immunocompetent cells from the lower respiratory tract of normal human lungs. J Clin Invest 1925; 56:986.

23. Boyum A. Isolation of mononuclear cells and granulocytes from human blood. Scand J Clin Invest 1968; 21:77–82.

24. Weiner MS, Bianco C, Nussenzweig V. Enhanced binding of neuraminidase-treated sheep erythrocytes to human T-lymphocytes. Blood 1976; 42:939–44.

25. Papamichail M, Brown JC, Holborow EJ. Immunoglobulins in the surface of human lymphocytes. Lancet 1971; 2:850–52.

26. Wybran JM, Carr C, Fudenberg HH. The human rosette-forming cell as a marker of a population of thymus-derived cells. J Clin Invest 1972; 51:2537–42.

27. Katoh AK, Charoensiri S. The formation of stable E-rosettes by human T-lymphocytes activated by photohemagglutinin. J Immunol 1977; 118:2291–94.

28. Yu DTY. Human lymphocyte subpopulations: suspension-sheep-red-blood cell rosettes. Clin Immunol Immunopathol 1977; 8:190–6.

29. Hunninghake GW, Fauci AS. Immunological reactivity of the lung. I. A guinea pig model for the study of pulmonary mononuclear cell subpopulations. Cell Immunol 1976; 26:89–97.

30. Bienenstock J, Clancy RL, Perey DY. Bronchus associated lymphoid tissue (BALT), its relationship to mucosal immunity. In: Kirkpatrick CH, Reynolds HY, eds, Immunologic and infectious reactions in the lung. New York: Marcel Dekker, 1976:29–58.

31. Reynolds HY. The importance of lymphocytes in pulmonary health and disease. Lung 1978; 155:225–42.

32. Gee JBL, Bodel PT, Zorn SK, Hinman LM, Stevens CA, Matthay RA. Sarcoidosis and mononuclear phagocytes. Lung 1978; 115:243–53.

33. Danel C, Arnoux A, Marsac J, Basset F, Chretien J. Cellular data from bronchoalveolar lavages in various interstitial disease. Bull Eur Physiopathol Respir 1979; 15:42–3P.

34. Rossman MD, Daniele RP, Dauber JH. Bronchoalveolar lymphocytes in sarcoidosis. J Lab Clin Med 1979; 94:862–71.

35. Yeager H, Williams MC, Beckman JF, Bayly TC, Beaman BL, Hawley RJ. Sarcoidosis: analysis of cells obtained by bronchial lavage. Am Rev Respir Dis 1977; 116:951–5.

Mitral valve "anular" calcium forming a complete circle or "O" configuration: Clinical and necropsy observations

Attention is called to the occurrence of a complete circle or "O"-shaped ring of calcium at the mitral anular region in each of two women, aged 67 and 82 years. Extension of mitral anular calcium from behind the posterior mitral leaflet across the ventricular aspect of the anterior mitral leaflet to form a complete circle has not been reported previously. (Am Heart J 101:619, 1981.)

William C. Roberts, M.D., and Bruce F. Waller, M.D. *Bethesda, Md.*

Calcification of the mitral anulus is a common occurrence in hearts of older persons in the Western World. The anular calcific deposits on radiographs generally are "J," "C," or "U"-shaped because they are located nearly always entirely in or below the anulus of the posterior mitral leaflet. Recently, we encountered two patients in whom calcific deposits not only were located in and beneath the anulus of the *posterior* mitral leaflet, but they extended across the ventricular aspect of the *anterior* leaflet to form a complete calcific circle or "O." Because we have not encountered this "O" configuration in over 200 other patients with mitral anular calcium studied at necropsy in our laboratory[1] and because we have found no reports by others describing a complete circumferential calcific ring at the site of the mitral "anulus," a brief description of the clinical and morphologic findings in our two patients appeared warranted.

From the Pathology Branch, National Heart, Lung and Blood Institute, National Institutes of Health.

Received for publication Jan. 7, 1981; accepted Jan. 29, 1981.

Reprint requests: Dr. William C. Roberts, Bldg. 10A, Room 3E30, National Institutes of Health, Bethesda, MD 20205.

METHODS AND RESULTS

Pertinent clinical and morphologic features in the two patients are summarized in Table I. Both were older women who died of noncardiovascular conditions. Both had precordial murmurs consistent with mitral regurgitation and one had a murmur of aortic stenosis. Neither patient had chest pain consistent with myocardial ischemia and neither had evidence of congestive cardiac failure. One had systemic hypertension, diabetes mellitus (adult onset), and chronic atrial fibrillation. Chest radiographs (Fig. 1) in each disclosed heavy mitral anular calcific deposits.

At necropsy, the hearts of both were mildly increased in weight. Neither had dilated cardiac ventricles, but both had dilated atria. One had severe (> 75% in cross-sectional area) narrowing of all three major epicardial coronary arteries by atherosclerotic plaques. The mitral "anular" circular calcium in each is shown in Figs. 2 and 3. Patient No. 2 also had calcific deposits in the aortic valve cusps to an extent to produce aortic valve stenosis. Both also had relatively heavy calcific deposits in the aorta, arch and abdominal portions. Patient No. 1 had a small transmural left ventricular scar.

DISCUSSION

Extension of calcium from the anulus of the posterior mitral leaflet across the ventricular aspect

Table I. Clinical and morphologic findings in patients with circle "O" mitral anular calcium

Pt.	Age (yrs)	Associated disease	Murmurs MR	Murmurs AS	SH	DM	AF	Cause of death	Heart wt. (gm)	Calcium (0-4+) AV	Calcium (0-4+) CA	Calcium (0-4+) Ao	AS	CA > 75%
1	67	Habitual alcoholism	3/6	0	+	+	+	Werniche's encephalopathy	390	0	2+	3+	0	+
2	82	Paget's, bone	3/6	2/6	0	0	0	Caecal volvulus	400	3+	2+	2+	+	0

Abbreviations: AF = atrial fibrillation; Ao = aorta; AS = aortic valve stenosis; AV = aortic valve; CA = coronary arteries; DM = diabetes mellitus; MR = mitral regurgitation; SH = systemic hypertension.

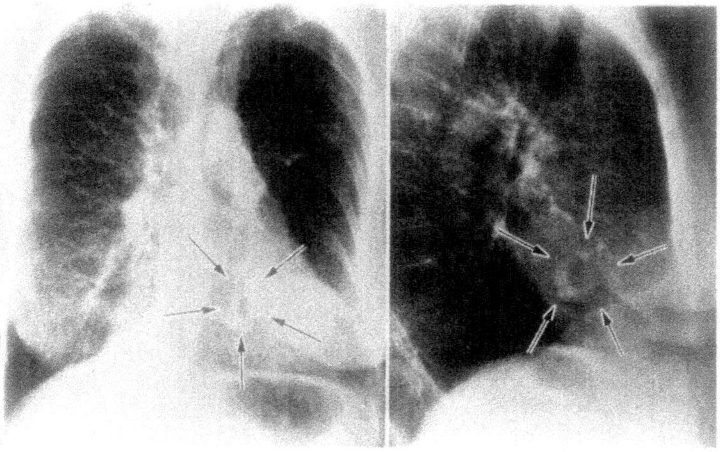

Fig. 1. Patient No. 1. Posteroanterior *(left)* and lateral *(right)* radiographs showing mitral anular calcium forming a complete circle *(arrows)*.

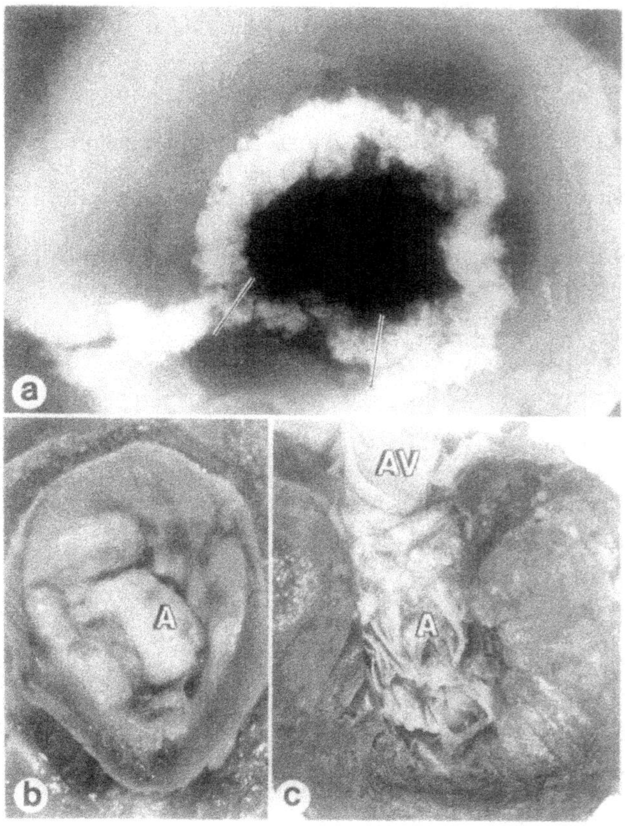

Fig. 2. Patient No. 1. Heart at necropsy. *a*, Radiograph of the heart specimen showing complete circle of "anular" calcium. The short distance between the lines designates the width of the anterior mitral leaflet. *b*, View of mitral valve from left atrium. *A* = anterior mitral leaflet. *c*, Opened left ventricular outflow tract and aortic valve *(AV)* showing calcium extending across the anterior *(A)* mitral leaflet.

of the *anterior* mitral leaflet to form a complete circle of calcium has not been reported previously to our knowledge. The stimulus to its extension across the anterior leaflet is unknown. It should be recalled that the anterior mitral leaflet does not have a true anulus because its ventricular aspect is continuous with the wall of the aorta and the aortic valve cusps and its atrial aspect is continuous with the mural endocardium of the atrial septum. The posterior mitral leaflet, in contrast, represents in effect the caudal extension of the mural endocardium of the entire free wall of left atrium. The site where the posterior mitral leaflet meets mural endocardium of left atrial free wall is the mitral anulus.

Calcium rarely is limited, however, to just the anulus, or if it were it would not be visible by radiography during life. Radiographically visible anular calcium in actuality is located primarily beneath the anulus, in the angle between posterior mitral leaflet and mural endocardium of left ventricle. The linear bar of calcium which extended across the anterior mitral leaflet in our two patients was located only on the ventricular aspect of the leaflet and at a level caudal to the anulus behind the posterior mitral leaflet. Thus because the anterior leaflet lacks a true anulus and because the calcium attached to it was located caudal to that behind posterior mitral leaflet, it is actually improper to designate the bar of calcium extending across anterior leaflet as "anular," although for convenience and to prevent confusion with leaflet calcium observed in patients with rheumatic mitral stenosis, calcium extending across the anterior leaflet and

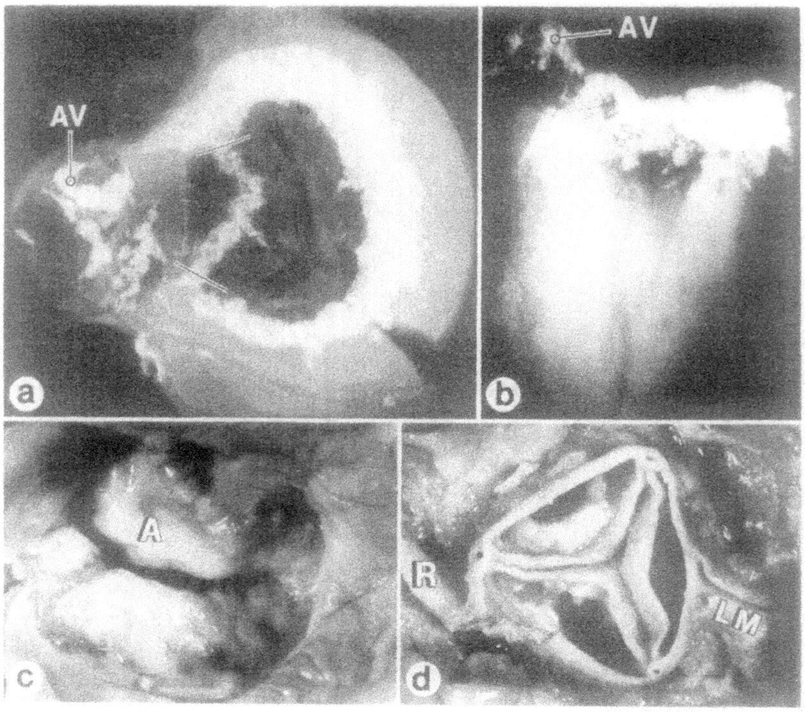

Fig. 3. Patient No. 2. Heart at necropsy. *a,* Radiograph of heart specimen. The short bar of calcium *between the lines* is that extending across the anterior mitral leaflet. Calcific deposits also are present in the aortic valve *(A V)* cusps and in coronary arterial atherosclerotic plaques. *b,* Radiograph of heart, lateral view, showing massive mitral anular calcific deposits. *c,* Mitral valve from left atrium. *A* = anterior mitral leaflet. *d,* Aortic valve from above showing calcific deposits on the aortic aspects of each of the three cusps. *R* = right and *LM* = left main coronary artery.

continuous with that in the angle behind posterior mitral leaflet might, nevertheless, be considered "anular."

Despite the circumferential nature of the mitral calcific deposits in our two patients, neither had functional (diastolic apical murmur or evidence of pulmonary venous or arterial hypertension) or anatomic evidence of mitral stenosis.

REFERENCE

1. Roberts WC, Perloff JK: Mitral valvular disease. A clinicopathologic survey of the conditions causing the mitral valve to function abnormally. Ann Intern Med **77**:939, 1972.

Selected Reports

Carcinoma of the Lung Causing Pulmonary Arterial Stenosis*

Bruce F. Waller, M.D., F.C.C.P.; Ross D. Fletcher, M.D.; and William C. Roberts, M.D., F.C.C.P.

A patient is described in whom carcinoma of the lung caused compression and obstruction of the left and right main pulmonary arteries and auscultatory features of peripheral pulmonary arterial stenosis.

Herein we describe findings in a man with carcinoma of the lung causing auscultatory features of peripheral pulmonary arterial stenosis. To our knowledge, such a patient has not been described previously.

Case Report

A 55-year-old man was healthy until January 1977 (11 months before death), when left anterior chest pain and dyspnea first appeared. He had smoked a package of cigarettes daily for 30 years. The mean jugular venous pressure was equivalent to about 6 cm of water, and a prominent A wave was visible. The carotid arterial pulse was normal. The breath sounds were decreased, and the percussion note was dull over the left chest. A right ventricular impulse was easily palpable. The second heart sound at the base was widely split on inspiration, and never became single during expiration (Fig 1). The pulmonary component of the second heart sound was increased in intensity. A third heart sound, S_3, was present over the right sternal border. A grade 3/6 systolic ejection murmur was heard over the precordium, both axillae and back, loudest over the second right and left intercostal spaces, and the murmur increased in intensity with inspiration, especially along the right sternal border and in the right axilla. No diastolic murmurs were heard. An ECG showed prominent left ventricular voltage and nonspecific ST segment and T wave changes. His chest roentgenogram (Fig 2) disclosed complete opacification of the left lung field. An echocardiogram was consistent with pulmonary hypertension.

Tissue obtained from the left main stem bronchus showed small-cell carcinoma. At right-sided cardiac catheterization, the pressures (in mm Hg) were as follows: right atrium, a = 8, v = 7); right ventricle, 55/10; pulmonary trunk, 55/10; proximal right pulmonary artery, 55/10, and distal right pulmonary artery, 22/10 (Fig 1). Right atrial angiogram (Fig 2) disclosed normal right atrial and ventricular cavities and pulmonary trunk, but severe narrowing of the left main and moderate narrowing of the right main pulmonary arteries.

The patient received chemotherapy and local irradiation, and a chest roentgenogram four weeks later showed considerable clearing of the left lung field. Moreover, the intensity of the systolic ejection murmur had decreased to grade 1/6.

*From the Pathology Branch, National Heart, Lung, and Blood Institute, National Institutes of Health, Bethesda, Md, and the Division of Cardiology, Department of Medicine, Veterans Administration Hospital, Washington, D.C.
Reprint requests: Dr. Roberts, Building 10A, Room 3E30, National Institutes of Health, Bethesda 20205

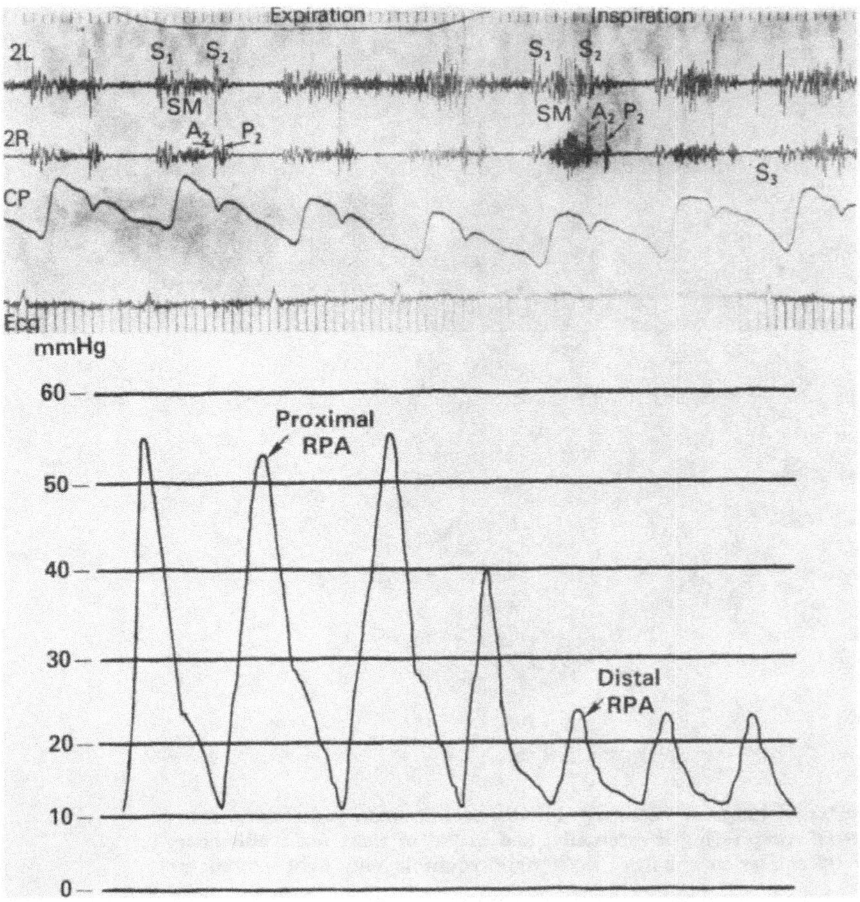

FIGURE 1. Phonocardiogram *(upper)* recorded at second left (2L) and right (2R) intercostal spaces showing systolic murmurs (SM) and a persistently split second heart sound (S_2). A_2= aortic component of S_2, CP=external carotid pulse; P_2=pulmonic component of S_2; S_1=first heart sound; S_3=third heart sound. Pressure tracing *(lower)* with pullback from distal to proximal right main pulmonary artery (RPA).

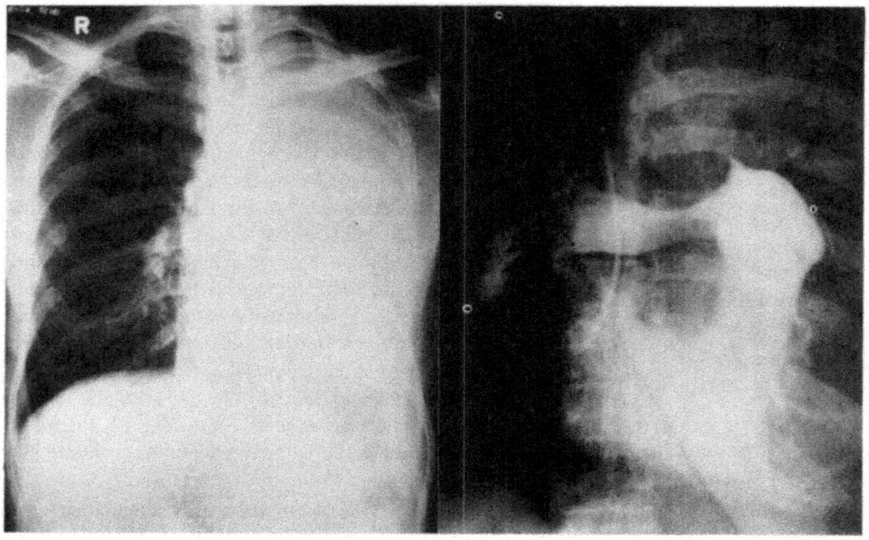

Figure 2. Posteroanterior chest roentgenogram *(left)* showing opacification of left lung field and angiogram *(right)* with injection into right atrium demonstrating severe luminal narrowing of left main and moderate narrowing of right main pulmonary arteries. Roentgenograms done 11 months before death.

He slowly deteriorated, however, and died ten months later (November 1977). His only evidence of right-sided congestive heart failure at any time was the presence of a third heart sound, which varied with respiration.

At necropsy, both right and left lung parenchyma and pleura were extensively replaced by carcinoma (Fig 3). The left main bronchus and pulmonary artery were severely compressed by tumor. The right main pulmonary artery was partially compressed by surrounding tumor. A large cavity filled with necrotic tumor was present in the upper left lobe. Histologic sections showed tumor invasion of the walls of the right and left main pulmonary arteries and intrapulmonary arteries. The heart weighed 420 g, and the right ventricle was dilated.

Discussion

Although many reports have described exterior compression of one or more major extrapulmonary pulmonary arteries by neoplasm, auscultatory evidence of obstruction to one or more major pulmonary arteries has not been documented previously. In our patient, total obstruction to the left main pulmonary artery and partial obstruction to the right main pulmonary artery was documented by both angiography (during life) and

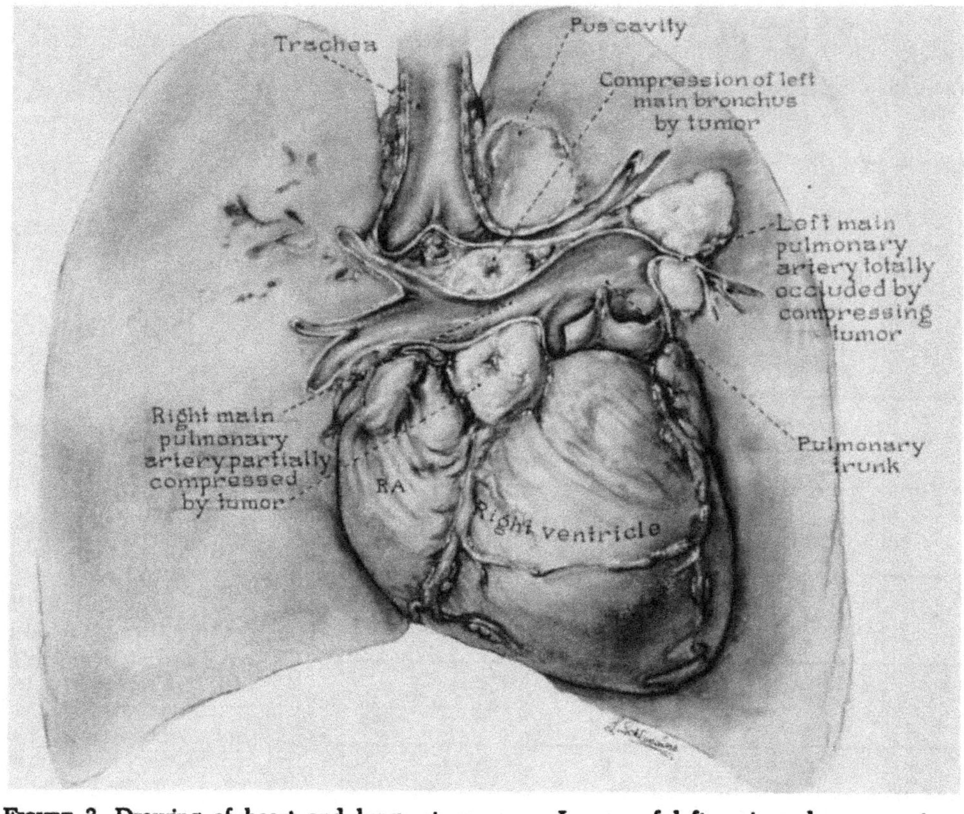

Figure 3. Drawing of heart and lungs at necropsy. Lumen of left main pulmonary artery totally occluded by carcinoma, compressing it externally, and lumen of right main pulmonary artery partially obstructed by similar mechanism. Both right ventricle and right atrium are dilated.

necropsy, and a 33 mm Hg peak systolic pressure gradient between proximal and distal right main pulmonary artery was found at catheterization. The wide splitting of the second heart sound at the cardiac base in our patient can be attributed to the peripheral pulmonary stenosis. There was not enough right ventricular failure (only a third heart sound) in the presence of the pulmonary hypertension in our patient to account for the wide splitting of the second heart sound.

ACKNOWLEDGMENT: The authors thank W. Proctor Harvey, M.D., Chief, Division of Cardiology, Department of Medicine, Georgetown University, Washington, D.C., for reviewing the manuscript and for making useful suggestions.

False Aneurysm of the Ascending Aorta Presenting as an Acute Myocardial Infarction*

A Late Complication of Aortocoronary Bypass

Martin Morissette, M.D.; Jean Lemire, M.D.; Normand Poirier, M.D.; and Paul Bettez, M.D.

After coronary bypass surgery, a 40-year-old man developed disruption of the site of cannulation of the ascending aorta. The false aneurysm which ensued presented as recurrent episodes of spontaneous angina and myocardial infarction ending in coronary death 48 days after surgery. The aortic origin of all three permeable coronary bypasses were strangulated by the hematoma. Awareness of this unusual potential hazard is essential, since an early suspicion would lead to proper diagnostic interventions and reoperation.

The surgical risk of aortocoronary bypass has progressively decreased from about 8 to less than 2 percent.[1,2] With the improvement of techniques and a better selection of patients, the relative frequency of unexpected death tends to increase.[3] We describe an unusual clinical presentation of a false aneurysm of the ascending aorta, provoking recurrent prolonged episodes of spontaneous angina, ending in coronary death 48 days after surgery.

Case Report

Ten months after an acute anteroseptal myocardial infarction, a 40-year-old man was readmitted for evaluation of angina pectoris refractory to conventional medical therapy. Selective coronary angiograms revealed severe three-vessel disease. The distal vascular bed was acceptable for coronary bypass. The left ventriculogram showed a small antero-apical dyskinetic area.

The surgery was performed under cardiopulmonary bypass and cryocardioplegia. The ascending aorta appeared normal macroscopically and was cannulated just proximal to the takeoff of the innominate artery. Six aortocoronary bypass grafts were completed, with three separate aortic ostia created for the saphenous vein. Each graft made a side-to-side before its end-to-side anastomosis. A thin antero-apical aneurysm was plicated. The site of cannulation of the ascending aorta was closed with 2-O silk using two pursestring sutures, one deep and one superficial. No Teflon felt was used. Before surgery and for the following two days, the patient received our routine antibiotics, consisting of prostaphyllin (2 gm intravenously every six hours) and streptomycin (0.5 gm intramuscularly every 12 hours).

The immediate postoperative course was unremarkable, despite a new myocardial infarction of the posteroinferior wall which was noted on the electrocardiogram. The patient was discharged on the ninth postoperative day.

Two weeks after surgery, the patient was readmitted after a 30-hour episode of supraventricular tachycardia. The rate was at 210 beats per minute at the time of admission. The patient had pulmonary edema. Electrocardioversion was performed. The congestive failure responded well to conventional medical therapy. The levels of cardiac enzymes did not rise. The patient returned home after ten days.

Three weeks later, the patient came to the emergency room, complaining of squeezing pain in the anterior portion of the chest similar to the pain of his previous myocardial infarction. The ECG revealed anterior subendocardial ischemia. The level of creatine phosphokinase was increased to more than twice normal. The patient became asymptomatic shortly after admission and remained so for 48 hours. He then sustained a severe pain in the anterior portion of the chest associated with

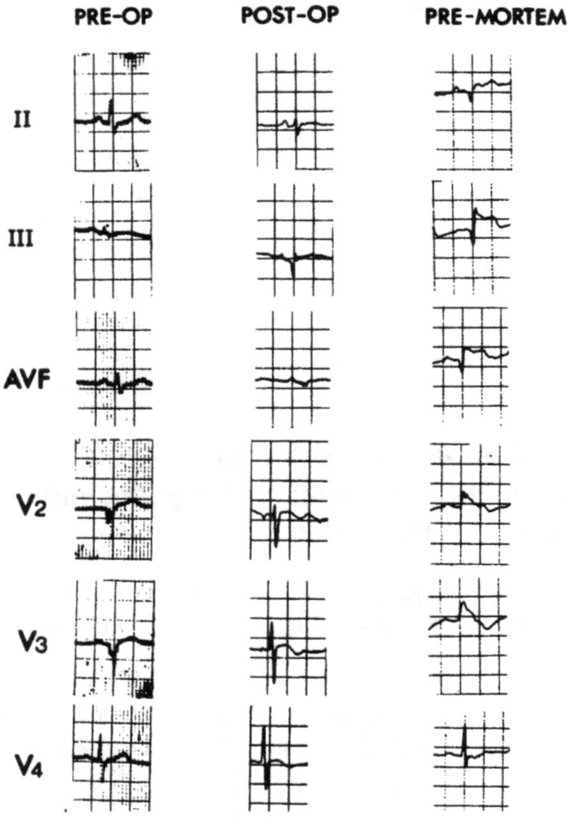

FIGURE 1. Evolution of ECGs. Postoperative tracing reveals presence of new infarction of posteroinferior wall. Premortem tracing shows acute anteroseptal and inferior subendocardial ischemia.

*From the Cardiovascular Division, Notre Dame Hospital, University of Montreal, Montreal, Quebec.
Reprint requests: Dr. Morissette, Notre Dame Hospital, 1560 Sherbrooke East, Montreal, Quebec, Canada H2L 4K8

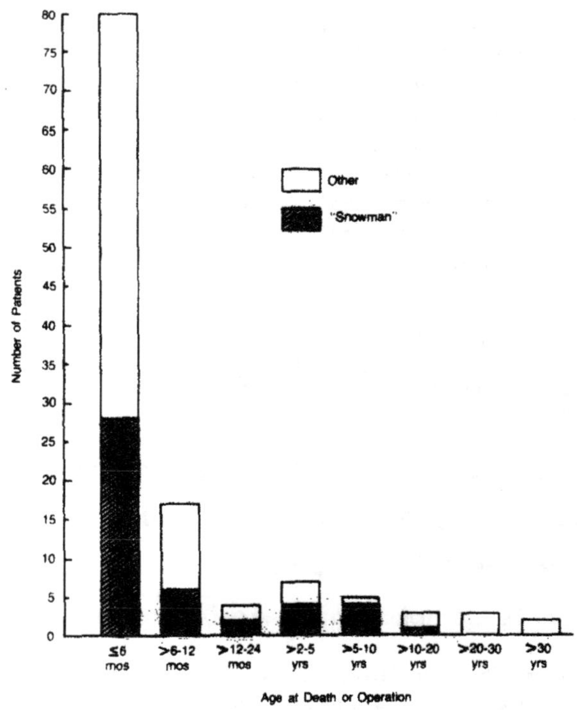

Fig. 1. Age at death or operation in 121 previously reported patients with isolated TAPVC.[1,2] Of those patients with the supracardiac "Snowman" type of TAPVC, 76% (34 of 45) had died or been operated upon by age 1 year, compared with 83% (63 of 76) of those with other types of TAPVC. Only five patients lived longer than 20 years of age and none of them had the "Snowman" type of pulmonary venous anomaly.

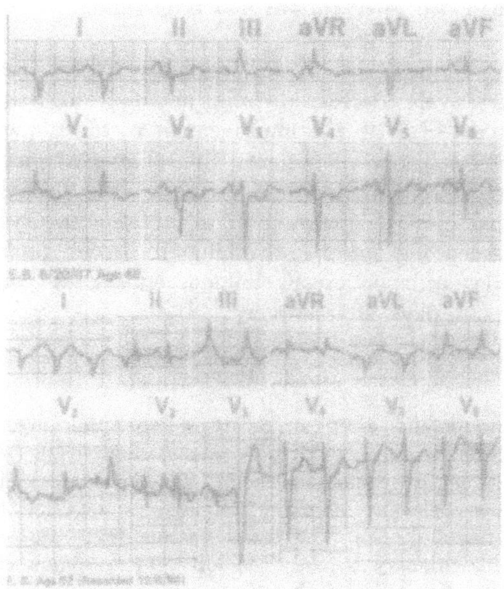

Fig. 2. Electrocardiograms at age 48 years, when the diagnosis of TAPVC was made initially, and at age 62 years, 2 days before death. On both occasions, sinus rhythm, right axis deviation, right atrial abnormality, and right ventricular hypertrophy are present.

Total anomalous pulmonary venous connection: Survival for 62 years without surgical intervention

Bruce M. McManus, M.D., Ph.D., Josef Luetzeler, M.D., and William C. Roberts, M.D. *Bethesda and Silver Spring, Md.*

Most patients with total anomalous pulmonary venous connection (TAPVC), irrespective of the drainage site,

From the Pathology Branch, National Heart, Lung and Blood Institute, National Institutes of Health; and the Department of Pathology, Holy Cross Hospital of Silver Spring.

Received for publication Sept. 28, 1981; accepted Oct. 6, 1981.

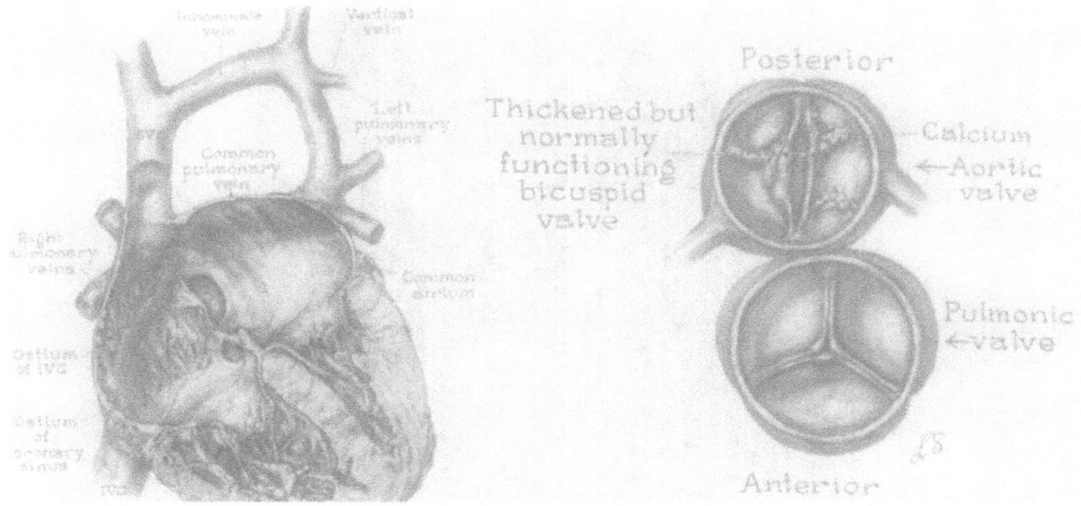

Fig. 3. Drawing of four-chamber view of the patient's heart illustrating the common atrium and anomalous pulmonary venous connection. Despite the presence of calcific deposits, the congenitally bicuspid aortic valve appears to have functioned normally. The anterior commissure of the aortic valve was not in apposition with the posterior commissure of the pulmonic valve as is normally the case. The pulmonic valve is normal, as was the right ventricular outflow tract.

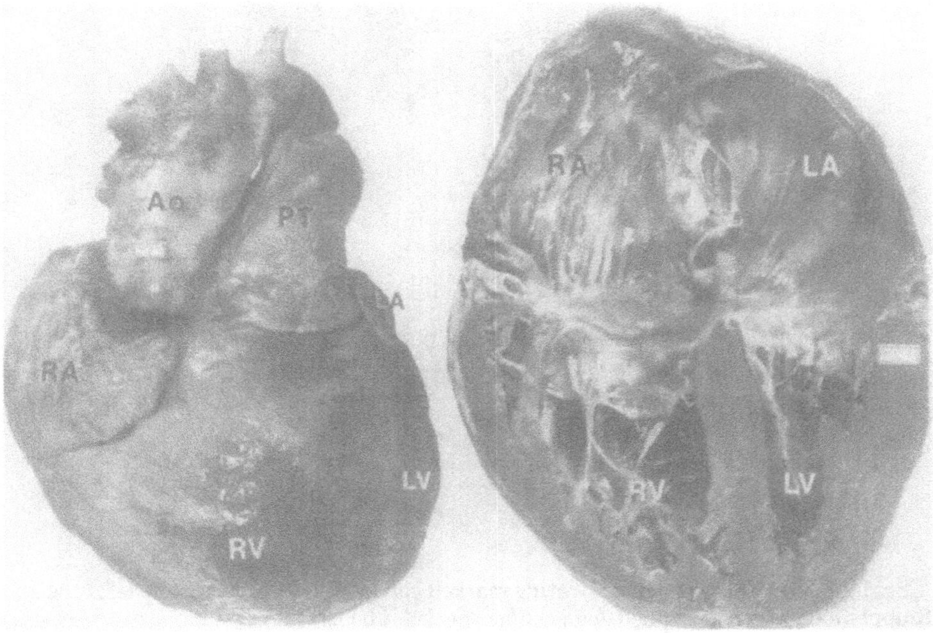

Fig. 4. Exterior *(left)* and interior *(right)* of heart. *Ao* = aorta; *LA* = left atrium; *LV* = left ventricle; *PT* = pulmonary trunk; *RA* = right atrium; *RV* = right ventricle. (Photographs by M.M.M. Moore)

live for less than 6 months.[1,2] Of reported nonoperated necropsy patients with TAPVC with drainage of a common pulmonary vein into the left innominate vein via a left vertical vein ("Snowman" type), none had survived as long as 10 years[1] (Fig. 1). The oldest reported patient with TAPVC of any type with necropsy verification was 39 years of age.[1] Recently, we studied at necropsy a 62-year-old man with unoperated TAPVC with drainage of a retroatrial common vein into the left innominate vein. He was cyanotic shortly after birth, acyanotic from about age 20 to 40 years, and cyanotic again during approximately his last 20 years. He was dyspneic on moderate exertion during his last 20 years. He had an acute febrile illness at age 48 years characterized by cough and excessive dyspnea. At that time chest roentgenogram disclosed cardiomegaly and a cavity in the left upper lobe. The pulmonic second sound was increased in intensity. After antibiotic therapy the signs suggestive of infection vanished. Because of cyanosis and cardiomegaly he underwent cardiac catheterization 6 months later. Pressures (mm Hg) and oxygen saturations (%) respectively were femoral artery (130/90, 78), left ventricle (110/3, 78), right ventri-

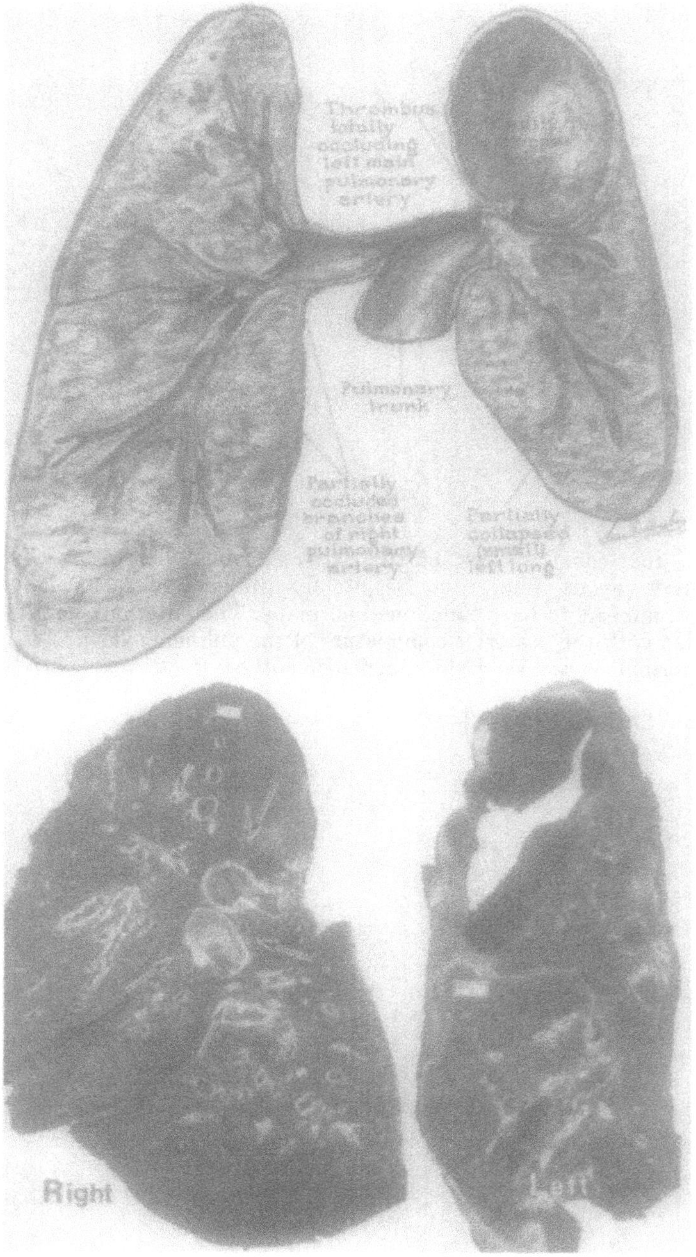

Fig. 5. The right and left lungs demonstrating marked collapse and fibrosis of the left lung and cavitation of the left upper lobe which contained *Aspergillus* species. The left main pulmonary artery was completely occluded by thrombus. Extensive thrombus also was present in the proximal branches of the right pulmonary artery *(arrows)*. The distal pulmonary arteries in the right lung are dilated.

cle (94/5, 78), left atrium (5, 76), right atrium (6, 78); oxygen saturations (%) superior vena cava (90), low left innominate vein (92), left subclavian vein (77), left brachial vein (59); and cardiac output 5.6 L/min. The ECG at that time and 2 days before death are shown in Fig. 2. He never had overt congestive cardiac failure or a precordial murmur. He died from complications of a perforated duodenal ulcer. The findings in the heart and lungs at necropsy are delineated in Figs. 3 to 6.

Besides lack of excessive pulmonary vascular resistance, survival in TAPVC appears to be dependent primarily on three factors: (1) the size of the defect in the atrial septum; (2) the length of the anomalous pulmonary veins(s), and (3) the degree of obstruction to flow in the anomalous pulmonary vein(s). Our patient appeared to have survived so long because of nearly ideal characteristics of each of these three factors. The atrial septum was virtually absent and therefore there was no interference to flow to the left side of the heart. The anomalous pulmonary vein was relatively short and free of any degree of obstruction. The cause of the total thrombotic occlusion of the left main pulmonary artery in our patient was not determined. It is

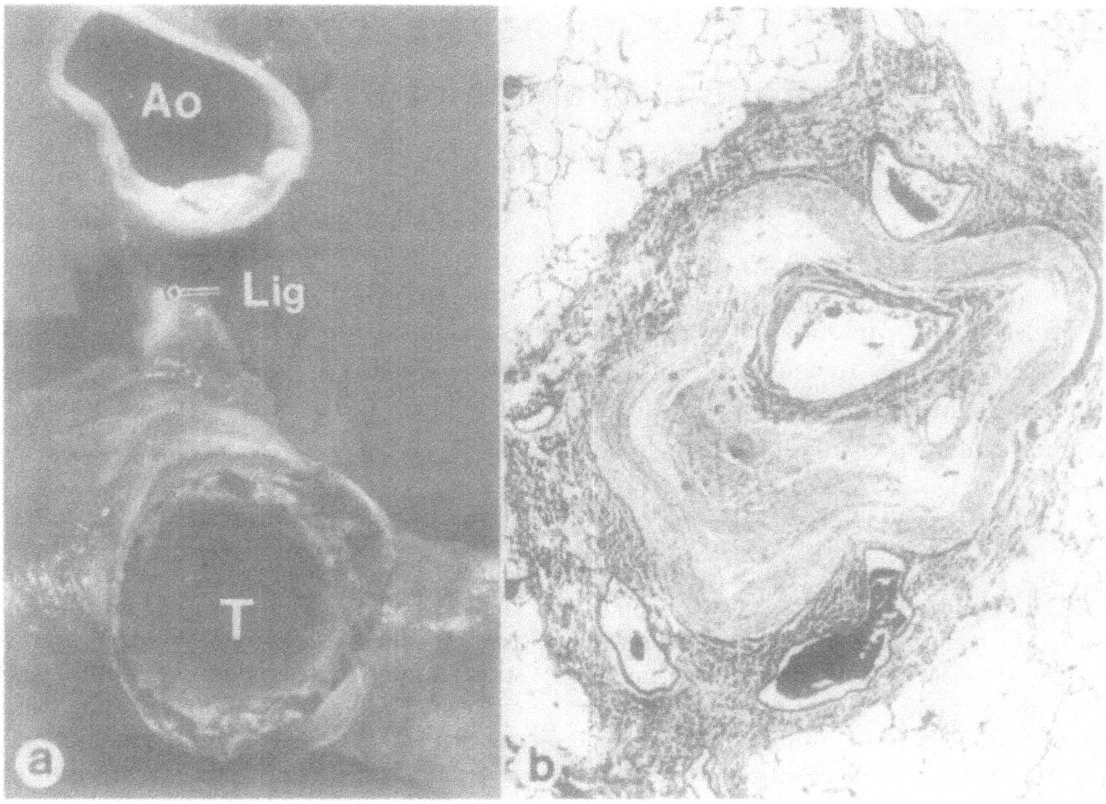

Fig. 6. *a*, View of the transected aorta *(Ao)* at its isthmus and left main pulmonary artery which is occluded by thrombus *(T)*. Extensive calcific deposits are present in the wall of the pulmonary artery. *Lig* = ligamentum arteriosum. *b*, Photomicrograph of a small pulmonary artery in the left lung with multiluminal channels presumably representing organized thrombus. Many such arteries were present. No plexiform lesions were present. (Movat stain; original magnification ×18.)

clear, however, that this artery was totally occluded for at least 13 years and maybe considerably longer. Its occlusion in the presence of the left-to-right shunt (via the TAPVC) may have further elevated the pulmonary arterial pressures.[3-7]

REFERENCES

1. Burroughs JT, Edwards JE: Total anomalous pulmonary venous connection. AM HEART J **59**:913, 1960.
2. Delisle G, Ando M, Calder AL, Zuberbuhler JR, Rochenmacher S, Alday LE, Mangini O, Van Praagh S, Van Praagh R: Total anomalous pulmonary venous connection: Report of 93 autopsied cases with emphasis on diagnostic and surgical considerations. AM HEART J **91**:99, 1976.
3. Harrison RW, Buehler WB, Thompson RG, Long ET, Carlson R, Charbon B, Adams WE: Cardiopulmonary reserve five to fifteen years following 50 percent or more reduction of lung volume. Surg Forum **8**:209, 1956.
4. Harrison RW, Adams WE, Beuhler WB, Long ET: Effects of acute and chronic reduction of lung volumes on cardiopulmonary reserve. Arch Surg **75**:546, 1957.
5. Harrison RW, Adams WE, Long ET, Burrows B, Reimann A: The clinical significance of cor pulmonale in the reduction of cardiopulmonary reserve following extensive pulmonary resection. J Thorac Surg **36**:352, 1958.
6. Rudolph AM, Neuhauser EBD, Golinko RJ, Auld PAM: Effects of pneumonectomy on pulmonary circulation in adult and young animals. Circ Res **9**:856, 1961.
7. Pool PE, Vogel JHK, Blount SG Jr: Congenital unilateral absence of a pulmonary artery. The importance of pulmonary hypertension. Am J Cardiol **10**:706, 1962.

Etiology of clinically isolated, severe, chronic, pure mitral regurgitation: Analysis of 97 patients over 30 years of age having mitral valve replacement

Bruce F. Waller, M.D.,* Andrew G. Morrow, M.D., Barry J. Maron, M.D., Albert A. Del Negro, M.D., Kenneth M. Kent, M.D., Francis J. McGrath, M.D., Robert B. Wallace, M.D., Charles L. McIntosh, M.D., and William C. Roberts, M.D.
Bethesda, Md., and Washington, D.C.

For many years rheumatic heart disease was considered the major cause of mitral regurgitation (MR) severe enough to necessitate mitral valve replacement (MVR). In most past studies of patients with mitral valvular disease, patients were subdivided on the basis of predominant mitral stenosis (MS) or predominant MR. This type of subdivision, however, does not provide as much information about etiology as can be obtained by dividing patients with mitral valve dysfunction into two groups based on the presence or absence of mitral valve obstruction. MS of any degree is recognized as usually having a rheumatic etiology. Likewise, most patients who have combined dysfunction of both mitral and aortic valves usually have a rheumatic etiology of their valvular lesions. The present study examines the etiology of the valvular disease in 97 patients over the age of 30 years in whom MVR was carried out for severe, chronic, pure MR unassociated with MS or aortic valve dysfunction.

PATIENTS STUDIED AND METHODOLOGY

Operatively excised mitral valves accessioned in the Pathology Branch, National Heart, Lung, and Blood Institute from July, 1968, through December, 1981, were reexamined and those which on anatomic grounds were purely regurgitant or possibly purely regurgitant were selected. The medical records including results of cardiac catheterization and angiographic procedures were then reviewed and the anatomic diagnosis of a purely regurgitant valve was substantiated by preoperative studies or the case was excluded. In addition to excluding patients with associated MS or aortic valve dysfunction, patients with intracardiac shunts or hypertrophic cardiomyopathy also were excluded.

After the exclusions noted, the study group comprised 97 patients (Table I). All fulfilled the following criteria: (1) severe (3+ or 4+/4+) MR by left ventricular (LV) angiography; (2) mean diastolic pressure gradient between left atrium (LA) (or pulmonary arterial wedge position) and LV of 2 mm Hg or less and no gradient at end-diastole between LA and LV; (3) no dysfunction (either stenosis or regurgitation or both) of the aortic valve; (4) age greater than 15 years (all patients were older than 30 years); and (5) clinical evidence of congestive heart failure (CHF) for 2 months or longer. Hereafter, the patients included in this study will be referred to as having *pure* MR, a word to signify the absence of associated MS, and *isolated* MR, a word to signify the absence of associated aortic valve stenosis or regurgitation.

The *circumference* (in centimeters) and *area* (in centimeters squared) of each excised mitral valve were determined in all 97 patients: the circumference, by measuring the length of the anulus of the excised mitral leaflets, and the area, by outlining the basal and distal margins of the leaflets on paper after opening the valve and then measuring the resulting area by videoplanimetry[1] (Fig. 1).

Criteria for etiologic subgrouping—Rheumatic. Both

From the Pathology, Surgery, and Cardiology Branches, National Heart, Lung and Blood Institute, National Institutes of Health; and the Departments of Medicine (Cardiology) and Surgery, Georgetown University Medical Center.

Received for publication Feb. 23, 1982; accepted March 2, 1982.

Reprint requests: William C. Roberts, M.D., Pathology Branch, NIH-NHLBI, Bldg. 10A, Room 3E-30, Bethesda, MD 20205.

*Present address: Department of Pathology, Indiana University Medical Center, Indianapolis, IN 46223.

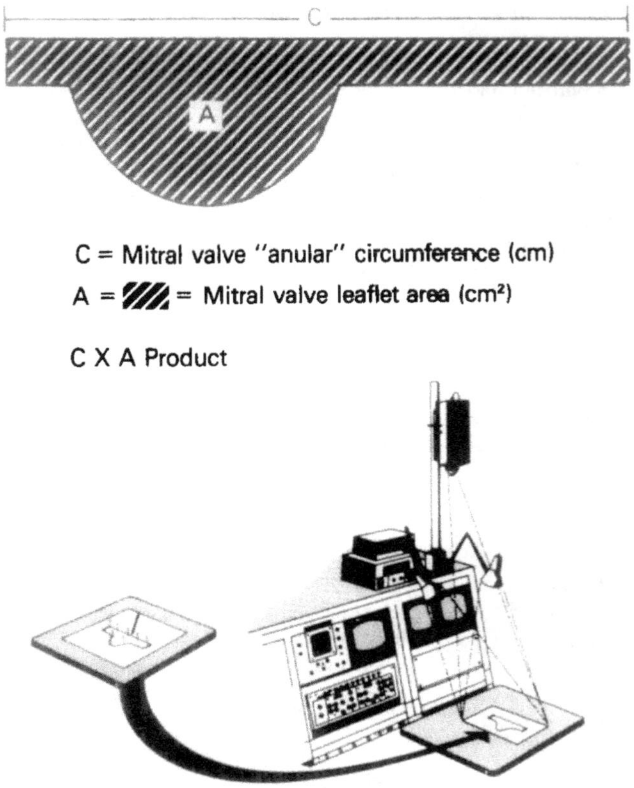

Fig. 1. Schematic drawing of opened operatively excised mitral valve showing methods of measuring the circumference and area. The videoplanimetry method of measuring leaflet area is shown in the lower drawing.

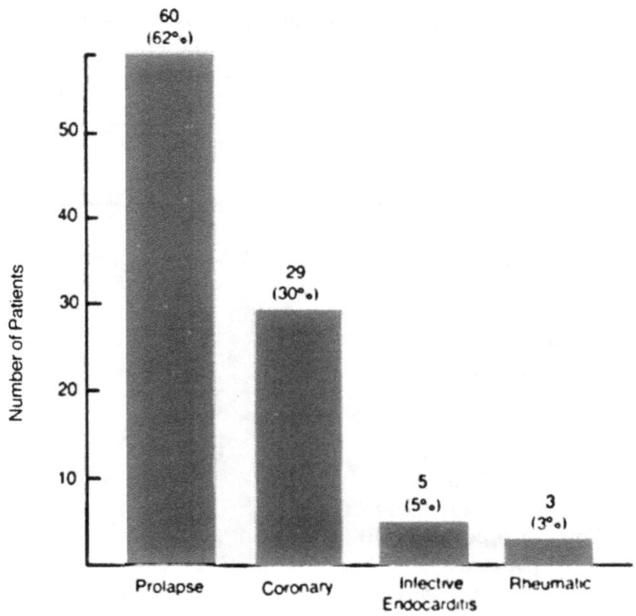

Fig. 2. Bar graph showing the four conditions causing chronic, isolated, pure, mitral regurgitation in the 97 patients with operatively excised valves.

mitral leaflets were diffusely thickened by fibrous tissue. The chordae tendineae may or may not have been abnormal.[2] Although the papillary muscles may have been focally scarred, neither was transmurally scarred. The mitral leaflet area was less than 12 cm^2 and the anular circumference was equal to or less than 11 cm.

Healed infective endocarditis on previously normal values. The major portion of leaflet and most chordae were normal. Several chordae, however, attached to one or both leaflets were absent or ruptured and the adjacent leaflet was thickened by fibrous tissue and a portion was either missing (indentation) or one or more perforations were present in one leaflet. The mitral leaflet area was less than 12 cm^2 and the mitral anular circumference was equal to or less than 11 cm.

Coronary heart disease with papillary muscle dysfunction. The mitral leaflets and chordae tendineae were either normal or only slightly and focally thickened. No leaflet indentation or perforations or ruptured or absent chordae tendineae were present. The mitral leaflet area was less than 12 cm^2 and the mitral circumference less than or equal to 11.5 cm. One or both papillary muscles were extensively scarred and usually atrophied.

Mitral valve prolapse with intact chordae tendineae. These valves had leaflet areas greater than 11 cm^2 and anular circumferences greater than 11 cm. The distance from basal attachment to distal margin in the posterior leaflet was not uniform in that one or more segments were elongated compared to other segments. No leaflet perforations or indentations were present and all chordae tendineae were intact.

Mitral valve prolapse with ruptured (or absent) chordae tendineae. These valves had focal thickening of one or both leaflets at sites of rupture of several chordae tendineae. Additionally, leaflet indentations or perforations were present. These values differed from those classified as "ruptured chordae tendineae on previously normal valves" by the presence of one or more elongated posterior leaflet segments as observed in the patients with mitral valve prolapse with intact chordae tendineae. Usually also the leaflet area and anular circumference were increased but neither was essential for classification in this subgroup.

OBSERVATIONS

Anatomic findings. Gross examinations of the 97 mitral valves revealed that the etiology of regurgita-

Table I. Certain clinical observations in 97 patients undergoing mitral valve replacement for isolated, severe, pure mitral regurgitation from various conditions

Item	Mitral valve prolapse (MVP) With RCT (n = 13)	Without RCT (n = 47)	Subtotal (n = 60)	Coronary (n = 29)[d]
1. Age (yr) at MVR	46-71 (57)	36-73 (55)	36-73 (55)	39-78 (56)
2. Men: Women	7(54%):6(46%)	22(47%):25(53%)	29(48%):31(52%)*	23(73%):6(27%)*
3. History of ARF	0	5 (11%)	5 (8%)	0
4. History of IE	4[a]	0	4 (7%)	0
5. History of AMI	0	2 (4%)	2 (3%)*	24 (83%)*
6. Angina pectoris	0	0	0[b]	19 (66%)
7. Systolic click(s)	0[c]	0	0	0
8. Duration (yr) MR, m	2-20 (8)	2-22 (9.5)	2-22 (9)	1-6 (4)
9. Duration (mo) CHF	6-24 (16)*	4-60 (31)*	4-60 (25)	10-36 (20)
10. Atrial fibrillation	0	4 (8%)	4 (7%)*	7 (24%)*
11. Abnormal Q waves on ECG	0	4 (8%)	4 (7%)*	29*
12. Total cholesterol (mg/dl) No. patients	4	25	25	13
Values (range [mean])	195-243 (221)	177-263 (234)	177-263 (228)*	242-305 (277)*
13. MVP by E only/total No. E	3/11	16/32 (50%)	19/43 (44%)	2/22 (9%)
14. MVP by A only/total No. A	0/13	3/47 (6%)	3/60 (5%)	0/29
15. MVP by both E and A/total No. with both E + A	3/11	10/32 (31%)	13/43 (30%)	0/22
16. Pressures (mm Hg)				
PAW: range (avg)				
a	10-18 (15)	9-20 (14)	9-20 (14)	10-16 (15)
v	18-48 (35)	16-42 (32)	16-48 (33)	18-34 (26)
mean	16-24 (19)	12-24 (18)	12-24 (18)	14-24 (19)
LV: range (avg)				
systolic	115-168 (149)	120-165 (131)	115-168 (137)	120-165 (146)
diastolic	16-24 (25)	12-24 (18)	12-24 (18)	14-24 (19)
SA: range (avg)				
systolic	115-168 (149)	120-165 (131)	115-168 (137)	120-165 (146)
diastolic	70-88 (81)	84-90 (83)	70-90 (82)	70-90 (86)
17. Direct systolic SAP > 140 or diastolic SAP > 90 mm Hg	11 (85%)*	11 (23%)*	22 (37%)	9 (31%)
18. One or more major CA narrowed > 50% in D by A/total No. A	0/1	3[g]/22 (14%)	3[g]/23 (13%)	29/29 (100%)

—(horizontal only) = $p < 0.05$.
[a]The four patients with MVP and RCT with a history of active IE were included in the prolapse group rather than in the IE group because MV function was abnormal before the active IE.
[b]Three patients had chest pain not judged to be angina pectoris unassociated with AMI.
[c]One patient had a systolic click and a late systolic murmur about 4 months before developing active IE murmur but the precordial murmur became holosystolic and the click disappeared.
[d]Of 29 patients, 28 (97%) had MVR with aortocoronary bypass grafting and one (3%) had MVR with LV aneurysmectomy. Only 1 of the 29 had neither angina pectoris nor past evidence of AMI.
[e]Healed in all.
[f]One patient with opiate abuse was treated for active IE 15 months before MVR. Both anterior and posterior MV leaflets were diffusely thickened by fibrous tissue, indicating underlying rheumatic mitral disease.
[g]Only the right coronary artery was narrowed in each patient, only one of whom had chest pain which was nonanginal in type.
Abbreviations: A = angiogram; ARF = acute rheumatic fever; AMI = acute myocardial infarction; CA = coronary arteries; CHF = congestive heart failure; D = diameter; E = echocardiogram; ECG = electrocardiogram; IE = infective endocarditis; LV = left ventricular; m = precordial murmur; mo = months; MR = mitral regurgitation; MVR = mitral valve replacement; PAW = pulmonary arterial wedge; RCT = ruptured chordae tendineae; SA = systemic artery; SAP = systemic artery pressure; yr = years.

tion was leaflet prolapse in 60 patients (62%); 13 of these 60 valves had ruptured chordae tendineae (Fig. 2) while in the other 47 the chordae were intact (Figs. 3, 4, and 5). In 29 patients (30%), the MR resulted from papillary muscle dysfunction secondary to coronary heart disease; neither the chordae nor papillary muscles were ruptured (Figs. 2 and 6). In five patients (5%) the regurgitation occurred after infective endocarditis involving an apparently normal mitral valve, and in all five patients the

Infective endocarditis (n = 5)[e]	Rheumatic (n = 3)	Totals (n = 97)
33-56 (42)	32,35,52, (40)	32-78 (54)
3:2	2:1	57(59%):40(41%)
0	2	7 (7%)
4	1[f]	9 (9%)
0	0	26 (27%)
0	0	19 (20%)
0	0	0
0.8-1.8(1.3)	1.3,14,20(12)	1-22 (10)
3-5 (3.8)	1.3,4,5(3.4)	2-60 (23)
1	1	13 (13%)
0	0	33 (34%)
4	3	49 (51%)
224-226 (241)	226,232,243(234)	177-305(248)
0/5	0/2	21/72 (29%)
0/5	0/3	3/97 (3%)
0/5	0/2	13/72 (18%)
10-14 (12)	-,10,27 (19)	9-27 (14)
18-36 (32)	21,24,40 (28)	16-48 (31)
16-18 (17)	10,18,27 (18)	12-27 (18)
140-155 (147)	130,145,160(145)	115-168 (143)
16-18 (17)	10,18,27 (18)	12-27 (18)
140-155 (147)	130,145,160(145)	115-168 (143)
75-90 (79)	70,78,85 (78)	70-90 (83)
4	2	37 (38%)
0/1	-/0	32/53 (60%)

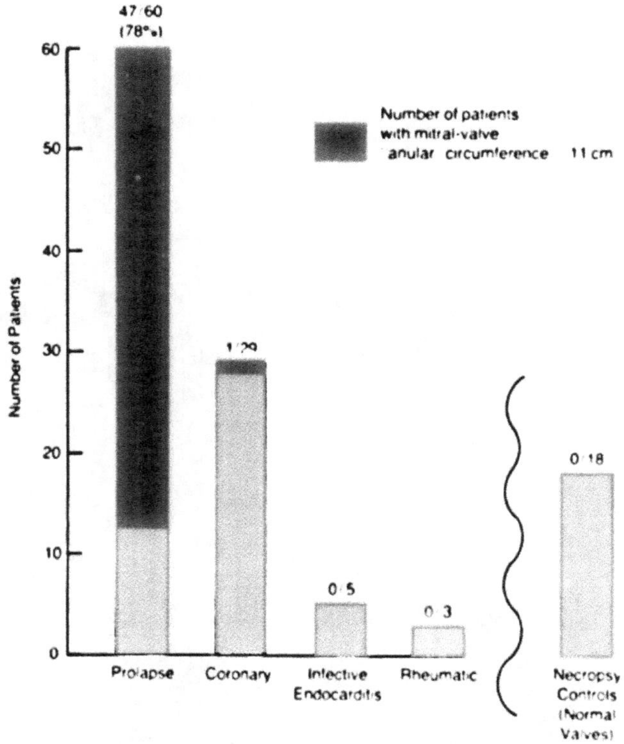

Fig. 3. Bar graph showing the frequency of mitral valve "anular" circumference of greater than 11 cm in the four conditions causing chronic, isolated, pure, mitral regurgitation in the 97 patients with operatively excised valves. The normal mitral valves used as controls were excised from hearts of 18 necropsy patients who had no cardiac abnormalities. The frequency of men and women and age range was similar in the control and study patients.

chordae were ruptured (Figs. 2 and 7). The remaining three patients had MR as the result of rheumatic heart disease (Figs. 2 and 8).

Anular circumference. The circumferences of the mitral anuli measured in the 18 control patients without heart disease ranged from 8.0 to 10.5 cm (average 9.4) (Table II, Fig. 9). Anular circumferences were not significantly different in the valves rendered regurgitant by coronary heart disease, infective endocarditis, rheumatic fever, or in prolapsed valves with ruptured chordae (Figs. 10 and 11). The anular circumferences of the prolapsed valves without chordae rupture were significantly larger than those of all other groups.

Leaflet area. In the 18 control patients, the areas of the excised leaflets ranged from 7.0 to 12.5 cm^2 (average 9.5) (Table II, Fig. 12). In 59 of the 60 patients with mitral valve prolapse, the leaflet area was greater than 11.0 cm^2; in the remaining patient, the area was 10.6 cm^2. In the patients with prolapse and ruptured chordae the leaflet areas were 10.6 to 18.4 cm^2 and averaged 14.3 cm^2. In those with prolapse and intact chordae, the leaflet areas ranged from 11.7 to 27.5 cm^2 (average 18.3). The leaflet areas of both groups of prolapsed valves were significantly larger than the valves rendered incompetent by coronary heart disease, infective endocarditis, or rheumatic heart disease (Fig. 12).

Product of valve circumference and area. The product of the circumference (in centimeters) times the area (in centimeters squared) calculated for the normal valves ranged from 45 to 140 cm^3 (average 91) (Fig. 13). The average product was 150 cm^3 in the prolapsed valves with ruptured chordae, and much larger, 273 cm^3, in the prolapsed valves with intact chordae (Table II). The products were 87, 93, and 106 cm^3, respectively, in the valves regurgitant because of papillary muscle dysfunction, infective endocarditis, or rheumatic disease, and these prod-

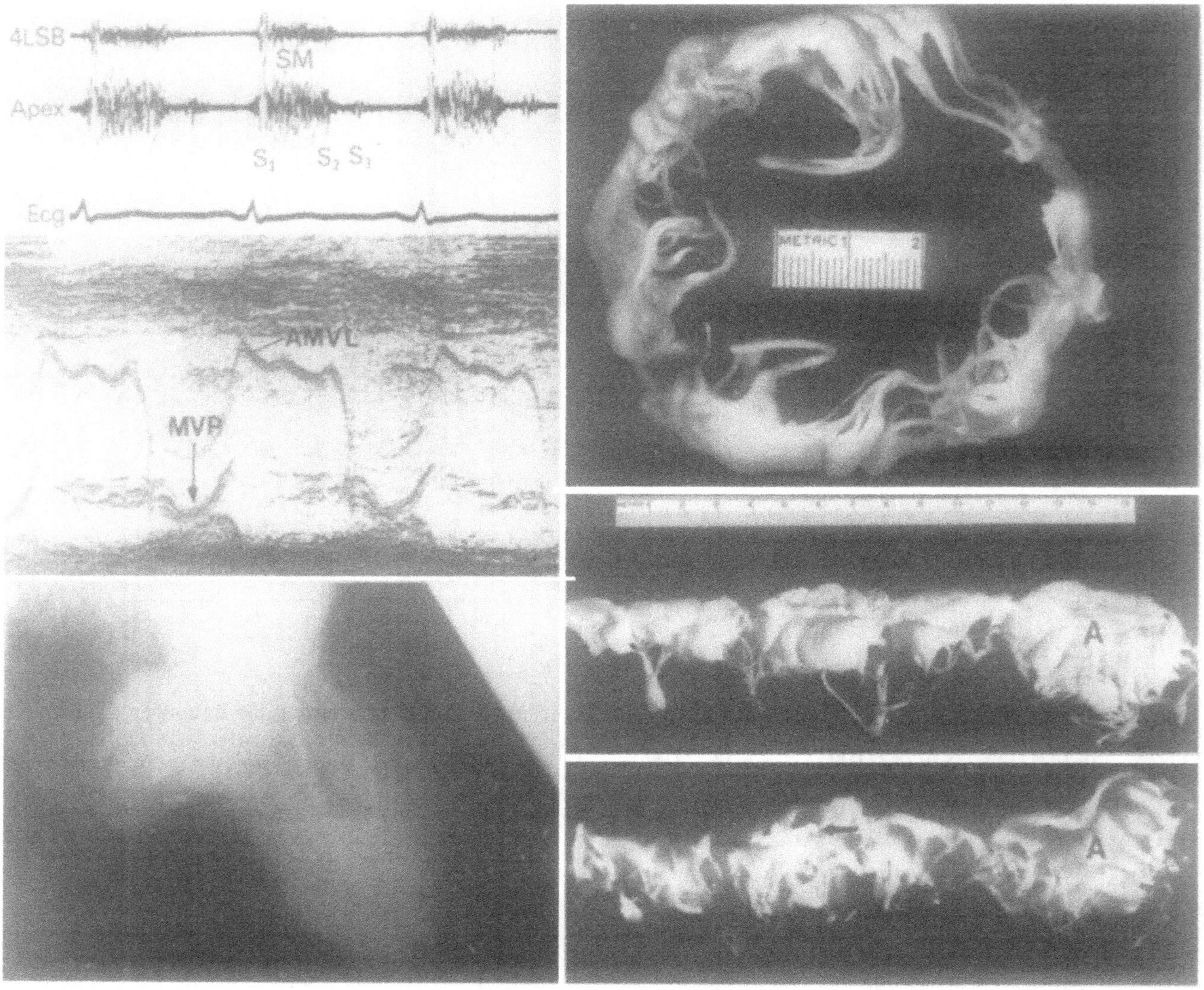

Fig. 4. Preoperative data and operatively excised mitral valve from a 51-year-old woman (S80-33) with *mitral valve prolapse* causing severe, isolated, pure mitral regurgitation. *Left upper,* Phonocardiogram recorded at the fourth left sternal border *(LSB)* and apex showing a holosystolic murmur *(SM)* and third heart sound *(S_3)*. *Ecg* = electrocardiogram; S_1 and S_2 = *first and second heart sounds. Left middle,* Echocardiogram of anterior *(A)* and posterior mitral valve leaflets *(MVL)* showing prolapse *(MVP)* during ventricular systole. *Left lower,* Frame from left ventricular angiogram showing mitral valve prolapse. *Right upper,* Operatively excised mitral valve with an "anular" circumference of 17 cm. *Right middle,* Opened mitral valve showing areas of focal fibrous thickening and an elongated posterior leaflet. *A* = anterior leaflet. *Right lower,* Postmortem radiogram showing focal and minimal calcific deposits *(between arrows)*.

ucts did not differ from those of the normal valves (Fig. 13).

COMMENTS

The cause of the pure MR in these 97 patients was determined by examination of the operatively excised mitral valves, but the correct etiology of the MR was usually predictable from the *history alone.* Of the 29 patients with papillary muscle dysfunction from atherosclerotic coronary heart disease, all have clinical evidence of myocardial ischemia: history of acute myocardial infarction which had healed in 24, a LV aneurysm from a silent infarction in one, and angina pectoris in four. Of the five patients found to have MR secondary to infective endocarditis, four had well-documented episodes of infection, which had been cured by antibiotic therapy, and none had evidence of valvular dysfunction before the episode of infective endocarditis. Of the three patients with MR secondary to a clinical rheumatic etiology, two

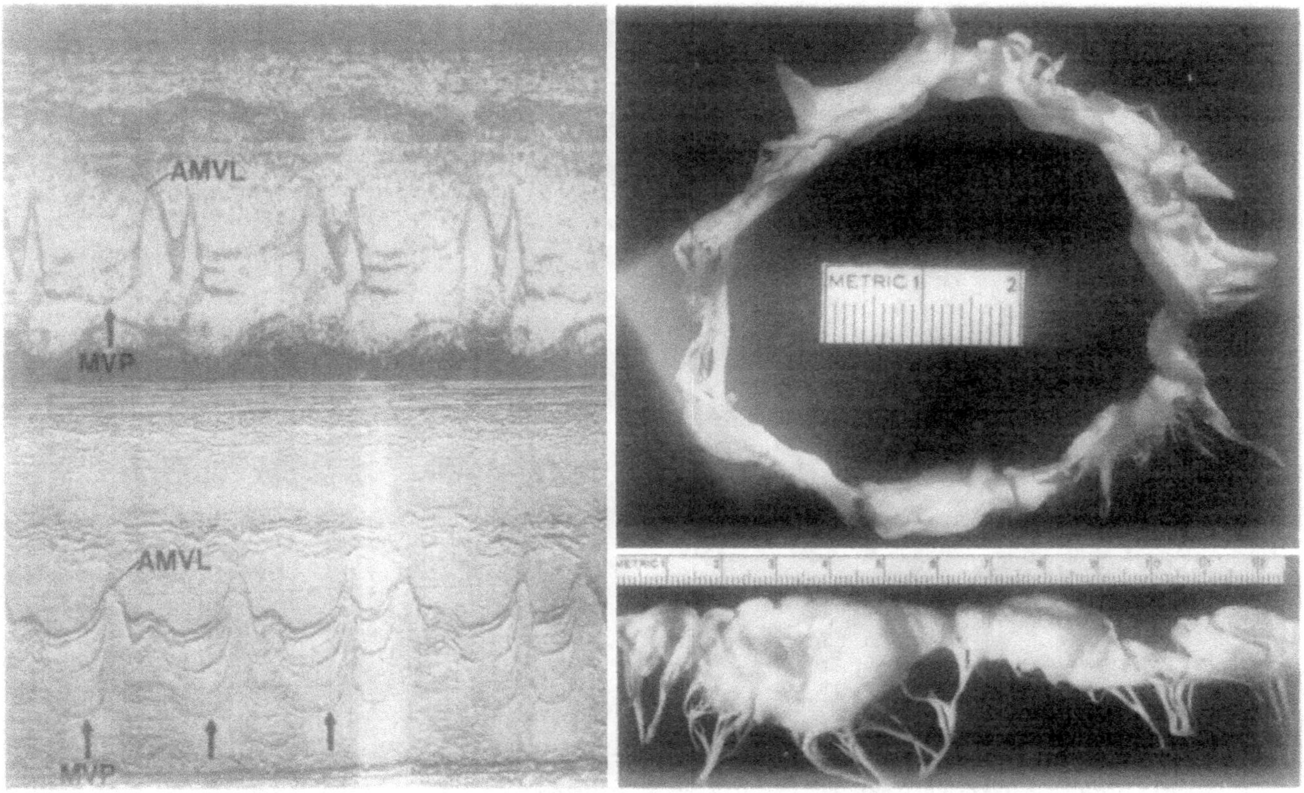

Fig. 5. Operatively excised mitral valve from a 52-year-old man (S80-17) with *mitral valve prolapse* causing chronic, severe, isolated, pure mitral regurgitation. *Left upper,* Echocardiogram of the anterior *(A)* and posterior mitral valve leaflets *(MVL)* obtained 7 years before operation showing prolapse *(MVP). Left lower,* Echocardiogram obtained 2 months before operation showing more severe mitral valve prolapse *(arrows). Right upper,* Operatively excised mitral valve showing a dilated "anular" circumference measuring 12.5 cm. *Right lower,* Opened mitral valve showing areas of focal fibrous thickening.

had a history of acute rheumatic fever, whereas this item was positive in only five of the other 94 patients. Clinical diagnosis of mitral valve prolapse was by a process of exclusion. Only two (3%) of these 60 patients had historical evidence of previous acute myocardial infarction; five (11%) had histories of acute rheumatic fever, and four (7%) had histories of active infective endocarditis. Compared to the five patients classified as having ruptured chordae tendineae on previously normal valves (four of whom had histories of infective endocarditis), the four patients with healed infective endocarditis and mitral prolapse were older (mean age 61 years vs 42 years), had previous systolic murmurs of MR before the episode of infective endocarditis (four of four vs none of five), and had a longer mean duration of CHF (11 months vs 4 months). Thus, of the 60 patients with prolapse, 51 (85%) had no historical evidence of myocardial ischemia, acute rheumatic fever, or infective endocarditis.

The etiology of the MR also was suggested preoperatively by more objective means. The *electrocardiogram* was most useful in delineating the patients with MR secondary to coronary heart disease. Of these 29 patients, all had abnormal Q waves whereas abnormal Q waves were present in only 4 of the 60 patients with mitral valve prolapse, and in none of the eight patients in whom the regurgitation resulted from either infective endocarditis or rheumatic disease. Atrial fibrillation was significantly ($P < 0.05$) more frequent in the patients in whom the MR resulted from coronary heart disease. It was present in seven (24%) of these 29 patients whereas it occurred in only four (7%) of the 60 patients with mitral valve prolapse and in two of the eight patients with either infective endocarditis or a rheumatic etiology.

The *M-mode echocardiogram* was helpful in delineating the patients in whom the MR resulted from mitral valve prolapse. Of the 60 patients with mitral valve prolapse, 43 had an M-mode echocardiogram performed and in 32 (74%) of them it

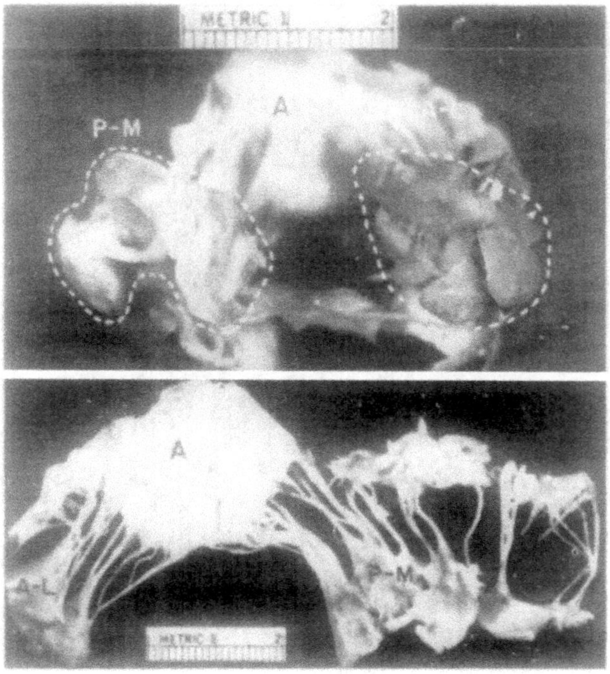

Fig. 6. Operatively excised mitral valve from a 53-year-old man who had chronic, pure mitral regurgitation from *papillary muscle dysfunction secondary to coronary heart disease. Upper,* Photography of cut surfaces of portions of the anterolateral *(A-L)* and posteromedial *(P-M)* papillary muscle showing extensive scarring of the P-M papillary muscle. *A* = anterior leaflet. *Lower,* Opened mitral valve showing anatomically normal leaflets and "anular" circumference of 7 cm.

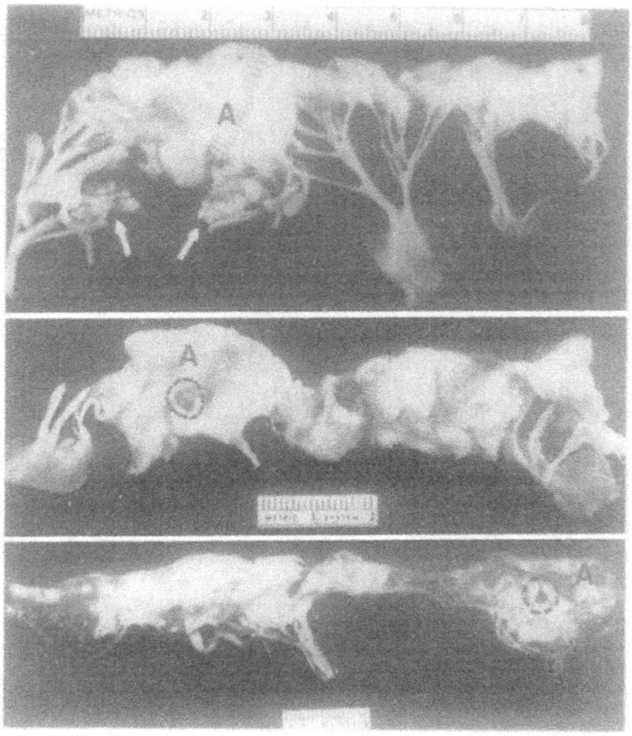

Fig. 7. Operatively excised mitral valves from three patients with chronic, isolated, pure mitral regurgitation from *healed infective endocarditis* occurring on previously anatomically and functionallly normal valves. *Upper,* Valve from a 32-year-old man (S80-131) showing a focally thickened anterior *(A)* leaflet with ruptured chordae tendineae *(arrows). Middle,* Valve from a 48-year-old man (S74-54) showing a perforation *(dashed circle)* in the anterior leaflet. *Lower,* Valve from a 42-year-old man (S79-38) showing a perforation *(dashed circle)* in the anterior leaflet.

indicated the presence of mitral prolapse. In contrast, of the 29 patients with MR secondary to coronary heart disease, M-mode echocardiograms were done in 22 and only two (9%) indicated the presence of mitral prolapse. M-mode echocardiograms were performed in seven of the eight patients with infective endocarditis and rheumatic etiologies and in none of them was mitral prolapse present by this procedure.

Left ventriculograms were performed in all 97 patients. Mitral prolapse was present by this procedure in 16 (27%) of the 60 patients in whom the MR was caused by mitral valve prolapse and in none of the other 37 patients with coronary or infective endocarditis or rheumatic etiologies.

Selective coronary angiograms were performed in 53 (55%) patients. All 29 with MR secondary to coronary heart disease had significant (> 50% diameter reduction) coronary narrowing demonstrated angiographically and 24 of them had evidence of past acute myocardial infarction and the others had other clinical evidences of myocardial ischemia. In 23 (38%) of the 60 patients with mitral valve prolapse coronary angiograms were performed and three (13%) had significant coronary narrowing, limited in each to one (right) coronary artery. In contrast, all 29 patients with MR from papillary muscle dysfunction had two or three of the three major coronary systems with significant narrowing.

Auscultation and hemodynamics at *cardiac catheterization* were not helpful in delineating the etiology of the MR. None of the 97 patients—including the 60 classified as mitral valve prolapse—had systolic clicks on precordial examination, and the systolic precordial murmurs in all 97 patients were holosystolic immediately before MVR. The average pulmonary arterial, LA (or pulmonary arterial wedge), and LV pressures were similar in all four etiologic groups. The systolic systemic arterial pressures, however, were significantly higher in the patients with mitral valve prolapse and ruptured chordae tendineae than in those with mitral valve prolapse with intact chordae tendineae.

Table II. Morphologic observations of operatively excised mitral valves in 97 patients with isolated, pure mitral regurgitation and in 18 normal necropsy valves

	Mitral valve prolapse						
Mitral valve observation	*With RCT (n = 13)*	*Without RCT (n = 47)*	*Subtotals (n = 60)*	*Coronary (n = 29)*	*Infective endocarditis (n = 5)*	*Rheumatic (n = 3)*	*Necropsy controls (n = 18)*
Circumference (C)(cm)	9.5-11.0 (10.5)†	11.5-19.5 (14.8)‡	9.5-19.5 (13.4)‡	8.0-11.5 (9.7)†	9.0-10.5 (9.7)†	9.5,10.5,11.0 (10.5)†	8.0-10.5 (9.4)†
Leaflet area (A) (cm^2)	10.6-18.4 (14.3)†	11.7-27.5 (18.3)‡	10.6-27.5 (16.8)‡	5.5-11.1 (8.9)*	9.2-10.6 (9.7)*	9.5,10.2,10.6 (10.1)*	7.0-12.5 (9.5)*
C x A product (cm^3)	111-225 (150)†	128-536 (273)§	111-536 (268)§	45-112 (87)*	87-111 (93)*	90,112,116 (106)*	45-140 (91)*
No. with C > 11 cm	0	13	47	1	0	0	0
No. with ruptured chordae tendineae (RCT)	13	0	13	0	5	0	0
No. with calcific deposits	0	3[a]	3[a]	0	0	1	0

[a]Primarily in the mitral valve anulus.
—, †—†,§—§(horizontal) = p = ns.
‡—‡(horizontal) = $p < 0.05$.
*—†, *—‡, †—‡, †—§ (horizontal) = $p < 0.01$.

Table III. Summary of causes of mitral regurgitation in 230 patients reported by Selzer and Katayama (Medicine 51:337, 1972)

Etiology	*No. (%) pts.*	*Ages (yr) range (mean)*	*MV op*	*No. without or only mild symptoms of CD*	*Probable no. with MS*	*AF*	*M:F*
1. Rheumatic	88[a] (38)	< 10-> 60 (43)	61	22	42[b]	50 (57%)[c]	26:62 (29%):(71%)
2. Rupture chordae tendineae[d]	44 (19)	21-> 60 (~ 55)	31	11	0	10 (23%)	36:8 (82%):(18%)
3. Late systolic murmur with or without click	28[e] (12)	17-72 (~ 40)	0	28	0	0	10:18 (35%):(65%)
4. Coronary (Post-myocardial infarct)	26 (11)	40-70 (~ 55)	11	2	0	2 (8%)	23:3 (88%):(12%)
5. Congenital[f]	23 (10)	1-56 (-)	11	0	0	4	11:12 (48%):(52%)
6. Infective endocarditis[g]	11 (5)	30-72 (-)	7	3	0	1	7:4
7. Miscellaneous	10[h] (5)	10-64 (45)	4[i]	4	0	1	0:10
Totals	230 (100)	1-72[j] (-)	125 (54%)	70 (30%)	0	68 (30%)	113:117 (49%):(51%)

[a]The MR in eight was attributed entirely to infective endocarditis. Probably several of them had previous mitral stenosis.
[b]Five patients had MR only after mitral valve commissurotomy for mitral stenosis. Of the 61 having mitral valve operations, 20 had calcific deposits on the valve observed at operation. Of the 27 patients not undergoing mitral valve operations, 13 appear to have had calcific deposits on the mitral valve observed radiographically. Probably at least four of the eight with infective endocarditis had previous mitral stenosis.
[c]Of the 61 patients having mitral valve operation, 46 (75%) had atrial fibrillation. Thus, only four (15%) of the 27 without mitral valve operations had atrial fibrillation.
[d]Defined by three characteristics: (1) sudden onset, (2) selective involvement of chordae supporting the posterior leaflet, and (3) a normal mitral valve except for the localized loss of chordal support. Ten of the 44 patients with isolated chordae rupture had mitral valve prolapse by LV angiogram.
[e]All were asymptomatic.
[f]Precordial murmur before age 3. At least two had associated atrial septal defect. Most had more than one congenital cardiovascular anomaly. Thirteen were under 18 years of age.
[g]None had previous evidence of cardiac disease.
[h]Of the 10, at least four had prolapsed mitral valves, two had left atrial myxomas, and in the other four clinical clues suggesting the proper cause were absent and operations were not performed.
[i]Two additional patients had left atrial myxomas excised.
[j]This is a minimal age, possibly older.
Abbreviations: AF = atrial fibrillation; CD = cardiac dysfunction; F = female; M = male; MS = mitral stenosis; MV = mitral valve; op = operation; pts = patients; yr = years.

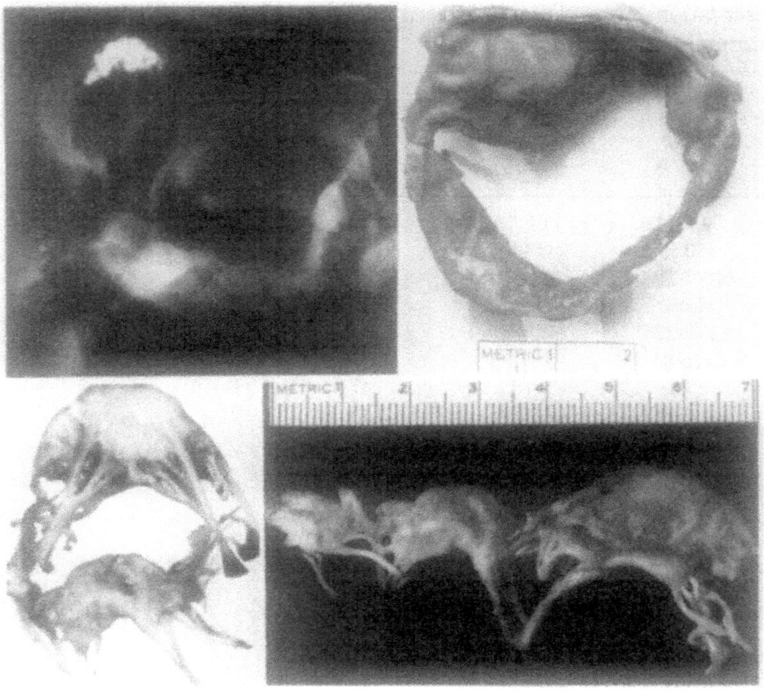

Fig. 8. Operatively excised mitral valves from two patients with chronic, isolated, pure mitral regurgitation from *rheumatic heart disease. Upper left,* Postmortem radiogram of the excised mitral valve from a 35-year-old man (S75-5148) showing focal and minimal calcific deposits. *Upper right,* Valve from the patient showing diffuse fibrous thickening of the anterior and posterior leaflets with an "anular" circumference of 11 cm. *Lower left,* Excised mitral valve from a 52-year-old woman (S78-8). *Lower right,* View of opened valve from the same patient showing diffuse fibrous thickening of both leaflets and a circumference of 7 cm.

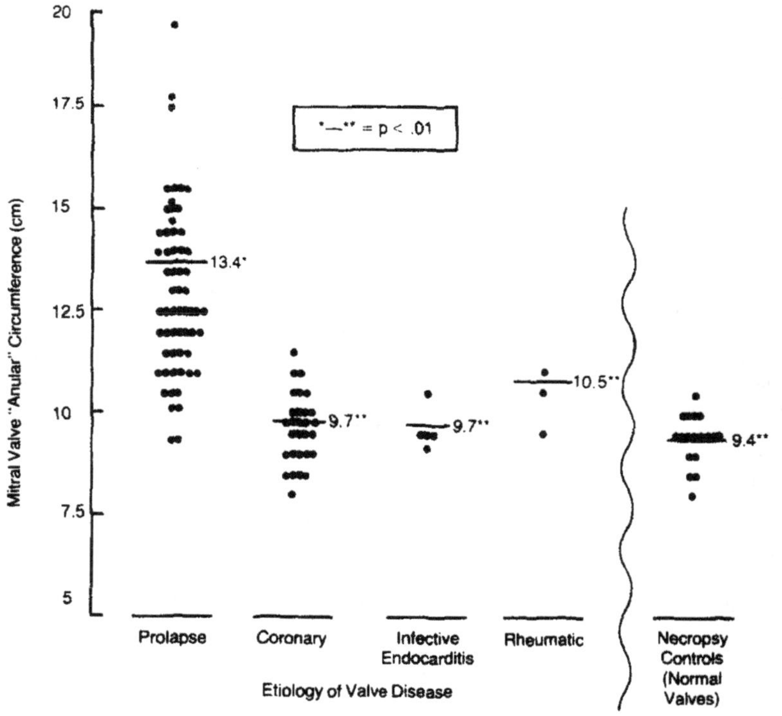

Fig. 9. Graph showing mitral valve "anular" circumference (in cm) in each of the 97 patients with operatively excised mitral valves in the four conditions causing chronic, isolated, pure mitral regurgitation, and in 18 necropsy control valves.

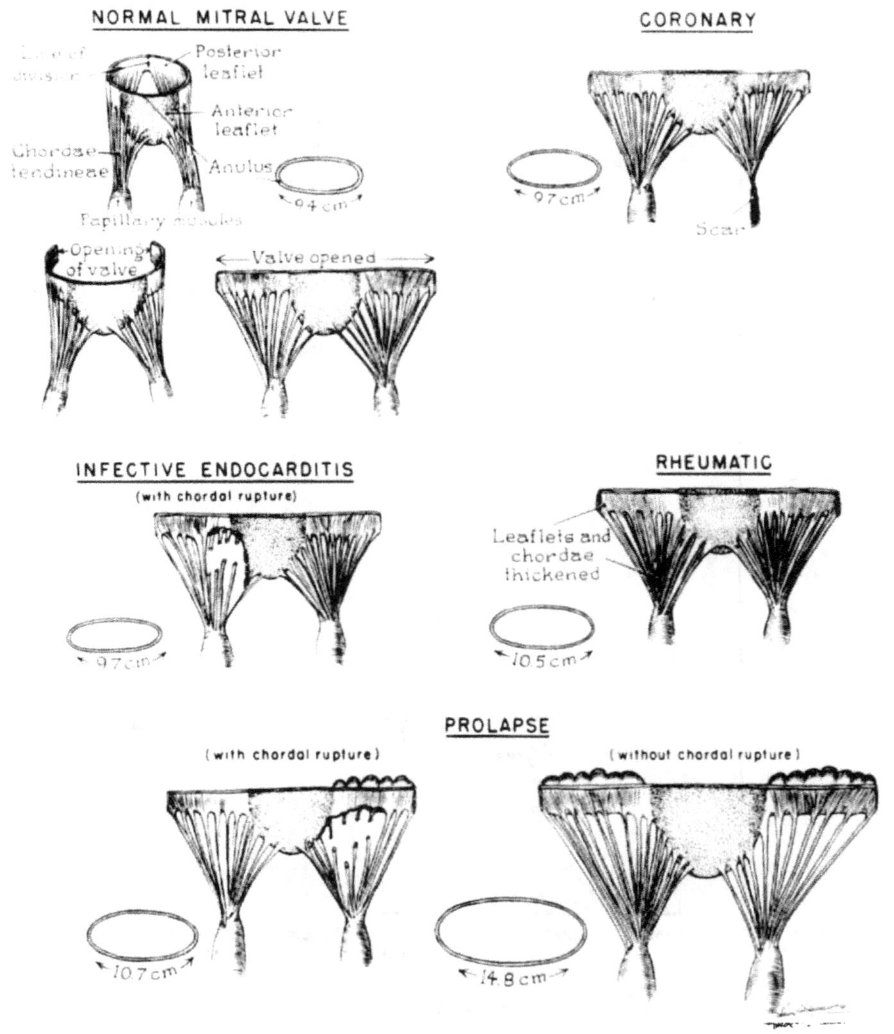

Fig. 10. Diagram showing morphologic variations in mitral valve "anular" circumference and leaflet area in four conditions causing isolated, pure mitral regurgitation.

Surprisingly few reports are available describing the various causes of MR in large numbers of patients. Furthermore, we were unable to find any reports concerning the etiology of pure MR in groups of patients in whom any associated MS or aortic valve dysfunction had been excluded by appropriate hemodynamic and angiographic studies.

The most frequently cited paper describing patients with MR appears to be that by Selzer and Katayama,[3] who summarized findings in 230 patients (Table III). Although 212 of their 230 patients had pure MR defined as the "absence of a late diastolic gradient across the valve . . . except in tachycardia . . . " at the time of cardiac catheterization, some of their patients had MS at other times. Of their 230 patients, 88 were classified as rheumatic in etiology, and we suspect that of them nearly half (42 patients) had MS at some time in their course:

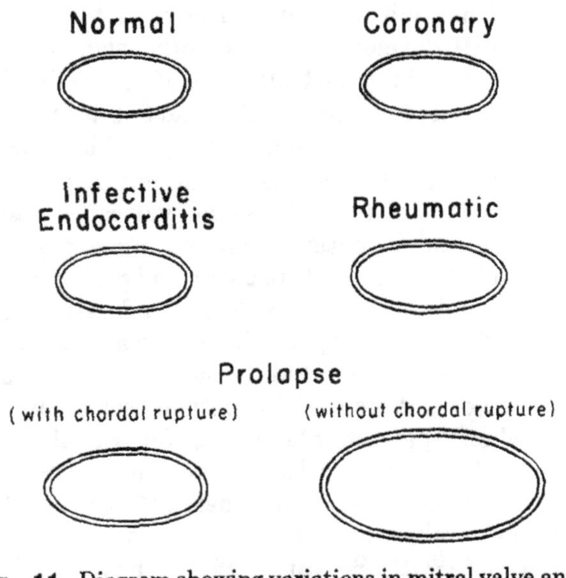

Fig. 11. Diagram showing variations in mitral valve anuli in conditions causing isolated, pure mitral regurgitation.

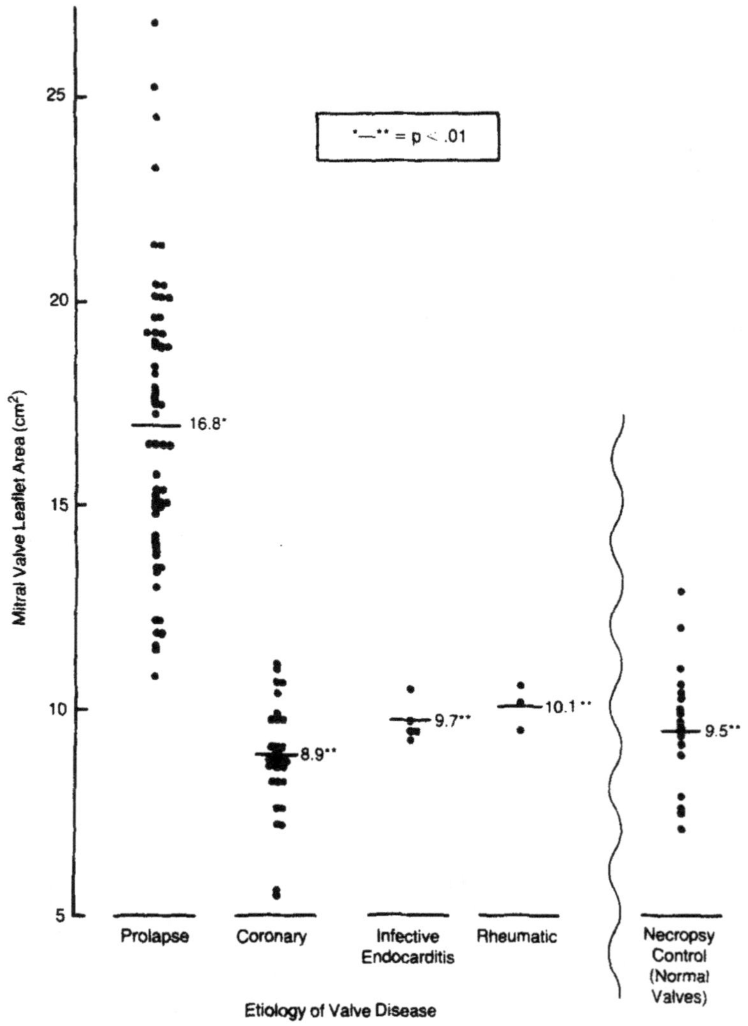

Fig. 12. Graph showing mitral valve leaflet area (in cm^2) in each of the 97 patients with operatively excised mitral valves in the four conditions causing chronic, isolated, pure mitral regurgitation and in 18 necropsy control valves.

five had had mitral commissurotomies for MS and severe MR developed subsequently; eight of their rheumatic patients had MR only after the development of infective endocarditis, and it is probable that one or more of them previously had had MS; 33 (38%) of their 88 rheumatic patients had sizable calcific deposits in their mitral valves, a finding quite unusual in patients without some degree of MS. (Only four of our 97 patients had grossly visible calcific deposits in their excised mitral valves.) It is also difficult to compare the observations in our patients to those reported by Selzer and Katayama because of differences in patient selection. We studied only patients who were in functional classes III and IV (New York Heart Association classification) because of CHF; all underwent MVR and all had their valves examined by the same observers (BFW and WCR). Seventy (30%) of the 230 patients reported by Selzer and Katayama were in functional classes I or II, and mitral valve operations were performed in just over half of the 230 patients. Additionally, they included children, which we did not. Finally, we excluded patients with any aortic valve dysfunction, which may or may not have been the case in the study by Selzer and Katayama.

In the past rheumatic heart disease has been considered the most common cause of severe MR, but it is likely that most or many patients so classified in older studies had some degree of MS. Because there has been such a strong tendency in the past to believe that severe MR was frequently the result of rheumatic heart disease, other etiologies commonly have not been sought and definitions of "rheumatic mitral regurgitation" have not been precisely stated. Before 1963, most prolapsing or floppy mitral valves almost certainly were called

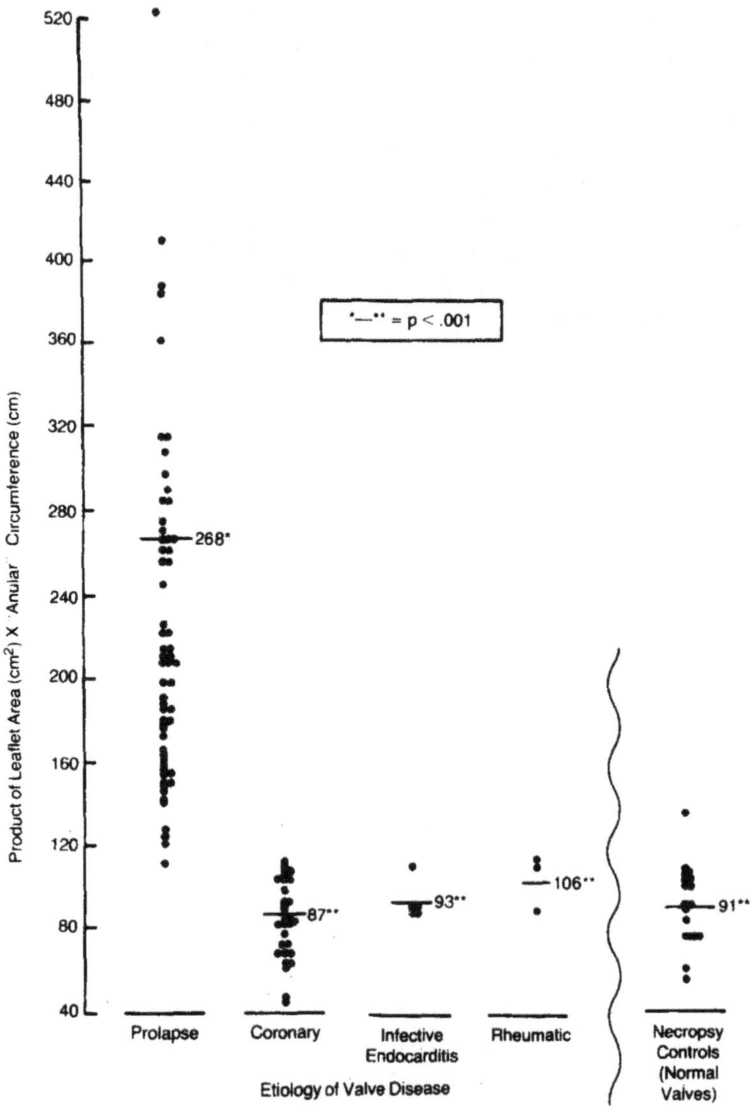

Fig. 13. Graph showing product of mitral valve leaflet area (in cm^2) times the "anular" circumference (in centimeters) in each of the 97 patients with operatively excised mitral valves in the four conditions causing chronic, isolated, pure mitral regurgitation, and in 18 necropsy control valves.

"rheumatic" in origin at necropsy or operation. The present report defines morphologically a prolapsed mitral valve which can cause severe MR: its anular circumference and leaflet area are clearly increased over that of other valves causing MR, except when the chordae tendineae of the prolapsing valve are ruptured. It is hoped that this definition will prevent indiscriminate labeling of mitral disease in the future as "rheumatic" when other evidences of previous rheumatic carditis are lacking.

CONCLUSIONS

The etiology of clinically isolated, severe, pure mitral regurgitation was determined in 97 patients over 30 years of age by examination of the operatively excised mitral valves. None had any degree of mitral stenosis or a dysfunctioning aortic valve as determined by preoperative catheterization. The etiology of the MR was leaflet *prolapse* in 60 patients (62%), *papillary muscle dysfunction* from coronary heart disease in 29 (30%), *infective endocarditis* on previously normally functioning valves in five (5%), and *rheumatic heart disease* in three (3%). Thus, nonrheumatic conditions caused the MR in 94 (97%) of the 97 patients. The history alone (previous acute myocardial infarction, rheumatic fever, active infective endocarditis) usually provided adequate information in the patients with coronary, infective endocarditis and rheumatic etiologies to predict accurately the cause of the MR preoperatively; conversely, the lack of a history of one of these other three conditions strongly suggested mitral valve prolapse as the cause of the MR preoperatively. All 60 patients with mitral valve prolapse had increased mitral valve circumferences, leaflet areas, and/or products of the circumference times the area. In contrast, only one of the 37 patients in whom the MR was due to another cause had increased mitral circumference, increased area, or the product of the two. A systolic click was not heard preoperatively in any of the 97 patients including the 60 with mitral valve prolapse.

REFERENCES

1. Dvorak JA, Schuette WH, Whitehouse WC: A simple video method for the quantification of microscopic objects. J Microsc **102**:71, 1974.
2. Roberts WC, Virmani R: Aschoff bodies at necropsy in valvular heart disease. Evidence from an analysis of 543 patients over 14 years of age that rheumatic heart disease, at least anatomically, is a disease of the mitral valve. Circulation **57**:803, 1978.
3. Selzer A, Katayama F: Mitral regurgitation: Clinical patterns, pathophysiology, natural history. Medicine **51**:337, 1972.

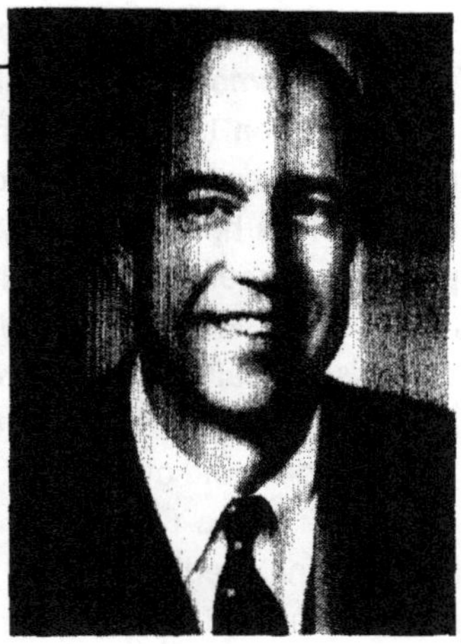

Mitral Commissurotomy—Still a Good Operation

Recently, I examined an operatively excised, severely stenotic mitral valve that was free of calcific deposits (by radiography of the excised valve) and of associated mitral regurgitation (by left ventricular angiography). The patient had no evidence of dysfunction of either the tricuspid or aortic valves. I asked the surgeon who had performed the mitral valve replacement (MVR) why that procedure was performed rather than mitral valve commissurotomy (MVC). I was surprised to hear that he "rarely did MVC anymore" and that he had "more confidence in MVR than in MVC." He had used a mechanical prosthesis for the MVR, which necessitated anticoagulant therapy for the rest of this 36-year-old woman's life. When I mentioned that chronic anticoagulant therapy would not have been necessary had MVC been performed, he responded that "MVR was still worth the difference." I disagree, and so does Bonchek[1] in the editorial in this issue.

In 1978, Lachman and I[2] radiographed 164 operatively excised stenotic mitral valves and quantitated the amount of calcific deposits in them. Of the 164 valves, 14 had absent and 43 minimal calcific deposits on x-ray examination of the excised valve. Of the 57 patients with absent or minimal calcific deposits, 37 had moderate to severe mitral regurgitation, and therefore, each clearly warranted MVR. The remaining 20 had absent or minimal calcific deposits and absent or minimal mitral regurgitation as determined by left ventricular angiography; nevertheless, MVR had been performed. We analyzed retrospectively those 20 patients to examine if MVR was preferable to MVC.[3]

To answer this question unequivocally, the stenotic mitral valves in patients who had only commissurotomy would have to be studied morphologically and radiographically in the same manner as those that were excised and replaced. Obviously, the nonexcised valve cannot be examined in the same manner as the excised valve. Nevertheless, the ideal valve for MVC in the past has been considered to be the stenotic one that is free of calcific deposits, free of significant mitral regurgitation, and mobile. The excised mitral valves in the 20 patients whom we[3] analyzed were free of calcific deposits by preoperative examination (or nearly so by radiography of the excised valve, a far more sensitive technique than x-ray or fluoroscopy through the chest wall), and none had significant regurgitation by left ventricular angiography. The degree of mobility was infrequently described in the operative note. All 20 patients analyzed would probably have been acceptable candidates for MVC in the pre–valve replacement era. Why, then, might valve replacement be performed with its prosthetic- or bioprosthetic-related complications rather than MVC in this circumstance?

Of the 20 patients studied by Lachman and me,[3] several reasons appeared to account for MVR rather than MVC: (1) *Another cardiac valve was also replaced* (13 patients). Therefore, if the patient is required to have anticoagulant therapy for a prosthesis in the tricuspid or aortic valve position, MVR may be the more reasonable procedure and will avoid the risk of significant regurgitation or incomplete relief of the stenosis by MVC. (2) *Cardiopulmonary bypass was used* (all 20 patients). This procedure obviously allows visual inspection of the valve, something not possible when MVC is done as a "closed" procedure. I suspect that the visually inspected stenotic mitral valve is more frightening to the observer than is the palpated stenotic valve. Thus, visual inspection alone, particularly when valve replacement is a reasonable and uncriticized option, may push the surgeon toward replacement rather than simple commissurotomy in some patients. (3) *Some surgeons had relatively little experience with MVC* (17 patients). Of the 20 patients we analyzed, 17 were operated on by surgeons <40 years old when the operation was done. As pointed out by Bonchek,[1] younger surgeons have had much less *with attempted MVC* (3 patients). (5) *Previous MVC had been performed* (11 patients). Although there is disagreement on this point, a mitral valve that has had a commissurotomy and later becomes severely stenotic can nevertheless have another MVC as long as calcific deposits are absent and regurgitation is absent or minimal. (6) *Incorrect identification of mitral calcific deposits* (2 patients). A calcific deposit was described in the mitral leaflets at operation, but x-ray of the excised valve showed that it was devoid of calcium.

Each of these 6 factors contributed in ≥1 of the 20 patients analyzed to the final operative decision of MVC rather than MVR. Even though MVC has been performed for >30 years, the mere alternative of MVR appears to have somewhat altered the definition of the mitral valve to the earlier definition of the ideal mitral valve suitable for MVC.

References

1. **Bonchek LI.** Current status of mitral commissurotomy: indications, techniques and results. Am J Cardiol 1983;52:411–414.
2. **Lachman AS, Roberts WC.** Calcific deposits in stenotic mitral valves. Extent and relationship to age, sex, degree of stenosis, cardiac rhythm, previous commissurotomy and left atrial body thrombus from study of 164 operatively-excised valves. Circulation 1978;57:808–815.
3. **Roberts WC, Lachman AS.** Mitral valve *commissurotomy* versus *replacement.* Considerations based on examination of operatively excised stenotic mitral valves. Am Heart J 1979;98:56–62.

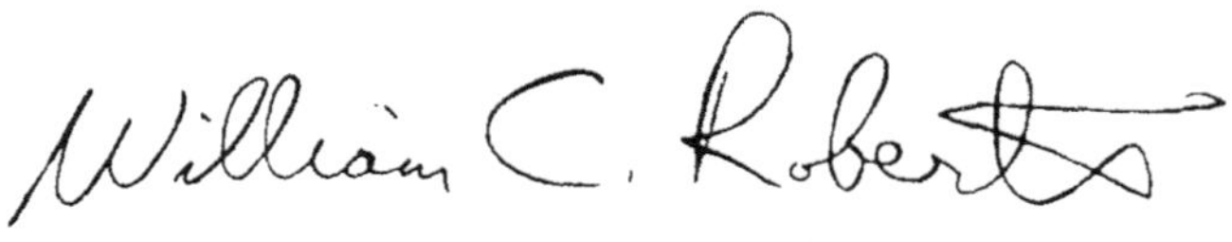

William C. Roberts, MD
Editor-in-Chief

Frequency and Significance of M-Mode Echocardiographic Evidence of Mitral Valve Prolapse In Clinically Isolated Pure Mitral Regurgitation: Analysis of 65 Patients Having Mitral Valve Replacement

BRUCE F. WALLER, MD, BARRY J. MARON, MD, ALBERT A. DEL NEGRO, MD, JOHN S. GOTTDIENER, MD, and WILLIAM C. ROBERTS, MD

To assess the reliability of M-mode echocardiographic patterns of mitral valve prolapse (MVP) (echo MVP) in detection of morphologic evidence of MVP (morphologic MVP), operatively excised mitral valves and corresponding M-mode echocardiograms from 65 patients with chronic, severe, isolated, pure mitral regurgitation (MR) were studied. Of the 65 patients, 45 (69%) had echo MVP (either holosystolic or mid-to-late systolic prolapse patterns on preoperative M-mode echograms) and 42 (93%) of them had morphologic MVP; of the 3 without morphologic MVP, 2 had ruptured chordae tendineae from infective endocarditis and 1 had papillary muscle dysfunction from atherosclerotic coronary heart disease. Of the 20 patients without echo MVP, 14 (70%) had no morphologic MVP (9 had papillary muscle dysfunction from coronary heart disease, 4 had infective endocarditis on previous normal valves and 1 had rheumatic heart disease). Of the 48 patients with morphologic MVP, 42 (88%) had echo MVP and most had considerably dilated mitral anulae; the other 6 had ruptured chordae tendineae with less degrees of anular dilatation. Of the 17 patients without morphologic MVP, 3 had echo MVP (coronary artery disease in 1 and infective endocarditis on a previous normal valve in 2); of the 14 with neither echo nor morphologic MVP, 9 had papillary muscle dysfunction from coronary artery disease, 4 had infective endocarditis on previously normal valves and 1 had rheumatic heart disease. The patients with very dilated mitral anuli and leaflet areas generally had holosystolic (hammocking) patterns on echo; the patients with small anuli and leaflet areas usually had mid-to-late systolic (buckling) prolapse patterns.

(Am J Cardiol 1984;53:139–147)

Numerous clinical, echocardiographic (echo) and angiographic studies have attempted to establish criteria for the diagnosis of mitral valve prolapse (MVP). The echo signs of MVP have usually been established by auscultatory or angiographic signs, or both, considered diagnostic of MVP, and the echo signs of MVP infrequently have been compared to valves that possess characteristic morphologic features of MVP.[1–4] To assess the reliability of M-mode echo patterns of MVP (echo MVP) in detecting morphologic evidence of MVP (morphologic MVP), preoperative M-mode echocardiograms and operatively excised mitral valves were analyzed from 65 patients undergoing mitral valve replacement for isolated, pure mitral regurgitation (MR) associated with normally functioning aortic valves.

From the Pathology and Cardiology Branches, National Heart, Lung, and Blood Institute, National Institutes of Health, Bethesda, Maryland, and the Department of Medicine (Cardiology), Georgetown University Medical Center, Washington, D.C. Manuscript received and accepted August 22, 1983.

Address for reprints: Bruce F. Waller, MD, Department of Pathology, Indiana University School of Medicine, University Hospital, N-340, Indianapolis, Indiana 46223.

Methods

Patients studied: Operatively excised purely regurgitant mitral valves accessioned in the Pathology Branch of the National Heart, Lung, and Blood Institute from December 1973 through August 1982 were examined. Preoperative precordial auscultatory, cardiac catheterization pressure and angiographic observations substantiated the anatomic diagnosis of a purely regurgitant valve. Patients with associated mitral stenosis, aortic valve dysfunction, intracardiac shunts or hypertrophic cardiomyopathy were excluded. After these exclusions, 97 patients had clinically *isolated, severe, chronic* and *pure* MR and each met the following criteria[5]: (1) severe (3+ or 4+/4+) MR by left ventricular angiography; (2) mean diastolic pressure gradient between the left atrium or pulmonary arterial wedge position and left ventricle of ≤2 mm

Hg, and no gradient at end-diastole between the left atrium and left ventricle; (3) no stenosis or regurgitation of the aortic valve; and (4) clinical evidence of congestive heart failure for ≥2 months. Of the 97 patients (described earlier[5]), 65 had preoperative echocardiograms available for review, and they constitute the study group.

Morphologic criteria for etiologic subgrouping: The circumference (in cm), by measuring the length of the anulus of the excised mitral valve, and the leaflet area, by outlining the basal and distal margins of the opened leaflets and measuring the area by videoplanimetry, were determined in all patients.[5] The patients were divided into 4 groups based upon "anular" circumference, leaflet area, status of the chordae tendineae and attached portions of papillary muscles (Tables I, II and III).

Morphologic mitral valve prolapse: These valves had leaflet areas >11 cm^2 and the distance from basal attachment to leaflet free margin of the posterior leaflet was focally increased in that ≥1 segment was elongated compared to other segments. Valves with intact chordae tendineae had circumferences of >11 cm, while the valves with absent or ruptured chordae tendineae had circumferences of >10 cm. The valves with ruptured chordae had focal thickening of 1 or both leaflets at sites of the ruptured chordae. Additionally, a portion of leaflet was missing (indented) or perforated.

Healed infective endocarditis on previously normal valves: The major portion of leaflet and most chordae tendineae in these valves were normal. The valve leaflet area was <11 cm^2 and the "anular" circumference was <11 cm. Several chordae attached to 1 or both leaflets were ruptured (or absent), and the adjacent leaflet was thickened by fibrous tissue and a portion was either indented or perforated. These valves differed from those classified as "prolapsed mitral valves with ruptured chordae tendineae" by the *absence* of ≥1 elongated posterior leaflet segment and smaller total leaflet areas.

Atherosclerotic coronary heart disease with papillary muscle dysfunction: The mitral leaflets and chordae tendineae were either normal or only slightly and focally thickened, the leaflet areas were <11 cm^2, the "anular" circumferences ≤10 cm, and no leaflet indentations, perforations or ruptured chordae were present and 1 or both papillary muscles was extensively scarred and usually atrophied.

Rheumatic: Both mitral leaflets were diffusely thickened by fibrous tissue and the chordae tendineae may or may not have been abnormal.[6] The mitral leaflet areas and "anular" circumferences were <11 cm^2 and <11 cm, respectively.

Echocardiographic techniques: Preoperative M-mode echocardiograms from the 65 patients were retrospectively and independently reviewed by 2 echocardiographers (BJM, AADN) who had no knowledge of the morphologic classification. M-mode echocardiograms were performed using a 2.25-MHz, 1.25-cm-diameter transducer and either a Hoffrel 201, Smith-Kline Ekoline or Irex ultrasound receiver interfaced with a Honeywell or Irex strip-chart recorder. Mitral valve echocardiograms were recorded using an ultrasound window at the left sternal border with the transducer perpendicular to the anterior chest wall. Each M-mode echocardiogram was analyzed for the presence or absence of the following 4 mitral valve echo signs or patterns: prolapse (mid-to-late systolic ["buckling"], holosystolic ["hammocking"]), ruptured chordae tendineae and vegetations.

Characterization of prolapse: Two echo patterns of MVP were observed: mid-to-late systolic and holosystolic. Mid-to-late systolic prolapse ("buckling") was defined as posterior motion of 1 or both mitral leaflets beginning at or during the latter half of ventricular systole. Holosystolic ("hammocking")

TABLE I Clinical Observations in 65 Patients with Mitral Valve Replacement for Isolated, Pure Mitral Regurgitation

Observation	Floppy: With RCT (n = 13)	Floppy: Without RCT (n = 35)	Floppy: Total (n = 48)	Coronary (n = 10)‡	Infective Endocarditis (n = 6)‖	Rheumatic (n = 1)
1. Age (yr) at MVR (range, mean)	48–69 (58)	26–74 (56)	24–74 (57)	47–78 (61)	32–56 (41)	53
2. Men (%))/Women (%)	9 (69):4 (31)	17 (49):18 (51)	26 (54):22 (46)	8:2	5:1	0:1
3. History of IE	4	0	4 (6%)	0	5	0
4. Systolic clicks	0*	0	0	0	0	0
5. Duration (yr) MR mur	2–20 (8)	2–22 (9)	2–22 (8.5)	1–5 (4)	0.8–1.8 (1.2)	12
6. Direct SAP (mm Hg) (range, mean)	115–160 (140) 70–85 (82)	110–168 (136) 62–90 (76)	110–168 (138) 62–90 (79)	100–160 (129) 75–88 (81)	138–155 (146) 65–88 (80)	160 90
7. Direct systolic SAP >140 or diastolic >90 mm Hg	6 (46%)	9 (28%)	15 (31%)	2	4	1
8. MVP by E/total no. E	7/13	35/35	42/48 (88%)	1/10	2/6	0
9. E pattern of MVP						
Holosystolic	6/7	20/35 (57%)	26/42 (62%)	1/1	1/2	0
Mid-to-late systolic	1/7	15/35 (43%)	16/42 (38%)	0	1/2	0
10. E pattern of RCT	10/13	5/35 (14%)	15/48 (31%)	0	4/6	0
(No. with both RCT + MVP patterns)	(4/10)	(5/5)	(9/15 [60%])		2/4	
11. E pattern of vegetation	5	6 (17%)	11 (23%)	0	2	0
12. Interval (days) from E to MVR (range, avg)	3–406 (47)	6–377 (94)	3–406 (82)	8–26 (18)	13–156 (43)	83
13. One or more major CA narrowed >50% in D by angio/total no. angio	0/1	3/22 (14%)†	3–23 (13%)†	10/10§	0/1	—

* One patient had a systolic click and late systolic murmur 4 months before active IE developed but the precordial murmur became holosystolic and the click disappeared.

† Only the right coronary artery was narrowed in each patient and only 1 had anginal pain.

‡ Of 10 patients, 9 had MVR with aortocoronary bypass grafting and 1 had MVR with left ventricular aneurysmectomy. All 10 patients had angina pectoris and evidence of past myocardial infarction.

§ All 3 major coronary arteries (left anterior descending, left circumflex and right) were narrowed in each patient and each patient had at least one and most 2 artery systems bypassed.

‖ Healed in all.

Angio = angiogram; CA = coronary arteries; D = diameter; Da = days; E = M-mode echocardiogram; IE = infective endocarditis; MR = mitral regurgitation; Mur = precordial murmur; MVP = mitral valve prolapse; MVR = mitral valve replacement; RCT = ruptured (or absent) chordae tendineae; SAP = systemic arterial pressure.

TABLE II Morphologic Criteria for Etiologic Subgrouping or Purely Regurgitant Mitral Valves

	Floppy				
	+RCT	−RCT	Coronary	Infective Endocarditis	Rheumatic
1. Leaflets					
A. Elongated (distance from basal attachment to distal margin of closure)	+	+	0	0	0
B. Increased area (anterior plus posterior >11 cm^2)	+	+	0	0	0
C. Indented or perforated	+	0	0	+	0
D. Diffuse fibrous thickening	0	0	0	0	+
2. Anular circumference >11 cm	0*	+	0	0	0
3. Chordae tendineae ruptured	+	0	0	+	0
4. Papillary muscles scarred	0	0	+	0	0

* Anular circumference ≥10.5 cm but ≤11.0 cm.
+ = present; 0 = absent.

prolapse was defined as posterior motion of 1 or both leaflets beginning at the onset of and continuing throughout ventricular systole with posterior excursion from the CD line of ≥3 mm. The echo prolapse pattern was observed on multiple recordings. Three patients had both late systolic and holosystolic patterns of MVP on the same recording, but the holosystolic pattern was the predominant one, and thus, each patient was classified under the holosystolic subgroup.

Characterization of ruptured chordae tendineae: Rupture of mitral chordae tendineae was diagnosed echocardiographically if ≥1 of the following patterns was observed: (1) abnormal echoes in the left atrium during ventricular systole; (2) coarse, irregular, erratic diastolic fluttering of the anterior or posterior leaflets; (3) systolic fluttering of 1 or both leaflets; and (4) early and sustained diastolic, anterior ("paradoxical") motion of the posterior leaflet.

Characterization of leaflet vegetations: The M-mode echo diagnosis of mitral valve leaflet "vegetation" was based on the presence of thick, irregularly bordered ("shaggy") echoes that involved the anterior or posterior leaflet, or both, in ventricular systole or diastole, or both, without significant impairment of leaflet movement.

TABLE III Morphologic Observations and M-Mode Echocardiographic Patterns of Operatively Excised Mitral Valves in 65 Patients with Isolated Pure Mitral Regurgitation and in 18 Necropsy Valves

	Floppy						
Mitral Valve (MV) Observation	With RCT (n = 13)	Without RCT (n = 35)	Total (n = 48)	Coronary (n = 10)	Infective Endocarditis (n = 6)	Rheumatic (n = 1)	Necropsy Controls (n = 18)
1. Circumference (C) (cm)	10.5–11.0 (10.9)*	11.5–16.0 (13.4)**	10.5–16.0 (12.8)**	8.5–10.0 (9.4)*	9.5–10.5 (9.7)*	10.5 ...	8.0–10.5 (9.4)*
2. Leaflet area (A) (cm^2)	11.6–16.0 (14.0)*	11.9–25.2 (17.5)**	11.6–25.2 (16.6)**	8.8–10.9 (9.9)***	9.2–10.6 (9.7)***	10.6 ...	7.0–12.5 (9.5)***
3. C × A product (cm^3)	128–178 (152)*	149–391 (240)**	128–391 (216)**	81–107 (94)***	87–113 (95)***	111 ...	45–140 (91)***
4. No. with C >11 cm	0	35	35 (73%)	0	0	0	0
5. No. with ruptured chordae tendineae (RCT)	13	0	13 (27%)	0	6	0	0
6. No. with vegetations	0‡	0§	0	0	0‖	0	0
7. Echo(E) pattern of mitral valve prolapse (MVP) *only*	3/13	30/35 (86%)	33/48 (69%)	1	0	0	...
C	11.0 (11.0*)	11.5–16.0 (13.4**)	11.0–16.0 (14.1**)†	9.5***			
A	15.4–16.2 (15.9)*	11.9–23.2 (17.2*)†	11.9–23.2 (17.1)*	9.7***			
C × A Product	165–178 (171)*	149–360 (235)**†	149–360 (229)**	92***			
8. E pattern of RTC *only*	6/13	0/35	6/48	0	2	0	...
C	10.5–11.0 (10.8)		10.5–11.0 (10.8)		9.5 (9.5)		
A	11.6–13.4 (12.6)		11.6–13.4 (12.6)		9.2,9.8 (9.5)		
C × A product	128–147 (136)		128–147 (136)		87,93 (90)		
9. E pattern of *both* MVP + RCT	4/13	5/35	9/48	0	2	0	...
C	10.5–11.0 (11.0)	12.5–15.5 (13.9)	10.5–15.5 (12.5)†		9.5,10.5 (10.0)		
A	14.6–15.3 (15.0)	13.4–25.2 (19.1)†	13.4–25.2 (17.1)		10.6,9.5 (10.1)		
C × A product	161–176 (165)	161–391 (266)†	161–391 (216)		90,113 (102)		

*-** (Horizontal only) = p <.01.
*-***,**-*** (Horizontal only) = p <0.001.
†-† (vertical only) = p <.05.
‡ Five patients had echocardiographic patterns of leaflet vegetations. All 5 valves were free of vegetations but had focal areas of leaflet fibrous thickening and indentation at sites of ruptured chords.
§ Six patients had echocardiographic patterns of leaflet vegetations. All 6 valves were free of vegetations but had large leaflet areas ("redundant") with focal sites of fibrous thickening.
‖ Two patients had echocardiographic patterns of vegetations but both operatively excised valves were free of vegetations and each had focal areas of fibrous thickening and leaflet indentation at sites of ruptured chords.

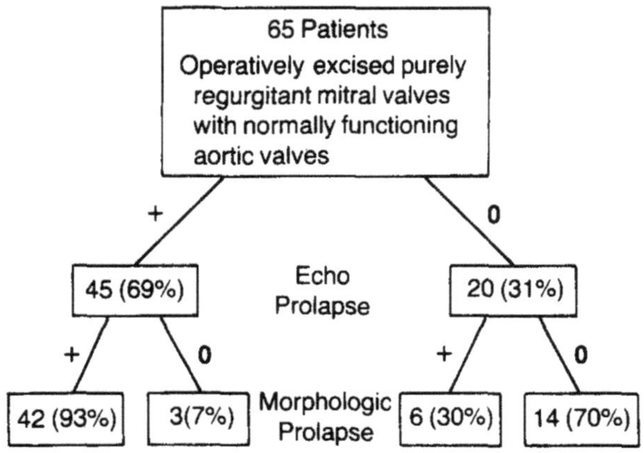

FIGURE 1. The frequency of echocardiographic (Echo) and morphologic mitral valve prolapse in the 65 patients with clinically isolated pure mitral regurgitation.

Temporal relation of echocardiogram to mitral valve replacement: The echocardiograms were recorded 3 to 406 days (mean 82) before MVR. Of 48 patients with morphologic MVP, the echocardiogram was performed within 30 days (mean 15) of operation in 26 patients, within 31 to 60 days (mean 43) in 6, 61 to 180 days (mean 104) in 7, and 6 to 12 months (mean 9) before operation in 8 patients. Two patients had echocardiograms done 377 and 406 days, respectively, before valve replacement; neither had ruptured chordae tendineae echocardiographically or morphologically. Patients with infective endocarditis on previously normal valves had echocardiograms recorded 13 to 156 days (mean 43) before valve replacement; patients with papillary muscle dysfunction had echograms 8 to 26 days (mean 18) preoperatively, and the only patient with rheumatic heart disease had an echocardiogram 83 days before valve replacement.

Statistical analysis: Data were compared using the chi-square test or unpaired *t* test, with statistical significance achieved if p was <0.05. The extent of agreement between the 2 independent echocardiographers was evaluated for each of the echo signs or patterns analyzed. Of 48 interpretations for the presence or absence of each of 3 patterns, 11 interobserver differences occurred, as follows: echo MVP, 5 patients (10%); ruptured chordae tendineae, 4 (8%); and leaflet vegetation, 2 (4%). These differences were then resolved by the third echocardiographer (JSG), who was unaware of the morphologic classification of the valve disease.

Results

Morphologic observations: Gross examination of the 65 mitral valves (Fig. 1) disclosed 48 with (Fig. 2) and 17 without (Fig. 3) morphologic MVP. In 10 patients (15%), the MR resulted from papillary muscle dysfunction secondary to atherosclerotic coronary heart disease (neither the chordae nor papillary muscles were ruptured); in 6 patients (9%), the cause was infective endocarditis that involved an apparently normal mitral valve (in all 6 valves the chordae were ruptured and the leaflets perforated or indented), and 1 patient had MR from rheumatic heart disease (Fig. 4). Results of morphologic measurements of anular circumference, leaflet area and circumference-area product for each subgroup are summarized in Table III. None of the 65 valves had vegetations of active infective endocarditis, but 19 valves (13 with morphologic MVP) with ruptured chordae tendineae had focal fibrous thickening of 1 or both leaflets at sites of ruptured chordae, and leaflet indentations or perforations indicative of healed infective endocarditis.[7]

Echocardiographic observations: Of the 65 patients, 45 (69%) had echo MVP, 42 (93%) of whom had morphologic MVP (Fig. 1); of the other 3 patients, 2 had healed infective endocarditis on previously normal valves and 1 had papillary muscle dysfunction from atherosclerotic coronary heart disease. Of the 20 patients without echo MVP, 6 (30%), nevertheless, had morphologic MVP and 14 (70%) did not (Fig. 1). Of the 48 patients with morphologic MVP (Fig. 2), 42 patients (88%) had echo MVP, and 7 of them had ruptured chordae; of the 6 patients with morphologic MVP without echo MVP, each had ruptured chordae tendineae. Of the 17 patients without morphologic MVP, 14 (82%) had no echo MVP; of the other 3 patients, 1 had papillary muscle dysfunction and 2 had healed infective endocarditis on previously normal valves (Fig. 3).

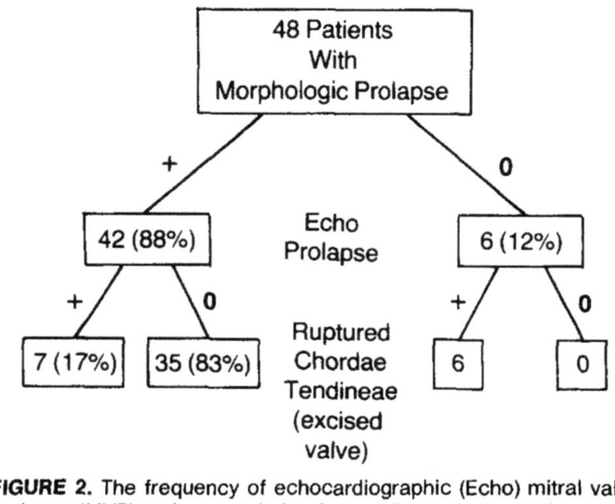

FIGURE 2. The frequency of echocardiographic (Echo) mitral valve prolapse (MVP) and ruptured chordae tendineae in the patients with morphologic MVP.

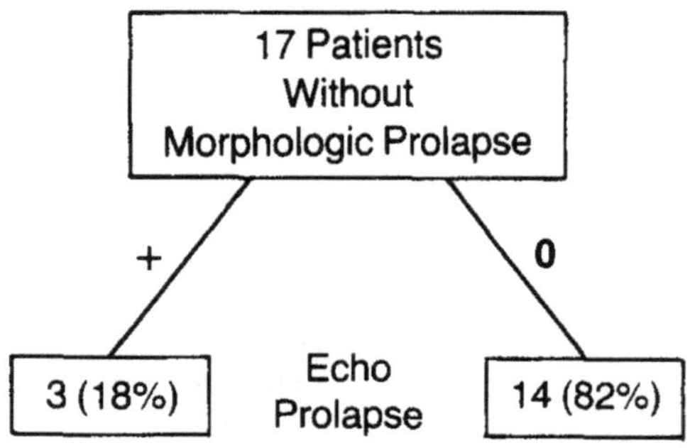

FIGURE 3. The frequency of echocardiographic (Echo) mitral valve prolapse (MVP) among the patients without morphologic MVP. Of the 3 patients with echo MVP, 1 had papillary muscle dysfunction from coronary heart disease and 2 had healed infective endocarditis on a previously normal mitral valve. Of the 14 patients without echo MVP, 9 had MR from coronary heart disease, 9 had healed infective endocarditis on previously normal valves, and 1 patient had rheumatic heart disease.

The 48 patients with morphologic MVP were divided into 3 groups: those with holosystolic echo MVP (26 patients) (Fig. 5 to 9), those with mid-to-late systolic echo MVP (16 patients) (Fig. 5–7 and 10) and those without echo MVP (6 patients) (Fig. 5, 6, 7 and 11). The mean mitral anular circumferences (Fig. 5), leaflet areas (Fig. 6) and the products of the leaflet areas (in cm^2) times the anular circumferences (in cm) (Fig. 7) were significantly different in each of the 3 groups of morphologic MVP. The 13 patients with morphologic MVP with ruptured chordae tendineae (7 with and 6 without echo MVP) are displayed in the dashed boxes in Figures 5 to 7. Of the 7 valves with echo MVP, 6 had holosystolic patterns. The 7 patients with ruptured chordae and combined echo and morphologic MVP had similar average "anular" circumferences (Fig. 5), but significantly different mean leaflet areas (Fig. 6) and circumference-area products (Fig. 7) than did the 6 patients with ruptured chordae and morphologic MVP without echo MVP.

M-mode echo patterns of ruptured chordae tendineae were observed in 19 patients (29%); 15 (79%) had morphologic MVP (Fig. 11) and 4 (21%) had infective endocarditis without morphologic MVP (Fig. 12). Of 15 patients with morphologic MVP and echo patterns of ruptured chordae (Table I), 10 had morphologically confirmed ruptured chordae and 5 had intact chordae

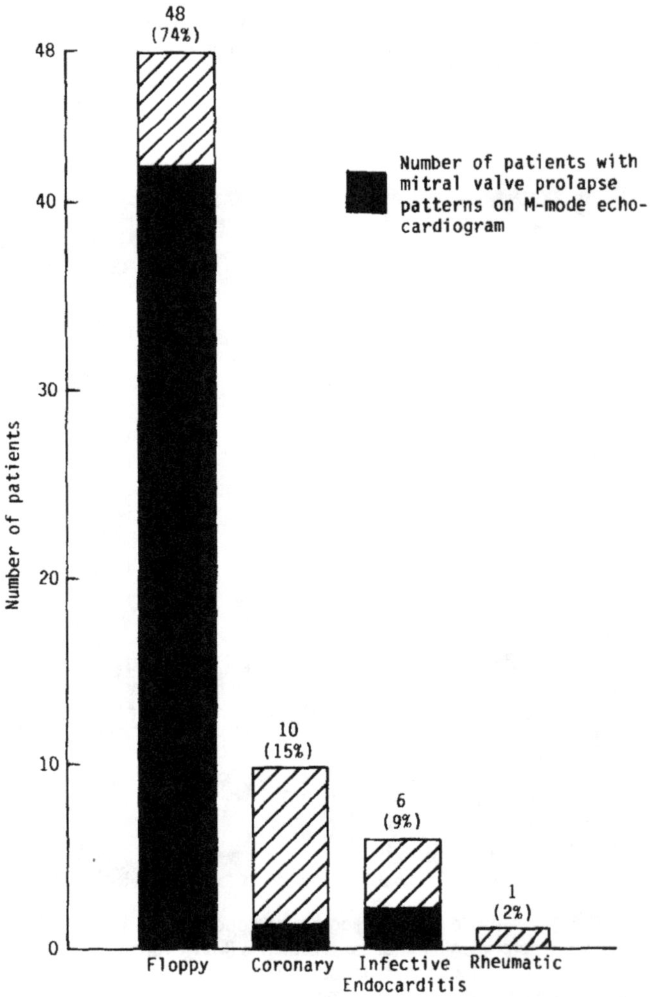

FIGURE 4. The etiology of isolated pure mitral regurgitation and number of patients and frequency of echocardiographic mitral valve prolapse in the 65 patients.

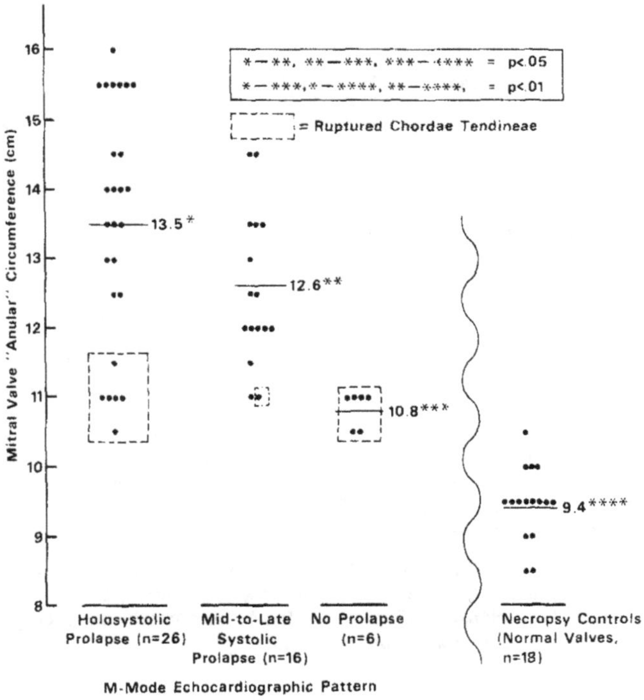

FIGURE 5. The relation of mitral valve anular circumference to M-mode mitral valve prolapse (MVP) patterns in the 48 patients with morphologic MVP and in 18 necropsy control valves.

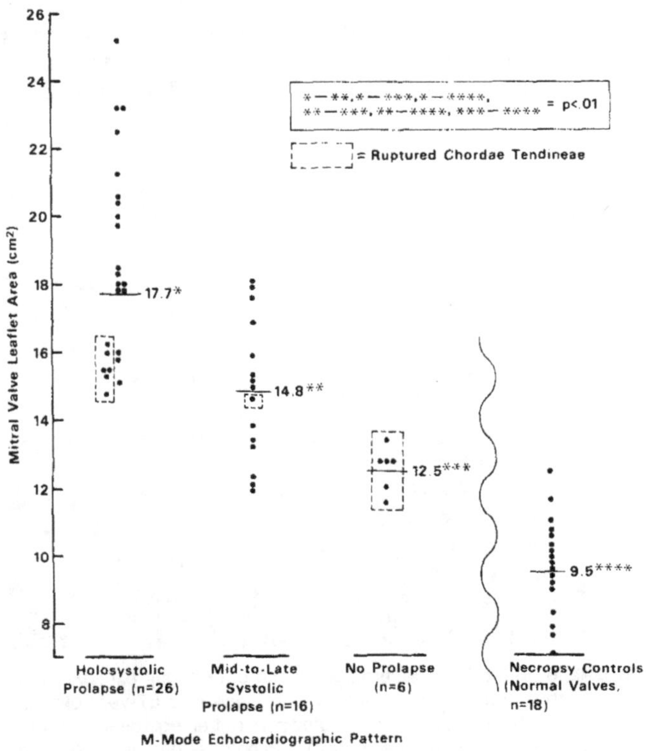

FIGURE 6. The relation of mitral valve leaflet area (in cm^2) to M-mode echocardiographic mitral valve prolapse (MVP) pattern in the 48 patients with morphologic MVP and in 18 necropsy control valves.

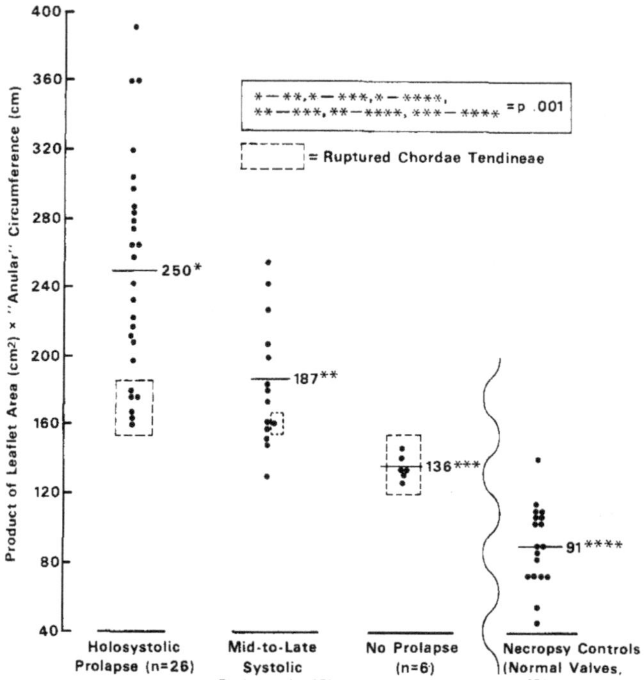

FIGURE 7. The relation of product of mitral valve leaflet area (in cm^2) times "anular" circumference (in cm) to M-mode echocardiographic mitral valve prolapse (MVP) pattern in the 48 patients with morphologic MVP and in 18 necropsy control valves.

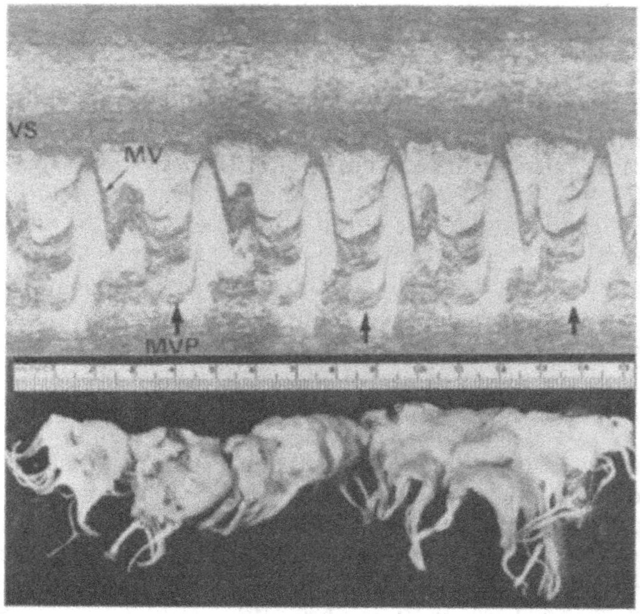

FIGURE 9. M-mode echocardiogram and operatively excised prolapsed mitral valve from a 60-year-old man (S79–119) with isolated pure MR. **Upper,** echocardiogram of mitral valve (MV) showing holosystolic echocardiographic mitral valve prolapse (MVP) during ventricular systole and thickened leaflets suggesting leaflet vegetation. VS = ventricular septum. **Lower,** operatively excised mitral valve showing an "anular" circumference of 15 cm, leaflet area of 18 cm^2 and extensive areas of leaflet fibrous thickening. No leaflet vegetations or ruptured chordae tendineae were present.

tendineae. Of 13 patients with morphologic MVP with ruptured chordae, 10 had echo patterns of ruptured chordae (Table I). Of 6 patients without morphologic MVP but with ruptured chordae, 4 had echo patterns of ruptured chordae. The 5 false-positive echograms were from patients with morphologic MVP with large anuli (14.0 to 15.5 cm) (Fig. 1) and leaflet areas (20 to

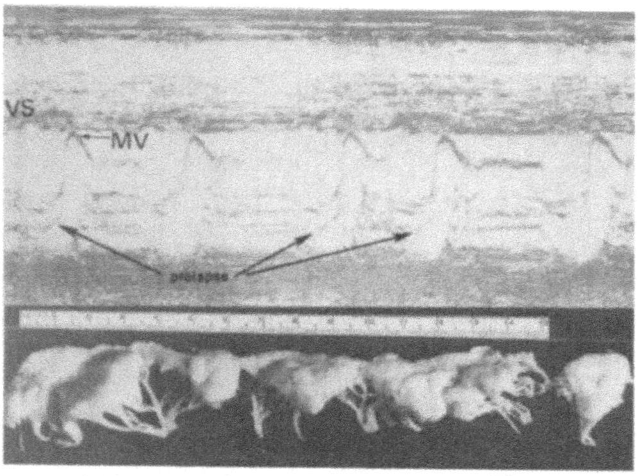

FIGURE 8. M-mode echocardiogram and operatively excised mitral valve with morphologic mitral valve prolapse in a 67-year-old man (S80-172) with chronic, severe, isolated pure mitral regurgitation. **Upper,** echocardiogram of mitral valve (MV) with holosystolic prolapse of the posterior leaflet during ventricular systole. VS = ventricular septum. **Lower,** operatively excised valve with an "anular" circumference of 16 cm and a leaflet area of 18 cm^2.

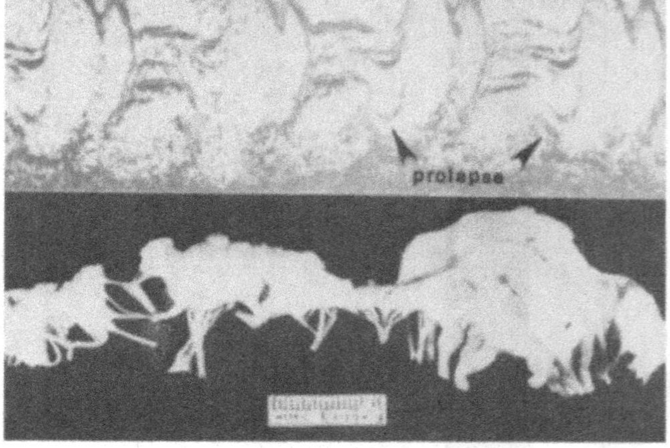

FIGURE 10. M-mode echocardiogram and operatively excised mitral valve with morphologic mitral valve prolapse (MVP) from a 45-year-old woman (S78–142) with chronic, severe, isolated pure mitral regurgitation. **Upper,** echocardiogram of mitral valve (MV) showing late systolic MVP of the posterior mitral leaflet during ventricular systole. RV = right ventricular cavity; VS = ventricular septum. **Lower,** operatively excised valve with an anulus of 14 cm and a leaflet area of 15 cm^2.

23 cm^2) (Fig. 2). Of the 5 false-negative echo patterns, 3 occurred in patients with morphologic MVP and holosystolic echo patterns; the other 2 were in patients without echo or morphologic MVP and without echo patterns of ruptured chordae (Table I).

M-mode echo patterns of leaflet "vegetations" of infective endocarditis were observed in 13 patients (20%) (11 with and 2 without morphologic MVP) (Fig. 9). In none of the 13 were the "vegetations" active. Of the 13 patients, 7 (5 with and 2 without morphologic MVP) had focal areas of leaflet indentation and fibrous thickening at sites of healed ruptured chordae indicative of healed infective endocarditis; the other 6 had mitral valves without morphologic MVP but with intact chordae tendineae, valves similar to the remaining 29 valves with morphologic MVP with intact chordae whose echograms did not have "vegetation" patterns.

Discussion

Considerable variation exists in the sensitivity of echo in detecting morphologic MVP because of the lack of consistent diagnostic criteria of morphologic MVP using auscultatory, angiographic or morphologic standards. Waller et al[5] recently reported a morphologic definition of MVP producing MR severe enough to warrent mitral valve replacement. The definition was based on mitral anular circumference and leaflet area. Operatively excised valves with morphologic MVP had anular circumferences or leaflet areas clearly increased over that of other mitral valve conditions causing severe, pure MR. Except when associated with ruptured chordae tendineae, anular circumferences >11 cm served to separate valves with from those without morphologic MVP. Valves with morphologic MVP and ruptured chordae had mitral circumferences usually increased above normal, but the additional measurement of increased leaflet area was necessary to clearly distinguish the valves with from those without morphologic MVP. With these morphologic criteria established, it became possible to assess the reliability of echo MVP using morphologic standards.

The combined sensitivity of holosystolic (hammocking) and late systolic (buckling) MVP patterns in diagnosing morphologic MVP in the present study was 88%. Of the 48 patients with morphologic MVP, 6 had false-negative M-mode echocardiograms of MVP and

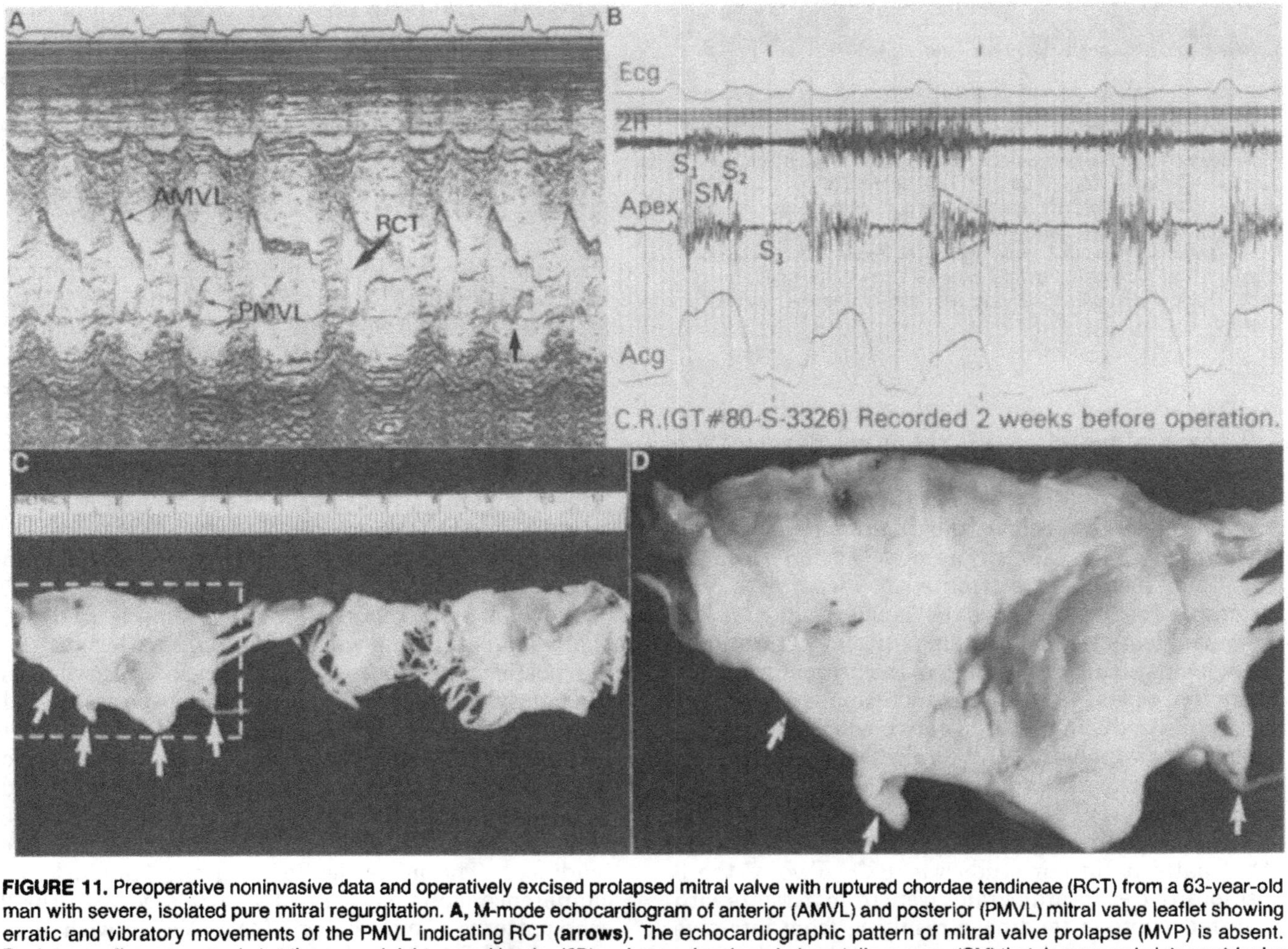

FIGURE 11. Preoperative noninvasive data and operatively excised prolapsed mitral valve with ruptured chordae tendineae (RCT) from a 63-year-old man with severe, isolated pure mitral regurgitation. **A,** M-mode echocardiogram of anterior (AMVL) and posterior (PMVL) mitral valve leaflet showing erratic and vibratory movements of the PMVL indicating RCT (**arrows**). The echocardiographic pattern of mitral valve prolapse (MVP) is absent. **B,** phonocardiogram recorded at the second right sternal border (2R) and apex showing a holosystolic murmur (SM) that decreases in late ventricular systole (**dashed lines**). Acg = apexcardiogram; Ecg = electrocardiogram; S_1, S_2, and S_3 = first, second and third heart sounds. **C,** operatively excised valve with morphologic MVP and an "anular" circumference of 11.5 cm and a leaflet area of 12 cm^2. Multiple chordae tendineae to an elongated posterior leaflet (**dashed box**) are missing (**arrows**). **D,** blow-up of leaflet in dashed box showing multiple RCT (**arrows**).

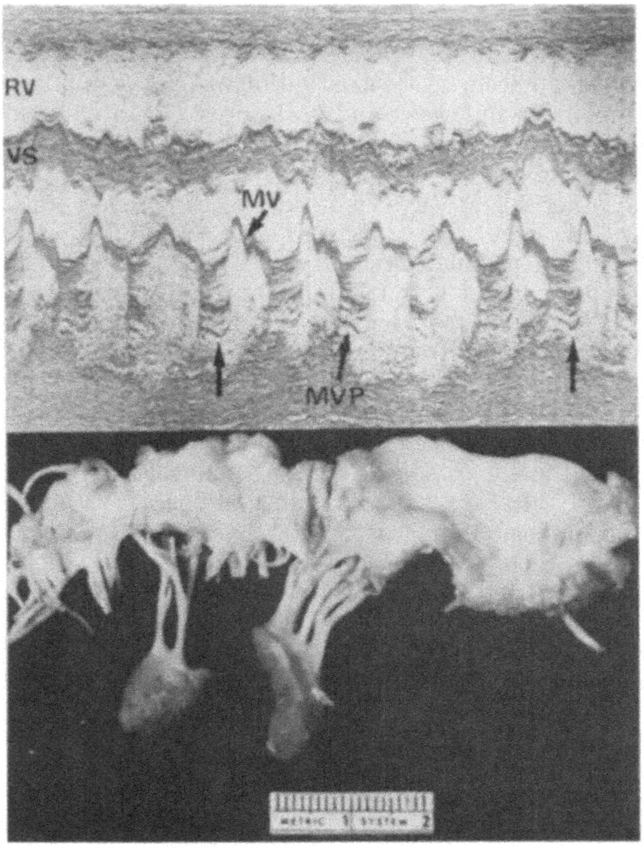

FIGURE 12. M-mode echocardiogram and operatively excised valve without morphologic mitral valve prolapse (MVP) from a 56-year-old man (GT 77S–5736) with chronic, isolated, pure mitral regurgitation from healed infective endocarditis on a previously anatomically and functionally normal valve. **Upper,** echocardiogram of mitral valve (MV) showing MVP and vibratory motion of portions of the posterior leaflet indicating ruptured chordae tendineae. RV = right ventricular cavity; VS = ventricular septum. **Lower,** operatively excised mitral valve with normal mitral "anular" circumference (9.5 cm) and leaflet area (9.8 cm^2). Multiple chordae tendineae are absent and the leaflets are scarred.

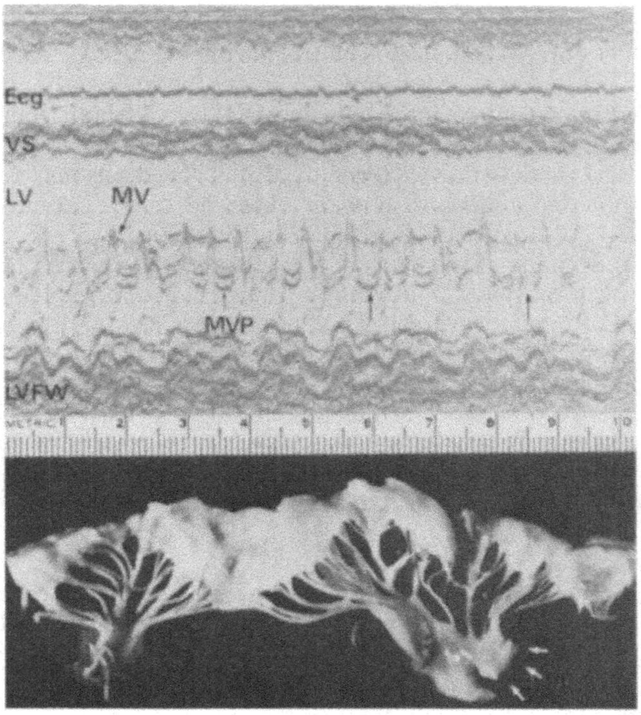

FIGURE 13. M-mode echocardiogram and operatively excised mitral valve without morphologic mitral valve prolapse (MVP) from a 54-year-old man (GT81-S-2186) with severe, chronic, pure mitral regurgitation from papillary muscle dysfunction secondary to atherosclerotic coronary heart disease. **Upper,** echocardiogram showing a dilated left ventricular (LV) cavity, increased E-to-septal distance, and holosystolic MVP. Ecg = electrocardiogram; LVFW = left ventricular free wall; MV = mitral valve; VS = ventricular septum. **Lower,** operatively excised valve with normal circumference (10.3 cm) and leaflet area (10.2 cm^2) but scarred and atrophied papillary muscle (**arrows**).

each had ruptured chordae tendineae. In the 42 patients with true-positive echo MVP, the mitral circumference leaflet areas and/or circumference area products were greater than that of the 6 valves with morphologic MVP and false-negative echocardiograms. Previously reported causes of false-negative MVP on M-mode echograms have been attributed to incomplete echo "scanning" of the mitral valve ("single-beam view" of the mitral leaflets), improperly positioned transducer or low-gain settings.[9] The data in the present study indicate that mitral valve anulus and leaflet sizes also are factors in producing false-negative echograms in patients with morphologic MVP. Valves with morphologic MVP but with small anuli and leaflet areas may not produce echo MVP.

The combined diagnostic specificity of the 2 echo MVP patterns in our study was 82%. Two of the 3 false-positive echocardiograms were from patients with ruptured chordae tendineae resulting from infective endocarditis on previously normal valves; each of the 2 valves had normal mitral anuli and leaflet areas. The third patient with false-positive echo MVP had papillary muscle dysfunction from atherosclerotic coronary heart disease and the mitral valve anulus and leaflet area also were normal (Fig. 13). Previously reported causes of false-positive MVP on M-mode echograms have been observed in patients with papillary muscle dysfunction from coronary artery disease,[10] "flail leaflets" associated with infective endocarditis,[4] mitral anular calcium,[11] inferior transducer angulation[12] and large pericardial effusions.[13] Thus, valves without morphologic MVP may produce echo MVP that is indistinguishable from that produced by valves with morphologic MVP.

Previous echo reports[2,17,21] have emphasized the sharp, midsystolic, posterior buckling pattern as the diagnostic cornerstones of morphologic MVP, whereas the holosystolic hammock pattern has been associated with ruptured chordae tendineae ("flail leaflet") and had been less reliable in the diagnosis of morphologic MVP. In the present study, holosystolic MVP was found in 26 (54%) of 48 patients with morphologic MVP: 6 (23%) had ruptured and 20 (77%) had intact chordae tendineae. The mitral leaflet area and "anular" circumference, however, generally correlated with the 2 echo patterns of morphologic MVP. Valves with morphologic MVP and very large circumferences (>14.5 cm) and leaflet areas (>18 cm^2) had holosystolic echo MVP. Excluding valves with ruptured chordae, valves with morphologic MVP and smaller anuli (<12.5 cm) and leaflet areas (<14.5 cm^2) had mid-to-late systolic echo MVP. DeMaria et al[22] also reported holosystolic echo MVP as the most frequent echocardiographic pattern of MVP in 26 patients with angiographic evidence of prolapse, but none of the valves from their patients was studied morphologically.

References

1. **Burgess J, Clark, R, Kamigaki M, Cohn K.** Echocardiographic findings in different types of mitral regurgitation. Circulation 1973;48:97–106.
2. **Popp RL, Brown OR, Silverman JF, Harrison DC.** Echocardiographic abnormalities in the mitral valve prolapse syndrome. Circulation 1974;49:428–433.
3. **Corrigall D, Bolen J, Hancock EW, Popp RL.** Mitral valve prolapse and infective endocarditis. Am J Med 1977;63:215–222.
4. **Child JS, Skorton DJ, Taylor RD, Krivokapich J, Abbasi AS, Wong M, Shah PD.** M-mode and cross-sectional echocardiographic features of flail posterior mitral leaflets. Am J Cardiol 1979;44:1383–1390.
5. **Waller BF, Morrow AG, Maron BJ, Del Negro AA, Ken KM, McGrath FJ, Wallace RB, McIntosh CL, Roberts WC.** Etiology of clinically isolated, severe, chronic, pure mitral regurgitation: analysis of 97 patients over 30 years of age having mitral valve replacement. Am Heart J 1982;104:276–288.
6. **Roberts WC, Virmani R.** Aschoff bodies at necropsy in valvular heart disease. Evidence from analysis of 543 patients over 14 years of age that rheumatic heart disease, at least anatomically, is a disease of the mitral valve. Circulation 1978;57:803–812.
7. **Roberts WC, Buchbinder NA.** Healed left-sided infective endocarditis: a clinicopathologic study of 59 patients. Am J Cardiol 1977;40:876–888.
8. **Haikal M, Alpert MA, Whiting RB, Ahmad M, Kelly D.** Sensitivity and specificity of M-mode echocardiographic signs of mitral valve prolapse. Am J Cardiol 1982;50:185–190.
9. **Feigenbaum H.** Echocardiography. 2nd Ed. Philadelphia: Lea & Febiger, 1976:119–130.
10. **Aranda JM, Befeler B, Lazzara R, Embi A, Machado H.** Mitral valve prolapse and coronary artery disease. Circulation 1975;52:245–253.
11. **Dashkoff N, Karacuschansky M, Come PC, Fortuin NJ.** Echocardiographic features of mitral annulus calcification. Am Heart J 1977;94:585–592.
12. **Sahn DJ, Allen HD, Goldberg SJ, Friedman WF.** Echocardiographic spectrum of mitral valve motion in children with and without mitral valve prolapse: the nature of false positive diagnosis. Am J Cardiol 1977;39:422–431.
13. **Levisman JA, Abbasi AS.** Abnormal motion of the mitral valve with pericardial effusion: pseudo-prolapse of the mitral valve. Am Heart J 1976;91:18–20.
14. **Criley JM, Kissel GL.** Prolapse of the mitral valve: the click and late systolic murmur syndrome. In: Goodwin J, Yu PN, eds. Progress in Cardiology. Vol. 4. Philadelphia: Lea & Febiger, 1976:23–26.
15. **Wann LS, Dillon JC, Weyman AE, Feigenbaum H.** Echocardiography in bacterial endocarditis. N Engl J Med 1976;295:135–139.
16. **Chandraratna PAN, Lagevin E.** Limitations of the echogram in diagnosing valvular vegetations in patients with mitral valve prolapse. Circulation 1977;56:436–438.
17. **Dillon JC, Haine CL, Chang S, Feigenbaum H.** Use of echocardiography in patients with prolapsed mitral valve. Circulation 1971;43:503–507.
18. **Kerber RE, Isaeff DM, Hancock EW.** Echocardiographic patterns in patients with the syndrome of systolic click and late systolic murmur. N Engl J Med 1971;284:691–693.
19. **Markiewicz W, Stoner J, London E, Hunt SA, Popp RL.** Mitral valve prolapse in one hundred presumably healthy young females. Circulation 1976;54:464–473.
20. **Higgens CB, Reinke RT, Gosink BB, Leopold GR.** The significance of mitral valve prolapse in middle-aged and elderly men. Am Heart J 1976;91:292–296.
21. **DeMaria AN, Neumann A, Lee G, Mason D.** Echocardiographic identification of the mitral valve prolapse syndrome. Am J Med 1977;62:819–829.
22. **DeMaria AN, King JF, Borgren HJ, Lies JE.** The variable spectrum of echocardiographic manifestations of the mitral valve prolapse syndrome. Circulation 1974;50:33–41.

Acquired Left Ventricular Endocardial Constriction From Massive Mural Calcific Deposits: A Newly Recognized Cause of Impairment to Left Ventricular Filling

MARC A. SILVER, MD
ROBERT O. BONOW, MD
STUART M. DEGLIN, MD
BARRY J. MARON, MD
RICHARD O. CANNON, III, MD
WILLIAM C. ROBERTS, MD

Impairment to left ventricular (LV) filling may result from left-sided cardiovascular conditions proximal to the left ventricle (mitral stenosis, cor triatriatum, pulmonary venous obstruction),[1] from LV myocardial conditions (including hypertrophic cardiomyopathy,[2] amyloidosis[3] and hemosiderosis[4]), from pericardial constriction (of several causes),[5] and from LV endomyocardial fibrosis with or without eosinophilia.[6] The last condition, which occurs mainly in Africa, causes extensive LV endocardial fibrosis located primarily in the LV inflow tract and is associated with little or no mural endocardial calcific deposits. The common denominator of all of these conditions is a normal-sized or small LV cavity. This report describes a hitherto unreported cause of impairment to LV filling: massive LV endocardial calcific deposits associated with LV hypertrophy of undetermined origin.

M.L., a 56-year-old white woman (CC #15-01-89-6), was well until age 49 years, when exertional dyspnea and substernal chest pain developed. She underwent the first of 4 cardiac catheterizations (Table I). In each, the LV end-diastolic and pulmonary arterial wedge pressures were elevated; cardiac output was normal; LV angiography (4 times) disclosed a normal-sized to small LV cavity and no mitral regurgitation, and coronary angiography (2 times) disclosed no abnormalities. By age 54 years, the dyspnea and chest pain were occurring at rest and LV calcific deposits were visible. During the next 2 years she remained in functional class IV (New York Heart Association classification) and had periodic episodes of acute pulmonary edema despite therapy with β-blocking and calcium-channel blocking agents, nitrates, furosemide and procainamide. Examination 3 months before death disclosed a grade 3/6 apical systolic precordial murmur that did not vary in intensity with maneuvers. The electrocardiogram had changes consistent with LV hypertrophy with strain (Fig. 1), and the 2-dimensional echocardiogram showed a large, echo-dense mass that measured about 3 × 4 cm and occupied most of the midportion of LV cavity (Fig. 2). Chest radiographs and LV angiograms revealed a small, hypercontractile LV cavity (Fig. 3). Radionuclide angiography disclosed an LV filling rate of 1.3 end-diastolic volumes/s (normal ≥2.5). Pulmonary function studies, summarized in Table II, revealed changes consistent with mixed obstructive and restrictive pulmonary disease. The patient had been in sinus rhythm until atrial fibrillation appeared intermittently about 2.5 months before death. She died on July 14, 1983, after another episode of acute pulmonary edema.

At necropsy, the heart weighed 560 g (the patient weighed 58 kg). The LV wall (including ventricular septum) was thick, its cavity small and many LV mural endocardial calcific deposits were present (Fig. 4). No LV foci of fibrosis, necrosis or myocardial fiber disorganization were present. Both intramural and extramural coronary arteries were normal or nearly normal. Both atria were dilated. Analysis of the LV calcific deposit disclosed that the deposit consisted of calcium phosphate (carbonate form) (60%), and blood and protein matrix (40%). The pulmonary veins were considerably dilated and their walls and those of the pulmonary arteries were mildly thickened. The pulmonary parenchyma had changes consistent entirely with those that result from chronic pulmonary venous hypertension. A primary parenchymal pulmonary disorder was absent.

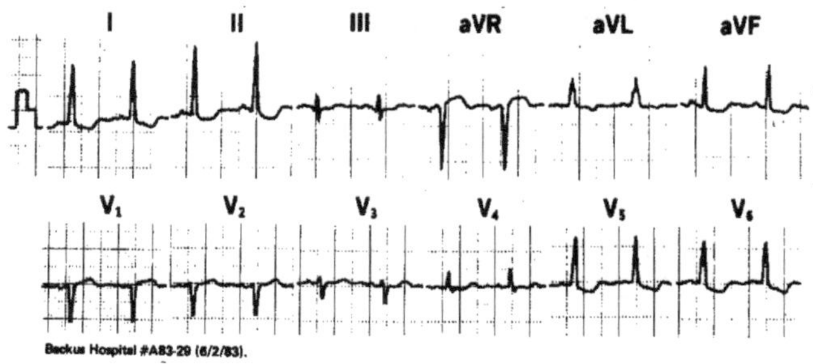

FIGURE 1. Electrocardiogram of patient taken 42 days before death. Leads V_1 to V_6 are recorded at one-half standard.

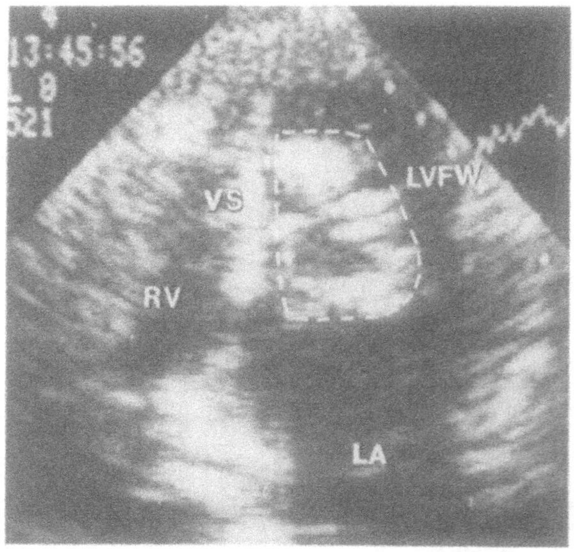

FIGURE 2. Two-dimensional echocardiogram obtained in the apical 4-chamber view. Left ventricular (LV) apex is to the **top** and the base is to the **bottom.** Calcific mass (within the **broken line**) occupies much of the LV cavity and appears to adhere to the LV free wall (LVFW), but not the ventricular septum (VS). LA = left atrium; RV = right ventricle. Calibration dots are 1 cm apart.

From the Pathology and Cardiology Branches, National Heart, Lung, and Blood Institute, National Institutes of Health, Bethesda, Maryland, and the Department of Medicine, Yale University School of Medicine, New Haven, Connecticut. Manuscript received and accepted February 15, 1984.

TABLE I Hemodynamic Data in Patient M.L.

Pressures (mm Hg)	3/15/76 (Age 49 yr)	8/13/81 (Age 54 yr)	8/21/81 (Age 54 yr)	4/8/83 (Age 56 yr)
Pulmonary artery wedge mean	26	24	25	35
Pulmonary artery (s/d)	50/20	58/25	55/25	75/35
Right ventricle (s/d)	50/10	50/11	55/9	75/11
Right atrial mean	12	6	3	7
Left ventricle (s/d)	130/32	118/31	130/40	145/40
Systemic artery (s/d)	130/75	120/65	130/65	165/75
Cardiac index (l/min/m²)	. . .	2.6	4.4	3.7

s/d = peak systole/end-diastole.

TABLE II Pulmonary Function Data in Patient M.L.

	8/12/81 (Age 54 yr)			4/15/83 (Age 56 yr)		
	Predicted	Actual	% Predicted	Predicted	Actual	% Predicted
Total lung capacity (liters)	4.2	3.9	92	4.0	2.7	68
Forced vital capacity (FVC)	2.7	1.5	54	2.6	1.0	39
Forced expired volume at 1 second (FEV_1)	2.0	0.8	41	1.9	0.7	34
FEV_1/FVC (%)	75	57	76	75	66	88
Maximal midexpiratory flow (liters/sec)	2.5	0.4	15	2.4	0.4	17
Peak flow (liters/min)	338	192	57	333	97	29
Diffusing capacity (CO)	14	12	89	20	3	15

CO = carbon monoxide.

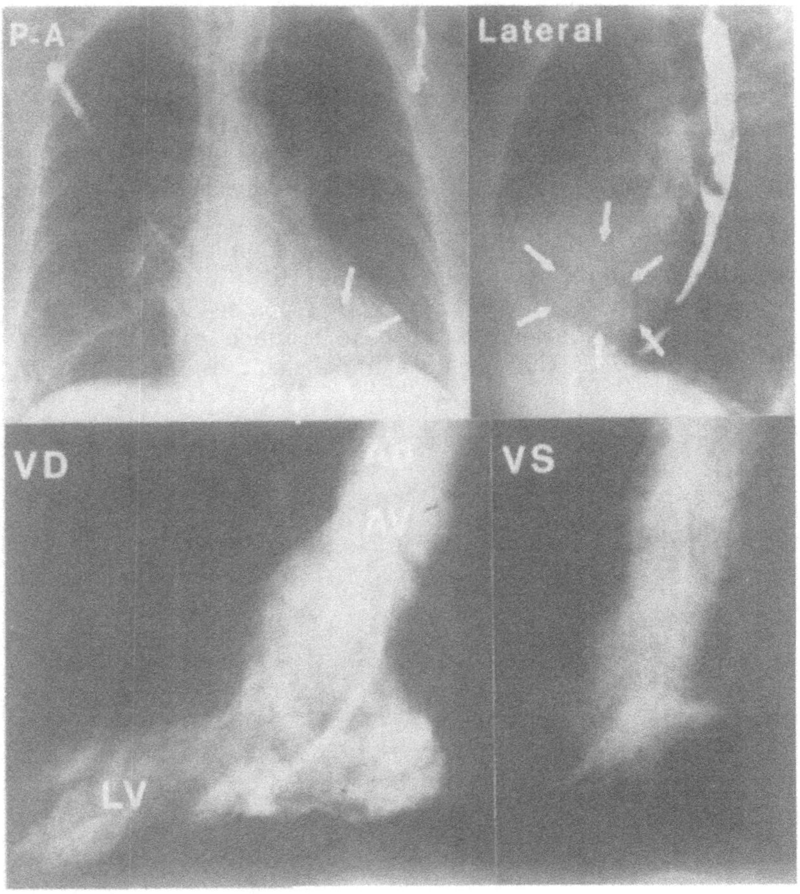

FIGURE 3. Upper, posteroanterior (P-A) and lateral chest roentgenograms. The **arrows** delineate the calcific deposits. **Lower,** cineangiographic frames of the left ventricle (LV) in ventricular diastole (VD) and in ventricular systole (VS). Ao = aorta; AV = aortic valve.

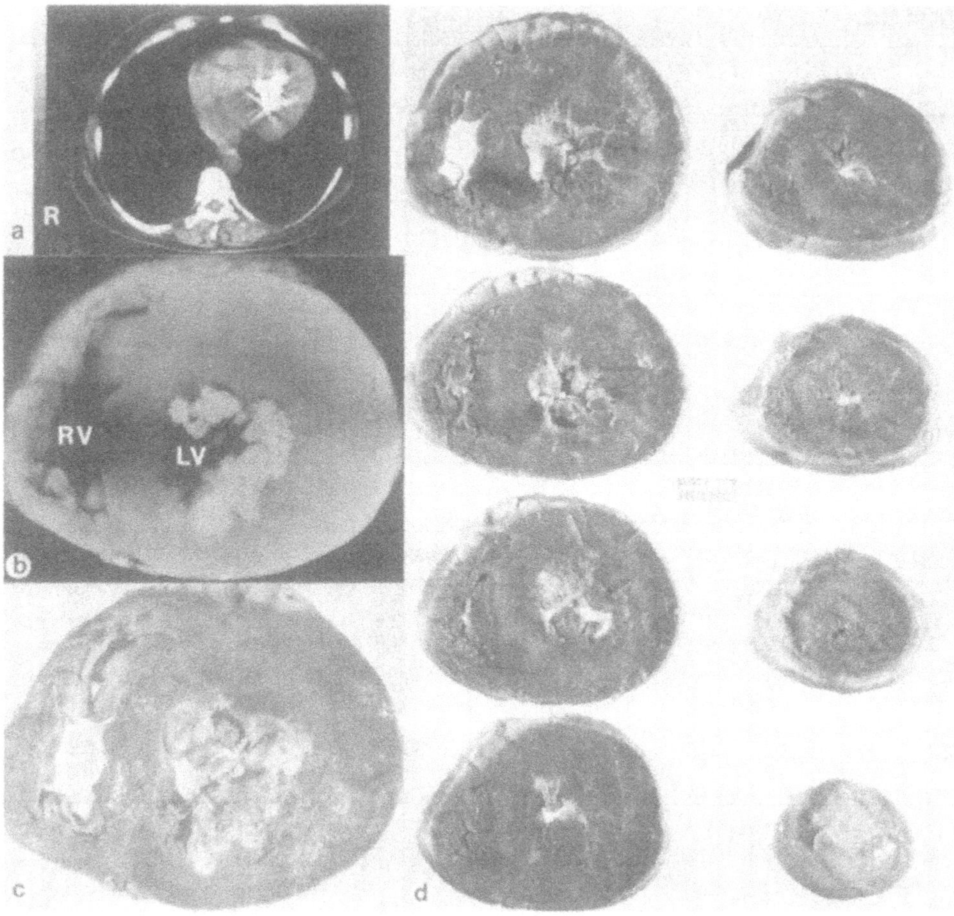

FIGURE 4. Transverse cuts of the cardiac ventricles showing left ventricular (LV) endocardial calcific deposits in a small LV cavity. **a,** computerized tomographic image showing dense calcific deposits nearly filling the LV cavity. **b,** radiograph of most basal transverse section of cardiac ventricles delineating the calcific deposits. **c,** most basal slice from which the radiograph in **b** was taken. **d,** other transverse sections of cardiac ventricles, base to apex, with calcific deposits in the more basal sections. R = right side; RV = right ventricle.

The cause of the LV mural endocardial calcific deposits and the associated LV hypertrophy in the above described patient is uncertain. The lack of blood eosinophilia at any time, the presence of considerable LV hypertrophy and the presence of the extensive, widely distributed calcific deposits within the LV cavity clearly distinguishes our patient from those who have "endomyocardial fibrosis with or without eosinophilia" or "Loffler's fibroplastic parietal endocarditis." Irrespective of its cause, however, the entity, "massive LV endocardial calcific deposits" needs to be added to the list of conditions that produce impairment of LV filling.

References

1. **Glancy DL, Roberts WC.** Congenital obstructive lesions involving the major pulmonary veins, left atrium, or mitral valve: a clinical, laboratory, and morphologic survey. Cathet Cardiovasc Diagn 1976;2:215–252.
2. **Bonow RO, Frederic TM, Bacharach SL, Green MV, Goose PW, Maron BJ, Rosing DR.** Atrial systole and left ventricular filling in hypertrophic cardiomyopathy: effect of verapamil. Am J Cardiol 1983;51:1386–1391.
3. **Roberts WC, Waller BF.** Cardiac amyloidosis causing cardiac dysfunction: analysis of 54 necropsy patients. Am J Cardiol 1983;52:137–146.
4. **Cutler DJ, Isner JM, Bracey AW, Hufnagel CA, Conrad PW, Roberts WC, Kerwin DM, Weintraub AM.** Hemochromatosis heart disease: an unemphasized cause of potentially reversible restrictive cardiomyopathy. Am J Med 1980;69:923–928.
5. **Roberts WC, Spray TL.** Pericardial heart disease. Curr Probl Cardiol 1977;2:1–71.
6. **Fauci AS, Harley JB, Roberts WC, Ferrans VJ, Gralnick HR, Bjornson BH.** The idiopathic hypereosinophilic syndrome. Clinical, pathophysiologic, and therapeutic considerations. Ann Intern Med 1982;97:78–92.

Atrioventricular Septal Defect (Primum Atrial Septal Defect) with Prolonged Survival (Despite Severe Mitral Regurgitation and Pulmonary Hypertension) and Associated Cardiac Calcification (Mitral Anulus, Coronary Artery and Pulmonary Trunk)

CAROLE A. WARNES, MB, BS, MRCP
GERALD I. SHUGOLL, MD
ROBERT B. WALLACE, MD
WILLIAM C. ROBERTS, MD

Atrioventricular (AV) septal defect (formerly called AV canal or endocardial cushion defect or primum atrial septal defect [ASD] with cleft mitral valve) may be either complete (single AV valve) or partial (2 well formed AV valves). Patients with complete AV septal defect rarely survive for more than a few years without operation. However, patients with partial AV septal defect often survive for many years, but not as long as patients with secundum ASD. Prolonged survival with partial AV septal defect (primum ASD), however, is unusual, particularly in the presence of severe mitral regurgitation and pulmonary hypertension, but such was the case in the patient described herein.

S.C., a 59-year-old woman, was found to have a precordial murmur in childhood. Episodic palpitations began at age 20 years and an episode of atrial fibrillation was documented when she was 37 years old. Although easily fatigued, she performed housework until her early 50s, when palpitations associated with dyspnea became more frequent and pedal edema developed. At age 59 years, orthopnea and angina pectoris appeared. The blood pressure was 110/70 mm Hg. A right ventricular lift was palpated, P_2 was loud and the interval between A_2 and P_2 was wider than normal and did not vary with respiration. A grade 3/6 systolic murmur was present at the apex and it radiated into the left axilla. A grade 2/6 systolic murmur along the lower left sternal border increased in intensity with inspiration. The electrocardiogram showed sinus rhythm with prolonged PR interval (0.24 s), right bundle branch block and left-axis deviation. The Holter monitor tracing showed both supraventricular and ventricular ectopic complexes with episodes of bigeminy and a 4-beat run of ventricular tachycardia. Chest radiography showed cardiomegaly with pulmonary congestion. The findings on cardiac catheterization are summarized in Table I. Left ventriculography demonstrated a normally contracting left ventricle, a narrowed outflow tract with the characteristic "goose-neck" deformity, no ventricular septal

---

From the Pathology Branch, National Heart, Lung, and Blood Institute, National Institutes of Health, Bethesda, Maryland, and Georgetown University Medical Center, Washington, D.C. Manuscript received May 8, 1984, accepted May 16, 1984.

TABLE I Hemodynamic Data

Chamber	Pressure (mm Hg) s/d	Oxygen Saturation (%)
IVC	...	69
SVC	...	53
RA mean	22	70
RV (s/d)	95/15	77
PA (s/d)	95/30	77
LA mean	20	85
LV (s/d)	120/20	83
Aorta (s/d)	120/65	83

IVC = inferior vena cava; LA = left atrium; LV = left ventricle; PA = pulmonary artery; RA = right atrium; RV = right ventricle; s/d = peak systole/end-diastole; SVC = superior vena cava.

defect, severe (grade 3+/4+) mitral regurgitation, and thickened, deformed, relatively immobile mitral leaflets. Calcium was visible in the mitral anular region. Pulmonary venogram demonstrated an ostium primum ASD. The pulmonary to systemic flow ratio was 1.7 and the net left-to-right shunt was 2.5 liters/min. The pulmonary resistance was 7 Wood units/m² and the systemic resistance was 28 Wood units/m². Coronary arteriography and, later, necropsy demonstrated a 50 to 75% diameter reduction in the midportion of the left anterior descending coronary artery. The ostium of the right coronary artery was located in the left coronary sinus (confirmed at necropsy).

On January 26, 1984, the deformed mitral valve was replaced with a 3M Starr-Edwards prosthesis, the primum ASD was closed with a pericardial patch, a de Vega tricuspid valve anuloplasty was performed, and a saphenous vein was inserted between the aorta and left anterior descending coronary artery (done first). Although atrial fibrillation developed, the early postoperative course was uneventful. She went home on February 4, 1984. Two days later she had an acute episode of dyspnea, and she died about 12 hours later.

At necropsy, the heart weighed 650 g. The defect (4 cm in maximal diameter) in the lower most portion of the atrial septum had been closed securely, 1 of the 4 stents of the prosthesis in the mitral position contacted the left ventricular wall, and the aortocoronary conduit was patent (Fig. 1 and 2). Heavy calcific deposits were present in the mitral anulus, pulmonary trunk and left anterior descending coronary artery (Fig. 3). No clear anatomic cause of death was discernible at necropsy.

Few reported patients with partial AV septal defect have survived for more than 50 years. One man with this defect, confirmed at necropsy, lived 69 years.[1] Hynes et al[2] reported 52 such patients aged 20 years or older, 18 of whom were 45 years or older and 6 of whom were 60 years or older. Pulmonary hypertension was rare; the highest mean pulmonary artery pressure was 55 mm Hg. Somerville[3] reported 14 patients aged 30 years or older with primum ASD, 2 of whom had pulmonary hypertension (pulmonary vascular resistance ≥3 Wood units). Severe mitral regurgitation also was unusual in the patients of Hynes et al: Of 33 patients who underwent left ventricular angiography, mitral regurgitation was found in 4 (12%). In Somerville's 14 patients, severe mitral regurgitation was present in 2. Martin et al[4] described 7 adults, aged 34 to 48 years, with primum ASD; 1 had an elevated pulmonary artery pressure (86/33 mm

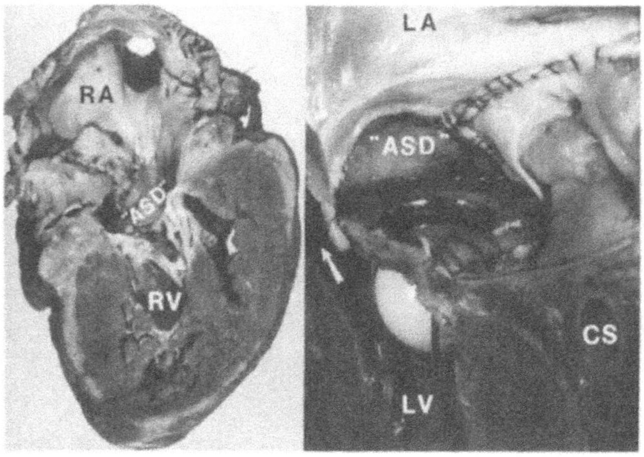

FIGURE 1. Opened right side of the heart (**left**) exposing the operatively closed atrial septal defect ("ASD"). The right atrium (RA) is dilated and the wall of right ventricle (RV) is markedly thickened. **Right,** opened left atrium (LA) showing the operatively closed ASD with a portion of the prosthetic ring attached to the most caudal margin of the ASD. The **arrow** points toward the aortic valve. CS = coronary sinus; LV = left ventricle.

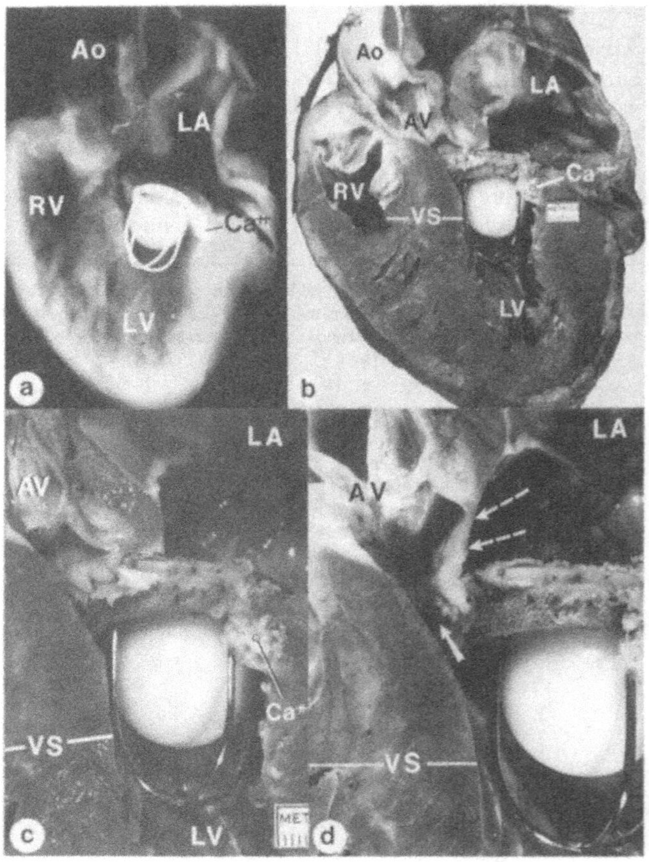

FIGURE 2. Left side of the heart. **a,** radiograph. Calcium (Ca^{++}) is present in the mitral anular region. **b,** long-axis view showing relative sizes of the right ventricle (RV), left ventricle (LV), left atrium (LA) and the relative thicknesses of the ventricular walls. The aortocoronary artery conduit is visible. **c,** close-up of the prosthesis. **d,** close-up of left ventricular outflow tract. The anterior mitral leaflet (**broken arrows**) is displaced anteriorly toward the ventricular septum (VS), and this displacement appears to have diminished the area of left ventricular outflow (**solid arrow**). Ao = ascending aorta; AV = aortic valve.

Hg), and mitral regurgitation was minimal in all 7. Goodman et al[5] reported 12 patients aged 15 to 53 years (mean 30) with primum ASD: 1 had a pulmonary artery systolic pressure >50 mm Hg, and 2 had severe mitral regurgitation.

Although recognized as frequent in patients with mitral valve prolapse, which in turn is recognized as frequent in older patients with secundum type ASD, mitral anular calcium is infrequent in patients with secundum ASD,[6] (presumably because survival longer than 65 years is relatively uncommon) and it has never been reported in a patient with primum ASD. The occurrence of significant coronary atherosclerosis, also present in our patient, has not been described previously in a patient with primum ASD, and obviously, aortocoronary bypass grafting, as performed on our patient, has not been reported previously in such a case. Moreover, the occurrence of a calcified mass in the pulmonary trunk has not been reported previously in a patient with primum ASD. Thus, the patient described herein is unusual on 7 counts (prolonged survival, severe mitral regurgitation, severe pulmonary hypertension, mitral anular calcium, pulmonary truncal calcium, coronary arterial calcium and severe coronary atherosclerosis necessitating aortocoronary bypass grafting).

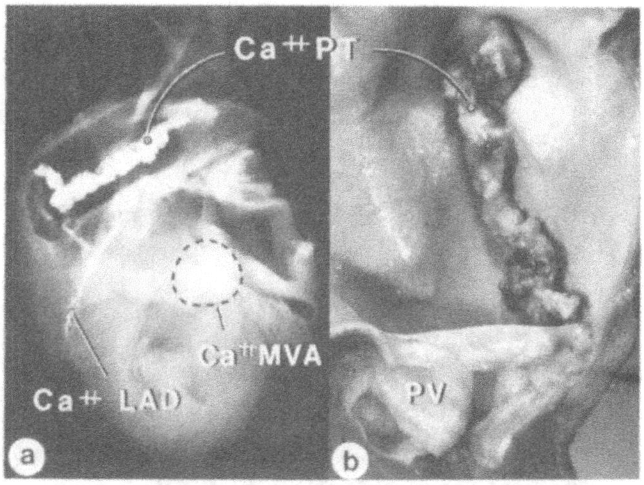

FIGURE 3. a, calcific deposit (Ca^{++}) in pulmonary trunk (PT), probably originally a thrombus, and in the mitral valve anulus (MVA) and left anterior descending coronary artery (LAD). **b,** close-up of the calcific deposit in the pulmonary trunk located just above the pulmonic valve (PV).

References

1. **Heath D.** Long survival in partial persistent common atrioventricular canal. Br J Dis Chest 1968;62:207–210.
2. **Hynes JK, Tajik AJ, Seward JB, Fuster V, Ritter DG, Brandenburg RO, Puga FJ, Danielson GK, McGoon DC.** Partial atrioventricular canal defect in adults. Circulation 1982;66:284–287.
3. **Somerville J.** Ostium primum defect: factors causing deterioration in the natural history. Br Heart J 1965;27:413–419.
4. **Martin CE, Thomas CS, Bender HW.** Ostium primum atrial septal defect in the adult. South Med J 1976;69:1058–1060.
5. **Goodman DJ, Harrison DC, Schroeder JS.** Ostium primum defect in the adult: postoperative follow-up studies. Chest 1975;67:185–189.
6. **Roberts WC.** Morphologic features of the normal and abnormal mitral valve. Am J Cardiol 1983;51:1005–1028.

Mitral Valve Cleft Without Cardiac Septal Defect Causing Severe Mitral Regurgitation but Allowing Long Survival

CHARLES W. BARTH, III, MD
JAMES D. DIBDIN, MD, LLB
WILLIAM C. ROBERTS, MD

From the Pathology Branch, National Heart, Lung, and Blood Institute, National Institutes of Health, Bethesda, Maryland 20205, and The Medical Examiner's Office, Washington, D.C. Manuscript received December 19, 1984, accepted December 31, 1984.

Partial atrioventricular "defect" includes a spectrum of 5 anatomic anomalies. Some patients have all 5 and others have only 1 or 2. The 5 are the following: (1) defect in the lower portion of the atrial septum, so-called primum atrial septal defect; (2) defect in, or absence of, the posterobasal portion of ventricular septum; (3) cleft, anterior mitral leaflet; (4) anomalous chordae tendineae from the anterior mitral leaflet to the crest of the ventricular septum; and (5) partial or complete absence of the septal tricuspid valve leaflet. There are at least 4 potential functional consequences of these 5 anatomic anomalies: (1) shunt at the atrial level, (2) shunt at the ventricular level, (3) mitral regurgitation (MR), and (4) obstruction to left ventricular outflow. Well over 95% of patients with partial atrioventricular defect have a primum type atrial septal defect, and most of those without a primum defect have a shunt at the ventricular

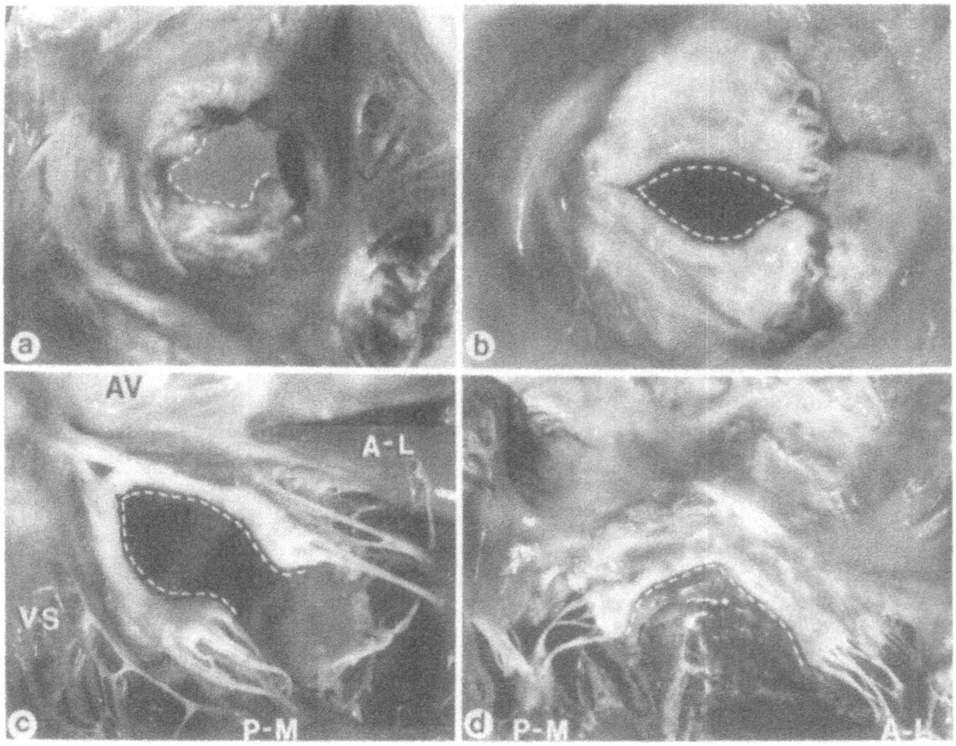

FIGURE 1. Mitral valve in the patient described. In each of the 4 views the space bordering the cleft in the anterior mitral leaflet is designated by **dashed lines. a,** view from left atrium during simulated ventricular diastole; **b,** close-up view from left atrium during simulated ventricular systole; **c,** view from left ventricle. The apex of the cleft inserts into the crest of the ventricular septum (VS) just caudal to the opened aortic valve (AV). The anterolateral (A-L) papillary muscle actually inserts into the anterior one-half of the cleft anterior mitral leaflet; **d,** opened left atrium, mitral valve and left ventricle. The large amount of anterior mitral leaflet actually missing, i.e., that space bordered by the **dashed lines,** is huge. The circumference of the mitral anulus is about twice normal. P-M = posteromedial papillary muscle. (Photographs by M.M.M. Moore.)

level. The occurrence of MR from a cleft in the anterior mitral leaflet unassociated with a defect in either atrial or ventricular septa is extremely rare. Such was the case, however, in the patient to be described herein.

B.P., a 27-year-old man, was found to have a precordial murmur consistent with MR at age 16 years. Atrial fibrillation was also present. Left ventricular angiogram at the time showed 2+/4+ MR. He continued to play recreational basketball and work as a service station attendant without difficulty. At age 27, five months before death, he had a respiratory infection followed by evidence of congestive heart failure. A grade 4/6 holosystolic murmur consistent with MR and a third heart sound were heard. M-mode echocardiogram showed thickened but mobile mitral leaflets; the left atrial dimension was 70 mm, and the left ventricular cavity was 82 mm in diastole and 58 mm in systole. The electrocardiogram showed atrial fibrillation, QRS voltage of left ventricular hypertrophy and inverted T waves in leads II, III and aVF. The pressures in mm Hg were as follows: pulmonary artery wedge mean 15, v wave 16; pulmonary artery 28/14 (mean 18); right ventricle 28/5; right atrial mean 5; left ventricle 120/8; and aorta 120/80 (mean 90). Cardiac index (thermodilution) was 2.3 liters/min/m^2. Left ventricular angiography now disclosed 4+/4+ MR. After discharge he returned to an active life. He died suddenly from an overdose of cocaine and phencyclidine.

At necropsy the heart weighed 900 g. All 4 cardiac chambers were dilated. A huge cleft was present in the anterior mitral leaflet (Fig. 1). The mitral anulus measured 17 cm in circumference and the tricuspid anulus measured 15 cm. The edges of the cleft were thick. The atrial and ventricular septa were intact. The tricuspid, pulmonary and aortic valve leaflets were normal.

We found studies describing 10 patients at necropsy with a cleft in the anterior mitral leaflet unassociated with a defect in either the atrial or ventricular septum.[1–4] Information on age and gender was available in 6 of the 10 patients: All were males; 5 were younger than age 10 years and 1 was 74 years old. Of the 10 patients, some degree of MR was present in 9; only the 74-year-old man had no MR.[3] Only 2 of the 10 patients were known to have a large cleft—such as occurred in our patient—and both had severe MR and progressive, eventually fatal congestive heart failure.

Our 27-year-old patient appears to be the oldest necropsy patient thus far reported with severe MR from a cleft in the anterior mitral leaflet. Although he had evidence of congestive heart failure for a few months before death, his death was not the result of cardiac disease. What allowed his relatively long survival? Although he had MR during his entire 27 years, the degree of MR worsened through the years. Initially, MR was probably due entirely to the regurgitation through the cleft in the anterior mitral leaflet, but with time the mitral anulus progressively dilated, and this huge anular dilation contributed to the degree of MR, as occurs in patients with mitral valve prolapse.[5]

It is likely that our patient was able to tolerate the MR well because the huge size of the left atrial cavity was able to "absorb" the left ventricular systolic pressure and prevent its reflection into the pulmonary veins and from there into the pulmonary arteries. More than 2 decades ago, Braunwald and Awe[6] demonstrated that patients with pure MR in whom huge left atrial cavities develop do not have pulmonary venous and subsequently pulmonary arterial hypertension; in contrast, those patients with severe MR whose left atrial cavities do not dilate do have severe elevation of their pulmonary venous and pulmonary arterial pressures.[7] The courses in the former group are long and those in the latter group are short. The present patient had a huge left atrial cavity, nearly normal pulmonary wedge pressures and normal pulmonary arterial pressures, and therefore prolonged survival.

References

1. **Edwards JE, Dry TJ, Parker RL, Burchell HB, Wood EH, Bulbulian AH.** An Atlas of Congenital Anomalies of the Heart and Great Vessels. Springfield, IL: Charles C Thomas, 1954:41–42.
2. **Berghuis J, Kirklin JW, Edwards JE, Titus JL.** The surgical anatomy of isolated congenital mitral insufficiency. J Thorac Cardiovasc Surg 1964;47:791–798.
3. **Di Segni E, Edwards JE.** Cleft anterior leaflet of the mitral valve with intact septa. A study of 20 cases. Am J Cardiol 1983;51:919–926.
4. **Sellers RD, Lillehei CW, Edwards JE.** Subaortic stenosis caused by anomalies of the atrioventriclular valves. J Thorac Cardiovasc Surg 1964;48:289–302.
5. **Waller BF, Morrow AG, Maron BJ, Del Negro AA, Kent KM, McGrath FJ, Wallace RB, McIntosh CL, Roberts WC.** Etiology of clinically isolated, severe, chronic, pure mitral regurgitation. Analysis of 97 patients over 30 years of age having mitral valve replacement. Am Heart J 1982;104:276–288.
6. **Braunwald E, Awe WC.** The syndrome of severe mitral regurgitation with normal left atrial pressure. Circulation 1963;27:29–35.
7. **Roberts WC, Braunwald E, Morrow Ag.** Acute severe mitral regurgitation secondary to ruptured chordae tendineae. Clinical, hemodynamic, and pathologic considerations. Circulation 1966;33:58–70.

A Simple Histologic Classification of Pulmonary Arterial Hypertension

For many years students of congenital heart disease were unable to explain the differences in survival patterns in patients with similar-sized isolated communications between systemic and pulmonary circulations. In 1927 Moschcowitz[1] suggested that the explanation may be the presence of pulmonary hypertension in some patients with shunts and its absence in others. In 1935, Brenner[2] described histologic features of the normal pulmonary arteries and veins. In 1936, Parker and Weiss[3] at the Boston City Hospital described changes in the parenchyma and vessels of lungs in patients with mitral stenosis. In the late 1940s, Edwards,[4] who also trained at the Boston City Hospital in the late 1930s, began describing anatomic changes in the pulmonary vasculature in patients with congenital heart disease, and he too attributed the changes to the effects of pulmonary hypertension. In 1958, Heath and Edwards[5] proposed an anatomic classification of hypertensive pulmonary changes (Fig. 1). Their classification was based primarily on observations of necropsy patients with large ventricular septal defect or patent ductus arteriosus having *pulmonary hypertension from birth*, but a few patients had primary pulmonary hypertension.

Although the Heath and Edwards classification brought organization to a complex subject, reevaluation nearly 30 years later indicates that their classification has certain deficiencies. Considerable overlap exists between their grades 2 and 3 and grades 4 and 5. *Alveolar hemosiderosis* (grade 5) does not concern a pulmonary artery and it may occur in patients without pulmonary arterial hypertension. In my view, a classification of pulmonary arterial changes should not include changes in alveolar spaces (hemosiderosis). Their grade 6 category implies that grades 1 through 5 are prerequisites, when, in actuality, necrotizing vasculitis may occur in the absence of grades 1 to 5 and it may occur in the absence of pulmonary hypertension. A classification of hypertensive changes in the pulmonary arteries should be applicable, of course, to all patients with pulmonary hypertension irrespective of its cause and irrespective of whether the hypertension is congenital or acquired in origin.

Basis of Grades of Hypertensive Pulmonary Vascular Disease Found in Association with Large Ventricular Septal Defects and Functionally Related Diseases

	Grade of hypertensive pulmonary vascular disease					
	1	2	3	4	5	6
Type of intimal reaction	←None→					
		← Cellular →				
			← Fibrous and fibroelastic →			
				← Plexiform lesion →		
State of media of arteries and arterioles	← Hypertrophied →					
			← Some generalized dilatation →			
				← Local "dilatation lesions"* →		
					← Pulmonary hemosiderosis† →	
						←Necrotizing arteritis→

*Vein-like branches of hypertrophied muscular pulmonary arteries, angiomatoid lesion, and cavernous lesion

†Associated with distended, thin-walled, arterial vessels throughout the lung

FIGURE 1. Classification of hypertensive pulmonary vascular changes by Heath and Edwards in 1958.[5] Reproduced with permission of the publisher.

The classification of pulmonary arterial changes recommended herein consists of only 3 grades, and is based on histologic alterations irrespective of the etiology of or the time of appearance of the pulmonary arterial hypertension. The major changes in the pulmonary arteries include: (1) *medial thickening* (MT), (2) *intimal thickening* (IT), and (3) *plexiform lesion* (PL) (Fig. 2). Grade I includes MT only; grade II, MT plus IT; and grade III, MT plus IT plus PL (Fig. 3). Neither arteritis (vasculitis) nor hemosiderosis are included in the grading system.

Medial thickening: This indicates an increase in the thickness of the media of a pulmonary artery or of a pulmonary arteriole, or both. Whether this occurs entirely from hypertrophy of smooth muscle cells or from both hypertrophy and hyperplasia is unclear. Thus, the reason for the phrase *medial thickening* rather than *medial hypertrophy*.

Intimal thickening: There are 2 types of intimal thickening: the cellular variety, in which the proliferated intima consists primarily of smooth-muscle cells with collagen in between, and the acellular variety, which consists mostly of dense fibrous (collagen) tissue with minimal or no smooth muscle cells.

Plexiform lesion: This is an aneurysmal or glomus-like structure that emerges at more-or-less right angles to a muscular pulmonary artery. Just after origin of the right-angle branch it suddenly bulges into a plexus of channels, the walls of which consist primarily of fibrous tissue covered by endo-

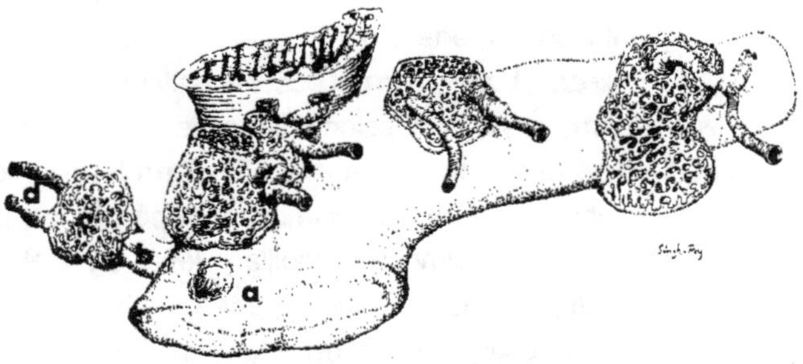

FIGURE 2. Drawing from Moschcowitz et al[10] of plexiform lesions arising from a muscular pulmonary artery. Reproduced with permission of the publisher.

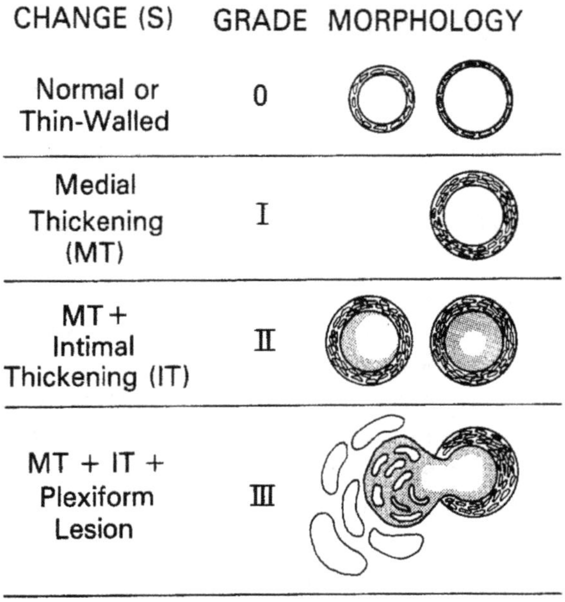

FIGURE 3. Types of grading of the morphologic pulmonary artery changes from Virmani and Roberts.[12] Reproduced with permission of the publisher.

thelial cells. The PL gives rise to thin-walled channels, probably dilated arterioles, which rapidly branch into alveolar septal capillaries. These thin-walled channels when considerably dilated have been called *dilatation lesions.*

Proposed causes: *Medial thickening* is a response of the arterial wall to increased pressure and therefore occurs only in patients with pulmonary arterial hypertension. Medial thickening is never simply a normal consequence of aging. *Intimal thickening* is not necessarily the consequence of pulmonary arterial hypertension, but it is accelerated by elevation of pulmonary arterial pressure. Cellular and acellular IT is frequently observed in older persons, most of whom have normal pulmonary arterial pressures.[6] The occurrence of IT combined with MT, however, is indicative of pulmonary hypertension. *Plexiform lesions* occur only in patients with severe pulmonary hypertension, but most patients with severe pulmonary hypertension do not have them. Plexiform lesions occur in patients with large intravascular shunts or primary pulmonary hypertension or pulmonary embolic or thrombotic disease, but they do not occur in patients in whom the severe pulmonary hypertension is secondary to left-sided cardiac disease (e.g., mitral stenosis). Plexiform lesions do not occur if the cause of the pulmonary hypertension is located distal to the pulmonary capillary level or, stated differently, if the pulmonary arterial hypertension is the consequence of pulmonary venous hypertension. For a PL to occur, the cause of the hypertension must originate at the capillary or recapillary level.[7]

The exact cause of PLs is unknown. Serial sections of lung at sites of a PL generally show extreme narrowing or almost total obstruction of the lumen of the muscular pulmonary artery distal to the origin of the small muscular pulmonary artery or arteriole which is the site of the PL. Kanjuh and colleagues[8] suggested that the PL was a consequence of a *jet lesion* caused by blood rapidly changing its course because of the distal obstruction of the relatively large muscular pulmonary artery distal to the site of the PL. Thus, the PL might act as a dissipator of the extremely high pulmonary arterial pressure. Others have suggested that the PL represents a site of *anastomoses of pulmonary arteries and veins*[9] or it is a *congenital malformation.*[10] PL, however, has never been observed in the lungs at birth; the earliest it has been observed is at 2 months of age.[11] The PL may represent an aneurysm formed at sites of *congenitally underdeveloped or weak media* (analogous to the formation of an intracerebral berry aneurysm in systemic hypertension), the aneurysm later being filled by thrombus, which organizes into multiple minute vascular channels.[12,13] Wagenvoort and Wagenvoort[14] proposed that the PL represents a site of healed necrotizing arteritis. The inflammation weakens the arterial wall, which focally expands, fibrin and platelets are deposited in the aneurysm, and organization of the thrombus produces multiluminal channels lined by endothelial cells.

Whatever its cause, the PL represents irreversible pulmonary hypertension, whereas MT alone or MT plus IT indicates that the pulmonary hypertension is reversible.

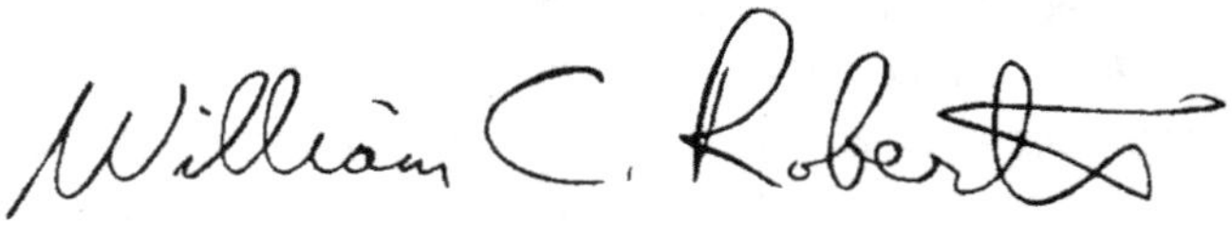

William C. Roberts, MD
Editor in Chief

References

1. Moschcowitz E. Hypertension of the pulmonary circulation; its causes, dynamics and relation to other circulatory states. Am J Med Sci 1927;174:388–406.
2. Brenner O. Pathology of the vessels of the pulmonary circulation. Arch Intern Med 1935;56:211–237, 457–497, 724–752, 976–1014, 1189–1241.
3. Parker F, Weiss S. The nature and significance of the structural changes in the lungs in mitral stenosis. Am J Pathol 1936;12:573–598.
4. Edwards JE. Functional pathology of the pulmonary vascular tree in congenital cardiac disease. Circulation 1957;15:164–196.
5. Heath D, Edwards JE. The pathology of hypertensive pulmonary vascular disease. A description of six grades of structural changes in the pulmonary arteries with special reference to congenital cardiac septal defects. Circulation 1958;18:533–547.
6. Wagenvoort CA, Wagenvoort N. Age changes in muscular pulmonary arteries and arterioles. Arch Pathol 1965;79:524–528.
7. Roberts WC, Fredrickson DS. Gaucher's disease of the lung causing severe pulmonary hypertension with associated acute recurrent pericarditis. Circulation 1967;35:783–789.
8. Kanjuh VI, Sellers RD, Edwards JE. Pulmonary vascular plexiform lesion. Arch Pathol 1964;78:513–522.
9. Hufner RF, McNicol CA. The pathologic physiology of microscopic pulmonary vascular shunts. AMA Arch Pathol 1958;65:554–560.
10. Moschcowitz E, Rubin E, Strauss L. Hypertension of the pulmonary circulation due to congenital glomoid obstruction of the pulmonary arteries. Am J Pathol 1961;39:75–93.
11. Hruban Z, Humphreys EM. Congenital anomalies associated with pulmonary hypertension in an infant. Arch Pathol 1960;70:766–779.
12. Virmani R, Roberts WC. Pulmonary arteries in congenital heart disease: a structure-function analysis. In: Roberts WC, ed. Adult Congenital Heart Disease. Philadelphia: FA Davis, 1987:77–131.
13. Naeye RL, Vennart GP. Structure and significance of pulmonary plexiform structures. Am J Pathol 1960;36:593–621.
14. Wagenvoort CA, Wagenvoort N. Pathology of Pulmonary Hypertension. New York: Wiley & Sons, 1977.

Pulmonary Arterial and Venous Hypertension and Left Ventricular Calcification of Undetermined Etiology

DEBORAH J. BARBOUR, MD
THOMAS V. INGLESBY, MD
JOEL A. ROTH, MD
WILLIAM C. ROBERTS, MD

In patients with severe pulmonary hypertension, the cause can nearly always be determined clinically or, if not, by necropsy examination. We recently studied a young woman with severe pulmonary hypertension and, despite cardiac catheterization, echocardiography, radionuclide angiography, pulmonary function studies, and, finally, necropsy, the cause of the severe pulmonary hypertension could not be determined. A description of the findings in this unusual patient is the purpose of this report.

From the Pathology Branch, National Heart, Lung, and Blood Institute, National Institutes of Health, Bethesda, Maryland, and the Departments of Medicine (Cardiology) and Pathology, Overlook Hospital, Summit, New Jersey. Manuscript received and accepted March 6, 1986.

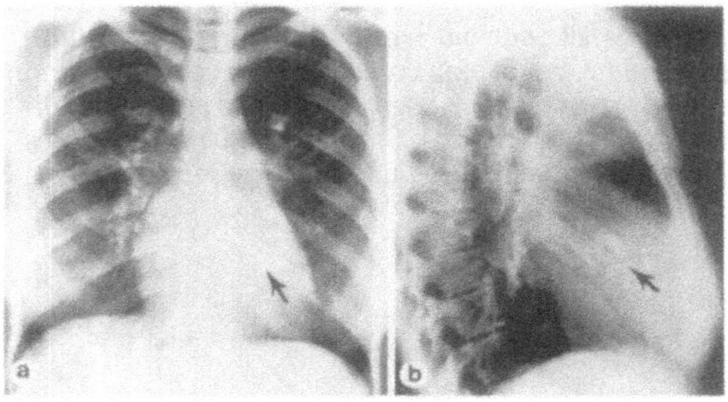

FIGURE 1. Posteroanterior and lateral chest radiographs taken 19 months before the patient's death showing mild cardiomegaly and an intracardiac calcific density (*arrows*) variously interpreted at the time as involving the aortic or mitral valve but which, at necropsy, was present in the ventricular septum.

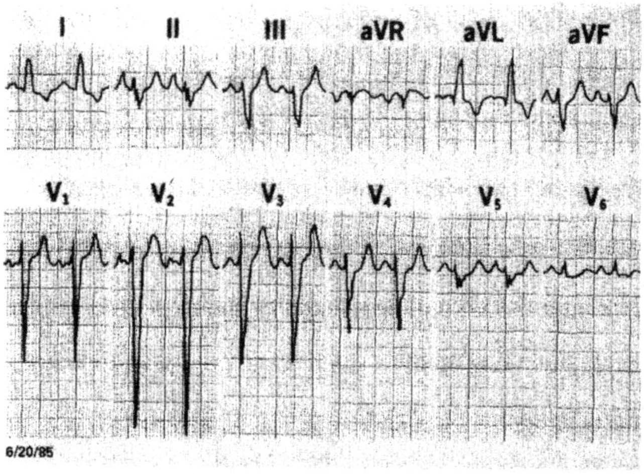

FIGURE 2. Twelve-lead electrocardiogram taken 3 months before death. The QRS axis is leftward (−40°), there is an intraventricular conduction delay and right atrial abnormality.

M.B., a 20-year-old white woman, was well until age 14 years, when exertional dyspnea developed and gradually worsened. At age 18, she had several respiratory infections (Fig. 1). She was evaluated 2 months before death and severe pulmonary hypertension was found. Cyanosis was absent and her lungs were clear. Precordial murmurs were absent; S_2 was loud, the interval between A_2 and P_2 did not vary with respiration, and both S_3 and S_4 gallops were present. The electrocardiogram is shown in Figure 2. A radionuclide angiogram revealed right ventricular enlargement and the left ventricular ejection fraction was 52%. On echocardiogram, the left atrial dimension was 42 mm, the left ventricular dimensions were 45 mm in diastole and 22 mm in systole; left ventricular wall thickness and motion and the cardiac valves were normal. Pulmonary function tests showed severe impairment of diffusion capacity, mild obstruction

TABLE I Hemodynamic Data Recorded Two Months Before Death

Pressures (mm Hg) (s/d = peak systole/end diastole)	
Pulmonary artery (PA) (s/d)	145/62
Right ventricle (s/d)	130/16
Right atrium (mean)	9
PA wedge (mean)	22
Left ventricle (s/d)	100/20
Systemic artery (s/d)	100/68
Cardiac index (liters/min/m^2)	1.9
Pulmonary vascular resistance (dynes s cm^{-5})	200

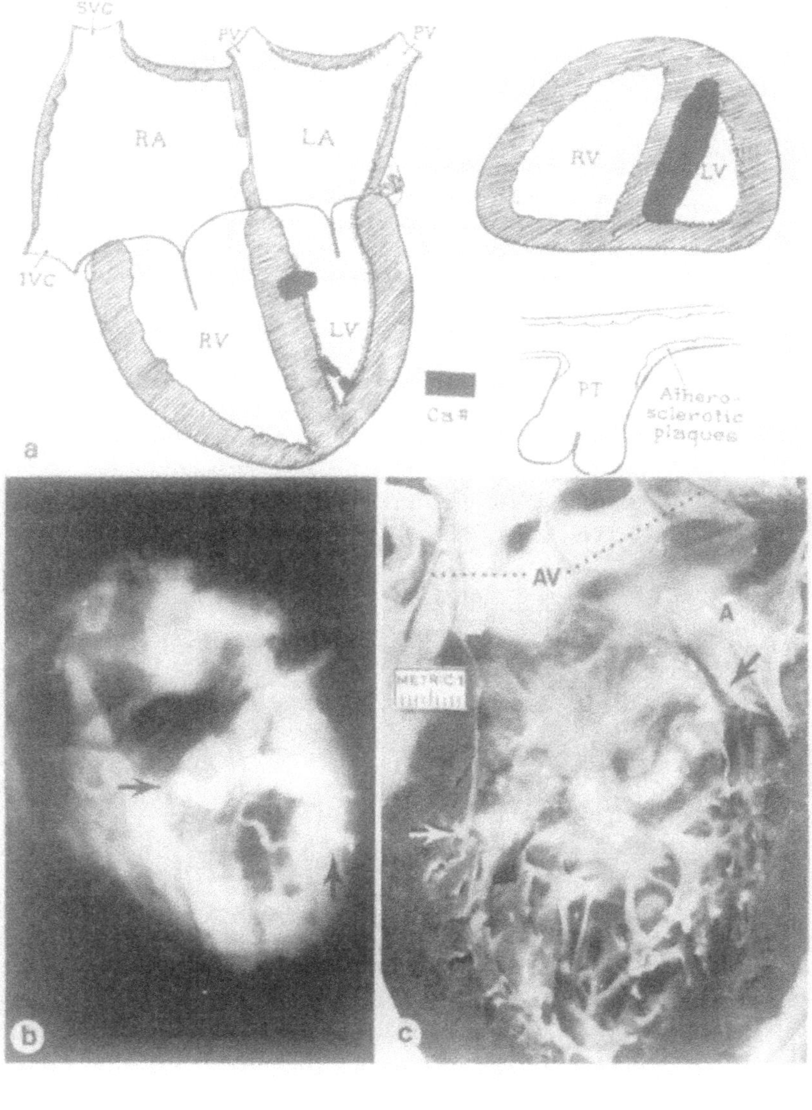

FIGURE 3. Heart. *a* (*left*), schematic representation of longitudinal section through the heart showing calcific bar on ventricular septum and calcified trabeculae within the left ventricular (LV) cavity. *Stippling* indicates thickened endocardium localized to left atrium (LA) and ventricle. The right atrium and ventricle (RA, RV) are dilated. Atherosclerotic plaques are present in the pulmonary trunk (PT) and right and left main pulmonary arteries. *b*, radiograph of the heart at necropsy showing a dense calcific bar (*between arrows*) extending across the ventricular septum and several calcified left ventricular trabeculae. *c*, a long axial cut showing the left ventricular aspect of the ventricular septum, opened aortic valve (AV) and anterior (A) mitral leaflet. The calcific bar (*between arrows*) extends across the ventricular septum. IVC = inferior vena cava; PV = pulmonary valve; SVC = superior vena cava.

and a vital capacity 58% of predicted. Data obtained at cardiac catheterization are summarized in Table I. Plans were made for combined heart and lung transplantation but she died of pneumonia while waiting.

At necropsy, the heart weighed 360 g and the right atrium and ventricle were dilated. The left atrial endocardium was diffusely thickened and the left ventricular endocardium was focally thickened. A dense, calcific bar extended transversely for approximately 4.5 cm in the ventricular septum and protruded approximately 1 cm into the left ventricular cavity (Fig. 3). Several left ventricular trabeculae also were calcified. The valves and coronary arteries were normal. Histologic sections of myocardium disclosed only myocyte hypertrophy.

Atherosclerotic plaques were present in the intima of the pulmonary trunk and in the extraparenchymal pulmonary arteries (Fig. 4). Histologic examination of both ascending aorta and pulmonary trunk (stained for elastic tissue) showed normal configuration of the elastic fibers in the pulmonary trunk (adult pattern).[1] Plexiform lesions were absent in all 16 sections of lung examined. The pulmonary veins were thickened and dilated, the alveolar septae were focally fibrotic and many but not all of the muscular pulmonary arteries had thickened media and in a few the intima was thickened by fibrous tissue. Many hemosiderin laden macrophages were present in alveolar spaces and the alveolar lining cells were cuboidal in shape and increased in number. The interlobular septa were thickened by fluid, fibrous tissue and dilated lymphatic channels.

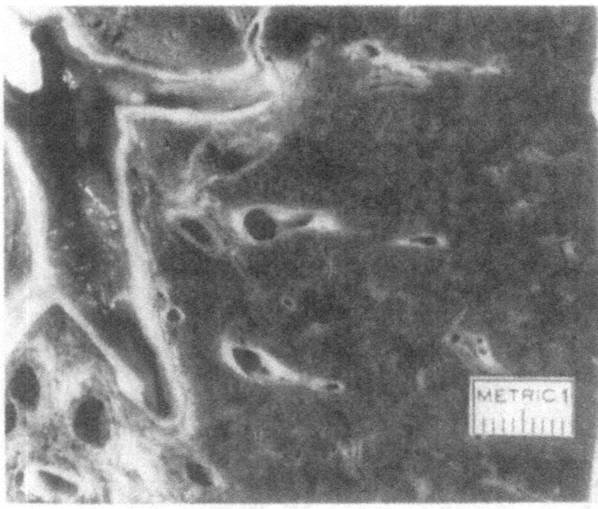

FIGURE 4. Close-up view of a longitudinal section of the lung showing a thickened large pulmonary artery. The aorta was free of atherosclerosis.

During life this patient was believed to have primary pulmonary hypertension, but at necropsy no plexiform lesions were present in the lungs, a finding essential for this diagnosis.[2] The medial thickening of the pulmonary arteries is simply an anatomic manifestation of severe pulmonary hypertension and not an indication of its cause. Study at necropsy of histologic sections of the wall of the pulmonary trunk indicated an adult configuration of the medial elastic fibers, a finding that indicates that the pulmonary hypertension was acquired rather than having persisted from birth.[1] The calcific bar in the ventricular septum and left ventricular free wall, of course, is not observed in patients with primary pulmonary hypertension, but again, its cause was not revealed by anatomic study. Thus, both the cause of the severe pulmonary arterial and venous hypertension and of the cardiac ventricular calcific deposit remain unexplained.

References

1. Heath D, Wood EH, DuShane JW, Edwards JE. *The structure of the pulmonary trunk at different ages and in cases of pulmonary hypetension and pulmonary stenosis. J Path Bact 1959;77:443–456.*

2. Wagenvoort CA, Wagenvoort N. *Primary pulmonary hypertension: a pathologic study of the lung vessels in 156 clinically diagnosed cases. Circulation 1970;42:1163–1184.*

Aneurysm of the Pulmonary Trunk Unassociated with Intracardiac or Great Vessel Left-to-Right Shunting

DEBORAH J. BARBOUR, MD
WILLIAM C. ROBERTS, MD

In contrast to aneurysm of the aorta, which is fairly common, aneurysmal dilation of the pulmonary trunk (PT) or of the right or left main pulmonary arteries is rare except in congenital heart disease with an intracardiac or great artery shunt. During the past 27 years we have studied at necropsy 3 patients with aneurysms (diameter more than 4 cm) of the PT and of 1 or both of its 2 major branches unassociated with congenital heart disease. This report describes findings in these 3 patients and summarizes findings in 3 previously reported necropsy patients with PT aneurysms unassociated with congenital heart disease.[1-3]

Certain findings in our 3 patients are summarized in Table I. All were women aged 40, 58 and 63 years. Patient 1 had hypertrophic cardiomyopathy (Fig. 1) and a pulmonary arterial systolic pressure of 54, 51 and 35 mm Hg on 3 occasions in the last 2 years of life. Patient 2 had systemic sarcoidosis and scleroderma with interstitial pulmonary fibrosis (Fig. 2) and a pulmonary arterial systolic pressure of 85 mm Hg. In patient 3, the cause of the PT aneurysm, which contained a large intraaneurysmal thrombus, could not be determined (Fig. 3). The PT aneurysms were 5, 7 and 7 cm in maximal diameter. Histologic study of the wall of the aneurysm disclosed it to be abnormal in patients 2 and 3 and normal in patient 1. The numbers of elastic fibers in the media in patients 2 and 3 clearly were decreased compared with normal (Fig. 3). Histologic study of 34 sections of lung in these 3 patients disclosed the pulmonary arterial intima and media to be thickened in all, but none had plexiform lesions (indicative of irreversible pulmonary hypertension).

Three previously reported patients with PT aneurysms unassociated with shunts included a 57-year-old man and 45- and 64-year-old women. The man had chronic lung disease and was an opium smoker; 1 woman was presumed to have primary pulmonary hypertension with pulmonary plexiform lesions and a pulmonary arterial mean pressure of 66 mm Hg; the other woman had no apparent explanation for the PT aneurysm which, like our patient 3, had an intraaneurysmal thrombus. All 3 had decreased numbers (compared with normal) of elastic fibers in the media of the PT.

From the Pathology Branch, National Heart, Lung, Blood Institute, National Institutes of Health, Bethesda, Maryland 20892.
Manuscript received and accepted June 18, 1986.

Aneurysms of the PT have been reported by other investigators in patients with primary pulmonary hypertension,[2] mitral stenosis,[4] the Marfan syndrome[5–7] and syphilis.[4–8] Since 1959, approximately 8,000 hearts have been examined in our laboratory and only the 3 patients included herein had aneurysms of the PT unassociated with left-to-right shunts. Of our 435 patients studied at necropsy with mitral stenosis, of 25 with primary pulmonary hypertension, and of 26 with the Marfan syndrome, none had an aneurysm of the PT.

The mechanism of development of PT aneurysm unassociated with left-to-right shunting is unclear. Pulmonary hypertension is usually present but it does not have to be severe as seen in our patient 1. The wall of the aneurysm may be abnormal as demonstrated by loss of elastic fibers in the media, but the wall may not be abnormal as was observed in our patient 1.

1. Shilkin KB, Low LP, Chen BTM. *Dissecting aneurysm of the pulmonary artery. J Pathol 1969;98:25–29.*
2. Luchtrath H. *Dissecting aneurysm of the pulmonary artery.* Virchows Arch *(Pathol Anat) 1981;391:241–147.*
3. Chiu B, Magil A. *Idiopathic pulmonary arterial trunk aneurysm presenting as cor pulmonale: report of a case. Hum Pathol 1985;16:947–949.*
4. Deterling RA, Clagett OT. *Aneurysm of the pulmonary artery: review of the literature and report of a case. Am Heart J 1947;34:471–499.*
5. Tung HL, Liebow AA. *Marfan's syndrome. Observations at necropsy: with special reference to medionecrosis of the great vessels. Lab Invest 1952;1:382–405.*

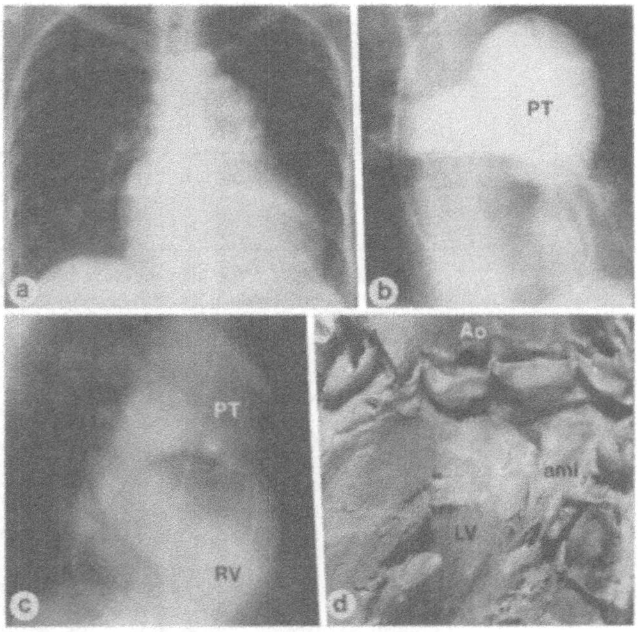

FIGURE 1. Patient 1 (Table I). Heart and radiograph. *a*, posteroanterior chest radiogram showing marked dilatation of the pulmonary trunk. *b*, posteroanterior angiogram with injection of contrast material into the huge pulmonary trunk (PT). *c*, lateral view of the same angiogram demonstrating aneurysm. *d*, opened left ventricular (LV) outflow tract showing a mural endocardial plaque in opposition to the anterior mitral leaflet (AMI) and a normal aortic valve. The mural endocardial plaque is typical of hypertrophic cardiomyopathy. Ao = ascending aorta; RV = right ventricle.

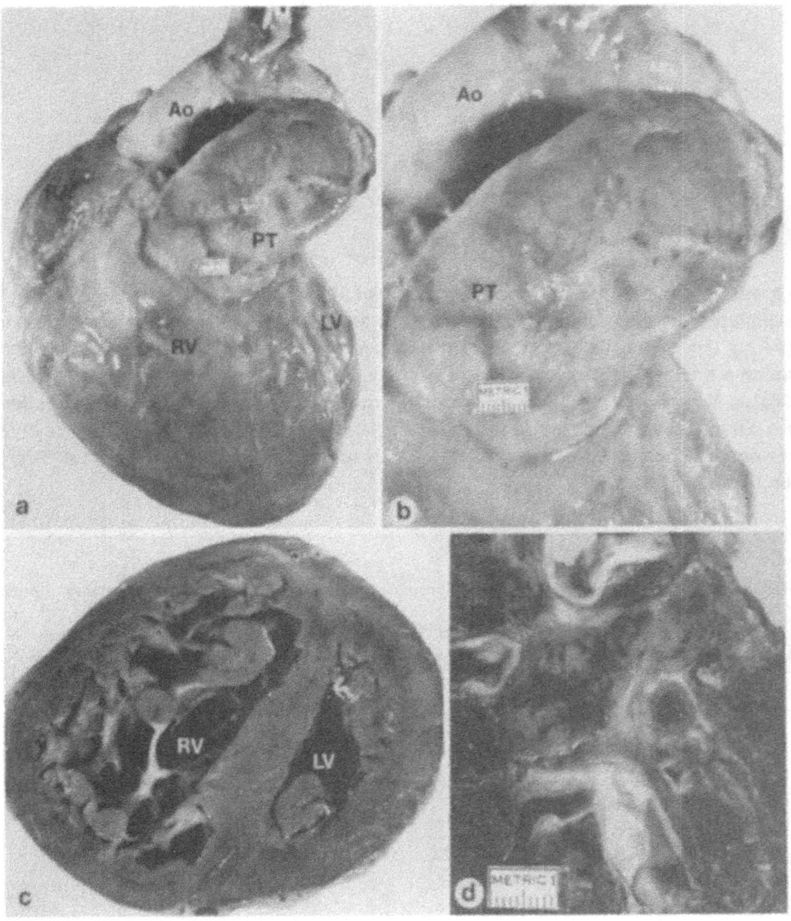

FIGURE 2. Heart and lung. *a* and *b*, exterior view of the anterior surface of the heart at necropsy showing the severely dilated pulmonary trunk (PT). The right ventricular (RV) cavity is much larger than the left ventricular (LV) cavity. *c*, transverse section through the ventricles at the level of the papillary muscles showing severe right ventricular (RV) wall thickening. *d*, longitudinal section through the lung near the hilum showing atherosclerotic plaques in the pulmonary arteries and enlarged perihilar lymph nodes containing noncaseating granulomas typical of sarcoidosis. Ao = aorta; RA = right atrium.

TABLE I Clinical Findings in Three Patients

Case	Necropsy Number	Age (yr)	PA (s/d)	RV (s/d)	RA (m)	SA (s/d)	LV (s/d)	Diameter (cm) PT Aneurysm	↓EF in PT
			Pressures (mm Hg)						
1	A63-77	40	35/17	35/5	4	130/85	125/12	7	0
2	A86-14	58	85/32	85/9	...	140/60	...	7	++
3	A85-29	63	...	...	...	...	...	5	+

EF = elastic fibers; LV = left ventricle; m = mean; PA = pulmonary artery; PT = pulmonary trunk; RA = right atrium; RV = right ventricle; SA = systemic artery; s/d = systolic/diastolic.

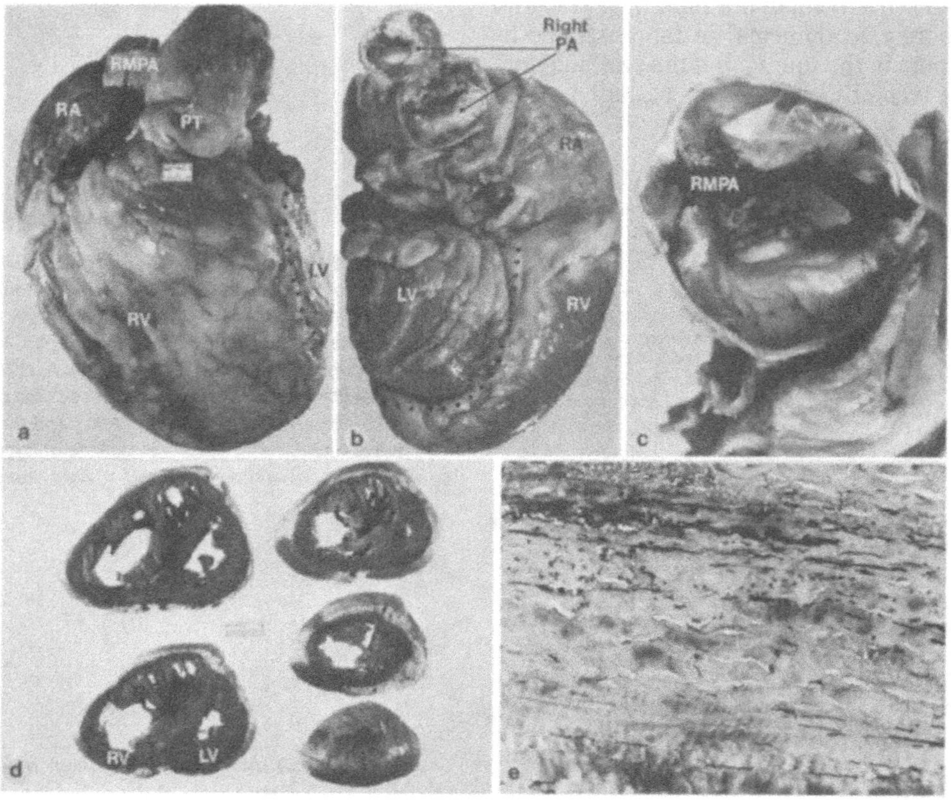

FIGURE 3. Patient 3. Heart (*a, b and d*) and pulmonary trunk (*b, c and e*). *a*, anterior view of the heart at necropsy. The right ventricle (RV) is massively enlarged and forms the cardiac apex. The pulmonary trunk (PT) and right main pulmonary artery (RMPA) are markedly dilated. *b*, posterior view of heart and right pulmonary artery (PA) at the level of its bifurcation showing extension of the PT aneurysm into the right upper and lower lobe main arterial branches, both of which are filled with organized mural thrombus. *c*, cross section through the right main pulmonary artery (RMPA) showing the aneurysmally dilated lumen to be markedly narrowed by organized thrombus. *d*, transverse sections through right (RV) and left ventricular (LV) chambers extending from base (*top left*) to apex (*bottom right*). The right ventricular cavity is markedly dilated while the left ventricular cavity is of normal dimension. No myocardial necrosis or fibrosis was present. *e*, photomicrograph of portion of wall of PT showing severe depletion of elastic fibers.

6. Headley RN, Carpenter HM, Sawyer CG. *Unusual features of Marfan's syndrome including two postmortem studies. Am J Cardiol 1963;11:259–266.*
7. Roberts WC, Honig HS. *The spectrum of cardiovascular disease in the Marfan syndrome: a clinicomorphologic study of 18 necropsy patients and comparison to 151 previously reported necropsy patients. Am Heart J 1982;104:115–135.*
8. Boyd LJ, McGavack TH. *Aneurysm of the pulmonary artery. A review of the literature and report of two new cases. Am Heart J 1939;18:562–578.*

Mechanisms of severe mitral regurgitation in mitral valve prolapse determined from analysis of operatively excised valves

Certain clinical and mitral valvular morphologic findings are described in 83 patients (age 26 to 79 years [mean, 60]; 26 women [31%] and 57 men [69%]) with mitral valve prolapse (MVP) and mitral regurgitation (MR) severe enough to warrant mitral valve replacement. All 83 operatively excised valves were examined by the same person, and all excised valves had been purely regurgitant (no element of stenosis). No patients had hemodynamic evidence of dysfunction of the aortic valve. In each valve a portion of the posterior mitral leaflet was elongated such that the distance from the distal margin to basal attachment of this leaflet was similar to the distance from the distal margin of the anterior leaflet to its basal attachment to the left atrial wall. Two major mechanisms for the severe MR were found: (1) dilatation of the mitral anulus with or without rupture of chordae tendineae and (2) rupture of chordae tendineae with or without dilatation of the mitral anulus. Of the 83 patients, 48 (58%) had both dilated anuli (>11 cm in circumference) and ruptured chordae tendineae; 16 (19%) had dilated anuli without ruptured chordae, and 16 (19%) had ruptured chordae without significant anular dilatation. In three patients the anulus was not dilated, nor were chordae ruptured, and therefore the mechanism of the MR is uncertain. Mitral chordal rupture was nearly as frequent in the 64 patients with clearly dilated anular circumferences as in the 19 patients with normal or insignificantly dilated anular circumferences (≤11 cm). (AM HEART J 1987;113:1316.)

William C. Roberts, M.D., Charles L. McIntosh, M.D., Robert B. Wallace, M.D.,
Bethesda, Md. and Washington, D.C.

Mitral valve prolapse (MVP) is recognized to occur clinically in about 5% of persons over 20 years of age. In the United States, approximately 160 million persons are over 20 years of age, 8 million of whom have MVP. In most persons with clinical evidence of MVP, no symptoms are produced by the prolapsed valve. Although many persons with MVP have auscultatory evidence of minimal or mild mitral regurgitation (MR), the development of severe MR, severe enough to require operative intervention, is uncommon. This article describes certain findings in 83 patients who had MVP and MR severe enough to warrant mitral valve replacement.

PATIENTS STUDIED

The surgical pathology files of the Pathology Branch, National Heart, Lung, and Blood Institute, were searched for persons who had had mitral valve excision for pure MR. All valves had been so classified initially by W.C.R. Nearly 300 cases were so classified. Many cases were eliminated because either the operatively excised valve was no longer available or photographs of the operatively excised valve were unavailable. Some cases were eliminated because it was apparent that the cause of the pure MR was the following: (1) *rheumatic heart disease* (diffuse fibrosis of both mitral leaflets without elongation of the basal to distal margin of the posterior leaflet), (2) *infective endocarditis* involving a previously normal valve or one previously affected by rheumatic heart disease, (3) *papillary muscle dysfunction* from coronary artery disease (necrotic or fibrotic papillary muscle in the absence of either significant mitral anular dilatation or posterior mitral leaflet elongation), (4) *hypertrophic cardiomyopathy* or (5) *systemic lupus erythematosus* or *hypereosinophilic syndrome*. Some cases were eliminated because the aortic valve had also been excised simultaneously or because the aortic valve was found to have functioned abnormally: either stenotic or regurgitant or both. A few cases were eliminated because on review of preoperative hemody-

From the Pathology and Surgery Branches, National Heart, Lung, and Blood Institute, National Institutes of Health, and the Department of Surgery, Georgetown University.

Reprint requests: William C. Roberts, M.D., Pathology Branch, Bldg. 10A, Room 3E-30, National Heart, Lung, and Blood Institute, National Institutes of Health, Bethesda, MD 20892.

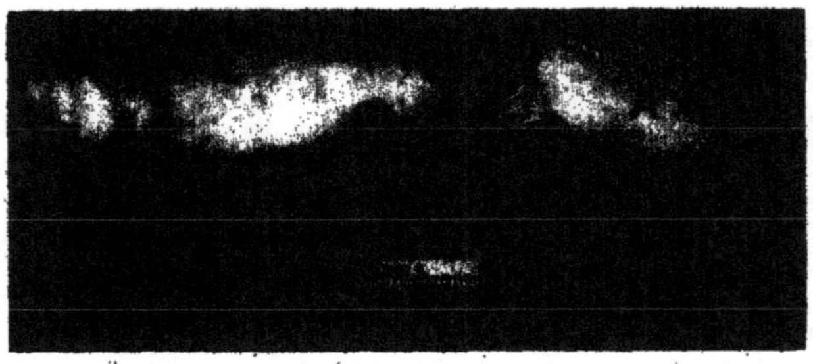

Fig. 1. Operatively excised mitral valve in a 56-year-old man (S68-4175). The anular circumference measures about 11 cm. Some chordae tendineae from the posterior leaflet are missing. The distance from site of attachment (anulus) to distal margin of both posterior and anterior *(A)* leaflets is similar. The atrial surface of the leaflets is shown.

namic data a small mean diastolic gradient had been recorded between the left atrium or pulmonary arterial wedge position and the left ventricle, and therefore the patient did not have "pure" MR.

A total of 83 cases were collected in which preoperative cardiac catheterization had indicated that the hemodynamic lesion involving the mitral valve was *pure* regurgitation, that the aortic valve had functioned normally (no element of either stenosis or regurgitation), and that examination of the operatively excised mitral valve had indicated that it fulfilled the following morphologic definition of MVP: in a portion of the posterior mitral leaflet the distance from its distal margin to its attachment at the mitral anulus was clearly elongated, a finding not observed in patients in whom the MR resulted from other causes, namely, rheumatic, infective endocarditis, coronary artery disease, hypertrophic cardiomyopathy, systemic lupus erythematosus, or hypereosinophilic syndrome. Usually at some point the distance from basal attachment to distal margin of the posterior mitral leaflet was similar to the distance from the distal margin of the anterior mitral leaflet to the point where the left atrial wall contacted it. The elongation of the posterior mitral leaflet caused an increase in the area of this leaflet. Many patients also had dilated mitral anuli, and the chordae in many patients appeared to be longer than usual. This latter finding, however, could not be systematically evaluated because many of the operatively excised mitral valves did not include attached papillary muscles. Photographs of the operatively excised mitral valves were available in 81 (98%) of the 83 patients. Of the 83 cases, 42 (51%) had been included in a previous publication concerning the various causes of pure MR severe enough to warrant mitral valve replacement.[1] Moreover, 25 (30%) of the 83 cases had been included in a previous publication concerning the frequency of calcific deposits in mitral valves excised because of pure MR.[2]

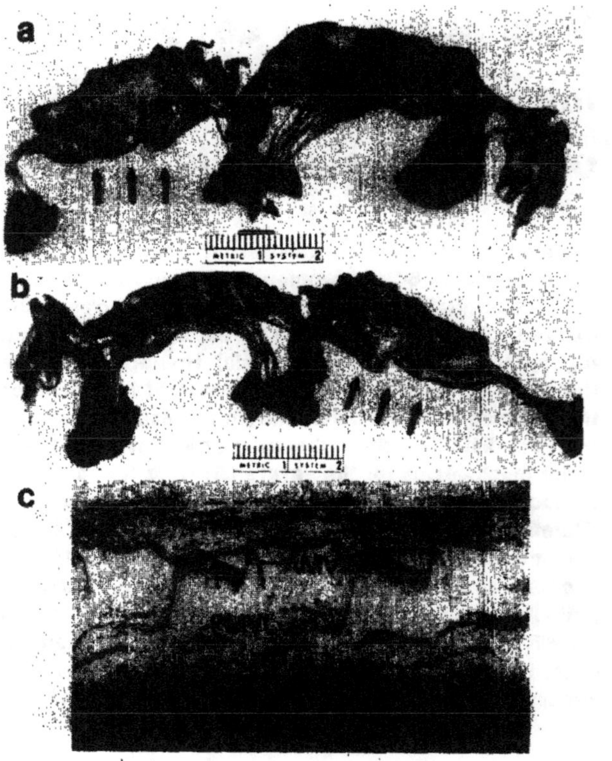

Fig. 2. Operatively excised mitral valve (*a* and *b*) and echocardiogram *(c)* recorded 1 month before valve replacement in a 43-year-old man (S70-3086). *a,* Atrial surface; *b,* Ventricular surface. Chordae are missing from the posterior leaflet *(arrows)*. The distance from the site of attachment to distal margin of both anterior *(A)* and posterior leaflets is similar. *c,* The echocardiogram shows prolapse of the posterior leaflet. AMVL = anterior mitral valve leaflet; PMVL = posterior mitral valve leaflet; VS = ventricular septum.

The operation to replace the mitral valve in the 83 patients had been performed at four different medical centers, and the operatively excised valve in each was thereafter submitted to the Pathology Branch of the National Heart, Lung, and Blood Institute for examination. The valve was weighed, its anular circumference was measured, and a determination was made whether chordae tendineae attached to both leaflets were "disrupted" or "missing" or neither. Chordae were considered "disrupted" if detached chordae had rounded or blunted distal ends that were thicker than normal, often thicker than the more proximal portions of the same chordae. Chordae were considered "missing" if none extended caudally beneath the ventricular surfaces of a portion of either or both leaflets. Both "dis-

Fig. 3. Operatively excised mitral valve in a 55-year-old woman (S76-35). The anulus measures about 12 cm in circumference. Most chordae from the posterior leaflet are missing *(arrows)*. *a,* Ventricular aspect of valve. *b,* Ventricular aspect of posterior leaflet. *c,* Atrial aspect of posterior leaflet.

Fig. 4. Operatively excised mitral valve *(a)* showing its atrial aspect and lateral radiographs showing a C-shaped calcific deposit before *(b)* and after *(c)* valve replacement in a 47-year-old woman (S76-156). Some chordae from the posterior leaflet are missing. A = anterior leaflet.

rupted" and "missing" chordae were considered "ruptured" chordae.

RESULTS

The 83 patients included 26 women (31%) and 57 men (69%). The women at the time of mitral valve replacement ranged in age from 42 to 79 years (mean, 61 years) and the men ranged from 26 to 77 years (mean, 59 years). The 26-year-old man had the Marfan syndrome. The next youngest patient was 42 years old. Of the 83 patients, 15 (18%) were younger than 51 years old, and 68 patients (82%) were older than 50 years of age at the time of mitral valve replacement. The excised valves (Figs. 1 to 18) ranged in weight from 4.0 to 14.5 gm (mean, 6.7 gm). The larger weights were in the valves in which one or both papillary muscles had usually been excised. Calcific deposits were present in 28 valves (34%). The calcific deposits involved primarily the mitral anular region in 19 patients (68%), one or both mitral leaflets without anular involvement in three patients (11%), one or more chordae tendineae only in four patients (14%), and papillary muscle only in two patients (7%). The calcific deposits were focal and small in all patients.

The circumference of the mitral anulus in the 26 women ranged from 9 to 15 cm (mean, 12). It was ≤11 cm in 10 patients (38%), and nine (90%) had missing or disrupted chordae tendineae. The circumference was >11 cm in 16 women (62%), and 13 (81%) had missing or disrupted chordae. Of the 26 women, 22 (85%) had ruptured chordae. In the 57 men, the mitral anular circumference ranged from 10 to 18 cm (mean, 14). It was ≤11 cm in nine patients (16%), and seven of the nine had missing or disrupted chordae. It was >11 cm in 48 men (84%), and 35 (73%) had missing or disrupted chordae. Of the 57 men, 42 (74%) had ruptured chordae. Of the entire 83 patients, 64 (77%) had missing or disrupted chordae: in 16 (84%) of the 19 patients in whom the anular circumference was ≤11 cm and in 48 (75%) of the 64 in whom the anular circumference was >11 cm.

Of the 64 (77%) patients with missing or disrupted chordae or both, the missing or disrupted

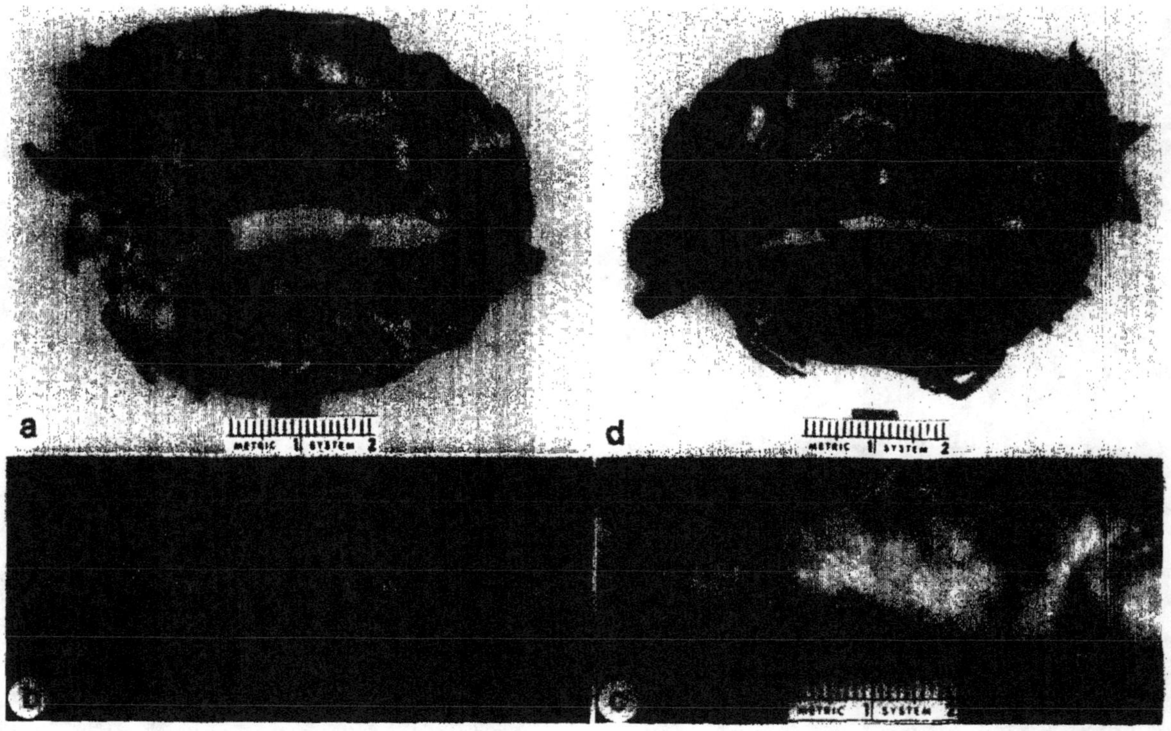

Fig. 5. Operatively excised mitral valve in a 60-year-old man (S77-157). *a-c* Atrial aspect. *d*, Ventricular aspect. Both anterior *(A)* and posterior leaflets are of similar size. Chordae from the posterior leaflet are both missing and disrupted. The disrupted chord is designated by the arrow. *c*, A close-up of the posterior leaflet. (Reproduced with permission from Byram MT and Roberts WC. Frequencies and extent of calcific deposits in purely regurgitant mitral valves: analysis of 108 operatively excised valves. Am J Cardiol 1983;52:1059-61.)

chordae involved the posterior leaflet only in 57 patients (90%), the anterior leaflet only in three patients (5%), and both leaflets in three patients (5%). In all 57 patients in whom only chordae to the posterior leaflet were affected, the chordae were considered missing in each. In the three patients in whom only chordae to the anterior leaflet were affected, the chordae were considered disrupted in one, missing in one, and both disrupted and missing in one. Finally in the three patients in whom chordae from both leaflets were affected, in each some chordae were disrupted and some were missing. No patient with missing chordae had historical evidence of infective endocarditis that had healed, and therefore the chordal rupture in them is considered "spontaneous." Of the eight patients with disrupted chordae with or without missing chordae, five had historical evidence of infective endocarditis that had healed.

DISCUSSION

The above data indicate that there are two major mechanisms for development of severe MR in MVP: (1) dilatation of the mitral anulus with or without rupture of chordae tendineae and (2) rupture of chordae tendineae with or without dilatation of the mitral anulus. Of our 83 patients with MVP, severe MR, and mitral valve replacement, 48 (58%) had both dilated anuli (>11 cm in circumference) and ruptured chordae tendineae; 16 (19%) had dilated anuli without rupture of chordae, and 16 (19%) had ruptured chordae without significant anular dilatation. In three of the 83 patients, the anulus was not dilated, nor were chordae ruptured. Therefore the mechanism of the severe MR in these three patients is unclear. Mitral chordal rupture was nearly as frequent in the 64 patients with clearly dilated mitral anuli (circumference >11 cm) as in the 19 patients with normal or insignificantly dilated anuli (circumference ≤11 cm) (75% [48/64] vs 84% [16/19]).

The reported frequencies of rupture of chordae tendineae in operatively excised prolapsed (floppy) mitral valves have not been as high as in the present study. The explanation almost surely lies in differing definitions of the term "ruptured chordae tendineae." In the present study only nine patients (11%) had easily identifiable, unequivocally disrupted

Fig. 6. Operatively excised mitral valve (*a* and *b*) and preoperative echocardiogram *(c)* in a 64-year-old man (S80-64). The anulus is nearly 15 cm in circumference. Chordae from the posterior leaflet are missing *(arrows)*. *c*, Echocardiogram showing prolapse *(arrows)*. A = anterior leaflet; VS = ventricular septum.

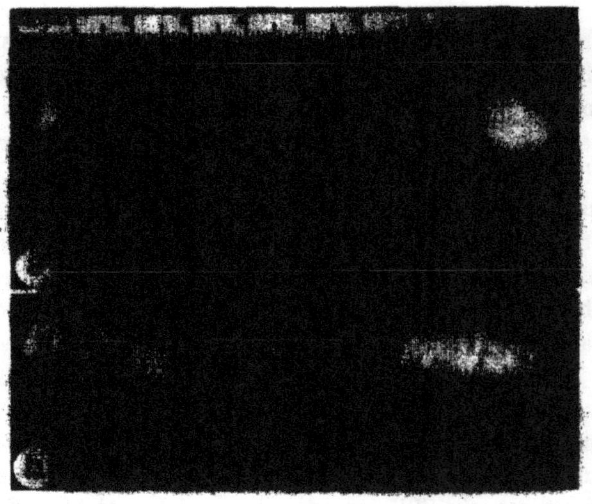

Fig. 7. Atrial *(a)* and ventricular *(b)* aspects of the excised mitral valve in a 70-year-old woman (S80-162). The anulus is only about 10 cm in circumference. Many chordae from the posterior leaflet are missing *(arrows)*.

Fig. 8. Intact *(a)* and opened *(b)* operatively excised mitral valve in a 67-year-old man (S80-172). The anulus is enormously dilated (17 cm). Some chordae from the posterior leaflet are missing. A = anterior leaflet.

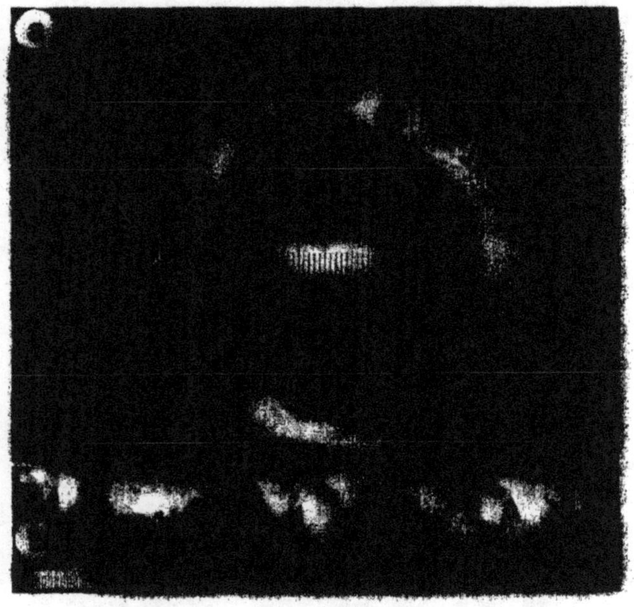

Fig. 9. Intact *(a)* and opened *(b)* operatively excised valve in a 26-year-old man (S82-1) who had the Marfan syndrome. This patient was the youngest in this study. The anulus is enormously dilated (about 18 cm). The chordae appear to be intact. A = anterior leaflet.

chordae. In contrast, 61 (73%) had no identifiable disrupted chordae, but portions of the posterior leaflet were devoid of chordae. These patients were considered to have "missing" chordae, a situation equivalent to disrupted chordae. Of the nine patients with disrupted chordae, seven also had

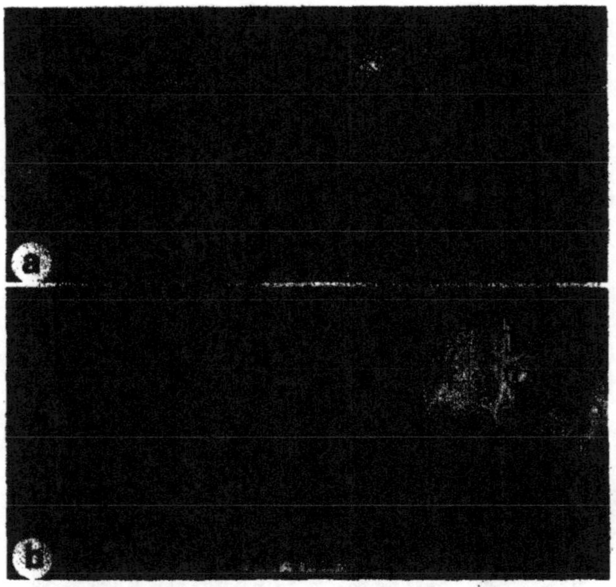

Fig. 10. Opened mitral valve showing the atrial *(a)* and ventricular *(b)* aspects in a 42-year-old woman (77S-3497). Both anterior *(A)* and posterior leaflets are of similar size. Many chordae from the posterior leaflet are missing. The anulus is about 13 cm in circumference.

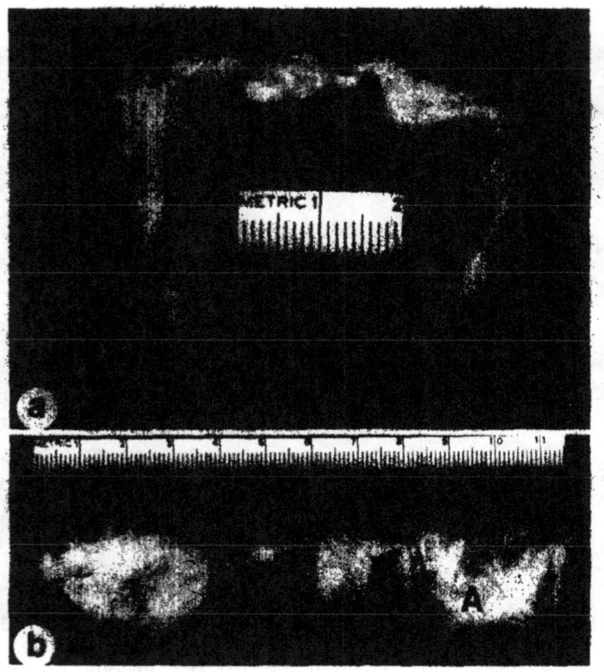

Fig. 11. Intact *(a)* and opened *(b)* mitral valve in a 65-year-old man (80-S-3326). The anulus is about 12 cm in circumference. Most chordae from the posterior leaflet are missing. A = anterior leaflet.

missing chordae. Of the 61 patients with missing chordae, seven also had disrupted chordae. Thus, only two of the 83 patients had disrupted without missing chordae.

The cause of the chordal rupture was not determined in 59 (92%) of the 64 patients, and therefore

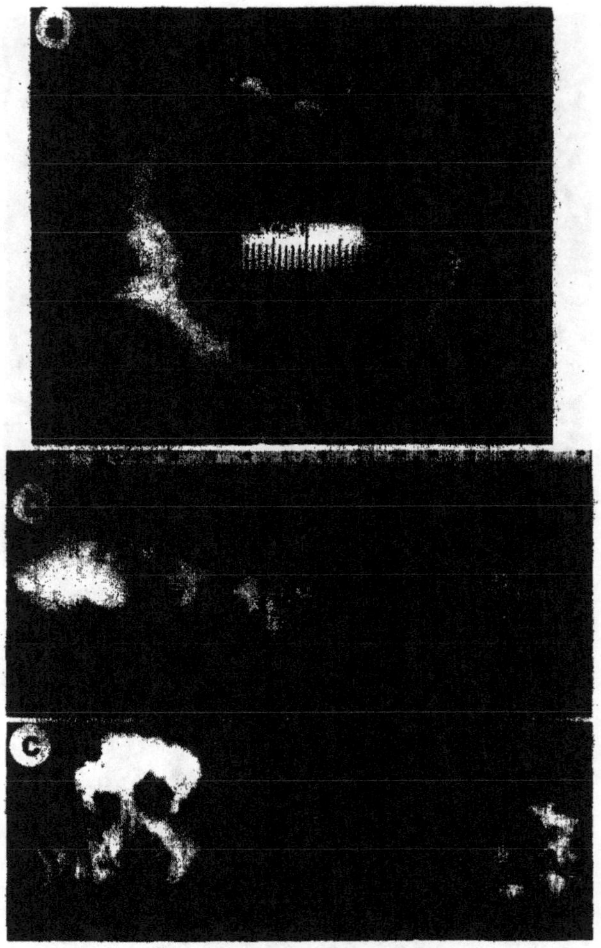

Fig. 12. Intact *(a)* and opened *(b)* mitral valve and a radiograph *(c)* of the valve in a 73-year-old man (81-S-2245). The anulus is about 14 cm in circumference. A large calcific deposit *(arrow)* is located at the anulus (site of attachment) of the largest scallop of the posterior leaflet. Chordae from the posterior leaflet are missing. A = anterior leaflet.

their chordal rupture is considered "spontaneous." It is now recognized that spontaneous rupture of mitral chordae tendineae is nearly always in the setting of MVP.[3-7] Of the 83 patients studied, at least six had a history of active infective endocarditis that had healed: five had disrupted mitral chordae and one had no disrupted or missing chordae. None of the 54 patients with missing but without disrupted chordae had had a history of active infective endocarditis.

Although MVP appears to be more common in women than in men, severe MR caused by MVP is more common in men. Of our 83 patients with MVR and MR severe enough to warrant mitral replacement, nearly 70% were men. In 23 patients with MVP and MR severe enough to warrant mitral valve replacement and reported by Jeresaty et al.,[3] at least 13 and probably 15 (65%) were men. Of 18 patients

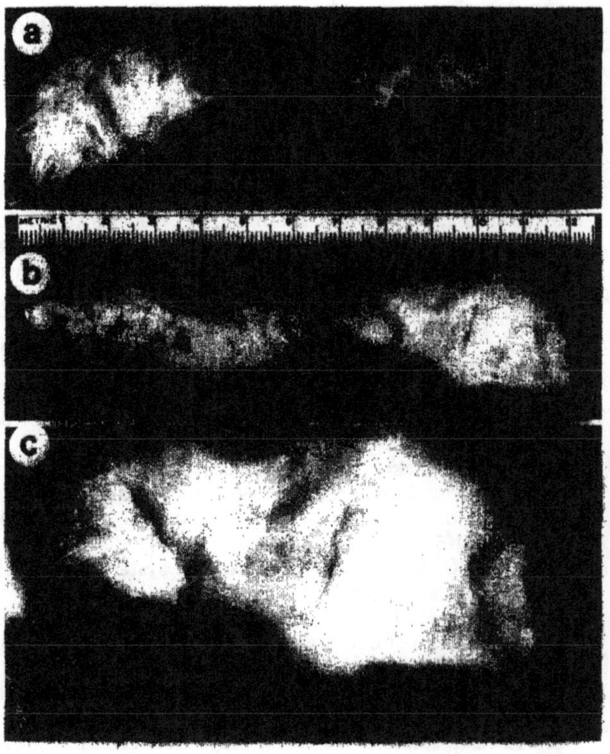

Fig. 13. Opened mitral valve (*a* and *b*) and close-up of portion of posterior leaflet *(c)* in a 58-year-old woman (83-S-3077). *a*, Ventricular aspect. *b*, Atrial aspect. *c*, Atrial aspect. The anulus is about 14 cm in circumference. Many chordae from the posterior leaflet are missing. A = anterior leaflet.

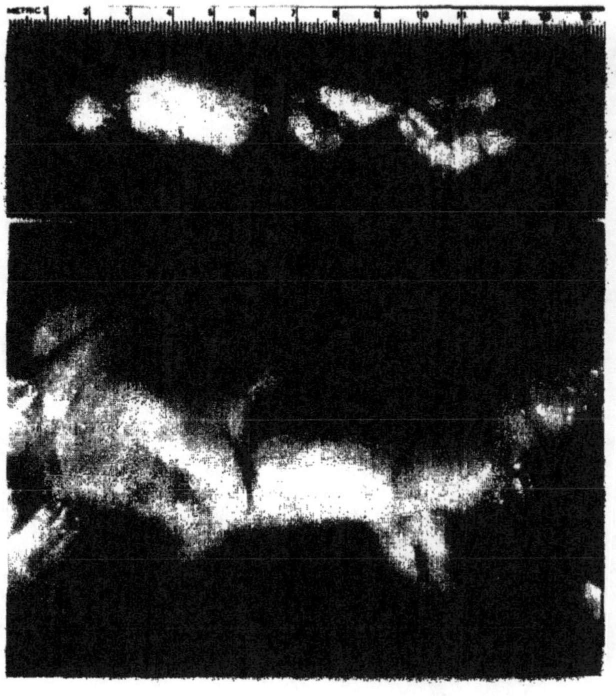

Fig. 14. Opened mitral valve from the atrial aspect in a 64-year-old woman (84-S-325). The anulus is nearly 14 cm in circumference. Many chordae from the posterior leaflet are missing *(arrows)*. A close-up of a portion of posterior leaflet is shown in the lower panel.

Fig. 15. Opened mitral valve showing its atrial aspects in a 65-year-old woman (84-S-3509). Many chordae from the posterior leaflet are missing *(arrows)*. The anulus is about 14 cm in circumference. A = anterior leaflet.

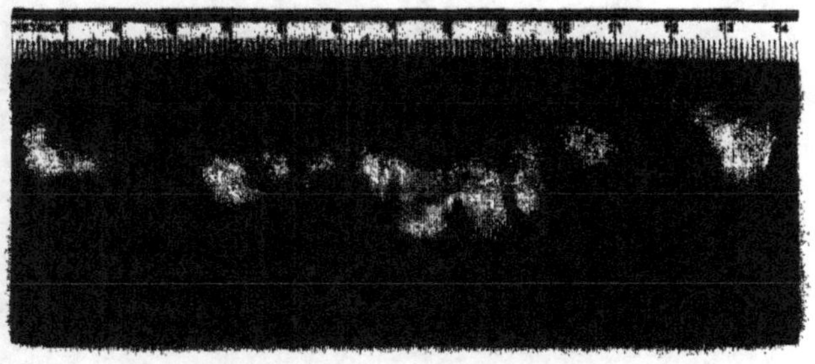

Fig. 16. Opened mitral valve showing its atrial aspect in a 71-year-old woman (84-S-7903). The anulus is about 14 cm in circumference. The chordae appear to be intact. A = anterior leaflet.

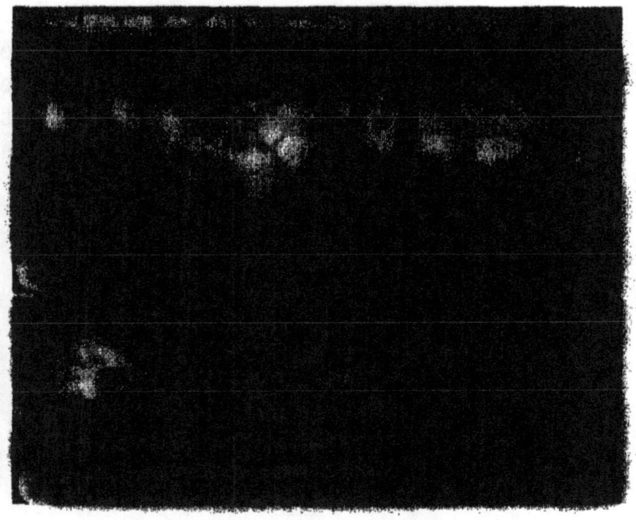

Fig. 17. Opened mitral valve showing its atrial *(a)* and ventricular *(b)* aspects in a 44-year-old man (85-S-971). The anulus is about 15 cm in circumference. Chordae from the posterior leaflet appear to be both missing and others disrupted. A = anterior leaflet.

with MVP and MR severe enough to warrant mitral replacement and reported by Olson et al.,[7] 14 (78%) were men. Of 11 patients ≥60 years of age with MVP and MR severe enough to warrant mitral replacement and reported by Naggar et al.,[8] six (55%) were men.

Finally, opportunities to study systematically

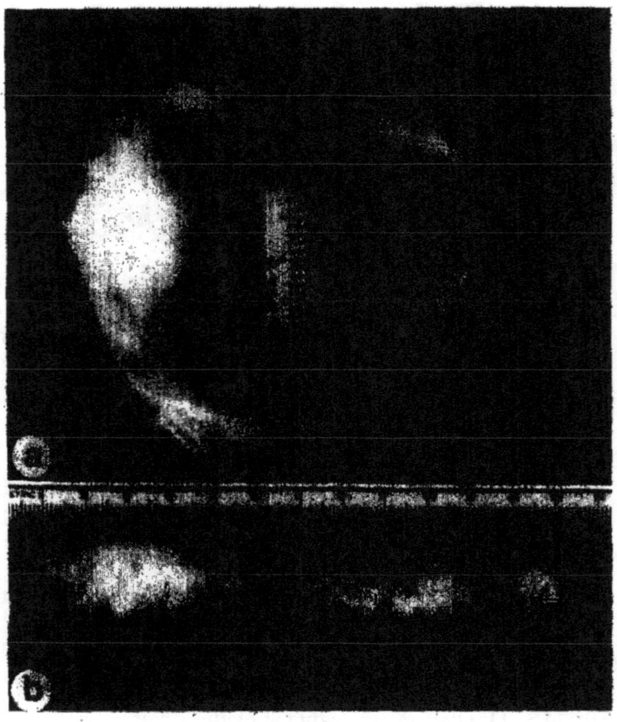

Fig. 18. Unopened *(a)* and opened *(b)* mitral valve in a 66-year-old man (85-S-2575). The anulus is about 14 cm in circumference. Many chordae from the posterior leaflet are missing *(arrows)*. A = anterior leaflet.

operatively excised prolapsed mitral valves in the future will almost surely diminish because of a move away from replacement in favor of repair procedures for patients with severe MR caused by MVP. Thus the data collected in the present study will not likely be collected again in a relatively short period of time.

REFERENCES

1. Waller BF, Morrow AG, Maron BJ, Del Negro AA, Kent KM, McGrath FJ, Wallace RB, McIntosh CL, Roberts WC. Etiology of clinically isolated, severe, chronic, pure mitral regurgitation: Analysis of 97 patients over 30 years of age having mitral valve replacement. Am Heart J 1982;104:276-88.
2. Byram MT, Roberts WC. Frequency and extent of calcific deposits in purely regurgitant mitral valves: analysis of 108 operatively excised valves. Am J Cardiol 1983;52:1059-61.
3. Jeresaty RM, Edwards JE, Chawla SK. Mitral valve prolapse and ruptured chordae tendineae. Am J Cardiol 1985;55:138-42.
4. Hickey AJ, Wicker Del, Wright JS, Warren BA. Primary (spontaneous) chordal rupture: relation to myxomatous valve disease and mitral valve prolapse. J Am Coll Cardiol 1985;5:1341-6.
5. Roberts WC. Mitral valve prolapse and systemic hypertension. Am J Cardiol 1985;56:703.
6. Aronson RJ, Hoffman M, Algueti-Margulis A, Yust I. Spontaneous rupture of mitral chordae tendineae in hypertension. Am J Cardiol (In press, 1987)
7. Olson LJ, Subramanian R, Ackerman DM, Orszulak TA, Edwards WD. Surgical pathology of the mitral valve: a study of 712 cases spanning 21 years. Mayo Clin Proc 1987;62:22-34.
8. Naggar CZ, Pearson WN, Seljan MP. Frequency of complications of mitral valve prolapse in subjects aged 60 years and older. Am J Cardiol 1986;58:1209-12.

PULMONARY ARTERIES IN CONGENITAL HEART DISEASE: A STRUCTURE-FUNCTION ANALYSIS

Renu Virmani, M.D.
William C. Roberts, M.D.

For many years, students of congenital heart disease were unable to explain the lack of survival patterns in patients with similar-sized, isolated communications between systemic and pulmonary circulations. Although in 1927 Moschcowitz[1] suggested that the explanation may be the result of pulmonary hypertension, hemodynamic and histologic studies during the past 30 years of the pulmonary vessels have helped enormously in explaining these differences. In 1935 Oscar Brenner in Birmingham, England, described histologic features of the normal pulmonary arteries and veins.[2] A year later Parker and Weiss,[3] at Boston City Hospital, described changes in the lungs and blood vessels in patients with mitral stenosis. Jesse Edwards, who also trained at Boston City Hospital in the late 1930s, began describing anatomic changes in the pulmonary vasculature in patients with congenital heart disease in the late 1940s: he too attributed the changes to the effects of pulmonary hypertension. Edwards, his colleagues, and many others described changes in a variety of congenital cardiac diseases,[4–45] and by 1958 a classification of the hypertensive pulmonary changes was formulated.[13] The recognition of the intimate association between the lung and the heart has been a major contribution to the understanding of congenital heart disease. Today it is well known that the state of the lung is the primary determinant of operability in a patient with a shunt. This chapter describes changes observed in the pulmonary vessels of adults with certain congenital cardiovascular malformations.

ANATOMIC CLASSIFICATION OF PULMONARY ARTERIAL HYPERTENSIVE CHANGES IN CONGENITAL HEART DISEASE

The anatomic classification of pulmonary hypertensive changes by Heath and Edwards[13] was based primarily on observations of patients with large ventricular septal defects, but it also was based on studies of a few patients with large patent ductus arteriosus and other defects associated with a free communication between the systemic and pulmonary circulations, which causes pulmonary hypertension

Table 1. Classification of hypertensive pulmonary vascular changes by Heath and Edwards in 1958.[13] (Reproduced with permission.)

	Grade of hypertensive pulmonary vascular disease					
	1	2	3	4	5	6
Type of intimal reaction	←None→	← Cellular	→	→	→	→
			← Fibrous and fibroelastic	→	→	→
				← Plexiform lesion	→	→
State of media of arteries and arterioles	← Hypertrophied	→	→	→	→	→
			← Some generalized dilatation	→	→	→
				← Local "dilatation lesions"*	→	→
					← Pulmonary hemosiderosis†	→
						←Necrotizing arteritis→

*Vein-like branches of hypertrophied muscular pulmonary arteries, angiomatoid lesion, and cavernous lesion

†Associated with distended, thin-walled, arterial vessels throughout the lung

from birth.* Their study also included a few patients with primary pulmonary hypertension.

The classification of Heath and Edwards is reproduced in Table 1. Although their classification of histologic changes observed in the pulmonary arteries in patients with pulmonary hypertension brought organization to a complex, previously unorganized subject, on re-evaluation, it is now apparent, 30 years later, that their classification has certain deficiencies. Considerable overlap exists between their grades 2 and 3, and between their grades 4 and 5. *Alveolar hemosiderosis* (grade 5) does not concern a pulmonary artery and is common in patients without pulmonary arterial hypertension. In our view, a classification of pulmonary arterial changes should not include changes in alveolar spaces (hemosiderosis). The grade 6 category implies that grades 1 through 5 are prerequisites, when, in actuality, necrotizing vasculitis may occur in the absence of grades 1 to 5. It seems to us that a classification of hypertensive changes in the pulmonary arteries should be applicable to all patients with pulmonary hypertension irrespective of the cause and irrespective of whether the hypertension is congenital or acquired.

Recently by a new quantitative method of analysis, additional features of pulmonary vascular changes associated with congenital heart disease have been described.[46–51] This method was first described by Davies and Reid[46] and applied to the study of lungs in which the pulmonary arteries were injected with a barium gelatin mixture and the brachial tree inflated with formalin and the following characteristics noted: (1) The degree of muscle extension in the small arteries in relation to the bronchial tree; (2) the thickness of the arterial medial muscular coat; and (3) the concentration of small peripheral arteries per unit area, judged in relation to the alveolar concentration. The degree of muscle extension is an age-related process (Fig. 1): at birth the muscle coat of the artery accompanying the respiratory unit extends up to terminal bronchiole (i.e., pre-acinar) and at the level of the respiratory bronchiole it is partially muscular. The wall thickness also varies. However, in the fetus, the arteries that are muscular have a thicker wall in relation to their size than in the adult, but the intra-acinar region has virtually no muscular arteries in the fetus. The

*This classic paper by Heath and Edwards included 27 photomicrographs of lung from 22 patients, only 5 of whom had ventricular septal defect. Of particular interest is that 17 of the 22 patients were over 20 years of age.

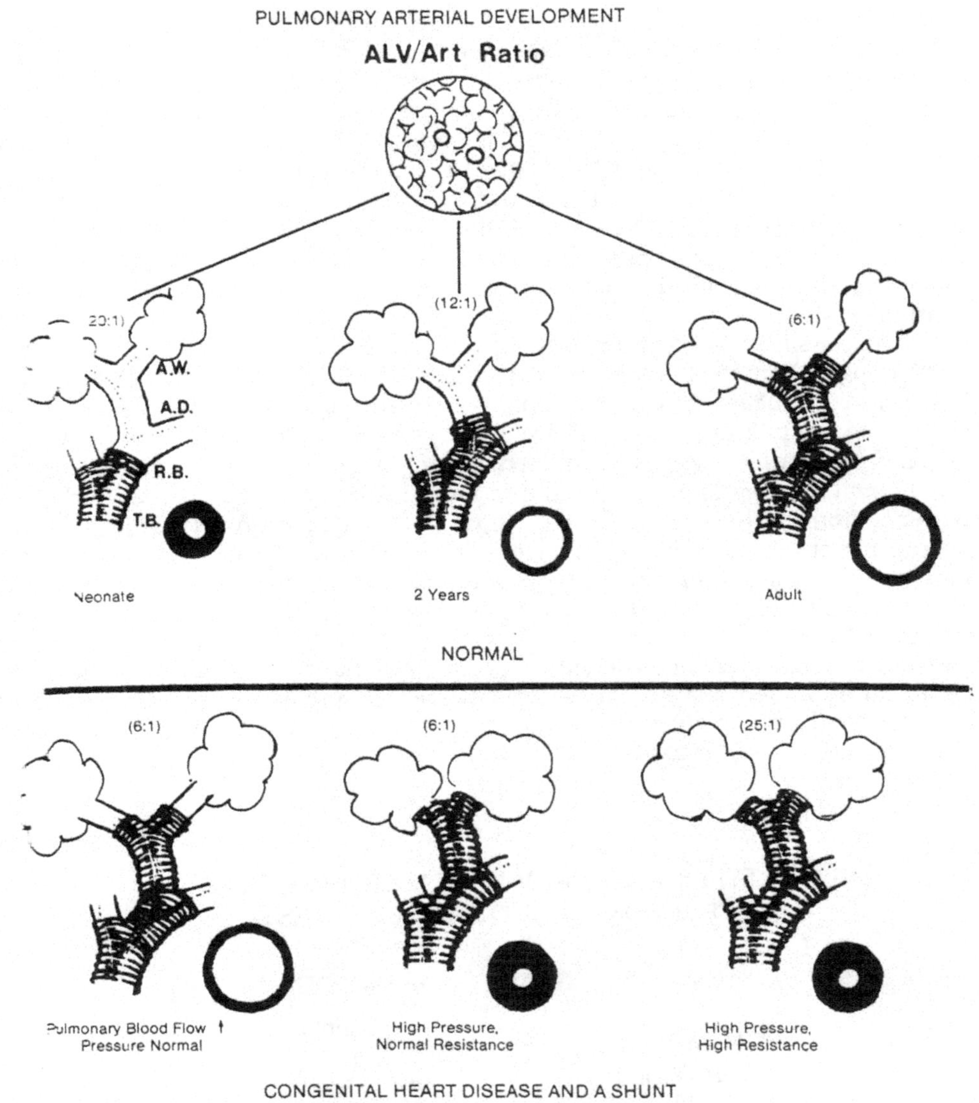

FIGURE 1. Diagram illustrating the pulmonary vascular pathway, that is, extension of muscle into peripheral arteries in relation to the bronchial tree, wall thickness of pulmonary arteries, and alveolar arteriolar (ALV/Art) ratio. The top panel demonstrates the normal development, whereas the lower panel relates structural changes with pulmonary arterial pressure, blood flow, and vascular resistance as seen in patients with congenital heart disease and a shunt. A.D. = alveolar duct; A.W. = alveolar wall; R.B. = respiratory bronchiolus; T.B. = terminal bronchiolus. Modified from Rabinowitch et al.[50]

drop in pressure that occurs rapidly at birth is associated with a change in compliance of the small muscular arteries (< 300 μm, in diameter). The vascular bed shows an increase in external diameter and a decrease in wall thickness within hours of birth. The larger arteries fall to adult value over the first few months after birth, and gradually during childhood and into adolescence, the muscle extends to the intra-acinar region into the alveolar duct (see Fig. 1). This has been related to the increase in the pressor response to hypoxia which occurs with increasing age.

At birth the ratio of alveoli to arteries is about 20:1; and as part of the fall in pressure in the postnatal period, there is an increase in the number of peripheral arteries so that by adult life the ratio of alveoli to arteries is 6:1. With persistent pulmonary hypertension as occurs in congenital heart disease with shunts, there is a reduction in the number of arteries and the ratio increases. Meyrick and Reid[51] have described that in the distended and fixed state of the pulmonary arteries the size of the vessel can be related to the structure. Human adult arteries greater than 2000 μm in diameter are elastic, and those between 150 and 2000 μm are muscular. Those less than 150 μm are a "mixed population"—muscular, partially muscular, or non-muscular—and these are intra-acinar in location. In the fetal and young lung, the mixed population is pre-acinar in position. Reid and Meyrick[51] suggest that the smallest muscular and the partially muscular arteries represent the resistance arteries.

The classification of pulmonary arterial changes used herein is based entirely on histologic alterations observed independent of etiology, time of appearance, and hemodynamic documentation of the pulmonary arterial pressure (Fig. 2). The major changes in the pulmonary arteries include (1) *medial thickening,* (2) *intimal thickening,* and (3) *plexiform lesions.* Only medial thickening is grade I; medial thickening and intimal thickening are grade II; and medial thickening and intimal thickening with plexiform lesions are grade III. We do not include arteritis (vasculitis), either necrotizing or non-necrotizing, in the grading system since pulmonary arteritis may occur in the absence of pulmonary hypertension. The classification of Reid and coworkers has been derived from the study of young infants who died with congenital heart disease and shunt within the first year of life with the pulmonary arteries fixed under high pressure. Therefore, the changes may be a reflection of underdevelopment, or there may be excessive dilatation of pulmonary arteries and these changes would not apply to the study of the adult lung in patients with congenital heart disease whose lungs were not pressure fixed.

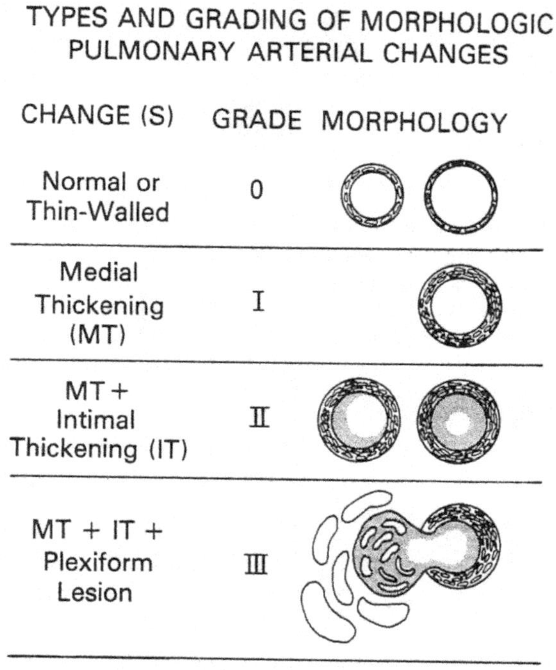

FIGURE 2. Types and grading of the morphologic pulmonary arterial changes in the patients studied (see text). From Virmani R, Roberts WC. Pulmonary arteries in congenital heart disease: A structure-function analysis. Cardiovasc Clin 1979; 10(1):457, with permission.

TABLE 2. Histologic Features of Normal Pulmonary Vessels in Adults

		MEDIA			LUMEN DIAMETER ÷ WALL THICKNESS	INTERNAL ELASTIC MEMBRANE	EXTERNAL ELASTIC MEMBRANE	ADVENTITIA (0–4)
	EXTERNAL DIAMETER	ELASTIC FIBERS (0–4)	SM CELLS (0–4)	COLLAGEN (0–4)				
Extrapulmonary Arteries								
Pulmonary trunk	1.6 cm	++++	++	+		+	+	+
Right main PA	1.3 cm	++++	++	+		+	+	+
Left main PA	1.3 cm	++++	++	+		+	+	+
Intrapulmonary Vessels								
Elastic arteries	>1000μ	+++	++	+	10	+	+	+
Muscular arteries	100–1000μ	+	++++	+	4	+	+	+
Arterioles	<100μ	0	0*	0	6	+	0	++
Capillaries	<10μ	0	0	0		0**	0	0
Venules	10–100μ	0	0	0		+	0	++
Veins	>100μ	++	+	++	4	+	0	+++
Bronchial arteries	100–300μ	+	++++	+	4	+	±	+
Bronchial veins		0	+	+	2	+	0	+
Lymphatic channels		0	0	0		0***	0	0

*A thin muscular media is present in its most proximal portion

**Endothelial layer plus basement membranes

***Actually an endothelial lining rather than an internal elastic membrane

SM = smooth muscle

From Virmani R, Roberts WC. Pulmonary arteries in congenital heart disease: A structure-function analysis. Cardiovasc Clin 1979; 10(1): 458, with permission.

HISTOLOGIC FEATURES OF NORMAL PULMONARY VESSELS

Much has been written on this subject.[1,9,13,25,45,52,53] Table 2 summarizes some of the features of normal adult pulmonary vessels. The extrapulmonary arteries, that is, the pulmonary trunk and right and left main pulmonary arteries, are elastic arteries. At birth the media of the pulmonary trunk consists of parallel elastic lamellae that are identical in number and configuration to those in the media of ascending aorta (Fig. 3). If the pulmonary arterial pressure falls to its normal level in the first few weeks

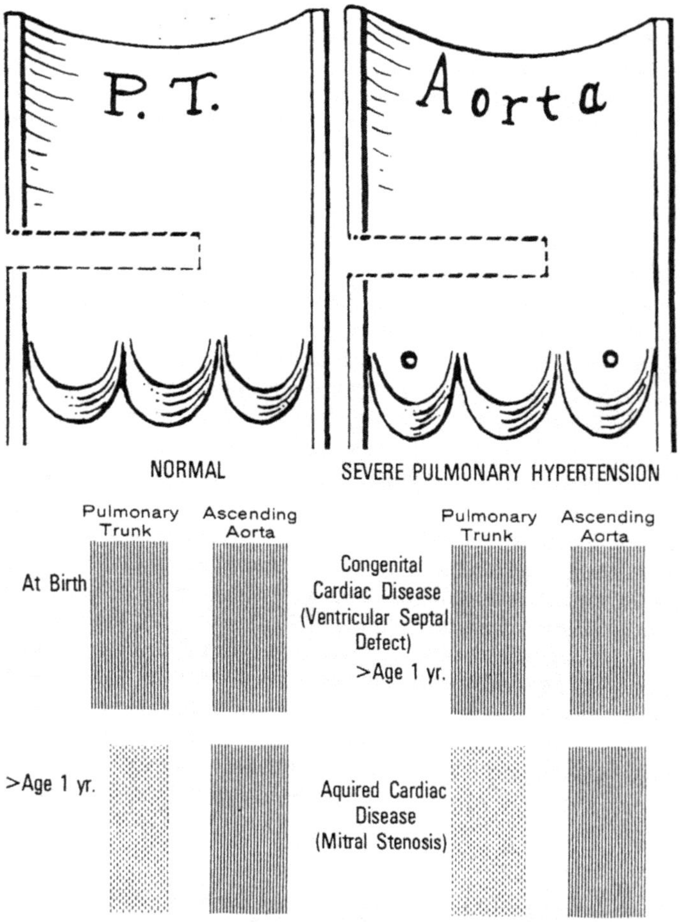

FIGURE 3. Configuration of elastic fibers in the pulmonary trunk at birth, after 1 year of age, with pulmonary hypertension from birth (ventricular septal defect), and with an acquired condition (mitral stenosis). The sketch (top) shows the sites in the pulmonary trunk (P.T.) and aorta at which the sections for histologic examination were taken. At birth the configuration of the elastic fibers in both the pulmonary trunk and ascending aorta are identical and wall thicknesses are similar. Normally, after a year of age the numbers of elastic fibers in the pulmonary trunk diminishes considerably to reach an "adult configuration," and the thickness of the wall also diminishes. If a large ventricular septal defect or aortic pulmonary defect is present from birth, both the configuration of the elastic fibers and wall thickness of the pulmonary trunk remain similar to that of the ascending aorta ("fetal configuration"). If pulmonary hypertension is acquired later in life, however, as in mitral stenosis, the configuration of the elastic fibers of the pulmonary trunk remains like that of the normal adult but wall thickness increases. The information on the configuration of elastic fibers in the pulmonary trunk is based on original work by Heath and associates.[85] From Virmani R, Roberts WC. Pulmonary arteries in congenital heart disease: A structure-function analysis. Cardiovasc Clin 1979; 10(1):459, with permission.

of life, the thickness of the wall of the pulmonary trunk and its branches diminishes, and the number of elastic lamellae decreases; those which remain are disrupted (see Fig. 3). Between the elastic fibers are smooth muscle cells and collagen fibrils. The integrity of the elastic pulmonary arteries in adults is dependent not on the disrupted elastic fibers but on the integrity of the smooth muscle cells and collagen. The elastic pulmonary arteries extend into the lungs to the levels of the intrapulmonary cartilaginous bronchi.

The *muscular* pulmonary arteries begin, obviously, where the elastic arteries end. Although it contains occasional elastic and collagenous fibrils, the media consists predominantly of smooth muscle cells bordered by internal and external elastic membranes. The muscular arteries and/or arterioles are adjacent to or associated with the terminal bronchioles, respiratory bronchioles, and alveolar ducts.

The pulmonary *arterioles* are branches of the muscular arteries. Except at their origin from the muscular arteries—where they have a thin muscular media between internal and external elastic membranes—the media is absent. An easily discernible elastic membrane covered by a single layer of endothelial cells borders the lumen. The arteriole divides into *capillaries*, which course directly into the alveolar septum rather than running parallel to the lining of the adjacent alveolus, as was originally believed.[3]

The capillaries drain into the pulmonary venules, which are larger than, but virtually identical in structure to, the capillaries: they consist of an endothelial layer covered by an elastic membrane. The *veins* have a thicker internal elastic membrane and are bordered by several irregularly arranged bundles of smooth muscle cells interspersed with collagenous fibrils and elastic fibrils.

The *bronchial arteries* are located within the walls of the bronchi but otherwise are similar to the muscular pulmonary arteries. The *bronchial veins* also are in the bronchial walls and have thinner walls and larger lumens than the bronchial arteries. *Lymphatics* are present adjacent to pulmonary arteries and bronchi and in the interlobular septa and subpleural areas.

HISTOLOGIC FEATURES AND PROPOSED CAUSES OF ABNORMAL PULMONARY ARTERIES

MEDIAL THICKENING

Medial thickening applies to an increase in the thickness of the media, either in the wall of the pulmonary artery or in the proximal portion of the pulmonary arteriole. Whether this occurs entirely from hypertrophy of smooth muscle cells or whether both hypertrophy and hyperplasia cause the thickening is unclear.

INTIMAL THICKENING

There are two types of intimal thickening—cellular and acellular. In the cellular variety, the proliferated intima consists primarily of strap cells with collagen in between. The strap cells appear to be primarily smooth muscle cells. The acellular variety consists mostly of dense fibrous tissue (collagen) with minimal smooth muscle cells or none at all.

PLEXIFORM LESION

A plexiform lesion is an aneurysmal or glomus-like structure that emerges at a right angle from a muscular pulmonary artery. The beginning of the right-angle branch is usually apparent; from there it rapidly dilates into a plexus of channels, the walls of which consist primarily of fibrous tissue covered by endothelial cells. The plexiform structure ends by giving off thin-walled channels, which probably are dilated arterioles; these branch quickly into alveolar septal capillaries. When these thin-walled channels are considerably dilated, they are sometimes called *dilatation lesions*. By electron microscopic examination, the thin-walled channels of the plexiform lesions are lined by cells resembling endothelium, but no Weibel-Palade bodies or careolae intracellulares have been demonstrated. Between the vessels is a matrix of proteoglycan ground substance. Interspersed in the matrix are fibrillary cells and myofibroblasts.[54]

PROPOSED CAUSES

Medial thickening is a response of the arterial wall to increased pressure and therefore occurs only in patients with pulmonary arterial hypertension. As mentioned earlier, whether the thickening of the media is a consequence of hypertrophy alone, or hypertrophy and hyperplasia, or hyperplasia alone is unclear. Medial thickening is never simply a normal consequence of aging.

Intimal thickening, be it cellular or acellular, is not necessarily the consequence of pulmonary arterial hypertension, but it is accelerated by elevation of pulmonary arterial pressure. Cellular and acellular intimal proliferation is observed commonly in older persons, most of whom have normal pulmonary arterial pressures.[53] The occurrence of intimal thickening combined with medial thickening, however, is indicative of pulmonary hypertension.

Plexiform lesions occur only in patients with severe pulmonary hypertension, although some patients with severe pulmonary hypertension do not have them. These lesions can occur in patients with large left-to-right shunts or primary pulmonary hypertension, but they do not occur in patients with severe pulmonary hypertension secondary only to left-sided cardiac disease (i.e., mitral stenosis). Plexiform lesions do not occur if the cause of the pulmonary hypertension is located distal to the pulmonary capillary level or, stated differently, if the pulmonary arterial hypertension is the consequence of pulmonary venous hypertension. For plexiform lesions to occur, the cause of the hypertension must originate at the capillary or precapillary level.[55]

The exact cause of plexiform lesions is unknown. Serial sections of lung at sites of plexiform lesions generally show extreme narrowing or almost total obstruction of the lumen of the muscular pulmonary artery distal to the origin of the small muscular pulmonary artery or arteriole which is the site of the lesions.[25] Kanjuh and colleagues[30] have speculated that the plexiform lesion is a consequence of a *jet lesion* caused by blood rapidly changing its course because of the distal obstruction of the relatively large muscular pulmonary artery distal to the site of the plexiform lesion. Thus, the plexiform lesion might act as a dissipater of the extremely high pulmonary arterial pressure.

Other proposed causes of plexiform lesions are that they represent *sites of anastomoses of pulmonary arteries and veins*[56–59] or that they are a *congenital malformation*.[60,61] The latter theory appears particularly unlikely because plexiform lesions have never been observed in the lungs at birth. The earliest these pulmonary lesions have been observed is 2 months of age;[25,30,62,63] they are rare, however, under the age of 5 years. Another proposal is that the plexiform lesions represent *sites of thrombosis that have subsequently recanalized*.[64,65] Recently, Wagenvoort[45] proposed that plexiform lesions represent sites of necrotizing arteritis and, therefore, *represent healing of a necrotizing inflammatory process*. The arteritis weakens the arterial wall which becomes focally aneurysmal. Fibrin and platelets are deposited in the aneurysm and organization of the resulting thrombus produces multiluminal channels lined by endothelial cells.

We believe that plexiform lesions may represent aneurysms formed at sites of *congenitally underdeveloped or weak media* (analogous to the formation of intracerebral berry aneurysms in systemic hypertension) and that the aneurysm is filled by thrombus, which organizes into multiple minute vascular channels. Distal to the weak or thin media, the lumen of the muscular artery is obliterated.

NECROPSY OBSERVATIONS OF PATIENTS OVER AGE 15 YEARS WITH CONGENITAL HEART DISEASE

To secure information on the lungs of adults with congenital cardiovascular anomalies, we reviewed clinical records accessioned in the Pathology Branch of the National Heart, Lung, and Blood Institute of the National Institutes of Health, often re-examining the heart itself and histologic sections of lung. All patients over age 15 with major anomalies of the heart and great vessels associated with a communication between pulmonary and systemic circulations were examined. A few cases were eliminated because histologic sections of lung were not available; a total of 87 patients was analyzed. At least five blocks of lung portions (all larger than 2 × 2 cm) had been processed in alcohol and xylene and embedded in paraffin from each patient. At least one section of lung from these paraffin blocks was stained by hematoxylin and eosin, and at least one additional section from each paraffin block was stained for elastic fibers by either Van Gieson or the Movat method. The status of the intrapulmonary pulmonary arteries was determined by histologic examination of each of the stained sections of lung, and the presence or absence of medial thickening, intimal thickening, plexiform lesions, and luminal thrombus was recorded. The presence and frequency of cholesterol-ester granulomas were also recorded.

OPERATED AND UNOPERATED PATIENTS

Certain clinical and morphologic observations in the 87 study patients are summarized in Tables 3 to 10, and Tables 13 to 15. The 87 patients ranged in age from 16 to 83 (mean 34); 47 (54%) were women and 40 (46%) were men. One or more cardiovascular operations had been performed in 65 patients (75%), and observations in this group are summarized in Table 3. The other 22 patients (25%) never had a cardiovascular operation, and observations in this group are summarized in Table 4. The 22 unoperated patients ranged in age from 16 to 33 (mean 36), and the 65 operated patients were between 16 and 64 years old (mean 33). In Tables 3 and 4, the patients are grouped by the type of congenital cardiovascular malformation present. Patients with multiple nonobligatory anomalies—those who presumably represent more than a single embryologic defect—are grouped together under the term "complex anomaly;" observations in them are summarized in Table 5.

PATIENTS WITH ABNORMAL PULMONARY ARTERIES

Medial thickening with or without intimal thickening or plexiform lesions was observed in the intrapulmonary pulmonary arteries by examination of lung sections of 44 (50%) of the 87 patients. The abnormalities consisted entirely of medial thick-

TABLE 3. Observations in 65 Necropsy Patients With Various Congenital Cardiovascular Malformations and One or More Cardiovascular Operations

MALFORMATION: SEX OF PATIENTS/ AGE RANGE/MEAN AGE	PA SYSTOLIC PRESSURE, mm Hg					SHUNTS			PULMONARY ARTERIAL CHANGES				
	<30	30–60	61–90	>90	U	L→R	R→L	BOTH	NONE	MT ONLY	MT + IT	PL	T
ASD													
Fossa ovale: 8F/43–64/61	1	4	2	1	0	8	0	0	4	1	3	0	4
Partial AV canal: 5F/21–54/38	1	3	0	0	1	4	0	1	2	1	2	0	2
Sinus venosus: 1M/37	1	0	0	0	0	1	0	0	1	0	0	0	0
VSD: 4F, 2M/16–54/29	0	1	4	1	0	4	1	1	1	2	2	1	2
Patent ductus arteriosus: 2F, 5M/16–44/30	0	0	1	6	0	5	2	0	0	0	1	6	1
VSD + PS (TOF): 5F, 10M/16–53/29	9	0	0	0	6	1	11	3	14	0	0	1	5
VSD + PV atresia: 1F/22	0	0	0	0	1	0	0	1	1	0	0	0	1
Complete transposition + VSD													
With PS: 3F/21–59/32	1	0	0	0	2	0	2	1	3	0	0	0	0
Without PS:0													
Corrected transposition + VSD: 1M/38	0	0	1	0	0	0	0	1	0	0	1	0	1
Double outlet right ventricle: 1F/24	0	1	0	0	0	1	0	0	0	0	1	0	0
Ebstein's anomaly + ASD: 1F, 1M/20–31/25	1	0	0	0	1	0	1	1	0	0	2	0	1
PS with intact VS + ASD: 3F/28–43/36	2	0	0	0	1	0	3	0	3	0	0	0	1
Tricuspid atresia: 1M/27	0	0	0	0	1	0	1	0	1	0	0	0	0
Parachute MV syndrome: 1F/24	0	0	0	1	0	1	0	0	0	0	1	0	0
Complex anomaly: 5F, 5M/16–39/27*	4	0	1	1	4	2	3	5	7	0	2	1	2
TOTALS: 39F, 26M/16–64/33	20	9	9	10	17	27	24	14	37	4	15	9	20

*See Table 5 for additional information on these cases.

ASD = atrial septal defect; AV = atrioventricular; F = female; IT = intimal thickening; L = left; M = male; MT = medial thickening; MV = mitral valve; PA = pulmonary artery; PL = plexiform lesions + MT + IT; PS = pulmonic stenosis; PV = pulmonic valve; R = right; T = thrombi; TOF = tetralogy of Fallot; U = unknown; VS = ventricular septum; VSD = ventricular septal defect.

From Virmani R, Roberts WC. Pulmonary arteries in congenital heart disease: A structure-function analysis. Cardiovasc Clin 1979; 10(1):462, with permission.

TABLE 4. Observations in 22 Unoperated Necropsy Patients With Various Congenital Cardiovascular Malformations*

MALFORMATION: SEX OF PATIENTS/AGE RANGE/MEAN AGE	PA SYSTOLIC PRESSURE, mm Hg					SHUNTS			PULMONARY ARTERIAL CHANGES				
	<30	30–60	61–90	>90	U	L→R	R→L	BOTH	NONE	MT ONLY	MT + IT	PL	T
ASD													
Fossa ovale: 5F, 2M/29–83/55	0	1	1	1	4	6	0	1	3	1	2	1	4
Partial AV canal: 0													
Sinus venosus: 1M/58	0	0	0	1†	0	1	0	0	0	0	1	0	1
VSD: 2M/16–37/27	1	0	0	0	1	2	0	0	1	0	1	0	0
PDA: 3F/17–34/21	0	0	0	2	1	0	1	2	0	1	0	2	1
VSD + PS (TOF): 1M/22	0	0	0	0	1	0	1	0	1	0	0	0	1
VSD + PV atresia: 1M/28	0	0	0	0	1	0	0	1	1	0	0	0	0
Complete transposition + VSD													
With PS: 0													
Without PS: 1F, 1M/21–39/30	0	0	0	0	2	1	0	1	0	0	2	0	1
Complex anomaly: 5M, / 20–41/26**	0	1	0	1	3	2	2	1	0	0	4	1	3
TOTALS: 9F, 13m/16–83/36	1	2	1	5	13	12	4	6	6	2	10	4	11

*Abbreviations listed in Table 3.

**See Table 5 for additional information on these cases.

†This patient died of carcinoma of the lung; some of this elevation probably is the result of the severe pulmonary cancer.

From Virmani R, Roberts WC. Pulmonary arteries in congenital heart disease:A structure-function analysis. Cardiovasc Clin 1979; 10(1):463, with permission.

TABLE 5. Observations in 15 Necropsy Patients With Complex Anomalies*

PATIENT AGE (YEARS)/SEX	MALFORMATION				PA PRESSURE mm Hg (s/d)	SA PRESSURE mm Hg (s/d)	SHUNT		SA O_2 SAT., %	OP	PULMONARY ARTERIAL CHANGES				
	PS	VSD	ASD	OTHER			L→R	R→L			NONE	MT ONLY	MT + IT	PL	T
WITHOUT RIGHT VENTRICULAR OUTFLOW OBSTRUCTION															
31/F	0	+	0	CS→LA	75 /25	130/75	+	0	81	+	0	0	+	0	+
39/M	0	+	0	COA	105/54	152/64	+	+	87	+	0	0	0	+	0
41/M	0	+	0	PDA + CT + IAA		120/70	0	+		0	0	0	0	+	0
21/M	0	+	0	DORV + CT	92 /48	104/64	+	0	90	0	0	0	+	0	0
21/M	0	+	0	DORV + CT		102/64	+	0	90	0	0	0	+	0	0
WITH RIGHT VENTRICULAR OUTFLOW OBSTRUCTION															
33/M	+	0	+	AS		80 /62	+	+	81	+	+	0	0	0	0
19/M	+	0	+	RPV→RA	18 /9	144/78	+	+	97	+	+	0	0	0	0
20/M	+	0	+	AV canal		180/100	0	+		0	0	0	+	0	+
25/F	+	+	+	AS		100/65	0	+	61	+	+	0	0	0	+
38/F	+	+	0	CT		125/48	0	+	62	+	0	0	+	0	0
17/M	+**	+	+	DORV, CT	20 /12	90 /60	+	0	93	+	+	0	0	0	0
22/F	+**	+	0	SV	15 /6	100/65	+	+	81	+	+	0	0	0	0
16/M	+**	+	0	SV + CT		100/75	+	+	51	+	+	0	0	0	0
25/M	+	0	+	TAPVC	55 /20	110/50	+	+	72	0	0	0	+	0	0
17/M	+**	0	+	TAPVC	20 /8	95 /60	0	+	92	+	+	0	0	0	+

*Last category in Tables 3 and 4.

**Subvalvular

AS = aortic stenosis; ASD = atrial septal defect; AV = atrioventricular; COA = coarctation of aorta; CS = coronary sinus; CT = corrected transposition; DORV = double outlet right ventricle; F = female; IT = intimal thickening; L = left; LA = left atrium; M = male; MT = medial thickening; OP = cardiovascular operation; PA = pulmonary artery; PDA = patent ductus arteriosus; PL = plexiform lesion + MT + IT; PS = pulmonic stenosis; R = right; RA = right atrium; RPV = right pulmonic vein; RV = right ventricle; SA = systemic artery; SAT. = saturation; s/d = systolic/diastolic; SV = single ventricle; T = thrombi; TAPVC = total anomalous pulmonary venous connection; VSD = ventricular septal defect.

From Virmani R, Roberts WC. Pulmonary arteries in congenital heart disease: A structure-function analysis. Cardiovasc Clin 1979; 10(1):464, with permission.

TABLE 6. Observations in 87 Necropsy Patients Over Age 15 With Congenital Cardiovascular Malformations

DIRECTION OF SHUNT	TOTALS	L→R	R→L	BOTH	L→R	R→L	BOTH	PULMONARY ARTERIAL CHANGES				
								NONE	MT ONLY	MT + IT	PL	T
No. Patients	87	3	22	11	36	6	9	43	6	25	13	31
RV Outflow Obst.		3	22	11	0	0	0					
PA systolic Pressure (mm Hg)												
≤30	21	2	9	5	3	0	2	20	0	1	0	5
31–60	11	0	0	1	9	0	1	5	1	5	0	2
61–90	10	1	0	0	8	0	1	1	3	6	0	5
>90	15	0	0	0	8	4	3	0	0	5	10	7
Unknown (U)	30	0	13	5	8	2	2	17	2	8	3	12
Morphologic changes in PAs												
None	43	3	19	10	10	0	1					
MI alone	6	0	0	0	6	0	0					
MT + IT	25	0	2	1	17	1	4					
PL	13	0	1	0	3	5	4					
Thrombi	31	1	8	2	13	2	5					

IT = intimal thickening; L = left; MT = medial thickening; obst = obstruction; PA = pulmonary artery; PL = plexiform lesions + MT + IT; R = right; RV = right ventricle; T = thrombi

From Virmani R, Roberts WC. Pulmonary arteries in congenital heart disease: A structure-function analysis. Cardiovasc Clin 1979; 10(1):466, with permission.

TABLE 7. Observations in 36 Necropsy Patients Over Age 15 With Right Ventricular Outflow or Inflow Obstruction

MALFORMATION: SEX OF PATIENTS/AGE RANGE/MEAN AGE	PA SYSTOLIC PRESSURES (mm Hg)						SA O_2 SAT. (%)	PULMONARY ARTERIAL CHANGES						
	<30	31–60	61–90	>90	U	OP		NONE	H	IT ONLY	MT ONLY	MT + IT	ARL	T
LEFT-TO-RIGHT SHUNT ONLY														
VSD + PS(TOF):1M/22	1	0	0	0	0	1	92	1	0	0	0	0	0	1
VSD + RVOTO: 1F/25	0	0	1	0	0	1	91	1	0	0	0	0	0	0
Complex anomaly: 1M/17	1	0	0	0	0	1	93	0	1	0	0	0	0	0
RIGHT-TO-LEFT SHUNT ONLY														
VSD + PS(TOF): 5F, 7M/17–36/27	5	0	0	0	7	11	9(82)	2	7	6	0	1(PL)	5	5
CT + PS + VSD + DORV: 1F/55	1	0	0	0	0	1		0	1	1	0	0	0	0
CT + PS + VSD + ASD: 1M/21	0	0	0	0	1	1		0	1	1	0	0	0	0
TVA + ASD: 1M/27	0	0	0	0	1	1	83	0	0	1	0	0	0	0
PS + IVS + ASD: 3F/28–43/36	2	0	0	0	1	3	2(75)	1	3	1	0	0	0	1
Complex anomaly: 2F, 2M/17–38/34	1	0	0	0	3	3	3(72)	1	1	2	0	2	0	3
BOTH LEFT-TO-RIGHT AND RIGHT-TO-LEFT SHUNTS														
VSD + PS(TOF): 3M/16–53/37	3	0	0	0	0	3	3(81)	0	1	2	0	0	2	0
VSD + PVA: 1F, 1M/22–28/25	0	0	0	0	2	1	2(67)	0	0	2	0	0	1	1
CT + VSD + PS: 1M/21	0	0	0	0	1	1	71	0	0	1	0	0	1	1
Complex anomaly: 1F, 4M/16–33/23	2	1	0	0	2	4	4(83)	1	1	2	0	1	0	0

ARL = Arnold Rich lesions; ASD = atrial septal defect; CT = corrected transpositon; DORV = double outlet right ventricle; F = female; H = hypoplastic; IT = intimal thickening; M = male; MT = medial thickening; OP = cardiovascular operation; PA = pulmonary artery; PL = plexiform lesions + MT and IT; PS = pulmonic stenosis; PVA = pulmonic valve atresia; RVTO = right ventricular outflow tract obstruction; SA = systemic artery; SAT. = saturation; T = thrombus; TOF = tetralogy of Fallot; TVA = tricuspid valve atresia; U = unknown; IVS = intact ventricular septum; VSD = ventricular septal defect.

From Virmani R, Roberts WC. Pulmonary arteries in congenital heart disease: A structure-function analysis. Cardiovasc Clin 1979 10(1):467, with permission.

TABLE 8. Clinical and Morphologic Observations in 36 Necropsy Patients Over Age 15 With CHD, L-R Shunts, and No Right Ventricular Outflow or Inflow Obstruction

MALFORMATION SEX OF PATIENTS/AGE RANGE/ MEAN AGE	PA SYSTOLIC PRESSURE (mm Hg)						PULMONARY ARTERIAL CHANGES				
	<30	31–60	61–90	>90	U	OP	NONE	MT ONLY	MT + IT	PL	T
ASD											
Fossa ovale: 13F, 1M/43–83/57	1	5	3	1	4	8	7	2	5	0	7
Partial AV canal: 4M/21–54/39	0	3	0	0	1	4	1	1	2	0	2
Sinus venosus: 2M/37–58/48	1	0	0	1	0	1	1	0	1	0	1
VSD: 2F, 3M/16–54/28	1	0	3	0	1	4	1	2	2	0	1
PDA: 1F, 4M/16–44/28	0	0	1	4	0	5	0	1	1	3	0
Complete transposition with VSD: 1F/39	0	0	0	0	1	0	0	0	1	0	0
DORV: 1F/24	0	1	0	0	0	1	0	0	1	0	0
Parachute MV syndromes: 1F/24	0	0	0	1	0	1	0	0	1	0	0
Complex anomaly: 1F, 2M/21–31/26	0	0	1	1	1	1	0	0	3	0	2
TOTALS: 20F, 16M/16–83/42	3	9	8	8	8	27	10	6	17	3	13

Abbreviations as in Tables 3, 5, and 6.

From Virmani R, Roberts WC. Pulmonary arteries in congenital heart disease: A structure-function analysis. Cardiovasc Clin 1979 10(1):468, with permission.

TABLE 9. Clinical and Morphologic Observations in 15 Necropsy Patients Over Age 15 With CHD and R-L Shunts Only or Both R-L and L-R Shunts, Without Right Ventricular Outflow or Inflow Obstruction

	F	M	ASD	VSD	PDA	OTHER	PA SYSTOLIC PRESSURE mm Hg	OP	PA LESIONS
						RIGHT-TO-LEFT SHUNT ONLY			
17	+	0	0	0	+	0	120	0	PL,T
20	+	0	+	0	0	Ebstein's + LSVC	U	+	MT + IT
25	+	0	0	+	0	0	98	+	PL
33	0	+	0	+	+	0	106	+	PL,T
40	+	0	0	0	+	0	132	+	PL
41	0	+	0	+	+	IAA + CT	U	0	PL
						BOTH RIGHT-TO-LEFT AND LEFT-TO-RIGHT SHUNTS			
16	+	0	0	+	0	0	60	+	MT + IT,T
21	+	0	0	+	+	0	138	0	PL,T
21	0	+	+	+	0	Comp T	U	0	MT + IT
24	+	0	0	0	+	0	U	0	PL
29	+	0	+	0	0	0	110	0	PL,T
31	0	+	+	0	0	Ebstein's	22	+	MT + IT,T
38	0	+	0	+	0	CT	83	+	MT + IT,T
39	0	+	0	+	0	COA	108	+	PL
40	+	0	+	0	0	TAPVC	20	+	O

Abbreviations as in Table 5 and 6; EA = Ebstein's anomaly.

From Virmani R, Roberts WC. Pulmonary arteries in congenital heart disease: A structure-function analysis. Cardiovasc Clin 1979; 10(1):470, with permission.

ening in 6 patients (14%), medial and intimal thickening in 25 patients (57%), and medial and intimal thickening with plexiform lesions in 13 patients (29%). In addition, fibrin or fibrin–platelet thrombi were observed in the lumen of one or more small pulmonary arteries in 31 patients: 12 (39%) had neither medial nor intimal thickening, nor plexiform lesions; one or more of these three lesions were present in 19 (61%).

PULMONARY ARTERIAL SYSTOLIC PRESSURE AND SHUNT DIRECTION

Of the 57 patients in whom pulmonary arterial pressures were recorded, the systolic pressure was ≤ 30 mm Hg in 21 (37%); 30 to 60 mm Hg in 11 (19%); 61 to 90 mm Hg in 10 (18%); and > 90 mm Hg in 15 (26%). All 87 patients had one or more communications between systemic and pulmonary circulations and were comprised as follows: (1) 39 patients with left-to-right shunt only (Tables 6 through 8); (2) 28 patients with right-to-left shunts (Tables 6, 7, and 9); and (3) 20 patients with both left-to-right and right-to-left shunts (Tables 6, 7, and 9). Right ventricular outflow obstruction occurred in 36 (41%) of the 87 patients, including 18 of the 57 patients in whom pulmonary arterial systolic pressures were recorded. Pulmonary arterial systolic pressures were ≤ 30 mm Hg in 5 (13%) of the 39 patients without right ventricular outflow obstruction, and in 16 (89%) of the 18 patients with obstruction. Conversely, the pulmonary arterial systolic pressure was elevated to (> 30 mm Hg) in 34 (87%) of 39 patients without right ventricular outflow obstruction and in 2 (11%) of the 18 patients with obstruction (Tables 6, 8, and 9).

ANATOMIC FEATURES OF THE PULMONARY VESSELS

Figures 4 to 14 illustrate some of the anatomic features observed in the pulmonary vessels of the study patients.

Left-to-Right Shunts

Of these 39 patients, the pulmonary arterial pressure had been recorded in 31: 4 patients (13%) had only medial thickening; 13 patients (42%) had medial and intimal thickening; 3 patients (10%) had medial and intimal thickening with plexiform lesions; and 11 patients (35%) had none of these changes. The pulmonary arterial

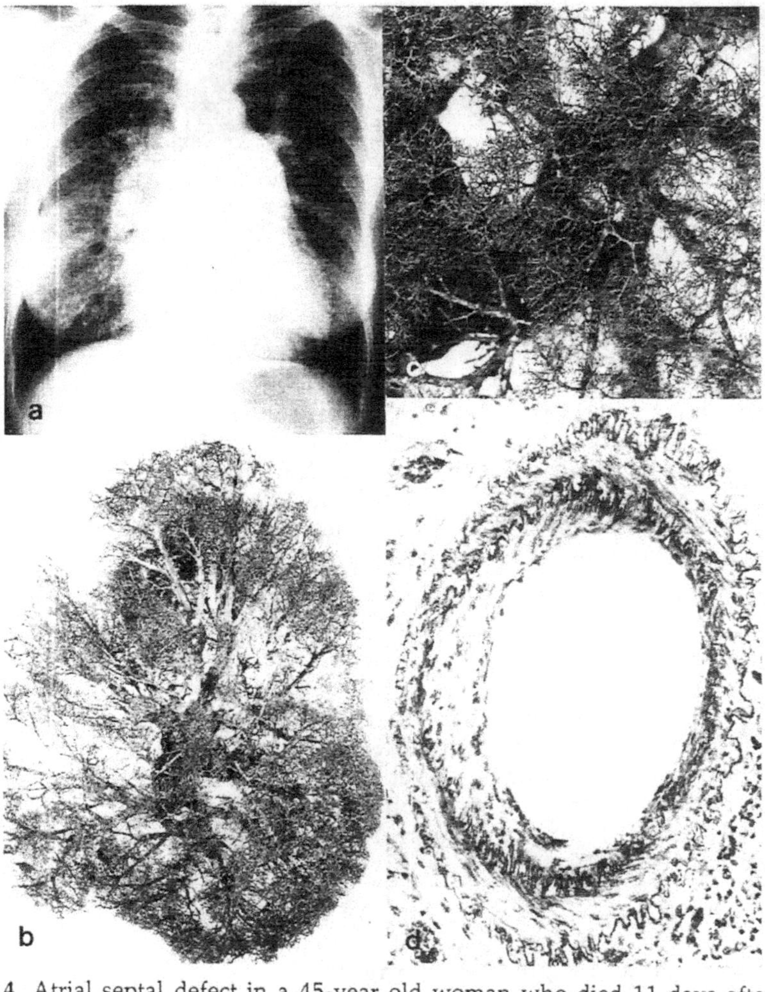

FIGURE 4. Atrial septal defect in a 45-year old woman who died 11 days after operative closure. Preoperative pulmonary arterial pressure was 40/14 mm Hg; left-to-right shunt was [illegible] to 1; and pulmonary to systemic resistance was 0.17 to 1. *a*, Radiograph immediately before operation. *b*, Mold of pulmonary arteries in one lung. *c*, Close-up of wide-open arteries. *d*, Typical muscular pulmonary artery showing mild medial and intimal thickening. (Movat stain. × 252; reduced 30%.) From Virmani R, Roberts WC. Pulmonary arteries in congenital heart disease: A structure-function analysis. Cardiovasc Clin 1979; 10(1):469, with permission.

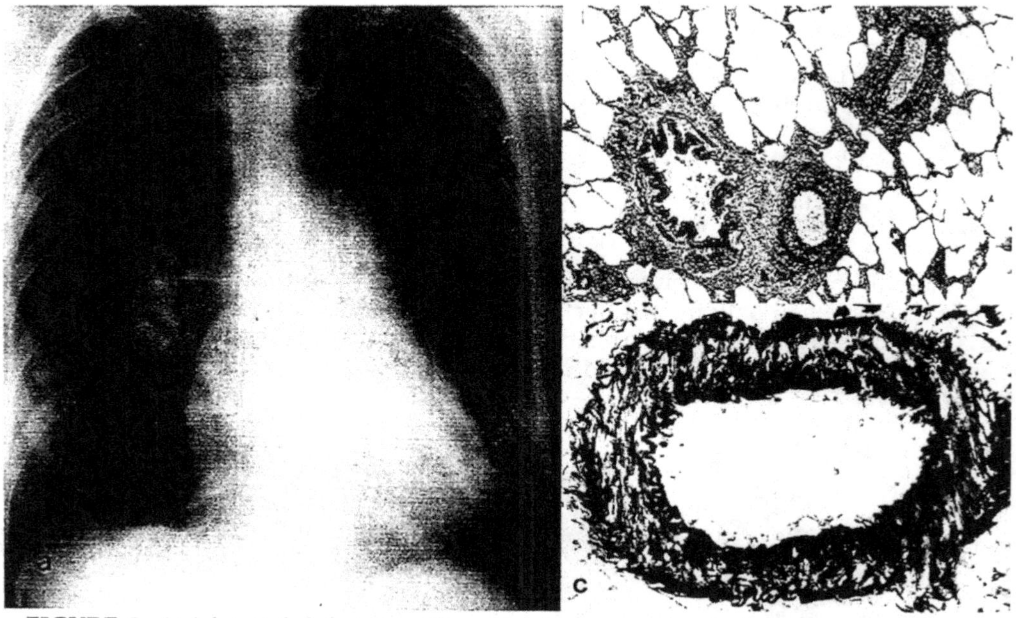

FIGURE 5. Atrial septal defect in a 50-year-old woman who died 11 days after operative closure of the defect. Preoperative pulmonary arterial pressure was 95/30 mm Hg; the shunt was entirely left-to-right. *a*, Radiograph immediately before operation. *b*, Two muscular pulmonary arteries with thickened media (× 60). *c*, Close-up (× 330) of one of the two muscular pulmonary arteries shown in *b*. (Movat stains; reduced 30%.) From Virmani R, Roberts WC. Pulmonary arteries in congenital heart disease: A structure-function analysis. Cardiovasc Clin. 1979; 10(1):470, with permission.

systolic pressures in the 11 patients ranged from 10 to 63 mm Hg (mean 36 mm Hg): in 5 it was ≤ 30 mm Hg. In the 4 patients with medial thickening only, this pressure ranged from 58 to 80 mm Hg (mean 70 mm Hg). In the 13 patients with medial and intimal thickening, pressures ranged from 37 to 118 mm Hg (mean 81 mm Hg). In the 3 patients with plexiform lesions, pulmonary arterial systolic pressure was 120 mm Hg in 2 and 136 mm Hg in the other.

Right-to-Left Shunts

Of these 13 patients, 9 had pulmonary arterial systolic pressures ≤ 30 mm Hg (mean 15 mm Hg) from right ventricular outflow obstruction, and none of them had morphologic changes in the pulmonary arteries. The 4 other patients who had no right ventricular outflow obstruction had pulmonary arterial systolic pressures ranging from 98 to 132 mm Hg (mean 114 mm Hg), and all had plexiform lesions in the pulmonary arteries.

Both Left-to-Right and Right-to-Left Shunts

Of these 13 patients, 6 had right ventricular outflow obstruction and 7 did not. There were no morphologic changes in the pulmonary arteries in 6 patients whose pressures ranged from 15 to 20 mm Hg (mean 15 mm Hg); 4 had medial and intimal thickening and their pressures ranged from 22 to 83 mm Hg (mean 55 mm Hg). The 3 patients with plexiform lesions had pressures of 108, 110, and 138 mm Hg.

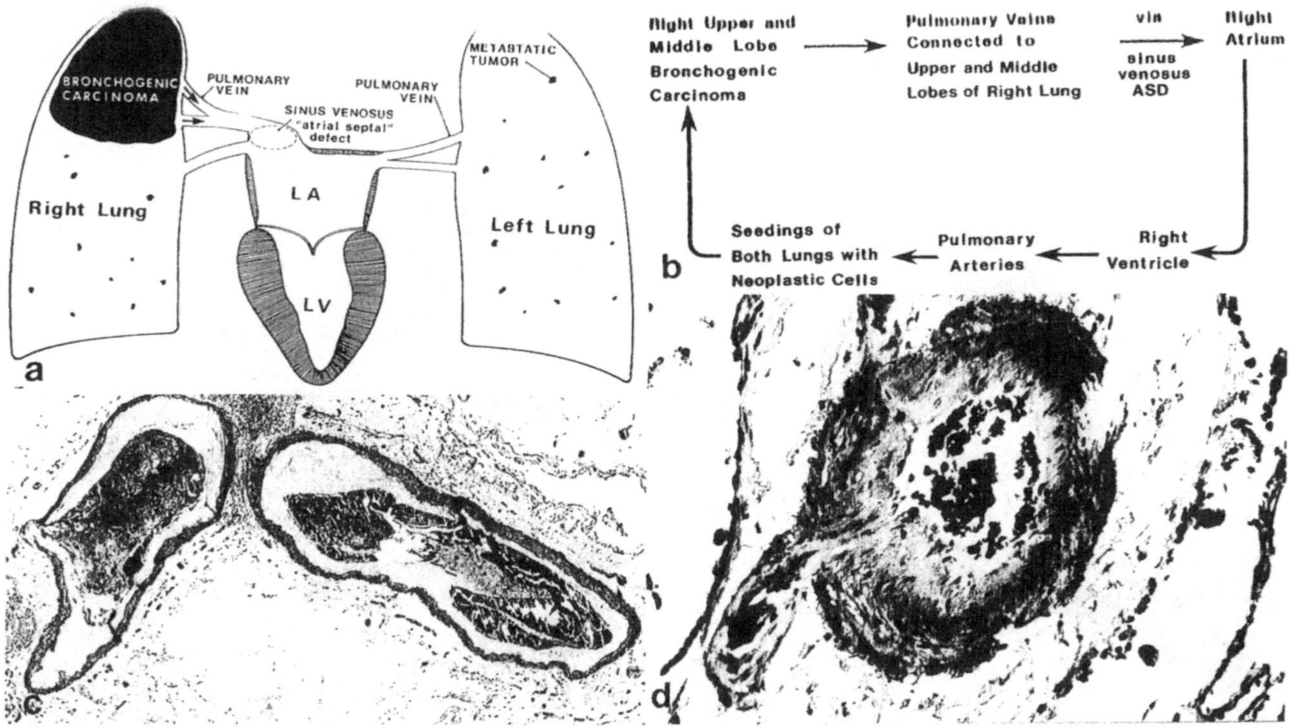

FIGURE 6. Sinus venosus–type atrial septal defect with anomalous pulmonary venous return from the right lung associated with bronchogenic carcinoma in a 58-year-old man. Three years before he died, his pulmonary arterial pressure was 100/22 mm Hg and left-to-right shunt was 1.5 to 1. *a*, Diagram of the heart and lungs. LA = left atrium; LV = left ventricle. *b*, Path of metastatic spread of the tumor in both lungs. *c*, Large pulmonary arteries with thickened intima and antemortem blood clot (× 85). *d*, Typical muscular artery and branching arteriole with thickened media and intima (× 200). (Movat stains; reduced 12%.) From Virmani R, Roberts WC. Pulmonary arteries in congenital heart disease: A structure-function analysis. Cardiovasc Clin 1979; 10(1):471, with permission.

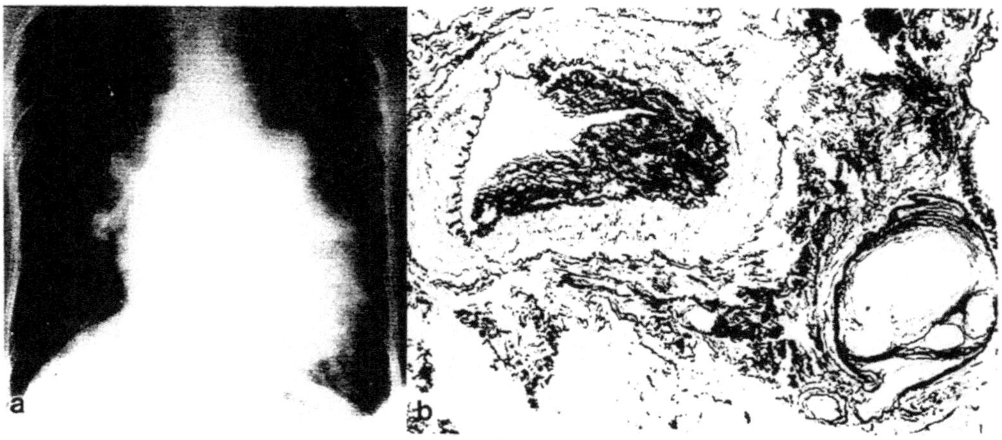

FIGURE 7. Patent ductus arteriosus in a 36-year-old man who died during attempted closure of the calcified ductus. Preoperative pulmonary arterial pressure (136/96 mm Hg). The shunt was entirely left to right. *a*, Radiograph immediately before operation. *b*, Muscular pulmonary artery showing marked medial and intimal thickening and a plexiform lesion. (Elastic Van Gieson stain; × 220; reduced 30%.) From Virmani R, Roberts WC. Pulmonary arteries in congenital cardiac disease: A structure-function analysis. Cardiovasc Clin 1979; 10(1):472, with permission.

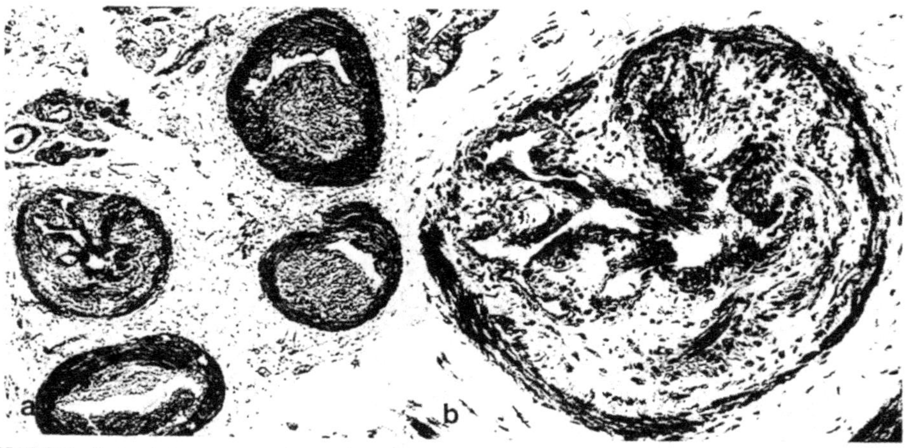

FIGURE 8. Patent ductus arteriosus in a 40-year-old woman who died during attempted operative closure. Simultaneous pulmonary arterial and femoral arterial pressures were 110/58 (mean 80) and 128/46 mm Hg (mean 80), respectively. The shunt was right-to-left, femoral arterial oxygen saturation was 70 percent, and blood hematocrit was 46 percent. *a*, Muscular pulmonary arteries wtih thickened media and intima and narrowed lumens (× 80). *b*, Plexiform lesions (× 240). (Movat stains; reduced 30%.) From Virmani R, Roberts WC. Pulmonary arteries in congenital heart disease: A structure-function analysis. Cardiovasc Clin 1979; 10(1):472, with permission.

FIGURE 10. Combined patent ductus arteriosus and ventricular septal defect in a 21-year-old woman who died soon after catheterization. The pulmonary and systemic arterial pressures were both 138/86 mm Hg (mean 107). The shunt through the ductus was mainly right-to-left, and the shunt through the ventricular septal defect was minute. Oxygen saturation was 89 percent in the brachial artery and 75 percent in the femoral artery; blood hematocrit was 66 percent. *a*, Chest radiograph. *b*, Intrapulmonary elastic artery (× 27). *c*, Plexiform lesion (× 225). (Hematoxylin and eosin stains; reduced 40%). From Virmani R, Roberts WC. Pulmonary arteries in congenital heart disease: A structure-function analysis. Cardiovasc Clin 1979; 10(1):473, with permission.

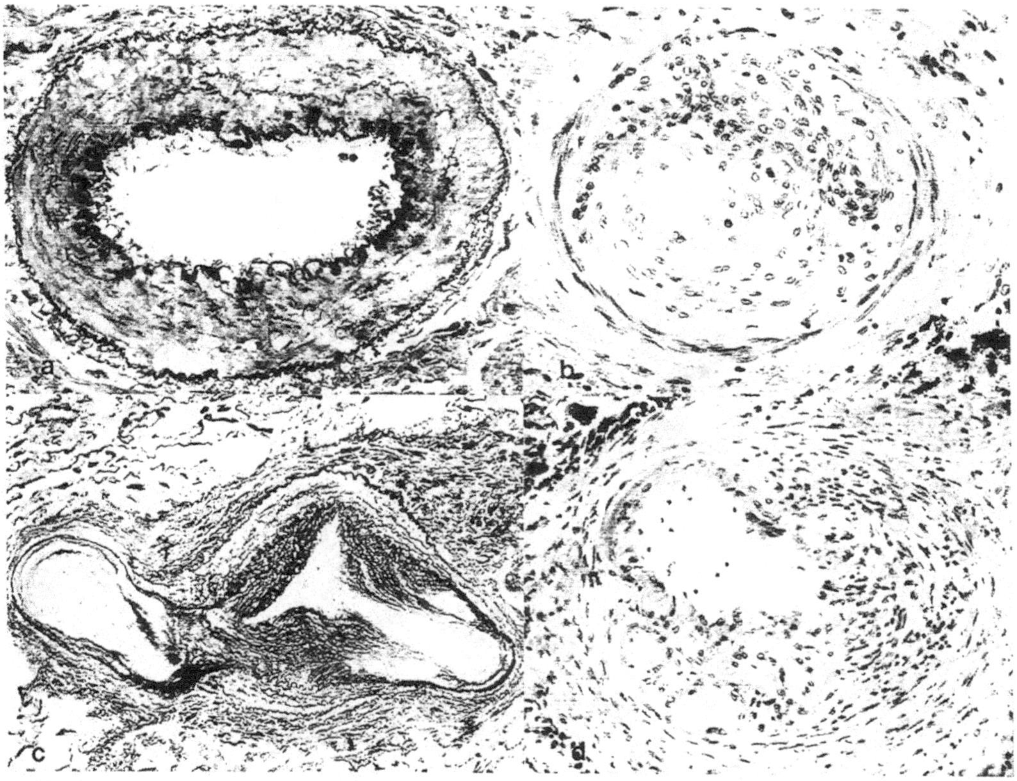

FIGURE 9. Combined patent ductus arteriosus and discrete subaortic stenosis in a 17-year-old boy. Peak systolic pressure gradient between left ventricle and brachial artery was 78 mm Hg. Pulmonary arterial pressure was 128/70 mm Hg, and the shunt was entirely left-to-right. Muscular pulmonary arteries (*a* through *d*) show severe medial hypertrophy and luminal narrowing by intimal thickening. *c, d,* Plexiform lesions. (Elastic Van Gieson stains: × 255 (*a*) and × 65 (*c*); hematoxylin and eosin stains: × 375 (*b*) and × 240 (*d*); reduced 34%.) From Virmani R, Roberts WC. Pulmonary arteries in congenital heart disease: A structure-function analysis. Cardiovasc Clin 1979 10(1):473, with permission.

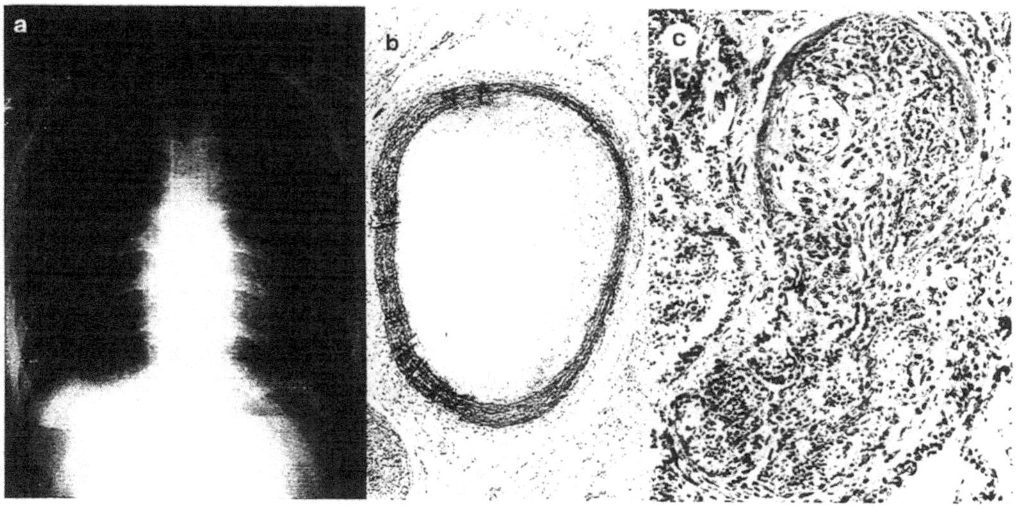

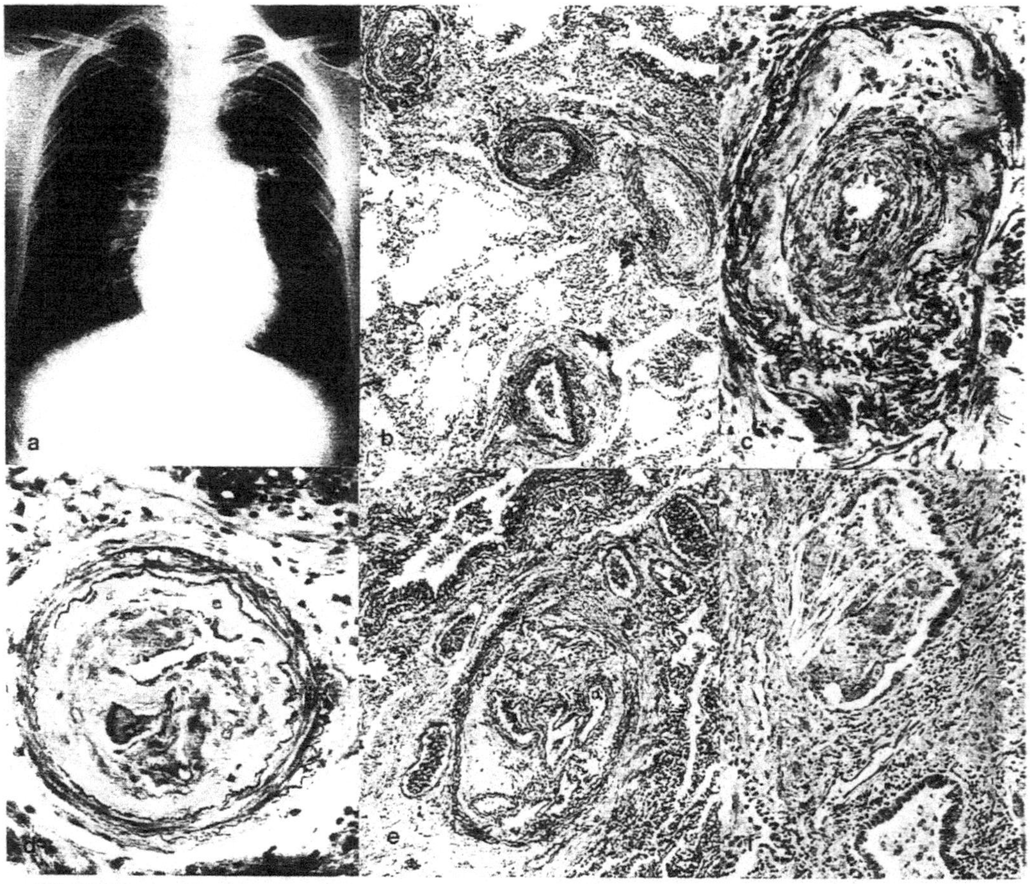

FIGURE 11. Combined patent ductus arteriosus and ventricular septal defect in a 33-year-old man who died during attempted operative closure of the ductus. Simultaneous pulmonary and femoral arterial pressures were 106/64 and 132/52 mm Hg, respectively. The femoral and brachial arterial oxygen saturations were 69 and 80%, respectively. Blood hematocrit was 54%, but severe iron deficiency anemia was present. The shunt at the ductus was primarily right-to-left, and no shunt was detected at the ventricular level. *a*, Chest radiograph immediately before operation. *b, c, d*, Severe medial and intimal thickening with luminal narrowing (× 95, × 380, × 385, respectively.) *e*, Plexiform lesions (× 130). *f*, Cholesterol-ester granuloma (× 160). (Movat stains: *b, c, d, e*; hematoxylin and eosin stain: *f*; reduced 42%.) From Virmani R, Roberts WC. Pulmonary arteries in congenital heart disease: A structure-function analysis. Cardiovasc Clin 1979; 10(1):474, with permission.

MORPHOLOGIC CHANGES IN THE PULMONARY ARTERIES: THE EFFECTS OF PULMONARY ARTERIAL SYSTOLIC PRESSURE, DIRECTION AND LOCATION OF SHUNT, AND PATIENT AGE

The observations described above and presented in detail in Tables 3 through 10 and 13 to 15 indicate that the crucial determinant of anatomic change in the muscular pulmonary arteries of patients over age 15 with congenital cardiac disease is the *level of the pulmonary arterial pressure*. These observations in our 57 necropsy patients in whom pulmonary arterial pressures were recorded are summarized in Figure 15. Of the 26 patients without morphologic pulmonary arterial changes, the average pulmonary arterial systolic pressure was 25 mm Hg (range 9 to 63 mm Hg), and only 6

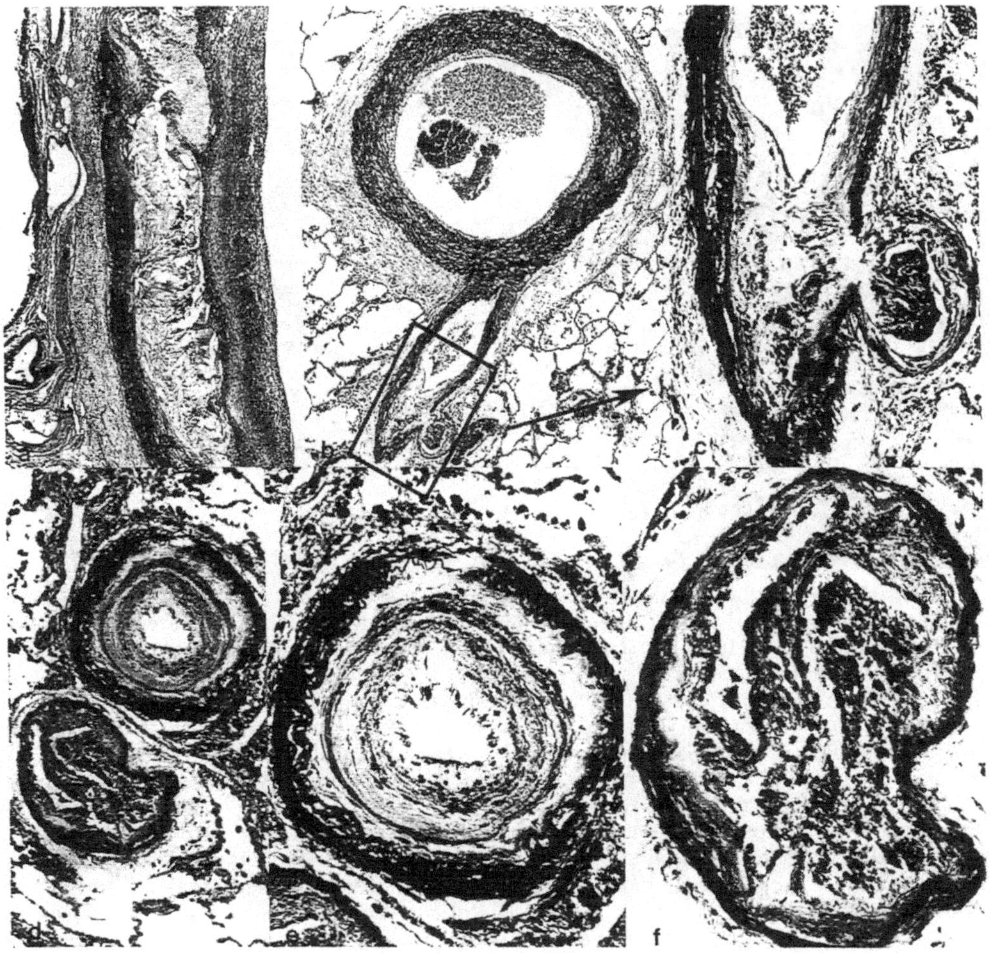

FIGURE 12. Combined ventricular septal defect and coarctation of aorta in a 39-year-old man who died 24 hours after operative closure of the defect. Simultaneous pulmonary arterial and aortic pressures were 131/76 (mean 93) and 144/84 (mean 100) mm Hg, respectively. Left brachial arterial oxygen saturation was 87%, blood hematocrit was 54%, and the shunt was bidirectional, but predominantly left-to-right. The pulmonary arteries had thick media, thick intima, narrowed lumens, and plexiform lesions. *a*, Intrapulmonary elastic artery (media stains black), with a huge atherosclerotic plaque (× 40). *b*, Large pulmonary artery with a muscular branch which has an obliterated lumen (× 60). *c*, Close-up of the area in brackets shown in *b* (× 155). This is a plexiform lesion. *d*, Muscular pulmonary artery (× 130). *e*, Close-up of artery shown in *d* (× 248). *f*, Close-up of plexiform lesion shown in *d* (× 330). (Movat stains; reduced 40%.) From Virmani R, Roberts WC. Pulmonary arteries in congenital heart disease: A structure-function analysis. Cardiovasc Clin 1979; 10(1):475, with permission.

patients had pressures > 30 mm Hg. In contrast, of the 10 patients with plexiform lesions, the average pulmonary arterial systolic pressure was 119 mm Hg (range 98 to 138 mm Hg; $p < .01$). The 21 patients with medial thickening only or medial and intimal thickening had similar average pulmonary arterial systolic pressures (70 and 75 mm Hg, respectively). The average pulmonary arterial systolic pressure in the patients with medial thickening with or without intimal thickening was significantly ($p < .01$) different than the pressures of patients without morphologic pulmonary arterial changes and patients with plexiform lesions (see Fig. 15).

The *direction of the intravascular shunt* appeared to have only indirect effect on the pulmonary arteries. As shown in Figures 15 through 17, 15 of the 26 patients

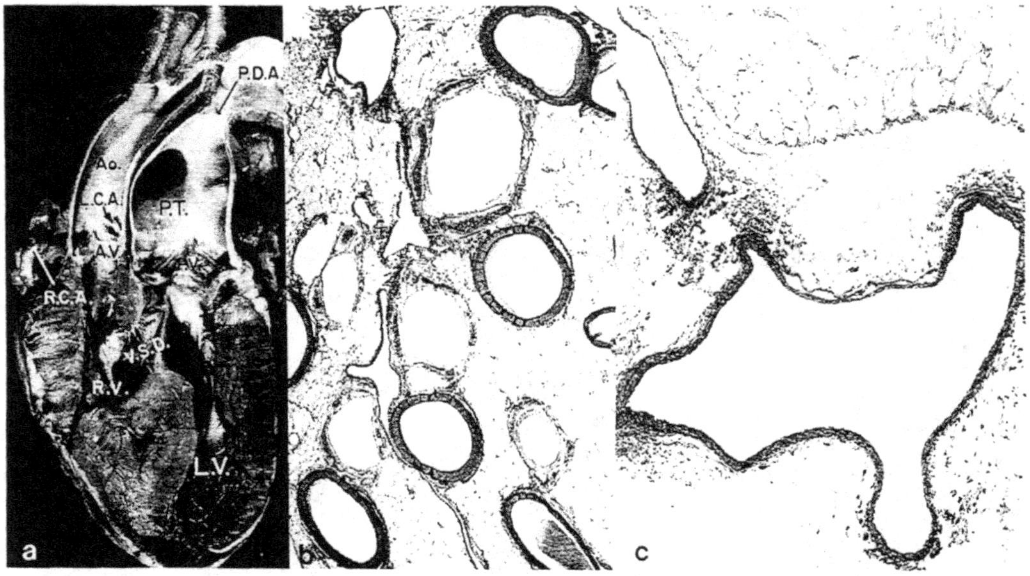

FIGURE 13. Ventricular septal defect and patent ductus arteriosus associated with the Taussig-Bing malformation in a 39-year-old woman described in detail elsewhere.[56] Pulmonary arterial pressure was 91/58 mm Hg; brachial arterial pressure, 93/56 mm Hg. Blood hematocrit was 75%; systemic arterial oxygen saturation, 47%. *a*, Longitudinal view of heart showing the pulmonary trunk (P.T.) and pulmonic valve (P.V.) overriding a large ventricular septal defect (V.S.D.). The aorta (A) arises anteriorly and from the right ventricle (R.V.). The patent ductus arteriosus (P.D.A.) Is large. L.V. = left ventricle; L.C.A. = ostium of left coronary artery; R.C.A. = right coronary artery. *b*, Greatly dilated pulmonary arteries near hilum of 1 lung (× 5). Media is thickened but intima is normal or only minimally thickened. The pulmonary arteries in this patient were everywhere wide open and dilated. *c*, Dilated pulmonary veins (× 40). Despite the balanced pulmonary and systemic arterial pressures maintained over many years, the anatomic pulmonary arterial changes were mild. (Elastic Van Gieson and Movat stains; reduced 33%). From Virmani R, Roberts WC. Pulmonary arteries in congenital heart disease: A structure-function analysis. Cardiovasc Clin 1979; 10(1):476, with permission.

without structural pulmonary arterial abnormalities (average pulmonary arterial systolic pressure = 15 mm Hg) had right-to-left or bidirectional shunts, and 7 of the 10 patients with plexiform lesions (average pulmonary arterial systolic pressure = 116 mm Hg) (see Fig. 16) also had right-to-left or bidirectional shunts. Thus, the pressure and not the direction of the shunt determines anatomic pulmonary arterial changes in these patients. As shown in Figure 17, patients with left-to-right shunts only also had all degrees of anatomic change in the muscular pulmonary arteries, again demonstrating that structural changes in these patients depend on the pulmonary arterial pressure.

The anatomic changes in the muscular pulmonary arteries were only secondarily dependent on the *location of the shunt* in the heart or great arteries. Among our 40 patients with isolated artrial septal defect or ventricular septal defect or patent ductus arteriosus (see Tables 3 and 4), 33 had pulmonary arterial pressures recorded at catheterization. As shown in Figures 18 and 19, the anatomic changes in the muscular pulmonary arteries in these 33 patients depended not on the location of the shunt but on the pressure in the pulmonary artery. Of course, the location of the communication played a major role in determining the pulmonary arterial pressure. Thus, the average pulmonary arterial systolic pressure in our patients was highest (118 mm Hg) (see Fig. 18) in the 9 patients with patent ductus arteriosus, lowest (58 mm Hg) in the 17 patients with atrial septal defect, and intermediate (68 mm Hg) in the 7 patients with isolated ventricular septal defect. Surprisingly, no significant difference in average pulmonary arterial systolic pressure was observed between the

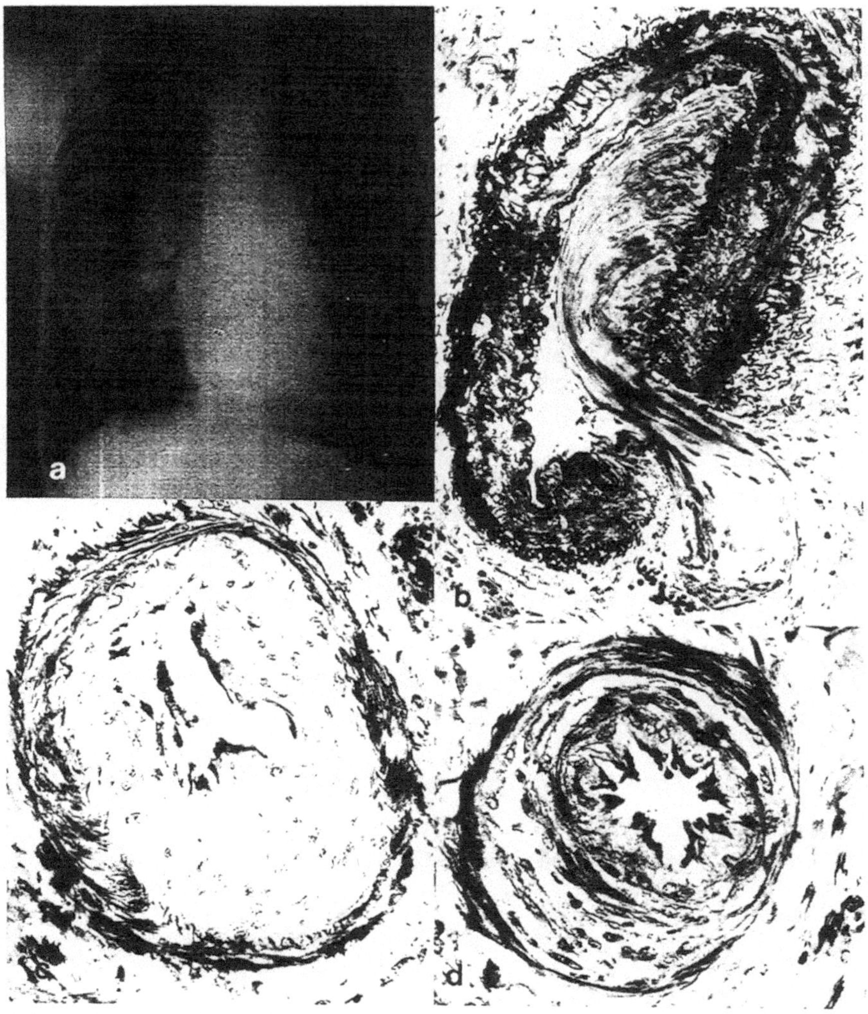

FIGURE 14. Congenital mitral stenosis, ventricular aseptal defect, patent ductus arteriosus, and coarctation of aorta in a 25-year-old asymptomatic woman.[87] Pulmonary arterial pressure was 104/60 mm Hg (mean 82); left ventricular pressure, 122/4 mm Hg. Left atrial to left ventricular end-diastolic gradient was 20 mm Hg and cardiac output was normal. *a*, Preoperative chest radiograph. A mitral commissurotomy was performed, but considerable mitral regurgitation resulted; the ventricular septal defect was closed by direct suture, and an unsuspected ductus was ligated. The patient died 20 hours after operation. *b* (× 220), *c* (× 330), *d* (× 435), Pulmonary arteries show severe intimal and medial thickening with luminal narrowing, and pulmonary venous and alveolar septal lesions are typical of mitral stenosis.[88–91] (Movat stains; reduced 25%.) From Virmani R, Roberts WC. Pulmonary arteries in congenital heart disease: A structure-function analysis. Cardiovasc Clin 1979; 10(1):477, with permission.

17 patients with isolated atrial septal defect and the 7 patients with isolated ventricular septal defect (see Fig. 18). The average pulmonary arterial systolic pressure in the 9 patients with isolated patent ductus arteriosus was nearly twice that of the patients with either atrial septal defect or ventricular septal defect, and this difference was highly significant ($p < .001$).

Plexiform lesions were observed in 1 of the 17 patients with atrial septal defect, and 1 of the 7 with ventricular septal defect, and in 7 of the 9 with patent ductus arteriosus. All 9 patients with plexiform lesions had pulmonary arterial systolic pressures > 90 mm Hg.

TABLE 10. Observations in 18 Necropsy Patients Over Age 15 With CHD, Pulmonary Arterial Systolic Pressures >90 mm Hg, and No Right Ventricular Outflow or Inflow Obstruction

PATIENT AGE, SEX MALFORMATION	PA PRESSURE (mm Hg, s/d)	SA PRESSURE (mm Hg, s/d)	SHUNT	SA O_2 SAT. (%)	CARDIAC OPERATION	INTERVAL (DAYS) OP TO DEATH
WITH PLEXIFORM LESIONS						
29 F/ASD, RPV→SVC	110/60	110/60	both		none	
25 F/VSD	98/62	104/66	R-L	88	VSD closed	1
33 M/VSD, PDA	106/64	136/68	R-L	61	PDA closed	0
21 F/VSD, PDA	138/86	140/88	both	89	none	
39 M/VSD, COA	108/54	152/64	both	87	VSD closed	1
41 M/VSD, PDA, IAA + CT		120/70	none	*	none	
40 F/PDA	132/64	128/68	R-L	70	PDA closed	0
24 F/PDA		128/70	none	*	none	
28 M/PDA	120/60	120/60	L-R	96	PDA closed	1
17 F/PDA	120/65	110/60	R-L	*	none	
36 M/PDA	136/96	136/96	L-R	95	PDA closed	0
17 M/PDA, SS	120/65	122/65	L-R	97	PDA closed; SS resectioned	1
19 F/TOF	105/—	108/78	R-L	70	right PA-DA anastomosis	14 yrs.
WITHOUT PLEXIFORM LESIONS						
50 F/ASD	95/30	105/80	L-R	96	ASD closed	11
58 M/ASD	100/22	140/90	L-R		none	
44 F/PDA	118/52	150/70	L-R	92**	PDA closed	7
24 F/VSD, PDA, MS + COA	104/60	118/70	L-R		PDA and VSD closed; MVC	1
21 M/VSD DORV + CT	92/48	102/64	L-R	90	none	0

*Central cyanosis present.

**Right brachial artery; 89 percent in femoral artery.

Abbreviations as in Tables 5 and 6; DA = descending aorta; IAA = interrupted aortic arch; MVC = mitral valve commissurotomy; MS = mitral stenosis; SS = subaortic stenosis; SVC = superior vena cava.

From Virmani R, Roberts WC. Pulmonary arteries in congenital heart disease: A structure-function analysis. Cardiovasc Clin 1979 10(1):486, with permission.

Age was not an important determinant of anatomic changes in the muscular pulmonary arteries (Fig. 20). Among the 40 patients with isolated atrial septal defect or ventricular septal defect or patent ductus arteriosus, the group with atrial septal defect was oldest (mean 51 years), and yet they had the least severe pulmonary arterial anatomic changes. Furthermore, the patients with ventricular septal defect and patent ductus arteriosus were younger and had the same mean age (28 years); yet the anatomic pulmonary arterial changes were far worse among the patients with patent ductus arteriosus ($p < .001$). The lack of severe morphologic pulmonary arterial changes in the patients with atrial septal defect appears to explain the much longer survival among these patients than among those with either isolated ventricular septal defect or patent ductus arteriosus (see Fig. 20).

OBSERVATIONS OF OTHER INVESTIGATORS

Although several investigators have described previously the effect of pressure, direction and location of shunt, and age on the anatomic changes in the pulmonary

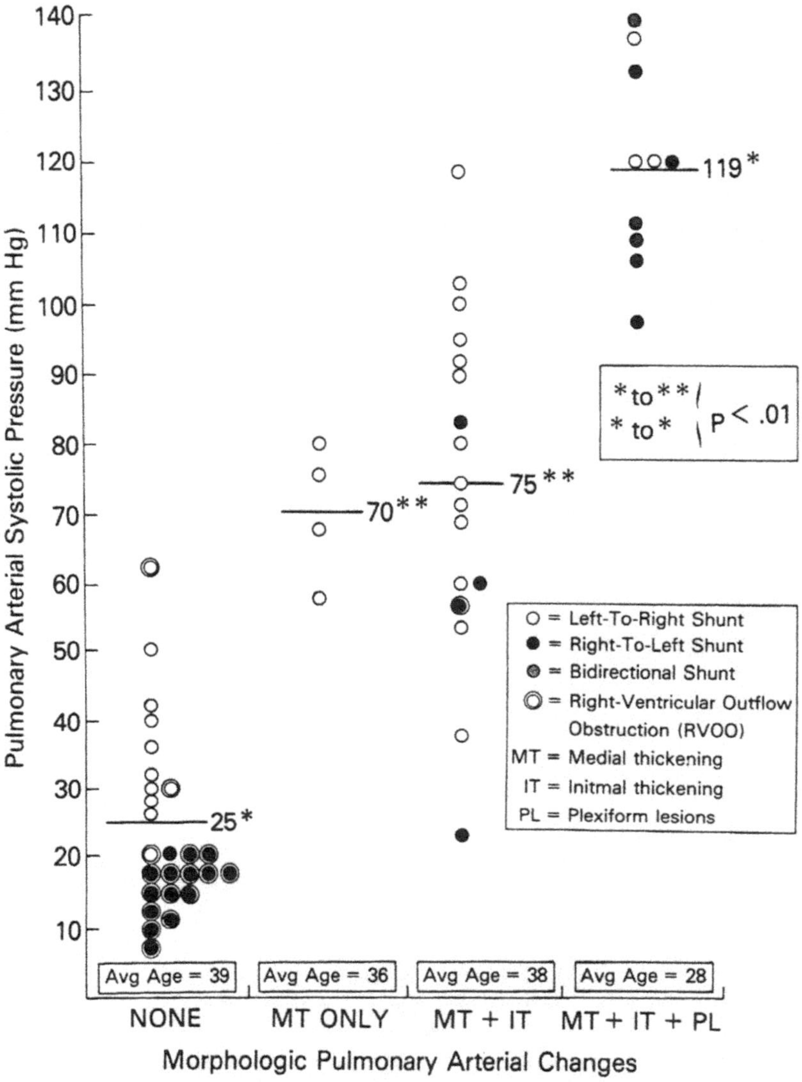

FIGURE 15. Morphologic pulmonary arterial changes, pulmonary arterial systolic pressure, and direction of shunt in 57 necropsy patients over age 15 with congenital heart disease. In 26 patients the media of the pulmonary arterial wall was normal or thinner than normal, in 4 there was medial thickening only, in 17 there was both medial and intimal thickening, and in 10 there was medial and intimal thickening with plexiform lesions. The average pulmonary arterial systolic pressure in the patients with medial thickening with or without intimal thickening was significantly ($p > .01$) different from the average pressure in patients without any morphologic changes and from the average pressure in those with plexiform lesions. From Virmani R, Roberts WC. Pulmonary arteries in congenital heart disease: A structure-function analysis. Cardiovasc Clin 1979; 10(1):478, with permission.

arteries, the only previous study that allows direct comparison with ours is the one by Heath and associates.[14] Among their 40 patients with isolated atrial septal defect or ventricular septal defect or patent ductus arteriosus, 23 were over 15 years of age (range 17 to 55; mean 32), and pulmonary arterial systolic pressures were available in all patients. Figures 21 to 23 show our plotting of their observations in 23 patients in the same way we plotted our own observations (see Figs. 18 through 20). As shown in Figure 22, the pulmonary arterial systolic pressures were significantly ($p < .01$) lower in patients in whom the morphologic pulmonary arterial changes con-

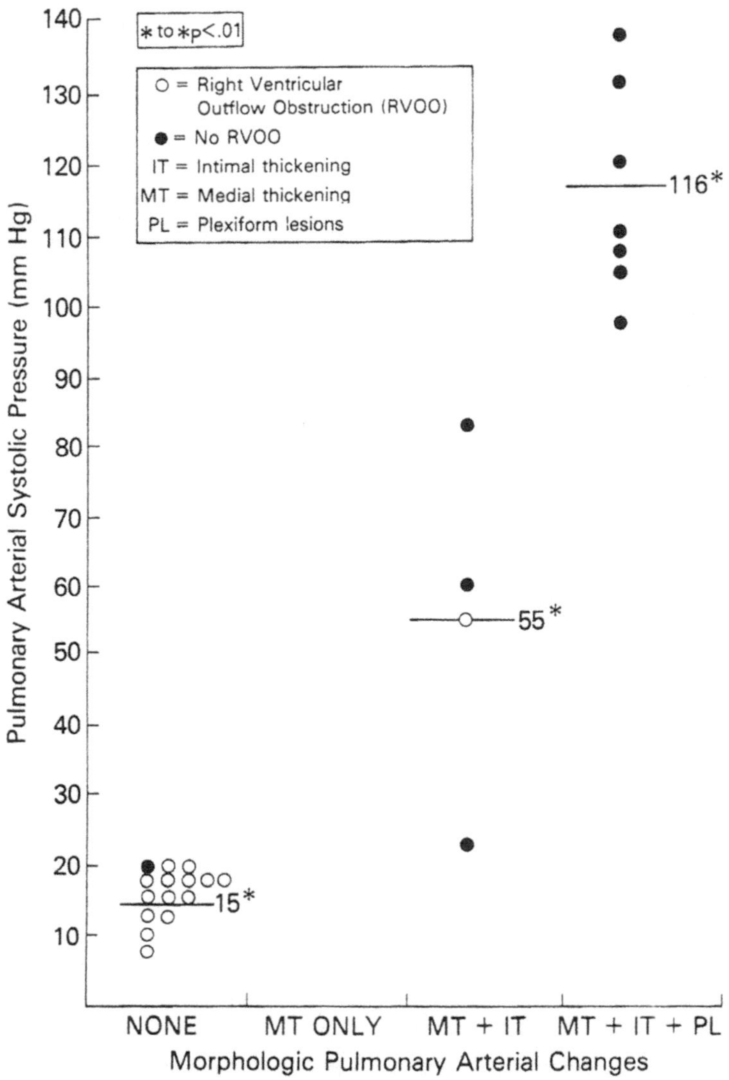

FIGURE 16. Morphologic pulmonary arterial changes and pulmonary arterial systolic pressure in 26 necropsy patients over age 15 with right-to-left or bidirectional shunts. In 15 patients the media of the pulmonary arteries was normal or thinner than normal; 4 patients had both medial and intimal thickening; 7 patients had both medial and intimal thickening with plexiform lesions. The average pulmonary arterial systolic pressure increased significantly as morphologic pulmonary arterial changes worsened. From Virmani R, Roberts WC. Pulmonary arteries in congenital heart disease: A structure-function analysis. Cardiovasc Clin 1979; 10(1):479, with permission.

sist only of medial thickening. Surprisingly, in contrast to our patients, no significant differences in these average pressures were observed between the patients with medial and intimal thickening and the patients with plexiform lesions. Furthermore, the average systolic pressure in their patients with isolated atrial septal defect was only slightly lower—although significantly ($p < 0.01$)—than the average pressures in their patients with either ventricular septal defect or patent ductus arteriosus (see Fig. 21).

As in our patients, their patients with atrial septal defect were significantly older than their patients with either ventricular septal defect or patent ductus arte-

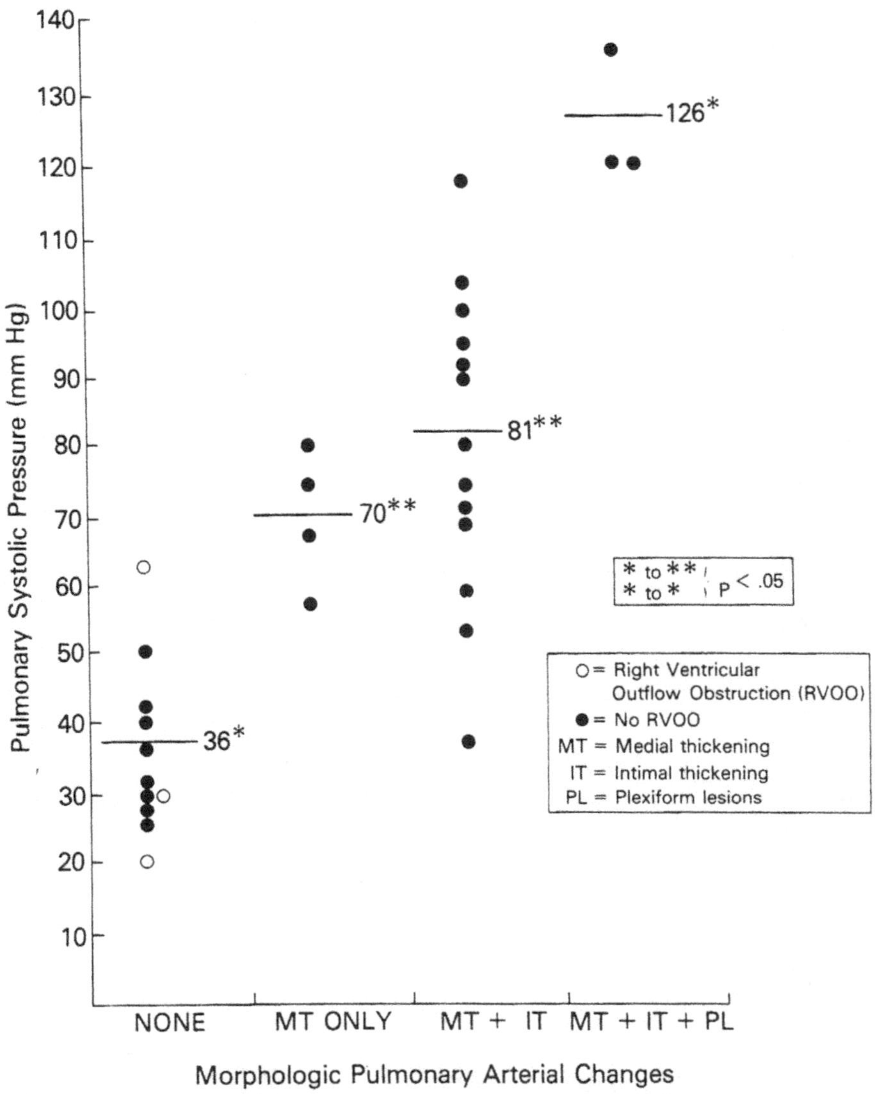

FIGURE 17. Morphologic pulmonary arterial changes and pulmonary arterial systolic pressure in 31 necropsy patients over age 15 with only left-to-right shunts. In 11 patients the media of the pulmonary arteries was normal or thinner than normal; 4 patients had only medial thickening; 13 patients had both medial and intimal thickening; 3 patients had both medial and intimal thickening with plexiform lesions. The average pulmonary arterial systolic pressure in the patients with medial thickening with or without intimal thickening was significantly ($p < .05$) different from the average pressure in patients without morphologic changes and from the average pressure in those with plexiform changes. From Virmani R, Roberts WC. Pulmonary arteries in congenital heart disease: A structure-function analysis. Cardiovasc Clin 1979; 10(1):480, with permission.

riosus, even though their pulmonary arterial systolic pressures were significantly lower. As pointed out by Heath and associates,[14] however, in patients with large ventricular septal defect or patent ductus arteriosus the systemic pressure is freely propagated into the pulmonary circulation from birth. Hence, the age of the patient is synonymous with the duration of the pulmonary arterial hypertension. As seen in Figure 23, there was an inverse correlation with the morphologic pulmonary arterial changes and the average age of their patients. In patients with medial thickening

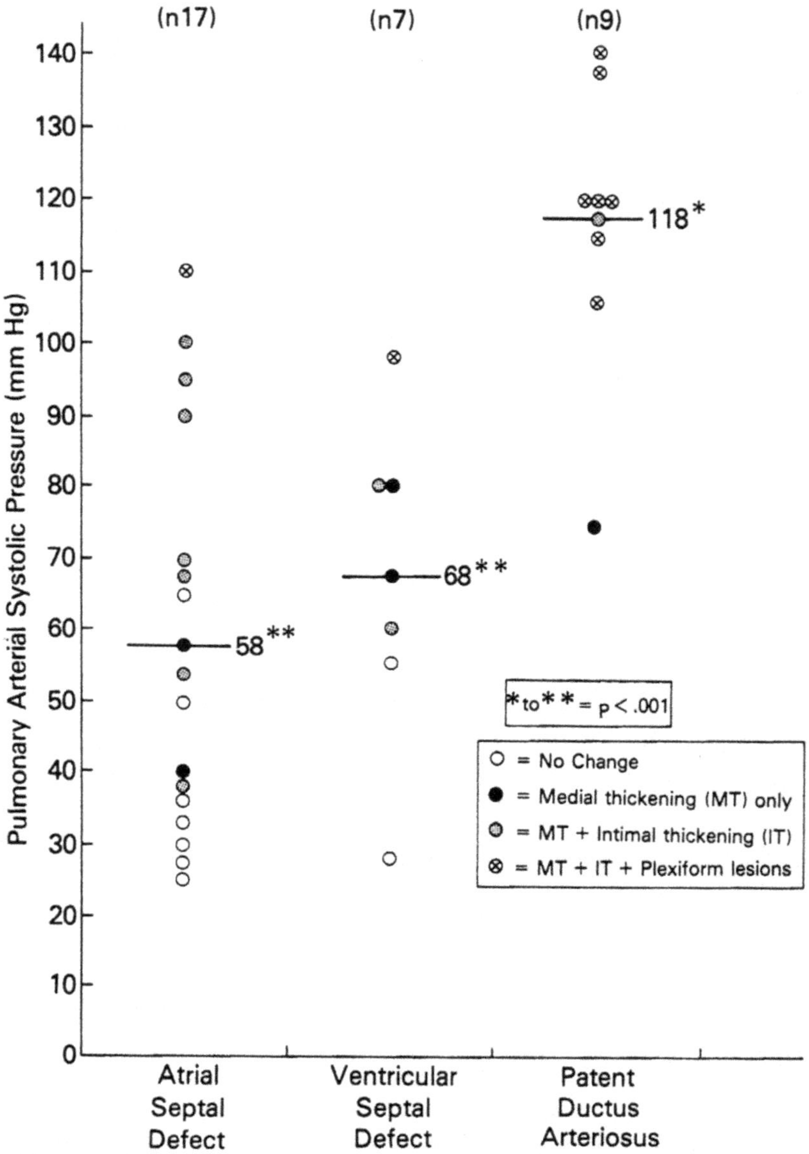

FIGURE 18. Interrelationship between type of isolated cardiovascular malformation, pulmonary arterial systolic pressure, and morphologic pulmonary arterial changes in 33 necropsy patients over age 15. There was no significant difference in the average systolic pressures in patients with atrial septal defect and ventricular septal defect, but both these averages were significantly ($p < .001$) different from the average pressure in patients with patent ductus arteriosus. From Virmani R, Roberts WC. Pulmonary arteries in congenital heart disease: A structure-function analysis. Cardiovasc Clin 1979; 10(1):481, with permission.

only, the average age was 37; in the group with medial and intimal thickening, the average age was 34; and in their patients with plexiform lesions, the average age was 29. A similar trend occurred in our patients (see Fig. 20).

The direction of the shunt, as shown in Figure 22, played a role in causing the morphologic pulmonary arterial changes, in that their patients with bidirectional or only right-to-left shunts had higher pulmonary arterial systolic pressures than those with only left-to-right shunts.

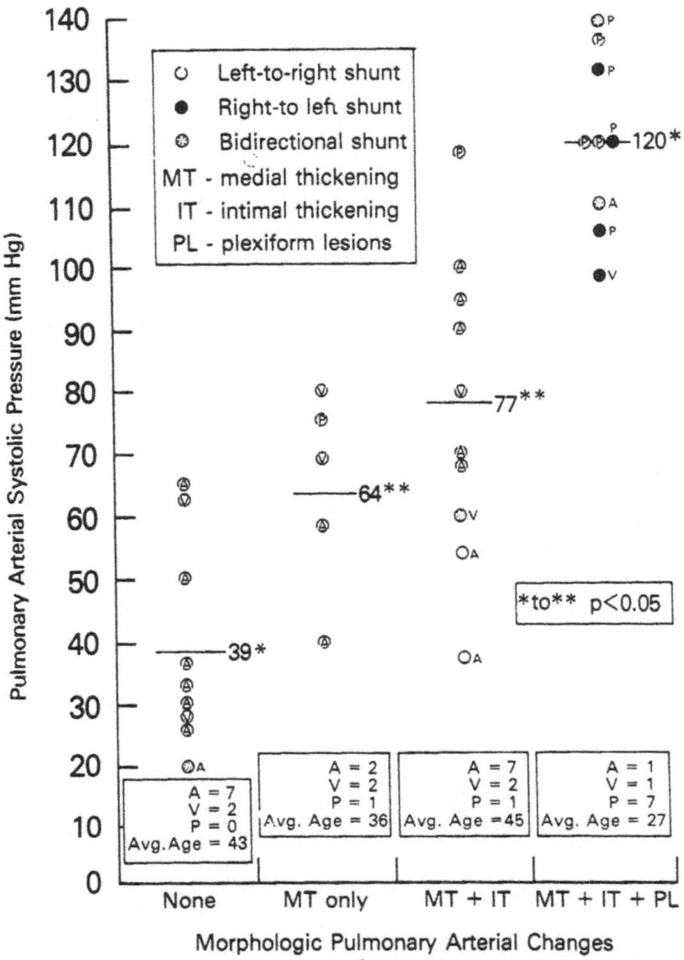

FIGURE 19. Morphologic pulmomary arterial changes, pulmonary arterial systolic pressure, and shunt direction in 33 necropsy patients over age 15 with isolated atrial septal defect or ventricular septal defect or patent ductus arteriosus. The pulmonary arteries were normal in 9 patients; 5 had medial thickening only; 10 had both medial and intimal thickening; 9 had both medial and intimal thickening with plexiform lesions. The average pulmonary arterial systolic pressures in the patients with medial thickening with or without intimal thickening was significantly ($p < .05$) different from average pressure in patients without morphologic changes and from the average pressure in those with plexiform changes. From Virmani R, Roberts WC. Pulmonary arteries in congenital heart disease: A structure-function analysis. Cardiovasc Clin 1979; 10(1):482, with permission.

Thus, the study of Heath and associates[14] showed no significant pulmonary arterial systolic pressure differences between patients with plexiform lesions and those with both medial and intimal thickening (see Fig. 22). Our study, in contrast, showed a significant difference in pulmonary arterial systolic pressure between these two anatomic groups (see Fig. 19). Their study showed a clear difference in pulmonary arterial systolic pressure in the patients with only medial thickening compared with those with both medial and intimal thickening and those with plexiform lesions (see Fig. 22). Our study (see Fig. 19), in contrast, showed no significant difference in the patients with medial thickening only as compared with those with both medial and intimal thickening.

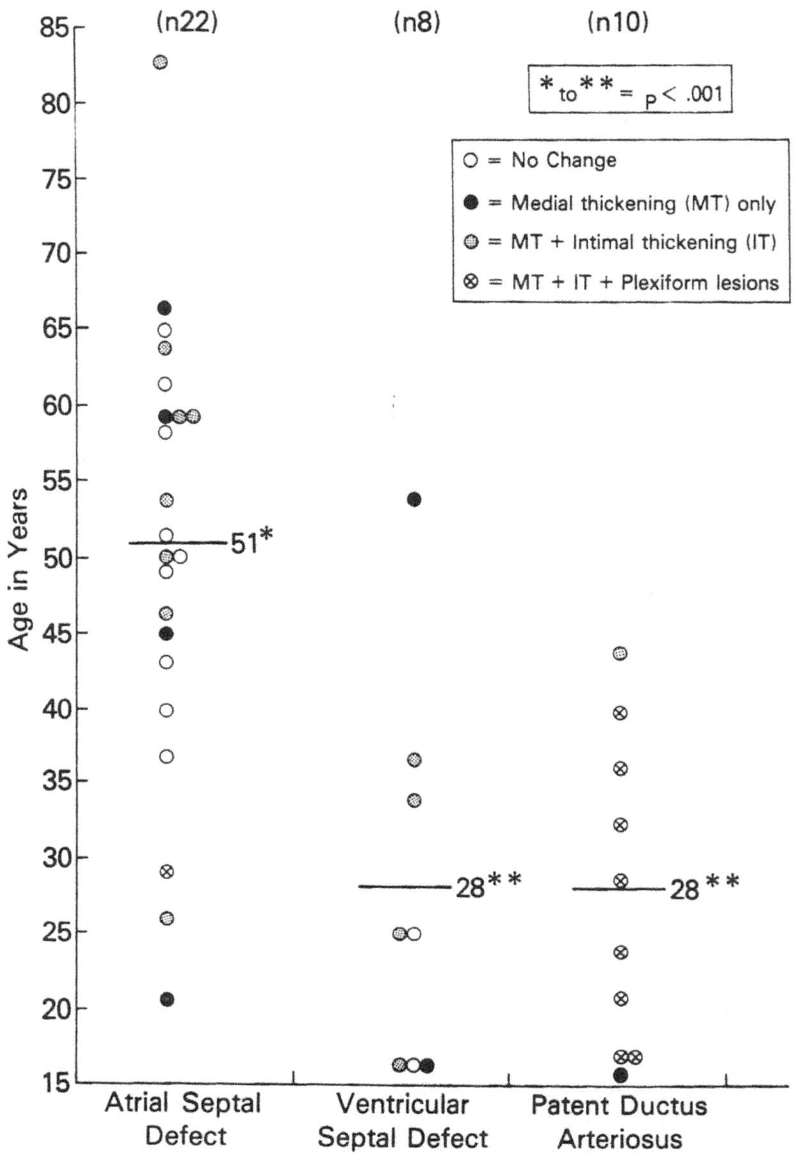

FIGURE 20. Interrelationship between type of isolated congenital cardiovascular malformation (atrial septal defect, n = 22; ventricular septal defect, n = 8; patent ductus arteriosus, n = 10) and morphologic pulmonary arterial changes in 40 necropsy patients over age 15. The average ages of patients with ventricular septal defect and patent ductus arteriosus are significantly ($p < .001$) different than the average set of patients with atrial septal defect. From Virmani R, Roberts WC. Pulmonary arteries in congenital heart disease: A structure-function analysis. Cardiovasc Clin 1979; 10(1):484, with permission.

When comparing pulmonary arterial systolic pressures to the location of the shunt, there was no significant difference in pulmonary pressures in their patients with ventricular septal defect and patent ductus arteriosus; there was a significant difference between the pressures of these two groups and pressures of patients with atrial septal defect (see Fig. 21). In contrast, our study showed a highly significant difference between average pulmonary systolic pressure in patients with patent ductus arteriosus and in those with ventricular septal defect, but no significant difference between patients with atrial septal defect and in those with ventricular septal defect (see Fig. 18).

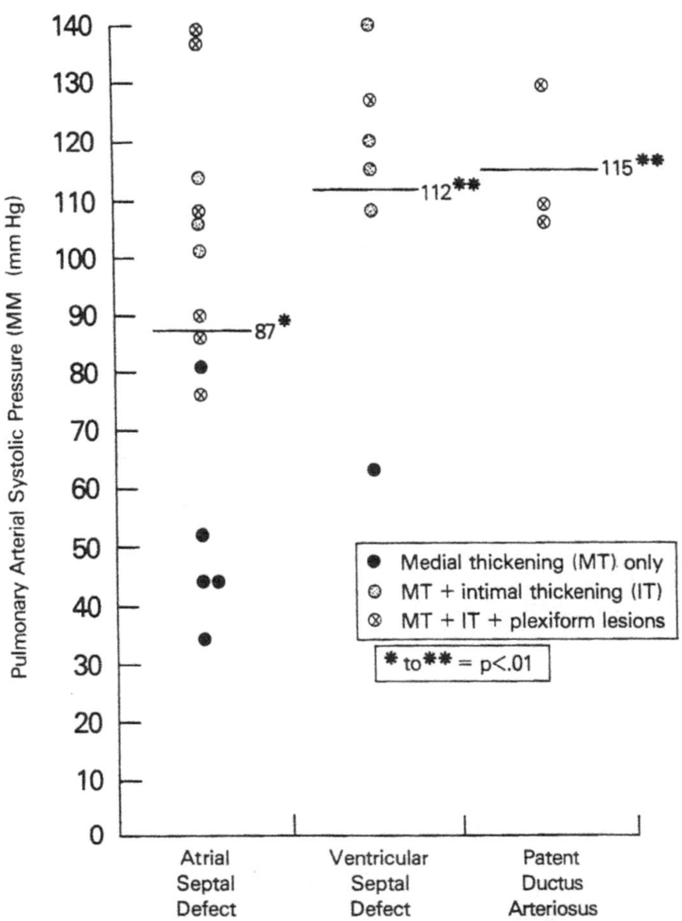

FIGURE 21. Data from Heath and associates[14] showing interrelationship between type of isolated congenital cardiovascular malformation (atrial septal defect, n = 14; ventricular septal defect, n = 6; patent ductus arteriosus, n = 3), pulmonary artery systolic pressure, and morphologic pulmonary arterial changes in 23 patients over age 15. There was no significant difference between the average pulmonary arterial systolic pressures in patients with ventricular septal defect and in patients with patent ductus arteriosus, but pressures in these two groups were significantly ($p < .01$) different from those in the patients with atrial septal defect. From Virmani R, Roberts WC. Pulmonary arteries in congenital heart disease: A structure-function analysis. Cardiovasc Clin 1979; 10(1):485, with permission.

The results of our study were similar to that of Heath and associates[14] in regard to age (see Figs. 20 and 23) and direction of the shunt.

How might the differences in the results of the two studies be explained? First, the patients were different. We studied only necropsy patients and many histologic sections from each patient. How many, if any, of their patients were studied at necropsy is not stated. It appears likely that the lung tissue in most of their patients was obtained at biopsy at the time of cardiac operation. Second, the investigators were different, and judgments of morphologic changes possibly were different. Third, the numbers of patients in each study were relatively small so the differences may have been magnified. Fourth, their study excluded patients without anatomic changes in the pulmonary arteries, whereas ours did not. Nevertheless, when we exclude our patients without anatomic pulmonary arterial changes, the differences between the two studies persist.

Recently pulmonary vascular changes were analyzed by Haworth[66] in the lungs of 10 patients with pulmonary hypertension (PA = 40–80/20–35) and isolated sec-

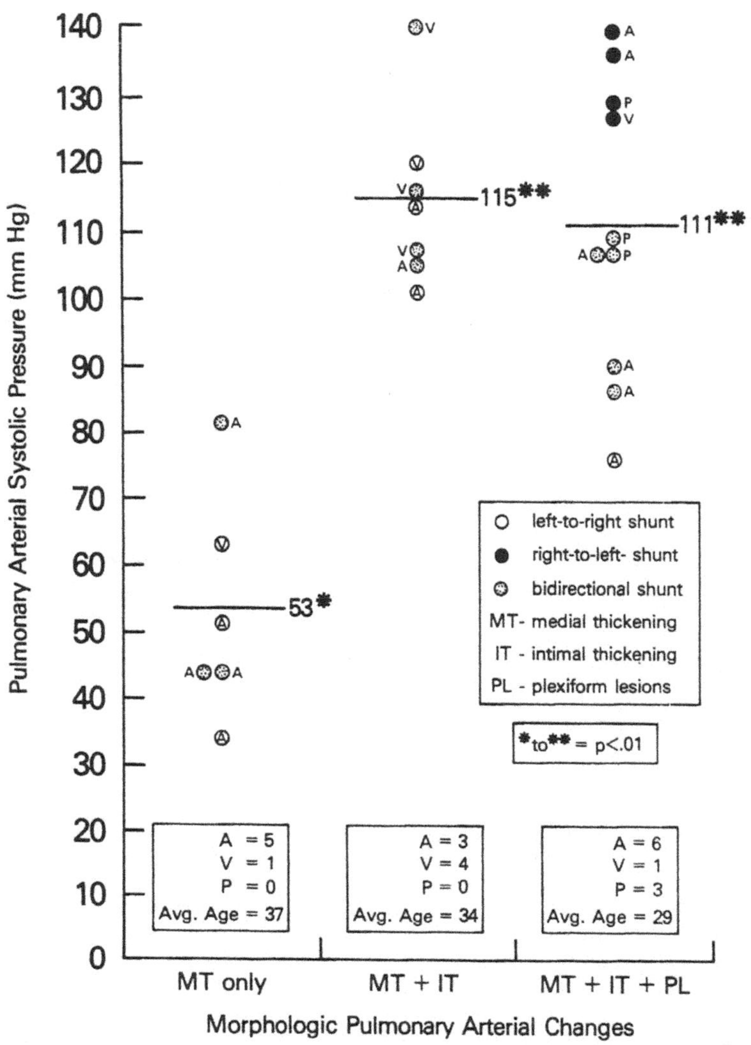

FIGURE 22. Data from Heath and associates[14] showing interrelationship between morphologic pulmonary arterial changes, pulmonary arterial systolic pressure, and direction of shunt in 23 patients over age 15 with isolated atrial septal defect or ventricular septal defect or patent ductus arteriosus. Medial thickening only occurred in 6 patients; 7 had medial and intimal thickening; 10 had both medial and intimal thickening with plexiform lesions. The average pulmonary arterial systolic pressures in the patients with medial and intimal thickening were not significantly different from those of patients who had medial and intimal thickening with plexiform lesions. Pressures in both of these groups were significantly ($p < .01$) different from pressures in patients with only medial thickening. From Virmani R, Roberts WC. Pulmonary arteries in congenital heart disease: A structure-function analysis. Cardiovasc Clin 1979; 10(1):487, with permission.

umdum atrial septal defect in 8, and in 2 patients atrial septal defect was associated with either ventricular septal defect or patent ductus arteriosus. The ages ranged from 3 months to 21 years, with 4 patients aged 6 months or less, 5 patients aged 2 to 9 years, and 1 aged 21 years. All patients had presented with heart failure. Five patients had open lung biopsies performed, and in 5 patients lungs were studied at autopsy. There was marked increase in pulmonary arterial smooth muscle, and fibrointimal proliferation was most marked in older children. Therefore, pulmonary hypertension develops rarely in secumdum atrial septal defect in childhood.

Wagenvoort and associates[33,40,41] studied lung tissue biopsied at the time of thoracotomy in patients with various congenital cardiovascular malformations. They

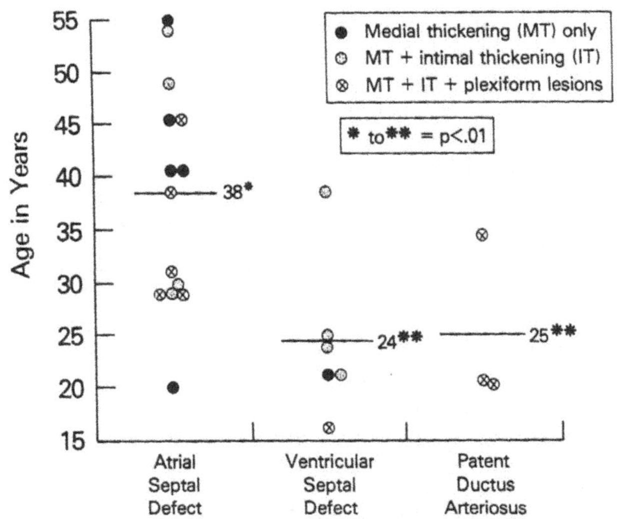

FIGURE 23. Data from Heath and associates[14] showing interrelationship between type of isolated congenital cardiovascular malformation (atrial septal defect, n = 14; ventricular septal defect, n = 6, patent ductus arteriosus, n = 3), age, and morphologic pulmonary arterial changes in 23 patients over age 15. The patients with ventricular septal defect and patent ductus arteriosus were significantly ($p < .01$) younger than those with atrial septal defect. From Virmani R, Roberts WC. Pulmonary arteries in congenital heart disease: A structure-function analysis. Cardiovasc Clin 1979; 10(1):488, with permission.

also have shown that the primary cause of anatomic pulmonary arterial changes is elevation of the pulmonary arterial pressure, and that the magnitude of pulmonary flow is not, in itself, a determinant of these anatomic changes. This group did find, however, that the location of the shunt was an important factor in determining the extent of the anatomic pulmonary arterial changes. Of 77 lung samples studied from patients with isolated atrial septal defect (mean age, 22 years), medial thickening occurred in only 22 (29%), intimal thickening occurred in only 14 (18%), and none had plexiform lesions. In contrast, of 44 patients with isolated ventricular septal defect (mean age, 9 years) and of 74 with isolated patent ductus arteriosus (mean age, 9 years), 44 (34%) had medial thickening, 36 (28%) had intimal thickening, and only 2 (2%) had plexiform lesions. Severe intimal thickening was not observed in any patient with atrial septal defect or patent ductus arteriosus but it occurred in 12 (27%) of the 44 patients with ventricular septal defect.

The Wagenvoort study emphasized that the pulmonary vessels of their patients with atrial septal defect (much younger than ours and Heath's) did not differ significantly from those of his "control subjects." Among Wagenvoort's 105 patients with left-to-right shunts and pulmonary arterial systolic pressures greater than 60 mm Hg, all had medial thickening and 74 (70%) had intimal thickening. In contrast, of his 45 patients with only right-to-left or bidirectional shunts, all had medial thickening and 44 (98%) had intimal thickening. Plexiform lesions were not described in any of these 150 patients but, again, they were much younger than our patients.

The presence of Eisenmenger syndrome is defined as "pulmonary hypertension at systemic level, due to a high pulmonary vascular resistance with reversal or bidirectional shunts at aorto-pulmonary, ventricular or atrial level." The size of the communication is large, usually 2 to 2.5 cm, and the arterial changes in the pulmonary circuit are usually extensive. The majority of patients with Eisenmenger syndrome have large ventricular septal defect, patent ductus arteriosus, alone or in combination with other congenital defects. Recent report by Warnes and associates[67] describes the longest survival in a 63-year-old man with unoperated large ventricular septal defect (2.5 cm) and PA pressure at last catheterization (51 years) of 150/70 mm Hg. At autopsy, the muscular pulmonary arteries were severely narrowed, medial thickening plus intimal thickening with occasional plexiform lesions. The average age at death in unoperated patients with an isolated (≥ 2 cm) ventricular septal defect is about 35 years. Complete necropsy reports are available in only 5 patients with an isolated, large (≥ 1.5 cm) ventricular septal defect who survived more than 40 years. Their ages ranged from 44 to 60 years (mean 51). Only 1 had cardiac catheterization, and the systemic arterial pressure was 180/120 mm Hg.

McManus and coworkers[68] recently described a 44-year-old man with a large (2.5 cm maximal diameter) ductus and PA pressure 90/25 mm Hg with systemic arterial pressure of 120/70 mm Hg. The muscular pulmonary arteries showed severe narrowing with medial and intimal thickening and occasional plexiform lesions. At least 23 other patients have been reported at necropsy, > 40 years of age (mean age 61) with unoperated patent ductus arteriosus. Fourteen of the patients died from the consequences of patent ductus arteriosus: 6 from chronic congestive heart failure; 4 from infective endocarditis or endarteritis; and 1 each from pulmonary artery rupture, aortic rupture, embolus, and pulmonary artery thrombus. Calcification in the wall of the patent ductus arteriosus was described in 7 patients.

Rabinovitch and colleagues[50] examined lung biopsies in 95 patients with ventricular septal defect (47 patients), d-transposition of great vessels (33 patients), and an atrioventricular canal defect (15 patients). The patients ranged in age from 2 days to 30 years (median 13 months). The pulmonary arteries were evaluated microscopically by quantitative morphologic techniques. Three grades of severity of changes were described: Grade A, abnormal extension of muscle into peripheral arteries only, pulmonary blood flow increased but pulmonary arterial pressure is normal; Grade B, increased medial wall thickness of the normal muscular arteries along with changes of Grade A and in these cases pulmonary artery pressure is also increased; Grade C, along with changes of Grade B there is reduction in the number of small peripheral arteries and in these cases the pulmonary vascular resistance is increased (see Fig. 1). In 21 patients, abnormal extension of muscle was the only abnormality (Grade A); of these, 20 had normal pulmonary arterial pressure, and in 1, the pressure was mildly elevated. Seventy-four patients had increased thickness of the medial wall of muscular arteries with a correlation coefficient between the percentage of wall thickness and the pulmonary artery pressure + .74 ($p < .005$). In 15 of the 74 patients there was also a reduction in the number of small peripheral arteries, and in all but 1 patient it was associated with elevation of pulmonary vascular resistance (≥ 3.5 μ per sq m). Rabinovitch and associates[50] have suggested that reduction in the number of small arteries may be a serious sign in children or adults with congenital heart disease. In this study the reduction in number of arteries was associated with Grade 1 changes of Health-Edward classification but was not seen in Grade 2, whereas this feature was always present with severe changes (Grade 3 or higher). Reid, Rabinovitch, and Meyrick[48,50,51] suggested that the reduction in the number of arteries is largely due to underdevelopment of pulmonary arterial tree or is due to a secondary loss of arteries from occlusive injury, and this correlates with high pulmonary vascular resistance. However, Mooi and Wagenvoort[69] and Takahashi and Wagenvoort[70] only rarely observed a significant decrease in the number of pulmonary arteries in patients with congenital heart disease with a shunt as long as the hypertensive pulmonary vascular disease had not advanced to a terminal stage. They caution about drawing conclusions from counting number of pulmonary blood vessels per field when only a very small area of the whole lung field is utilized for counting studies.

CHANGES IN PULMONARY ARTERIES IN PATIENTS WITH COMPLETE TRANSPOSITION OF GREAT ARTERIES AND PULMONARY HYPERTENSION

Ferencz,[31] Viles and coworkers,[36] and Newfeld and colleagues[39] have reported severe pulmonary vascular disease in complete transposition of the great arteries. Recently

Yauaki and Tezuka[71] studied 40 necropsy cases of transposition of the great arteries and compared the morphologic changes in the lungs with 22 necropsy cases of ventricular septal defect, and an index of pulmonary vascular disease was derived. Index of pulmonary vascular disease was based on the scores (1 to 4) obtained from histologic changes in the arteries according to the following findings: (1) no intimal reaction, (2) cellular intimal reaction, (3) fibrous and fibroelastic proliferation of intima, and (4) partial and total destruction of media. An index of pulmonary vascular disease was then defined by:

$$IPVD = \frac{(1 \times n_1 + (2 \times n_2) + (3 \times n_3) + (4 \times n_4)}{n_1 + n_2 + n_3 + n_4}$$

where n_1, n_2, n_3, and n_4 were the numbers of arterial sections bearing the score of 1, 2, 3, and 4, respectively. Positive correlation was observed between the index of pulmonary vascular disease and blood pressure of pulmonary circulation. No significant difference in index of pulmonary vascular disease was found between transposition of the great arteries and ventricular septal defect in the first 5 months of life, when cases of each disease were compared at similar blood pressure levels. Beyond that age, however, index of pulmonary vascular disease was much higher in transposition of the great arteries, and severe pulmonary vascular disease was demonstrated histologically. Morphometric analysis of medial hypertrophy of pulmonary arteries revealed decreased progress of medial thickening in cases of transposition of the great arteries older than 5 months and was only 70% of that of ventricular septal defect at the same blood pressure. Yamaki and Tezoka[71] regard suppression of the progress of medial hypertrophy to the stress of pulmonary pressure (i.e., relatively weak muscular coat) as one of the important factors precipitating severe pulmonary vascular disease in transposition of the great arteries. Wagenvoort and coworkers[35] suggested that dilatation of small pulmonary arteries with attenuated walls in transposition of the great arteries with intact ventricular septum is due to hyperxemia of pulmonary circulation and is characteristic of transposition of the great arteries.

Yamaski and Horiuchi[72] carried out quantitative analysis of postoperative changes of pulmonary arteries in 3 late deaths in patients with transposition of the great arteries with large ventricular septal defect and pulmonary hypertension. In the postoperative course of 2 of the 3 cases, extreme medial hypertrophy of small pulmonary arteries was noted along with severe pulmonary vascular disease. In the third case, thickening of the media was mild, and pulmonary vascular disease had not progressed owing to a residual ventricular septal defect. They concluded that in cases of transposition of the great arteries with severe pulmonary hypertension, marked hypertrophy of the media accompanied by pulmonary vascular disease developed after total correction, and this was brought about by vasoconstriction secondary to hypoxemia of the pulmonary circulation and probable release of intrinsic chemical mediators like catecholamines, histamine, prostaglandin, angiotensin, etc., compared with the preoperative state in transposition of the great arteries. Oxygen saturation of pulmonary arterial blood is markedly decreased postoperatively; therefore, it is possible that vasoconstriction of small pulmonary arteries occurs immediately after surgery, and in cases of sustained high pulmonary arterial pressure, this will further contribute to excessive hypertrophy of pulmonary arterial media and endothelium damage leading to pulmonary vascular disease. Consequently, when marked hypertrophy of the pulmonary arterial media is seen postoperatively, it is probably indicative of progressive pulmonary disease. In patients with transposition of the great arteries over the age of 6 months who have severe preoperative pulmonary hypertension, most have already severe pulmonary vascular disease, so that the pulmonary arterial pressure will probably remain high even after total correction. Because the degree of medial hypertrophy is proportional to the degree of intra-arterial blood pressure, the progression of pulmonary vascular disease is unavoidable, so that death in late postoperative period seems likely.

SIGNIFICANCE OF PLEXIFORM LESIONS IN PATIENTS WITH PRIMARY PULMONARY HYPERTENSION

Plexiform lesions in the lung are indicative of severe pulmonary arterial hypertension that is almost always irreversible. Of our 87 patients, 13 (15%) had plexiform lesions: they occurred in 12 (23%) of the 51 patients without and in 1 (3%) of the 36 patients with right ventricular outflow or inflow obstruction (see Table 10). The latter patient, however, developed plexiform lesions after operative creation of a large end-to-side communication between aorta and right main pulmonary artery. The pulmonary arterial systolic pressures were known in 11 of 13 patients with plexiform lesions, and in each this pressure was greater than 90 mm Hg (mean 118 mm Hg). Of the 13 patients with lesions, 12 had either ventricular septal defect or patent ductus arteriosus, and only 1 had isolated atrial septal defect; they were between 17 and 41 years old (mean 28).

Heath and associates[14] described plexiform lesions in 10 (43%) of their 23 patients over 15 years of age with isolated atrial septal defect or ventricular septal defect or patent ductus arteriosus (see Fig. 22). In their 10 patients with plexiform lesions, the pulmonary arterial systolic pressures ranged from 76 to 139 mm Hg (mean 111 mm Hg), and in 8 of the 10 this pressure was ≥ 90 mm Hg. These lesions were observed in 6 (43%) of their 14 patients with atrial septal defect, in 1 (17%) of 6 with ventricular septal defect, and all of the 3 with patent ductus arteriosus. Among our patients, in contrast, plexiform lesions were seen in 1 (6%) of 17 with atrial septal defect, in 1 (14%) of 7 with ventricular septal defect, and in 7 (78%) of 9 with patent ductus arteriosus. Except for the patients with atrial septal defect, the frequency of

TABLE 11. Observations in 16 Necropsy Patients With Primary Pulmonary Hypertension

PATIENT AGE, SEX	DURATION OF SYMPTOMS (MONTHS)	PRESSURES (mm Hg)		CI (ml/min/m²)	SA O^2 SAT. (%)	HEART WEIGHT (gm†)	PL	CEF-PT
		PA (s/d)	SA (s/d)					
8F*	24	190/100	90/55			160	+	A + F
17 F*	24	192/5	138/90	2.1	91	340	+	F
18 M	1	135/90	92/68	1.9	66	440	+	A
22 M**	36	88/54	100/60	1.5	86		+	A
25 F	30	92/39	130/78	2.0	98	460	+	A
25 F	54	122/49	122/80	2.7		360	+	A
25 F**	24	91/41	104/67	2.0	95		+	A
25 F	48	112/41	109/70	2.5			+	
28 M	24	108/58	127/80	3.2	92	630	+	A
29 F*	60	120/40	110/80	1.5	91	320	+	A
35 F*	84	101/38	108/72		86	400	0	A
38 M	144	138/88	138/88		↓†	880	+	F
39 F*	30	49/30	96/73		81†	390	0	A
39 F*	6	60/45	112/85			360	+	A
43 M	4	70/30	115/72	2.5		500	+	
56 M**	24		110/80				+	

*Death during or shortly after cardiac catheterization.

**Father-son-daughter relationship reported in detail elsewhere.[92]

†Right-to-left shunt via patent foramen ovale.

CEF-PT = configuration of elastic fibers of pulmonary trunk (A = adult; F = fetal); CI = cardiac index; PA = pulmonary artery; PL = plexiform lesion; SA = systemic artery; Sat. = saturation; s/d = systole diastole.

From Virmani R, Roberts WC. Pulmonary arteries in congenital heart disease: A structure-function analysis. Cardiovasc Clin 1979 10(1):488, with permission.

plexiform lesions in our patients was similar to that observed in the patients studied by Heath and associates.[14]

Plexiform lesions are observed in highest frequency not in patients with congenital cardiovascular malformations but in patients with primary or idiopathic pulmonary hypertension. Observations in 16 necropsy patients with this condition are summarized in Table 11. Fourteen (87%) of these 16 patients had plexiform lesions in the lungs; in 13, pulmonary arterial systolic pressures ranged from 60 to 192 mm Hg (mean 117 mm Hg). In 11 of these 13 patients, this pressure was > 90 mm Hg. In the 2 patients without plexiform lesions, pulmonary arterial systolic pressures were 49 and 101 mm Hg.

Of the 10 patients with primary pulmonary hypertension with plexiform lesions and known pulmonary arterial pressures reported by Walcott and associates,[7] the pulmonary arterial systolic pressures ranged from 76 to 168 mm Hg (mean = [illegible] mm Hg), and in only 2 patients was this pressure < 90 mm Hg.

Wagenvoort and Wagenvoort[74] summarized pulmonary morphologic observations in 110 patients (age range, infancy to 69 years; mean age, 23) with primary pulmonary hypertension, and 77 (70%) had plexiform lesions. Of their 110 patients,

TABLE 12. Clinical and Morphologic Observations in 31 Autopsy Patients with Primary Pulmonary Hypertension

SERIAL NO.	AGE (IN YEARS)	SEX	DURATION OF SYMPTOMS (IN MONTHS)	PA SYSTOLIC (mm Hg)	HEART WT (IN GRAMS)	MORPHOLOGIC CHANGES		MORPHOLOGIC ANALYSIS
						MT + IT	PL	
1	.41	M	2	↑	↑	+	0	0
2	.62	M	4	70	↑	+	0	0
3	5	M	14	↑	150	+	+	+
4	6	F	9	74	83	+	+	0
5	12	F	SD	—	125	+	+	+
6	17	M	—	110	520	+	+	0
7	21	F	96	90	260	+	+	+
8	22	F	4	↑	365	+	+	0
9	23	F	24	78	280	+	+	0
10	24	F	48	108	450	+	+	0
11	25	M	SD	—	380	+	+	+
12	25	M	SD	—	380	+	+	+
13	26	F	1	—	350	+	+	0
14	26	M	1	—	420	+	+	+
15	29	F	8	100	410	+	+	+
16	30	F	8	100	350	+	+	+
17	34	F	20	120	330	+	+	0
18	35	F	48	110	350	+	+	+
19	35	M	46	—	430	+	+	0
20	36	M	96	70	350	+	0	0
21	36	M	12	92	350	+	0	0
22	38	F	SD	—	250	+	+	+
23	40	F	48	110	400	+	+	+
24	43	M	48	—	575	+	+	+
25	46	M	48	93	450	+	0	0
26	47	F	48	—	470	+	+	+
27	47	M	—	—	620	+	+	0
28	48	M	1	—	475	+	+	0
29	50	F	10	115	450	+	+	+
30	51	M	24	↑↑	500	+	+	0
31	54	M	36	110	500	+	+	+

IT = intimal thickening; MT = medial thickening; PA = pulmonary artery; PL = plexiform lesions.

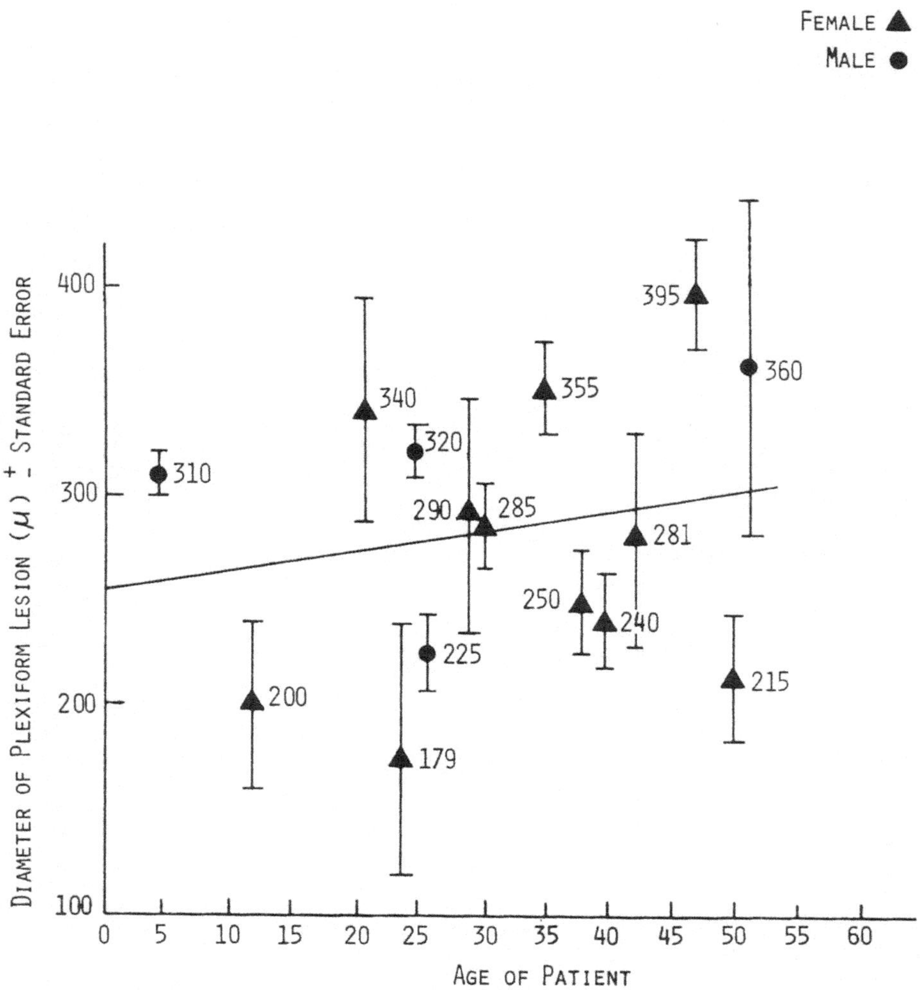

FIGURE 24. The relationship between the diameter of plexiform lesions and the age of the patient in years in 15 patients wtih primary pulmonary hypertension. The diameter is expressed as mean ± standard error in μm.

however, only 70 were 16 years of age or older; and of the remaining 39 patients, many were infants and young children. Had these authors included only patients over age 15, their frequency of plexiform lesions almost certainly would have been higher.

Recently, Bjornsson and Edwards[75] have reported 80 cases with clinical diagnosis of "primary (unexplained) pulmonary hypertension." Histopathologically, the World Health Organization has recognized primary pulmonary hypertension as at least 3 distinct entities: (1) thromboembolic pulmonary hypertension, (2) primary plexogenic pulmonary arteriopathy (primary pulmonary hypertension), and (3) pulmonary veno-occlusive disease, as the medical therapy may be different for the 3 types and open lung biopsy may be indicated to distinguish these 3 entities. These 80 cases include 73 autopsies, 6 open lung biopsies, and 1 with both biopsy and an autopsy. They excluded cases with congenital cardiac shunts, obstructive lesions of the left side of the heart (e.g. mitral stenosis), pulmonary parenchymal disease, clinical pulmonary emboli, and collagen vascular diseases (except Reynaud's phenomenon). The most common histologic type was thromboembolic pulmonary hypertension (45 of 80; 56%), was characterized by thrombi of various ages and by eccentric intimal proliferation and fibrosis. Primary plexogenic pulmonary arteriopathy (primary pulmonary hypertension) was present in 22 of 80 (28%) and histologically con-

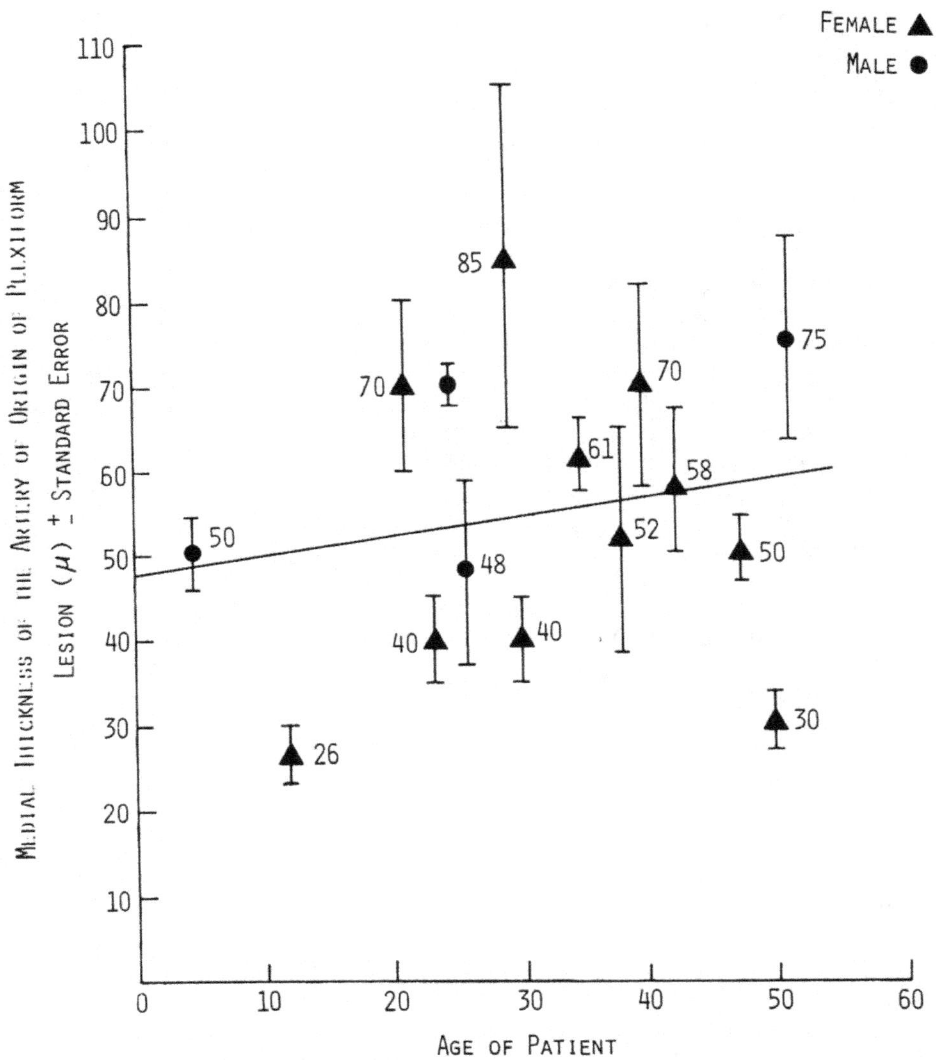

FIGURE 25. The relationship between the medial thickness of the artery of origin of the plexiform lesion and the age of the patient in years. The medial thickness of the artery is expressed as mean ± standard error in μm.

sisted of concentric intimal proliferation and fibroelastosis. Plexiform lesions consisted of aneurysmal dilatation of a muscular pulmonary artery with a cellular intimal proliferation, and their presence was required to include the case in this category. The researchers noted that plexiform lesions varied considerably in number and their extent did not correlate with pulmonary arterial pressure or duration of survival. The remaining 13 (16%) had pulmonary veno-occlusive disease (5 cases), primary medial hypertrophy (3 cases), primary pulmonary arteritis (3 cases), or changes consistent with pulmonary veno-occlusive hypertension (2 cases). The mean age varied from 16 to 45 years, with the mean age of 16 years for patients with arteritis and 30 and 41 years for plexogenic and thromboembolic disease. In all forms except pulmonary veno-occlusive disease and apparent pulmonary venous hypertension, the disease tended to occur twice as often in female patients as male patients. With the exception of pulmonary venous hypertension, patients with plexogenic pulmonary arteriopathy had the longest survival (63 months). Also, sudden death occurred most frequently in patients with plexogenic disease (45%).

We have recently reported 31 necropsy patients[76] (5 months to 54 years, mean 31 years) with primary pulmonary hypertension (Table 12). Presenting symptoms ranged from sudden death (4 patients) to an illness of 120 months (mean 20 months). Cardiac catheterization had been performed in 16 patients and the pulmonary arterial systolic pressure ranged from 70 to 120 mm Hg (mean 99 mm Hg). Pulmonary plexiform lesions were observed in 26 (84%) patients. The two youngest patients—5 and 7½ months—had only medial and intimal thickening of the pulmonary arteries, as did three of the older patients, two of whom were 36 years of age and one 46 years. The pulmonary arterial systolic pressures in the three older patients were 70, 92, and 93 mm Hg, respectively. Arteritis was present in only 2 patients, 5 and 30 years old.

Morphometric analysis was carried out in 15 patients with plexiform lesions. The diameter of all plexiform lesions and the diameter and the medial thickness of the artery of origin of the plexiform lesion were determined using Zeiss computerized planimeter. A minimum of 7 plexiform lesions and the artery of origin of each were measured per patient. The diameter of the plexiform lesions varied from 100 μm to 575 μm (average 282 μm). There was no statistically significant difference in the diameter of the plexiform lesions as age advanced in these 15 patients (Fig. 24). There was a large intrapatient variation in the diameter of the arteries of origin of the plexiform lesions. There was no statistically significant difference between the size of the artery of origin of the plexiform lesions in the younger patients as compared with that in the older patients (range 75 to 970 μm; mean 366 μm). This was also true of the thickness of the media of the arteries of origin of the plexiform lesions (10 to 100 μm; mean 55 μm) (Fig. 25). One may assume, therefore, that once the plexiform lesion is formed, the size of the lesion changes only very slightly if at all throughout the patient's illness.

TABLE 13. Observations in 13 Necropsy Patients Over Age 15 With Cholesterol-Ester Granulomas

PATIENT AGE, SEX	DIAGNOSIS	PRESSURE (mm Hg) PA (s/d)	PRESSURE (mm Hg) SA (s/d)	SHUNT	ANATOMIC GRADE OF PA CHANGES
29 F	ASD	110/60	110/60	both	III
33 M	VSD + PDA	106/60	136/68	R-L	III
21 F	VSD + PDA	138/86	140/88	both	III
38 M	VSD + CT	83/20	102/65	both	II
24 F	VSD + DORV	60/12	80/48	L-R	II
38 F	ASD + PS			R-L	0
24 F	VSD + PDA + MS + COA	104/60	118/70	L-R	II
25 F*	VSD + PS + AS		100/65	R-L	0
25 F	PPH	122/49	122/80	0	III
25 F	PPH	91/41	104/67	0	III
17 F	PPH	192/5**	138/90	0	III
38 M	PPH	138/88	138/88	0	III
39 F	PPH	50/30	96/73	L-R	II

*Patient also had pulmonary tuberculosis.

**Right ventricular pressure; pulmonary artery not entered.

AS = aortic stenosis; ASD = atrial septal defect; COA = coarctation of aorta; CT = corrected transposition; DORV = double outlet right ventricle; MS = mitral stenosis; PDA = patent ductus arteriosus; PPH = primary pulmonary hypertension; PS = pulmonic stenosis; PA = pulmonary artery; SA = systemic artery; s/d = systole/diastole; VSD = ventricular septal defect.

From Virmani R, Roberts, WC. Pulmonary arteries in congenital heart disease: A structure-function analysis. Cardiovasc Clin 1979; 10(1):489, with permission.

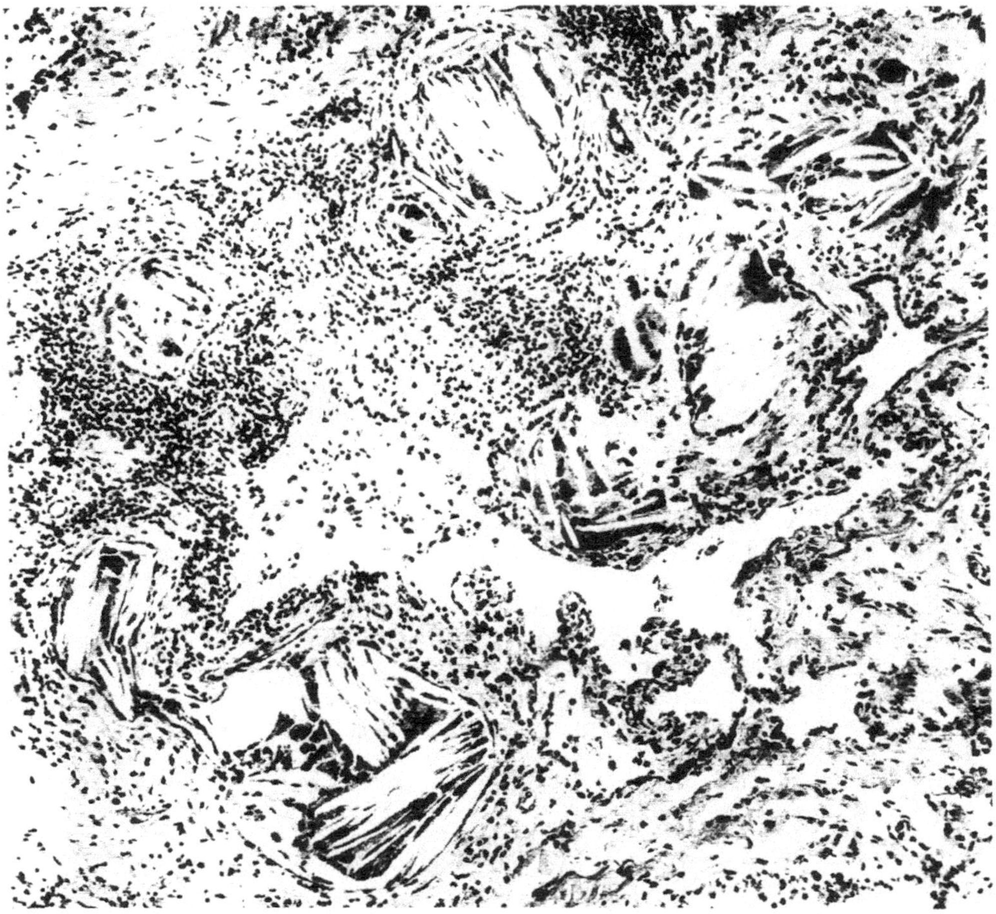

FIGURE 26. Multiple cholesterol-ester granulomas in the pulmonary parenchyma of a 38-year-old woman with ventricular septal defect and corrected transposition. She had severe pulmonary hypertension (83/20 mm Hg). Brachial arterial pressure was 102/65 mm Hg and the left-to-right shunt was 2.1:1. (Hematoxylin and eosin stain, × 82; reduced 30%.) From Virmani R, Roberts WC. Pulmonary arteries in congenital heart disease: A structure-function analysis. Cardiovasc Clin 1979; 10(1):490, with permission.

SIGNIFICANCE OF PULMONARY PARENCHYMAL CHOLESTEROL-ESTER GRANULOMAS

Among our 87 necropsy patients with various congenital cardiovascular malformations, 8 (11%) had pulmonary parenchymal cholesterol-ester granulomas (Table 13, Fig. 26). The cause of these granulomas is uncertain, but most patients who have them also have pulmonary hypertension.[77] We observed 13 necropsy patients with cholesterol-ester pulmonary granulomas (see Table 13): 11 had pulmonary arterial systolic pressures recorded, and these ranged from 50 to 138 mm Hg (mean 108 mm Hg). The other 2 patients have pulmonic stenosis and probably normal or only mildly elevated arterial pressures.

PULMONARY ARTERIAL HYPOTENSION

To this point we have discussed changes in pulmonary arteries primarily in patients with pulmonary *hyper*tension. Now we focus on patients with pulmonary arterial

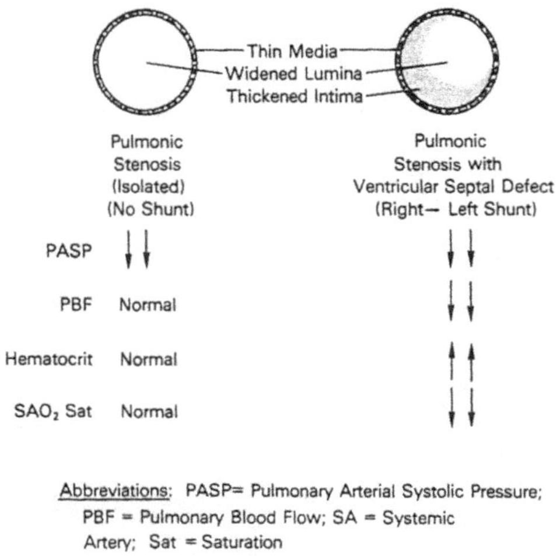

FIGURE 27. Diagram showing appearance of the pulmonary arteries in patients with pulmonary *hypo*tension. Patients with pulmonic stenosis have thinned media and wide lumina. If isolated, there is usually no thickening of the intima; but if pulmonic stenosis is combined with ventricular septal defect, the intima is usually thickened. From Virmani R, Roberts WC. Pulmonary arteries in congenital heart disease: A structure-function analysis. Cardiovasc Clin 1979; 10(1):490, with permission.

*hypo*tension. The media of the pulmonary arteries in the patients with chronic pulmonary hypertension is usually thicker than normal; the reverse is true in patients with chronic pulmonary hypotension in whom the media is thinner than normal. In addition, the lumens of these arteries, as well as those of the capillaries and pulmonary veins, are dilated.[45] The medial thinning and the luminal widening appear to be a consequence of the decreased pulmonary arterial pressure and not a consequence of decreased pulmonary arterial flow because these findings are present both in patients with isolated pulmonary stenosis (normal pulmonary flow) and in

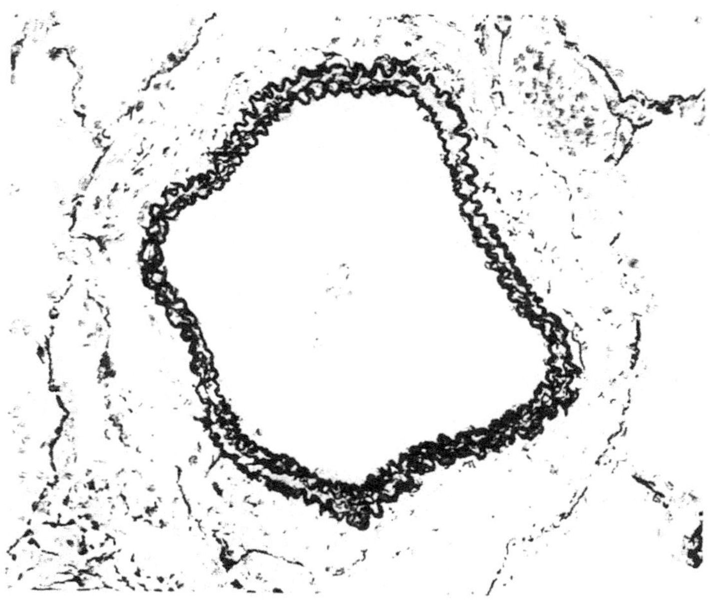

FIGURE 28. Pulmonic stenosis with atrial septal defect and anomalous drainage of the right pulmonary veins into the right atrium in a 19-year-old man who died three days after closure of the defect, pulmonic valvulotomy, and rerouting of the anomalous pulmonary veins. Preoperatively, pulmonary arterial pressure was 18/9 mm Hg (mean 15), right ventricular pressure was 78/6 mm Hg, brachial arterial pressure was 144/84 mm Hg (mean 100), pulmonary to systemic flow ratio was 1.6:1, and systemic arterial oxygen saturation was 97%. Pulmonary arteries in this patient had thin medial walls and no intimal thickening, changes typical of pulmonary *hypo*tension. (Elastic Van Gieson stain, × 272.) From Virmani R, Roberts WC. Pulmonary arteries in congenital heart disease: A structure-function analysis. Cardiovasc Clin 1979; 10(1):491, with permission.

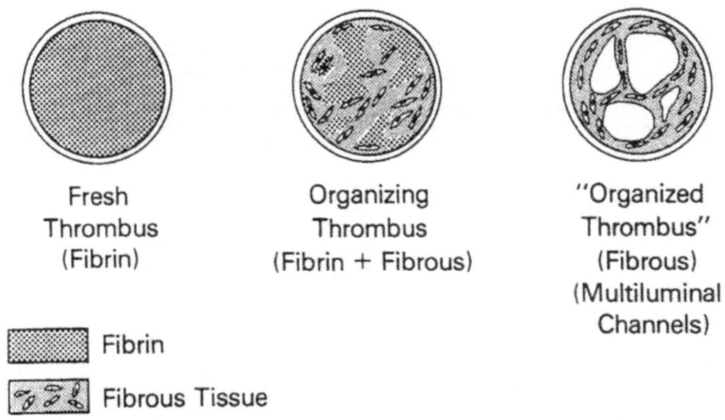

FIGURE 29. Diagram of Arnold Rich leisons occurring in patients with pulmonary hypotension and inadequate pulmonary blood flow. From Virmani R, Roberts WC. Pulmonary arteries in congenital heart disease: A structure-function analysis. Cardiovasc Clin 1979; 10(1):491, with permission.

patients with pulmonic stenosis associated with ventricular septal defect and right-to-left shunt (diminished pulmonary flow) (Figs. 27 and 28).

Another finding in some patients with pulmonary hypotension caused by congenital cardiovascular malformations is intimal fibrinous and fibrous changes. These intimal lesions were described initially by Arnold Rich[4] and are illustrated in Figure 29. Although pulmonary hypotension accompanies these lesions, it does not appear to be their cause. Evidence for this conclusion is provided by the fact that these lesions are rare in patients with pulmonic stenosis unassociated with communications between systemic and pulmonary circulations, but they are common in patients with pulmonic stenosis associated with ventricular septal defect and right-to-left shunts (Table 14). The cause for the intimal lesions, therefore, must be related to the decreased pulmonary blood flow and associated polycythemia. It is also possible that "sludging" of blood flowing through the pulmonary vascular bed plays a role. Our observations in necropsy patients over age 15 with pulmonic stenosis are summarized in Table 14.

TABLE 14. Observations in 9 Necropsy Patients Over Age 15 With Pulmonic Stenosis Associated With Either Patent Foramen Ovale or Ventricular Septal Defect

PATIENT AGE, SEX, ASSOCIATED DEFECT	PRESSURES (mm, Hg, s/d)			SA O_2 SAT. (%)	BLOOD HCT. (%)	OP	INTERVAL (DAYS) OP TO DEATH	PAs		
	PA	RV	SA					M	I	AR
28 F/PFO	9/4	170/4	123/70	67	61	PV	4	↓	nl	0
38 F/PFO						PV	60	↓	nl	0
43 F/PFO	13/8	172/12	130/70	83	65	PV	0	↓	↑	+
35 F/VSD	20/10	88/6		87	54	BT	21	↓	nl	0
22 M/VSD		145/9	148/105	88	71	0		↓	nl	0
53 M/VSD	17/8	95/8	110/65	77	69	TC	1	nl	↑	+
30 M/VSD	20/10	124/11	116/73	72	76	TC	45	↓	↑	+
23/M/VSD	12/4	112/4	131/85	68	72	TC	0	↓	↑	0
55 M/VSD	15/7	135/7	125/71	71	65	BT	6	↓	↑	0

AR = Arnold Rich lesions; Art = arterial; BT = Blalock-Taussig; Hct. = hematocrit; I = intima; nl = normal; M = media; OP = Cardiovascular operation; PA = pulmonary artery; PFO = patent foramen ovale; PV = pulmonic valvulotomy; RV = right ventricle; SA = systemic artery; Sat. = saturation; TC = total correction; ↓ = thinner than normal; ↑ = thickened; VSD = ventricular septal defect

From Virmani R, Roberts WC. Pulmonary arteries in congenital heart disease: A structure-function analysis. Cardiovasc Clin 1979; 10(1):492, with permission.

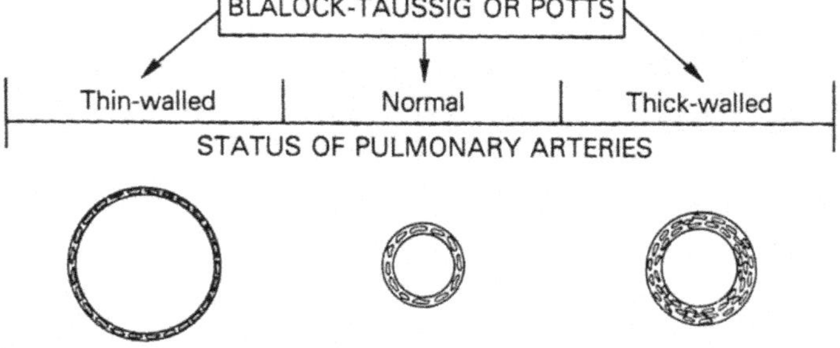

FIGURE 30. Diagram illustrating the effect of operative creation of systemic to pulmonary arterial communications on pulmonary arteries of patients wtih pulmonary *hypo*tension. The media of the pulmonary arteries may remain thin-walled and dilated (left), may increase to normal thickness (center), or may develop abnormally thickened media. From Virmani R, Roberts WC. Pulmonary arteries in congenital heart disease: A structure-function analysis. Cardiovasc Clin 1979; 10(1):492, with permission.

OPERATIVE CREATION OF SYSTEMIC-TO-PULMONIC ARTERIAL COMMUNICATIONS IN PATIENTS WITH PULMONARY HYPOTENSION

Although development of pulmonary arterial hypertension is a recognized complication of operative creation of pulmonary-to-systemic arterial anastomoses,[78–82] the actual occurrence of pulmonary hypertension is uncommon. Therefore, anatomic pulmonary arterial changes indicative of pulmonary hypertension are also uncommon (Figs. 30 through 33).

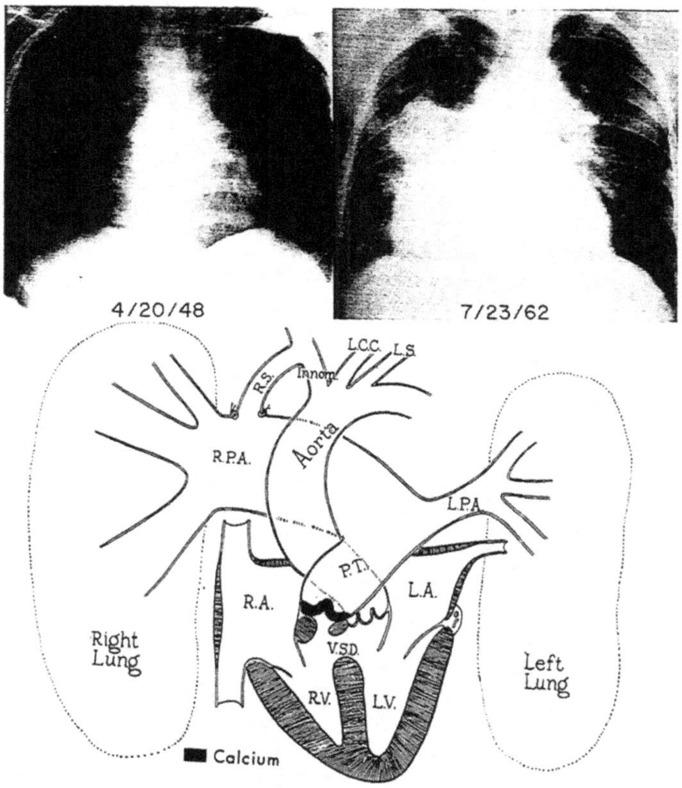

FIGURE 31. Tetralogy of Fallot in a 35-year-old man described in detail elsewhere.[81] By age 16 he was severely cyanotic and clubbed. Hemoglobin was 19.5 gm/100 ml. Chest radiograph (4/20/48) disclosed decreased pulmonary vascularity, and a subclavian-to-pulmonary arterial

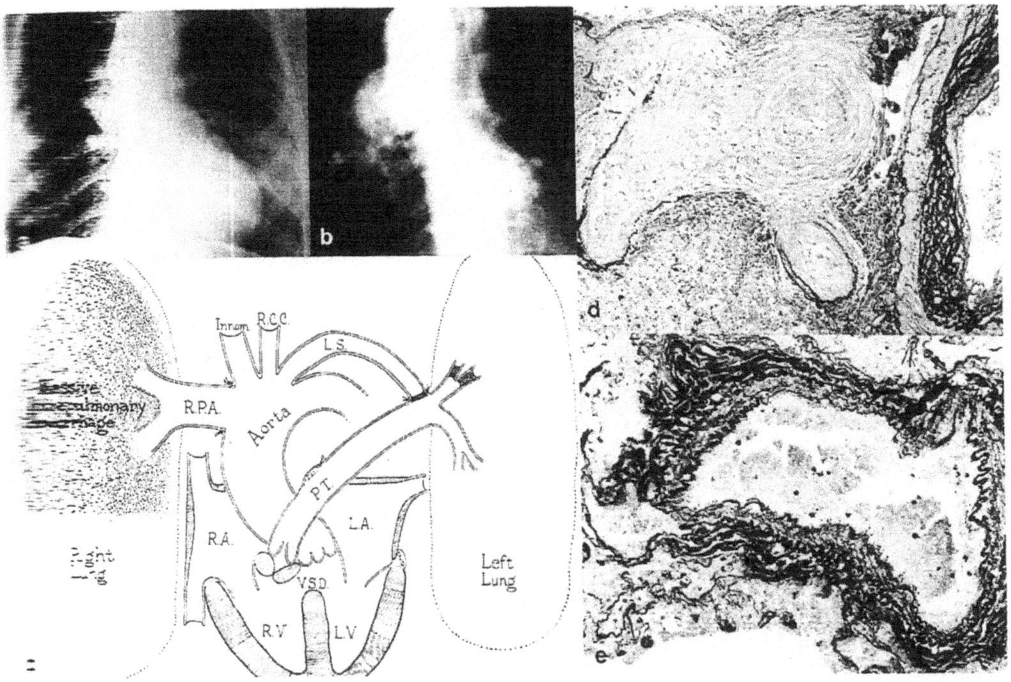

FIGURE 32. Tetralogy of Fallot in a 19-year-old woman described in detail elsewhere.[81] A left subclavian to left pulmonary arterial anastomosis was performed at age 3. There was little improvement, however, and an end-to-side anastomosis between aorta and right main pulmonary artery was performed 2 years later. She was nearly asymptomatic thereafter until age [illegible] when exercise tolerance diminished and cyanosis returned. At age 18 hematocrit was 80% a, Chest radiograph shows right aortic arch, decreased vascularity in the left lung, and increased vascular markings in the central portions of the right lung. The pulmonary trunk could not be entered by catheter from the right ventricle. Simultaneous right ventricular, femoral arterial, and right main pulmonary arterial systolic pressures were equal (108 mm Hg). Oxygen saturation in the femoral artery was 70%. *b*, At right ventricular angiography all contrast material was ejected into the aorta, and the lumens of the intrapulmonary branches of the right main pulmonary artery were severely narrowed. The left subclavian artery was occluded just proximal to its connection to the left main pulmonary artery. No contrast material entered the pulmonary trunk, left main pulmonary artery, or left lung. Because of systemic pressure in the right pulmonary arteries and absent blood flow to the left lung, the patient was considered inoperable. At age 19 she died suddenly of massive intrapulmonary hemorrhage. *c*, Diagram of findings in heart and lungs at necropsy (abbreviations in Fig. 31). *d*, A portion of wall of a right pulmonary artery. Arising from it (but not connected in this section) is a plexiform lesion. *e*, Left pulmonary artery is normal. (Elastic Van Gieson stain, × 160; reduced 41%). From Virmani R, Roberts WC. Pulmonary arteries in congenital heart disease: A structure-function analysis. Cardiovasc Clin 1979; 10(1):494, with permission.

---

anastomosis was performed. Postoperatively, exercise tolerance improved and cyanosis had disappeared. At age 26 he had the first of many episodes of rapid heart action; 3 years later a chest radiograph (7/23/62) showed aneurysmal dilatation of the right pulmonary artery; systemic blood pressure was 150/25 mm Hg. The patient died at age 35 of progressive right- and left-sided congestive heart failure. Shortly before death the hematocrit was 44%. The diagram of the heart and lungs at necropsy shows total obstruction of the pulmonic valve, ventricular septal defect (VSD), severely dilated pulmonary trunk (PT) and right main pulmonary artery (RPA), and widely patent right subclavian (RS) artery and anastomosis. LCC = left common carotid artery; LS = left subclavian artery; LPA = left pulmonary artery; LA = left atrium; LV = left ventricle; RA = right atrium; RV = right ventricle. Histologically, there was neither medial nor intimal thickening of the pulmonary arteries of either lung. From Virmani R, Roberts WC. Pulmonary arteries in congenital heart disease: A structure-function analysis. Cardiovasc Clin 1979; 10(1):493, with permission.

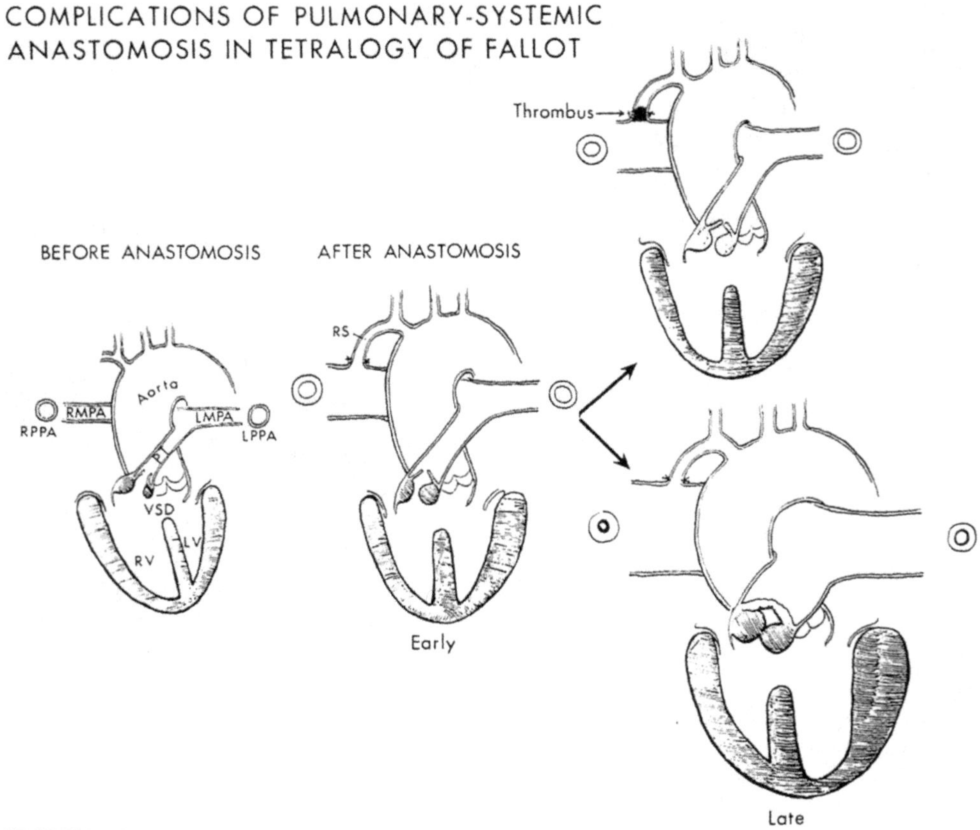

FIGURE 33. Diagram illustrating complications of pulmonary-systemic anastomosis in patients with tetralogy of Fallot. After anastomosis the early changes are related to the beneficial effects of increased blood flow to the lungs. With the shunt wide open, blood flow through the right ventricular outflow tract decreases and the amount of blood shunted from the right ventricular body to the left ventricle in diastole increases. As a result of the increased blood flow and pressure, the major pulmonary arteries widen and their wall thicknesses increase. Late complications include occlusion of the shunt and of the pulmonic valve or right ventricular infundibulum. LV = left ventricle; LPPA and RPPA = left and right peripheral pulmonary arteries; LMPA and RMPA = left and right main pulmonary arteries; RS = right subclavian artery; RV = right ventricle; VSD = ventricular septal defect. From Virmani R, Roberts WC. Pulmonary arteries in congenital heart disease: A structure-function analysis. Cardiovasc Clin 1979; 10(1):495, with permission.

Table 15 summarizes our observations in 10 necropsy patients over 15 years of age in whom pulmonary-to-systemic shunts had been created operatively between 3 and 23 years (mean 14 years) before death because of inadequate pulmonary blood flow. Nine patients had tetralogy of Fallot, and 1 had combined pulmonic stenosis and atrial septal defect. Surprisingly, 9 of the 10 patients showed neither pulmonary arterial or intimal thickening; 5 showed media of normal thickness and media thinner than normal. The 1 patient (see Table 15) who did have medial thickening also had plexiform lesions. This patient, reported elsewhere,[81] was the only 1 of the 10 patients who had a Potts[83] operation rather than a Blalock-Taussig[84] anastomosis. The anastomosis in her was an end-to-side connection between right pulmonary artery and aorta. The right lung consequently developed systemic pressures and plexiform lesions (see Fig. 32). It is now well appreciated that pulmonary hypertension and anatomic pulmonary arterial changes of pulmonary hypertension are far more likely to develop after Potts than after Blalock-Taussig anastomoses. The var-

TABLE 15. Observations in 10 Necropsy Patients Over Age 15 With Cyanotic CHD: Pulmonary Vascular Changes in Patients Having Operatively Created Systemic to Pulmonary Arterial Shunts for Inadequate Pulmonary Blood Flow (or Severe Systemic Arterial Desaturation)

PATIENT AGE, SEX	ANOMALIES	SA* O_2 SAT. (%)	RV PRESSURE (mm Hg, s/d) PRE-PO	PA PRESSURE (mm Hg, s/d) PRE-PO	SA PRESSURE (mm Hg, s/d) PRE-PO	TYPE OPERATIVE SHUNT CREATED	DIRECTION OF PO SHUNT R→L	DIRECTION OF PO SHUNT L→R	INTERVAL (YRS) OP-SHUNT TO DEATH	CAUSE OF DEATH/ STATUS OF OPERATIVE SHUNT	MORPHOLOGIC PULMONIC ARTERIAL CHANGES
19F	PS, VSD	70	NA-105/6	NA-108/78**	NA-108/78	(1)LSA→LPA (2)Ao→RPA	+	+	16 14	bleeding, lung/(1)C;(2)O	(1)H, (2)PL
35 M	PS, VSD		172/18-NA	20/10-NA	108/85-150/25	RSA→RPA	+	+	19	CHF/O	H, T
36M	PS, VSD		NA	NA	NA-104/63	Ao→LPA			20	reoperation	H, T
24 F	PS, VSD	89	NA-40/0	NA-14/4	NA-90/70	(1)RSA→RPA (2)RSA→RPA	+	0	18 23	reoperation/O↓↓	H
27 M	PS, VSD		NA	NA	NA	LSA→LPA	+	0	9	CHF/(1) + (2)O↓↓↓	H
21 M	PS, VSD, ASD, CT		NA	NA	NA-120/80	LSA→LPA	+	0	11	polycythemia/O↓↓↓	none
21 M	PS, VSD, CT	71	125/0-NA	NA	NA-125/80	(1)LSA→LPA (2)RSA→RPA	+	+	6 3	reoperation/(1)C, (2)O↓	(1)T, (2)none
33 M	PS, ASD	81	NA-130/10	NA	NA-80/55†	LSA→LPA	+	+	20	reoperation/O	none
27 M	PS, VSD, ASD, TA	88	NA	NA	NA-112/66	LSA→LPA	+	+	20	reoperation/O	none
22 F	PS, VSD	72	145/0-154/13	15/0-NA	120/65-196/75	LSA→LPA	+	0	8	reoperation C	none

*Last year of life

**Right pulmonary artery

†Left brachial artery; right femoral artery = 98/58

ASD = atrial septal defect; C = closed; CHF = congestive heart failure; CT = complete transposition; H = hypoplastic; LPA = left main pulmonary artery; LSA = left subclavian artery; NA = data not available; OP = cardiovascular operation; O = open; PA = pulmonary artery; PL = plexiform lesion + medial hypertrophy + intimal proliferation; PO = postoperative; PRE = preoperative; PS = pulmonic or subpulmonic stenosis; RPA = right pulmonary artery; RSA = right subclavian artery; RV = right ventricle; T = thrombi containing fibrin; TA = tricuspid atresia; SA = systemic artery; Sat. = saturation; s/d = systolic/diastolic; VSD = ventricular septal defect.

From Virmani R, Roberts WC. Pulmonary arteries in congenital heart disease: A structure-function analysis. Cardiovasc Clin 1979; 10(1):496, with permission.

ious changes may develop after creation of pulmonary-to-systemic anastomoses in patients with previous pulmonary hypotension are shown diagrammatically in Figure 33.

SUMMARY

Our 3-grade anatomic classification of pulmonary arterial changes for patients with pulmonary arterial hypertension is a modification of the classification of Heath and Edwards. Our new classification consists of medial thickening only, grade I; medial and intimal thickening, grade II; and both medial and intimal thickening plus plexiform lesions, grade III. These anatomic changes in the pulmonary arteries result entirely from pulmonary hypertension. Intimal thickening without medial thickening, however, is observed in older persons, and, in itself, is not a consequence of pulmonary hypertension.

Observations in our 87 necropsy patients over age 15 with major congenital cardiovascular malformations indicate that the changes in the pulmonary arteries are directly related to the level of pulmonary arterial pressure. Direction of the shunt, location of the shunt, and age of the patient were important only by their effect on the pulmonary arterial pressure. The patients with patent ductus arteriosus had the most severe changes in the pulmonary arteries and the highest average pulmonary arterial pressures.

Although not *all* patients with pulmonary arterial systolic pressures $>$ 90 mm Hg had them, plexiform lesions were observed only in patients in whom pulmonary artery systolic pressure was $>$ 90 mm Hg. Plexiform lesions indicate the irreversible nature of pulmonary hypertension and are more frequent in patients with primary pulmonary hypertension than in patients with congenital cardiovascular malformations.

The cause of plexiform lesions is unknown. We believe they are aneurysmal dilatations at sites of congenitally weak and/or thin walls of muscular pulmonary arteries. Distal to the weak or thin media, the lumen of the muscular artery is obliterated. The aneurysmal protrusion is filled with thrombus that organizes into multiluminal channels.

Cholesterol-ester granulomas in the lungs usually indicate the presence of pulmonary hypertension; their cause is also uncertain.

In patients with pulmonary *hypo*tension (isolated pulmonic stenosis) and in patients with pulmonic stenosis and ventricular septal defect (tetralogy of Fallot), the media of the pulmonary arteries is thinner than normal and the lumens are larger than normal. Intimal thickening is usually seen in patients with tetralogy of Fallot even though the media is not thickened.

Surgical creation of systemic-to-pulmonary arterial anastomoses may cause the pulmonary arterial media to thicken to normal widths or even to widths thicker than normal, but the development of pulmonary hypertension after such operations is infrequent.

REFERENCES

1. Moschcowitz E. Hypertension of the pulmonary circulation; its causes, dynamics and relation to other circulatory states. Am J Med Sci 1927; 174:388.
2. Brenner O. Pathology of the vessels of the pulmonary circulation. Arch Intern Med 1935; 56:211.

3. Parker F, Weiss S. The nature and significance of the structural changes in the lungs in mitral stenosis. Am J Pathol 1936; 12:573.
4. Rich AR. A hitherto unrecognized tendency to the development of widespread pulmonary vascular obstruction in patients with congenital pulmonary stenosis (tetralogy of Fallot). Bull Johns Hopkins Hosp 1948; 82:389.
5. Edwards JE, Douglas JM, Burchell HB, et al. Pathology of the intrapulmonary arteries and arterioles in coarctation of the aorta associated with patent ductus arteriosus. Am Heart J 1949; 38:208.
6. Civin WH, Edwards JE. Pathology of the pulmonary vascular tree. I. A comparison of intrapulmonary arteries in the Eisenmenger complex and in stenosis of ostium infundibuli associated with biventricular origin of the aorta. Circulation 1950; 21:545.
7. Heath D, Witaker W. The pulmonary vessels in patent ductus arteriosus. J Pathol Bacteriol 1955; 70:285.
8. Brewer DB. Fibrous occlusion and anastomosis of the pulmonary vessels in a case of pulmonary hypertension associated with patent ductus arteriosus. J Pathol Bacteriol 1955; 70:299.
9. Dammann JF, Ferencz C. The significance of the pulmonary vascular bed in congenital heart disease. I. Normal lungs. II. Malformation of the heart in which there is pulmonary stenosis. Am Heart J 1956; 52:7.
10. Dammann JF Jr, Ferencz C. The significance of pulmonary vascular bed in congenital heart disease. III. Defects between the ventricles or great vessels in which both increased pressure and blood flow may act upon the lungs in which there is a common ejectile force. Am Heart J 1956; 52:210.
11. Edwards JE. Functional pathology of the pulmonary vascular tree in congenital cardiac disease. Circulation 1957; 15:164.
12. Heath D, Dushane JW, Wood EH, et al. The etiology of pulmonary thrombosis in cyanotic congenital heart disease with pulmonary stenosis. Thorax 1958; 13:213.
13. Heath D, Edwards JE. The pathology of hypertensive pulmonary vascular disease. A description of six grades of structural changes in the pulmonary arteries with special reference to congenital cardiac defects. Circulation 1958; 18:533.
14. Heath D, Helmholz HF, Burchell HB, et al. Graded pulmonary vascular changes and hemodynamic findings in cases of atrial and ventricular septal defect and patent ductus arteriosus. Circulation 1958; 18:1155.
15. Heath D, Helmholtz HF, Burchell HB, et al. Relation between structural changes in the small pulmonary arteries and the immediate reversibility of pulmonary hypertension following closure of ventricular and atrial septal defects. Circulation 1958; 18:1167.
16. Wagenvoort CA. The morphology of certain vascular lesions in pulmonary hypertension. J Pathol Bacteriol 1959; 78:503.
17. Ferencz C. The pulmonary vascular bed in tetralogy of Fallot. I. Changes associated with pulmonic stenosis. Bull Johns Hopkins Hosp. 1960; 106:81.
18. Ferencz C. The pulmonary vascular bed in tetralogy of Fallot. II. Changes following a systemic-pulmonary arterial anastomosis. Bull Johns Hopkins Hosp 1960; 106:100.
19. Heath D. Pathology of the pulmonary vessels. Br J Dis Chest 1960; 54:182.
20. Wagenvoort CA, Dushane JW, Edwards JE. Hypertensive pulmonary arterial lesions as a result of anastomosis of systemic and pulmonary circulations. May Clin Proc 1960; 5:186.
21. Naeye RL. Perinatal changes in the pulmonary vascular bed with stenosis and atresia of the pulmonic valve. Am Heart J 1961; 61:586.
22. Wagenvoort CA, Neufeld HN, Dushane JW, et al. The pulmonary arterial tree in ventricular septal defect. A quantitative study of anatomic features in fetuses, infants, and children. Circulation 1961; 23:740.
23. Wagenvoort CA, Edwards JE. The pulmonary arterial tree in pulmonic atresia. Arch Pathol 1961; 71:646.
24. Wagenvoort CA. Pulmonary arteries in infants with ventricular septal defect. Med Thorac 1962; 19:354.
25. Harris P, Heath D. The Human Pulmonary Circulation. Its Forms and Functions in Health and Disease. London: E & S Livingstone, 1962.
26. Thomas MA. Pulmonary vascular changes in pulmonary stenosis with and without ventricular septal defect. Br Heart J 1964; 26:655.
27. Ferencz C. Pulmonary vascular changes in tetralogy of Fallot. Dis Chest 1964; 46:664.
28. Wagenvoort CA, Heath D, Edwards JE. The Pathology of the Pulmonary Vasculature. Springfield, Ill: Charles C Thomas, 1964.

29. Thomas MA. Pulmonary vascular changes in pulmonary stenosis with and without ventricular septal defect. Br Heart J 1964; 26:655.
30. Kanjuh VI, Sellers RD, Edwards JE. Pulmonary vascular plexiform lesion. Arch Pathol 1964; 78:513.
31. Ferencz C. Transposition of the great vessels: pathophysiologic consideration based upon a study of the lungs. Circulation 1966; 33:232.
32. Anderson RA, Levy AM, Naeye RL, et al. Rapidly progressive pulmonary vascular obstructive disease. Association with ventricular septal defects during early childhood. Am J Cardiol 1967; 19:854.
33. Wagenvoort CA, Nauta J, Van Der Schaar PJ, et al. Effect of flow and pressure on pulmonary vessels. A semiquantitative study based on lung biopsies. Circulation 1967; 35:1028.
34. Wagenvoort CA, Nauta J, Van Der Scharr PJ, et al. Vascular changes in pulmonic stenosis and tetralogy of Fallot studied in lung biopsies. Circulation 1967; 36:624.
35. Wagenvoort CA, Nauta J, Van Der Schaar PJ, et al. The pulmonary vasculature in complete transposition of the great vessels judged from lung biopsies. Circulation 1968; 38:746.
36. Viles PH, Ongley PA, Titus JL. The spectrum of pulmonary vascular disease in transposition of the great arteries. Circulation 1969; 40:31.
37. Wagenvoort CA. Hypertensive pulmonary vascular disease complicating congenital heart disease: A review. Cardiovasc Clin 1973; 5:43.
38. Hislop A, Reid L. Structural changes in the pulmonary arteries and veins in tetralogy of Fallot. Br Heart J 1973; 35:1178.
39. Newfeld EA, Paul MH, Muster AJ, et al. Pulmonary vascular disease in complete transposition of the great arteries: A study of 200 patients. Am J Cardiol 1974, 34:75.
40. Wagenvoort CA. Classification of pulmonary vascular lesions in congenital and acquired heart disease. Adv Cardiol 1974; 11:48.
41. Wagenvoort CA, Wagenvoort N. Pathology of the Eisenmenger syndrome and primary pulmonary hypertension. Adv Cardiol 1974; 11:123.
42. Hoffmeister HE, Apitz J, Backmann R. The correlation between pulmonary hypertension and histological findings of the pulmonary vessels in congenital heart disease. Thoraxchir Vask Chir 1975; 23:436.
43. Bessinger FB, Blieden LC, Edwards JE: Hypertensive pulmonary vascular disease associated with patent ductus arteriosus. Primary or secondary? Circulation 1975; 52:157.
44. Newfeld EA, Sher M, Paul MH, et al. Pulmonary vascular disease in complete artrioventricular canal defect. Am J Cardiol 1977; 39:721.
45. Wagenvoort CA, Wagenvoort N. Pathology of Pulmonary Hypertension. New York: John Wiley & Sons, 1977.
46. Davies G, Reid L. Growth of the alveoli and pulmonary arteries in childhood. Thorax 1970; 25:669.
47. Hislop A, Reid L. Pulmonary arterial development during childhood: branching pattern and structure. Thorax 1973; 28:129.
48. Rabinovitch M, Haworth S, Castaneda AR, Nadas AS, et al. Lung biopsy in congenital heart disease: a morphometric approach to pulmonary vascular disease. Circulation 1978; 58:1107.
49. Murphy JD, Rabinovitch M, Goldstein JD, et al. The structural basis of persistent pulmonary hypertension of the newborn infant. J Pediatr 1981; 98:962.
50. Rabinovitch M, Haworth S, Vance Z, et al. Early pulmonary vascular changes in congenital heart disease studied in biopsy tissue. Hum Pathol 1980; 11:499.
51. Meyrick B, Reid L. Pulmonary hypertension: anatomic and physiologic correlates. Clinics in Chest Medicine 1983; 4(2):199.
52. Civin WH, Edwards JE. The postnatal structural changes in the intrapulmonary arteries and arterioles. Arch Pathol 1951; 51:192.
53. Wagenvoort CA, Wagenvoort N. Age changes in muscular pulmonary arteries. Arch Pathol 1965; 79:524.
54. Heath D, Smith P. Electron microscopy of hypertensive vascular disease. Br J Dis Chest 1983; 77:1.
55. Roberts WC, Frederickson DS. Gaucher's disease of the lung causing severe pulmonary hypertension with associated acute recurrent pericarditis. Circulation 1967; 35:783.
56. Spencer H. Primary pulmonary hypertension and related vascular changes in the lungs. J Pathol Bacteriol 1950; 62:75.

57. Gordon AJ, Donoso E, Kuhn CLA, et al. Patent ductus arteriosus with reversal of flow. N Engl J Med 1954; 251:923.
58. Hufner RF, McNicol CA. The pathologic physiology of microscopic pulmonary vascular shunts. AMA Arch Pathol 1958; 65:554.
59. Rossall RE, Thompson H. Formation of new vascular channels in the lungs of a patient with secondary pulmonary hypertension. J Pathol Bacteriol 1958; 76:593.
60. Plant A. Hemangioendothelioma of the lung. Report of two cases. Arch Pathol 1940; 29:517.
61. Moschcowitz E, Rubin E, Strauss L. Hypertension of the pulmonary circulation due to congenital glomoid obstruction of the pulmonary arteries. Am J Pathol 1961; 39:75.
62. Cross KR, Kobayashi CK. Primary pulmonary vascular sclerosis: Report of a case. Am J Clin Pathol 1947; 17:155.
63. Hruban Z, Humphreys EM. Congenital anomalies associated with pulmonary hypertension in an infant. Arch Pathol 1960; 70:766.
64. Naeye RL, Vennart GP. Structure and significance of pulmonary plexiform structures. Am J Pathol 1960; 36:593.
65. Kapanci Y. Hypertensive pulmonary vascular disease. Endothelial hyperplasia and its relations to intravascular fibrin precipitation. Am J Pathol 1965; 48:665.
66. Haworth SG. Pulmonary vascular disease in secundum atrial septal defect in childhood. Am J Cardiol 1983; 51:265.
67. Warnes CA, Boger JE, Roberts WC. Eisenmenger ventricular septal defect with prolonged survival. Am J Cardiol 1984; 54:460.
68. McManus BM, Hahn PF, Smith JA, et al. Eisenmenger ductus arteriosus with prolonged survival. Am J Cardiol 1984; 54:462.
69. Mooi W, Wagenvoort CA. Decreased numbers of pulmonary blood vessels: reality or artifact? J Pathol 1983; 141:411.
70. Takahashi T, Wagenvoort CA. Density of muscularized arteries in the lung: Its role in congenital heart disease and its clinical significance. Arch Pathol Lab Med 1983; 107:23.
71. Yamaki S, Tezuka F. Quantitative analysis of pulmonary vascular disease in complete transposition of the great arteries. Circulation 1976; 54:805.
72. Yamaki S, Horiuchi T. Quantitative analysis of postoperative changes of pulmonary artery in patients with complete transposition of the great arteries and pulmonary hypertension. Am J Cardiol 1979; 44:284.
73. Walcott G, Burchell HB, Brown AL. Primary pulmonary hypertension. Am J Med 1970; 49:70.
74. Wagenvoort CA, Wagenvoort N. Primary pulmonary hypertension. A patholytic study of the lung vessels in 156 clinically diagnosed cases. Circulation 1970; 42:1163.
75. Bjornsson J, Edwards WD. Primary pulmonary hypertension: a histopathologic study of 80 cases. Mayo Clin Proc 1985; 60:16.
76. Virmani R, Robinowitz M, McAllister HA Jr. Primary pulmonary hypertension: quantitation of the size of plexiform lesions with uniformity in size irrespective of age. Lab Invest 1980; 42:61.
77. Glancy DL, Frazier PD, Roberts WC. Pulmonary parenchymal cholesterol-ester granulomas in patients with pulmonary hypertension. Am J Med 1968; 45:198.
78. Ross RS, Taussig HB, Evans MH. Late hemodynamic complications of anastomotic surgery for the treatment of the tetralogy of Fallot. Circulation 1958; 18:553.
79. Paul MH, Miller RA, Potts WJ. Long-term results of aortic-pulmonary anastomosis for tetralogy of Fallot: An analysis of the first 100 cases eleven to thirteen years after operation. Circulation 1961; 23:525.
80. McCagg CJ, Ross RS, Braunwald E. The development of elevated pulmonary vascular resistance in man following increased pulmonary blood flow from systemic pulmonary anastomoses. Am J Med 1962; 33:201.
81. Roberts WC, Friesinger GC, Cohen LS, et al. Acquired pulmonic atresia. Total obstruction to right ventricular outflow after systemic to pulmonary arterial anastomoses for cyanotic congenital cardiac disease. Am J Cardiol 1969; 24:335.
82. Newfeld EA, Waldman JD, Paul MH, et al. Pulmonary vascular disease after systemic-pulmonary arterial shunt operations. Am J Cardiol 1977; 39:715.
83. Potts WJ, Smith S, Gibson S. Anastomosis of the aorta to a pulmonary artery. Certain types in congenital heart disease. JAMA 1946; 132:627.
84. Blalock A, Taussig HB. Surgical treatment of malformations of the heart in which there is a pulmonary stenosis or pulmonary atresia. JAMA 1945; 128:189.

85. Heath D, Dushane JW, Wood EH, et al. The structure of the pulmonary trunk at different ages and in cases of pulmonary hypertension and pulmonary stenosis. J Pathol Bacteriol 1959; 77:443.
86. Perloff JK, Urschell CW, Roberts WC, et al. Aneurysmal dilatation of the coronary arteries in cyanotic congenital cardiac disease. Am J Med 1968; 45:802.
87. Glancy DL, Roberts WC. Congenital obstructive lesions involving the major pulmonary veins, left atrium, or mitral valve: A clinical, laboratory, and morphologic survey. Cathet Cardiovasc Diagn 1976; 2:215.
88. Parker F Jr, Weiss S. The nature and significance of the structural changes in the lungs in mitral stenosis. Am J Pathol 1936; 12:573.
89. Heath D, Whitaker W. The pulmonary vessels in mitral stenosis. J Pathol Bacteriol 1955; 70:291.
90. Aber CP, Campbell JA, Meecham J. Arterial patterns in mitral stenosis. Br Heart J 1963; 25:109.
91. Tandon HD, Kasturi J. Pulmonary vascular changes associated with isolated mitral stenosis in India. Br Heart J 1975; 37:26.
92. Kingdon HS, Cohen LS, Roberts WC, et al. Familial occurrence of primary pulmonary hypertension. Arch Intern Med 1966; 118:422.

Hemodynamic Confirmation of Peripheral Pulmonary Stenosis Caused by Aortic Dissection

William C. Roberts, MD, Lowell F. Satler, MD,
and Robert B. Wallace, MD

In aortic dissection, the intimal and medial tear most commonly is located in the ascending aorta. The dissecting channel is located in the outer one half or the outer one third of the aortic media.[1] As a consequence, the thickness of the medial wall separating the true and false channels is always greater than the thickness of the medial wall forming the outer wall of the false channel. Because the outer medial wall of the false channel is thin and the thinned wall is subjected to a systemic intra-aortic pressure, additional tearing of the media of the outer wall commonly occurs in the vicinity of the initial intimal-medial aortic tear. The further tearing of the outer aortic wall may lead to extravasation of intra-aortic blood into the adventitia of the

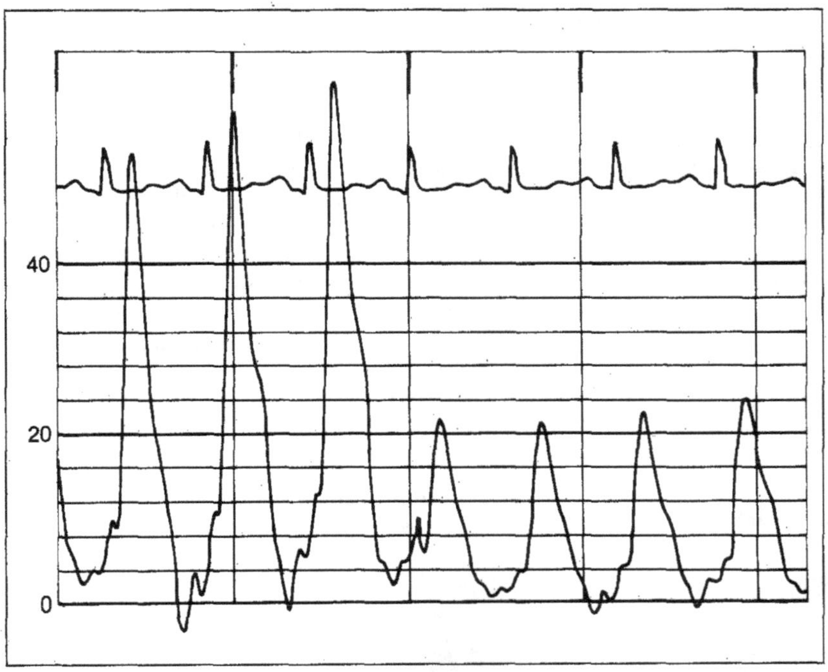

FIGURE 1. Pressure tracing with catheter tip in right ventricular cavity (*left*) and in pulmonary arterial lumen (*right*) immediately before operation. The peak systolic pressure gradient is approximately 25 mm Hg.

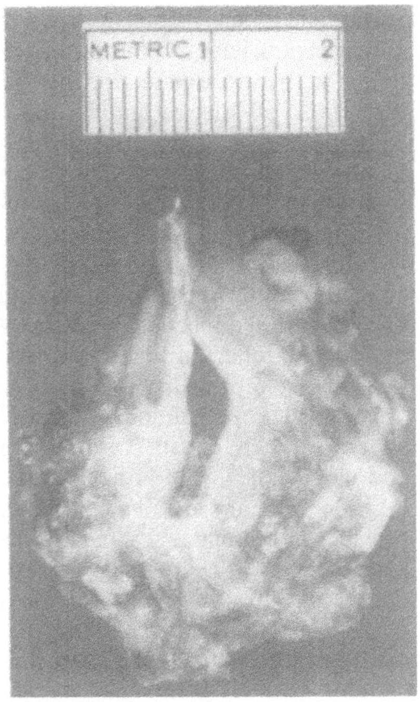

FIGURE 2. Operatively excised, heavily calcified, severely stenotic, unicuspid aortic valve.

From the Pathology Branch, National Heart, Lung, and Blood Institute, National Institutes of Health, Bethesda, Maryland 20892, and the Division of Cardiology, Department of Medicine, and Department of Surgery, Georgetown University Medical Center, Washington, DC.
Manuscript received February 6, 1989; revised manuscript received and accepted March 13, 1989.

aorta. The ascending aorta and pulmonary trunk have a common adventitia, and therefore dissection into the adventitia of the ascending aorta commonly extends into the adventitia of the pulmonary trunk and from there into the right and left main pulmonary arteries and their branches. Because the intraluminal pulmonary arterial pressure is relatively low and the adventitial dissection in both aorta and pulmonary arteries is driven by a systemic pressure, the extravasated blood in the pulmonary arterial adventitia can cause compression and narrowing of the lumens of the major pulmonary arteries. Although peripheral pulmonary stenosis has been observed at necropsy as a consequence of adventitia dissection from initial aortic medial dissection, hemodynamic proof of peripheral pulmonary stenosis from this mechanism has not been reported. Such is the purpose of this report.

W.D., a 45-year-old white male roofer, was well until about 60 hours before death when he developed substernal chest pain that radiated into his neck while sitting drinking a beer. Shortly thereafter he began sweating profusely and when he stood up he fainted. He was taken to a local hospital. On examination, a grade 4/6 systolic ejection murmur was heard over the precordium, loudest in the second right intercostal space, with radiation into the neck. Because of intermittent persistence of the chest pain, he was transferred to Georgetown University Hospital 24 hours before death. The chest pain had worsened, but repeated electrocardiograms did not disclose evidence of myocardial ischemia. Doppler echocardiogram showed a peak systolic pressure gradient across the aortic valve of approximately 80 mm Hg. Cardiac catheterization disclosed a 25-mm Hg peak systolic pressure gradient between right ventricle and an intrapulmonary pulmonary artery (Figure 1). The mean pulmonary artery wedge pressure was 10 mm Hg. On retrograde aortic catheterization, the stenotic aortic valve could not be crossed by the catheter and neither coronary ostium could be entered. Injection of contrast material into the ascending aorta disclosed true and false aortic lumens. Because of severe hypotension an aortic balloon pump was inserted and the patient was taken to the operating room. After median sternotomy and incision of the parietal pericardium, blood was found in the pericardial sac. The outer wall of the entire ascending aorta, pulmonary trunk and main right and left main pulmonary arteries was found to be bloody, the consequence of dissection into their adventitia. The ascending aorta measured about 10 cm in diameter. After institution of cardiopulmonary bypass, the ascending aorta was incised and thrombus was found in the false lumen. The entrance tear was located about 2 cm cephalad to the aortic valve, which was severely stenotic, heavily calcified and unicuspid (Figure 2). The aortic valve and a portion of ascending aorta were excised and replaced with a woven Dacron conduit containing a mechanical valve. The portions of aorta containing the ostia of the right and left main coronary artery were inserted into the Dacron graft. Attempts to separate

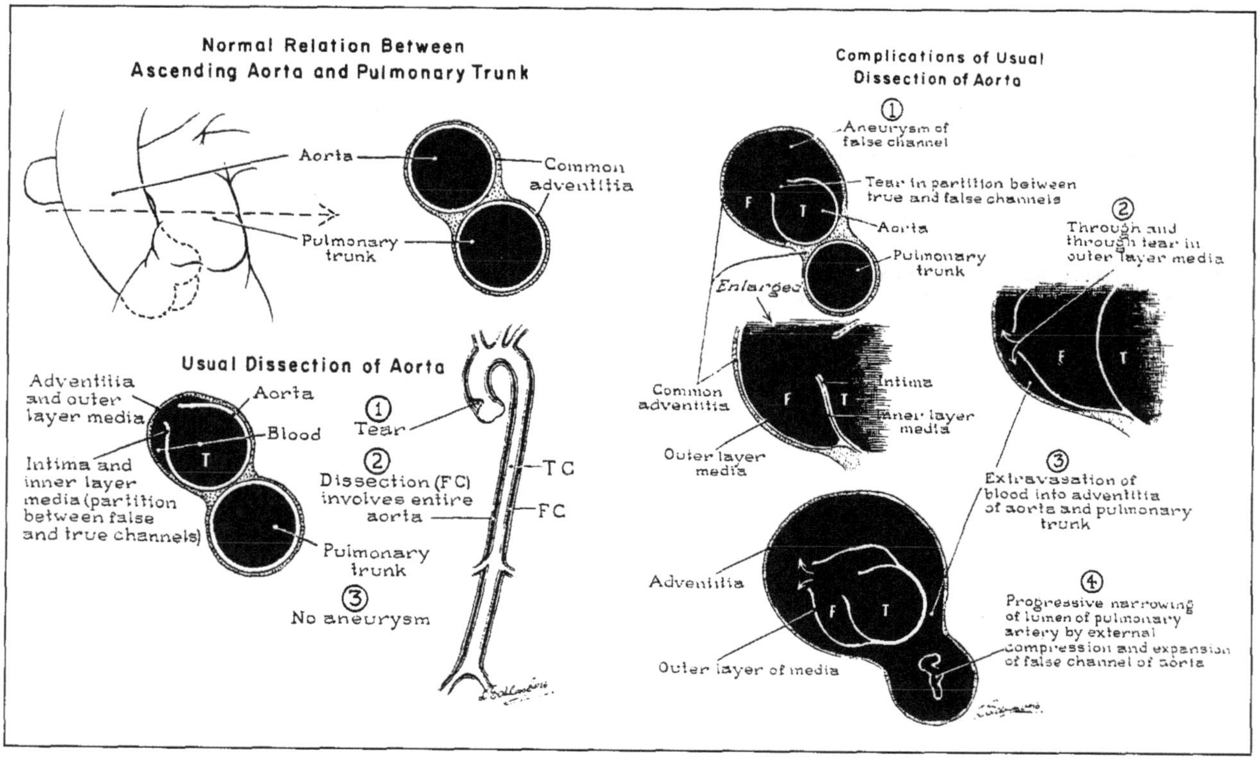

FIGURE 3. The relation between the adventitia of the ascending aorta and pulmonary trunk, the usual aortic dissection and a major complication of aortic dissection, namely adventitial pulmonary dissection with pulmonary arterial narrowing. Reproduced with permission from Roberts WC.[1]

the patient from cardiopulmonary bypass were unsuccessful.

The presence of firm infiltrates of blood in the adventitia of the major pulmonary arteries as observed at operation is strong evidence that the right ventricular outflow obstruction observed at cardiac catheterization preoperatively in this patient was the consequence of luminal compression by adventitial blood by the mechanism illustrated in Figure 3. Although suspected from anatomic studies previously,[1,2] hemodynamic confirmation of peripheral pulmonic stenosis from complications of aortic dissection has not been demonstrated previously.

1. Roberts WC. Aortic dissection: anatomy, consequences, and causes. *Am Heart J 1981;101:195–214.*
2. Buja LM, Ali N, Fletcher RD, Roberts WC. Stenosis of the right pulmonary artery: a complication of acute dissecting aneurysm of the ascending aorta. *Am Heart J 1972;83:89–92.*

Huge, Unattached Left Atrial Thrombus in Mitral Stenosis

C. S. Roberts, M.D., W. C. Roberts, M.D.

Surgery and Pathology Branches, National Heart, Lung, and Blood Institute, National Institutes of Health, Bethesda, Maryland, USA

Summary: We describe certain clinical and morphologic findings in a 75-year-old woman in whom a large, spherical, nonadherent, clinically undetected thrombus developed in the left atrium in association with mitral stenosis.

Key words: left atrial thrombus, mitral stenosis, atrial fibrillation, abdominal aortic aneurysm

Introduction

While thrombus isolated to the appendage of the left atrium is common, its presence in the body of the left atrium is infrequent, occurring nearly always in association with mitral stenosis. When thrombus is located in the body of the left atrium and attached to its mural endocardium, similar attached thrombus is virtually always present in the appendage. Nonadherent thrombus in the body of the left atrium is rare, and when it occurs, thrombus is usually absent in the appendage. Wood,[1] in 1814, observed at necropsy an unattached, spherical thrombus in the left atrial body of a 15-year-old girl with mitral stenosis. Abramson,[2] in 1924, found 19 reported necropsy cases aged 15 to 49 years (mean 36) of unattached left atrial thrombus and all 19 patients had associated mitral stenosis. In the last 35 years, only 3 cases of unattached left atrial body thrombus observed at necropsy have been reported. In 1955, Read and associates[3] described a 62-year-old man with a spherical 5 cm left atrial thrombus without associated mitral stenosis. In 1976, Lie and Entman[4] described an 83-year-old woman with a 3.8 cm spherical left atrial thrombus with associated mitral stenosis. In 1981, Söogaard[5] reported a 76-year-old woman with a 4.5 cm left atrial thrombus without associated mitral stenosis. The rarity of unattached left atrial body thrombus prompted the present report.

Address for reprints:

Charles Stewart Roberts, M.D.
Surgery Branch
National Heart, Lung and Blood Institute
National Institutes of Health
Bethesda, MD 20892, USA

Received: November 7, 1989
Accepted with revision: January 2, 1990

Case Report

LC, a 75-year-old white woman, who had acute rheumatic fever at age 20 years, was well until age 60 when atrial fibrillation and systemic hypertension were detected. Soon thereafter she had a stroke, resulting in permanent right hemiplegia. At age 75 she had acute onset of aphasia. On examination the next day, she was obese and semiconscious (responded only to painful stimuli). Blood pressure was 140/90 mmHg and arterial pulse was 100 beats/min. A grade 1/6 systolic precordial murmur was recorded. No diastolic precordial murmur was described. The patient's legs were cool and pale and no femoral, popliteal, dorsalis pedal, or posterior tibial arterial pulses were palpated. The electrocardiogram showed atrial flutter with 2:1 atrioventricular block, left anterior hemiblock, and nonspecific ST-segment changes. Translumbar aortogram showed near complete occlusion of the aorta at the level of the renal arteries and distally. She was anuric and acidotic. Bilateral femoral endarterectomy was performed and peritoneal dialysis started, but she died 6 days later.

At necropsy, the heart weighted 500 g. Both atria were dilated. The myocardium was free of grossly visible foci of necrosis or fibrosis. The tricuspid, pulmonic, and aortic valves were normal. The mitral leaflets and chordae

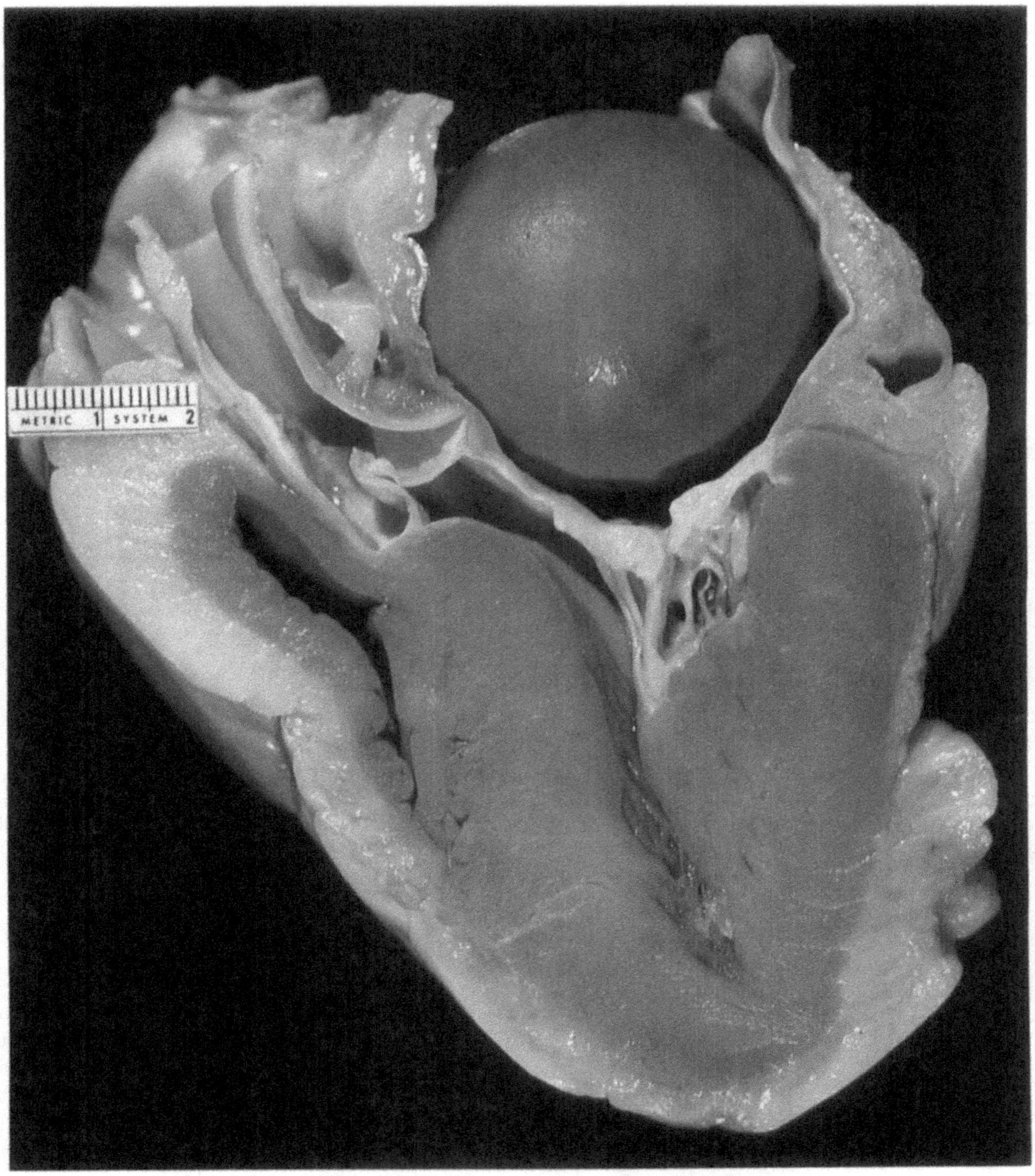

FIG. 1. Longitudinal view of heart showing the large unattached, smooth-surfaced thrombus in the left atrial chamber and a stenotic mitral valve. The left ventricular cavity is not dilated but its wall is thicker than normal.

tendineae were diffusely fibrotic and the mitral orifice was severely stenotic (Figs. 1, 2). The body of the left atrium contained a nonadherent, smooth-surfaced, spherical thrombus weighing 53 g and measuring 4.6 cm in diameter. The abdominal aorta was severely atherosclerotic and aneurysmal, and its lumen was filled with thrombus which obstructed the ostia of both renal arteries, the inferior mesenteric artery, and both common iliac arteries (Fig. 3). Both kidneys had multiple cortical infarcts. An old infarct was found in the left cerebral hemisphere. (It is likely that the thrombi in these various systemic arteries were not embolic in nature.)

Discussion

The most unusual features of the aforementioned patient are the huge size of the left atrial thrombus and its

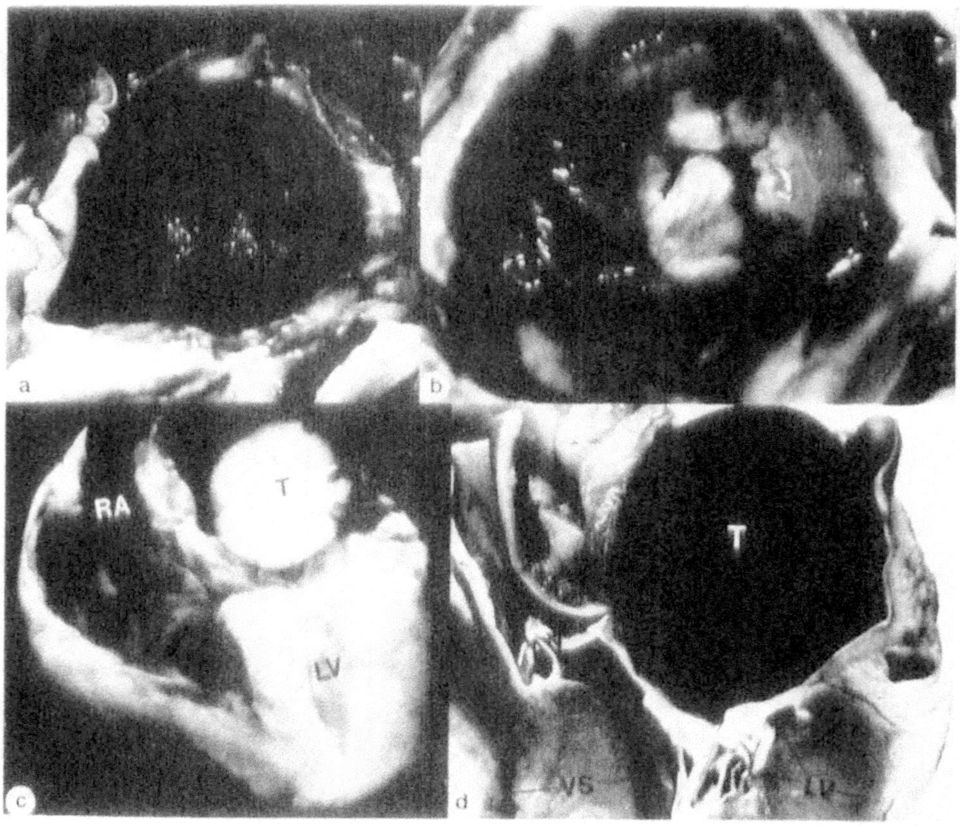

FIG. 2. (A) View of thrombus from above after incising the wall from a right pulmonary vein to a left pulmonary vein. (B) View of opened left atrium from above after removing the thrombus. The valve is stenotic and the mural endocardium is smooth. (C) Radiograph of the heart at necropsy showing the four chambers and the left atrial thrombus. RA = right atrial cavity; RV = right ventricular cavity; T = thrombus. (D) Longitudinal view of left side of the heart after cutting the thrombus in half. The thrombus histologically consisted virtually entirely of fibrin. Ao = aorta; LV = left ventricular wall; VS = ventricular septum.

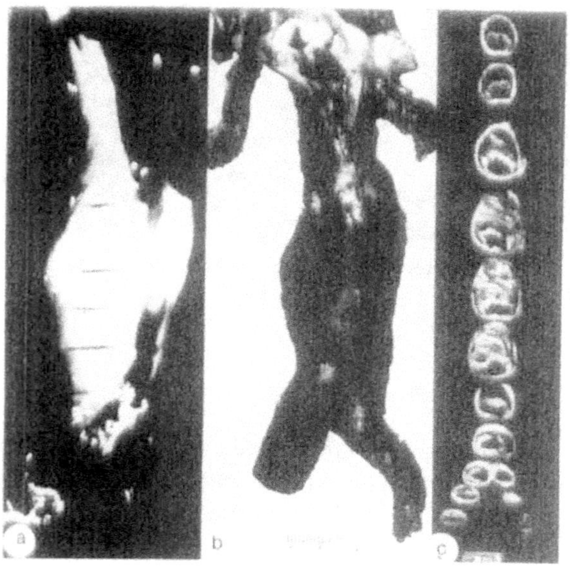

FIG. 3. Abdominal aorta. (A) Radiograph of the abdominal aorta showing an aneurysm, intraaneurysmal thrombus-narrowed lumen, and calcific deposits. (B) Abdominal aorta itself. (C) Transverse sections of the abdominal aorta showing the narrowed lumen due entirely to thrombus.

nonadherence to left atrial endocardium. There were no left atrial endocardial lesions to suggest that the thrombus had at one time been attached. We have never observed thrombus in the body of left atrium, in contrast to that in appendage only, without associated mitral stenosis, but most thrombi in this chamber, of course, are attached to its mural endocardium. How the left atrial thrombus in the present patient could have developed to such a large size without its ever having become attached is unknown.

References

1. Wood W: Letter enclosing the history and dissection of a case in which a foreign body was found within the heart. *Edinburgh Med Surg J* 10, 50 (1814)
2. Abramson JL: Ball thrombi of the heart. *Ann Clin Med* 3, 327 (1924)
3. Read JL, Porter RR, Russi S, Kriz JR: Occlusive avricular thrombi. *Circulation* 12, 250 (1955)
4. Lie JT, Entman ML: "Hole-in-one" sudden death: Mitral stenosis and left atrial ball thrombus. *Am Heart J* 91, 798 (1976)
5. Söogaard PE: Free ball thrombus of the left atrium. *Eur J Cardiol* 12, 177 (1981)

Primary Sarcoma of the Heart Causing Mitral Stenosis

Michael J. Domanski, MD, Thomas F. Delaney, MD, David E. Kleiner, Jr., MD, Mary Goswitz, MD, Arthur Agatston, MD, Eben Tucker, MD, Michael Johnson, MD, and William C. Roberts, MD

Cardiac sarcomas are rare and mitral stenosis caused by this neoplasm in the left atrium is even rarer. Such was the case, however, in the patient to be described herein.

A 46-year-old woman (CC no. 22-72-58-1) who died on January 7, 1990, had been well until April 1989, when she had an episode of dizziness and right eye blindness that resolved spontaneously. In June 1989, she had a transient episode of right lower arm numbness and right eye blindness that resolved spontaneously. In September 1989, she developed orthopnea, dyspnea with walking, syncope and easy fatigability. In October 1989, examination by a cardiologist disclosed a loud first heart sound, a grade 1/6 systolic ejection murmur at the left sternal border and apex that radiated into the axilla and a grade 2/6 systolic murmur at the right sternal border that increased with inspiration. Chest radiograph suggested a dilated left atrium and was consistent with congestive heart failure. An echocardiogram disclosed severe mitral stenosis, mild mitral regurgitation, a dilated right atrium and right ventricle, pericardial effusion and a large mass in the region of the posterior mitral leaflet protruding into and obstructing the mitral orifice (Figure 1). Cardiac catheterization revealed the following pressures (in mm Hg): right atrial mean, 20; right ventricular, 105/18; pulmonary artery wedge mean, 35; left ventricular, 125/18; and aortic, 125/80. The pulmonary artery wedge—left ventricular mean diastolic gradient was 20 mm Hg. The left ventricle contracted normally. By angiography, neither mitral nor aortic valve regurgitation was present and the epicardial coronary arteries were normal. Thoracotomy was performed and a "lemon"-sized mass involving the basal portion of the left ventricular wall was found. Computed tomography after operation localized the mass to the region of the posterior mitral leaflet. Electrocardiogram showed changes of right ventricular hypertrophy, incomplete right bundle branch block and left atrial abnormality. Echocardiogram showed a large mass in the region of the mitral valve and it extended into the left atrium and left ventricle. By Doppler, the estimated mean mitral pressure gradient was 18 mm Hg. Magnetic resonance imaging (Figure 2) confirmed these findings. The patient received radiation therapy, but died suddenly.

At necropsy (A90-2), the heart with the neoplasm weighed 530 g. The visceral and parietal pericardia

From the Cardiology and Pathology Branches, National Heart, Lung, and Blood Institute, the Radiation-Oncology Branch and Laboratory of Pathology, National Cancer Institute, Bethesda, Maryland; the Division of Cardiology, Georgetown University Hospital, Washington, D.C.; the Division of Cardiology, Mount Sinai Medical Center, Miami, Florida; and the National Institutes of Health, Building 10, Room 7B15, Bethesda, Maryland 20892. Manuscript received and accepted May 24, 1990.

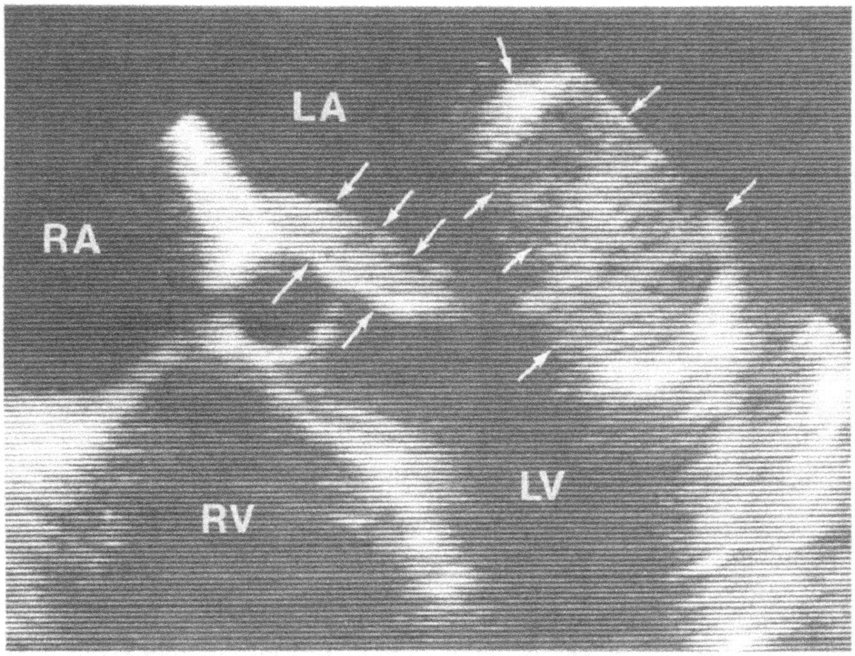

FIGURE 1. Transesophageal echocardiogram showing the tumors *(arrows)* in the left atrial (LA) wall. LV = left ventricle; RA = right atrium; RV = right ventricle.

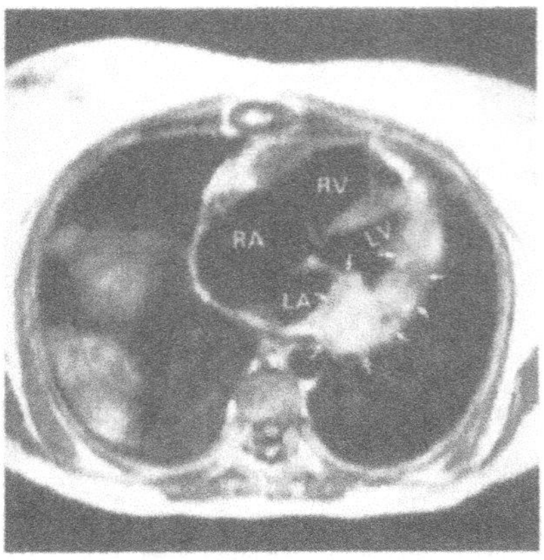

FIGURE 2. Magnetic resonance image of thorax showing the tumor in the walls of left atrium (LA) and left ventricle (LV) and pulmonary infarcts in 1 lung from occlusion of several pulmonary arteries by sarcoma from the right atrium. Abbreviations as in Figure 1.

were adhered to one another by fibrous and neoplastic adhesions. The neoplasm in the wall of the left atrium caused severe obstruction to the mitral orifice (Figure 3) and also to the left pulmonary veins. The neoplasm also invaded the coronary sinus, basal portion of the left ventricular wall and a single tumor deposit was present in the right atrial cavity at the orifice of the coronary sinus. The only body organ containing the neoplasm other than the heart was the lung; a tumor was present in several pulmonary arteries with resulting pulmonary infarcts. Histologically, the neoplasm was a spindle-cell sarcoma. Both pleural spaces (approximately 1,000 ml each) and the peritoneal cavity (1,400 ml) contained dark, amber-colored watery fluid.

The aforementioned patient had sarcoma involving the left atrium and the tumor extended into the mitral orifice producing severe mitral stenosis. We found 7 previously reported cases of left atrial sarcoma causing mitral stenosis and pertinent observations in them are listed in Table I.[1–7] Only 1 of the previously reported cases had the mitral obstruction confirmed by catheterization,

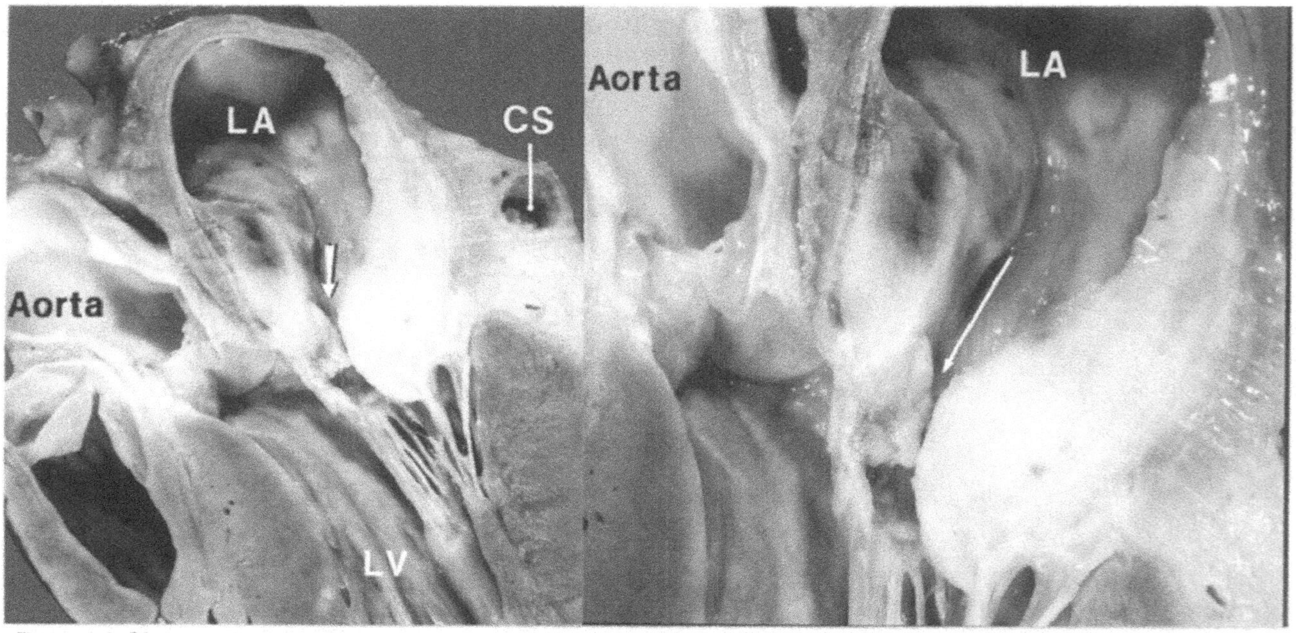

FIGURE 3. Photographs of longitudinal views of the heart showing large tumor deposits in the wall of left atrium (LA) with resulting severe obstruction *(arrows)* to the mitral valve orifice. Tumor also invaded the coronary sinus (CS). Abbreviations as in Figure 1.

TABLE I Observations in Previously Reported Patients with Left Atrial Sarcoma Causing Mitral Stenosis

Case	First Author	Year	Age (yr) & Sex	Duration of Symptoms (months)	DM	OS	P_2	PAW-LV MDG (mm Hg)	Echocardiographic Evidence of MS	Type of Sarcoma
1	Muir	1966	50 F	3	0	—	—	—	—	Chondrosarcoma
2	Dutschmann	1974	39 F	7	+(4/6)	+	+	—	—	Rhabdomyosarcoma
3	Shuh	1978	37* F		+(2/6)	+	+	—	—	Fibrous histiocytoma
4	Frendsen	1981	39 F	0.5	+	—	—	—	—	Mesenchymoma
5	Terashima	1983	27 F	5	—	—	—	—	—	Fibrous histiocytoma
6	Ormerod	1984	48 M	"Weeks"	+	—	—	—	+	Angiosarcoma
7	Villasenor	1985	82 F		+(2/6)	+	—	28	+	Rhabdomyosarcoma

* Only patient still alive at follow-up.
DM = diastolic murmur; LV = left ventricle; MDG = mean diastolic gradient; MS = mitral stenosis; OS = opening snap; PAW = pulmonary arterial wedge; P_2 = pulmonary component of second heart sound; ↑ = increased; + = present; 0 = negative; — = no informatiion.

but all had clear anatomic evidence of mitral obstruction by the neoplasm. Another unusual feature of this sarcoma was invasion of the coronary sinus by the neoplasm and migration (embolization) of the neoplasm from the lumen of the coronary sinus into the right atrium. Portions of the right atrial tumor migrated into several peripheral pulmonary arteries (another embolism), causing neoplastic pulmonary infarcts.

1. Muir CS, Seah CS. Primary chondrosarcomatous mesenchymoma of the mitral valve. *Thorax 1966; 21:254–262.*

2. Dutschmann L, Duarte S, Da Costa JN. Rhabdomyosarcoma of the heart (a case of unusual localization). *Angiology 1974;25:186–196.*

3. Shah AA, Churg A, Sbarbarao JA, Shepard JM, Lamberti J. Malignant fibrous histiocytoma of the heart presenting atrial myxoma. *Cancer 1978;42: 2466–2471.*

4. Frandsen NE, Andersen G, Nielsen JR. Malignant mesenchymoma of the heart presenting as mitral stenosis. *Acta Med Scand 1981;209:235–237.*

5. Terashima T, Aoyama K, Nihei K, Nito T, Imai Y, Takahashi K, Shichibei D. Malignant fibrous histiocytoma of the heart. *Cancer 1983;52:1919–1926.*

6. Omerod OJ, Spratt PM, Lewis NP, Wallwork J. Primary angiosarcoma of the heart mimicking a left atrial myxoma. *Thorax 1984;39:798–799.*

7. Villasenor HR, Fuentes F, Walker WE. Left atrial rhabdomyosarcoma mimicking mitral valve stenosis. *Tex Heart Inst J 1985;12:107–110.*

Morphologic Comparison of Patients With Mitral Valve Prolapse Who Died Suddenly With Patients Who Died From Severe Valvular Dysfunction or Other Conditions

ALLEN L. DOLLAR, MD,* WILLIAM C. ROBERTS, MD, FACC

Bethesda, Maryland

Clinical and necropsy findings are described in 56 patients with mitral valve prolapse: 15 patients, aged 16 to 69 years (mean 39), died suddenly and mitral valve prolapse was the only cardiac condition found at necropsy (hereafter called isolated mitral valve prolapse); the remaining 41 patients had other conditions that were capable of being fatal. Of the latter 41 patients, 7, aged 17 to 59 years (mean 45), had associated congenital heart disease, and 34 patients, aged 17 to 70 years (mean 52), had no associated congenital cardiac abnormalities.

Compared with the 34 patients without associated congenital heart disease and with nonmitral valve prolapse conditions capable in themselves of being fatal, the 15 patients who died suddenly with isolated mitral valve prolapse were younger (mean age 39 ± 17 versus 52 ± 15 years; p = 0.01), more often women (67% versus 26%; p = 0.008) and had a lower frequency of mitral regurgitation (7% versus 38%; p = 0.02). The 15 patients dying suddenly with isolated mitral valve prolapse also were less likely to have evidence of ruptured chordae tendineae (29% versus 67%; p = 0.04).

The frequency of increased heart weight (67% versus 59%), a dilated mitral valve anulus (80% versus 81%), a dilated tricuspid valve anulus (17% versus 17%), an elongated anterior mitral leaflet (86% versus 54%), an elongated posterior mitral leaflet (79% versus 77%) and fibrous endocardial plaque under the posterior mitral leaflet (73% versus 63%) was similar between the two groups. The severity of the prolapse (mild 20% versus 11%; moderate 27% versus 58%; severe 53% versus 32%) also was similar between the two groups.

Thus, persons with mitral valve prolapse dying suddenly without another recognized condition tend to be relatively young women without mitral regurgitation.

(J Am Coll Cardiol 1991;17:921–31)

Mitral valve prolapse is a common condition affecting an estimated 5% of the U.S. population (1). A rare but much-feared occurrence in persons with mitral valve prolapse is sudden death. Although only a small number of patients with mitral valve prolapse die suddenly (without other potentially fatal conditions), mitral valve prolapse accounts for a substantial proportion of sudden deaths in persons without other clear causes of death. One study (2) of 50 persons, aged 7 to 35 years, dying suddenly and unexpectedly found mitral valve prolapse to be present in 12 (24%). Several necropsy studies (3–23) have reported on individuals or small groups of patients with sudden death associated with mitral valve prolapse.

No study has compared morphologic findings in patients with mitral valve prolapse unassociated with another potentially fatal condition (hereafter called isolated mitral valve prolapse) with those patients with mitral valve prolapse associated with another potentially fatal condition. Such a comparison is the purpose of this study.

Methods

Inclusion criteria. For a patient to be included in this study, three criteria had to be met: 1) the patient's heart was examined by the Pathology Branch, National Heart, Lung, and Blood Institute, and was classified by us as "mitral valve prolapse"; 2) at death, the patient was 16 to 70 years of age; and 3) the patient's heart (or photographs if the heart was unavailable) possessed morphologic features for the diagnosis of mitral valve prolapse used in this study (to be discussed subsequently). In cases where mitral valve replacement had been performed, the operatively excised mitral valve or photographs of it had to be available to reconfirm the diagnosis of mitral valve prolapse.

Sources of cases. From January 1956 to February 1990, the hearts of 101 patients were classified as "mitral valve prolapse" by the Pathology Branch, National Heart, Lung, and Blood Institute. Of these 101 heart specimens, 81 were available for reexamination by both authors and photographs of the hearts were available in the other 20 cases. Of the 101 cases, review of medical necropsy records disclosed that 21 patients were >70 years of age and that 2 were <16 years of

From the Pathology Branch, National Heart, Lung, and Blood Institute, National Institutes of Health, Bethesda, Maryland.

*Present address: Division of Cardiology, Department of Medicine, The Washington Hospital Center, Washington, DC

Manuscript received August 7, 1990; revised manuscript received October 2, 1990, accepted October 14, 1990.

Address for reprints: William C. Roberts, MD, Pathology Branch, Building 10, Room 2N258, National Institutes of Health, Bethesda, Maryland 20892.

Table 1. Clinical and Morphologic Features of Mitral Valve Prolapse at Necropsy Unassociated With Other Congenital Cardiovascular Anomalies (49 patients aged 16 to 70 years)

Patient Category	+SCD −MR −CAD	+SCD +MR −CAD	+SCD −MR +CAD	−SCD +MR −CAD	−SCD −MR −CAD	Total (%)
No. of patients	14	3	3	10	19	49
Mean age (yr)	38 ± 17	50 ± 17	65 ± 3	55 ± 13	49 ± 17	48 ± 17
Women/men	10/4	0/3	0/3	3/7	6/13	19/30
Heart weight (g)	379 ± 96	770 ± 105	462 ± 103	577 ± 180	397 ± 131	458 ± 167
MV anulus >10 cm	11/14	1/1	2/3	8/8	6/10	29/36 (81)
TV anulus >14 cm	1/13	1/2	0/3	2/9	1/10	5/37 (14)
AML length >2.0 cm	11/13	1/1	2/3	2/4	3/6	19/27 (70)
PML length >1.5 cm	10/13	1/1	3/3	4/4	3/6	21/27 (78)
Absent chordae	4/12	0/1	2/2	6/8	2/6	14/29 (48)
LV cavity dilated (grade 3/4 or 4/4)	0/14	1/3	0/3	3/9	1/19	5/48 (10)
CA narrowed >75% in CSA	0/14	0/3	3/3	3/9	1/15	7/44 (16)
LV necrosis	0/14	0/3	1/3	0/10	0/18	1/48 (2)
LV fibrosis	0/14	1/3	1/3	2/10	1/18	5/48 (10)
Grade of MVP						
Mild	3/14	0/1	0/3	0/5	2/11	5/34 (15)
Moderate	4/14	0/1	2/3	2/5	7/11	15/34 (44)
Severe	7/14	1/1	1/3	3/5	2/11	14/34 (41)
Endocardial fibrous plaque under PML	10/14	1/1	1/3	6/7	5/9	23/34 (68)
Mitral annular calcium						
Grade 1–2/4	3/14	0/2	1/3	1/7	2/17	7/43 (16)
Grade 3–4/4	1/14	0/2	0/3	2/7	2/17	5/43 (12)
Valvular competent PFO	3/11	1/3	1/3	1/5	1/8	7/31 (23)
Redundant FO membrane	3/11	0/3	1/3	2/5	0/7	6/30 (20)
SCD due to MVP	14/14	1/3	0/3	0/10	0/19	15/49 (31)
The Marfan syndrome	2/14	0/3	0/3	2/10	4/19	8/49 (16)
Mitral valve replacement	0/14	2/3	0/3	1/10	0/19	3/49 (6)

AML = anterior mitral leaflet; CA = coronary artery; CAD = fatal coronary artery disease; CSA = cross-sectional area; FO = fossa ovale; LV = left ventricular; MR = severe mitral regurgitation; MV = mitral valve; MVP = mitral valve prolapse; PFO = patent foramen ovale; PML = posterior mitral leaflet; SCD = sudden cardiac death; TV = tricuspid valve; − = absent; + = present.

age and, therefore, these 23 cases were excluded. The children were excluded because morphologic comparisons with measurements in adults, such as heart weight, leaflet length and anular circumference, would be meaningless. Persons >70 years of age were excluded because some age-related changes in the mitral leaflets of elderly persons are similar to features of mitral valve prolapse, including leaflet thickening, especially in the portions adjacent to the posteromedial commissure, and the thickened portions often protrude toward the left atrium. Although several hearts in the elderly patients clearly had unequivocal features of mitral valve prolapse, many did not. To avoid including patients who did not have mitral valve prolapse, the older patients were excluded.

On reexamination of the remaining 78 patients, 22 were determined not to have morphologic features (to be discussed subsequently) of mitral valve prolapse. After these exclusions, 56 patients, aged 16 to 70 years (mean 48), remained and all had unequivocal morphologic features of mitral valve prolapse.

Definitions. *Sudden cardiac death* was defined as death occurring within 6 h of the onset of symptoms of cardiac dysfunction or myocardial ischemia. *Sudden death* associated with mitral valve prolapse (isolated mitral valve prolapse) was defined as sudden cardiac death where mitral valve prolapse was present and no other cardiac or noncardiac condition was present at autopsy to explain death. Sudden death associated with *coronary artery disease* was defined as sudden cardiac death with >75% cross-sectional area luminal narrowing of one or more of the four major epicardial coronary arteries. If both mitral valve prolapse and significant coronary arterial narrowing was present, death was attributed to coronary artery disease.

Significant mitral regurgitation was defined as the presence of at least "moderate" or grade 3/4 or 4/4 mitral regurgitation by left ventricular angiography or Doppler echocardiography. If no objective assessment of mitral regurgitation was made during life, significant mitral regurgitation was presumed to have been present if the left atrium and ventricle were significantly (grade >2/4) dilated in the absence of another cause of chamber enlargement.

Morphologic criteria of mitral valve prolapse. Morphologic criteria used for the diagnosis of mitral valve prolapse were: 1) elongation of a portion of the posterior mitral leaflet such that the distance from distal margin to its attachment at

Table 2. Clinical and Morphologic Features in 15 Patients Dying Suddenly Secondary to Mitral Valve Prolapse

Pt No.	Age (yr)	Race	Gender	MVP Diagnosed Clinically	The Marfan Syndrome	Location of Death	Last Activity	Auscultatory Findings SC	Auscultatory Findings SM	SH	CHF	VPCs on ECG	HW (g)	MV Anulus (cm)	TV Anulus (cm)	AML Length (cm)	PML Length (cm)	Chords Missing	Grade of MVP (1-3+)	Plaque Under PML	MAC (0-4+)	VC PFO	Redundant FO Membrane
1	16	W	M	+	+	Basketball court	Sitting after playing	–	+	0	0	+	325	12.5	12	3	2.5	+	2	0	0	–	–
2	18	W	F	+	0	Home	Arguing	–	0	0	0	+*	220	9.6	11.5	2	1.5	0	1	+	0	0	0
3	21	W	F	+	0	Work	Talking on phone	–	–	0	0	–	360	14	—	3	1.5	+	2	0	1	–	–
4	23	W	F	+	0	Work	Drinking water	+	+	0	0	–	280	10	9	2.5	2	0	3	+	0	+	+
5	26	W	F	+	0	Work	Talking	+	+	0	0	0†	265	12	11	3	3	0	3	+	0	+	+
6	30	B	M	0	0	Work	Sitting alone	–	–	–	0	–	570	15.5	13	3	2.5	0	3	+	0	0	0
7	30	W	M	0	0	Golf course	Playing golf	–	–	0	0	–	475	10	11	3	2	0	1	+	0	0	0
8	40	W	F	0	–	Home	Playing with children	–	–	0	0	–	355	13	12	–	–	+	2	0	2	–	+
9	47	W	F	0	0	Home	Gardening	–	–	0	0	+	445	12.5	12.5	2.5	2	0	3	+	0	0	0
10	51	W	M	+	0	Restaurant	Sitting after last dancing	+	+	0	0	0	500	10.5	12	2	1.5	0	1	0	0	0	0
11	53	W	F	+	0	Church	Sitting	–	–	0	0	+	325	12.6	10.5	2.5	3	0	2	+	3	0	0
12	53	W	F	0	0	Restaurant	Getting up to dance	–	–	–	0	–	390	13.6	11	3.5	3	0	3	+	1	+	+
13	55	W	F	+	0	Home	Standing	+	+	0	0	+	390	13	13	3	2.5	+	3	–	0	0	0
14	55	W	M	+	0	Home	Sleeping	–	+	0	+	+	670	>12	14	3.5	2	0	3	+	0	+	0
15	69	W	F	0	0	Home	…	–	–	–	0	–	400	15.4	14.5	2.5	3	+	3	+	0	0	0

*This patient had survived a cardiac arrest 2 years earlier; †this patient had a history of paroxysmal atrial tachycardia. AML = anterior mitral leaflet; B = black; CHF = congestive heart failure; F = female; FO = fossa ovale; HW = heart weight; M = male; MVP = mitral valve prolapse; MAC = mitral annular calcification; PFO = patent foramen ovale; PML = posterior mitral leaflet; Pt = patient; SC = systolic click; SH = systemic hypertension; SM = systolic murmur; TV = tricuspid valve; VC = valvular competent; VPC = ventricular premature complex; W = white; + = present; 0 = absent; – = no information available.

the mitral anulus was >1.5 cm; or 2) presence of mitral leaflet protrusion toward the left atrium, usually also associated with missing chordae tendineae, and the prolapsed portion of the leaflet involving >50% of the anterior leaflet and >33% of the posterior leaflet. Others (9,23) have referred to this leaflet prolapse as "interchordal hooding."

Morphologic measurements. All morphologic measurements and observations were performed by one or both authors. The length of the mitral leaflets was measured from the line of attachment of the leaflet to its free margin at the longest portion of each leaflet. Chordae tendineae were considered "missing" if none extended caudally from the ventricular surface of a portion of either or both leaflets or if detached chordae that had rounded or blunted distal ends were present. ("Missing" chordae were considered to represent sites of previously ruptured chordae [24]). The severity of mitral valve prolapse was subjectively graded as mild, moderate or severe.

Determination of normal measurement values. Normal values for various morphologic measurements were determined

Figure 1. Patient 1. The heart of a 16 year old boy (Suffolk County Medical Examiner #84-4276, Hauppauge, NY) who had skeletal features of Marfan syndrome (examination of his aorta did not reveal "cystic medial necrosis"). He had a systolic murmur and mitral valve prolapse was diagnosed by echocardiography. His rest electrocardiogram showed occasional uniform premature ventricular complexes that disappeared with exercise. He died suddenly in a locker room after playing basketball. **Top,** View of the opened mitral valve, showing mild changes of mitral valve prolapse in the anterior leaflet (A) and more severe changes in the posterior leaflet. **Bottom,** Close-up view of the posterior leaflet.

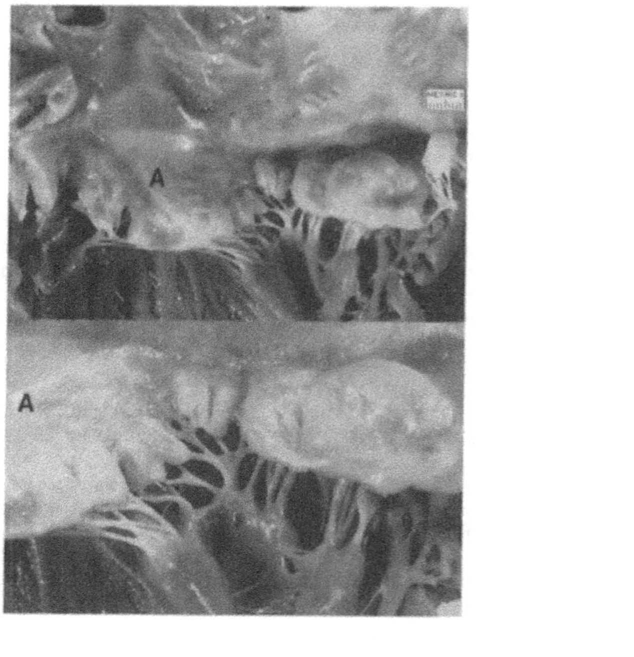

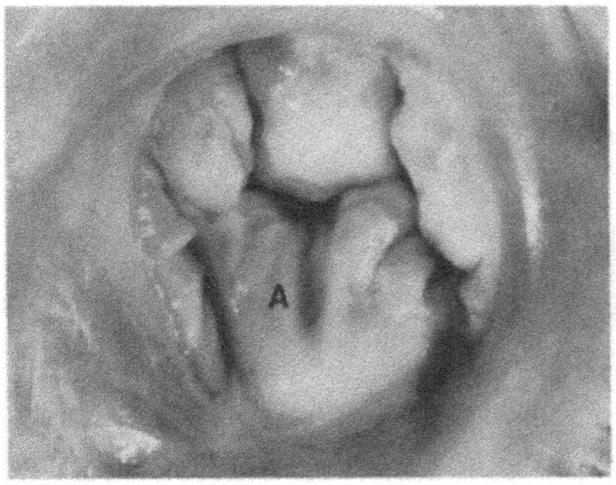

Figure 2. Patient 2. View of the intact mitral valve from the left atrium, showing a normal-appearing anterior leaflet (A) and prolapse of the posterior leaflets from the heart of an 18 year old woman (Rockford Memorial Hospital #A85-6, Rockford, IL) who was the daughter of a physician. Twenty-seven months before death, she had a cardiac arrest from which she was resuscitated. Evaluation included electrocardiography, coronary angiography, echocardiography, exercise stress testing, electrophysiologic studies and right ventricular endomyocardial biopsy. These examinations revealed mitral valve prolapse, a slightly prolonged QTc interval (0.46 s) and ventricular premature complexes that became more frequent and complex (couplets and triplets) during the recovery phase after exercise. She did not have mitral regurgitation. She was taking propranolol and mexiletine at the time of death, which occurred during an emotional argument.

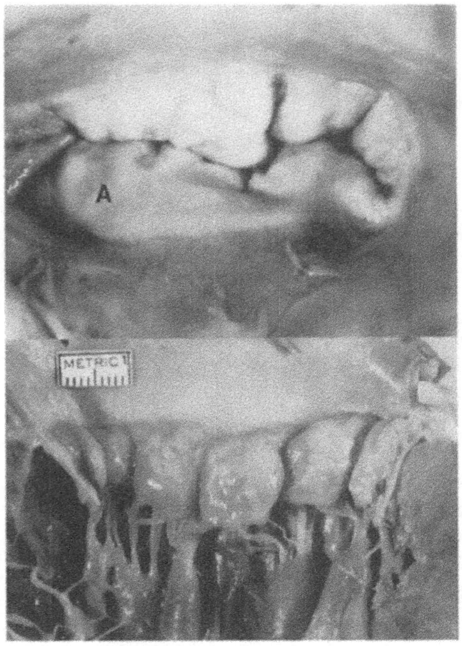

Figure 3. Patient 4. The heart of a 21 year old woman (York Hospital #81AX-132, York, PA) who had the diagnosis of mitral valve prolapse at age 16 years. One year before death, while pregnant, she complained of palpitation and substernal pressure. She died suddenly at a water fountain. **Top.** View of the intact mitral valve from the left atrium, showing prolapse of several scallops of the posterior leaflet, but the valve does not appear regurgitant. **Bottom.** View of the posterior leaflet of the opened mitral valve, showing extensive "hooding" and elongation of the leaflet. A = anterior leaflet.

by measurements in 20 normal hearts from persons aged 15 to 70 years (mean 47). The 95% confidence intervals derived from these measurements of normal hearts were: mitral anular circumference 7.8 to 8.5 cm, tricuspid valve anulus 8.4 to 11.4 cm, anterior mitral leaflet length 1.5 to 1.8 cm and posterior mitral leaflet length 1.1 to 1.3 cm. The following upper limits therefore were used: mitral anular circumference 10 cm; tricuspid valve anular circumference 14 cm; anterior mitral leaflet length 2 cm and posterior mitral length 1.5 cm.

Histologic studies. One or more of the following histologic sections (stained by hematoxylin and eosin or Movat stain) were prepared from each heart: 1) at least two sections of left ventricular myocardium extending from endocardium to epicardium; and 2) a transverse section of the ascending aorta about 1 cm cephalad to the sinotubular junction.

Results

Subgroupings of the patients with mitral valve prolapse without congenital heart disease. Table 1 summarizes clinical and morphologic findings in the 49 patients without congenital heart disease. The 49 patients were divided into five subgroups on the basis of the presence or absence of sudden cardiac death (SCD) (from any cause), regurgitation (MR) (as determined by objective studies during the patient's life and morphologic evidence of significant mitral regurgitation) and fatal coronary artery disease (CAD). Fourteen of the 15 patients who had sudden death associated with mitral valve prolapse (isolated mitral valve prolapse) comprise the category *+SCD, −MR, −CAD*, and the 1 patient with sudden death due to mitral valve prolapse but who had mitral regurgitation is in the category *+SCD, +MR, −CAD*. No patient had a history or morphologic evidence of infective endocarditis.

Characteristics of the 15 patients dying suddenly from mitral valve prolapse. Of the total group of 56 patients, 22 died suddenly from a cardiac cause: 4 had significant coronary artery disease (>75% cross-sectional area narrowing of at least one major epicardial coronary artery), 2 had had mitral valve replacement, 1 had cyanotic congenital heart disease and 15 (Table 2) had no explanation for death other than mitral valve prolapse. The age of the latter 15 patients ranged from 16 to 69 years (mean 39); 10 (67%) were women.

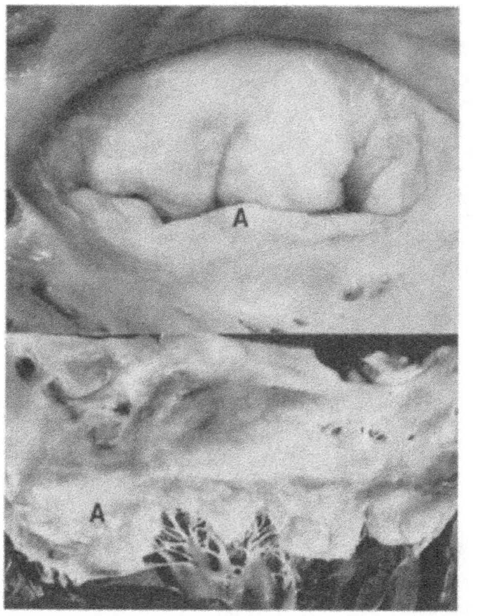

Figure 4. Patient 5. The heart of a 26 year old woman (District of Columbia Medical Examiner's Office #87-07-681) who was a lawyer. She had palpitation associated with paroxysmal atrial tachycardia beginning at age 9 years and had mitral valve prolapse diagnosed by echocardiography at age 15 years. She was started on propranolol therapy at 15 years of age and changed to atenolol 2 years before death. She had an episode of atrial tachycardia about once each 3 months, and it resolved promptly with the Valsalva maneuver. While talking with two colleagues she collapsed suddenly and died. **Top**, View of the intact mitral valve from the left atrium, showing pronounced prolapse of the posterior leaflet. **Bottom**, View of the opened mitral valve, showing pronounced "hooding" of the posterior leaflet. The anterior leaflet (A) is relatively uninvolved.

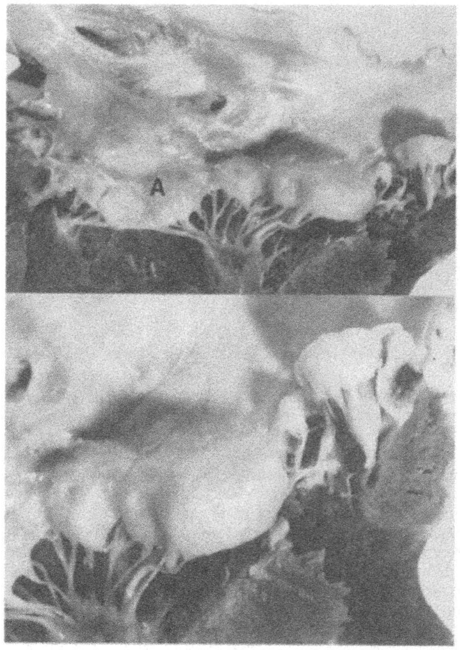

Figure 5. Patient 8. The heart of a 40 year old woman (Suffolk County Medical Examiner #84-4578, Hauppauge, NY) who had Marfan syndrome. She had a history of "valve problems," but no echocardiography was ever done. She was asymptomatic and on no medication. She collapsed suddenly and died while playing with neighborhood children. **Top**, View of the opened mitral valve, showing a mildly abnormal anterior leaflet (A) and a very abnormal posterior leaflet. **Bottom**, Close-up view of a portion of the posterior leaflet, showing a scallop of this leaflet, which is severely prolapsed toward the left atrium. This heart weighed 355 g and no chamber was dilated.

Diagnosis of mitral valve prolapse was made during life in eight (53%); Marfan syndrome was diagnosed in two (13%). Of seven patients whose electrocardiographic (ECG) data were available, six had ventricular premature complexes on their rest ECG, including one patient who had nonfatal cardiac arrest 2 years before death. Four patients were known to be on medication at the time of death: one woman who had nonfatal cardiac arrest was taking propranolol and mexiletine; one woman with paroxysmal atrial tachycardia was taking atenolol; one woman with frequent ventricular premature complexes was taking nadolol and one woman was taking thyroxine. Four patients died suddenly during or shortly after physical exertion and one patient died after an emotional argument.

Certain cardiac morphologic findings in some of the 15 patients who died suddenly from mitral valve prolapse are illustrated in Figures 1 to 7. In the 15 patients, the heart weight ranged from 220 to 670 g (mean 398); in the 5 men, four hearts weighed >400 g; in the 10 women, six hearts weighed >350 g. The mitral valve anulus was dilated (>10 cm in circumference) in 12 of the 15 patients (mean anular circumference 12.4 ± 1.9 cm). The anterior mitral leaflet was elongated (>2 cm from margin of attachment to free margin) in 12 of 14 patients, and the posterior leaflet was elongated (>1.5 cm) in 11 of 14 patients. In none of the 15 hearts was any major epicardial coronary artery narrowed >25% in cross-sectional area and none had gross or microscopic foci of myocardial necrosis or fibrosis. By visual inspection, the cardiac chambers were of normal size in eight patients, only mildly dilated in six and moderately dilated in one. Fibrous thickening of the mural endocardium (endocardial plaque) behind the posterior mitral leaflet was present in 11 of the 15 patients. The presence or absence of mitral

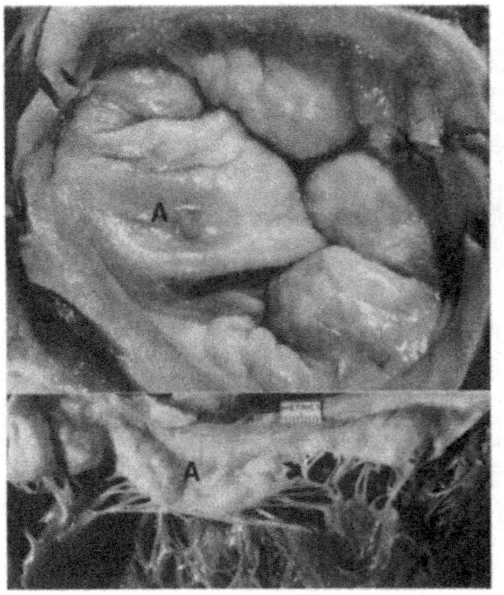

Figure 6. Patient 9. The heart of a 47 year old woman (District of Columbia Medical Examiner's Office #80-06-485) who was a psychiatrist. She had been dieting for 2 weeks before death and was taking thyroid supplements to aid in her weight loss. She was found dead in her yard, dressed in jogging clothes. Her only known cardiac problem was ventricular premature complexes noted by her physician husband. **Top.** View of the intact mitral valve from the left atrium, showing both the anterior (A) and posterior leaflets to be redundant. **Bottom.** The opened mitral valve, showing the posterior leaflet to be elongated.

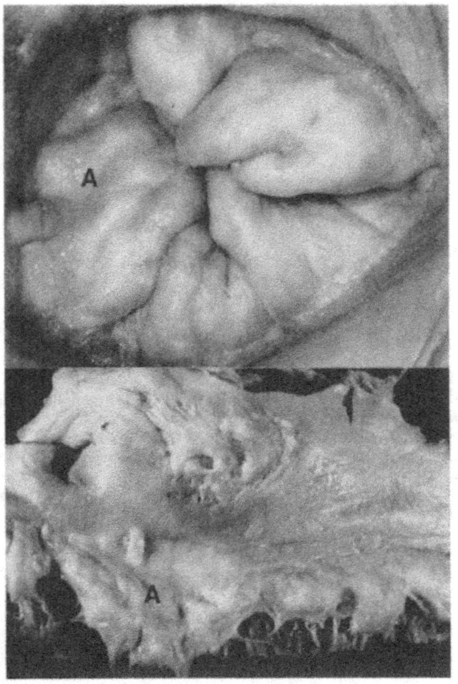

Figure 7. Patient 12. The heart of a 53 year old woman (District of Columbia Medical Examiner's Office #88-09-961) who was the wife of a plastic surgeon. She was out with her husband, got up to dance and suddenly collapsed and died. **Top.** View of the intact mitral valve from the left atrium, showing prolapse of the posterior leaflet above the anterior leaflet (A). **Bottom.** The opened mitral valve, showing a very large anterior leaflet (A) and an elongated redundant posterior leaflet.

regurgitation was documented during life by objective testing in three patients: echocardiography showed trace mitral regurgitation in one patient; left ventricular angiography showed no regurgitation in one patient and moderate regurgitation in another. The latter patient's heart weighed 670 g and all four cardiac chambers were moderately dilated.

Comparison of patients dying suddenly with isolated mitral valve prolapse with other patients with mitral valve prolapse without congenital heart disease. Comparison of the 15 patients in whom sudden death was associated with isolated mitral valve prolapse (14 patients from the group *+SCD, −MR, −CAD* and 1 patient with mitral regurgitation from the group *+SCD, +MR, −CAD*) with the other patients with mitral valve prolapse without associated congenital heart disease (Table 1) disclosed the following differences: 1) a lower mean age at death (39 ± 17 versus 52 ± 15 years; $p = 0.01$); 2) a preponderance of women (10 [67%] of 15 versus 9 [26%] of 34; $p = 0.008$); 3) a lower frequency of mitral regurgitation (1 [7%] of 15 versus 13 [38%] of 34; $p = 0.02$); and 4) a lower frequency of having evidence of ruptured chordae tendineae (4 [29%] of 14 versus 10 [67%] of 15; $p = 0.04$). No significant differences were noted between the patients dying suddenly with mitral valve prolapse and the other patients with mitral valve prolapse with regard to heart weight, circumference of the mitral or tricuspid anulus, length of the anterior or posterior mitral leaflet, presence of missing chordae tendineae, grade of mitral valve prolapse, presence of endocardial fibrous plaque under the posterior mitral leaflet or presence of a patent foramen ovale or redundant fossa ovale membrane. Cardiac morphologic findings in two patients from the group *−SCD, +MR, −CAD* are illustrated in Figures 8 and 9 and two patients from the group *−SCD, −MR, −CAD* are illustrated in Figures 10 and 11.

Mitral valve prolapse associated with congenital heart disease. Congenital heart disease was present in 7 of the 56 patients (Table 3). These congenital abnormalities included *ostium secundum atrial septal defect* (four patients), *bicuspid aortic valve* (three patients), *coarctation of the aorta* (one patient), *Ebstein's anomaly* (one patient), *partial atrio-*

ventricular canal (one patient) and *sinus of Valsalva aneurysm* (one patient). The patient with total anomalous pulmonary venous connection and one patient with a severely stenotic bicuspid aortic valve died suddenly.

Mitral valve prolapse associated with the Marfan syndrome. Eight patients had the Marfan syndrome, two of whom died suddenly without a clear cause. Three had rupture of the ascending aorta, one had congestive heart failure with severe aortic and mitral regurgitation and two died of noncardiac causes. Histologic sections of ascending aorta were available in six of the eight patients: four had

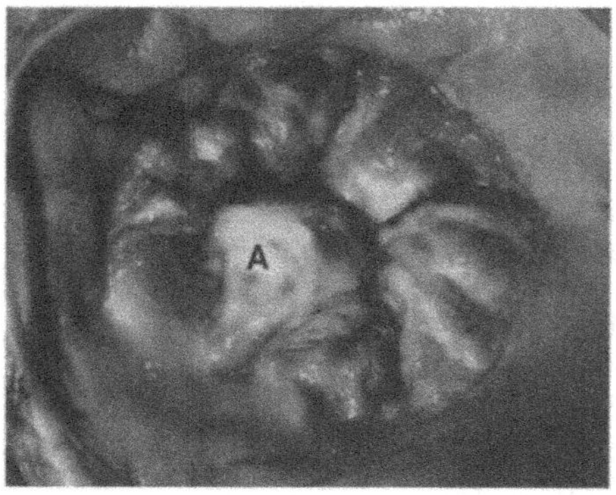

Figure 8. Patient from *−SCD, +MR, −CAD* group. The heart of a 65 year old woman (Georgetown University Hospital #81A-122, Washington, DC) who had chronic congestive heart failure and severe mitral regurgitation. She died in cardiogenic shock. View of the intact mitral valve from the left atrium, showing prolapse of both the anterior (A) and posterior mitral leaflets. CAD = fatal coronary artery disease; MR = mitral regurgitation; SCD = sudden cardiac death; − = absent; + = present.

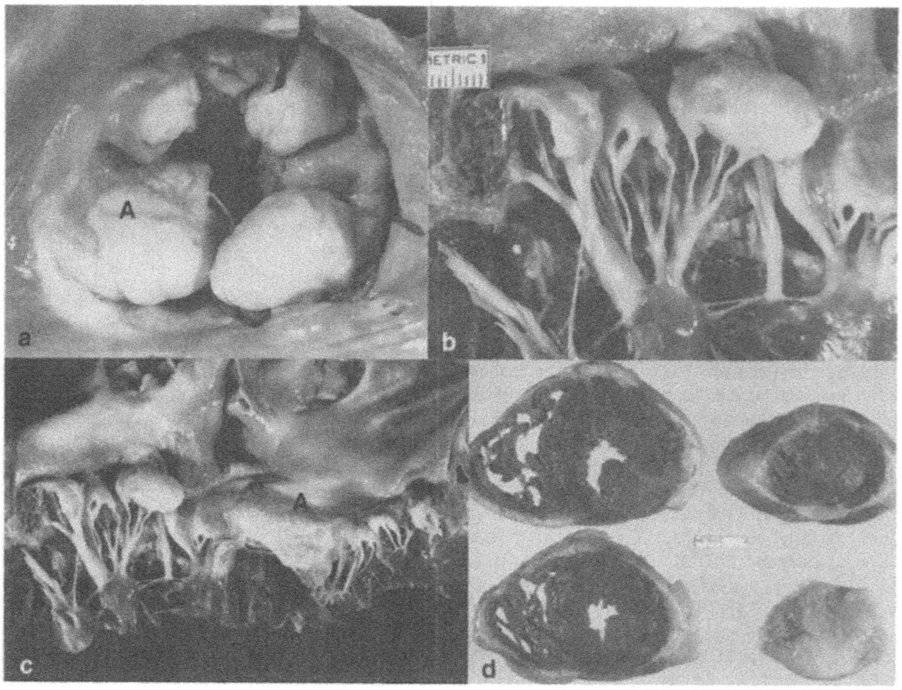

Figure 9. Patient from *−SCD, +MR, −CAD* group. The heart of a 54 year old man (District of Columbia Veterans Administration Hospital #83A-84, Washington, DC) with grade 3/4 chronic atrial fibrillation and mitral regurgitation by ventriculography. He died of a cerebral embolic event. **a.** View of the intact mitral valve from the left atrium, showing a patulous mitral valve with a very dilated anulus (15 cm). **b.** Close-up view of the posterior leaflet of the opened mitral valve, showing pronounced hooding of each of the scallops of the leaflet. **c.** The opened mitral valve. **d.** Transverse slices of the ventricles, showing a surprising lack of left ventricular dilation given the degree of mitral regurgitation present. Abbreviations as in Figure 8.

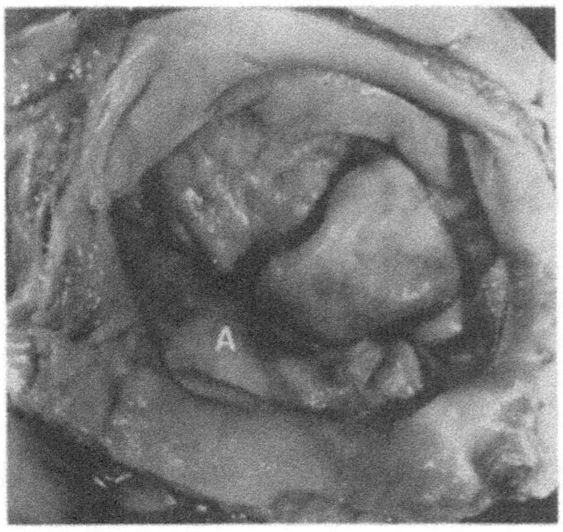

Figure 10. Patient from *−SCD, −MR, −CAD* group. The heart of a 63 year old woman (Georgetown University Hospital #79A-100. Washington, D.C.) who died of cancer. View of the intact mitral valve from the left atrium, showing herniation of the posterior leaflet above the anterior leaflet (A). Abbreviations as in Figure 8.

classic "medial cystic necrosis" with massive degeneration of elastic fibers and two had a normal configuration of elastic fibers in the aortic media. At least one histologic section of ascending aorta stained for elastic fibers was examined in 22 patients with mitral valve prolapse unassociated with the Marfan syndrome, and the aortic media in each appeared normal.

Discussion

Major findings in the present study. Several differences were observed in the 15 patients with sudden death associated with isolated mitral valve prolapse (without the pres-

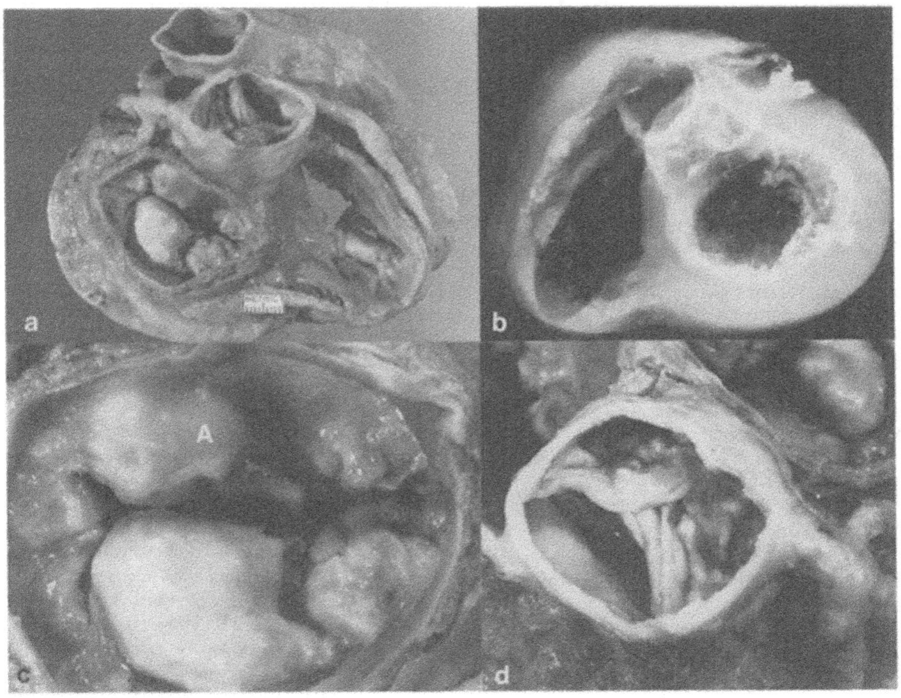

Figure 11. Patient from *−SCD, −MR, −CAD* group. The heart of a 63 year old man (Georgetown University Hospital #82A-04, Washington, DC) who died of cancer. **a.** View of the heart from above after removal of the atria. **b.** Radiograph of the base of the heart, showing massive calcium deposits in the anulus of the mitral valve, aortic valve and epicardial coronary arteries. **c.** Close-up view of the intact mitral valve as viewed from the left atrium showing pronounced enlargement of the posterior leaflet. **d.** View of the aortic valve from above, showing a stenotic tricuspid valve with calcium deposits and no fusion of the commissures. Abbreviations as in Figure 8.

Table 3. Clinical Features of Seven Adult Patients With Congenital Heart Disease With Morphologic Features of Mitral Valve Prolapse Studied at Necropsy

Pt No.	Congenital Abnormality	Age (yr)/ Gender	MVP Diagnosed Clinically	MR	Cardiac Operation	Mode of Death
1	ASD (secundum), Ebstein's anomaly	17/F	0	–	0	Noncardiac (cancer)
2	Aortic coarctation, BAV (AR)	30/M	+	+	Coarctectomy, AVR, MVR	Cardiac operation
3	ASD (secundum), TAPVC	42/M	0	–	0	Sudden (cardiac)
4	Atrioventricular canal (partial)	55/F	+	–	0	Noncardiac (pneumonia)
5	BAV, valvular aortic stenosis	56/M	–		Coronary bypass	Sudden (CAD + AS)
6	ASD (secundum), BAV, SV aneurysm	57/F	0	–	0	Rupture of SV aneurysm
7	ASD (secundum)	59/F	+	+	ASD closure, MVR	Cardiac operation

ASD = atrial septal defect; AVR = aortic valve replacement; BAV = bicuspid aortic valve; MVR = mitral valve replacement; SV = sinus of Valsalva; TAPVC = total anomalous pulmonary venous connection; + = present; 0 = absent; – = no information available; other abbreviations as in Tables 1 and 2.

ence of other potentially fatal conditions) compared with the patients with mitral valve prolapse with other potentially fatal causes of death and without other congenital cardiac malformations: the patients who died suddenly with isolated mitral valve prolapse were younger, more likely to be women and less likely to have mitral regurgitation or evidence of ruptured chordae tendineae.

Severe mitral regurgitation was infrequent (1 of 15 patients) in the patients with mitral valve prolapse who died suddenly without associated significant coronary artery disease or other congenital cardiac anomalies. There have been conflicting views regarding the importance of mitral regurgitation as a predisposing factor for sudden death in patients with mitral valve prolapse. Some investigators (25,26) emphasized the importance of mitral regurgitation as a risk factor for sudden death in patients with mitral valve prolapse, going so far as to calculate an estimated annual mortality rate from sudden death due to mitral valve prolapse in patients with and without mitral regurgitation. Their estimates were based primarily on a study by Davies et al. (15), who reported on 13 patients at necropsy who died suddenly and had mitral valve prolapse. At least 4 of their 13 patients, however, had an etiology for the mitral regurgitation and sudden death other than mitral valve prolapse: 2 patients had bacterial endocarditis, 1 had a previous myocardial infarction and 1 patient, a 79 year old man, had chronic lung disease. After reviewing 25 previously reported patients with mitral valve prolapse who died suddenly, Jeresaty (27) concluded that the typical patient with mitral valve prolapse who dies suddenly has only minimal to moderate mitral regurgitation.

Frequency of mural endocardial fibrous plaque in patients dying suddenly with mitral valve prolapse. The presence of mural endocardial fibrous plaque beneath the posterior mitral leaflet has been noted previously in necropsy studies of patients dying suddenly from mitral valve prolapse. Chesler et al. (22) suggested that the friction between chordae tendineae and the underlying left ventricular mural endocardium, presumably the mechanism of formation of this endocardial plaque, may cause ventricular arrhythmias. We found a high frequency of such plaque, both in patients whose death was attributed to isolated mitral valve prolapse (11 of 15) and patients whose death was attributed to other causes (12 of 19).

Abnormalities of the fossa ovale membrane in patients with mitral valve prolapse. Secundum atrial septal defect is associated with mitral valve prolapse (28,29). Four of our seven patients with mitral valve prolapse and congenital heart disease had ostium secundum atrial septal defect. Redundancy (aneurysm) of the fossa ovale membrane also has been noted (30) in association with mitral valve prolapse at necropsy, and a recent report (31) found a higher prevalence of atrial septal aneurysm diagnosed by echocardiography in patients with mitral valve prolapse (9.5%) compared with those without (3.1%). We found a 20% frequency of redundancy of the fossa ovale membrane among the 49 patients with mitral valve prolapse without congenital cardiovascular anomalies. Probe-patent valvular-competent foramen ovale occurred in 7 (23%) of 31 patients among the entire group. This frequency, however, is similar to that of valvular-competent patent foramen ovale in normal adult hearts (30). Neither redundancy of the fossa ovale membrane nor probe-patency of the foramen ovale was more common among the sudden death group compared with the other patients with mitral valve prolapse.

Previously reported studies on patients who died suddenly from mitral valve prolapse. We searched for published reports of patients with mitral valve prolapse who died suddenly and who had no other condition present at autopsy to explain death. A total of 63 patients (3–14,16–23) were found, of whom 39 had individualized clinical data (3–14, 16–22) (Table 4). These previously reported patients were similar in many respects to our group of 15 patients dying suddenly with mitral valve prolapse. The mean age of the previously published patients was 33 ± 14 years; 27 (71%) of 38 were women and the mean heart weight was 306 ± 76 g. Severe mitral regurgitation was uncommon: only one patient had a heart weight above normal (≤350 g for women and ≤400 g for men) and only one other patient (whose heart weighed 340 g) had dilated cardiac chambers. Only six patients had results of cineangiocardiography: mitral regur-

Table 4. Clinical Information in 39 Previously Reported Patients Studied at Necropsy Who Died Suddenly With Mitral Valve Prolapse as the Only Explanation for Death

								Auscultatory Findings					MR by LV Cine	ECG Findings							Abnormal MV Leaflet		
Reference (first author)	Year	Age (yr)/ Gender	MVP Diagnosed Clinically	P	D	S	CP	MR	SH	CHF	SC	SM	(0–3+)	Rhythm	QTc (ms)	T Wave Inversion	VPCs	Last Activity	Medication	HW (g)	AML	PML	Plaque Under PML
Hancock (3)	1966	29/F	+	+	0	0	0	–	0	0	+	+	–	S	45	+(A,I)	+	—	Quinidine	–	–	–	–
Barlow (4)	1968	39/M	+	–	–	–	–		–	–	+	+	–		–	–	+	Mowing lawn	—	–	–	–	–
Trent (5)	1970	63/F	+	+	0	0	+	Y	0	+	0	+	++	S	–	–	0	—	Digoxin	340	+	+	–
Jeresaty (6)	1973	62/F	+	–	–	–	–	–	–	–	0	+	++	AF	N	+(A,I)	+	Sleeping	—	–	–	–	–
Shappell (7)	1973	27/F	+	0	0	+	0	N	0	0	+	+	0	S	45–47	+(I)	0	Arguing	Propranolol	310	+	+	–
Marshall (8)	1974	36/F	+	+	+	0	0	–	0	0	–	–	–	–	–	–	–	Sitting		350	+	+	–
Guthrie* (9)	1976	20/F	+	0	0	0	0		–	0	+	0	–		N	0	+	—	0	–	–	–	–
Guthrie* (9)	1976	25/F	+	+	+	+	+		–	–	+	+	+		–	–	+	—	Quinidine, propranolol	–	–	–	–
Guthrie* (9)	1976	29/M	0	0	0	0	0		–	0	0	+	–		–	–	–	Sitting at desk	—	–	–	–	–
Jeresaty (10)	1976	39/F	+	0	0	0	0	Y	0	0	+	+	+	S	N	+(I)	0	—	Furosemide	–	+	+	–
Kleid (11)	1976	38/F	–	+	0	0	0	N	0	0	0	+	–	S	–	–	+	—	0	–	–	–	–
Koch (12)	1976	9/–	+	–	–	–	–	–	–	–	–	–	–	–	–	–	†	—	—	–	–	–	–
Koch (12)	1976	30/–	+	–	–	–	–	–	–	–	–	–	–	–	–	–	†	—	—	–	–	–	–
Koch (12)	1976	32/–	+	–	–	–	–	–	–	–	–	–	–	–	–	–	†	—	—	–	–	–	–
Koch (12)	1976	50/–	+	–	–	–	–	–	–	–	–	–	–	–	–	–	†	—	—	–	–	–	–
Koch (12)	1976	64/–	+	–	–	–	–	–	–	–	–	–	–	–	–	–	†	—	—	–	–	–	–
Mills (14)	1977	58/M	+	–	+	–	–		–	+	0	+	–		–	+	+	—	Quinidine	–	–	–	–
Mair (16)	1980	25/F	+	+	0	+	0	–	0	0	+	+	–	–	–	–	–	Driving	0	230	+	+	+
Mair (16)	1980	29/F	+	–	–	+	–	–	0	0	+	0	–	–	–	–	–	Lying in bed	0	250	+	+	+
Mair (16)	1980	35/F	–	+	+	0	0	–	0	0	–	–	–	–	–	–	–	Conversing	0	270	+	+	+
Bharati (17)	1981	17/M	0	–	–	–	–	–	–	0	–	–	–	–	–	–	–	Playing football	—	–	–	–	–
Bharati (17)	1981	19/F	0	–	–	–	–	–	–	–	–	–	–	–	–	–	–	—	—	–	–	–	–
Bharati (18)	1981	45/M	+	+	–	–	–	–	–	–	+	+	–	S	N	–	+	—	0	–	–	+	–
Dupasquier (19)	1981	43/M	+	+		+	0	Y	0	0	0	+	–	S	N	+(I)	0	Driving	0	550	–	–	–
Salmela (20)	1981	27/M	+	–	+	+	0	–	0	0	+	+	–	S	N	+(I)	+	Watching television	Digoxin	–	–	+	–
Pocock (21)	1984	24/F	+	+	0	0	0	Y	0	0	+	+	+	S	N	+(I)	+	Conversing	Disopromide, acebutolol	–	0	+	+
Chesler (22)	1983	14/F	0	0	0	0	0	0	–	–	–	–	–	–	–	–	–	—	Methyldopa	230	+	+	+
Chesler (22)	1983	19/F	–	–	–	–	–		–	–	–	–	–	–	–	–	–	—	—	230	0	–	+
Chesler (22)	1983	19/M	+	0	0	0	0	0	–	–	+	+	–	–	–	–	–	—	Steroid inhaler	220	+	–	+
Chesler (22)	1983	21/F	+	0	0	0	0	0	–	–	+	0	–	–	–	–	–	—	Primidone	260	0	–	0
Chesler (22)	1983	21/F	+	+	0	0	0	0	–	–	+	+	–	–	–	–	–	—	0	290	+	–	+
Chesler (22)	1983	24/F	–	0	0	0	0	0	–	–	0	+	–	–	–	–	–	—	0	350	+	–	+
Chesler (22)	1983	25/F	+	+	+	0	+		–	–	+	+	–	–	–	–	–	—	Propranolol	220	+	–	+
Chesler (22)	1983	26/F	–	–	–	–	–		–	–	–	–	–	–	–	–	–	—	—	340	+	–	+
Chesler (22)	1983	27/F	–	0	0	0	0	0	–	–	0	+	–	–	–	–	–	—	0	325	+	+	+
Chesler (22)	1983	29/M	–	+	0	0	0	0	–	–	0	+	–	–	–	–	–	—	0	365	–	+	+
Chesler (22)	1983	30/M	+	0	0	0	0	0	–	–	+	0	–	–	–	–	–	—	0	325	+	+	+
Chesler (22)	1983	39/F	0	0	0	0	0	0	–	–	0	0	–	–	–	–	–	—	0	348	+	+	0
Chesler (22)	1983	59/F	0	0	0	0	0	0	–	–	–	–	–	–	–	–	–	—	0	320	0	+	+

*Some of the details of these cases were not in the original report but were provided in Jeresaty (6); †two of these five patients had multiform ventricular premature complexes (VPCs) on their electrocardiogram. A = anterior; AF = atrial fibrillation; CP = chest pain; D = dizziness; I = inferior; LV Cine = left ventricular cineangiogram; N = normal; P = palpitation; QTc = QT interval corrected for rate; S = syncope; Y = yes; other abbreviations as in Tables 1 and 2.

gitation was absent in one, mild in three and moderate in two.

Previously reported patients with mitral valve prolapse who survived potentially lethal ventricular arrhythmias. Several studies (33–35) have detailed the characteristics of patients with mitral valve prolapse who had life-threatening ventricular tachyarrhythmias or who survived cardiac arrest. Winkle et al. (33) reported on seven patients (five women, mean age 49 years) with mitral valve prolapse who had survived one or more episodes of life-threatening ventricular arrhythmias: six patients had a systolic click or systolic murmur, or both. Mitral regurgitation was objectively diagnosed or excluded in only three of the seven patients (by left ventricular angiography): mitral regurgitation was absent in two and moderate in one. Wei et al. (34) reported on 10 patients with mitral valve prolapse (7 women, mean age 47 years) with symptomatic recurrent ventricular tachyarrhythmias refractory to conventional drug therapy. Although left ventricular angiography was performed in all patients, there was no specific mention of mitral regurgitation. Boudoulas et al. (33) reported on nine patients with mitral valve prolapse who had cardiac arrest (seven women, mean age 33 years) of whom seven survived. All seven had cardiac catheterization, but mitral regurgitation was not mentioned.

References

1. Savage DD, Garrison RJ, Devereux RB, et al. Mitral valve prolapse in the general population. 1. Epidemiologic features: the Framingham Study. Am Heart J 1983;106:571–6.
2. Topaz O, Edwards JE. Pathologic features of sudden death in children, adolescents, and young adults. Chest 1985;87:476–82.
3. Hancock EW, Cohn K. The syndrome associated with midsystolic click and late systolic murmur. Am J Med 1966;41:183–96.
4. Barlow JB, Bosman CK, Pocock WA, Marchand P. Late systolic murmurs and non-ejection ("mid-late") systolic clicks: an analysis of 90 patients. Br Heart J 1968;30:203–18.
5. Trent JK, Adelman AG, Wigle ED, Silverman MD. Morphology of a prolapsed posterior mitral valve leaflet. Am Heart J 1970;79:539–43.
6. Jeresaty RM. Mitral valve prolapse-click syndrome. Prog Cardiovasc Dis 1973;15:623–52.
7. Shappell SD, Marshall CE, Brown RE, Bruce T. Sudden death and the familial occurrence of mid-systolic click, late systolic murmur syndrome. Circulation 1973;48:1128–34.
8. Marshall CE, Shappell SD. Sudden death and the ballooning posterior leaflet syndrome: detailed anatomic and histochemical investigation. Arch Pathol 1974;98:134–8.
9. Guthrie RB, Edwards JE. Pathology of the myxomatous mitral valve: nature, secondary changes and complications. Minn Med 1976;59:637–47.
10. Jeresaty RM. Sudden death and the mitral valve prolapse-click syndrome. Am J Cardiol 1976;37:317–8.
11. Kleid JJ. Sudden death and the floppy mitral valve syndrome. Angiology 1976;27:734–7.
12. Koch FH, Hancock EW. Ten year follow up of forty patients with the mid-systolic click/late systolic murmur syndrome (abstr). Am J Cardiol 1976;37:149.
13. Allen H, Harris A, Leatham A. Significance and prognosis of an isolated late systolic murmur: a 9-to-22-year follow-up. Br Heart J 1974;36:525–32.
14. Mills P, Rose J, Hollingsworth J, Amara I, Craige E. Long-term prognosis of mitral-valve prolapse. N Engl J Med 1977;297:13–8.
15. Davies MJ, Moore BP, Braimbridge MV. The floppy mitral valve: study of incidence, pathology, and complications in surgical, necropsy, and forensic material. Br Heart J 1978;40:468–81.
16. Mair WJ. Sudden death in young females with floppy mitral valve syndrome. Aust N Z J Med 1980;10:221–3.
17. Bharati S, Granston AS, Liebson PR, Loeb HS, Rosen KM, Lev M. The conduction system in mitral valve prolapse syndrome with sudden death. Am Heart J 1981;101:667–70.
18. Bharati S, Rosen KM, Miller LB, Strasberg B, Lev M. Sudden death in three teenagers (abstr). Circulation 1981;64(suppl IV):IV-72.
19. Dupasquier E, Bernoy JL. Le syndrome du prolapsus valvulaire mitral: deux complications rares: la mort subite, l'embolie cerebrale. Schweiz Med Wochenschr 1981;111:73–81.
20. Salmela PI, Ikaheimo M, Juustila H. Fatal ventricular fibrillation after treatment with digoxin in a 27-year-old man with mitral leaflet prolapse syndrome. Br Heart J 1981;46:338–41.
21. Pocock W, Bosman CK, Chesler E, Barlow JB, Edwards JE. Sudden death in primary mitral valve prolapse. Am Heart J 1984;107:378–82.
22. Chesler E, King RA, Edwards JE. The myxomatous mitral valve and sudden death. Circulation 1983;67:632–9.
23. Virmani R, Atkinson JB, Forman MB, Rabinowitz M. Mitral valve prolapse. Hum Pathol 1987;18:596–602.
24. Roberts WC, McIntosh CL, Wallace RB. Mechanisms of severe mitral regurgitation in mitral valve prolapse determined from analysis of operatively excised valves. Am Heart J 1987;113:1316–23.
25. Kligfield P, Levy D, Devereux RB, Savage DD. Arrhythmias and sudden death in mitral valve prolapse. Am Heart J 1987;113:1298–307.
26. Devereux RB, Kramer-Fox R, Kligfield P. Mitral valve prolapse: causes, clinical manifestations, and management. Ann Intern Med 1989;111:305–17.
27. Jeresaty RM. Mitral Valve Prolapse. New York: Raven, 1979:209–21.
28. Betriu A, Wigle ED, Felderhof CH, McLoughlin MJ. Prolapse of the posterior leaflet of the mitral valve associated with secundum atrial septal defect. Am J Cardiol 1975;35:363–9.
29. Leachman RD, Cokkinos DV, Cooley DA. Association of ostium secundum septal defects with mitral valve prolapse. Am J Cardiol 1976;38:167–9.
30. Roberts WC. Aneurysm (redundancy) of the atrial septum (fossa ovale membrane) and prolapse (redundancy) of the mitral valve. Am J Cardiol 1984;54:1153–4.
31. Rahko PS, Xu QB. Increased prevalence of atrial septal aneurysm in mitral valve prolapse (abstr). Circulation 1989;80(suppl II):II-10.
32. Barry A, Patten BM. The structure of the adult heart. In: Gould SE, ed. Pathology of the Heart and Blood Vessels. Springfield, IL: Charles C Thomas, 1968:91–130.
33. Winkle RA, Lopes MG, Popp RL, Hancock EW. Life-threatening arrhythmias in the mitral valve prolapse syndrome. Am J Med 1976;60:961–7.
34. Wei JY, Bulkley BH, Schaeffer AH, Greene HL, Reid PR. Mitral-valve prolapse syndrome and recurrent ventricular tachyarrhythmias. Ann Intern Med 1978;89:6–9.
35. Boudoulas H, Schaal SF, Stang JM, Fontana ME, Kolibash AJ, Wooley CF. Mitral valve prolapse–sudden death with long term survival (abstr). J Am Coll Cardiol 1986;7:29A.

Appearance of or Persistence of Severe Mitral Regurgitation Without Left Ventricular Outflow Obstruction After Partial Ventricular Septal Myotomy-Myectomy in Hypertrophic Cardiomyopathy

Charles Stewart Roberts, MD, S. David Gertz, MD, Heinrich G. Klues, MD, Richard O. Cannon III, MD, Barry J. Maron, MD, Charles L. McIntosh, MD, and William Clifford Roberts, MD

At the National Heart, Lung, and Blood Institute from 1959 through October 1989, 626 patients underwent operative treatment of obstructive hypertrophic cardiomyopathy: ventricular septal myotomy-partial myectomy alone in 539 patients; mitral valve replacement alone in 68 patients; and both procedures, not necessarily simultaneously, in 27 patients. The septal myotomy-myectomy procedure in most patients provided clinical improvement, but in some patients the results of this procedure have been unsatisfactory and reoperation has been performed.[1] In the 27 patients who underwent reoperation after septal myotomy-myectomy, the indication was persistent left ventricular outflow obstruction in 24 patients[2] and pure mitral regurgitation, without outflow obstruction, in 3 patients. This report describes certain clinical and morphologic features in the latter 3 patients.

Certain clinical and operative findings in the 3 patients are summarized in Table I. All 3 patients had peak systolic pressure gradients at rest or with provocation between left ventricle and systemic artery >50 mm Hg before the myotomy-myectomy operation, and 1 patient (no. 2) had a large (61 mm Hg) gradient across the right ventricular outflow tract. All 3 patients also had mitral regurgitation before the myotomy-myectomy operation performed through an aortotomy. Mitral regurgitation in patient 1 was only mild before the myotomy-myectomy operation but severe afterwards; in patient 2, mitral regurgitation was severe both before and after the initial operation (Figure 1), and in patient 3 it was of moderate degree before myotomy-myectomy and severe afterwards. All 3 patients had complete relief of left ventricular outflow obstruction by the myotomy-myectomy operation; nevertheless, severe symptoms of cardiac dysfunction persisted. At reoperation, ruptured mitral chordae tendineae were found in patients 1 and 2 and severe posterior mitral leaflet systolic anterior motion in patient 3. In none of the 3 patients was the mitral anulus dilated. The operatively excised mitral valves are shown in Figure 2. After mitral replacement, symptoms of cardiac dysfunction less-

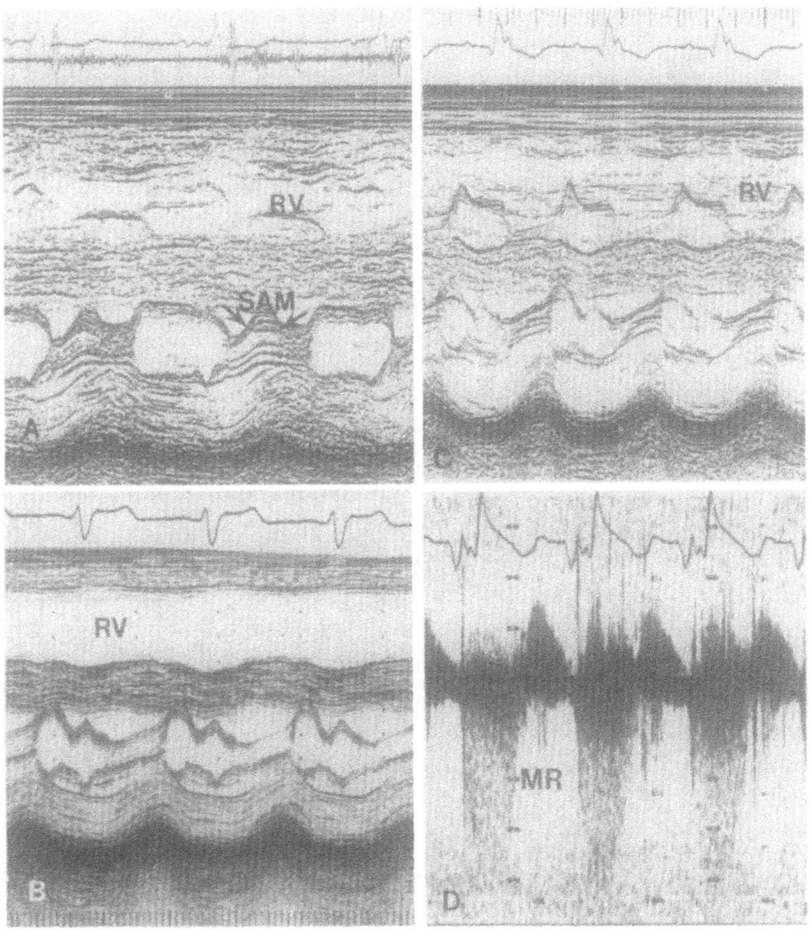

FIGURE 1. M-mode echocardiograms from patient 2 (CW). *A*, preoperative. Systolic anterior motion (SAM) of the mitral valve with mitral valve–septal contact. *B and C*, 6 and 25 months after septal myotomy-myectomy operation. SAM is now absent and the ventricular septum is thinner. *D*, postoperative. Continuous-wave Doppler tracing obtained from left ventricular apex showing mitral regurgitation (MR). RV = right ventricle.

From the Surgery, Pathology, and Cardiology Branches, National Heart, Lung, and Blood Institute, National Institutes of Health, Bethesda, Maryland. Manuscript received July 9, 1991; revised manuscript received and accepted August 14, 1991.

TABLE I Observations in Three Patients with Hypertrophic Cardiomyopathy Who Had Ventricular Myotomy–Myectomy for Left and/or Right Ventricular Outflow Obstruction Followed Later by Mitral Valve Replacement for Pure Mitral Regurgitation

	Patient 1 (MS)				Patient 2 (CW)				Patient 3 (AM)			
	Before M&M	Six Months After M&M	Shortly Before MVR	Six Months After MVR	Before M&M	Six Months After M&M	Shortly Before MVR	Six Months After MVR	Before M&M	Six Months After M&M	Shortly Before MVR	Six Months After MVR
Age (years)	23	23	34	34	22	22	24	25	55	55	60	60
Functional class (I–IV) (NYHA)	3	1	3	2	3	2	3	2	4	2	4	2
Atrial fibrillation	0	0	0	0	0	0	0	0	+	+	+	+
Echocardiographic findings												
Systolic anterior motion	+	–	0	–	+	0	0	–	+	0	0	–
Right ventricular cavity (mm)	28	–	35	34	30	36	42	40	22	30	29	28
Left atrial cavity (mm)	56	–	66	64	46	55	55	60	45	50	62	57
Left ventricular cavity (mm) (s/d)	38/–	–	50/38	50/40	31/21	41/24	46/34	45/	38/24	42/32	42/30	44/32
Ascending aorta (mm)	33	–	32	32	26	28	29	–	25	25	28	29
Ventricular septum (mm)	21	–	10	10	34	19	14	–	21	11	12	12
Left ventricular free wall (mm)	14	–	14	14	18	18	18	–	10	10	10	10
Intravascular pressures (mm Hg)												
Pulmonary artery wedge, V (m)	12 (9)	14 (11)	26 (18)	10 (7)	20 (15)	36 (29)	–	–	25 (18)	–	30 (24)	32 (21)
Right ventricle (s/d)	28/6	26/6	33/7	26/9	95/18	56/24	–	–	48/4	–	65/12	67/18
Pulmonary artery (s/d)	26/18	26/10	33/12	26/4	34/24	57/29	–	–	48/20	–	65/30	67/25
Left ventricle (s/d)	90/13	110/28	93/22	95/6	125/20	102/37	–	–	150/6	–	122/17	115/16
Aorta (s/d)	90/55	120/60	93/57	100/58	125/78	115/75	–	–	96/60	–	122/60	120/60
LV–aorta peak systolic gradient												
Rest	0	0	0	0	0*	0	–	–	54	–	0	0
Provocation	91	0	0	0	70	0	–	–	96	–	–	0
Cardiac index (liters/min/m²)	2.9	2.9	1.7	2.6	2.9	1.8	–	–	1.9	–	2.7	1.7
Mitral regurgitation (0.4+), LV cine	1+	–	4+	1+	3+	3+	3+	–	2+	–	3+	0
Interval (mo) M&M to MVR		128					25			73		
Interval (mo) MVR to March 1990				44				21 →				97‡ →
Date of M&M (month–year)	11–1975	–	–	–	6–1986	–	–	–	2–1976	–	–	–
Date of MVR (month–year)	–	–	7–1986	–	–	–	6–1988	–	–	–	2–1982	–
Type (size [mm]) substitute valve	–	–	B-S (27)	–	–	–	SJM (31)	–	–	–	Hancock (27)	–
Operative findings												
Weight VS excised (g)	9.6	–	–	–	10.2†	–	–	–	0.6	–	–	–
Ruptured mitral CT	–	–	+	–	–	–	0	–	–	–	0	–
Prolapsed PML	–	–	0	–	–	–	0	–	–	–	+	–
Thickened AML + CT	–	–	+	–	–	–	+	–	–	–	+	–

*Immediately before provocation, peak systolic gradient at rest was 50 mm Hg. Note that this patient had a 61 mm Hg systolic pressure gradient at rest between right ventricle and a major pulmonary artery.
†Includes myocardium from both right and left ventricular outflow tracts.
‡This patient died suddenly 97 months after mitral valve replacement. A necropsy was not performed.
AML = anterior mitral leaflet; B-S = Bjork-Shiley prosthesis; cine = cineangiography; CT = chordae tendineae; LV = left ventricular; M&M = myotomy and myectomy (partial); MVR = mitral valve replacement; NYHA = New York Heart Association classification; PML = posterior mitral leaflet; s/d = peak systolic/end diastolic; SJM = St. Jude Medical prosthesis; V = peak V wave; VS = ventricular septum; – = no information available or not done.

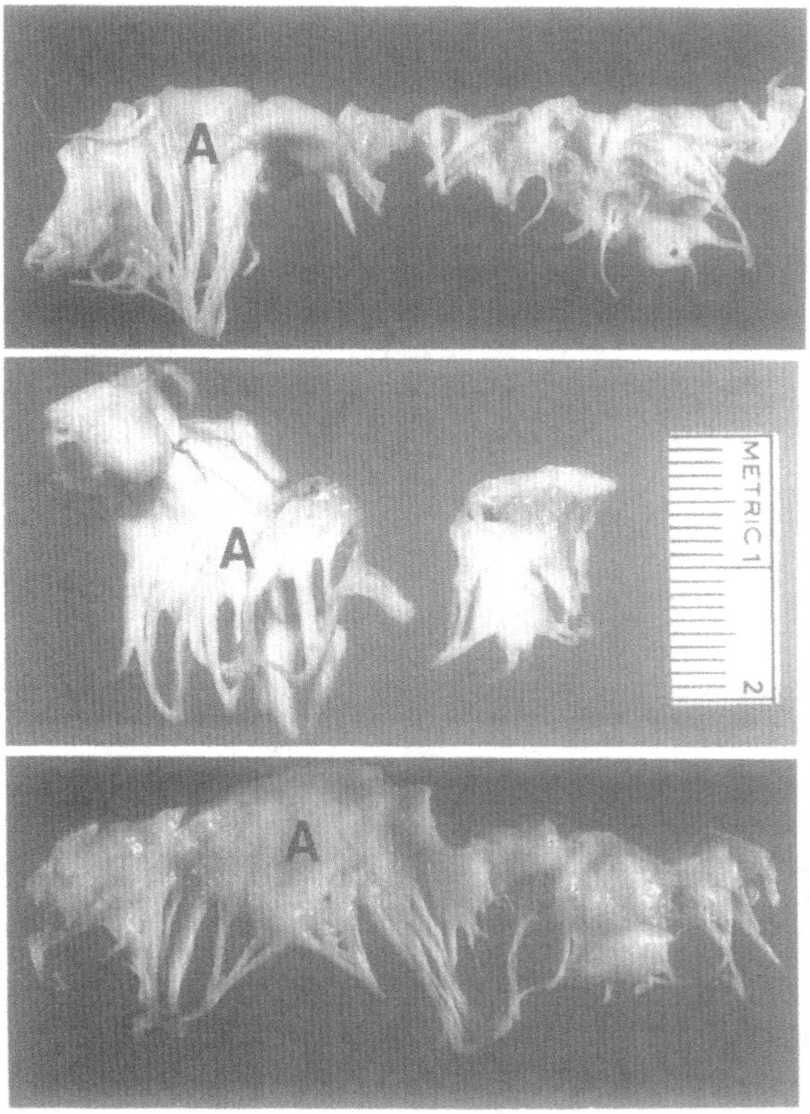

FIGURE 2. Operatively excised mitral valves from each of the 3 patients. *Upper*, patient 1 (MS) showing ruptured chordae tendineae from the anterior half of the anterior (A) mitral leaflet. A portion of the posterior leaflet is elongated. *Middle*, patient 2 (CW). Chordae from the anterior (A) half of the anterior leaflet also are absent (ruptured). *Bottom*, patient 3 (AM). No chordae are ruptured or missing but a portion of posterior leaflet is elongated. The *bottom* photograph is reproduced with permission from the American Heart Association, from Maron BJ, Harding AM, Spirito P, Roberts WC, and Waller BF. Systolic anterior motion of the posterior mitral leaflets: a previously unrecognized cause of dynamic subaortic obstruction in patients with hypertrophic cardiomyopathy. *Circulation* 1983;68:282–293.

ened by 1 New York Heart Association functional class in patients 1 and 2 and by 2 functional classes in patient 3 late postoperatively.

Almost every patient who undergoes ventricular septal myotomy-myectomy for left ventricular outflow obstruction has some degree of mitral regurgitation preoperatively. This operative procedure usually reduces the degree of mitral regurgitation, and it also usually relieves left ventricular outflow obstruction.[3] Reoperation is seldom necessary in obstructive hypertrophic cardiomyopathy and when it is performed, the indication is usually persistent left ventricular outflow obstruction. Rare is the postoperative patient who has pure mitral regurgitation producing significant symptoms without any associated left ventricular outflow obstruction. Such was the case, however, in our 3 patients.

The causes of the worsening or persistence of pure mitral regurgitation in patients 1 and 2 appear to have been inadvertent severance of several mitral chordae tendineae at the time of the myotomy-myectomy operation. This technical complication was unrecognized at operation. Retrospective review of the intraoperative echocardiogram before and after the septal myectomy, however, clearly indicates that several chordae tendineae were severed. Patient 3 was known to have systolic anterior motion of a portion of posterior mitral leaflet before myotomy-myectomy and this systolic anterior motion persisted after the initial operation. Why the mitral regurgitation worsened, however, after relief of left ventricular outflow obstruction was not discernible from study of the operatively excised mitral valve.

This study indicates that damage may occur to the mitral valve at the time of ventricular septectomy-septotomy in obstructive hypertrophic cardiomyopathy, and that this damage may cause worsening of or persistence of mitral regurgitation postoperatively.

1. McIntosh CL, Maron BJ. Current operative treatment of obstructive hypertrophic cardiomyopathy. *Circulation* 1988;78:487–495.

2. Roberts CS, McIntosh CL, Brown PS Jr, Cannon RO III, Gertz SD, Clark RE. Reoperation for persistent outflow obstruction in hypertrophic cardiomyopathy. *Ann Thorac Surg* 1991;51:455–460.

3. Cooper MM, Tucker E, McIntosh CL, Cannon RO III, Clark RE. Effect of left ventricular septal myectomy on concurrent mitral regurgitation. *Ann Thorac Surg* 1989;48:251–256.

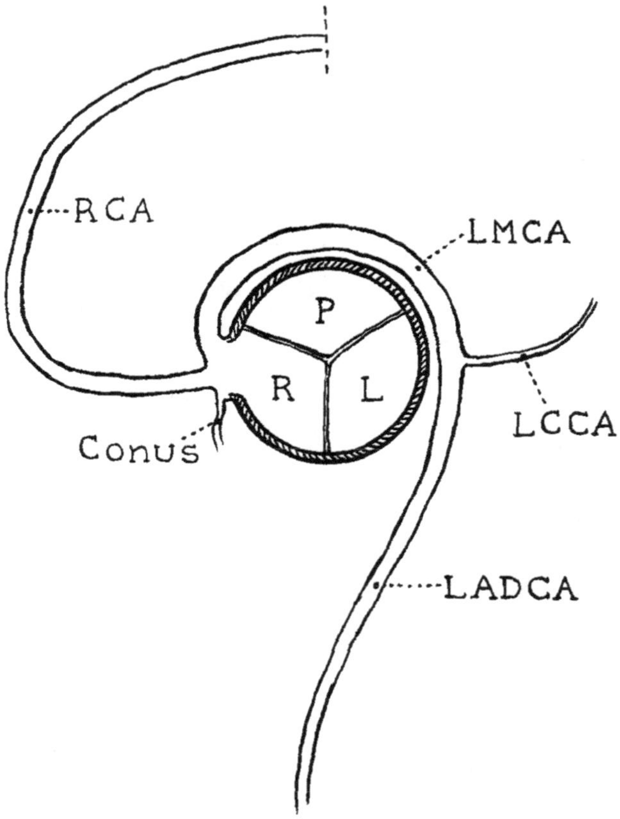

Fig. 1. Diagram showing anomalous origin of left main coronary artery from right aortic sinus with retroaortic coursing of anomalistically arising artery.

Origin of the left main coronary artery from the right aortic sinus with retroaortic course of the anomalistically arising artery

Jamshid Shirani, MD, and William C. Roberts, MD
Bethesda, Md.

Anomalous origin of the left circumflex coronary artery from the right aortic sinus or from the right coronary artery with retroaortic coursing of the anomalistically arising artery is the most common congenital coronary artery anomaly; it occurs in approximately one of every 300 human hearts.[1] In this laboratory we have studied 17 hearts with anomalously arising left circumflex coronary artery with retroaortic coursing. Anomalous origin of the left main coronary artery from the right aortic sinus or from the right coronary artery with retroaortic coursing of the anomalistically arising artery (Fig. 1), in contrast, is less common. In this laboratory we have studied four hearts with this latter anomaly. A description of the clinical and cardiac morphologic findings in these four patients is the purpose of this report.

From the Pathology Branch, National Heart, Lung, and Blood Institute, National Institutes of Health.

Reprint requests: Pathology Branch, NHLBI—Bldg. 10, Room 2N258, Bethesda, MD 20892.

4/4/39803

Certain findings in the four patients (three men and one woman) are summarized in Table I. The patients were 32, 45, 57, and 69 years of age (mean age 51 years) at the time of death. In none of the four patients did the coronary anomaly cause cardiac dysfunction or myocardial ischemia, and in none was it a factor in causing death. Three patients, one of whom has been reported previously,[2] died of noncardiac causes; the fourth died suddenly of consequences of atherosclerotic coronary artery disease. The left main and right coronary arteries each arose from a separate ostium, which was located in the right sinus of Valsalva in three patients; in the fourth patient a single ostium was present in the right aortic sinus, and the left main coronary artery arose as the first branch of the right coronary artery. In all four patients the left main coronary artery coursed posterior to the aorta and then branched at the usual site into the left anterior descending and left circumflex coronary arteries. The length of the left main coronary artery measured from the point of its origin in the right aortic sinus or from the right coronary artery to the site of its bifurcation into the left anterior descending and left circumflex coronary arteries was 3.3 to 4.5 cm (mean 3.6). The right coronary artery coursed to the crux and was much larger and longer than the left circumflex coronary artery

Table I. Clinical and morphologic findings in four patients with origin of the left main coronary artery from the right aortic sinus or right coronary artery with retroaortic course of the anomalistically arising artery

Patient number	*Age (yr)*	*Sex*	*Mode of death*	*Heart weight (gm)*	*Number of ostia in right aortic sinus*	*Length of left main coronary artery (cm)*	*RCA > LCCA*	*No. of major coronary arteries >75% ↓ by plaque*	*LV scar*
1	32	M	Trauma	325	2	3.3	0	0	0
2	45	M	Atherosclerotic CAD	580	2	4.5	+	1*	+
3	57	F	Infection	300	2	3.6	+	0	0
4	69	M	Forme fruste Marfan syndrome	685	1	3.0	+	0	0

CAD, Coronary artery disease; *LCCA*, left circumflex coronary artery; *LV*, left ventricular; *RCA*, right coronary artery.
*Left main coronary artery.

in three patients; in the fourth patient the left circumflex coronary artery coursed to the crux, and it was much larger and longer than the right coronary artery.

Origin of the left main coronary artery from the right aortic sinus or proximal portion of the right coronary artery was observed by Yamanaka and Hobbs[3] in 22 of 126,595 coronary angiograms performed at the Cleveland Clinic from 1960 to 1988. The course of the anomalistically arising coronary artery in these 22 patients, however, was not described.

Although none of our four patients had evidence of myocardial ischemia as a result of the coronary anomaly, Murphy et al.[4] reported a 12-year-old girl with a similar coronary anomaly who had acute dyspnea, central chest discomfort, and loss of consciousness on two occasions 7 months apart. The first episode occurred during a school soccer game and the second while she was competing in a one-mile race. During hospitalization after the second episode, she had evidence of an anterior wall acute myocardial infarction as determined by electrocardiogram and cardiac enzyme levels. A saphenous vein conduit was placed between the aorta and left anterior descending coronary artery.

REFERENCES

1. White NK, Edwards JE. Anomalies of the coronary arteries. Report of four cases. Arch Pathol 1984;45:766-71.
2. Waller BF, Reis RL, McIntosh CL, Epstein SE, Roberts WC. The Marfan cardiovascular disease without the Marfan syndrome. Chest 1980;77:533-40.
3. Yamanaka O, Hobbs RE. Coronary artery anomalies in 126,595 patients undergoing coronary arteriography. Cathet Cardiovasc Diagn 1990;21:28-40.
4. Murphy DA, Roy DL, Sohal M, Chandler BM. Anomalous origin of left main coronary artery from anterior sinus of valsalva with myocardial infarction. J Thorac Cardiovasc Surg 1978;75:282-5.

Fatal Cor Pulmonale Caused by Extensive Tumor Emboli in the Small Pulmonary Arteries Without Emboli in the Major Pulmonary Arteries or Metastases in the Pulmonary Parenchyma

Michael J. Domanski, MD, Robert E. Cunnion, MD, Daniel J. Fernicola, MD, and William C. Roberts, MD

Microscopic-sized tumor emboli are an uncommon cause of cor pulmonale.[1–4] We report 2 patients who had precipitous terminal courses of respiratory insufficiency caused by extensive tumor emboli in the small pulmonary arteries.

Both patients were young (aged 38 and 27 years), both had recognized cancers (breast and pancreas) for short periods (12 and 9 months), and both had acute dyspnea for the first time beginning a short time before death (17 days and 1 day) with tachypnea and tachycardia. During the final acute dyspneic period, both had clear lung fields by chest radiographs and no neoplasm in the lung parenchyma at necropsy; both had elevated pulmonary arterial pressures (58/38 and 68/40 mm Hg), normal-sized cardiac silhouettes on chest radiograph and normal-sized hearts at necropsy (270 and 330 g); both had dilated right ventricular cavities (with normal-sized left ventricular cavities) and severe tricuspid regurgitation by echocardiogram; both had hypoxemia and respiratory alkalosis, and both had thrombocytopenia (40,000 and 44,000 cu mm) and anemia (hematocrits 33 and 27%). One patient (case 2) had schistocytes in peripheral blood. Pulmonary arteriogram (recorded only in patient 1) was normal (Figure 1); perfusion lung scan (recorded only in patient 2) was normal; cytology of pulmonary venous blood (analyzed only in patient 2) was positive for cancer cells. At necropsy, both had numerous small pulmonary arteries containing tumor emboli (Figure 2) without emboli in the major pulmonary arteries and without metastases in the pulmonary parenchyma, and both had widespread metastases in liver, lymph node and bone.

From the Clinical Trials and Cardiology and Pathology Branches, National Heart, Lung, and Blood Institute, and the Critical Care Medicine Department, National Institutes of Health, Bethesda, Maryland 20892.
Manuscript received December 31, 1992, and accepted February 6, 1993.

The 2 patients described in this study had rapidly progressive pulmonary and cardiovascular compromise resulting from extensive tumor emboli in the small pulmonary arteries. Diagnosis of this mechanism of dyspnea is rarely suspected antemortem.[2,3] Adenocarcinomas and trophoblastic neoplasms are the most frequently reported causes but other malignancies have been implicated.[3,5] Gastric carcinoma is the neoplasm giving rise most frequently to this syndrome.[5]

Patients generally present with dyspnea, tachypnea, tachycardia and hypoxemia with a normal chest radiograph and a nondiagnostic pulmonary arteriogram.[2,3,6] Progressive pulmonary hypertension is typical. Treatment is usually unsuccessful.[6] In our patient 1, a correct presumptive diagnosis was made based upon the clinical picture and the exclusion of large-artery thromboembolism by arteriography. Cytologic examination of pulmonary venous blood withdrawn through a wedged pulmonary artery catheter can be diagnostic,[7] as was the case in the second patient.

Small artery tumor emboli should be considered whenever a patient with a known malignancy presents

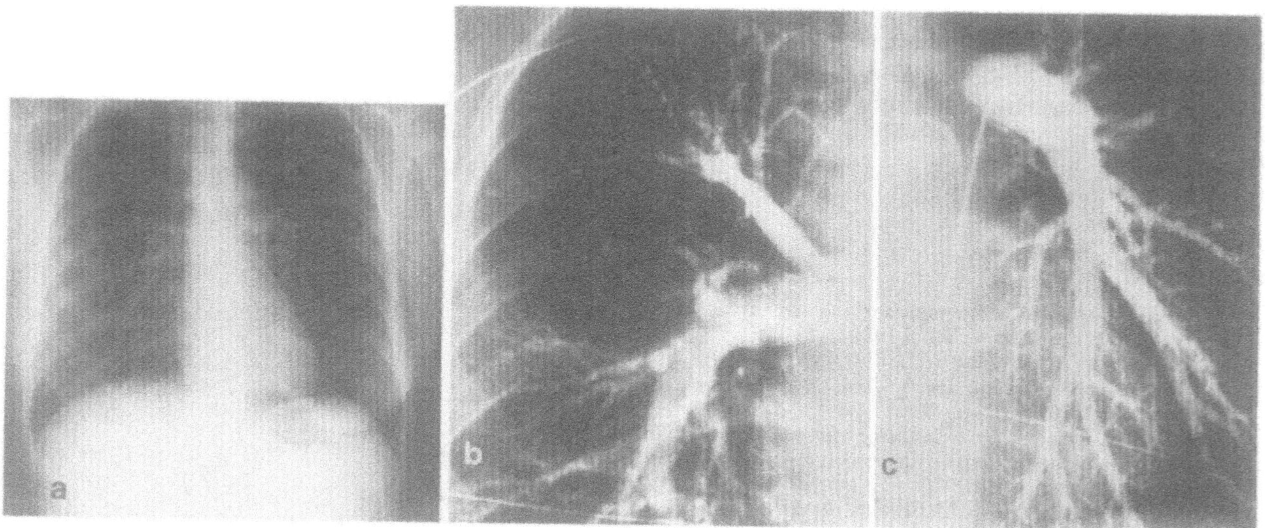

FIGURE 1. Case 1. Posteroanterior chest radiograph and pulmonary arteriograms. The chest radiograph *(a)*, obtained 2 days before death, is normal. No filling defects are seen on right *(b)* or left *(c)* pulmonary arteriograms obtained 1 day before death.

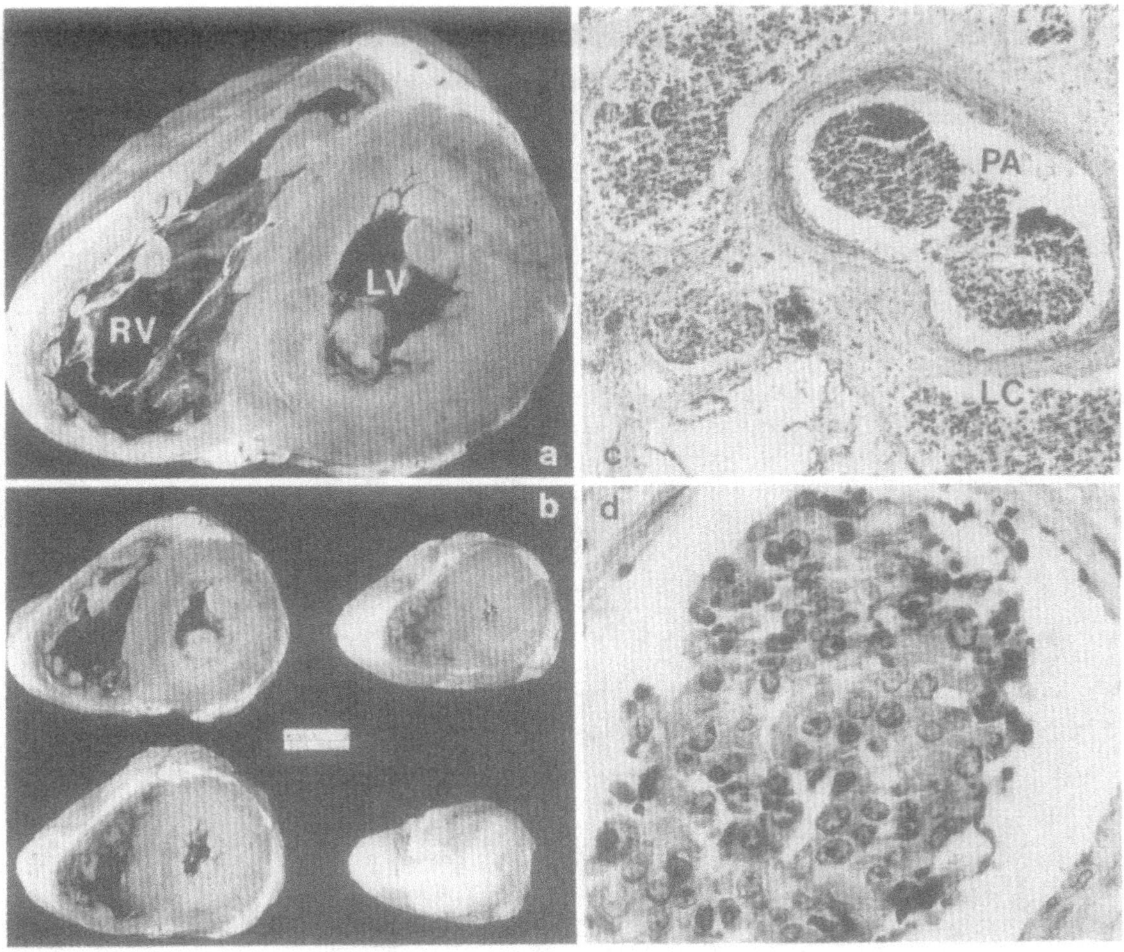

FIGURE 2. Case 1. Transverse cuts of the cardiac ventricles *(a and b)* showing a dilated right ventricle (RV) and a normal-sized left ventricle (LV). Microscopic sections of the lung show tumor emboli in *(c and d)* small pulmonary arteries (PA) and metastatic tumor in *(c)* lymphatic channels (LC). Hematoxylin-eosin stain × 100 *(c)*; Movat stain × 630 *(d)*; both reduced by 29%.

with progressive, unexplained dyspnea or pulmonary hypertension. Cytology of pulmonary venous blood may be diagnostic and antineoplastic therapy may be useful.

1. Kane RD, Hawkins HK, Miller JA, Noce PS. Microscopic pulmonary tumor emboli associated with dyspnea. *Cancer* 1975;36:1473–1482.

2. Marini JJ, Bilnoski W, Huseby JS. Acute cor pulmonale resulting from tumor microembolism. *West J Med* 1980;132:77–80.

3. Schriner RW, Ryu JH, Edwards WD. Microscopic pulmonary tumor embolism causing subacute cor pulmonale: a difficult antemortem diagnosis. *Mayo Clin Proc* 1991;66:143–148.

4. von Herbay A, Illes A, Waldherr R, Otto HF. Pulmonary tumor thrombotic microangiopathy with pulmonary hypertension. *Cancer* 1990;66:587–592.

5. Scully RE, ed. Case records of the Massachusetts General Hospital: case 30-1987. *N Engl J Med* 1987;317:225–235.

6. Altemus L, Lee R. Carcinomatosis of the lung with pulmonary hypertension: pathoradiologic spectrum. *Arch Intern Med* 1967;119:32–38.

7. Masson RG, Krikorian J, Lukl P, Evans GL, McGrath J. Pulmonary microvascular cytology in the diagnosis of lymphangitic carcinomatosis. *N Engl J Med* 1989; 321:71–76.

The Heart at Necropsy in Massive Obesity (>300 pounds or >136 kilograms)

A 52-year-old African-American man, who weighed 580 pounds (264 kg) and was 72 inches tall (body mass index = 79 kg/m^2!), was hospitalized because of increasing dyspnea. He had been known to have systemic hypertension, sleep apnea, and diabetes mellitus. He never had symptoms or objective evidence of myocardial ischemia. The serum total cholesterol was 142, low-density lipoprotein cholesterol 40, high-density lipoprotein cholesterol 17, and triglycerides 242 mg/dl. An echocardiogram disclosed the left ventricular ejection fraction to be 62%. Twelve days after admission he was found dead in bed. Autopsy disclosed massive pulmonary embolism without pulmonary infarction. The heart weighed 780 g, but did not float in water. The epicardium and the 4 cardiac valves were normal. The walls of the ventricles were devoid of foci of necrosis and fibrosis. The major epicardial coronary arteries were all large and devoid of atherosclerotic plaques. Likewise, the aorta contained few atherosclerotic plaques.

There are relatively few necropsy data on the status of the heart at necropsy in massively obese subjects. Amad et al,[1] in 1965, described findings at necropsy in 6 patients aged 35 to 65 years (mean 47), who weighed from 308 to 495 pounds (140 to 225 kg): the hearts in the 3 women weighed 400, 500, and 620 g and the hearts in the 3 men, 450, 900, and 1,100 g. The weights had been taken from autopsy reports. These authors excluded patients "who had clinical signs or pathologic evidence of coronary atherosclerosis or who had systemic arterial pressures ≥150/90 mm Hg." The number of patients excluded was not described. By gross examination, none of their patients had fatty infiltration into myocardium or grossly visible foci of myocardial necrosis or fibrosis.

Warnes and Roberts,[2] in 1984, described 12 patients at necropsy aged 25 to 59 years (mean 37; 5 women and 7 men) who weighed from 312 to >500 pounds (mean 381). Five patients had died suddenly, 2 of chronic congestive heart failure, 1 of acute myocardial infarction, 1 of aortic dissection, 1 of an intracerebral bleed, 1 of drug overdose, and 1 shortly after ileal bypass. Only 2 of the 12 patients had 1 or more epicardial coronary arteries narrowed >75% in cross-sectional area by atherosclerotic plaque and those 2 were the only 2 with left ventricular foci of either necrosis or fibrosis. Of the 2 patients with narrowing 76% to 100% in cross-sectional area by plaque, each patient had both the right and left anterior descending coronary arteries narrowed to this degree. Of the 48 major epicardial coronary arteries in the 12 patients (4/patient), 4 were narrowed at some point 76% to 100% in cross-sectional area by atherosclerotic plaque. A total of 664 five-mm segments were examined from 11 hearts (mean 60/patient). Only 2 patients had any 5-mm segments narrowed 76% to 100% in cross-sectional area. Of the 664 five-mm coronary segments, 431 (65%) were narrowed 0% to 25% in cross-sectional area; 143 (21%), 26% to 50%; 73 (11%), 51% to 75%; and 17 (3%) were narrowed 76% to 100%. The hearts in the 12 patients were all heavier than normal (380 to 990 g [mean 616]). The subepicardial adipose tissue by visual inspection appeared to be increased in 9 of the 12 patients, but in no patient did the heart float in water.

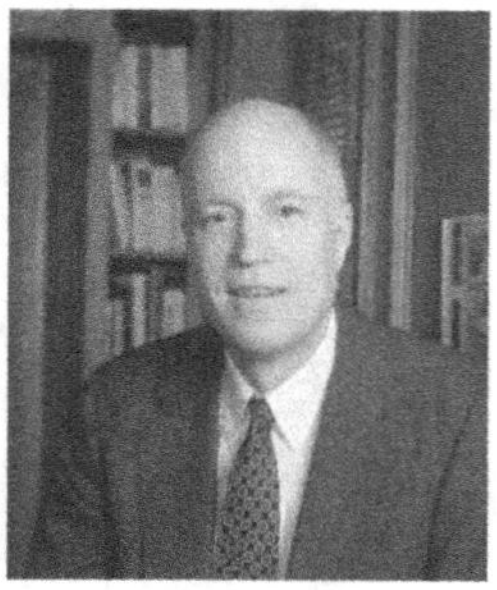

The average age of death in the 12 patients described by Warnes and Roberts was only 37 and only 1 patient was >50 years of age. That fact may be a major reason for the mild amount of coronary atherosclerosis found in these patients. The 2 with symptomatic fatal coronary disease were aged 42 and 59 years. In none of the 12 patients reported by Warnes and Roberts or in the 6 patients reported by Amad et al were serum cholesterol values available.

No other reports on the heart at necropsy in massively obese persons have appeared since 1984. It appears that the massively obese person usually dies from a noncoronary cause before significant coronary atherosclerosis has had time to develop.

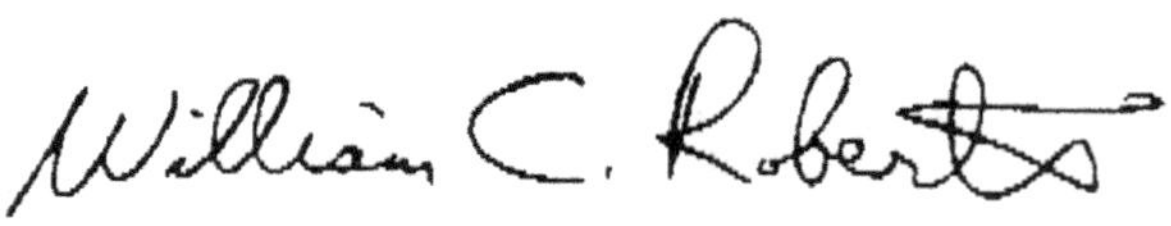

William Clifford Roberts, MD
Editor in Chief
Baylor Heart & Vascular Institute
Baylor University Medical Center
Dallas, Texas

1. Amad KH, Brennan JC, Alexander JK. The cardiac pathology of chronic exogenous obesity. *Circulation* 1965;32:740–745.
2. Warnes CA, Roberts WC. The heart in massive (more than 300 pounds or 136 kilograms) obesity: Analysis of 12 patients studied at necropsy. *Am J Cardiol* 1984;54:1087–1091.

Pulmonary talc granulomas, pulmonary fibrosis, and pulmonary hypertension resulting from intravenous injection of talc-containing drugs intended for oral use

William Clifford Roberts, MD

Talcosis or talc pneumoconiosis is an uncommon form of pulmonary dust disease first recognized over 100 years ago. Talcosis may follow inhalation of relatively low concentrations of talc dust over a long period or exposure to very high concentrations of the dust over a short time (1, 2). In an infant, death occurred within 20 hours of accidental inhalation of talcum powder containing approximately 93% talc (3). Baby powder, consisting mainly of talc powder, is insoluble and, if inhaled in large amounts, dries the tracheobronchial mucous membrane and prevents normal ciliary function. The small air passages then fill with retained mucus.

Talc, or hydrated magnesium silicate, is formed during the breakdown and weathering of serpentine, tremolite, and anthrophyllite rock (1). The fibrogenic properties of talc are attributed to these impurities, especially anthrophyllite and tremolite, which are members of the asbestos group of minerals.

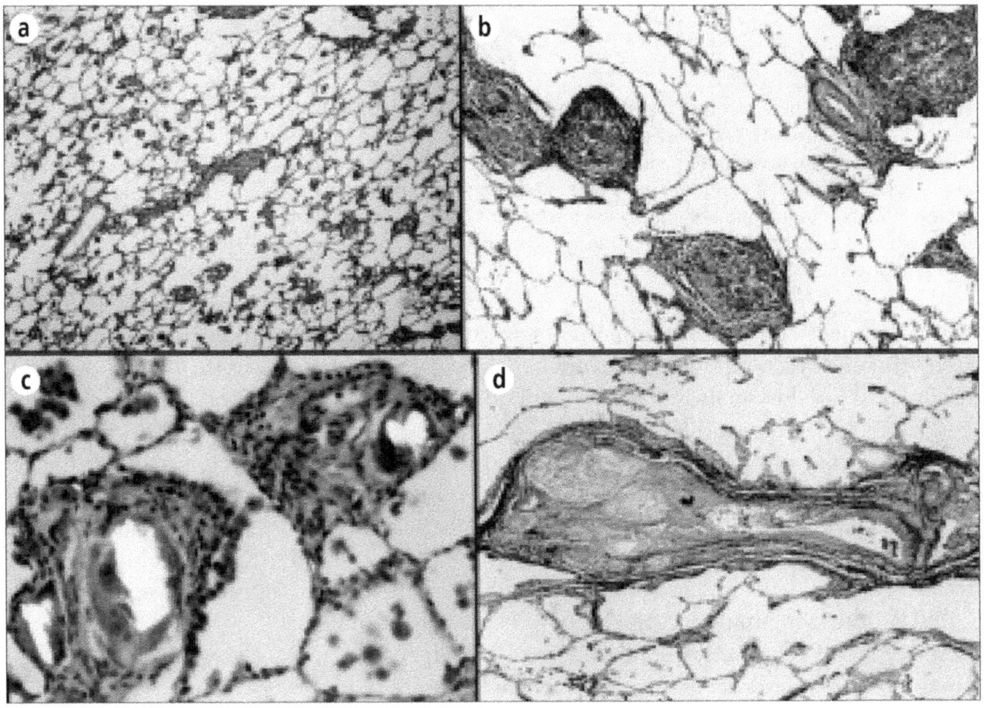

Figure 1. Histologic sections from the excised left lower lobe of the lung of a 23-year-old man who had been an intravenous drug addict (heroin, methadone, and methylphenidate tablets) since age 18. Interstitial talc granulomas are shown in **(a)**, **(b)**, and **(c)** at progressively higher magnifications. The refractile talc is best seen in **(c)**. Intra-arterial granuloma, shown in **(d)**, is an unusual occurrence in this patient. **(a, b, c)** Hematoxylin and eosin stains; **(d)** elastic van Gieson stain. Original magnification: **(a)** ×16; **(b)** ×54; **(c)** ×160, and **(d)** ×80. Reprinted from reference 4, copyright 1976, with permission from Excerpta Medica Inc.

Talc pneumoconiosis has been described in persons in several occupations, including talc mining and milling; manufacture of rubber cable and tires, accumulator plates, cosmetics, soaps, paints, and textiles; and sailing, since sailors dust life rafts with talc.

A new form of talc pulmonary disease, described initially in the 1960s, occurs in intravenous drug addicts who also inject tablets intended for oral use (4–10). Because most tablets (including phenmetrazine and methylphenidate) contain talc, which is used to hold the components of the medication together in tablet form, this practice can cause arterial obstruction by this foreign material. When these talc-containing drugs are injected into blood vessels rather than swallowed, foreign-body granulomatous reactions occur (*Figure 1*). Injection of these talc-containing drugs into a peripheral artery may cause ischemic necrosis of portions of the distal extremities or another organ (4). The more common practice of injecting these drugs into peripheral veins results in foreign-body granulomas in the lungs.

The exact percentage of addicts who follow this practice is uncertain (4). As shown in *Figure 2*, however, it is probably about 1% of nonalcohol drug addicts. Among intravenous drug addicts, all appear to inject opiates and probably none inject only tablets. It is probable that only a small percentage of opiate addicts frequently inject tablets. Thus, of all the intravenous drug users, pulmonary talc granulomas develop in only about 5%, i.e., those

From the Baylor Heart and Vascular Institute, the Department of Pathology, and the Section of Cardiology, Department of Internal Medicine, Baylor University Medical Center, Dallas, Texas.

Corresponding author: William Clifford Roberts, MD, Baylor Heart and Vascular Institute, Baylor University Medical Center, 3500 Gaston Avenue, Dallas, Texas 75246 (e-mail: wc.roberts@BaylorHealth.edu).

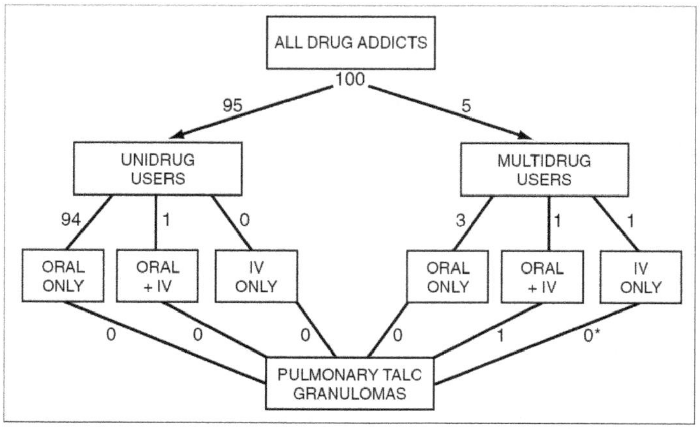

Figure 2. Among all persons who abuse drugs, those who use only one drug constitute the great majority, and those who abuse many drugs, the minority. Virtually all intravenous drug abusers appear to fall into the multidrug group. Talc granulomas form only in multidrug users because the intravenous injectors of tablets intended for oral use also usually use intravenous opiates and/or ingest drugs orally as well. Reprinted from reference 4, copyright 1976, with permission from Excerpta Medica Inc.

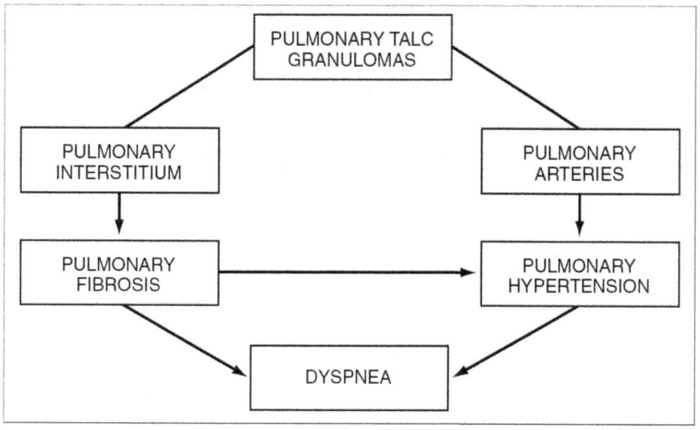

Figure 3. The effect of pulmonary talc granulomas located in pulmonary interstitium or in lumens of pulmonary arteries. Reprinted from reference 4, copyright 1976, with permission from Excerpta Medica Inc.

who also inject oral tablets. Pulmonary talc granulomas do not result from intravenous injection of opiates alone, because these drugs are diluted by maltose, lactose, and quinine, called "fillers," all of which are readily soluble.

Of reported intravenous drug addicts with pulmonary talc granulomas confirmed morphologically by lung biopsy or necropsy, virtually all had repeatedly injected medications intended for oral use. Six different medications have been reported to be associated with talc granulomas in addicts: methylphenidate (Ritalin), methadone, tripelennamine (Pyribenzamine), propoxyphene (Darvon), phenmetrazine (Preludin), and amphetamines; all contain talc. The foreign material present in the granulomas is morphologically consistent with talc, and in several reported patients, x-ray diffraction studies positively identified the material as talc (1). Additionally, when various components of drugs associated with granulomas are injected into experimental animals, only talc produces granulomas. Thus, talc, long known to cause foreign-body granulomatous reactions when applied to serosal surfaces and similar granulomatous reactions in the lungs when inhaled over prolonged periods, also produces foreign-body granulomas when injected intravenously as part of a dissolved oral medication.

The reaction to talc, however, is variable *(Figure 3)*. In some patients, widespread granulomas develop in the interstitium of the lung but relatively few in the pulmonary arteries. In other patients, this interstitial reaction may eventually lead to interstitial pulmonary fibrosis and to clinical evidence of restrictive lung disease. Other patients, after intravenous injection of oral medications, have talc granulomas predominantly in the lumens of small pulmonary arteries rather than in the interstitium. The result in these patients is pulmonary arterial hypertension rather than interstitial pulmonary disease. The pulmonary hypertension causes medial hypertrophy of the pulmonary arteries, often intimal fibrous thickening, and occasionally plexiform lesions in the lungs. The occurrence of plexiform lesions indicates that the pulmonary hypertension is irreversible (11).

Why the pulmonary talc granulomas are located predominantly in the interstitium in some patients and predominantly in the lumens of the pulmonary arteries in others is unclear. The total amount of injected talc must be important, but quantity may not be the only factor. It is unlikely that the type of tablet injected plays an important role, because a number of reported patients with severe pulmonary hypertension and predominantly intravascular granulomas injected different talc-containing drugs. Conceivably, there are differences in the talc itself, or possibly people react differently to injections of identical talc.

1. Miller A, Teirstein AS, Bader ME, Bader RA, Selikoff IJ. Talc pneumoconiosis. Significance of sublight microscopic mineral particles. *Am J Med* 1971;50:395–402.
2. Fine LJ, Peters JM, Burgess WA, Di Berardinis LJ. Studies of respiratory morbidity in rubber workers. Part IV. Respiratory morbidity in talc workers. *Arch Environ Health* 1976;31:195–200.
3. Molnar JJ, Nathenson G, Edberg S. Fatal aspiration of talcum powder by a child. Report of a case. *N Engl J Med* 1962;266:36–37.
4. Arnett EN, Battle WE, Russo JV, Roberts WC. Intravenous injection of talc-containing drugs intended for oral use. A cause of pulmonary granulomatosis and pulmonary hypertension. *Am J Med* 1976;60:711–718.
5. Paré JAP, Fraser RG, Hogg JC, Howlett JG, Murphy SB. Pulmonary "mainline" granulomatosis: talcosis of intravenous methadone abuse. *Medicine (Baltimore)* 1979;58:229–239.
6. Farber HW, Fairman RP, Glauser FL. Talc granulomatosis: laboratory findings similar to sarcoidosis. *Am Rev Respir Dis* 1982;125:258–261.
7. Paré JP, Cote G, Fraser RS. Long-term follow-up of drug abusers with intravenous talcosis. *Am Rev Respir Dis* 1989;139:233–241.
8. Schmidt RA, Glenny RW, Godwin JD, Hampson NB, Cantino ME, Reichenbach DD. Panlobular emphysema in young intravenous Ritalin abusers. *Am Rev Respir Dis* 1991;143:649–656.
9. Yohay DA, Oddone EZ. Intravenous drug use fools us again. The importance of open lung biopsy in evaluating a patient with progressive interstitial lung disease presenting with pneumothorax. *N C Med J* 1991;52:357–358.
10. Nan DN, Fernandez-Ayala M, Iglesias L, Garcia-Palomo D, Parra JA, Farinas MC. Talc granulomatosis. A differential diagnosis of interstitial lung disease in HIV patients. *Chest* 2000;118:258–260.
11. Roberts WC. A simple histologic classification of pulmonary arterial hypertension. *Am J Cardiol* 1986;58:385–386.

Mitral "Annular" Calcium Forming a Complete Circle "O" Causing Mitral Stenosis in Association With a Stenotic Congenitally Bicuspid Aortic Valve and Severe Coronary Artery Disease

Kevin P. Theleman, MD;[1,3] Paul A. Grayburn, MD;[1,3] William C. Roberts, MD[1,2,3]
From the Departments of Medicine (Division of Cardiology)[1] and Pathology[2] and the Baylor Heart and Vascular Institute,[3] Baylor University Medical Center, Dallas, TX
Address for correspondence: William C. Roberts, MD, Baylor Heart and Vascular Institute, Baylor University Medical Center, 621 North Hall Street, Suite H-030, Dallas, TX 75226
E-mail: wcroberts@baylorhealth.edu

Calcific deposits in the epicardial arteries, mitral valve annulus, and aortic valve cusps are common in older persons in the Western world.[1] Recently, we encountered a patient with massive mitral annular calcium causing mitral stenosis in association with a stenotic congenitally bicuspid aortic valve and heavy coronary calcific deposits. The extent of the cardiac calcific deposits is unusual and prompted this report.

A 73-year-old man had an orthotopic liver transplant for alcoholic cirrhosis at age 60, a renal transplant at age 65, a dual-chamber pacemaker inserted for sick sinus syndrome at age 72, and had corticosteroid-induced diabetes mellitus and systemic hypertension. The present examination was prompted by the recent onset of pedal edema. A grade 2/6 systolic ejection murmur that was loudest over the right base of the precordium was present. His body mass index was 22 kg/m^2. Echocardiography disclosed a 6-mm Hg mean diastolic gradient at the mitral orifice and a left ventricular ejection fraction of about 55% (Figure 1). Cardiac catheterization revealed a peak systolic pressure gradient between the left ventricle and aorta of 50 mm Hg (mean gradient, 38 mm Hg) and an aortic valve area of 0.6 cm^2. The left anterior descending artery was narrowed up to 70% in diameter proximally, the second diagonal artery up to 80% proximally, and the ramus intermedius artery up to 80% proximally. The left main coronary artery was widely patent. The dominant left circumflex artery was narrowed up to 50% in diameter and was heavily calcified. The nondominant right coronary artery was free of narrowing.

The aortic valve was replaced with a 21-mm Medtronic Mosaic (Medtronic, Inc., Mineapolis, MN) bioprosthesis. The surgically removed aortic valve was congenitally bicuspid (Figure 2). Aortosaphenous vein grafts were placed to the left anterior descending and the first marginal coronary arteries. An intra-aortic balloon pump was placed intraoperatively. Aortic cross-clamp time was 149 minutes. The postoperative course was complicated by the low cardiac output syndrome, and death occurred 5 days postoperatively.

At necropsy, the coronary arteries and mitral annular region were massively calcified (Figure 3). The ventricular cavities were not dilated (Figure 4). The bioprosthesis in the aortic valve position appeared to have functioned normally. The venous conduits to the left anterior descending and obtuse marginal arteries were patent.

The most prevalent site of cardiac calcific deposits is the epicardial coronary arteries, followed by the mitral annular area and aortic valve cusps. The apical portions of the left papillary

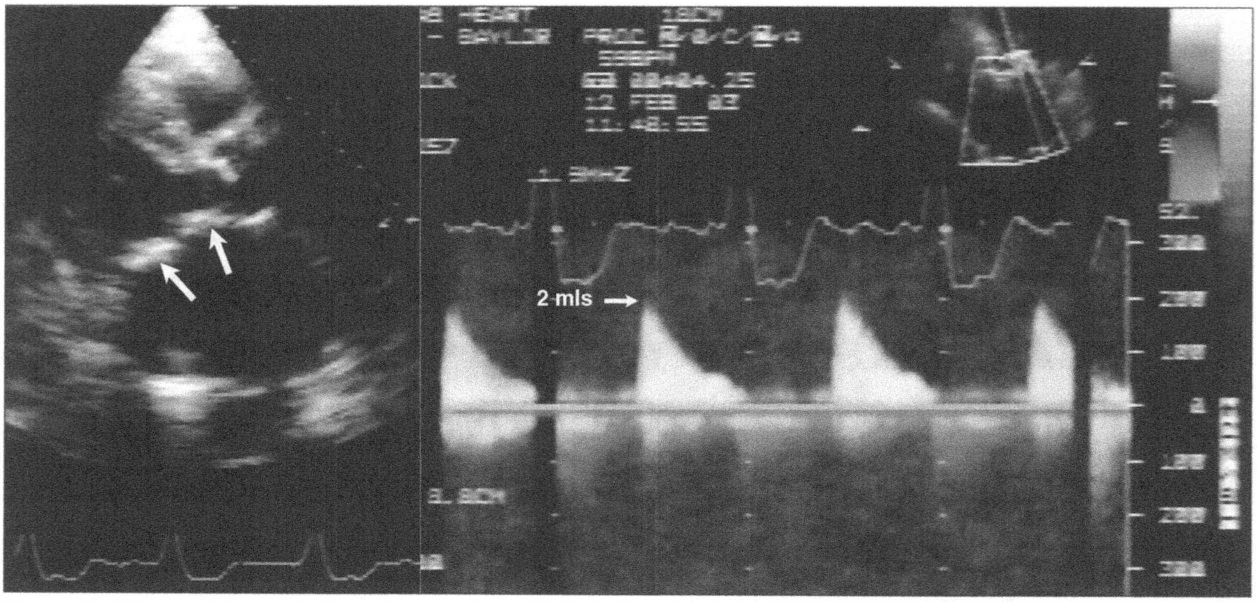

Figure 1. Echocardiogram. Left panel: parasternal long-axis view showing extensive calcification deposits of the mitral annulus (arrows) and aortic valve; right panel: transmitral Doppler inflow showing a peak velocity of 2.0 m/sec and a mean gradient of 6 mm Hg

muscles are the fourth most common area of the heart to have calcific deposits.[1] The term "mitral annular calcium" is not accurate in that the calcium deposits are actually located between the ventricular surface of the posterior mitral valve leaflet and the mural endocardium of the left ventricle. When the calcium deposits are extensive, a "C"-shaped or "J"-shaped configuration can appear on radiograph. In rare cases, the calcium extends across the anterior mitral leaflet forming an "O"-shaped configuration.[2] Mitral annular calcium is often associated with mild or moderate mitral regurgitation, but severe regurgitation due to the calcium deposits alone probably does not occur.[2] Significant mitral stenosis due to annular calcium has been reported only in the setting of left ventricular outflow obstruction, as occurred in the present patient.[3]

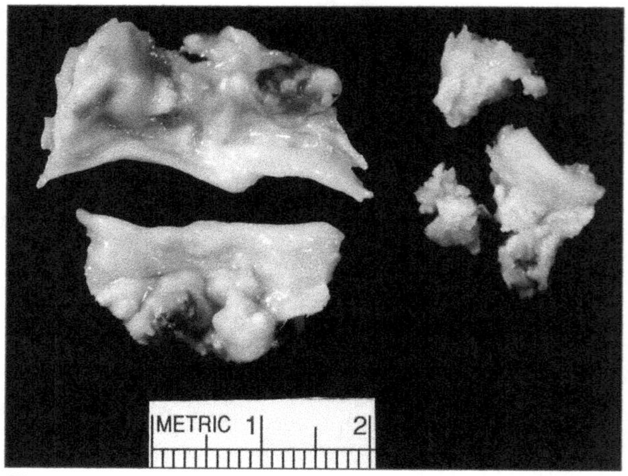

Figure 2. Photograph of the operatively excised focally calcified, stenotic, congenitally bicuspid aortic valve

References

1 Roberts WC. The senile cardiac calcification syndrome. *Am J Cardiol.* 1986;58:572–574.

2 Roberts WC, Waller BF. Mitral valve "annular" calcium forming a complete circle or "O" configuration: clinical and necropsy observations. *Am Heart J.* 1981;101:619–621.

3 Hammer WJ, Roberts WC, deLeon AC. "Mitral stenosis" secondary to combined "massive" mitral annular calcific deposits and small, hypertrophied left ventricles. Hemodynamic documentation in four patients. *Am J Med.* 1978;64:371–376.

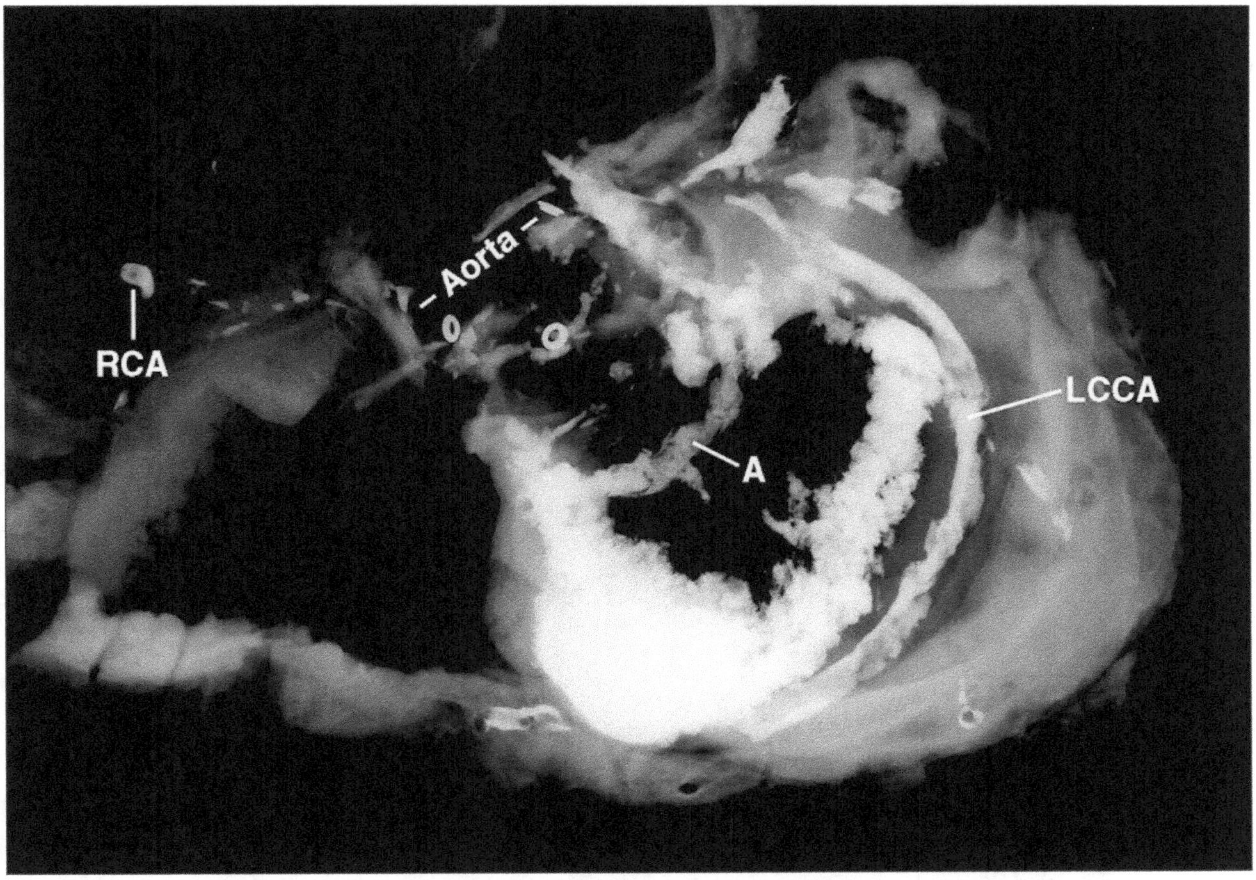

Figure 3. Radiograph of the heart at necropsy. A huge amount of calcium is located beneath the posterior mitral leaflet and extends across the anterior (A) mitral leaflet forming a circle "O." The left circumflex coronary artery (LCCA) is heavily and diffusely calcified (about 50% of patients with a congenitally bicuspid aortic valve have a dominant left circumflex rather than a dominant right coronary artery [RCA], the situation in about 90% of patients with a tricuspid aortic valve). Calcific deposits also are present in the left main and left anterior descending coronary arteries.

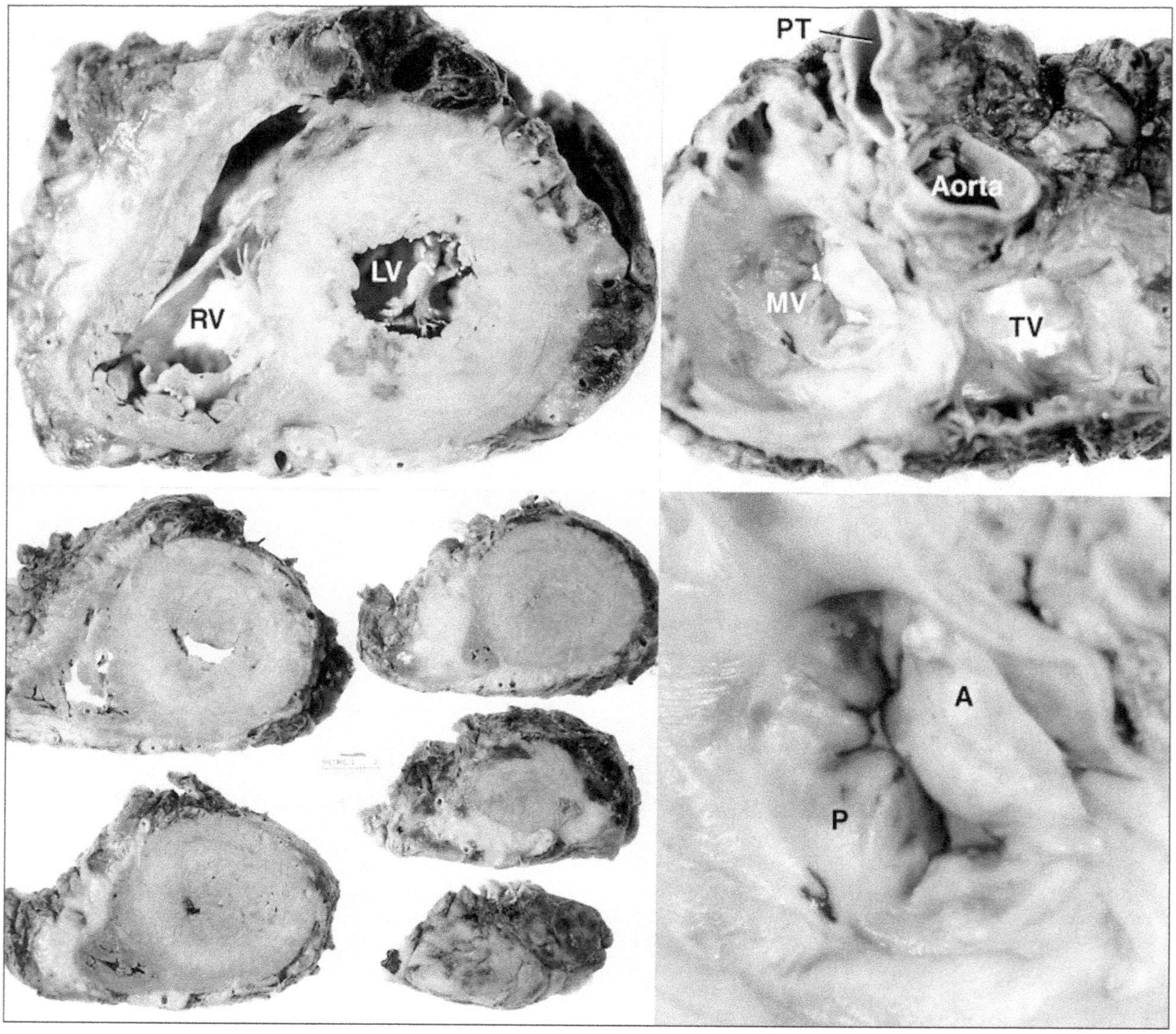

Figure 4. Photographs of the heart at necropsy. Upper left: view of left (LV) and right (RV) ventricles showing normal-sized cavities and a small area of myocardial necrosis in the posterior wall; lower left: transverse sections of the cardiac ventricles showing small cavities and no myocardial lesions; upper right: view of mitral (MV) and tricuspid valve (TV) orifices from the atrial aspects, with pulmonary trunk (PT); lower right: close-up view of the MV from the left atrium showing the anterior (A) and posterior (P) leaflets

Comparison of Findings in Patients With Versus Without Atrial Fibrillation Just Before Isolated Mitral Valve Replacement for Rheumatic Mitral Stenosis (With or Without Associated Mitral Regurgitation)

John Bryan Sims, MD[a,b], and William Clifford Roberts, MD[a,b,*]

Among 104 patients with mitral stenosis (MS) severe enough or symptomatic enough to warrant mitral valve replacement (MVR), 47 (45%) had atrial fibrillation (AF) and 57 (55%) had sinus rhythm just before the MVR. Of the latter 57 patients, 21 (37%) had had previous episodes compatible with AF. If these 21 patients were included with the 47 patients with electrocardiographic documentation of AF just before MVR, a total of 68 (65%) would have had ≥1 presumed episodes of AF before MVR. The 13 patients with previous mitral commissurotomy had a frequency of AF similar to that of the 91 whose first operation was MVR. Compared with the patients with sinus rhythm just before MVR, those with AF had more heart failure (functional class III or IV preoperatively, 79% vs 62%), larger left atria (6.0 vs 5.2 cm), larger left ventricles in peak systole (4.0 vs 2.6 cm), and more had 2 or 3 coronary arteries narrowed >50% in diameter (23% vs 10%).
(Am J Cardiol 2006;97:1035–1038)

The frequency of atrial fibrillation (AF) is higher in patients with mitral stenosis (MS) than in any other condition. In a study of 710 patients with unoperated MS seen in an outpatient clinic by Diker and associates[1] and unassociated with aortic valve disease, 343 (48%) had AF by electrocardiogram. The average age of those with chronic AF was 43 years and those with sinus rhythm, 33 years. The present study focuses on patients with MS who underwent mitral valve replacement (MVR) and compares those with AF to those without AF by electrocardiogram immediately before MVR.

• • •

Patients having isolated (no other cardiac valves replaced) MVR for MS at Baylor University Medical Center from May 1993 to January 2005 were reviewed. All operatively excised stenotic mitral valves submitted to the surgical pathology department during this period were examined by 1 of us (WCR). That the valves were stenotic was determined by gross examination of the operatively excised valve by 1 of us (WCR), and by examining the clinical and hemodynamic records to confirm the presence of MS with or without mitral regurgitation . Patients ≤20 years of age and patients having simultaneous aortic and/or tricuspid valve replacement were excluded. Cases in whom the MS was the result of mitral annular calcium also were excluded.

A total of 104 patients had MVR for MS (with or without mitral regurgitation) during the 128-month period of this study. Electrocardiographic data immediately before MVR were available in all patients. Echocardiographic data were available in 65 patients (63%), hemodynamic data in 74 patients (71%), and coronary arterial angiographic data in 91 patients (88%).

Statistical analysis was performed using SigmaStat (version 2.0; SPSS, Inc., Chicago, Illinois). Parametric tests were used for the analysis of the data, which passed the assumption tests for normality and equal variance: for continuous variables, unpaired *t* test was performed for 2 variable comparisons and 1-way analysis of variance for >2 variable comparisons. When the data did not pass the assumption tests, nonparametric tests, i.e., Man-Whitney Rank Sum test for 2 variable comparisons and Kruskal-Wallis 1-way analysis of variance on ranks test for >2 continuous variable comparisons, were used. To compare the percentages in 2 different groups, the z-test was used. To compare the percentages in >3 different groups, the chi-square test was used. A p value <0.05 was considered statistically significant.

Table 1 compares certain clinical, echocardiograpic, hemodynamic, and cineangiographic findings in the 13 patients with previous mitral commissurotomy to the 91 patients without previous mitral commissurotomy. The only difference observed between these 2 groups were higher pressures in the aorta in those with previous mitral commissurotomy versus those whose first mitral operation was MVR.

Table 2 excludes the 13 patients with previous mitral commissurotomy and compares the remaining 91 patients whose first cardiac operation was MVR. The 38 patients (42%) who had AF by electrocardiogram immediately before MVR compared with the 53 patients (58%) who were in sinus rhythm immediately before MVR had a higher

From the Departments of [a]Internal Medicine (Division of Cardiology) and [b]Pathology, and the Baylor Heart & Vascular Institute, Baylor University Medical Center, Dallas, Texas. Manuscript received October 11, 2005; revised manuscript received and accepted November 15, 2005.

* Corresponding author: Tel: 214-820-7911; fax: 212-820-7533.
E-mail address: wc.roberts@baylorhealth.edu (W.C. Roberts).

Table 1
Comparison of various variables in the 13 patients with previous mitral commissurotomy to the 91 patients without mitral commissurotomy

	Previous Mitral Commissurotomy		
Variable	No (n = 91)	Yes (n = 13)	p Value
Age (years)	33–80 (60)	35–70 (54)	0.09
White	63 (69%)	6 (46%)	0.49
Female	79 (87%)	12 (92%)	0.98
Atrial fibrillation immediately before mitral valve replacement by electrocardiogram	38 (42%)	9 (69%)	0.28
Atrial fibrillation (by history)	57 (62%)	10 (77%)	0.58
Systemic hypertension (by history)	48 (53%)	4 (31%)	0.75
Diabetes mellitus	15 (16%)	2 (15%)	0.32
Prior myocardial infarction	8 (8%)		0.42
Coronary bypass at time of mitral operation	23 (25%)	1 (8%)	0.23
New York Heart Association functional class			
I	1 (1%)		
II	27 (30%)	1 (8%)	
III	58 (64%)	12 (92%)	
IV	5 (5%)		
Number of major coronary arteries narrowed >50% in diameter			0.80
0	64 (70%)	10 (77%)	
1	14 (5%)	2 (15%)	
2	5 (5%)	1 (8%)	
3	6 (7%)	0 (0%)	
Left main	2 (2%)	0 (0%)	
Body mass index (kg/m^2): range (mean)	16–84 (30)	17–34 (26)	0.51
<25	34 (37%)	5 (85%)	0.21
26–30	31 (34%)	7 (54%)	
<30	26 (29%)	1 (8%)	
Days in hospital after mitral operation	4–36 (9)	5–18 (8)	0.25
Echocardiographic data: range (mean)			
Left atrium (mm)	38–66 (52)	45–92 (60)	0.08
Left ventricle, peak systole (mm)	20–52 (34)	32–42 (37)	0.73
Mitral valve area (cm^2)	0.7–1.6 (1.2)	0.8–1.6 (1.1)	0.14
Ejection fraction (%)	10–70 (56%)	50–65 (59%)	0.59
Cardiovascular direct pressures (mm Hg): range (mean)			
Mean diastolic gradient between pulmonary artery wedge and left ventricle	5–35 (16)	10–26 (15)	0.90
Pulmonary artery wedge	12–60 (25)	15–35 (23)	0.65
Right ventricular peak systole	27–170 (58)	30–64 (45)	0.09
Right ventricular end-diastole	1–36 (13)	12–14 (13)	0.86
Right atrium mean	1–35 (11)	8–12 (10)	0.84
Pulmonary artery peak systole	24–171 (55)	26–68 (46)	0.21
Pulmonary artery end-diastole	7–76 (25)	15–26 (20)	0.18
Pulmonary artery mean	13–115 (37)	21–40 (30)	0.10
Left ventricular systole	85–184 (129)	106–176 (140)	0.31
Left ventricular end-diastole	4–72 (15)	6–50 (21)	0.34
Aorta peak systole	90–179 (127)	125–187 (148)	0.04
Aorta end-diastole	32–100 (71)	70–90 (82)	0.04
Aorta mean	58–142 (96)	96–125 (110)	0.02
Other cardiac catheterization data:			
Valve area (cm^2)	0.5–2.1 (1.0)	0.8–1.2 (1.1)	0.40
Cardiac index ($L/min/m^2$)	1.5–3.3 (2.3)	1.8–3.2 (2.5)	0.42
Ejection fraction (%)	15–70 (58)	45–60 (54)	0.37
Associated mitral regurgitation	74 (81%)	9 (69%)	0.68
Maze procedure	17 (19%)	1 (8%)	0.29
Tricuspid valve annuloplasty	7 (8%)	2 (15%)	0.29
Patent foramen ovale closure	7 (8%)	2 (15%)	0.29

percentage of heart failure class III or IV (79% vs 62%), a higher percentage of narrowing >50% in diameter of 2 or 3 major epicardial coronary arteries (23% vs 10%), more days in the hospital after MVR (10 vs 9 days), larger left atria (5.7 vs 4.8 cm), larger left ventricular cavities in peak systole (4.0 vs 2.6 cm), smaller mitral valve areas (1.0 vs 1.3 cm), and lower mean pulmonary artery wedge pressures (22 vs 27 mm Hg). Comparison of various variables among the 20 patients who had had a history of an arrhythmia but had sinus rhythm by electrocardiogram immediately before

Table 2
Comparison of clinical findings in patients with and without atrial fibrillation (AF) by electrocardiogram just before mitral valve replacement (MVR) for mitral stenosis and never a previous mitral commissurotomy (n = 104)

Variable	Atrial Fibrillation by Electrocardiogram Immediately Before MVR: Yes (n = 38)	No* (n = 53)	p Value
Age (years)	42–80 (62)	33–78 (59)	0.22
White	27 (71%)	36 (68%)	0.098
Female/male	34 (89%)/4 (11%)	45 (85%)/8 (15%)	.098
Systemic hypertension (by history)	20 (53%)	28 (53%)	0.77
Diabetes mellitus	9 (24%)	6 (11%)	0.97
Prior myocardial infarction	5 (13%)	3 (6%)	0.38
Coronary bypass at time of mitral operation	11 (29%)	12 (23%)	0.88
New York Heart Association functional class			
I	0 (0%)	1 (2%)	0.31
II	8 (21%)	19 (36%)	
III	27 (71%)	31 (58%)	0.05
IV	3 (8%)	2 (4%)	
Number of major coronary arteries narrowed >50% in diameter			
0	25 (66%)	35 (66%)	0.14
1	4 (11%)	13 (25%)	
2	5 (12%)	2 (4%)	0.001
3	4 (11%)	3 (6%)	
Left main	1 (3%)	1 (2%)	
Body mass index (kg/m^2): range (mean)	16–43 (28)	16–48 (28)	0.29–0.75
<25	14 (36%)	21 (40%)	
26–30	12 (32%)	19 (36%)	
<30	12 (32%)	13 (25%)	
Days in hospital after mitral operation	4–36 (10)	4–25 (9)	0.03
Echocardiographic data: range (mean)			
Left atrium (mm)	43–60 (57)	33–65 (48)	0.002
Left ventricle, peak systole (mm)	32–52 (40)	20–30 (26)	0.02
Mitral valve area (cm^2)	0.7–1.4 (1.0)	1–1.6 (1.3)	0.007
Ejection fraction (%)	10–70 (54)	30–70 (57)	0.25
Cardiovascular direct pressures (mm Hg): range (mean)			
Mean diastolic gradient between pulmonary artery wedge and left ventricle	5–35 (15)	4–33 (18)	0.13
Pulmonary artery wedge	12–46 (22)	7–60 (27)	0.02
Right ventricular peak systole	27–170 (59)	31–119 (58)	0.61
Right ventricular end-diastole	2–25 (12)	1–46 (14)	0.36
Right atrium mean	3–26 (11)	1–35 (11)	0.77
Pulmonary artery peak systole	24–171 (55)	28–103 (54)	0.68
Pulmonary artery end-diastole	10–76 (27)	7–46 (23)	0.39
Pulmonary artery mean	15–115 (38)	13–64 (37)	0.55
Left ventricular systole	85–163 (125)	82–234 (131)	0.84
Left ventricular end-diastole	4–23 (13)	1–72 (17)	0.14
Aorta peak systole	90–171 (128)	87–225 (126)	0.90
Aorta end-diastole	32–100 (72)	5–100 (71)	0.72
			0.79
Other cardiac catheterization data:			
Mitral valve area (cm^2)	0.5–1.4 (0.9)	0.7–2.1 (1.1)	0.07
Cardiac index ($L/min/m^2$)	1.5–3.3 (2.2)	1.4–3.4 (2.3)	0.17
Ejection fraction (%)	15–65 (51)	25–70 (58)	0.06
Associated mitral regurgitation	29 (76%)	45 (85%)	0.51
Maze procedure	12 (32%)	5 (9%)	0.70
Tricuspid valve annuloplasty	5 (13%)	4 (8%)	0.40
Patent foramen ovale repair	1 (3%)	4 (8%)	0.04

* Of the 53 patients with sinus rhythm by electrocardiogram immediately before MVR, 20 (38%) had had previous episodes constantly with AF. Comparison of these 20 patients with paroxysmal AF to the 33 without disclosed only 1 significant difference: those with paroxysmal AF had a higher frequency of left atria >4.0 cm than the group who never had AF.

MVR showed only 1 significant difference between them, i.e., a higher percent of left atrial cavities (>4.0 cm) in the paroxysmal AF group by echocardiography.

• • •

The present study showed that among 104 patients with MS, 47 (45%) had AF and 57 (55%) had sinus rhythm by electrocardiogram immediately before MVR. The frequency of electrocardiographically documented AF just before MVR was similar in the 13 patients with previous mitral commissurotomy compared with the 91 patients in whom MVR was their first cardiac operation. Of the 57 patients among the total of 104 with sinus rhythm just before MVR, 21 (37%) had a history of a dysrhythmia, presumably AF. If these 21 patients were included with the 47 with electrocardiographic documentation of AF just before MVR, a total of 68 (65%) would have had ≥1 presumed episodes of AF before MVR.

Others have shown the left atrium to be larger in MS patients with AF compared with those in sinus rhythm. Probst et al[2] studied 135 patients with MS who had not undergone a mitral valve operation: 73 (54%) had AF (intermittent in 27 and persistent in 46) and 62 (46%) had persistent sinus rhythm. Compared with the sinus rhythm group, the AF patients were older (52 vs 42 years), had a higher frequency of "moderate" and "gross" left atrial enlargement by radiograph (41 of 73 [56%] vs 26 of 62 [42%]), and lower cardiac indexes (2.2 vs 2.8 L/min^2). Henry and associates[3] studied, by M-mode echocardiography, 85 patients with "isolated mitral valve disease" (at least 67 of whom had MS) and found AF in 47 (55%), 45 (96%) of whom had left atrial dimensions ≥40 mm. Of 733 unoperated MS patients studied by Diker et al,[1], the left atrial diameter averaged 5.7 ± 1.2 cm among the 355 patients (48%) with AF (unassociated with aortic valve disease) and 4.0 ± 7 cm among the 378 patients (52%) with sinus rhythm. The left atrium usually becomes smaller after a successful operation for MS.[4]

Acknowledgment: We are grateful to Jong Mi Ko, BS, for the superb help with the statistical analyses.

1. Diker E, Aydogdu S, Özdemir M, Kural T, Polat K, Cehreli S, Erdogan A, Göksel S. Prevalence and predictors of atrial fibrillation in rheumatic valvular heart disease. *Am J Cardiol* 1996;77:96–98.
2. Probst P, Goldschlager N, Selzer A. Left atrial size and atrial fibrillation in mitral stenosis. Factors influencing their relationship. *Circulation* 1973;48:1282–1287.
3. Henry WL, Morganroth J, Pearlman AS, Clark CE, Redwood DR, Itscoitz SB, Epstein SE. Relation between echocardiographically determined left atrial size and atrial fibrillation. *Circulation* 1976; 53:273–279.
4. Sherrid MV, Clark RD, Cohn K. Echocardiographic analysis of left atrial size before and after operation in mitral valve disease. *Am J Cardiol* 1979;43:171–178.

Frequency of Atrial Fibrillation in Patients Having Mitral Valve Repair or Replacement for Pure Mitral Regurgitation Secondary to Mitral Valve Prolapse

Rafic Fouad Berbarie, MD[a,b], and William Clifford Roberts, MD[a,b,c,*]

Relatively little attention has been paid to the frequency of atrial fibrillation (AF) in patients with mitral regurgitation (MR) secondary to mitral valve prolapse (MVP). We reviewed clinical, electrocardiographic, echocardiographic, hemodynamic, and angiographic findings in 246 patients aged 21 to 84 years (mean 61) (66% men) who had mitral valve repair or replacement for MR secondary to MVP. Immediately before the mitral operation by electrocardiogram, only 37 patients (15%) had AF and the other 209 patients were in sinus rhythm. Of the latter, 32 had had a history of AF that had reverted to sinus rhythm spontaneously or with antiarrhythmic therapy. Thus, a total of 69 patients (28%) had AF at some time. In conclusion, the frequency of AF in patients with MR secondary to MVP and sick enough to warrant a mitral valve operation have a relatively low frequency of AF (persistent in 15%, paroxysmal in another 13%), percentages considerably lower than that seen in patients with mitral stenosis just before a mitral commissurotomy or replacement. **(Am J Cardiol 2006;97:1039–1044)**

Since its initial description in 1963, numerous articles on various aspects of mitral valve prolapse (MVP) have appeared.[1] Indeed, from 1966 to 2000, a total of 3,772 articles on MVP were cited on a Medline search. Although many articles mentioned atrial fibrillation (AF), few have focused on its frequency. This report focuses on the frequency of AF in a large group of patients having either mitral valve repair or replacement for mitral regurgitation (MR) secondary to MVP. The hypothesis was that the frequency of AF preoperatively would be relatively small despite the frequency of relatively large atrial cavities.

Methods

From March 1993 to January 2005, a total of 274 patients had mitral valve repair or replacement for pure, i.e., no element of mitral stenosis, MR secondary to MVP at Baylor University Medical Center. All of these operatively excised valves or portions of the valves were examined by 1 of us (WCR), and the etiology of the MR was determined by gross (and often histologic) examination of the operatively excised valve tissue plus examination of the medical record.[2] Of the 274 patients, 28 were eliminated from the present study because of a previous cardiac operation (10 patients), having a pacemaker (5 patients), having a procedure performed simultaneously on the aortic valve (1 patient), or because the clinical chart was unavailable for review (12 patients). The remaining 246 patients were included in the present study. The mitral operation in these patients was their first cardiac operation; all were >20 years of age, none had tricuspid valve replacement, or a procedure performed on the aortic valve.

The electrocardiogram immediately before the mitral operation was reviewed in all 246 patients. Hemodynamic data from cardiac catheterization was available in 143 patients (58%); coronary angiographic data were also available in 217 patients (88%); and echocardiographic data were available in 94 patients (38%).

Statistical analysis was completed using GB-STAT version 10.0 (Dynamic Microsystems Inc., 2004). Variables are expressed as means, with corresponding ranges or frequencies, with corresponding percentages. Means and frequencies were compared with Student's *t* tests. The patients were divided and compared by preoperative rhythm, age, sex, and whether mitral repair or replacement was done. A p value <0.05 was considered statistically significant.

Results

The major findings in the 246 patients are listed in Table 1. The patients were divided into 2 groups: (1) those in whom the electrocardiogram immediately before the mitral valve operation disclosed sinus rhythm (n = 209; 85%); and (2) those in whom the electrocardiogram immediately preoperatively

From the [a]Baylor Heart & Vascular Institute, and the Departments of [b]Medicine (Division of Cardiology) and [c]Pathology, Baylor University Medical Center, Dallas, Texas. Manuscript received October 11, 2005; revised manuscript received and accepted November 4, 2005.

* Corresponding author: Tel: 214-820-7911; fax: 214-820-7533.
E-mail address: wc.roberts@baylorhealth.edu (W.C. Roberts).

Table 1
Preoperative clinical findings in 246 patients with and without pre-op atrial fibrillation by electrocardiogram immediately before mitral valve operation for mitral regurgitation secondary to mitral valve prolapse

Variable	Atrial Fibrillation		p Value
	No (n = 209) (85%)	Yes (n = 37) (15%)	
Age (years): range (mean)	21–81 (59)	34–84 (69)	<0.0001
White	191 (91%)	37 (100%)	<0.06
Men:women	143 (68%):66 (32%)	20 (54%):17 (46%)	0.10
Echocardiographic dimensions (mm) (mean)			
Left atrium	29–65 (50)	41–76 (54)	0.16
Left ventricular peak systole	13–48 (36)	17–50 (38)	0.53
Left ventricular end diastole	18–79 (60)	39–61 (56)	0.22
Pressures (mm Hg) (range) (mean)			
Pulmonary artery peak systole	17–87 (39)	41–76 (44)	0.12
Pulmonary artery mean	10–62 (25)	10–50 (29)	0.15
Left ventricular peak systole	68–198 (125)	89–190 (124)	0.92
Left ventricular end-diastole	3–36 (19)	9–39 (19)	0.99
Pulmonary artery wedge mean	3–43 (17)	5–31 (20)	<0.08
Right ventricular peak systole	12–83 (39)	20–71 (43)	0.14
Right ventricular end-diastole	2–24 (11)	4–25 (12)	0.52
Right atrial mean	1–35 (7)	1–20 (10)	<0.004
Aorta (peak systole)	68–200 (126)	87–199 (126)	0.90/0.67
(end diastole)	39–98 (70)	50–99 (71)	
Other hemodynamic			
Cardiac index (L/min/m^2)	1.4–5.4 (2.7)	1.5–4.1 (2.3)	<0.06
Ejection fraction (%)	30–75 (58)	25–70 (51)	0.0003
Body mass index (kg/m^2)(mean)	26	24	<0.006
≤25	109 (52%)	24 (65%)	0.15
26–30	77 (37%)	12 (32%)	0.56
>30	23 (11%)	1 (3%)	0.13
Systemic hypertension	106 (51%)	20 (54%)	0.74
Mean New York Heart Association functional class (mean)	2.4	2.9	<0.002
I	38 (18%)	3 (8%)	
II	74 (35%)	6 (16%)	<0.002
III	76 (36%)	20 (54%)	
IV	21 (11%)	8 (22%)	<0.002
Number of major coronary arteries narrowed >50% in diameter:	(n = 182)	(n = 35)	
0	139 (77%)	24 (69%)	0.31
1	20 (11%)	3 (9%)	
2	11 (6%)	0 (0%)	
3	8 (4%)	5 (13%)	0.31
Left main	4 (2%)	3 (9%)	
Coronary bypass	42 (20%)	10 (27%)	0.34

disclosed AF (n = 37; 15%). Of the 11 major variables analyzed in the 2 groups, 5 showed significant differences. In contrast to the sinus rhythm group, preoperatively, the AF patients were significantly older (69 vs 59 years), had a lower mean body mass index (24 vs 26 kg/m^2), had a higher New York Heart Association functional class (2.9 vs. 2.4), a higher mean right atrial pressure (10 vs 7 mm Hg), and lower mean ejection fraction (51% vs 58%).

Of the 209 patients with sinus rhythm by electrocardiogram immediately before the mitral valve operation, 32 (15%) had had previous episodes of AF that had either converted to sinus rhythm spontaneously or with use of antiarrhythmic drugs or electrical cardioversion. Thus, of the total 246 patients, 69 (28%) had had ≥1 episode of AF (persistent in 37 and paroxysmal in 32). Comparison of the various variables depicted in Table 1 between the 37 patients with persistent AF and the 32 patients with paroxysmal AF disclosed only 1 significant difference: the persistent group had a lower frequency of a history of systemic hypertension than the paroxysmal AF group (20 [54%] vs 23 [72%]; p = 0.01).

Comparison of 12 variables in the men versus the women are presented in Table 2. In contrast to the women, the men had significantly larger left ventricular cavities, lower left ventricular and aortic peak systolic pressures, lower ejection fractions, higher body mass indexes, more angiographic coronary arterial narrowing, and a higher frequency of simultaneous coronary arterial bypass grafting (at the time of the mitral operation).

Comparison of 13 variables in the 157 patients having mitral valve repair versus the 89 patients having mitral valve replacement are listed in Table 3; only 1 significant difference was found—the replacement group had a higher frequency of AF.

Table 2
Comparison of preoperative findings between the men and women who had mitral valve operations for mitral regurgitation secondary to mitral valve prolapse

Variable	Men (n = 163)	Women (n = 83)	p Value
Age (years)	21–84 (60)	27–84 (62)	0.21
White	156 (96%)	72 (87%)	<0.01
AF	20 (12%)	17 (20%)	0.095
Sinus rhythm + history of AF	22 (14%)	10 (12%)	0.66
Sinus rhythm − history of AF	121 (74%)	56 (68%)	0.32
Echocardiographic dimensions (mm)			
Left atrium	29–76 (51)	38–64 (49)	0.52
LV peak systole	13–48 (37)	17–50 (35)	0.36
LV end diastole	18–79 (61)	39–68 (56)	0.03
Pressures (mm Hg) (range)(mean)			
Pulmonary artery peak systole	17–87 (40)	17–86 (40)	0.99
Pulmonary artery mean	10–62 (26)	10–52 (26)	0.85
LV peak systole	68–163 (118)	94–198 (138)	<0.0001
LV end diastole	3–39 (19)	7–36 (18)	0.44
Pulmonary artery wedge mean	3–43 (18)	6–32 (16)	0.31
RV peak systole	12–71 (37)	22–83 (42)	0.05
RV end diastole	2–25 (11)	3–22 (11)	0.47
Right atrial mean	1–20 (7)	1–35 (7)	0.82
Aorta peak systole	68–177 (117)	91–200 (140)	<0.0001
Aorta end diastole	39–90 (67)	47–79 (74)	0.0001
Other hemodynamic data:			
Cardiac index (L/min/m^2)	1.5–5.4 (2.7)	1.5–4.6 (2.7)	0.98
Ejection fraction (%)	25–75 (55)	40–75 (60)	0.0007
Body mass index (kg/m^2) (mean)	26	25	<0.03
≤25	80 (49%)	53 (64%)	<0.03
26–30	65 (40%)	24 (29%)	0.09
>30	18 (11%)	6 (7%)	0.31
Systemic hypertension	79 (48%)	48 (58%)	0.14
Mean NYHA functional class (mean)	2.4	2.5	0.38
I	27 (17%)	14 (17%)	
II	58 (36%)	22 (27%)	0.18
III	60 (36%)	36 (43%)	
IV	18 (11%)	11 (13%)	0.18
No. of major coronary arteries narrowed >50% ↓ in diameter:	(n = 142)	(n = 75)	
0	99 (69%)	65 (80%)	
1	15 (11%)	7 (10%)	<0.004
2	11 (8%)	1 (1%)	
3	12 (8%)	1 (1%)	<0.004
Left main	5 (4%)	1 (1%)	
Coronary bypass	43 (26%)	8 (10%)	<0.004

AF = atrial fibrillation; LV = left ventricular; NYHA = New York Heart Association; RV = right ventricular.

Table 3
Comparison of preoperative findings between patients who had mitral valve repair versus replacement for mitral regurgitation secondary to mitral valve prolapse

Variable	Repair (n = 157)	Replacement (n = 89)	p Value
Age (years)	21–84 (59)	27–84 (62)	0.05
Men	106 (68%)	57 (64%)	0.52
White	147 (94%)	81 (91%)	0.38
AF	18 (11%)	19 (21%)	<0.04
Sinus rhythm + history of AF	26 (17%)	6 (7%)	<0.03
Sinus rhythm − history of AF	113 (72%)	64 (72%)	1.0
Echocardiographic dimensions (mm)			
Left atrium	38–65 (50)	27–76 (51)	0.58
LV peak systole	17–50 (38)	13–48 (34)	0.08
LV end diastole	39–79 (61)	18–79 (57)	0.12
Pressures (mm Hg)			
Pulmonary artery peak systole	17–77 (39)	18–87 (42)	0.15
Pulmonary artery mean	10–50 (25)	10–62 (27)	0.23
LV peak systole	94–83 (125)	68–198 (125)	0.83
LV end-systole	7–36 (19)	3–39 (18)	0.21
Pulmonary artery wedge mean	5–43 (17)	3–32 (18)	0.30
RV peak systole	12–71 (38)	22–83 (42)	0.13
RV end-diastole	3–25 (11)	2–22 (11)	0.79
Right atrial mean	1–35 (7)	1–20 (8)	0.36
Aorta peak systole	87–177 (126)	68–200 (125)	0.94
Aorta end diastole	39–97 (70)	49–99 (70)	0.98
Other hemodynamic data:			
Cardiac index (L/min/m^2)	1.4–4.7 (2.7)	1.5–5.4 (2.6)	0.80
Ejection fraction (%)	25–75 (57)	30–75 (57)	0.87
Body mass index (kg/m^2) (mean)	26	25	0.28
≤25	82 (52%)	50 (56%)	0.54
26–30	60 (38%)	30 (34%)	0.53
<30	15 (10%)	9 (10%)	1
Systemic hypertension	74 (47%)	53 (60%)	0.05
Mean NYHA functional class (mean)	2.4	2.5	0.45
I	26 (17%)	15 (17%)	
II	56 (36%)	24 (27%)	0.18
III	57 (36%)	39 (44%)	
IV	18 (11%)	11 (12%)	0.18
Major coronary arteries narrowed >50% ↓ in diameter:			
0	113/142 (79%)	54/75 (71%)	
1	14/142 (10%)	7/75 (9%)	0.19
2	7/142 (5%)	4/75 (5%)	
3	7/142 (5%)	6/75 (8%)	0.19
Left main	1/142 (1%)	5/75 (7%)	
Coronary bypass	27 (17%)	24 (27%)	0.06

Abbreviations as in Table 2.

Comparison of 13 variables in 3 different age groups (21 to 50 vs 51 to 70 vs >70 years) are listed in Table 4. In comparison to 1 or both of the younger age groups, the 59 patients >70 years of age had a higher frequency of AF, a higher percentage had mitral replacement (compared with repair), higher peak systolic and mean pulmonary arterial pressures, higher left ventricular peak systolic pressures, higher mean pulmonary arterial wedge pressures, higher right ventricular peak systolic pressures, higher peak systolic aortic pressures, lower cardiac indexes, higher New

Table 4
Comparison of the findings by age in patients undergoing mitral valve operation for mitral regurgitation secondary to mitral valve prolapse

Variable	Age Groups (years)			p Values		
	21–50 (n = 57)	51–70 (n = 130)	>70 (n = 59)	1 vs 2	2 vs 3	1 vs 3
Men:women	40 (70%):17 (30%)	89 (68%):41 (32%)	34 (58%):25 (42%)	0.79	0.18	0.18
White	51 (89%)	120 (92%)	57 (97%)	0.51	0.20	<0.10
AF	3 (5%)	12 (9%)	22 (37%)	0.35	0.0001	0.0001
Sinus rhythm (ECG) + history of AF	3 (5%)	24 (18%)	5 (8%)	<0.02	<0.08	0.51
Sinus rhythm (ECG) − history of AF	51 (90%)	94 (72%)	32 (55%)	<0.01	<0.03	0.001
Mitral repair/replacement	40 (70%)/17 (30%)	88 (68%)/42 (32%)	29 (49%)/30 (51%)	0.79	<0.02	<0.03
Echocardiographic dimension (mm):						
Left atrium	39–63 (48)	29–65 (50)	34–76 (51)	0.24	0.92	0.32
LV peak systole	36–47 (40)	13–48 (36)	17–50 (35)	0.18	0.74	<0.07
LV end diastole	56–78 (64)	18–79 (59)	39–73 (57)	0.13	0.39	<0.008
Pressures (mm Hg)						
Pulmonary artery peak systole	17–61 (31)	17–18 (41)	21–86 (44)	<0.002	0.25	0.0001
Pulmonary artery mean	10–44 (21)	10–62 (26)	14–52 (28)	<0.02	0.27	0.0005
LV peak systole	76–167 (118)	68–183 (121)	89–198 (137)	0.50	<0.002	<0.003
LV end-diastole	7–30 (17)	3–39 (19)	7–32 (18)	0.26	0.41	0.70
Pulmonary artery wedge mean	5–28 (13)	3–43 (18)	6–31 (19)	<0.02	0.61	<0.003
RV peak systole	20–66 (33)	20–83 (39)	12–81 (43)	<0.04	0.18	<0.005
RV end-diastole	2–24 (11)	3–22 (11)	3–25 (12)	0.75	0.30	0.62
Right atrial mean	1–12 (6)	1–35 (7)	1–20 (8)	0.30	0.20	<0.03
Aorta peak systole	91–163 (119)	68–177 (122)	87–200 (137)	0.61	<0.002	<0.004
Aorta end-diastole	52–98 (73)	47–94 (69)	39–99 (69)	<0.07	0.84	0.20
Other hemodynamic data:						
Cardiac index (L/min/m^2)	1.9–4.7 (3.0)	1.4–4.3 (2.6)	1.5–5.4 (2.5)	<0.05	0.51	<0.04
Ejection fraction (%)	30–70 (57)	35–75 (58)	25–75 (56)	0.91	0.25	0.47
Body mass index (kg/m^2)	20–41 (25)	17–46 (26)	18–34 (24)	0.11	<0.02	0.50
Systemic hypertension	18 (32%)	71 (55%)	37 (65%)	<0.005	0.20	0.0006
Mean NYHA functional class	2.1	2.4	2.8	<0.02	<0.02	0.0001
I	16 (30%)	19 (15%)	5 (8%)			
II	21 (37%)	46 (35%)	13 (22%)	<0.04	<0.02	0.0001
III	15 (26%)	51 (39%)	30 (51%)			
IV	4 (7%)	14 (11%)	11 (19%)	<0.04	<0.02	0.0001
No. of major coronary arteries narrowed >50% in diameter:	(n = 43)	(n = 120)	(n = 54)			
0	37 (86%)	93 (77%)	34 (63%)	0.21	<0.06	<0.02
1	3 (7%)	13 (11%)	6 (11%)			
2	1 (2%)	8 (7%)	3 (6%)			
3	2 (5%)	5 (4%)	6 (11%)			
Left main	0 (0%)	1 (1%)	5 (9%)			
Coronary bypass	5 (9%)	28 (22%)	18 (31%)	<0.04	0.19	<0.004

ECG = electrocardiogram; other abbreviations as in Table 2.

York Heart Association functional classes, and greater coronary arterial narrowing.

Discussion

The heretofore described data in 246 patients having mitral valve repair or replacement for MR due to MVP disclosed that the frequency of AF preoperatively was relatively low, namely, 15%. Compared with the 209 patients with sinus rhythm preoperatively, the 37 patients with AF were significantly older, less likely to be men, more likely to be lean, more likely to have severe heart failure, to have higher right atrial pressures and lower left ventricular ejection fractions. The frequency of AF in previously published reports of patients with MVP is listed in Table 5.[2–13]

The frequency of AF among patients with MR from MVP severe enough to warrant a mitral operation might logically be expected to be >15% because the disease process would appear to be in a relatively late stage. Earlier stages of MVP, for example, in cases picked up by community screening programs (auscultation, echocardiography) among asymptomatic MVP patients or early symptomatic patients, have an even lower frequency of MVP. Indeed, Freed and colleagues[10] reviewed echocardiograms in 3491 offspring cohorts of the Framingham Heart Study, and found 84 subjects (2.4%) to have MVP. Only 1 (1.2%) had AF. The subjects with MVP were leaner than the subjects without MVP. None had a mitral valve operation. Grigioni and associates[12] analyzed 360 patients (aged 65 ± 13 years; 74% men in the local Rochester, Minnesota, community)

Table 5
Previous publications of patients with mitral valve prolapse showing frequency of atrial fibrillation and other variables

First Author	Year of Publication	Method of Diagnosis of MVP	No. of Patients With MVP	Age (years) Range (mean)	Men	AF	Angiographic Coronary Disease	Mitral Valve Operation
Waller[2]	1982	Surgical	60	36–73 (55)	29 (48%)	4 (7%)	3/23 (13%)	69 (100%)
Ranganathan[3]	1973	S or Autopsy	16	37–69 (—)	9 (56%)	11 (69%)	—	Most
Higgins[4]	1976	Echo	40*	50–90 (65)	40* (100%)	14 (35%)	—	—
Kolibash[5]	1983	Au, Echo, An	62	60–81 (—)	25 (40%)	13 (21%)	4/26 (15%)	21 (34%)
Tresch[6]	1985	Operation	30	25–72 (60)	20 (67%)	13 (43%)	3/29 (10%)	30 (100%)
Penkoske[7]	1985	Operation	31	— (63)	17 (55%)	18 (58%)	9 (29%)	31† (100%)
Kolibash[8]	1986	Operation	86	26–82 (60)	53 (62%)	48 (56%)	8 (9%)	76 (88%)
Naggar[9]	1986	Echo	145	≥60	71 (49%)	27 (18%)	—	22 (15%)
Freed[10]	1999	Echo	84‡	26–84 (56)	34 (41%)	1 (1%)	—	1 (1%)
Ohki[11]	2001	Echo	118	32–68 (50)	69 (58%)	29 (25%)	—	—
Grigioni[12]	2002	Echo	89§	52–78 (65)	59 (66%)	19 (21%)	—	35 (39%)
Avierinos[13]	2002	Echo	833‖	29–71 (50)	300 (36%)	67 (8%)	—	65 (8%)

* Studied at a Veterans-Administration Hospital.
† Mitral-valve repair in each.
‡ Diagnosed from a general population survey (Framingham).
§ Focused on patients with sinus rhythm at diagnosis of "degenerative" mitral regurgitation and percent who developed AF at 5 and 10 years of follow-up.
‖ Focused on patients with asymptomatic MVP in a community (Rochester).
An = angiography; Au = auscultation; MVP = mitral valve prolapse; S = surgery; other abbreviation as in Table 2.

with MR due to flail mitral leaflet (n = 360) and patients with grade 3 or 4 MR secondary to MVP (n = 89). All 449 patients were in sinus rhythm at diagnosis. By 10 years after diagnosis, however, nearly 50% had developed AF. The patients who developed AF were older and had larger left atria than did those who remained in sinus rhythm.

It is well known that MVP tends to be more frequent in women than in men. It has been estimated that MVP is present in about 8 million adults in the USA. The MVP patients who develop enough MR to warrant mitral valve operation, however, are more often men than women. In the present study, 163 (66%) of the 246 patients were men. The reason for the dominance of men in this circumstance is unclear.

The ages of the patients included in the present study ranged from 21 to 84 years (mean 61). The mean age of these patients places them, of course, in a category where coronary artery disease is relatively frequent. Surprisingly, however, only 54 (22%) had angiographic evidence of narrowing >50% in diameter of ≥1 epicardial coronary artery. A possible explanation for this relatively low frequency of angiographically demonstrated coronary arterial narrowing may be the relatively high frequency of body mass indexes of ≤ 25 kg/m^2. Of the 246 patients, 134 (54%) had this relatively low body mass index and, furthermore, only 24 (10%) were obese (body mass index >30 kg/m^2).

Why AF appears to be less frequent in adults with MR from MVP than in similar aged adults with mitral stenosis has received virtually no attention. Mitral stenosis in adults is virtually always of rheumatic origin, a process which affects the left atrial wall as well as the mitral valve with or without involvement of other valves.[14] In contrast, MVP has no direct effect on the atrial walls other than the secondary hemodynamic consequences. In other words, the atrial walls are histologically abnormal in patients with mitral stenosis, whereas these walls are histologically normal, except for myofiber hypertrophy, in patients with MVP.

Like virtually all clinical investigations, this work has limitations. An important one is the lack of hemodynamic, angiographic, and echocardiographic data on all the patients included. Another limitation is almost certainly different standards regarding need for operative intervention among the multiple cardiologists referring these patients for cardiac operations. Additionally, some of the cardiac surgeons leaned more to mitral repair versus mitral replacement than did others.

1. Barlow JB, Pocock WA, Marchand P, Denny M. The significance of late systolic murmurs. *Am Heart J* 1963;66:443–452.
2. Waller BF, Morrow AG, Maron BJ, Del Negro AA, Kent KM, McGrath FJ, Wallace RB, McIntosh CL Roberts WC. Etiology of clinically isolated, severe, chronic, pure mitral regurgitation: analysis of 97 patients over 30 years of age having mitral valve replacement. *Am Heart J* 1982;104:276–288.
3. Ranganathan N, Silver MD, Robinson TI, Kostuk WJ, Felderhof CH, Patt NL, Wilson JK, Wigle ED. Angiographic-morphologic correlation in patients with severe mitral regurgitation due to prolapse of the posterior mitral valve leaflet. *Circulation* 1973;48:514–518.
4. Higgins CB, Reinke RT, Gosink BB, Leopold GR. The significance of mitral valve prolapse in middle-aged and elderly men. *Am Heart J* 1976;91:292–296.
5. Kolisbash AJ, Bush CA, Fontana MB, Ryan JM, Kilman J, Wooley CF. Mitral valve prolapse syndrome: analysis of 62 patients aged 60 years and older. *Am J Cardiol* 1983;52:534–539.
6. Tresch DD, Doyle TP, Boncheck LI, Siegel R, Keelan MH Jr, Olinger GN, Brooks HL. Mitral valve prolapse requiring surgery. Clinical and pathologic study. *Am J Med* 1985;78:245–250.

7. Penkoske PA, Ellis FH Jr, Alexander S, Watkins E Jr. Results of valve reconstruction for mitral regurgitation secondary to mitral valve prolapse. *Am J Cardiol* 1985;55:735–738.
8. Kolibash AJ Jr, Kilman JW, Bush CA, Ryan JM, Fontana ME, Wooley CF. Evidence for progression from mild to severe mitral regurgitation in mitral valve prolapse. *Am J Cardiol* 1986;58:762–767.
9. Naggar CZ, Pearson WN, Seljan MP, with the technical assistance of Mannock LK, Masrof S, Elwood DJ. Frequency of complications of mitral valve prolapse in subjects aged 60 years and older. *Am J Cardiol* 1986;58:1209–1212.
10. Freed LA, Levy D, Levine RA, Larson MG, Evans JC, Fuller DL, Lehman B, Benjamin EJ. Prevalence and clinical outcome of mitral-valve prolapse. *N Engl J Med* 1999;341:1–7.
11. Ohki R, Yamamoto K, Okayama M, Nonaka M, Suzuki C, Ikeda U, Shimada K. The site of mitral valve prolapse is a predictor of atrial fibrillation. *Am J Cardiol* 2001;88:811–813.
12. Grigioni F, Avierinos J-F, Ling LH, Scott CG, Bailey KR, Tajik AJ, Frye RL, Enriquez-Sarano M. Atrial fibrillation complicating the course of degenerative mitral regurgitation. Determinants of long-term outcome. *J Am Coll Cardiol* 2002;40:84–92.
13. Avierinos J-F, Gersh BJ, Melton LJ III, Bailey KR, Shub C, Nishimura RA, Tajik AJ, Enriquez-Sarano M. Natural history of asymptomatic mitral valve prolapse in the community. *Circulation* 2002;106:1355–1361.
14. Bailey GWH, Braniff BA, Hancock EW, Cohn KE. Relation of left atrial pathology to atrial fibrillation in mitral valve disease. *Ann Intern Med* 1968;69:13–20.

Cardiac Restriction Secondary to Massive Calcific Deposits in the Left Ventricular Cavity

William C. Roberts, MD[a,b,c,*], Randall L. Rosenblatt, MD[d], Jong Mi Ko, BA[a], Paul A. Grayburn, MD[a,c], Johannes J. Kuiper, MD[c], and Joseph M. Guileyardo, MD[b]

Described herein are clinical and necropsy findings in a 61-year-old woman with fatal left ventricular diastolic failure secondary to massive calcific deposits primarily within the left ventricular cavity. At age 3, an isthmic aortic coarctation was resected, and at age 44, a stenotic congenitally bicuspid aortic valve was replaced. The cause of the intracavitary calcific deposits remains unclear, but surgical resection of the deposits has been an effective form of therapy. **(Am J Cardiol 2014;113:1442–1446)**

Calcific deposits are common in the heart particularly in older individuals and especially in atherosclerotic plaques in coronary arteries, in aortic valve cusps, and in the mitral annulus.[1] These deposits may also occur but far less commonly in other areas of the heart. In 1984, Silver et al[2] described clinical and necropsy findings in a 56-year-old woman with numerous calcific deposits in the left ventricular cavity causing severe impairment to left ventricular filling. This report describes clinical and necropsy findings in a similar patient and reviews other reported cases of large, mainly intracavitary, left ventricular calcific deposits.

Case Report

This 61-year-old white woman had resection of an aortic isthmic coarctation at age 3. At age 44, she underwent an aortic valve replacement with a bileaflet mechanical prosthesis for a stenotic congenitally bicuspid aortic valve. At age 54 (2006), she experienced her first episode of acute pulmonary edema requiring mechanical ventilator. Coronary angiography showed significant narrowing of the left circumflex coronary artery and a stent was inserted. A year later (age 55), another acute episode of heart failure occurred. Repeat angiography disclosed that the lumen of the stent in the left circumflex coronary artery was partially thrombosed, the clot was extracted, and angioplasty was performed. Echocardiogram disclosed a left ventricular ejection fraction of about 30%, but the prosthesis in the aortic valve position was functioning well. She had another episode of acute pulmonary edema 1 year later.

Because of increasing fatigue and periodic evidence of worsening heart failure, she was admitted to the Baylor University Medical Center, Dallas, for the first time at age 59 (February 2011). An echocardiogram, at that time, disclosed severe left ventricular endocardial thickening with numerous intracavitary calcific deposits, a restrictive left ventricular filling pattern without respiratory variation, normal-sized right and left ventricular cavities, and a normally functioning aortic valve prosthesis. The cavitary calcific deposits were also seen by chest radiographs and by chest computed tomography. Right-sided cardiac catheterization showed the following pressures in mm Hg: pulmonary arterial wedge mean 20, a wave 26, v-wave 40, pulmonary artery 72/24, and right ventricle 78/15. The cardiac index was 2.25 L/min/m^2.

Over the next 2 years, the heart failure gradually worsened. Her body mass index was 17 kg/m^2. The pulmonary arterial pressure rose to 99/29, the right ventricular pressure to 99/0, and the pulmonary arterial wedge pressure to mean 30, a wave 38, and v wave 33 mm Hg. Echocardiogram (Figure 1) revealed findings similar to the one performed 2 years earlier. Repeat chest radiograph showed more left ventricular intracavitary calcific deposits (Figure 2) than had been seen 5 years earlier. Computed tomography (Figure 3) showed the calcific deposits filling the left ventricular cavity. An electrocardiogram a month before death is shown in Figure 4. Cardiopulmonary transplantation was deemed inappropriate and she died of heart failure in August 2013 at age 61.

Numerous serum calcium levels were available between June 2007 and August 2013 and ranged from 8.1 to 9.5 mg/dl. Several serum phosphorous levels in February 2008 ranged from 2.4 to 3.6 mg/dl.

At necropsy, the heart weighed 440 g. Huge calcific deposits were present in the left ventricular cavity from apex to base (Figures 5 and 6). The right ventricular and left ventricular walls and the ventricular septum were of similar thicknesses and free of grossly visible myocardial lesions, and neither ventricular cavity was dilated. Histologically, sections of the myocardium were normal except for enlargement of the myofibers. The discs of the mechanical prosthesis (St. Jude Medical) in the aortic valve position appeared to move properly without interference. Metallic stents were present in the left circumflex coronary artery (Figure 3). The right and left anterior descending coronary

[a]Baylor Heart and Vascular Institute, [b]Department of Pathology, and Divisions of [c]Cardiology and [d]Pulmonology, Department of Internal Medicine, Baylor University Medical Center, Dallas, Texas. Manuscript received December 19, 2013; revised manuscript received and accepted December 26, 2013.

The study was funded by the Baylor Health Care System Foundation, Dallas, Texas.

See page 1446 for disclosure information.

*Corresponding author: Tel: (214) 820-7911; fax: (214) 820-7533.

E-mail address: wc.roberts@baylorhealth.edu or ajc@baylorhealth.edu (W.C. Roberts).

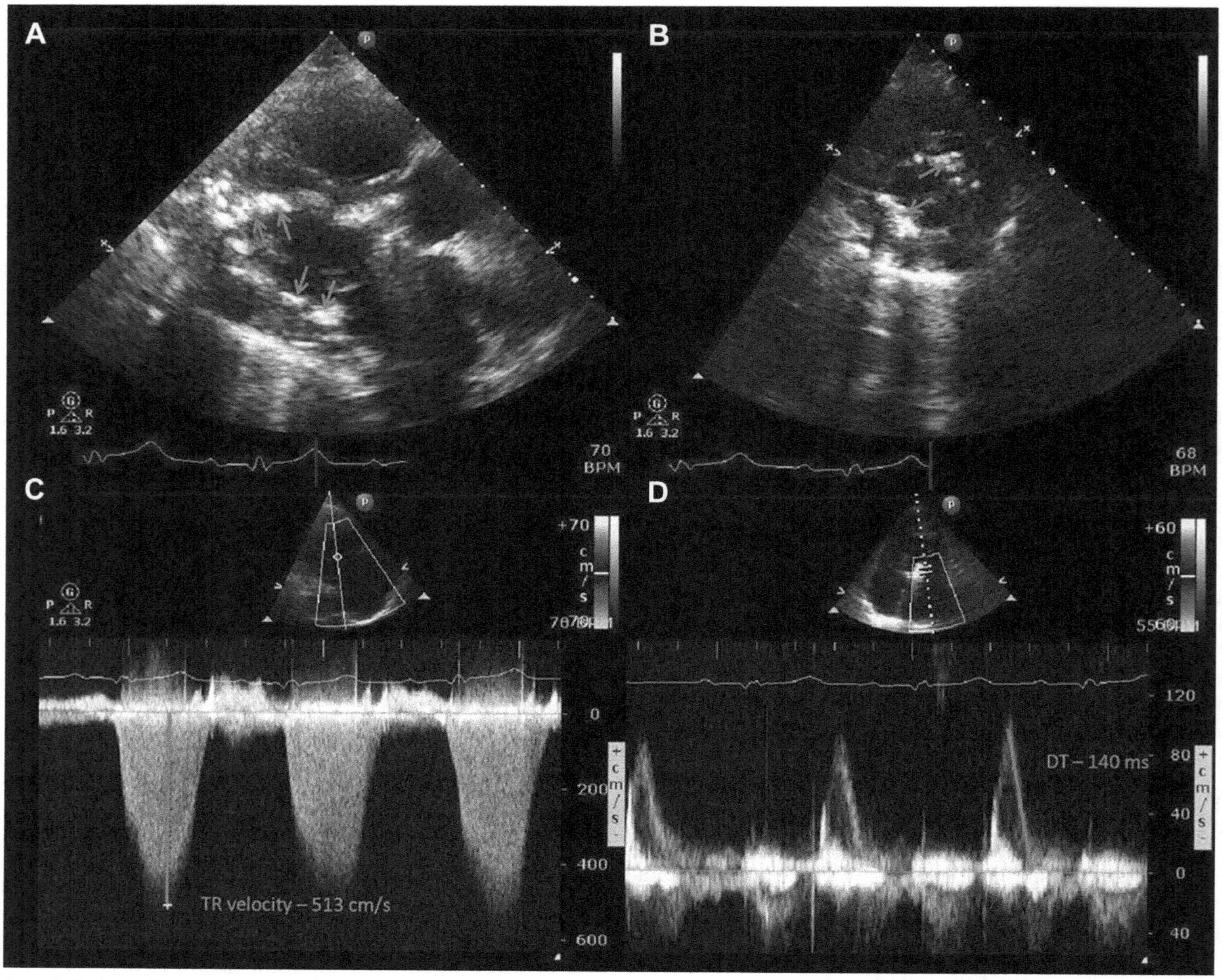

Figure 1. End-systolic frames *(A)* from parasternal long-axis view and *(B)* from short-axis view. *Arrows* point to dense endocardial calcium, which is bright white. *(C)* Continuous-wave Doppler profile from tricuspid regurgitation shows a peak velocity of 513 m/s, consistent with systemic pulmonary artery pressure. *(D)* Mitral inflow pattern exhibits a short deceleration time of 140 ms, consistent with restrictive filling.

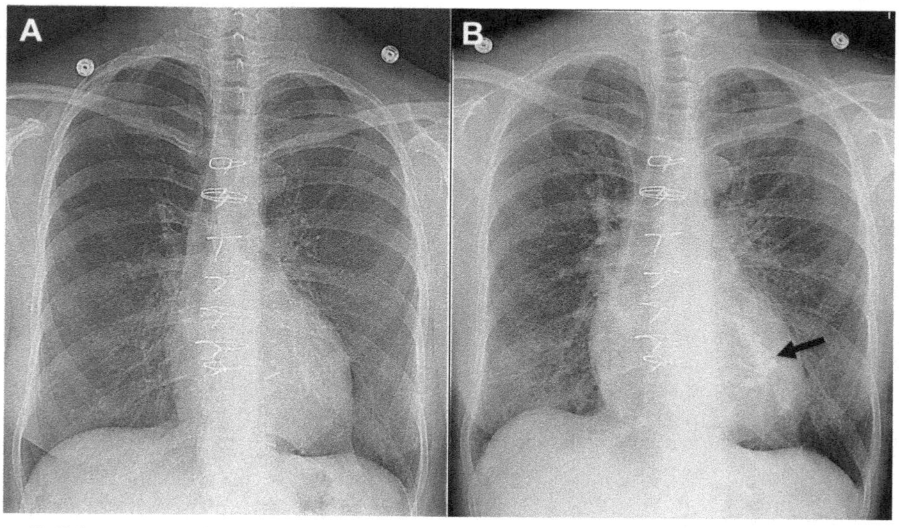

Figure 2. Chest radiographs. *(A)* Taken 5 years before death and *(B)* taken 4 months before death. The left ventricular intracavitary calcific deposits are visible in both, but they are larger *(arrow)* in the latest radiograph.

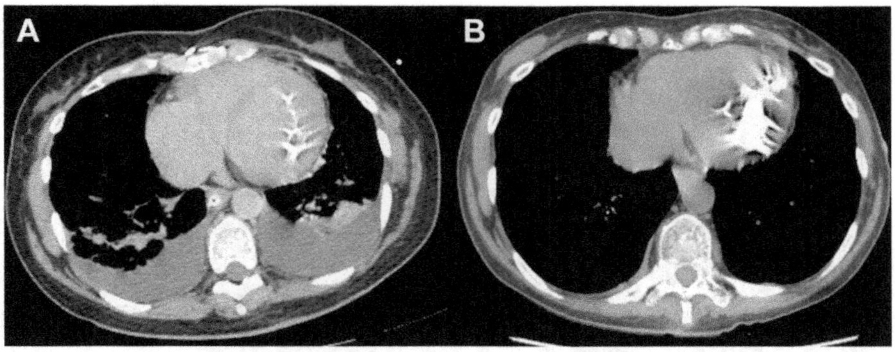

Figure 3. Computed tomographic studies. *(A)* Taken 6 years before death and *(B)* taken 4 months before death.

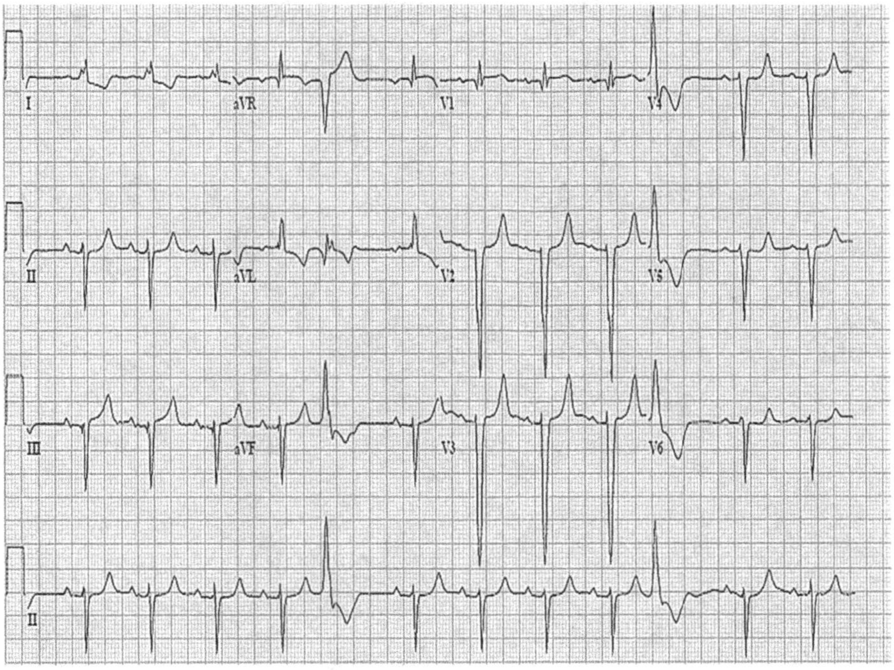

Figure 4. Electrocardiogram, recorded 3 months before death, showing changes of marked right ventricular hypertrophy and frequent ventricular premature complexes.

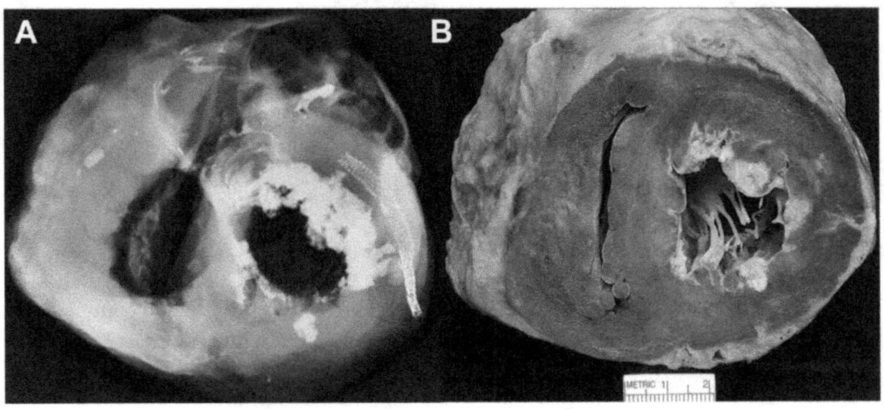

Figure 5. *(A)* Radiograph and *(B)* photograph of transverse section of the heart at the base showing extensive left ventricular endocardial calcific deposits and severe thickening of the right ventricular free wall.

arteries were virtually free of atherosclerotic plaques. The right atrium was larger than the left atrium. A saccular aneurysm with a very thin wall was present at the aortic anastomotic site where the isthmic aortic coarctation had been resected.

The right pleural space contained 750 ml and the left 950 ml of serous fluid. Sections of the lungs stained by the Movat method showed that the media of the pulmonary arteries were thickened, and many had mild thickening of the intima, but no plexiform lesions were present. The

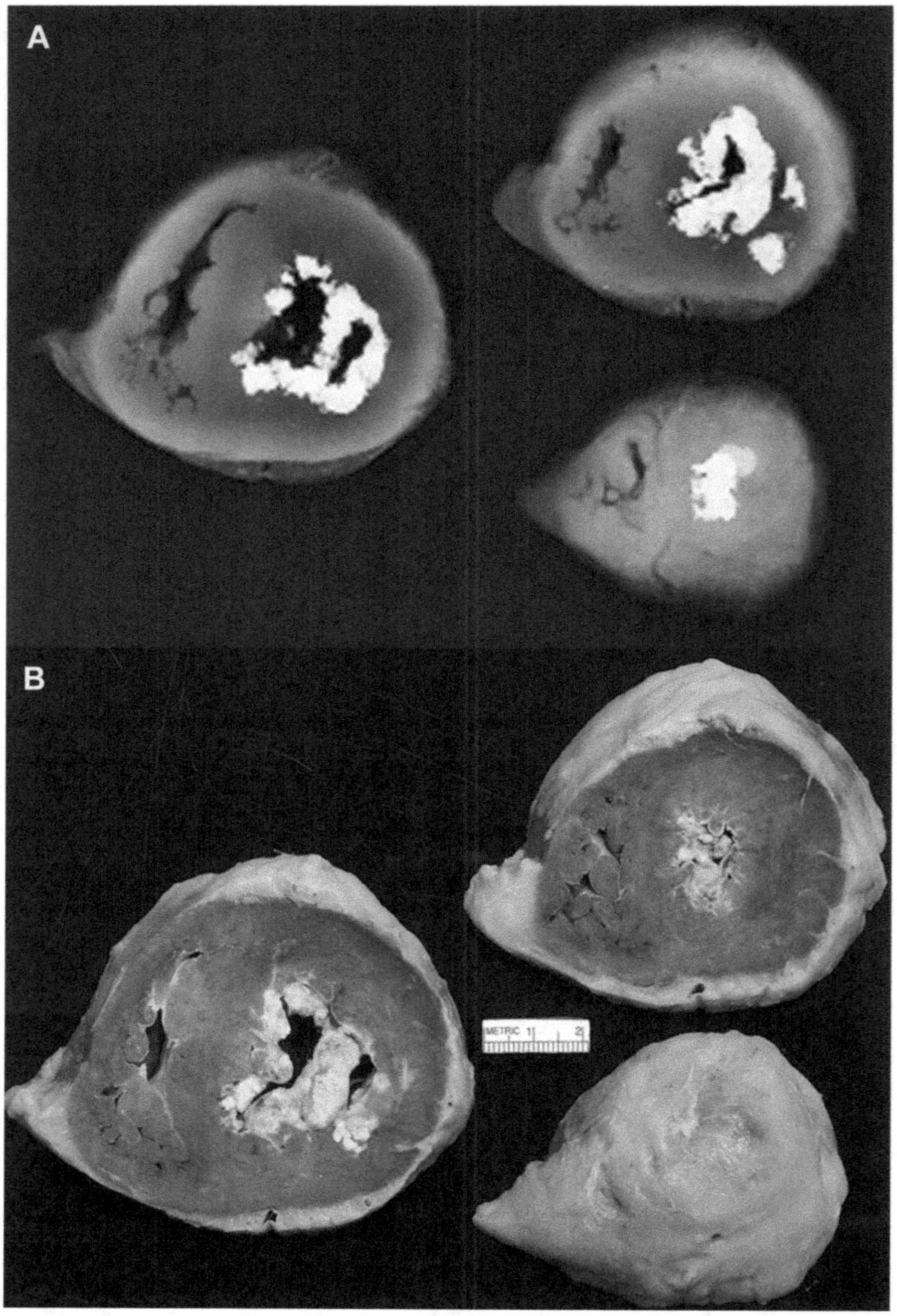

Figure 6. *(A)* Radiograph and *(B)* transverse views of the cardiac ventricles in the apical half again show the extent of the calcific deposits.

intrapulmonary pulmonary veins were dilated, the interlobular septa were thickened (Kerley B lines), and extravasated erythrocytes and hemosiderin-laden macrophages were present in some alveolar spaces. Although most were of normal thickness, some alveolar septa were thickened by fibrous tissue.

Discussion

The patient described herein is virtually identical to the one described in 1984 by Silver et al[2] with huge intracavitary left ventricular calcific deposits leading to extreme difficulty in filling the left ventricular cavity with resulting severe secondary pulmonary hypertension.

In recent years, a number of reports have appeared describing calcific deposits in 1 or more cardiac chambers.[3–20] Reynolds et al[5] in 1997 coined the phrase "calcified amorphous tumor of the heart" to characterize the cardiac calcific deposits because the individual calcific deposits are held together by an "amorphous material," mainly fibrous tissue. In our patient, the intracavitary calcific deposits were essentially "glued" together and to the mural endocardium by the "amorphous" material that prevented the left ventricular cavity from expanding much during ventricular diastole. Similar huge calcific deposits within the left ventricular and ventricular septal walls unassociated with similar intracavitary calcific deposits can result in similar restriction of left ventricular diastolic filling. A list of reported cases of left ventricular wall

Table 1
Previously reported patients with large left ventricular intracavitary calcific deposits

	First Author	Publication Year	Reference Number	Age (yrs)	Sex	Method of Diagnosis	ESRD	DM
1	Silver	1984	2	56	F	Necropsy	0	0
2	Reynolds	1997	5	30	M	Operation	0	0
3	Tom	2006	6	36	F	CT	+*	+
4	Ho	2008	9	44	M	CT	0	0
5	Kubota	2010	12	64	F	E	+	+
				44	M	CT†	+‡	0
6	Habib	2010	14	58	F	E	0	0
7	van Kruijsdijk	2011	15	56	M	CT	0	0
8	Segura	2011	18	20	M	CT§	0	0
9	Mana	2012	18	55	F	E	0	0
10	Nasli*	2013	19	54	F	CT†	0	0

CT = computed tomography; DM = diabetes mellitus; E = echocardiogram; ESRD = end-stage renal disease; F = female; M = male.
* Secondary hyperparathyroidism.
† The calcific deposits were successfully excised at operation.
‡ Patient had systemic lupus erythematosus.
§ Patient underwent successful cardiac transplantation.

and/or intracavitary huge calcific deposits is listed in Table 1. The calcific deposits in each of these patients were clearly visible by echocardiographic and/or computed tomographic studies. Cases in which the calcific deposits involved cardiac valves were excluded from the list.

The cause of "calcified amorphous tumor of the heart" unassociated with heavy calcific deposits involving 1 or more cardiac valves is unclear. At least 4 of the 10 patients listed in Table 1 had chronic renal disease with chronic hemodialysis and at least 1 had secondary hyperparathyroidism. The serum calcium levels in these patients were nearly always normal.

What is the proper management of patients with left ventricular diastolic heart failure secondary to huge intracavitary calcific deposits? The answer appears to be operative excision of the calcific deposits. Both Reynolds et al[5] and Kubota et al[12] have reported operative success by this procedure leading to complete resolution of the left ventricular diastolic heart failure. Cardiac transplantation has been also successful.[18]

Disclosures

The authors have no conflicts of interest to disclose.

1. Roberts WC. The senile cardiac calcification syndrome. *Am J Cardiol* 1986;58:572–574.
2. Silver MA, Bonow RO, Deglin SM, Maron BJ, Cannon RO III, Roberts WC. Acquired left ventricular endocardial constriction from massive mural calcific deposits: a newly recognized cause of impairment to left ventricular filling. *Am J Cardiol* 1984;53:1468–1470.
3. Dean DC, Pamukcoglu T, Roberts WC. Rocks in the right ventricle. A complication of congenital right ventricular infundibular obstruction associated with chronic pulmonary parenchymal disease. *Am J Cardiol* 1969;23:744–747.
4. Waller BF, Maron BJ, Morrow AG, Roberts WC. Hypertrophic cardiomyopathy mimicking pericardial constriction or myocardial restriction. *Am J Cardiol* 1981;102:790–792.
5. Reynolds C, Tazelaar HD, Edwards WD. Calcified amorphous tumor of the heart (cardiac CAT). *Hum Pathol* 1997;28:601–606.
6. Tom CW, Talreja DR. Heart of stone. *Mayo Clin Proc* 2006;81:335.
7. Lewin M, Nazarian S, Marine JE, Yuh DD, Argani P, Halushka MK. Fatal outcome of a calcified amorphous tumor of the heart (cardiac CAT). *Cardiovasc Pathol* 2006;15:299–302.
8. Fealey ME, Edwards WD, Reynolds CA, Pellikka PA, Dearani JA. Recurrent cardiac calcific amorphous tumor: the CAT had a kitten. *Cardiovasc Pathol* 2007;16:115–118.
9. Ho HH, Min JK, Lin F, Wong SC, Bergman G. Images in cardiovascular medicine. Calcified amorphous tumor of the heart. *Circulation* 2008;117:e171–e172.
10. Gutiérrez-Barrios A, Muriel-Cueto P, Lancho-Novillo C, Sancho-Jaldón M. Calcified amorphous tumor of the heart. *Rev Esp Cardiol* 2008;61: 892–893.
11. Vaideeswar P, Karunamurthy A, Patwardhan AM, Hira P, Raut AR. Cardiac calcified amorphous tumor. *J Card Surg* 2010;25:32–35.
12. Kubota H, Fujioka Y, Yoshino H, Koji H, Yoshihara K, Tonari K, Endo H, Tsuchiya H, Mera H, Soga Y, Taniai S, Sakata K, Sudo K. Cardiac swinging calcified amorphous tumors in end-stage renal failure patients. *Ann Thorac Surg* 2010;90:1692–1694.
13. Gupta R, Hote M, Ray R. Calcified amorphous tumor of the heart in an adult female: a case report. *J Med Case Rep* 2010;4:278.
14. Habib A, Friedman PA, Cooper LT, Suleiman M, Asirvatham SJ. Cardiac calcified amorphous tumor in a patient presenting for ventricular tachycardia ablation: intracardiac echocardiogram diagnosis and management. *J Interv Card Electrophysiol* 2010;29: 175–178.
15. van Kruijsdijk RC, van der Heijden JJ, Uijlings R, Otterspoor LC. Sepsis-related myocardial calcification. *Circ Heart Fail* 2011;4:e16–e18.
16. Greaney L, Chaubey S, Pomplun S, St Joseph E, Monaghan M, Wendler O. Calcified amorphous tumour of the heart: presentation of a rare case operated using minimal access cardiac surgery. *BMJ Case Rep* 2011. http://dx.doi.org/10.1136/bcr.02.2011.3882.
17. Vlasseros I, Katsi V, Tousoulis D, Tsiachris D, Bousiotou A, Souretis G, Stefanadis C, Kallikazaros I. Visual loss due to cardiac calcified amorphous tumor: a case report and brief review of the literature. *Int J Cardiol* 2011;152:e56–e57.
18. Segura AM, Radovancevic R, Connelly JH, Loyalka P, Gregoric ID, Buja LM. Endomyocardial nodular calcification as a cause of heart failure. *Cardiovasc Pathol* 2011;20:e185–e188.
19. Mana M, Sanguineti F, Unterseeh T, Bouvier E, Garot J. Petrified myocardium: the age of stone? *Circulation* 2012;126:1139–1142.
20. Nazli Y, Colak N, Atar IA, Alpay MF, Haltas H, Eryonucu B, Cakir O. Sudden unilateral vision loss arising from calcified amorphous tumor of the left ventricle. *Tex Heart Inst J* 2013;40: 453–458.

Clinical and Morphologic Features of Acute, Subacute and Chronic Cor Pulmonale (Pulmonary Heart Disease)

William Clifford Roberts, MD[a,b,c,*], Alexis E. Shafii, MD[d], Paul A. Grayburn, MD[a,b], Jong Mi Ko, BS[a], Matthew R. Weissenborn, MD[c], Randall L. Rosenblatt, MD[b], and Joseph M. Guileyardo, MD[c]

Described are certain clinical and morphologic features of one patient with *acute*, another with *subacute*, and one with *chronic* cor pulmonale. All 3 had evidence of severe pulmonary hypertension. The patient with acute cor pulmonale 4 days after coronary bypass for unstable angina pectoris suddenly developed severe breathlessness with cyanosis and had fatal cardiac arrest and necropsy disclosed massive pulmonary embolism. The patient with subacute cor pulmonale had severe right-sided heart failure for 5 weeks and necropsy disclosed microscopic-sized neoplastic pulmonary emboli from a gastric carcinoma without parenchymal pulmonary metastases. The patient with chronic cor pulmonale had evidence of right-sided heart failure for years, the result of primary or idiopathic pulmonary hypertension almost certainly present from birth because the pattern of elastic fibers in the pulmonary trunk was that seen in newborns where the pressure in the pulmonary trunk and ascending aorta are similar. The patient with chronic cor pulmonale had plexiform pulmonary lesions indicative of irreversible pulmonary hypertension. Neither the acute nor the subacute patient had chronic pulmonary vascular changes. All 3 patients had dilated right ventricular cavities and non-dilated left ventricular cavities and only the patient with chronic cor pulmonale had right ventricular hypertrophy. **(Am J Cardiol 2015;115:697−703)**

In Paul Dudley White's third edition of his *Heart Disease* published in 1951, sixteen pages were devoted to acute and chronic cor pulmonale.[1] In Braunwald's ninth edition of *Heart Disease* published in 2012, cor pulmonale was not mentioned in the index, although many pages were devoted to pulmonary hypertension,[2] the common denominator of acute, subacute, and chronic cor pulmonale. Cor pulmonale may be defined as dilatation of the right ventricular cavity without hypertrophy of its wall (*acute* and *subacute* cor pulmonale) or both dilatation of the right ventricular cavity and hypertrophy of its wall (*chronic* cor pulmonale), secondary to pulmonary hypertension not caused by a condition involving the left side of the heart. Although chronic cor pulmonale appears to have been recognized by Laennec by 1821,[3] acute cor pulmonale was not described until 1935 by McGinn and White[4] and the subacute form was described initially by Brill and Robertson in 1937.[5] Although the echocardiographic or computed tomographic features of acute cor pulmonale have been well described, we were unable to find any published reports describing clinical and morphologic features in patients with all 3 forms of cor pulmonale. Our purpose herein is simply to illustrate these characteristic features in 3 patients, 1 each with the acute, the subacute, and the chronic forms of cor pulmonale.

[a]Baylor Heart and Vascular Institute, Departments of [b]Internal Medicine, [c]Pathology, [d]Cardiothoracic Surgery, and [e]Radiology, Baylor University Medical Center, Dallas, Texas. Manuscript received November 6, 2014; revised manuscript received and accepted December 5, 2014.

Support for this investigation was provided by the Baylor Health Care System Foundation.

See page 703 for disclosure information.

*Corresponding author: Tel: (214) 820-7911; fax: (214) 820-7533.
E-mail address: wc.roberts@baylorhealth.edu (W.C. Roberts).

Table 1
Clinical and Morphologic Findings in the 3 Patients with Cor Pulmonale

Variable	Acute	Subacute	Chronic
Age (Years)	67	52	33
Sex	Man	Woman	Woman
Duration of symptoms of heart failure	< 1 hour	5 weeks	20 years
Cause of pulmonary hypertension	Massive PE	PE (Neoplastic)	PPH
Echocardiogram			
Dilated right ventricular cavity	-*	3+/4+	3+/4+
Dilated right atrial cavity	-*	0/4+	2+/4+
Thickened right ventricular wall	-*	0/4+	4+/4+
Left ventricular ejection fraction (%)	65	55	55
Pressures (mm Hg)			
Pulmonary artery wedge (a/v/mean)	-	6/10/6	16/18/14†
Pulmonary artery (s/d)	-	70/30	94/45†
Right ventricle (s/d)	-	70/14	94/31†
Right atrium (a/v/mean)	-	13/10/8	19/15/15†
Systemic artery (s/d)	-	115/70	90/50
Cardiac index (L/min/m^2)	-	1.7	-
Hematocrit (%)	43	37	41
Body mass index (Kg/m^2)	43	32	21
Children	1	3	0
Heart and lung transplant	0	0	+
Heart weight (g)	570	385	430
Floating heart‡	+	+	+

a = a wave; PE = pulmonary embolism; PPH = primary pulmonary hypertension; s/d = peak systolic/end diastolic; v = v wave.
* Unable to access because of severe obesity.
† At age 27 years.
‡ Indicative of severe cardiac adiposity.

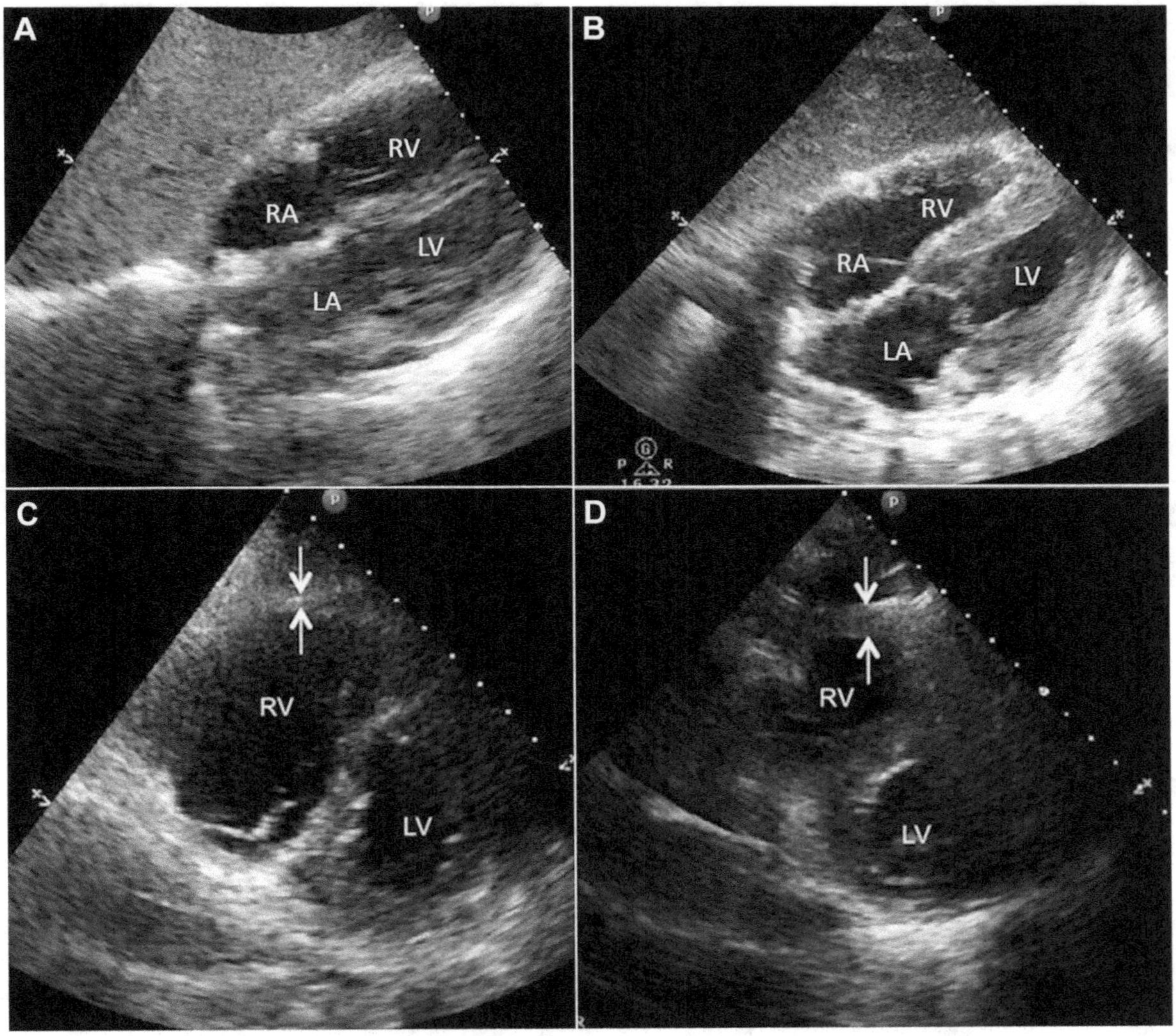

Figure 1. Echocardiograms in the patients with subacute (*A* and *C*) and chronic (*B* and *D*) cor pulmonale. *A* and *B* represent 4-chamber views and *C* and *D* represent cross-sectional views. The right ventricular (RV) cavity is dilated in both patients and the left ventricular (LV) cavity is not dilated in either patient. The RV wall is very thick in the patient with chronic cor pulmonale (*B* and *D*) but not in the patient with subacute cor pulmonale (*A* and *C*). LA = left atrium; RA = right atrium. The arrows indicate normal RV wall thickness in *C* and abnormally thick RV in *D*.

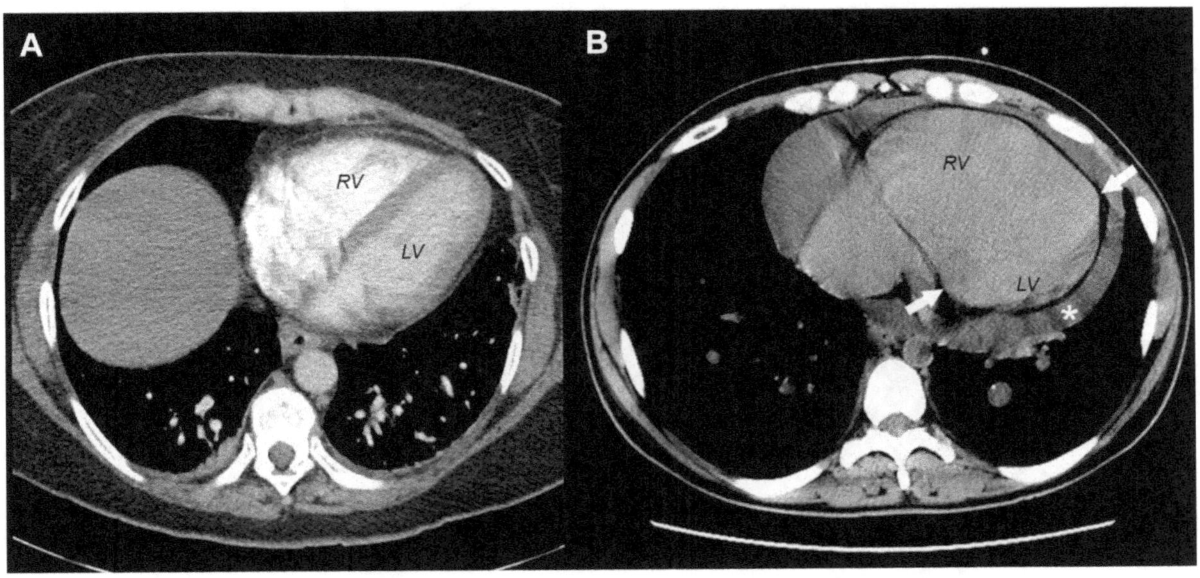

Figure 2. Computed tomographic pictures in the subacute patient (*A*) and in the chronic patient (*B*). The right ventricular cavity is greatly dilated. A pericardial effusion is present in *B*. The left ventricular cavity in *B* is minute. The arrows point to the ventricular septum. LV = left ventricle; RV = right ventricle; * = pericardial effusion.

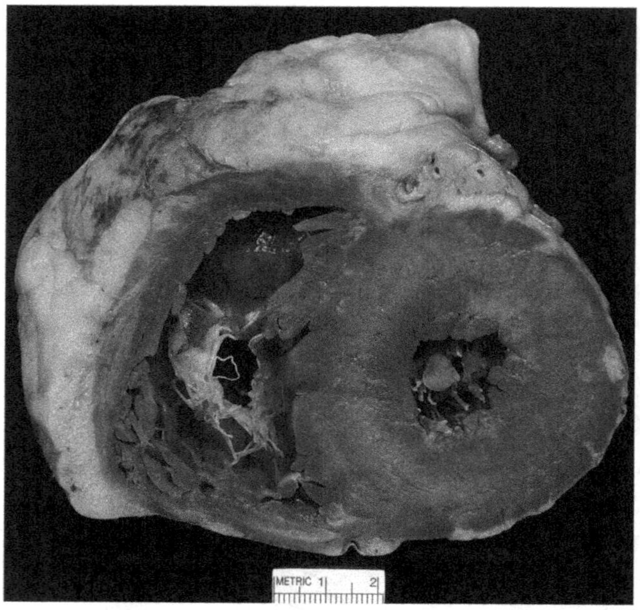

Figure 3. Acute cor pulmonale. Cross sections of the cardiac ventricles showing a dilated right ventricle and a normal size left ventricular cavity. The right ventricular wall is not thickened. The quantity of subepicardial adipose tissue is so extensive that the heart floated in a container of formaldehyde (body mass index 43 Kg/m^2).

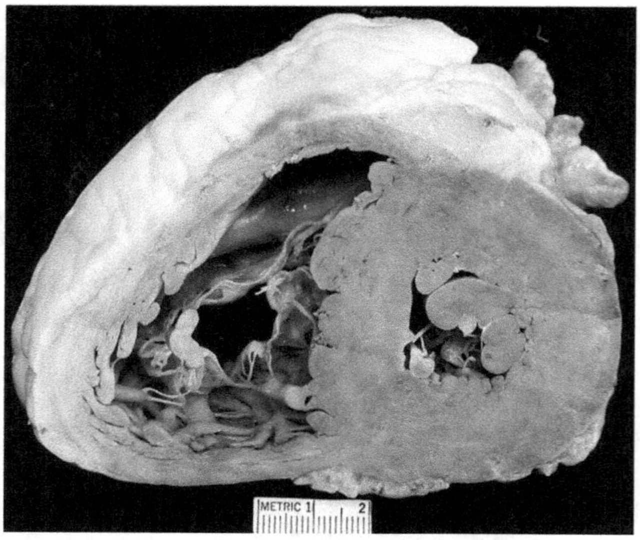

Figure 4. Subacute cor pulmonale. Transverse view of the ventricles showing the tricuspid valve and mitral valve. The right ventricular cavity is greatly dilated but the left ventricular cavity is not. The right ventricular wall is not thickened. The quantity of subepicardial adipose tissue is greatly increased such that the heart floated in a container of formaldehyde.

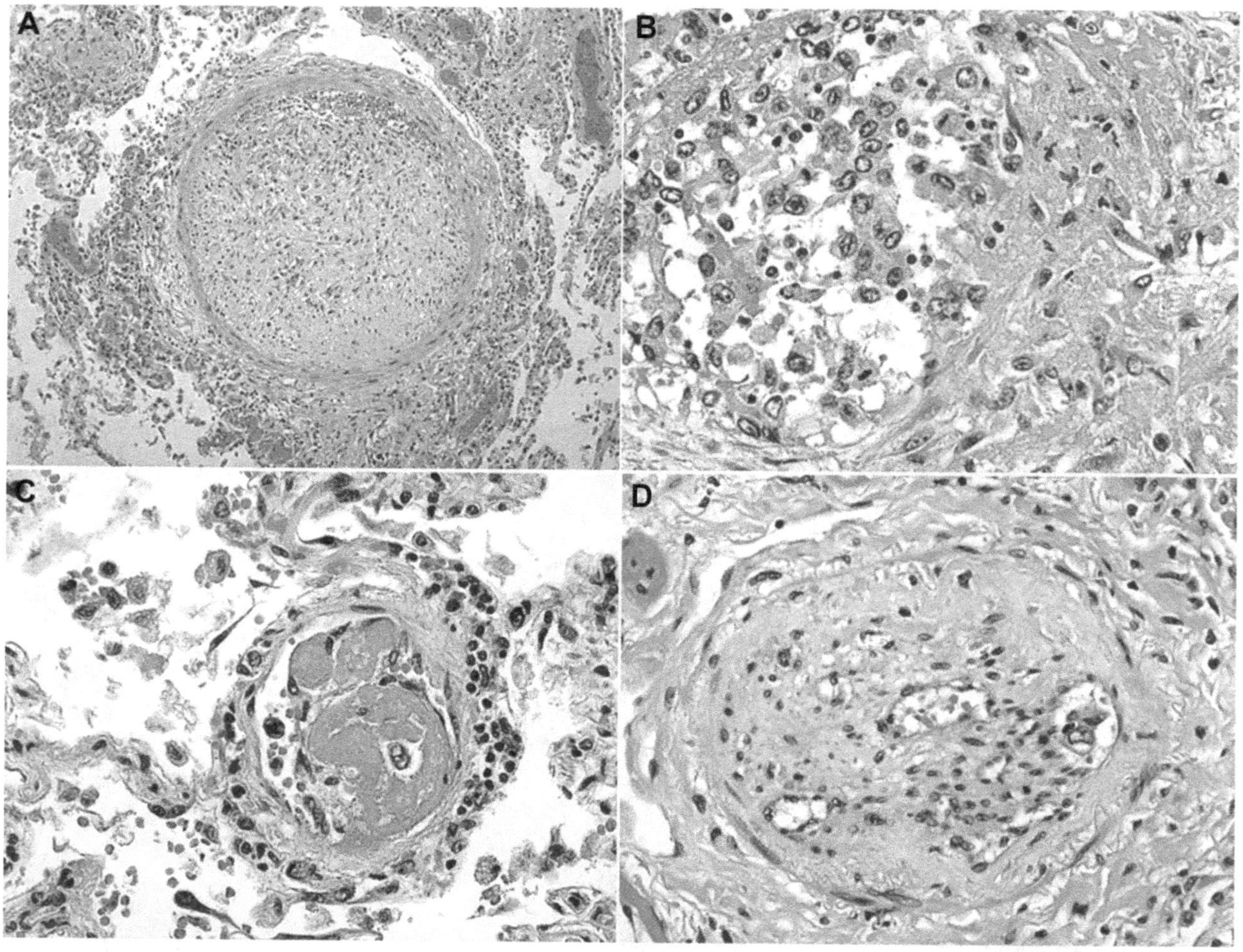

Figure 5. Subacute cor pulmonale. Photomicrographs of intrapulmonary arteries occluded or narrowed by metastatic cells within the lumen and with superimposed thrombus. The artery in *A* is virtually occluded. The gastric cancer cells are easily seen in the pulmonary artery illustrated in *B* and there is also some fibrin deposits within the lumen. *C* This small pulmonary artery is narrowed mainly by fibrin but a few gastric carcinoma cells are present. *D* This pulmonary artery contains organized thrombus and 4 small recanalized channels indicating that the emboli to the lungs probably occurred during the 5 symptomatic last weeks of this patient's life. Hematoxylin-eosin stains: X 100 *(A)*; X 400 *(B, C* and *D)*.

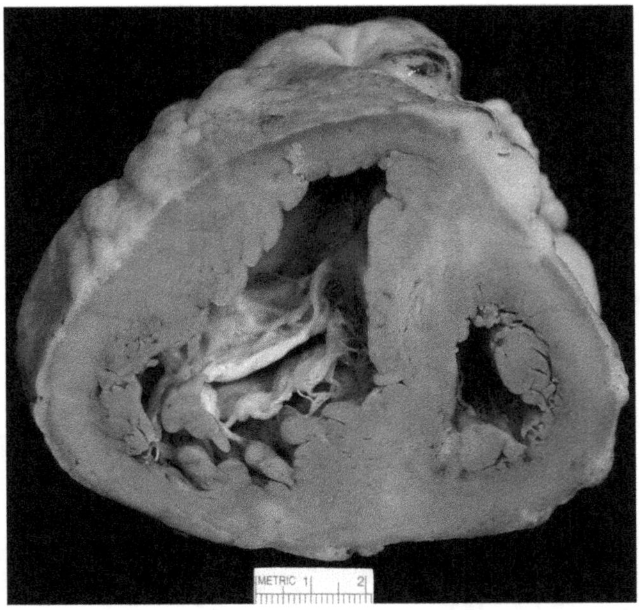

Figure 6. Chronic cor pulmonale. Transverse section of the ventricles in the patient with primary pulmonary hypertension. The right ventricular cavity is considerably dilated and the left ventricular is not. The right ventricular wall is about as thick as the left ventricular wall. The margins of the tricuspid valve leaflets are thickened, presumably the result of the very high closing pressure (peak right ventricular systolic pressure). The ventricular septum is thicker than either the right or left ventricular free walls.

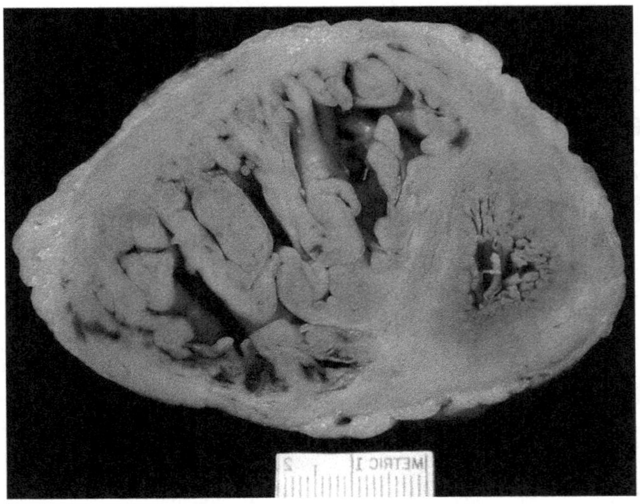

Figure 7. Chronic cor pulmonale. This view is a transverse cut in the apical half of the cardiac ventricles and it is shown to show how thick the pectinate muscles are in the right ventricular cavity. In this view the anterior and posterior right ventricular walls are really not thickened but the pectinate muscles are enormously thickened. Thickening of the pectinate muscles is one of the best signs of right ventricular hypertrophy, better than wall thickness. The left ventricular cavity is minute.

Patient Descriptions

Pertinent features of each of the 3 patients are summarized in Table 1. Echocardiographic and computed tomographic features in the subacute and chronic cases are shown in Figures 1 and 2. The acute patient, aged 67, had symptoms suggesting a respiratory catastrophe for only several minutes and necropsy disclosed massive pulmonary emboli (Figure 3); the subacute patient, aged 52, had symptoms for 5 weeks, determined at necropsy to be the result of multiple microscopic-sized pulmonary neoplastic emboli without parenchymal lung metastases from carcinoma of the stomach (Figures 4 and 5), and the chronic patient, only 33 years old, had symptoms of right-sided heart failure and periodic substernal chest pain for about 20 years (Figures 6–8). All 3 had very dilated right ventricular cavities, the acute and subacute patients without right ventricular wall thickening, and the chronic patient with both right ventricular dilatation and severe right ventricular wall thickening. The subacute and chronic patients had documented severely elevated right ventricular and pulmonary arterial peak systolic pressures (70 and 94 mm Hg, respectively), and the acute patient almost certainly did as well. Neither the acute nor the subacute patients had thickened walls of the pulmonary arteries and neither had plexiform lesions. The chronic patient, in contrast, had classic findings of primary pulmonary hypertension (medial and intimal thickening of the pulmonary arteries and numerous pulmonary plexiform lesions) (Figure 8). Sections of the pulmonary trunk in the acute and subacute patient disclosed a typical adult pattern of the medial elastic fibers whereas in the chronic patient the pattern was that present at birth and similar to the medial elastic fiber pattern of the aorta (Figures 9 and 10).

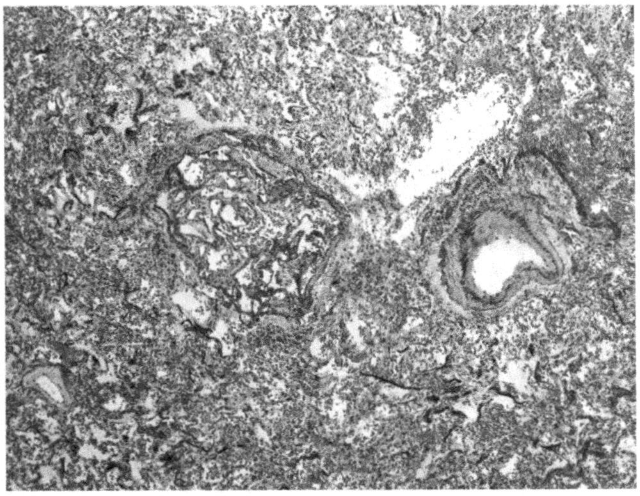

Figure 8. Chronic Cor pulmonale. Photomicrograph of a portion of lung showing a large plexiform lesion and a muscular pulmonary artery with thickening of its media and of its intima. Erythrocytes have entered most of the alveolar spaces. Movat stain, x100.

Discussion

Each of the 3 patients described herein fulfilled a definition of acute, subacute, and chronic cor pulmonale. The causes of the pulmonary hypertension in them, however, were quite different. The acute patient had a massive pulmonary embolus and died within a few minutes. The patient with the subacute syndrome had extensive neoplastic emboli to the small pulmonary arteries without emboli to the major pulmonary arteries or metastases from her gastric cancer to the pulmonary parenchyma and had symptoms of right-sided heart failure for

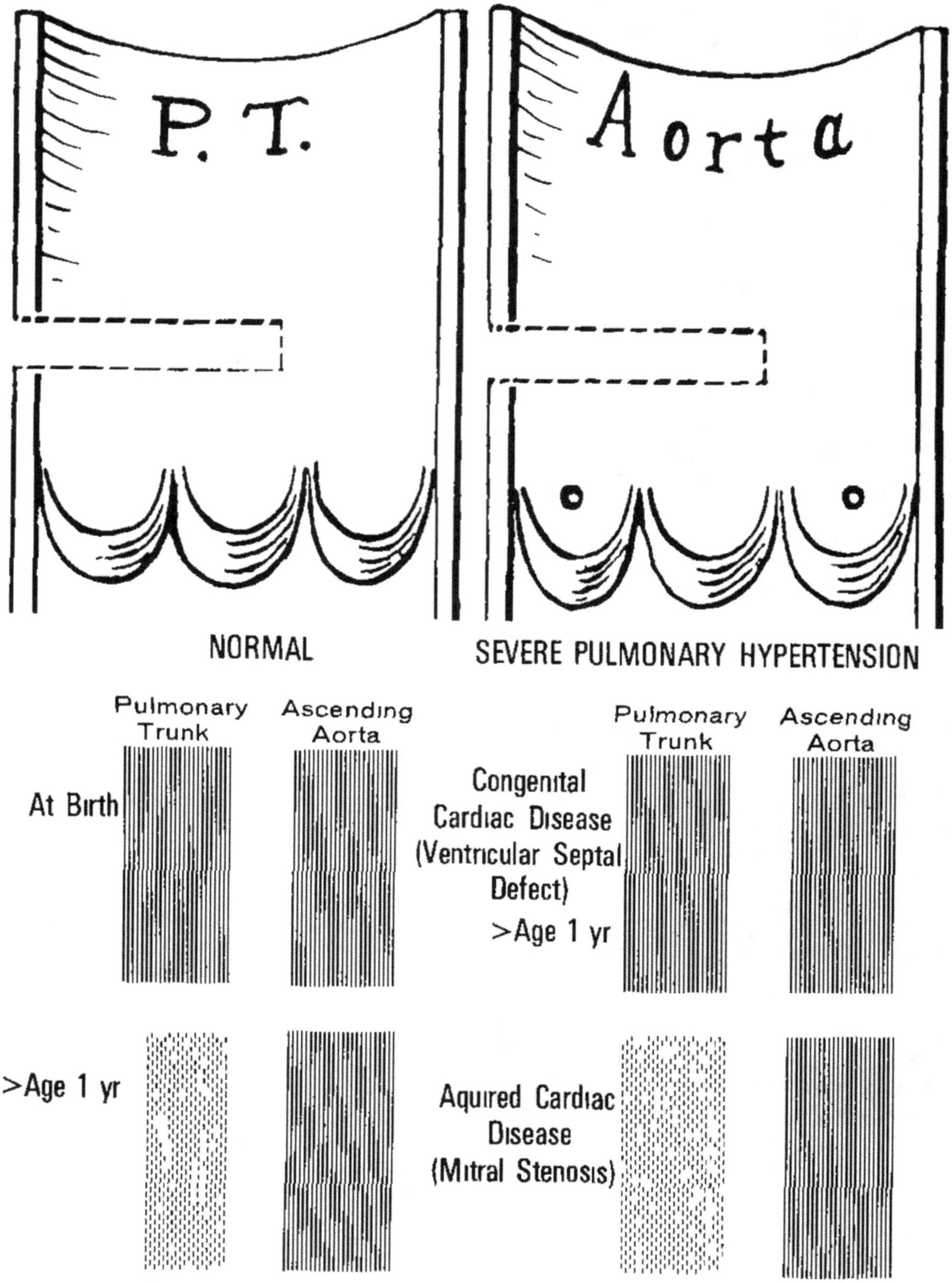

Figure 9. Configuration of elastic fibers in the pulmonary trunk at birth, after 1 year of age, with pulmonary *hypertension from birth* (VSD), and with an acquired condition (*mitral stenosis*). The sketch (*top*) shows the sites in the pulmonary trunk (PT) and aorta at which the sections for histologic examination were taken. At birth the configuration of the elastic fibers in both the pulmonary trunk and ascending aorta are identical and wall thicknesses are similar. Normally, after a year of age the number of elastic fibers in the pulmonary trunk diminishes considerably to reach an "adult configuration," and the thickness of the wall also diminishes. If a large ventricular septal defect or a aorticopulmonary defect is present from birth, both the configuration of the elastic fibers and wall thickness of the pulmonary trunk remains similar to that of the normal aorta. The information on the configuration of elastic fibers in the pulmonary trunk is based on original work by Heath and associates.[9,10]

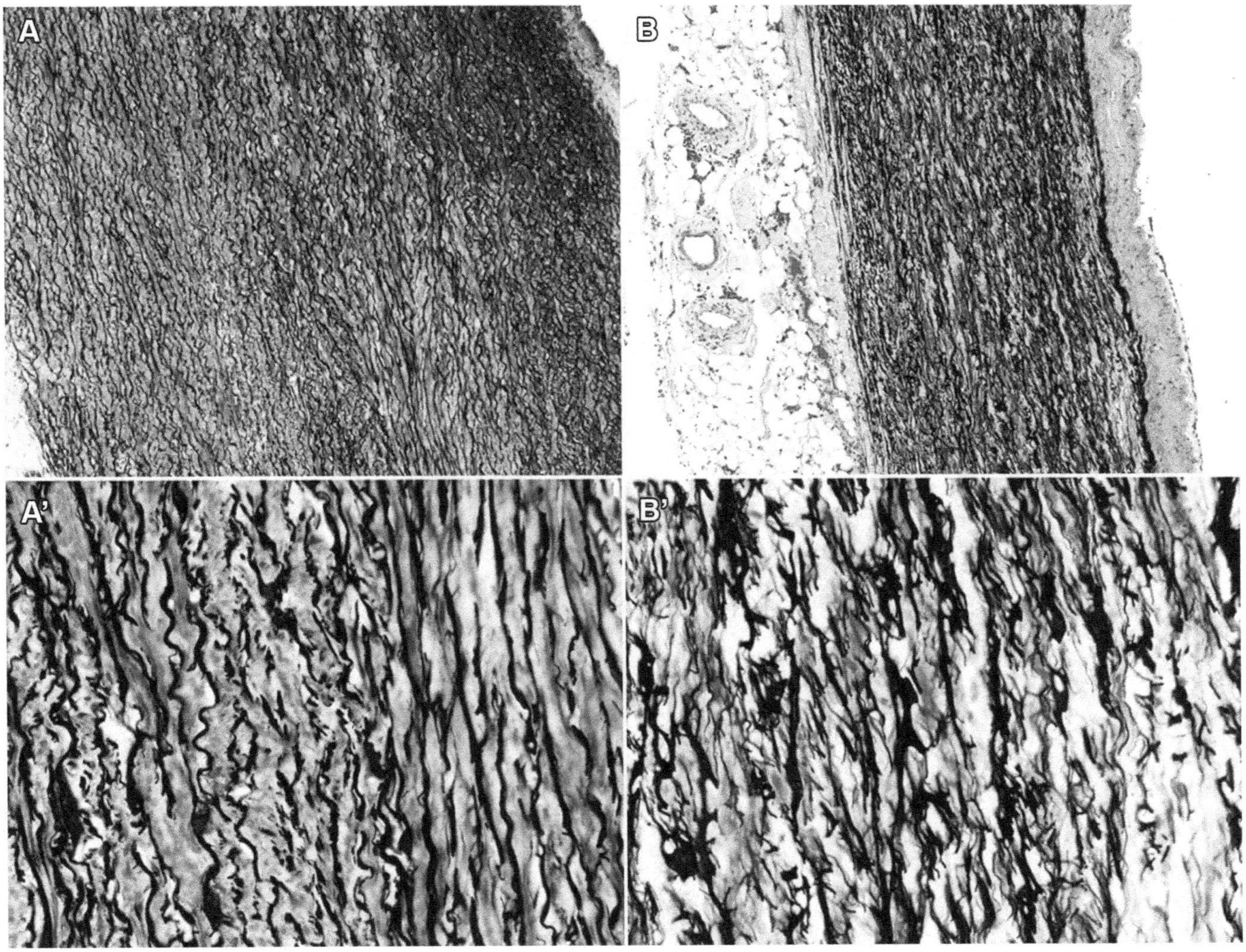

Figure 10. Chronic cor pulmonale. *A* and *A'* are sections of the ascending aorta stained for elastic fibers, and *B* and *B'* are sections of the pulmonary trunk stained for elastic fibers. The aorta is much thicker than is the pulmonary trunk but the configuration of the elastic fibers in the aorta and pulmonary trunk are similar, indicating that the pulmonary hypertension was almost certainly present from the time of birth. Movat stains X 100 *(A* and *B)*; X 400 *(A'* and *B')*.

5 weeks. Microscopic pulmonary neoplastic emboli without pulmonary parenchymal metastases was originally described by Brill and Robertson[5] in 1937 and they termed the condition "subacute cor pulmonale." Subsequently, a number of such cases has been reported.[6–8]

The patient with chronic cor pulmonale had primary or idiopathic pulmonary hypertension.[9] The unusual feature is that pulmonary hypertension appears to have been present from the time of birth. The evidence comes from studies by Heath and colleagues[10] and Heath and Edwards[11] who examined histologic sections of the pulmonary trunk and ascending aorta and found from study of patients with large left-to-right shunts (ventricular septal defect or patent ductus arteriosus) that the configuration of the elastic fibers in each of these arteries was similar when the pulmonary hypertension was present from birth, whereas in the patients who acquired pulmonary hypertension later in life (for example, from mitral stenosis) the pulmonary trunk had few elastic fibers and those present were disrupted (The aorta retains its fetal pattern of medial elastic fibers throughout life.). At birth, peak systolic pressures in the pulmonary trunk and ascending aorta are similar and therefore the configuration of elastic fibers in both pulmonary trunk and ascending aorta are similar. By one year of age, the peak systolic pressure in the pulmonary trunk has fallen to about one fifth of the peak systolic pressure in the ascending aorta and the elastic fibers have also decreased by approximately 80%, proportional to the reduction in peak systolic pressure.

Heath and Edwards[11] also found that some patients with primary pulmonary hypertension retain the fetal elastic pattern in the pulmonary trunk suggesting that the high pressure in the pulmonary circuit persisted from birth. A similar study by Roberts[12] in 1963 found the classic fetal pattern of elastic fibers in the pulmonary trunk in 1 and probably in 2 of 5 adults with primary pulmonary hypertension studied by him, again strongly suggesting that the high pulmonary pressure present at birth was retained into adulthood.

Neither our acute nor subacute cor pulmonale patient had medial or intimal thickening of the intrapulmonary

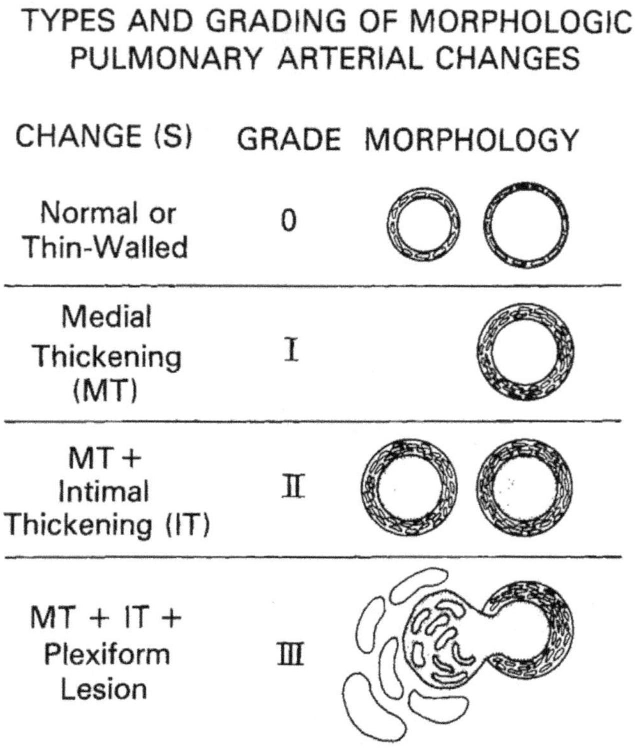

Figure 11. Diagram showing the types and grading of morphologic arterial changes in the lungs. Any elevation of pulmonary arterial pressure can cause medial thickening and if the pressure persists also intimal thickening. Plexiform lesions have occurred only in patients with severe pulmonary hypertension, usually pulmonary artery systolic pressures equivalent to aortic peak systolic pressures and indicate that the pulmonary hypertension is irreversible.

pulmonary arteries or plexiform lesion, whereas our chronic cor pulmonale patient had intrapulmonary arteries with thickened intima and media and numerous plexiform lesions (Figure 11). The plexiform lesions are indicative of irreversible pulmonary hypertension.[13]

Disclosures

The authors have no conflicts of interest to disclose.

1. White PD. Heart Disease. Fourth Edition. New York: The McMillan Company, 1951:1015.
2. Bonow RO, Mann DL, Zipes DP, Libby P, eds. Braunwald's HEART DISEASE. A Textbook of Cardiovascular Medicine. Ninth Edition. Philadelphia: Elsevier Saunders, 2012:1961.
3. Laennec RTH, Forbes J. A Treatise on the Diseases of the Chest and on Mediate Auscultation. London: Thomas & George Underwood, 1829: 736.
4. McGinn S, White PD. Acute cor pulmonale resulting from pulmonary embolism: its clinical recognition. *JAMA* 1935;104:1473–1480.
5. Brill IC, Robertson TD. Subacute cor pulmonale. *Arch Intern Med* 1937;60:1043–1057.
6. Mason DG. Subacute cor pulmonale. *Arch Intern Med* 1940;40: 1221–1229.
7. Schriner RW, Ryu JH, Edwards WD. Microscopic pulmonary tumor embolism causing subacute cor pulmonale: A difficult antemortem diagnosis. *Mayo Clin Proc* 1991;66:143–148.
8. Domanski MJ, Cunnion RE, Fernicola DJ, Roberts WC. Fatal cor pulmonale caused by extensive tumor emboli in the small pulmonary arteries without emboli in the major pulmonary arteries or metastases in the pulmonary parenchyma. *Am J Cardiol* 1993;72:233–234.
9. Simonneau G, Gatzoulis MA, Adatia I, Celermajer D, Denton C, Ghofrani A, Gomez Sanchez MA, Krishna Kumar R, Landzberg M, Machado RF, Olschewski H, Robbins IM, Souza R. Updated clinical classification of pulmonary hypertension. *J Am Coll Cardiol* 2013;62:D34–41.
10. Heath D, DeShane JW, Wood EH, Edwards JE. The structure of the pulmonary trunk at different ages and in case of pulmonary hypertension and pulmonary stenosis. *J Pathol Bacteriol* 1959;77:443.
11. Heath D, Edwards JE. Configuration of elastic tissue of pulmonary trunk in idiopathic pulmonary hypertension. *Circulation* 1960;21:59.
12. Roberts WC. The histologic structure of the pulmonary trunk in patients with "primary" pulmonary hypertension. *Am Heart J* 1963;65:230–236.
13. Roberts WC. A simple histologic classification of pulmonary arterial hypertension. *Am J Cardiol* 1986;58:385–386.

Case Reports

Large Patent Ductus Arteriosus in a 44-Year-Old Woman

Leading to Calcium Deposition in the Left Atrium and Mitral and Aortic Valves

Carey Camille Roberts, BS
William Clifford Roberts, MD

This report describes unusual autopsy findings in a 44-year-old woman who had a large, calcified patent ductus arteriosus that produced substantial left-to-right shunting. The patient died in 1962, 7 days after patch closure of the aortic orifice of the ductus. Numerous calcific deposits were present in the mural left atrial endocardium, the mitral valve leaflets and annulus, and the aortic valve cusps. The cause of the left-sided calcific deposits was perhaps related to the patient's several-decades-old giant aortopulmonary shunt, causing a major increase in the volume of blood passing through the left-sided cardiac chambers in comparison with the volume in the right side. To our knowledge, such findings in a patient with patent ductus arteriosus have not been reported previously. ***(Tex Heart Inst J 2015;42(3):262-4)***

Key words: *Adult; calcinosis/pathology; cardiomegaly/etiology/radiography; ductus arteriosus, patent/surgery; heart atria/pathology; heart diseases/physiopathology*

From: *Second-year medical student (Ms Roberts), Georgetown University School of Medicine, Washington, DC 20057; Baylor Heart and Vascular Institute (Dr. Roberts and Ms Roberts), Dallas, Texas 75246; Departments of Internal Medicine (Division of Cardiology) and Pathology (Dr. Roberts), Baylor University Medical Center; Dallas, Texas 75246; and Pathology Branch (Dr. Roberts), National Heart, Lung and Blood Institute, Bethesda, Maryland 20205*

Address for reprints: *William C. Roberts, MD, Baylor Heart and Vascular Institute, Baylor University Medical Center, 3500 Gaston Ave., Dallas, TX 75246*

E-mail: *wc.roberts@baylorhealth.edu*

A large patent ductus arteriosus (PDA) is now rarely seen in adults in the Western world; however, this was not necessarily the case 50 years ago. We describe noteworthy autopsy findings in a woman who had presented with symptoms after several decades of aortopulmonary shunting through a large PDA.

Case Report

A childless housewife was born in 1917 and died in 1962, at 44 years of age. A precordial murmur had been present since childhood, when she was diagnosed with rheumatic heart disease. She was asymptomatic until 40 years of age, when peripheral edema, abdominal swelling, and exertional dyspnea developed. The patient was seen initially in November 1959 at the National Heart Institute (Bethesda, Md), at 41 years of age. She was cachectic and in severe right-sided heart failure. Her neck veins were markedly distended. On auscultation, the following were heard: rales in the lung bases, an apical grade 4/6 blowing systolic murmur in association with a thrill that radiated into the left axilla, a diastolic rumble at the apex, a crescendo diastolic grade 3/6 blowing murmur along the left sternal border, and an accentuated P_2. A chest radiograph showed a greatly enlarged cardiac silhouette. An electrocardiogram, measured with normal 10-mm standardization (10 mm=1 mV), showed a total 12-lead QRS voltage of 315 mm (consistent with combined right and left ventricular hypertrophy); the rhythm was atrial fibrillation (Fig. 1).[1] Cardiac catheterization via the transbronchial route (involving endotracheal intubation, with the pressure-recording catheter inserted into the left atrium from the trachea) provided only the left-sided cardiac pressures (Table I). These findings were interpreted as showing "predominant mitral regurgitation." The patient's blood hematocrit was 34%. During her 6-week hospitalization, she was placed on a low-salt diet, chlorothiazide, and acetazolamide, and she lost 40 pounds from her already cachectic frame.

In June 1962, she was readmitted because of similar symptoms and signs. Table I also shows the findings from right-sided and transseptal left-sided cardiac catheterization. The ^{85}Kr and indocyanine green dye curves showed predominant left-to-right shunting (Fig. 2). The catheter was passed from the aorta into the major pulmonary arteries through a PDA, which a chest radiograph showed to contain calcific deposits. The patient's right brachial and femoral arterial oxygen saturations were 92% and 89%, respectively. After a course of diuretic therapy, her peripheral edema and ascites completely resolved. In July 1962, the PDA was closed via the surgical placement of a Teflon patch at the aortic entrance of the PDA, with use of extracorporeal circulation during the procedure.[2] Postoperative bleeding necessitated the evacuation of a left hemothorax the next day, at which time the right and left ventricular peak systolic pressures were 105 and 80 mmHg, respectively. Hypotension and renal, hepatic, respiratory, and cerebral failure developed thereafter, and the patient died 7 days after the PDA closure operation. (This patient would not have been a candidate for PDA closure today.)

At necropsy, the heart weighed approximately 520 g. The PDA was 1.5 cm in diameter, and its wall was heavily calcified. All 4 cardiac chambers were dilated and had thicker walls than normal: both the right and left ventricular free walls were approximately 1.3 cm thick. The left atrium was dilated much more than the right atrium. The pulmonary trunk and main right and left pulmonary arteries were very dilated.

Figure 3 shows the locations of calcific deposits in several structures: sprinkled within the mural left atrial endocardium, focal within the mitral and aortic valves (with more in the aortic cusps than in the mitral cusps), and in the mitral annular area behind the posterior mitral leaflet.

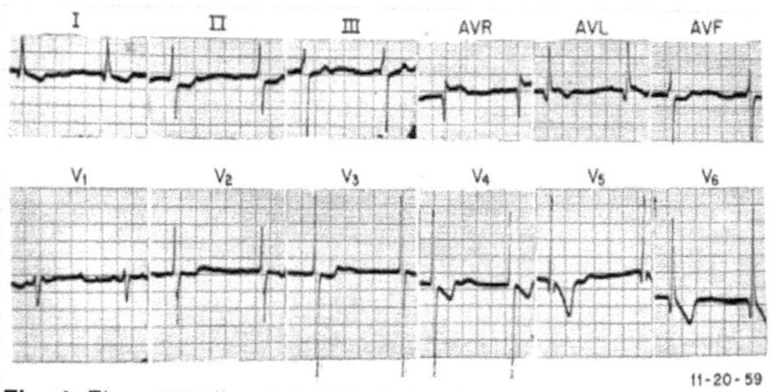

Fig. 1 *Electrocardiogram of the patient at 41 years of age shows atrial fibrillation and excessive QRS voltage consistent with both right and left ventricular hypertrophy.*

TABLE I. Cardiac Hemodynamic Values in the Patient

Pressure Variable (mmHg)	**December 1959**	**May 1962**
Pulmonary artery	—	118/52
Right ventricle	—	118/52
Right atrium		
Mean	—	21
V wave	—	25
Right brachial artery	—	144/60
Femoral artery	150/70	—
Left atrium		
Mean	22	18
V wave	32	27

Discussion

This case is unusual in several aspects. The PDA had been confused with valvular disease for more than 4 decades. The patient's first cardiac catheterization, in 1959, was via the transbronchial route and yielded pressures only in the left side of the heart; these data did not enable a diagnosis of PDA but were consistent with the admitting diagnosis of mitral regurgitation. The right-sided pressures were not determined until 2 years later, and at that time no echocardiography was available for making estimates. The wall of the PDA was heavily calcified at the time of diagnosis, when the patient was 44 years of age. Although the peak systolic pressures were similar in the major pulmonary arteries and in the brachial artery, the shunting through the PDA

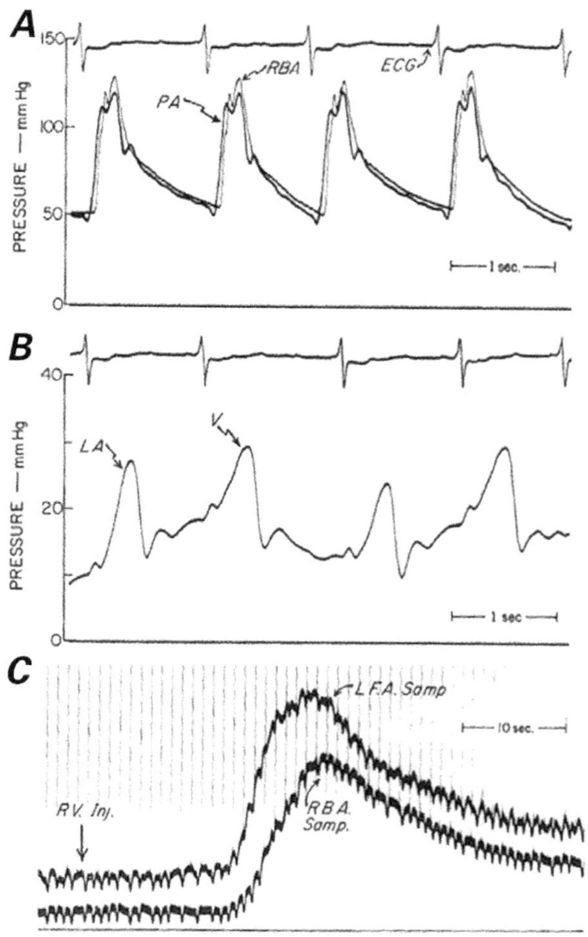

Fig. 2 *Diagrams show findings in June 1962, approximately one month before closure of the ductus.* ***A)*** *Simultaneous pressure tracings of the pulmonary artery (PA) and right brachial artery (RBA) show similar pressures in each vessel.* ***B)*** *Left atrial (LA) pressure tracing shows tall V waves.* ***C)*** *Drawing shows indocyanine green dye curves upon right ventricular injection (RV. Inj.) and sampling (Samp.) at simultaneous times in the left femoral artery (L.F.A.) and right brachial artery (R.B.A.).*

ECG = electrocardiogram

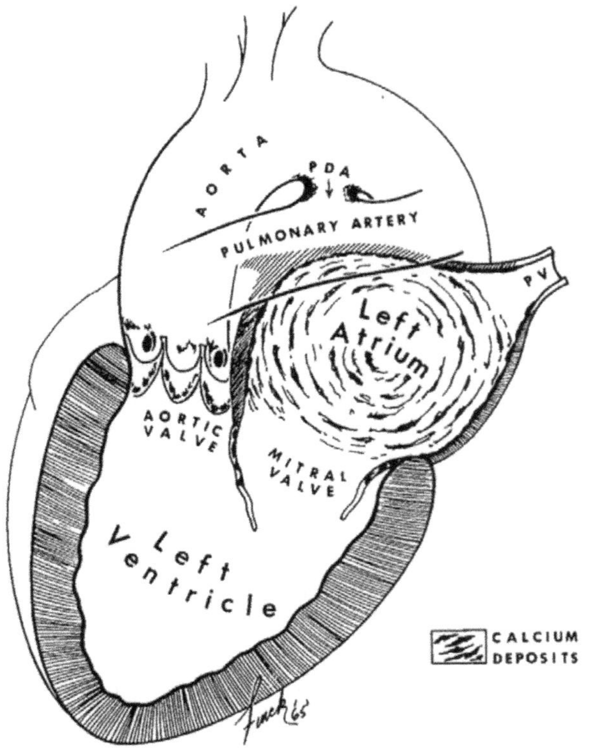

Fig. 3 Diagram shows locations of calcific deposits in the patent ductus arteriosus (PDA), mitral valve, aortic valve, and left atrial endocardium.

was overwhelmingly from left to right. Nevertheless, the heart failure was mainly right-sided. The method of closing the calcified PDA was new at the time: inserting a Teflon patch over the aortic entrance into the PDA, with use of extracorporeal circulation.[2] Finally, calcific deposits in the left atrial wall and in the leaflets of the mitral and aortic valves have not to our knowledge been reported previously in patients with PDA.

The reason for the deposits in the left atrial endocardium and in the mitral and aortic valves is unclear. The phenomenon might be explained by the massive volume overload on the left side of the heart—caused by the left-to-right shunting through the PDA—while much smaller volumes of blood passed through the right side of the heart. The increased volume and therefore increased work of the left side of the heart might have caused rapid aging, such that the condition of that side more resembled typical findings in an 85-year-old patient than those expected in a 44-year-old. The calcific deposits in the left atrial endocardium might have resulted in part from the considerable stretching of that chamber due to increased volume and pressure, and from the superimposed mitral regurgitation. In patients with mitral stenosis, calcific deposits have been seen in the left atrial endocardium when a thrombus has organized into calcific plaques; however, this patient never had evidence of left atrial thrombus.[3] Her PDA was heavily calcified, a finding in older patients with a large PDA.

References

1. Roberts WC, Filardo G, Ko JM, Siegel RJ, Dollar AL, Ross EM, Shirani J. Comparison of total 12-lead QRS voltage in a variety of cardiac conditions and its usefulness in predicting increased cardiac mass. Am J Cardiol 2013;112(6):904-9.
2. Morrow AG, Clark WD. Closure of the calcified patent ductus. A new operative method utilizing cardiopulmonary bypass. J Thorac Cardiovasc Surg 1966;51(4):534-8.
3. Roberts WC, Humphries JO, Morrow AG. Giant right atrium in rheumatic mitral stenosis. Atrial enlargement restricted by mural calcification. Am Heart J 1970;79(1):28-35.

www.ingramcontent.com/pod-product-compliance
Lightning Source LLC
LaVergne TN
LVHW062137200926
848484LV00007B/1827